Amy Marti

W9-CYY-628

Amy Marti

W9-CYY-628

Textbook of
RADIOGRAPHIC
POSITIONING
and
Related
Anatomy

**Third
Edition**

About the Author

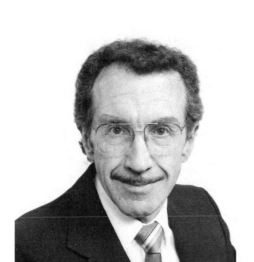

Kenneth L. Bontrager, M.A., RT(R), who was trained in radiologic technology at St. Luke's Hospital in Denver, received a B.A. degree from the University of Colorado, and an M.A. from the University of Northern Colorado. He has served as technical director and instructor of a hospital school of radiologic technology, administrative technologist in a large hospital and the director and instructor of an associate degree college program in radiologic technology.

Mr. Bontrager founded Multi-Media Publishing, Inc. in 1972 for the express purpose of developing educational resources for radiologic technology and other health care professions. Mr. Bontrager has mastered the techniques involved in the challenging field of writing and developing successful self-instructional audiovisual educational materials. Among his best known radiologic technology programs are an x-ray physics and technique series, a dental radiography series and a 21-unit Radiographic Anatomy and Positioning series. These self-instructional programs, student workbooks and textbooks are being used by literally thousands of students each year in the U.S., Canada and other countries.

Mr. Bontrager completed the second and third editions of this text in Phoenix, Arizona, where he moved with his family after selling Multi-Media Publishing, Inc. to the C. V. Mosby Company in 1985.

The work on this completely revised and expanded third edition began in 1989 with a national survey (described on following pages), and with a weekend conference in Phoenix by a selected group of RT educators. Using the results of the survey and the guidelines and suggestions of the focus group, Mr. Bontrager spent the next two and one-half years working full time on the revisions and additions to this text. During this time he worked with students and clinical instructors at local Phoenix area hospitals and with instructors at Gateway Community College in Phoenix testing new ideas for changes and additions.

Radiographic Anatomy & Positioning
A Self-Paced Multimedia Learning Series

by Kenneth L. Bontrager, M.A. RT(R)

Barry T. Anthony, R.T. (R)

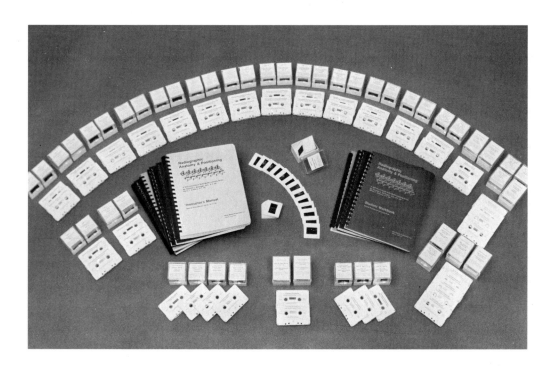

Content of the Audio-Visual Series

The anatomy and positioning audiovisual series covers those basic and common optional projections and procedures being done in general diagnostic radiology departments. The audiovisual units on cerebral pneumography, cerebral angiography and computed tomography are directed toward advanced, second-year students and practicing technologists. This information is presented in less depth in corresponding chapters of this textbook.

Each audiovisual unit contains a series of visuals accompanied by an audio tape narration. The student workbook contains review exercises and a self-administered test on the material presented in the unit. The instructor's manual that accompanies each unit contains a lesson evaluation to measure each student's mastery of the material.

The complete 21-unit series contains **1,536 slides**, **48 audio tapes**, a **three-volume student workbook** and a **five-volume set of instructor's manuals**.

Relationship of Audiovisual Series to Textbook

The textbook covers the anatomy and positioning information needed by students and can be used by itself, without the A-V series. The A-V series, however, provides an excellent adjunct to the text. The series presents the subject matter in the multimedia format of

seeing, hearing and doing. It has a proven history of increasing comprehension and retention, resulting in improved Registry and certification scores.

The A-V series with student workbooks can be used either as an individualized, self-paced learning program or as a teaching aid in classroom instruction. Either way it enhances the use of this text. A student may study a chapter of this textbook, then take the corresponding A-V unit to reinforce and expand knowledge in that area; or an instructor can use the visuals in the classroom to supplement and guide his/her lectures. Students can be assigned specific chapters in this text as preparation for the classroom presentation then individually complete review exercises in the student workbook for reinforcement.

Second Edition: An expanded second edition of this A-V series is under development. This includes certain new units to be in agreement with the revisions and new chapters in this textbook.

Availability of Audiovisual Series

This series is only available from the publisher. For ordering and pricing information, please write to Mosby-Year Book, Inc. 11830 Westline Industrial Drive, St. Louis, MO 63146, or call 800-325-4177.

Textbook of RADIOGRAPHIC POSITIONING and Related Anatomy

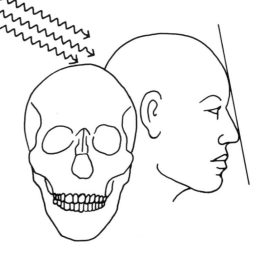

Expanded Third Edition
with 2076 Illustrations

Kenneth L. Bontrager
M.A., R.T. (R)

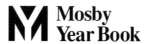

Mosby
Year Book

St. Louis Baltimore Boston Chicago London Philadelphia Sydney Toronto

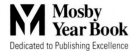
Mosby Year Book
Dedicated to Publishing Excellence

Publisher: Alison Miller

Editor: Dave Culverwell

Developmental Editor: Christi Mangold

Graphic Design and Page Layout: Neil Bontrager
Joan Lapre'

Data Entry and Proofreading: Mary Lou Bontrager

Illustrations for 3rd Edition: Debra Ravin
Joan Lapre'
Sally Schmitt

Photography: Ken Bontrager

Hospital Facilities for
3rd Edition Photography:
Energized Laboratory
Gateway Community College, Phoenix, Arizona

Phoenix Baptist Hospital and Medical Center
Phoenix, Arizona

St. Joseph's Hospital and Medical Center
Phoenix, Arizona

University of Iowa Hospitals and Medical Clinics
Iowa City, Iowa

Third Edition

Copyright © 1993 by Mosby-Year Book, Inc.
A Mosby imprint of Mosby–Year Book, Inc.

All rights reserved. No part of this publication may be reproduced, stored in a
retrieval system, or transmitted, in any form or by any means, electronic,
mechanical, photocopying, recording, or otherwise, without prior permission
from the publisher.

Permission to photocopy or reproduce solely for internal or personal use is
permitted for libraries or other users registered with the Copyright Clearance
Center, provided that the base fee of $4.00 per chapter plus $.10 per page is
paid directly to the Copyright Clearance Center, 27 Congress Street, Salem,
MA 01970. This consent does not extend to other kinds of copying , such as
copying for general distribution, for advertising, or promotional purposes, for
creating new collected works or for resale.

Pevious Editions copyrighted 1982, 1987.

Printed in the United States of America

Mosby-Year Book, Inc.
11830 Westline Industrial Drive, St. Louis   MO 63146

Library of Congress Cataloging in Publication Data

Bontrager, Kenneth L.
Textbook of radiographic positioning and related anatomy, third edition
Bibliography: p.
Includes index.
1. Radiography, Medical–Positioning.
2. Anatomy, Human
I. Title. (DNLM: 1. Technology, Radiologic.
WN 160 B722T)
RC 78.4.B66   1982   616.07'572   81-82006
ISBN 0-8015-0537-7

93 94 95 96 97 MPS/MV 9 8 7 6 5 4 3 2 1

Preface

Purpose

This book is designed to meet the need for a thorough, clearly illustrated, simply written anatomy and positioning textbook for student radiographers. This textbook is not another comprehensive reference atlas. Instead it encompasses in one volume explanations and illustrations of the anatomy and positioning that all radiographers must master. All of the basic or routine projections or positions commonly done throughout the U.S. for all body parts and systems are described and illustrated. The more common optional projections and/or positions are also covered.

Uniqueness of Book

What is unique about this book is the way that it incorporates the techniques of self-paced, multimedia instruction into a textbook format. The writing is concise and visually oriented. The content is programmed to build from known to unknown, simple to difficult. All anatomy and positioning descriptions are accompanied by extensive visuals. The author has taken much care and effort in the organization and layout of this material. Topics and sub-topics fit on individual pages with accompanying visuals always on the same page to enable the student to quickly comprehend the information being presented.

The author developed this writing style through many years of writing self-paced audiovisual programs for student radiographers. The testimony from students and instructors has shown that programmed self-paced, visually oriented instruction dramatically increases student comprehension and retention. A major purpose of this book is to provide the students with proven benefits of this method presented in textbook form.

Combining Anatomy & Positioning

The author firmly believes in the importance of learning anatomy and positioning concurrently. Unless they are studied together, positioning is often learned by simply memorizing body positions and central ray locations. A thorough understanding of body structures and anatomical relationships helps develop highly competent, "thinking" radiographers who can conceptually visualize each part being radiographed and thus can change or adapt positioning routines as needed.

This instructional approach and the combining of anatomy and positioning has also been used by the author in the accompanying audiovisual series. According to instructors from around the U.S. and Canada, this approach has resulted in dramatic improvements in anatomy and positioning scores on certification and registry exams.

Expanded Third Edition

Much planning and preparation preceded the writing of this third edition. The author received guidance and input from a focus group of RT educators and reviewers from across the country. Certain contributing authors were invited to submit information on more specialized chapters. A national survey, as described on the following pages, determined which procedures and/or projections should be included in this text. Careful planning by the author went into organizing all of this information into a visually oriented, logical and easy to understand format.

Acknowledgments

Determination of appropriate acknowledgments for this project is difficult because of the many persons who have contributed to this and earlier editions.

I want to first acknowledge and thank **Barry Anthony**, RT, for his contributions in the areas of anatomy and special procedures for the first edition of both this text and the associated audio-visual series which provided the foundation for the expanded third edition of this textbook.

I also want to thank all those educators and the clinical supervisors and/or instructors who took the time to complete the national survey which provided the basis for what information and which procedures were included in this new edition. I especially want to thank those manuscript reviewers who took the extra time to not only critique but to add positive and detailed suggestions as to what should be deleted or added. These included: **Michael Adams**, RT, **Gene Frank**, RT, **Laverne Gurley**, RT, **David Hall**, RT, **Penny Mays**, RT, **Fred Price**, RT, **Dennis Spragg**, RT, and **Andrew Woodward**, RT. I would also like to thank Anatomist, **Margaret Wilson Cascarano**, Ph.D. for her thorough review and suggestions on the anatomy sections.

I want to thank those contributing authors listed under specific chapters who submitted suggestions, radiographs, photographs and/or manuscript copy in their specific areas of expertise which I could incorporate into this edition. **Alex Backus, RT**, and **John Lampignano, RT**, from Gateway Community College provided much support and the use of their energized lab for testing techniques and for photography. **Karen Brown, RT**, clinical coordinator at St. Joseph's Hospital and Medical Center, was especially kind and helpful in assisting me in testing new projections including the new chest positioning methods. She also provided a valuable service in locating and copying hard-to-find radiographs. She and **Jeffrey Wrasper**, RT, also very graciously assisted me during many long sessions of positioning photography.

I would also like to thank **Jim Sanderson, RT,** and Valley Lutheran and Mesa Lutheran Hospitals of Mesa, AZ and **Bill Collins, RT,** of Maricopa County Hospital, Phoenix, AZ for their cooperation in helping me locate radiographs for this text.

I am very grateful to **Del Hershberger**, RT, Phoenix Baptist Hospital and Medical Center, for those many evenings that she helped us with positioning photography and in locating and copying radiographs. In addition I thank **Kathy Martensen**, RT, **Tom Mougin**, RT, and **Joan Radke**, RT, from the University of Iowa Hospitals and Clinics for their help with positioning photography for the skull, facial bones and MRI chapters, and for providing copies of radiographs and MRI scans for these chapters.

I thank **Dave Culverwell** from Mosby-Year Book, Inc. for his support and faith in me with this total project, especially in the stressful and frustrating times during the complex production phase when schedules needed to be extended. I also thank **Christi Mangold** for her help in coordinating reviewer's schedules and feedback. **Jerry Wood**, director of manufacturing at Mosby-Year Book and production editor **Mary Steuck** were very helpful in guiding me through the complex production process and in providing the necessary proof copies at various stages of production.

I also thank **Joan Lapre'** and **Sally Schmitt** of our production staff for their help and contributions with the art and graphics, especially those months when we all worked extra long days and evenings trying to meet production schedules.

Last and most important to me I want to thank my wife, **Mary Lou** and our two sons **Neil** and **Troy** for their love and support during the past three years. Mary Lou keyed in all the new pages and chapters, and most importantly proofed each page for content and spelling errors. Thank you, Mary Lou. You were truly my support and my partner in this project.

I thank you, Troy, for your understanding during those weekends home from college when I couldn't spend much time with you.

I especially want to thank you, Neil, for committing two years to this project. I realize and appreciate very much what you have given up to help me with "the book". In doing this however you learned much about radiographic anatomy and positioning! You laid out these 700 plus pages over and over again as I kept revising and changing the visuals or adding to the text. You demonstrated much patience and understanding with your perfectionist Dad who always wanted to make that "last" change or addition.

I also thank you Neil, for your willingness to be the positioning model for the MRI and the head chapters we photographed that cold snowy weekend in Iowa City!

KLB

Third Edition Changes

Anatomical Terms

Anatomical terms were updated to nationally accepted standards in agreement with those adopted by the 12th International Congress of Anatomists, For example the terms **upper** and **lower limbs** are used rather than the more common older terms upper and lower extremities. Other examples are the carpal and tarsal bones wherein the preferred names are listed first, with parentheses used to indicate those familiar terms more commonly used in the past.

Phonetic respelling is included in parentheses according to *Dorland's Illustrated Medical Dictionary,* 27th edition, after each unfamiliar word throughout the text to help students in correct pronunciation of these terms.

Chapter Additions

The introductory Chapter 1 was expanded to include a section on **basic imaging principles** including exposure factors, density, contrast and distortion as related to positioning. A new section was also added on **radiation protection**. Certain **new anatomy** and **new projections** were added throughout the text including the chapters on the cranium and facial bones.The section on **Mammography** was expanded and updated into a separate chapter. The MRI chapter was expanded to include more clinical applications and procedures.

Combining Chapters on Upper and Lower Limbs

The chapter on the hand and wrist was combined with the chapter on the forearm, elbow and humerus into a new single expanded chapter on the upper limb. The same was done with the lower limb, wherein two chapters were combined into one.

Positioning Page Additions

Evaluation criteria sections and more complete step by step positioning instructions were added to each positioning page. New model photographs and new radiographs and line drawings are incorporated throughout the text.

New Chapters & New Procedures

Two totally new chapters were added on **Pediatric Radiography** and **Conventional Tomography**. New procedures were added to special procedures chapters including arthrograms of the knee and shoulder and peripheral arteriograms and venograms.

Focus Group Members

Patrick Apfel, M.Ed., RT(R) University of Nevada, Las Vegas, NV.

Alex Backus, MS, RT(R) Gateway Community College, Phoenix, AZ.

Tom Baier, Ph.D., RT(R) Ommi-Dyne, Inc., Hilo, HI.

Joan Dickerson, BS, RT(R) Pima Medical Institute, Tempe, AZ.

Marilyn Faye, BS, RT(R) Joint Review Committee (ASRT), Chicago, IL.

Eugene D. Frank, MA, RT(R) FASRT Mayo Clinic, Rochester, MN.

Neta McKnight, BS, RT(R) Jackson State Community College, Jackson, TN.

Kathy Martensen, BS, RT(R) University of Iowa Hospitals & Clinics, Iowa City, IA.

Darrell McKay, Ph.D. RT(R) St. Louis Community College, St. Louis, MO.

Bob Parelli, BS, RT(R) Cypress College, Cypress, CA.

E. Russel Ritenour, Ph.D. University of Minnesota Hospitals, Minneapolis, MN.

Ken Rossel, BS, RT(R) Geisinger Medical Center, Danville, PA.

Carol Urbanski, BS, RT(R) Avila College, Kansas City, MO.

Contributors for Third Edition

Barry T. Anthony, RT(R) Swedish Medical Center, Englewood, CO.

Patrick Apfel, M.Ed, RT(R) University of Nevada, Las Vegas, NV.

Alex Backus, MS, RT(R) Gateway Community College, Phoenix, AZ.

Karen Brown, RT(R) St. Joseph's Hospital and Medical Center, Phoenix, AZ.

Claudia Calandrino, MPA, RT(R) Signa Health Plans of Calif., Los Angeles, CA.

Nancy Dickerson, RT(R)(M) Mayo Clinic, Rochester, MN.

Eugene D. Frank, MA, RT(R) FASRT, Mayo Clinic, Rochester, MN.

Jessie R. Harris, RT(R) Signa Health Plans of Calif., Los Angeles, CA.

John P. Lampignano, M.Ed, RT(R) Gateway Community College, Phoenix, AZ.

James D. Lipcamon, RT(R) Harbor-UCLA Diagnostic Imaging Center, Torrance, CA.

Kathy M. Martensen, BS, RT(R) University of Iowa Hospitals & Clinics, Iowa City, IA.

J. Fred Price, MS, RT(R) FASRT Garland County Community College, Hot Springs, AR.

Joan Radke, BS, RT(R) University of Iowa Hospitals & Clinics, Iowa City, IA.

E. Russel Ritenour, Ph.D. University of Minnesota Hospitals, Minneapolis, MN.

Mariane Tortorici, Ed.D, RT(R) University of Nevada, Las Vegas, NV.

National Survey Information

Purpose and Results

In November 1989, a questionnaire was sent to all clinical affiliated hospitals of Radiologic Technology Educational Programs in the United States. According to the AART and the Joint Review Committee on Education in Radiologic Technology, to their knowledge this type of survey had never been done before but was sorely needed. The purpose was to **determine a national standard or norm for all radiographic positioning.** This was needed by Mr. Bontrager and educators using this textbook and the accompanying A-V series and student workbooks to know which procedures and which basic **minimum** positioning routines should be taught by all schools nationwide and thus included in this textbook. In our mobile society it is important to prepare students who can function effectively in any hospital or clinical setting throughout the U.S. without extensive orientation or additional instruction. All students should have an awareness of which procedures and which projections are being done throughout the different regions of the U.S.

With the increased use of newer imaging modalities, certain radiographic procedures are being done less frequently and some not at all in most institutions. Therefore these no longer need to be included in basic student textbooks such as this.

Specific results of the survey which may be useful to readers of this text and to program directors and instructors are included in each chapter.

Summary: The following three things were accomplished by this survey as used in the writing of this text:

1. A national norm or standard was determined for **routine** or **basic projections** for all common radiographic procedures.

2. Determination was made of which **optional** or **extra projections** are most commonly taken throughout the different regions of the U.S., to better demonstrate specific anatomical parts or certain pathological conditions, or for those patients who cannot cooperate fully.

3. A determination was made of which radiographic procedures are still commonly done across the U.S. and at what frequency, and which have become obsolete and should no longer be included in this text.

Discontinued procedures

Following are the results for six procedures which are no longer included in the third edition of this textbook. (Pneumoencephalography had already been eliminated from the second edition.)

A breakdown as to responses by regions of the U.S. is included in each respective chapter along with other survey information. The questionnaire included questions on: I Quantity done yearly, II Estimate of a change in the quantity over the next 3-4 years, III should the procedure still be taught and included in this text.

Procedure	I. Quantity Done Yearly	II. Estimates of increase(+) decrease(-) No change(0)	III. Should not be included
1. Gallbladder, post fatty meal or CCK-PZ injection	0-4 = 55% 5-24 = 26% 25+ = 18%	7% + 43% - 51% 0	43%
2. IV Cholangiogram	0-3 = 81% 4-11 = 10% 12+ = 9%	2% + 34% - 64% 0	64%
3. Lymphogram or Lymphangiogram	0-4 = 65% 5-10 = 20% 11+ = 15%	3% + 35% - 62% 0	42%
4. Fetograms	0-3 = 77% 4-10 = 14% 11+ = 9%	2% + 27% - 71% 0	65%
5. Pelvimetry	0-3 = 60% 5-24 = 21% 25+ = 19%	3% + 38% - 57% 0	45%
6. Temporal Bone Survey	0-2 = 81% 3-20 = 10% 21+ = 9%	3% + 16% - 81% 0	62%

Survey Respondents by Regions

A total of 520 responses were received, of which 283 were from college program affiliates and 237 from hospital based programs. These responses were divided into three regions of the U.S. as follows:

Region	States	College Affiliates	Hospital Based	Total Respondents
1. West	7 States - AZ, CA, HI, ID, NM, OR, WA	52	19	71
2. Midwest	23 States - AL, AR, CO, IA, IL, IN, KS, LA, MI, MN, MO, MS, MT, ND, NE, NV, OH, OK, SD, TX, UT, WI, WY	128	123	251
3. East	18 States - CT, DE, FL, GA, KY, MA, MD, ME, NC, NH, NY, PA, RI, SC, TN, VA, WV	103	95	198
		283	237	520

Size & Type of Program

The size and type of radiologic technology educational programs responding to the survey by region were as follows:

Number of first year students	East	Midwest	West	Totals
1 - 7	24.4%	32.8%	11.8%	27.6%
8 - 11	27.6%	30.5%	17.6%	28.4%
12 - 17	24.4%	18.0%	5.9%	20.1%
18 - 62	23.6%	18.8%	64.7%	23.9%

Size of Clinical Institutions

The number of beds of the clinical institutions responding to the survey and the number of radiographic exams done per year were as follows:

Number of Exams / Year	25- 199 beds	200-300 beds	309-980 beds	481-2000 beds	Totals
75 - 30,000 exams	72.4%	17.6%	5.2%	3%	25.1%
30,001 - 53,738 exams	21.9%	50.9%	20.6%	5%	25.1%
53,739 - 79,000 exams	5.7%	24.1%	50.5%	19%	24.4%
79,001 - 999,999 exams	–	7.4%	23.7%	73%	25.4%

CONTENTS

Chapter 1

General Anatomy, Terminology, Imaging Principles, Radiation Protection and Positioning Principles

Contributions by: Kathy Martensen, BS, RT (R)
E. Russell Ritenour, Ph.D.
Barry Anthony, RT (R)

Contents

Part I General, Systemic and Skeletal Anatomy and Arthrology

General Anatomy

Anatomy is the science of the structure of the human body, while **physiology** deals with functions of the body, or how the body parts work. In the living subject, it is almost impossible to study anatomy without also studying some physiology. Radiographic study of the human body is primarily a study of the anatomy of the various systems with lesser emphasis on the physiology. Consequently, anatomy of the human system will be emphasized in this radiographic anatomy and positioning text.

Structural Organization

Several levels of structural organization compose the human body. The lowest level of organization is the **chemical level.** All of the chemicals necessary for maintaining life are composed of **atoms**, joined in various ways to form **molecules.** Various chemicals in the form of molecules are organized to form **cells.**

Cells: The cell is the basic structural and functional unit of the entire human being. Every single part of the body, whether muscle, bone, cartilage, fat, nerve, skin or blood, is composed of cells.

Tissues: Tissues are groups of similar cells which together with their intercellular material, perform a specific function. The four basic types of tissues are:

1. **Epithelial** *(ep'i-the'le-al)* - Tissue which covers internal and external surfaces of the body including lining of vessels and organs, such as the stomach and intestines.
2. **Connective** - Tissues which bind together and support the various structures.
3. **Muscular** - Tissues which make up the substances of a muscle.
4. **Nervous** - Tissues which make up the substance of nerves and nerve centers.

Organs: When various tissues are joined together to perform a specific function, the result is an organ. Organs usually have a specific shape. Some of the organs of the human body are the kidneys, heart, liver, lungs, stomach and brain.

System: A system consists of a group or association of organs that has a similar or a common function. The urinary system, consisting of kidneys, ureters, bladder and urethra, as described on page 4, is an example of a body system. There are ten individual body systems composing the total body.

Organism: All of the ten systems of the body functioning together constitute the total organism--one living being.

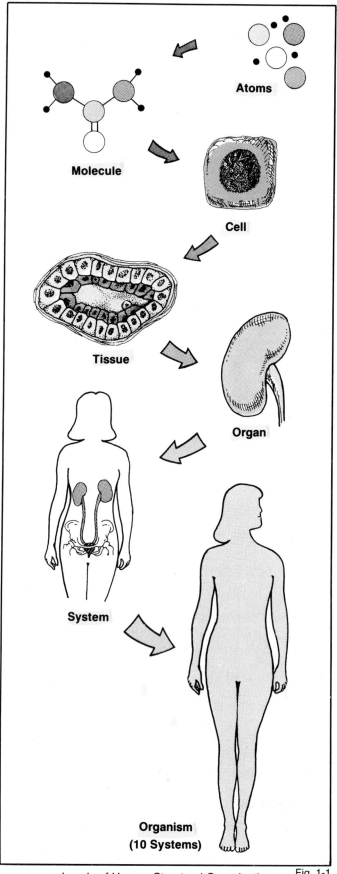

Levels of Human Structural Organization   Fig. 1-1

Systemic Anatomy

Body Systems

The human body is a structural and functional unit made up of ten lesser units termed systems. These ten systems are: (1) skeletal, (2) circulatory, (3) digestive, (4) respiratory, (5) urinary, (6) reproductive, (7) nervous, (8) muscular, (9) endocrine, and (10) integumentary.

1. Skeletal System: The skeletal system is an important system to be studied by the radiographer. The skeletal system includes the 206 separate bones of the body and their associated cartilages and joints. The study of bones is termed **osteology**, while the study of joints is termed **arthrology.**

Four functions of the skeletal system are to:
1. Support and protect the body
2. Allow movement by interacting with the muscles to form levers
3. Produce blood cells
4. Store calcium.

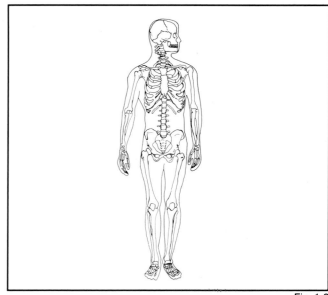

Skeletal System   Fig. 1-2

2. Circulatory System: The circulatory system is composed of the cardiovascular organs — heart, blood and blood vessels, and the lymphatic system — lymph nodes, lymph, lymph vessels and lymph glands.

Six functions of the circulatory system are to:
1. Distribute oxygen and nutrients to the cells of the body
2. Carry cell waste and carbon dioxide from the cells
3. Transport water, electrolytes, hormones and enzymes
4. Protect against disease
5. Prevent hemorrhage by forming blood clots
6. Help regulate body temperature.

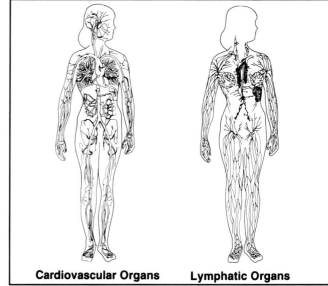

Cardiovascular Organs   **Lymphatic Organs**

Circulatory System   Fig. 1-3

3. Digestive System: The digestive system includes the alimentary canal and certain accessory organs. The alimentary canal is made up of the mouth, pharynx, esophagus, stomach, small intestine, large intestine and anus. Accessory organs of digestion include the salivary glands, liver, gall bladder and pancreas.

The twofold function of the digestive system is to:
1. Prepare food for absorption by the cells through numerous physical and chemical breakdown processes
2. Eliminate solid wastes from the body.

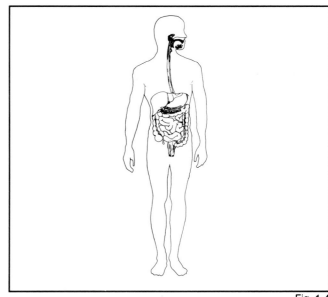

Digestive System   Fig. 1-4

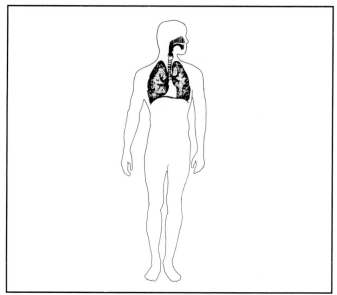

Respiratory System   Fig. 1-5

4. Respiratory System: The respiratory system is composed of two lungs and a series of passages connecting the lungs to the outside atmosphere. The structures making up the passageway from the exterior to the alveoli of the lung interior are the nose, mouth, pharynx, larynx, trachea and bronchial tree.

Three functions of the respiratory system are to:
1. Supply oxygen to the blood and eventually to the cells
2. Eliminate carbon dioxide from the blood
3. Assist in regulating the acid-base balance of the blood.

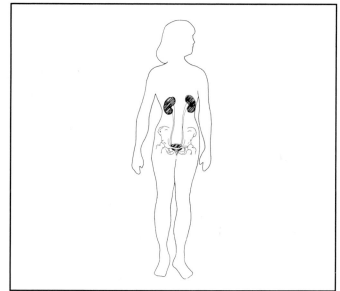

Urinary System   Fig. 1-6

5. Urinary System: The urinary system includes those organs that produce, collect and eliminate urine. The organs of the urinary system are the kidneys, ureters, bladder and urethra.

The urinary system functions to:
1. Regulate the chemical composition of the blood
2. Eliminate many waste products
3. Regulate fluid and electrolyte balance and volume
4. Maintain the acid-base balance of the body.

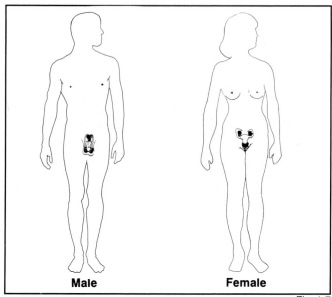

Male   **Female**

Reproductive System   Fig. 1-7

6. Reproductive System: The reproductive or genital system includes those organs that produce, transport and store the germ cells. The testes in the male and the ovaries in the female produce mature germ cells. Transport and storage organs of the male include the vas deferens, prostate gland and penis. Additional organs of reproduction in the female are the uterine tubes, uterus and vagina.

The function of the reproductive system is to reproduce the organism.

Systemic Anatomy continued

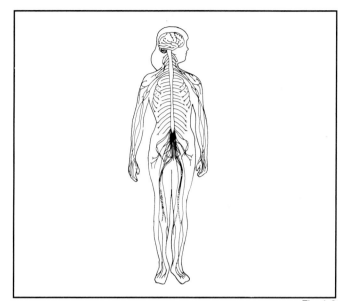

Nervous System   Fig. 1-8

7. Nervous System: The nervous system is composed of the brain, spinal cord, nerves, ganglia and special sense organs such as the eyes and ears.

The function of the nervous system is to regulate body activities with electrical impulses traveling along various nerves.

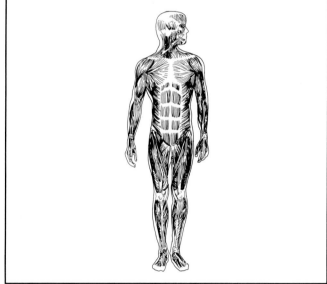

Muscular System   Fig. 1-9

8. Muscular System: The muscular system includes all muscle tissues of the body and is subdivided into three types: (1) skeletal, (2) visceral, and (3) cardiac. Most of the muscle mass of the body is skeletal muscle, which is striated and under voluntary control. The voluntary muscles act in conjunction with the skeleton to allow body movement. About 43 percent of the weight of the human body is composed of voluntary or striated skeletal muscle. Visceral muscle, which is smooth and involuntary, is located in the walls of hollow internal organs such as blood vessels, stomach and intestines. These muscles are termed involuntary because their contraction is usually not under voluntary or conscious control. Cardiac muscle is found only in the walls of the heart and is involuntary, but striated.

Three functions of muscle tissue are to:
1. Allow movement, such as locomotion of the body or movement of substances through the alimentary canal
2. Maintain posture
3. Produce heat.

9. Endocrine System: The endocrine system includes all of the ductless glands of the body. These glands include the testes, ovaries, pancreas, adrenals, thymus, thyroid, parathyroids, pineal and pituitary. The placenta acts as a temporary endocrine gland.

Hormones, which are the secretions of the endocrine glands, are released directly into the bloodstream.

The function of the endocrine system is to regulate bodily activities through the various hormones carried by the cardiovascular system.

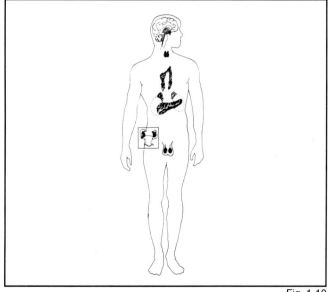

Endocrine System   Fig. 1-10

10. Integumentary System: The **integumentary** *(in-teg-u-men'tar-e)* system is composed of the skin and all structures derived from the skin. These derived structures include hair, nails, and sweat and oil glands. The skin is an organ that is essential to life. In fact, the skin is the largest organ of the body, covering a surface area of approximately 7,620 square centimeters in the average adult.

Four functions of the integumentary system are to:
1. Regulate body temperature
2. Protect the body
3. Eliminate waste products through perspiration
4. Receive certain stimuli such as temperature, pressure and pain.

Skeletal Anatomy

Since a large part of general diagnostic radiography involves examinations of the bones and joints, **osteology** *(os'te-ol'o-je)* (the study of bones) and **arthrology** *(ar-throl'o-je)* (the study of joints) are important subjects for the radiographer.

Osteology

The adult skeletal system is composed of 206 separate bones, forming the framework of the entire body. Certain cartilages, such as at the ends of long bones, are included in the skeletal system. These bones and cartilages are united by ligaments and provide surfaces to which the muscles attach. Since muscles and bones must combine to allow body movement, these two systems are sometimes collectively referred to as the locomotor system.

The adult human skeleton is divided into either the axial skeleton or the appendicular skeleton.

Axial Skeleton: The **axial** *(ak'se-al)* **skeleton** includes all bones that lie on or near the central axis of the body. The adult axial skeleton consists of 80 bones and includes the skull, vertebral column, ribs and sternum.

Adult Axial Skeleton

Skull
    Cranium 8
    Facial Bones 14
Hyoid 1
Auditory Ossicles ... 6
    (Small bones
    in each ear)
Vertebral column
    Cervical 7
    Thoracic.............. 12
    Lumbar................ 5
    Sacrum................ 1
    Coccyx................ 1
Thorax
    Sternum................ 1
    Ribs...................... 24

Total   80

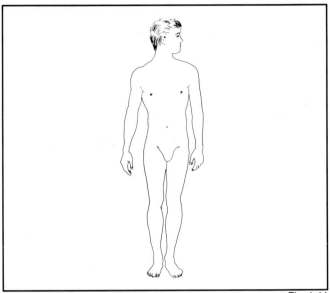

Integumentary System   Fig. 1-11

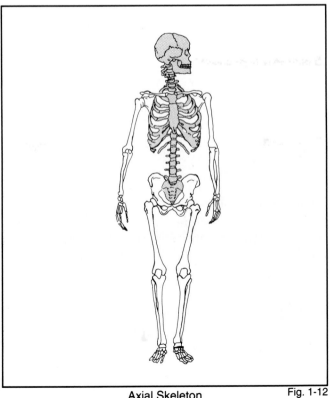

Axial Skeleton   Fig. 1-12

Appendicular Skeleton: The second division of the skeleton is the **appendicular** *(ap'en-dik'u-lar)* portion. This division consists of all bones of the upper and lower limbs (extremities), as well as the shoulder and pelvic girdles. There are 126 separate bones in the adult appendicular skeleton.

Adult Appendicular Skeleton

Shoulder Girdles
    Clavicle.................. 2
    Scapula.................. 2
Upper Limbs
    Humerus................ 2
    Ulna 2
    Radius................... 2
    Carpals.................. 16
    Metacarpals........... 10
    Phalanges.............. 28
Pelvic Girdle
    Hip Bone 2
Lower Limbs
    Femur 2
    Tibia 2
    Fibula 2
    Patella 2
    Tarsals 14
    Metatarsals 10
    Phalanges 28

Total 126

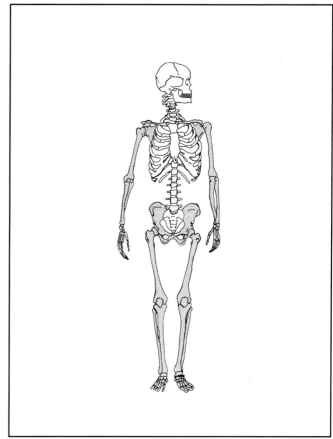

Appendicular Skeleton   Fig. 1-13

Classification of Bones

Each of the 206 bones of the body can be classified according to shape as a (1) long bone, (2) short bone, (3) flat bone, or (4) irregular bone.

1. Long Bones: Long bones consist of a shaft or **diaphysis** *(di-af'i-sis)*, and two ends or extremities. The ends of long bones articulate with other bones; thus the ends are enlarged, smooth and covered with hyaline cartilage.

    Hyaline *(hi'ah-lin)*, meaning glassy or clear, is a common type of cartilage or connecting tissue, also known as gristle. It's name comes from the fact that it is not visible with ordinary staining techniques, thus appearing as "clear" or glassy in lab studies. It is present in many places including the covering over ends of bones where it is called **articular cartilage**.

    Long bones are found only in the appendicular skeleton and are usually curved for strength. *Figure 1-14* is a radiograph of a humerus, a typical long bone.

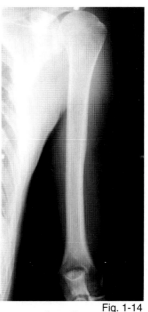

Fig. 1-14
Long Bone
(Humerus)

Long Bones continued

The outer shell of most bones is composed of hard or dense bone tissue known as **compact bone** or **cortex**, meaning an external layer. Compact bone has few intercellular empty spaces and serves to protect and support the entire bone. The **diaphysis** or **shaft** contains a thicker layer of compact bone than the ends to help resist the stress of the weight placed on them.

Inside the shell of compact bone, and especially at both ends of each long bone, is found **spongy** or **cancellous bone**. Cancellous bone is highly porous and usually contains red bone marrow, which is responsible for production of red blood cells.

The shaft of a long bone is hollow. This hollow portion is known as the **medullary cavity**. In the adult the medullary cavity usually contains fatty yellow marrow. A dense fibrous membrane, the **periosteum**, covers bone except at the articulating surfaces. The articulating surfaces are covered with a layer of cartilage. The periosteum is essential for bone growth, repair and nutrition. Bones are richly supplied with blood vessels that pass into them from the periosteum. Near the center of the shaft of long bones, a **nutrient artery** passes obliquely through the compact bone via a **nutrient foramen** into the medullary cavity.

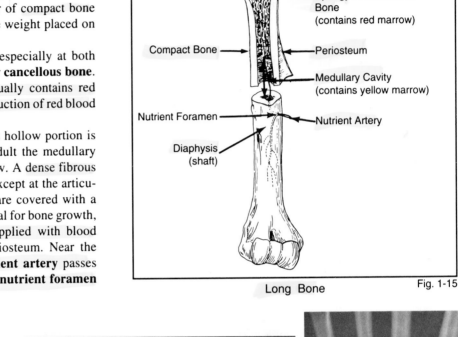

Long Bone   Fig. 1-15

2. **Short Bones:** Short bones are roughly cuboidal in shape and are only found in the wrists and ankles. Short bones consist mainly of cancellous tissue with a thin outer covering of compact bone. The eight carpal bones of each wrist and the seven tarsal bones of each ankle are all short bones.

3. **Flat Bones:** Flat bones consist of two plates of compact bone with cancellous bone and marrow between them. Examples of flat bones are the bones making up the calvarium (skull cap), sternum, ribs and scapulae. The narrow space between the inner and outer table of the flat bones of the cranium is known as diploe. Flat bones provide either protection or broad surfaces for muscle attachment.

4. **Irregular Bones:** Bones that have peculiar shapes are lumped into the final category of irregular bones. Vertebrae, facial bones, bones of the base of the cranium and bones of the pelvis are examples of irregular bones.

Blood Cell Production: It should be noted that in adults red blood cells (RBC) are produced by the red bone marrow of certain flat and irregular bones such as the sternum, ribs, vertebrae and pelvis.

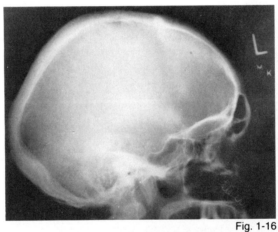

Fig. 1-16

Flat Bones (Calvarium)

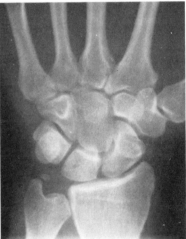

Fig. 1-17

Short Bones (Carpals)

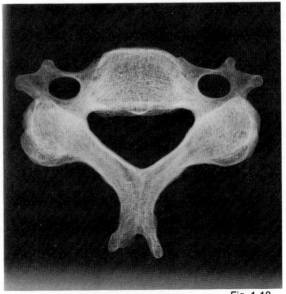

Irregular Bone (Vertebra)   Fig. 1-18

Development of Bones

The process by which bones form in the body is known as **ossification** *(os″i-fi-ka′shun)*. The embryonic skeleton is composed of fibrous membranes and hyaline cartilage. Ossification begins about the sixth embryonic week and continues until adulthood.

Two Kinds of Bone Formation

Two kinds of bone formation are known. When bone replaces membranes, the ossification is termed **intramembranous** *(in″trah-mem′brah-nus)*. When bone replaces cartilage, the result is **endochondral** *(en″do-kon′dral)* (intracartilaginous) ossification.

Intramembranous Ossification: Intramembranous ossification occurs rapidly and takes place in bones that are needed for protection, such as sutures of the flat bones of the skullcap which are centers of growth in early bone development.

Endochondral Ossification: Endochondral ossification occurs much slower than intramembranous ossification and occurs in most parts of the skeleton, especially in the long bones.

Primary and Secondary Centers of Endochondral Ossification

The first center of ossification is termed the **primary center** and occurs in the **midshaft area.** This primary center of ossification becomes the **diaphysis** *(di-af′i-sis)*.

Secondary centers of ossification appear near the ends of long bones. Most secondary centers appear after birth, while most primary centers appear before birth. **Each secondary center of ossification is termed an epiphysis** *(e-pif′i-sis)*. Epiphyses of the distal femur and the proximal tibia are the first to appear and may be present at birth in the term newborn. Cartilaginous plates termed **epiphyseal plates** are found between the diaphysis and each epiphysis until skeletal growth is complete.

Growth in the length of bones is due to a longitudinal increase in these epiphyseal cartilaginous plates. This is followed by progressive ossification through endochondral bone development until all of the cartilage has been replaced by bone at which time growth to the skeleton is complete. This process of epiphyseal fusion of the long bones occurs progressively from the age of puberty to full maturity which is about twenty-five years. However the time for each bone to complete growth varies for different regions of the body. In addition, the female skeleton usually matures more quickly than does the male skeleton. Extensive charts that list the normal growth patterns of the skeleton are available.

Radiograph demonstrating Bone Growth

Figure 1-20 shows a radiograph of a leg (tibia and fibula) of a young child. Primary and secondary centers of endochondral ossification or bone growth are well demonstrated and labeled.

Primary Centers: The primary centers of bone growth show well developed bone and include the (A) **diaphysis** or midshaft area.

Secondary Centers: The secondary centers of bone growth are the (C) **epiphyses** which are shown at both ends of the tibia, as well as the distal fibula at the ankle joint, and the distal femur at the knee joint. These epiphyses are separated from the main bone by a space or joint called an (B) **epiphyseal plate**. These are made up of cartilage which does not visualize on radiographs because there is no calcium in these areas at this stage of growth. Therefore, these epiphyseal plates disappear completely as cartilage is replaced with calcium when growth is completed.

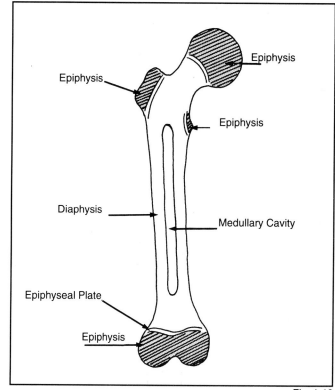

Endochondral Ossification

Fig. 1-19

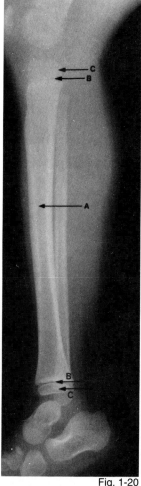

Fig. 1-20
Leg (Tibia and Fibula)
Courtesy of Joan Dickerson, RT

Arthrology (Joints)

The study of joints or articulations is called **arthrology**. In studying joints of the skeletal system it is first important to understand that movement does not occur in all joints. Indeed the first type of joints to be described are primarily immovable joints held together by several fibrous layers. These are joints adapted for growth rather than for movement. The second grouping of joints includes most joints of the body and are those adapted for movement.

Classification of Joints

Functional
Joints are often classified according to their function as to their mobility or lack of mobility. The three common functional classifications are as follows:

1. **Synarthrosis** *(sin″ar-thro′sis)* - immovable joints
2. **Amphiarthrosis** *(am″fe-ar-thro′sis)* - limited movement
3. **Diarthrosis** *(di″ar-thro′sis)* - freely movable joint

Structural
It has been a common practice in radiography to classify or group all joints or articulations of the body under the three functional classes. However, the primary classification system of joints, which is recognized by *NOMINA ANATOMICA* and which is used in this textbook, **is a structural classification** based on the **type of tissue which separates the ends of the bone**. Functional types (listed by description of movement type) are included under each of these structural classifications.

There are three structural classifications based on the **three types of tissues** which separate the ends of bones in the different joints. These three classifications by tissue types are listed below along with the sub classes.

A. **Fibrous** *(fi′brus)* **Joints**
1. Syndesmosis *(sin″des-mo′sis)*
2. Suture *(su′tur)*
   (Gomphysis *(gom-fo′sis)* - see NOTE below)

B. **Cartilaginous** *(kar″ti-laj′i-nus)* **Joints**
1. Symphysis *(sim′fi-sis)*
2. Synchondrosis *(sin″kon-dro′sis)*

C. **Synovial** *(si-no′ ve-al)* **Joints**

Each of these three classes and their subclasses will be described and illustrated with examples beginning with fibrous joints.

A. Fibrous Joints
Fibrous joints lack a joint cavity. The adjoining bones, which are nearly in direct contact to each other, are **held together by fibrous connective tissue**. Two types of fibrous joints are **syndesmoses**, which are slightly movable, and **sutures**, which are immovable *(Fig. 1-21)*.

1. Syndesmoses
The only true syndesmosis joint in the body is the distal tibiofibular joint.
Fibrous ligaments hold the distal tibia and fibula together at this joint which is only **slightly movable** or **amphiarthrodial.**

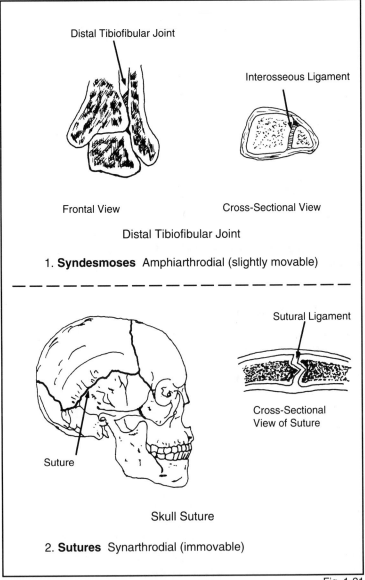

Distal Tibiofibular Joint

Interosseous Ligament

Frontal View

Cross-Sectional View

Distal Tibiofibular Joint

1. **Syndesmoses** Amphiarthrodial (slightly movable)

Sutural Ligament

Suture

Cross-Sectional View of Suture

Skull Suture

2. **Sutures** Synarthrodial (immovable)

A. Fibrous Joints   Fig. 1-21

2. Sutures
Sutures are found only between bones in the skull. These bones make contact with one another along interlocking or serrated edges and are **held together by layers of fibrous tissue or ligaments.** Therefore, there is very limited movement at these articulations and they are considered **immovable** or **synarthrodial joints.**

Some limited expansion-compression type movement at these sutures can occur in the infant skull such as during the birthing process, but upon reaching adulthood active bone deposition partially or completely obliterates these suture lines.

NOTE: A **gomphysis** joint is a third unique type of fibrous joint in which a conical process is inserted into a socket-like portion of a bone. The best example is the immovable type joint or fibrous union between the roots of the teeth and the alveoli of the mandible and maxillae as described in Chapter 12.

B. Cartilaginous Joints

Cartilaginous joints also lack a joint cavity and the articulating bones are **held tightly together by cartilage.** Like fibrous joints they allow little or no movement. Therefore, these joints are either synarthrodial or amphiarthrodial and are held together by two types of cartilage. They are as follows:

1. Symphyses

The essential feature of a symphysis type joint is **the presence of a broad, flattened disc of fibrocartilage** between two contiguous bony surfaces. These fibrocartilage discs form relatively thick pads which are capable of being compressed or displaced thereby allowing some movement of these bones, or **amphiarthrodial (slightly movable).**

Examples of such symphyses are the intervertebral discs (between bodies of the vertebrae) and the pubic symphysis (between the two pubic bones).

2. Synchondroses

A typical synchondrosis is a **temporary form of joint** wherein the connecting **hyaline cartilage** (which on long bones is called an epiphyseal plate) is converted into bone upon reaching adulthood. These temporary type of growth joints are considered **synarthrodial** or **immovable.**

Examples of such joints are between the epiphyses and diaphyses of long bones.

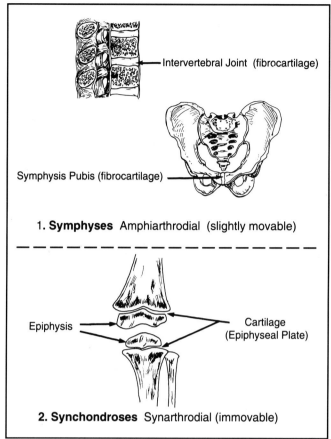

1. Symphyses Amphiarthrodial (slightly movable)

2. Synchondroses Synarthrodial (immovable)

B. Cartilaginous Joints   Fig. 1-22

C. Synovial Joints

The third classification of joints are synovial joints, those freely movable joints, mostly of the upper and lower limbs, characterized by **a fibrous capsule containing synovial fluid.** The ends of the bones making up a synovial joint may make contact but are completely separate and contain a joint space or cavity which allows for the wide range of movement at these joints. All synovial joints are **diarthrodial** or **freely movable.**

The exposed ends of these bones contain thin protective type coverings of **hyaline articular cartilage.** The **joint cavity**, which contains a viscous lubricating **synovial fluid**, is surrounded by a **fibrous capsule**, which is reinforced by strengthening **accessory ligaments**. These ligaments limit motion in undesirable directions. The inner surface of this fibrous capsule is thought to secrete the lubricating synovial fluid.

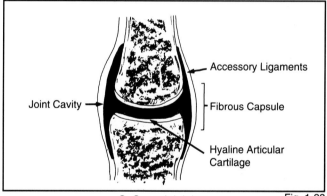

C. Synovial Joints   Fig. 1-23
Diarthrodial (freely movable)

Movement Types of Synovial Joints

Synovial joints occur in considerable number and variety and they are grouped according to the six types of movements they permit. These are listed in order from the least to the greatest permitted movement.

1. Gliding (Plane) Joints

This type of synovial joint permits the least movement, which as the name implies, is **a sliding or gliding motion between the articulating surfaces.**

Examples of such joints are the intermetacarpal, carpometacarpal and intercarpal joints of the hand and wrist.

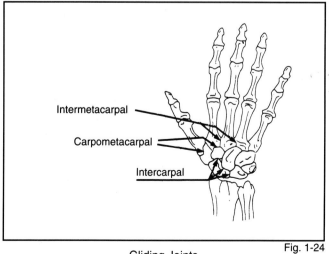

Gliding Joints   Fig. 1-24

2. Hinge (Ginglymus) Joints

The articular surfaces of a hinge joint are molded to each other in such a way to permit **flexion and extension movements** only. The articular fibrous capsule on this type of joint is thin on those surfaces where bending takes place but strong collateral ligaments firmly secure the bones at the lateral margins of the fibrous capsule.

Examples of such joints are the interphalangeal joints of both fingers and toes, the knee joint, the elbow joint and the ankle joint.

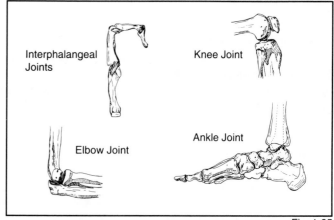

Hinge Joints   Fig. 1-25

3. Pivot (Trochoidal) Joints

The pivot joint is formed by a bony pivot-like process which is surrounded by a ring of ligaments and/or bony structure. This allows **rotational movements** around a single axis.

Examples of such joints are the proximal and distal radioulnar joints which demonstrate this pivot-like movement during pronation and supination. Another example is the joint between first and second cervical vertebrae. The dens of the axis (C2) forms the pivot, and the anterior arch of the atlas (C1) combined with posterior ligaments form the ring.

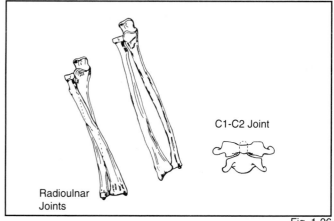

Pivot Joints   Fig. 1-26

4. Condyloid Joints

In the condyloid joint, movement occurs primarily in one plane combined with a slight degree of rotation at an axis which is at right angles to the primary plane of movement. The rotational movement is somewhat limited by associated ligaments and tendons.

This type of joint therefore allows primarily four directional movements of **flexion and extension** along with **abduction and adduction.** **Circumduction** movement also occurs which results from cone-like sequential movements of flexion, abduction, extension and adduction.

Examples of condyloid joints are the 2nd through 5th metacarpophalangeal joints of fingers and the wrist joint.

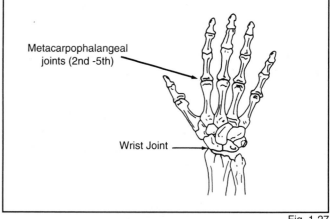

Condyloid Joints   Fig. 1-27

5. Saddle (Sellar) Joint

The term saddle describes this joint structure well as the ends of the bones are shaped concavoconvex or opposite to one another as illustrated in *Fig. 1-28*.

Movements of this biaxial type saddle joint are the same as for condyloid joints, namely **flexion, extension, adduction, abduction** and **circumduction**.

Examples of saddle joints are the first carpometacarpal and metacarpophalangeal joints of the thumb.

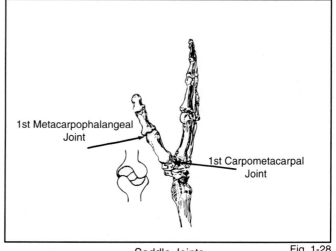

Saddle Joints   Fig. 1-28

6. Ball and Socket or **Spheroidal Joint**

The ball and socket or spheroidal joint allows the greatest freedom of motion. The distal bone making up the joint is capable of motion around an almost indefinite number of axes, with one common center.

The greater the depth of the socket, the more limited the movement. The joint however is stronger and more stable. For example, the hip joint is a much stronger and more stable joint than the shoulder joint, but the range of movement is also more limited in the hip.

Movements of ball and socket joints are **flexion, extension, abduction, adduction, circumduction, medial** and **lateral rotation.**

The two examples of ball and socket joints are the hip joint and the shoulder joint.

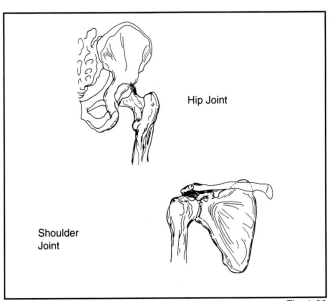

Ball and Socket or Spheroidal Joints   Fig. 1-29

Summary of Joint Classification

Joint Classification	Mobility Classification	Examples
A. Fibrous Joints		
1. Syndesmoses	Amphiarthrodial (slightly movable)	- Distal tibiofibular joint
2. Sutures	Synarthrodial (immovable)	- Skull sutures
B. Cartilaginous Joints		
1. Symphyses	Amphiarthrodial (slightly movable)	- Intervertebral discs - Pubic Symphysis
2. Synchondroses	Synarthrodial (immovable)	- Between ephiphyses and diaphyses of long bones.
C. Synovial Joints	Diarthrodial (freely movable)	
	Movement Type	
	1. Gliding (plane)	- Intercarpal and carpometacarpal joints
	2. Hinge (ginglymus)	- Interphalangeal joints of fingers and toes, knee, ankle and elbow joints
	3. Pivot (trochoidal)	- Proximal and distal radioulnar and between C1 and C2 vertebrae
	4. Condyloid	- Metacarpophalangeal and wrist joints
	5. Saddle (sellar)	- First carpometacarpal and metacarpophalangeal of thumb
	6. Ball & Socket (spheroidal)	- Hip and shoulder joints

Study of Arthrology Continues: Arthrology or the study of joints will continue throughout this text as specific anatomy including all joints of the human body is studied in more detail in following chapters.

Part II   Radiographic Terminology

It is essential that each person planning to work as a medical radiographer clearly understand the terminology commonly used in medical radiographic positioning. This part of Chapter 1 lists, describes and illustrates those commonly used terms consistent with the positioning and projection terminology as adopted and published by *The American Registry of Radiologic Technologists* in January, 1990.

Throughout this text the use of named positions (proper names of the person first describing a specific position or procedure) is generally avoided, except for the most common ones, such as Towne, Waters and Caldwell. Instead, the text contains standardized anatomic projection/position terminology, utilizing terms defined and illustrated in this chapter.

The anatomical terms used in this section and throughout this text are in agreement with the widely used standard as adopted in 1985 by the Twelfth International Congress of Anatomists in London, published in the sixth edition of *NOMINA ANATOMICA*.

General Terms

The following terms, commonly used in radiographic positioning, are defined in clear and precise language to allow easy understanding. Phonetic respelling (according to *Dorland's Illustrated Medical Dictionary,* 24th edition) is included in parentheses to aid in correct pronunciation for the more uncommon terms. Wherever possible, illustrations and examples are also included to further clarify meanings and definitions.

1. Radiograph *(ra´de-o-graf)* vs. **X-ray Film**
* An x-ray film containing an image of an anatomical part of a patient (produced by action of x-rays on x-ray film).

   Radiography *(ra˝de-og´rah-fe)* is the production of radiographs.

   NOTE: In practice, the terms **radiograph** and **x-ray film** are often used interchangeably. The x-ray film specifically refers to the physical piece of material upon which the radiographic image is exposed. The term radiograph includes the x-ray film **and** the image that is contained on it.

2. Radiographic Examination or Procedure
* A radiographer is shown positioning the patient for a routine chest exam or procedure.
   A radiographic examination of the chest includes five general functions as follows:
   (a) Positioning of the body part; and CR (central ray) alignment.
   (b) Selection of radiation protection measures.
   (c) Selection of exposure factors (radiographic technique) on control panel of x-ray machine.
   (d) Taking exposure.
   (e) Processing (developing) of the film.

3. Anatomical *(an˝ah-tom´e-kal)* **Position**
* An **upright position, arms adducted** (down), **palms forward, head and feet directed straight ahead.**
* This specific body position is used as a reference for other positioning terms.

   NOTE: When referring to one part of the body in relationship to other parts, one must always think of the person as **standing erect in the anatomical position,** even when describing parts of a patient who is lying down, otherwise confusion as to the meaning of the description may result.

   Viewing Radiographs: In the U.S. there is a generally accepted way of placing radiographs for viewing. This general rule in viewing radiographs is to display them so that **the patient is facing the viewer,** with the patient in the **anatomical position** (as if you were shaking hands with the patient). This places the patient's left on the viewer's right. This is true **for either AP or PA projections** of the chest, abdomen, spine, skull and proximal upper and lower limbs. (Exceptions to this rule are the distal upper and lower limbs such as radiographs of the hands and feet which generally are placed on the viewbox with the fingers and toes upward.)

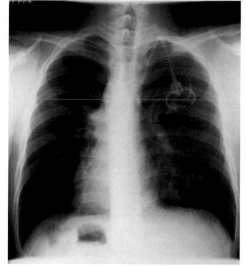

Chest Radiograph   Fig. 1-30

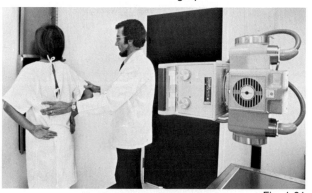

Radiographic Examination   Fig. 1-31

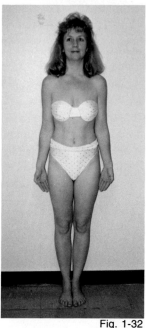

Fig. 1-32
Anatomical Position

Radiographic Projections

Body Surfaces

4. Posterior *(pos-te're-or)* (Dorsal) *(dor'sal)*
- Refers to the **back half** of patient, includes bottom of feet and back of hands. (See exception.)

5. Anterior *(an-te're-or)* (Ventral) *(ven'tral)*
- Refers to **front half** of patient, includes top of feet and front or palms of hands. (See exception.)

EXCEPTION: It should be noted that for the **hands,** the terms **palmar or volar** are sometimes substituted for ventral or anterior.
For the **foot** the posterior or sole of the foot is also commonly called the **plantar** surface and the top of the foot is called the **dorsal** or **dorsum** surface. (See terms numbered 45-47 for further descriptions of the surfaces of the hands and feet.

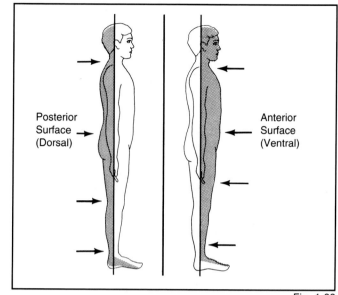

Posterior vs. Anterior · Fig. 1-33

Projections

Projection is an anatomical positioning term used to describe the path of the x-ray beam projecting an image on to radiographic film or other image receptor. Following are two of the most commonly used projection terms.

6. Posteroanterior *(pos"ter-o-an-te're-or)* (PA) **Projection**
- **A projection of the x-ray beam from posterior to anterior.**
- Combines these two terms, posterior and anterior, into one word.
- Refers to the direction which the x-ray beam travels, called a projection. The x-ray beam enters a posterior surface and exits an anterior surface (PA projection).

Body Position: This PA projection could also be called an **erect anterior position** of the chest, describing the body part closest to the film as defined under specific body positions on page 18. However, in practice it is more common to call this a PA projection rather than an anterior position.

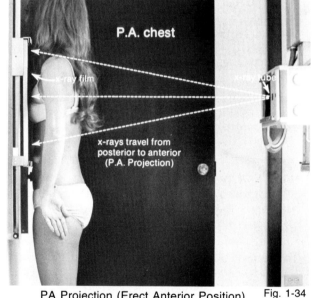

PA Projection (Erect Anterior Position) · Fig. 1-34

7. Anteroposterior *(an"ter-o-pos-te're-or)* (AP) **Projection**
- **A projection of the x-ray beam from anterior to posterior.**
- Combines these two terms, anterior and posterior, into one word.
- Describes the direction of travel of the x-ray beam, which enters at an anterior surface and exits at a posterior surface (AP projection).

Body Position: This AP projection of the chest could also correctly be called an **erect posterior position**, wherein the posterior portion of the chest is closest to the film. However, as noted above, in practice these PA and AP projections are more commonly described as projections rather than as body positions.

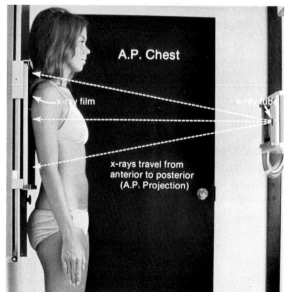

AP Projection
(Erect Posterior Position) · Fig. 1-35

Additional Projection Terms

Following are additional terms commonly used by practicing radiographers to describe projections. These terms, as shown by their definitions, are not as specific or as descriptive as other projection terms but generally refer to the path or projection of the x-ray beam. (Additional explanation and examples of the uses of the terms projection and position are included on page 29.)

8. Axial *(ak'se-al)*
- Axial refers to the **long axis** of a structure or part around which a rotating body turns or is arranged.

  The term, **cephalocaudal** describes the long axis or center line of the human body from the head to the feet.

Special Application: In positioning, the term axial is commonly used to describe **any angle of the central ray along the long axis of the body**. It should be noted however, in a true sense an axial projection would be directed along, or parallel to the long axis. The term "semi" axial or "partly" axial more accurately describes any angle along the axis that is not truly along or parallel to the long axis. However, for the sake of consistency with other references and to avoid confusion in practice, the term axial projection will be used throughout this text to describe both axial and semi-axial projections as defined above and as illustrated in *Figs. 1-36 and 37*.

Therefore the term axial as used in this text is a general term, describing **a projection** wherein there is some angling of the central ray along the long axis.

9. Tangential *(tan"jen'shal)*
- Means **touching a curve or surface at only one point.**
- A term to describe **a projection** that merely skims a body part to project it away from other body structures.

Examples: Following are three examples or applications of the term tangential as defined above:
- Zygomatic arch projection *(Fig. 1-38)*
- Trama skull projection for demonstrating impacted skull fracture. *(Fig. 1-39)*
- Special projection of patella *(Fig. 1-40)*.

10. Lordotic *(lor-dot'ik)* (Apical Lordotic Projection)
- A **specific AP chest projection** for demonstrating the apices of the lungs without superimposition by the clavicles.
- The term **lordotic** comes from **lordosis,** a term denoting the curvature of the spine with forward convexity. As the patient assumes this position *(Fig. 1-41)*, the lumbar lordotic curvature is exaggerated making this a descriptive term for this special chest projection.

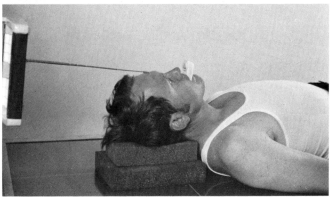

Axial (Supero-inferior) Projection   Fig. 1-36

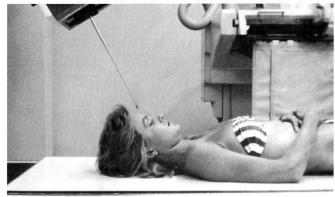

AP Axial (Semi-axial) Projection   Fig. 1-37

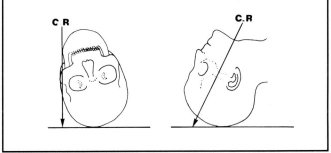

Tangential Projection   Fig. 1-38

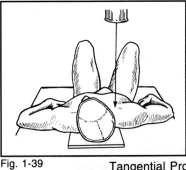

Fig. 1-39

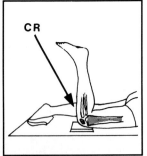

Tangential Projection   Fig. 1-40

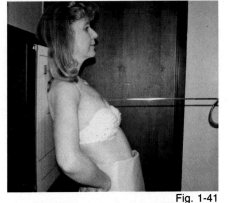

Fig. 1-41
AP Chest Lordotic Projection

Radiographic Positions

The term **position** in radiography is used to discuss the patient's physical position in two ways. First is a more general use of this term referring to **general body positions** such as **supine, prone, erect, recumbent** or **Trendelenburg** (terms 11-15).

General Body Positions

11. Supine *(su'pin)*
- A body position
- **Lying on back** with face directed upward (anteriorly).

12. Prone *(pron)*
- A body position
- **Lying on abdomen,** facing downward (head may be turned to one side).

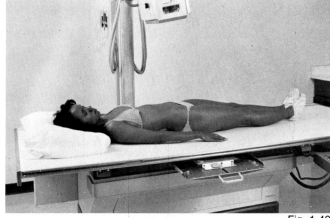

Supine   Fig. 1-42

13. Erect *(i'reckt')*
- A body position
- An **upright position,** to stand or sit erect.

14. Recumbent *(re-kum'bent)* (Reclining)
- A body position
- **Lying down in any position** (prone, supine, on side etc)
  - **Dorsal recumbent**, lying on back (supine)
  - **Ventral recumbent**, lying face down (prone)
  - **Lateral recumbent**, lying on side (right or left lateral).

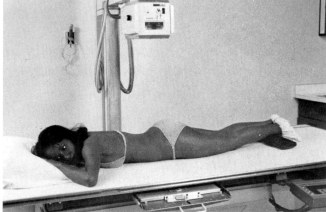

Prone   Fig. 1-43

15. Trendelenburg[1] *(Tren-del'en-berg)*
- A body position
- **A recumbent position** with body plane tilted so **head is lower than feet.**

NOTE: In radiology, the term Trendelenburg is commonly used to refer to any supine position wherein the head is lower than the feet, even though certain references state a specific amount of tilt that varies from 30 to 45 degrees.[2]

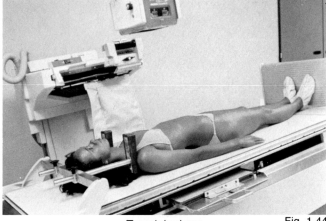

Trendelenburg   Fig. 1-44

[1]Friedrich *Trendelenburg*, a surgeon in Leipzig, 1844-1925.
[2]**Dorland's Illustrated Medical Dictionary**, 24th Edition.

Specific Body Positions

A second way the term **position** is used in radiography is to describe a **specific body position** wherein certain parts of the body are closest to the film, or by the surface on which the patient is lying (decubitus).

The term itself includes a description of **that body part which is closest to the film** (terms 16-21), or **the surface on which the patient is lying** (terms 23-26).

16. Lateral *(lat'er-al)* (Lat.) **Position**
- A body position
- Refers to **the side of,** a side view
- A true lateral will always be rotated 90° (1/4 turn) from a true AP or PA
- A true lateral is said to be perpendicular or at right angles to a true AP or PA.

    Right and left lateral positions: A **left lateral** position has the patient's **left side against the film**, and a **right lateral** has the **right side against the film,** as shown.

17. Oblique *(ob-lēk', ob-lik')*[1] (Obl.) **Position**
- A body position
- A position in which the coronal or frontal body plane is **not perpendicular** or at a right angle (Lat.) or is **not parallel** (PA or AP) to the film or recording medium, but is somewhere between a PA (AP) and Lat.

    The degree of obliquity or the amount of body rotation in an oblique position can vary as long as it is somewhere between a true lateral or a true PA or AP.

Specific oblique positions are described by **the part closest to the film** (terms 18-21).

18. Left Posterior Oblique (LPO) **Position**
- Describes that position in which the **left posterior** aspect of the body is closest to the film.

    This may be either in the erect (upright) body position, or the recumbent (reclining) position. *Figs. 1-47* and *48* both illustrate a 45° LPO position.

19. Right Posterior Oblique (RPO) **Position**
- Describes that position in which the **right posterior** part of the body is closest to the film.

    This may also be in either an erect or recumbent position. A 45° RPO is illustrated in *Figs. 1-49* and *50.*

---

[1] "Ob-lĕk" is the preferred pronunciation according to **Dorland's Illustrated Medical Dictionary** (24th Edition), the **New World Dictionary** (2nd College Edition) and the **American College Dictionary**. "Ob-lik" is the second pronunciation, as especially used in the military.

18

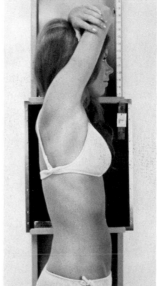
Fig. 1-45
Erect L Lat. Position

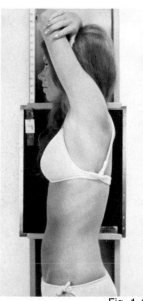
Fig. 1-46
Erect R Lat. Position

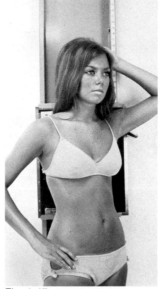
Fig. 1-47
Erect LPO Position

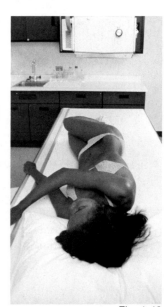
Fig. 1-48
Recument LPO Position

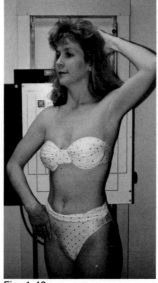
Fig. 1-49
Erect RPO Position

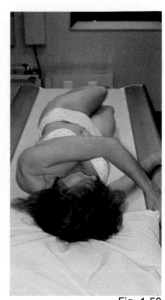
Fig. 1-50
Recumbent RPO Position

Specific Body Positions

20. Right Anterior Oblique (RAO) Position
* That position in which the **right anterior** aspect of body is closest to film.

  This may be in erect or recumbent position, as illustrated with the 45° RAO positions in *Figs. 1-51* and *52.*

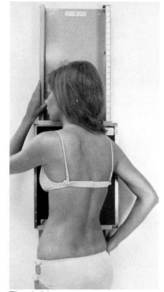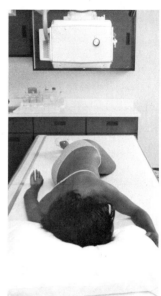

Fig. 1-51
Erect RAO Position

Fig. 1-52
Recumbent RAO Position

21. Left Anterior Oblique (LAO) Position
* That position in which the **left anterior** part of the body is closest to the film.

  This again is illustrated in the 45° LAO in both erect and recumbent positions. *(Figs. 1-53* and *54).*

NOTE: Two additional specific body positions are the anterior position and the posterior position wherein the anterior or posterior body part is closest to the film . These would fit the body position description for the PA and AP projections respectively, as described on page 15.

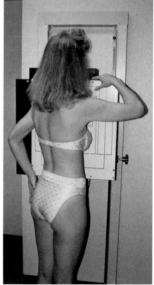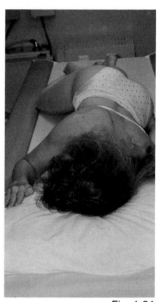

Fig. 1-53
Erect LAO Position

Fig. 1-54
Recumbent LAO Position

22. Decubitus (de-ku'bi-tus) (Decub.)
* A body position meaning to **lie on a horizontal surface,** designated according to that surface on which the body is resting.

  Therefore this refers to the patient **lying down** on one of the following body surfaces: back (dorsal), front (ventral), side (right or left lateral.)

  In **radiographic** positioning, decubitus is **always used with a horizontal x-ray beam.**

NOTE: When used in radiographic positioning, this term is used to denote **both** a recumbent body position and the use of a horizontal x-ray beam. Decubitus positions are used to detect air-fluid levels or free air in a body cavity such as in the chest or abdomen.

  Specific decubitus positions are described by the surface on which the patient is lying, remembering a horizontal x-ray beam is always used (terms 23-26).

23. Left Lateral Decubitus Position
* That body position wherein the patient **lies on the left side** and the **x-ray beam is directed horizontally.**

  This is similar to an AP projection or a left lateral position, however in this case the x-ray beam is directed horizontally and the patient is lying on the left side. Therefore the correct description for this position is a **left lateral decubitus (AP)**. The AP is added in parenthesis to denote that this is taken as an AP projection rather than a PA.

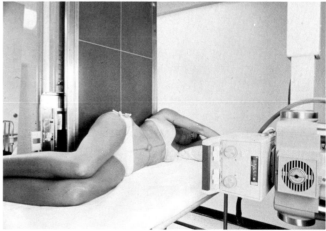

L Lat. Decub. (AP)

Fig. 1-55

Specific Body Positions continued

24. Right Lateral Decubitus Position

• That body position wherein the patient lies on the **right side** and the **x-ray beam is directed horizontally.**

   This is similar to a PA projection or a right lateral position, however since the x-ray beam is directed horizontally and patient is lying on her right side, the correct description for this position is a **right lateral decubitus (PA).** The PA is again added in parenthesis to denote a PA projection rather than an AP.

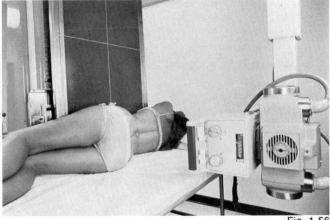

Right Lat. Decub. (PA)   Fig. 1-56

25. Dorsal Decubitus Position

• That body position described as **lying on the dorsal** (posterior) surface with the **x-ray beam directed horizontally.**

   This is similar to a supine or a left lateral position, however since the x-ray beam is directed horizontally and the image is lateral, this is correctly described as a **dorsal decubitus position (L Lat).** The left lateral is added in parenthesis to denote a left lateral rather than a right lateral position.

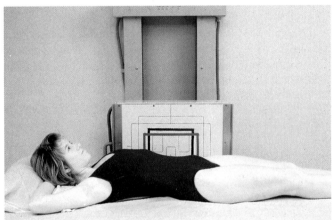

Dorsal Decub. (L Lat.)   Fig. 1-57

26. Ventral Decubitus Position

• That body position described as **lying on the ventral** (anterior) surface with the **x-ray beam directed horizontally.**

   This is similar to a prone position, **except** the x-ray beam is directed horizontally and the image is a lateral, therefore, the correct description is a **ventral decubitus position (R Lat).** The right lateral is again added in parenthesis to denote that this is a right lateral rather than a left lateral.

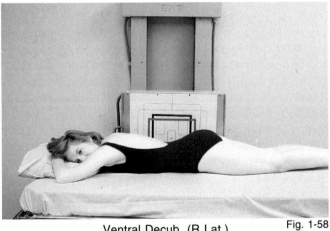

Ventral Decub. (R Lat.)   Fig. 1-58

Terminology

Relationship Terms

Following are paired positioning and/or anatomical terms describing relationships to parts of the body; the meanings of which are opposites:

27. Lateral *(lat'er-al)*
  • **Away from the center,** or away from median plane or midline of body.
  Example: In the anatomical position, the thumb is on the lateral aspect of the hand.

  vs.

28. Medial *(me'de-al)* or **Mesial** *(me'ze-al)*
  • **Toward the center,** or toward the median plane or midline.
  Example: In the anatomical position, the medial aspect of the ankle joint is the "inside" part closest to the median plane.

29. Proximal *(prok'si-mal)*
  • **Near the source** or beginning. In regard to the upper and lower limbs, it would be that part closest to the trunk, the source or beginning of that limb.
  Example: The elbow is proximal to wrist and the knee is proximal to the ankle.

  vs.

30. Distal *(dis'tal)*
  • **Away from the source** or beginning or away from the trunk.
  Example: The ankle is distal to the knee and the wrist is distal to the elbow.

31. Cephalad *(sef'ah-lad)* adv., **Cephalic** *(se-fal'ik)* adj. or **Superior**
  • **Toward head end** of body.
  A cephalic angle is an angle toward the head end of the body. (Cephalad or cephalic is a word element literally meaning "head"). The term **superior** means higher or above, and is sometimes used rather than cephalad for an angle toward the head end.

  vs.

32. Caudad *(kaw'dad)* adv., **Caudal** *(kaw'dal)* adj. or **Inferior**
  • **Away from head end** of body, toward the feet.
  Caudad or caudal comes from "cauda" literally meaning tail. In human anatomy it is the same as inferior or away from the head, toward the feet.
  The term **inferior** literally means lower in place or position and can be used rather than caudal for an angle toward the feet.

NOTE: These two terms are correctly used to describe the direction of angle for axial projections along the entire body, not just related to the head. For example, a routine AP projection for the sacrum includes a CR angle of 15° cephalad or superior (toward the head). A routine AP projection of the coccyx includes a 10° caudal or inferior angle (toward the feet).

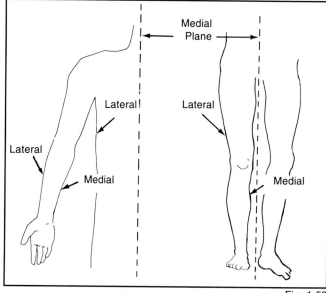

Lateral - Medial   Fig. 1-59

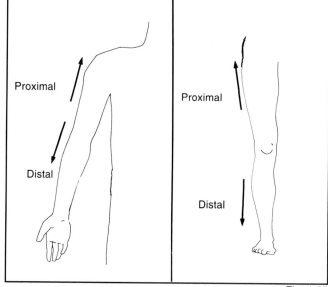

Proximal - Distal   Fig. 1-60

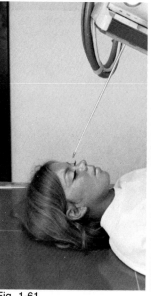

Fig. 1-61
Cephalic (or Superior)

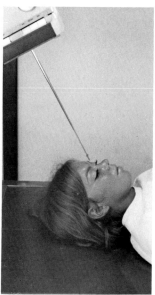

Fig. 1-62
Caudad (or Inferior)

Relationship Terms continued

33. Superficial
• Nearer to the skin surface.

vs.

34. Deep
• **Further from the skin surface** than other structures being compared.
   Example: The cross-sectional drawing in *Fig. 1-63* shows that the humerus is deep compared to the skin of the arm.

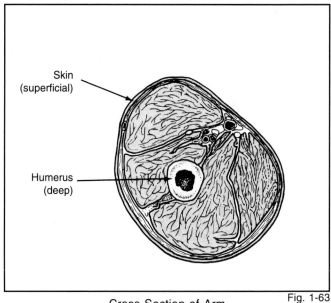

Cross Section of Arm   Fig. 1-63

35. Interior (Internal, Inside)
• **Inside** of something, **nearer to the center.**
   Prefix: **Intra**, meaning **within** or **inside.**
      (Intravenous - inside a vein)
   Prefix: **Inter,** meaning situated **between something.**
      (Intercostal - located between the ribs)

vs.

36. Exterior (External, Outer)
• **Situated** on or near the outside.
   Prefix: **Exo**, meaning **outside** or **outward.**
      (Exocardial - something developing or situated outside the heart)

Another example of the use of these two terms involves the circulatory system, wherein the internal carotid artery passes inside the cranium to the brain and the external carotid artery to the exterior parts of the head.

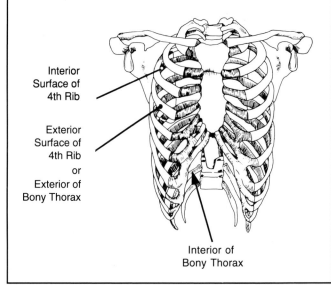

Bony Thorax   Fig. 1-64

37. Ipsilateral (ip″si-lat′er-al)
• **On the same side** of the body or part.

vs.

38. Contralateral (kon″trah-lat′er-al)
• **On the opposite side** of the body or part.
   Example: The right thumb and the right great toe are ipsilateral; the right foot and the left hand are contralateral.

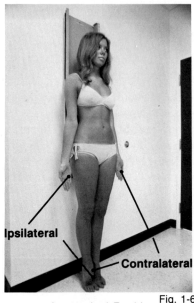

Anatomical Position   Fig. 1-65

Body Planes and Sections

Positioning terms describing central ray angles or relationships between body parts are often related to imaginary planes passing through the body in the **anatomical position**. Emphasis on cranial or whole body CT (computed tomography) requires knowledge of sectional anatomy, involving the following primary body planes and body sections:

39. Median *(me'de-an)* or Midsagittal *(mid-saj'i-tal)* Plane
- The vertical plane dividing the body into **right and left halves**.

    The median plane is also called the **midsagittal** plane because it passes through the sagittal suture of the skull. Therefore, any plane parallel to it is called a **sagittal** or **parasagittal** plane.

    These can also be described as anteroposterior planes which are parallel to the long axis of the body.

40. Coronal *(ko-ro'nal)* or Frontal Plane
- Any plane dividing the body into **anterior and posterior portions.**

    Since one of the frontal planes passes through the coronal suture of the skull, these are called **coronal** planes.

    These planes can also be described as side-to-side or lateral planes that are parallel to the long axis of the body and perpendicular to the median or midsagittal plane.

    Midcoronal or **midaxillary** are terms sometimes used to denote a plane that divides the body into anterior and posterior halves.

41. Transverse or Horizontal Plane
- Any plane passing through the body at **right angles to the sagittal or coronal planes**, dividing the body into superior and inferior portions.

    Therefore, a transverse or horizontal plane is a **cross section** of the part or body.

42. Longitudinal Sections
- Those sections running **lengthwise** in the direction of the long axis of the body or any of its parts, regardless of the position of the body (erect or recumbent).

    Longitudinal sections may be taken in the **sagittal** or **coronal** planes as shown in *Fig. 1-67* with longitudinal sections of the kidney.

    Vertical Sections: The same as longitudinal sections, except these sections denote that they were taken in the anatomical (erect) position.

43. Transverse (Cross) Sections
- Are taken **at right angles to the longitudinal axis** of the body or its parts.

44. Oblique Sections
- Those sections that are **not** taken in one of the main planes of the body or any of its parts.

    These oblique sections **slant** or **deviate** from the perpendicular or the horizontal, the longitudinal or the transverse.

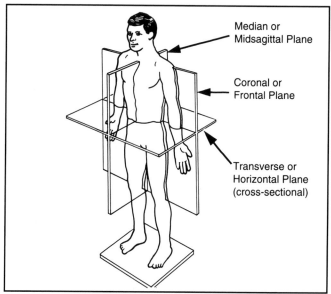

Fig. 1-66

Median, Coronal, and Transverse Body Planes

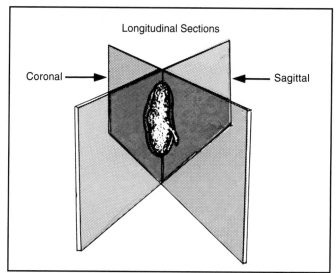

Longitudinal Sections of Kidney   Fig. 1-67

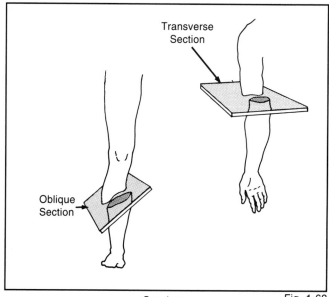

Sections   Fig. 1-68

Surfaces of Limbs (Extremities)

There are three terms used in radiography to describe specific surfaces of the upper and lower limbs. They are:

45. Plantar *(plan'tar)*
- Refers to the **sole** or **posterior** surface of the foot.

vs.

46. Dorsum *(dor'sum)* (Dorsum Pedis)
- Refers to the **top** or **anterior** surface of the foot.
  It should be noted that the term **dorsum or dorsal in general refers to the vertebral or posterior part** of the body. However, when used in relationship with the foot or toes, the term dorsum pedis specifically refers to the **anterior** part of the foot.

Examples
Dorsoplantar: The dorsoplantar projection is the same as an AP projection of the foot. The x-ray beam enters at the dorsum (anterior) of the foot and exits at the plantar (posterior) surface *(Fig. 1-69).*

Plantodorsal: The plantodorsal projection of the foot or toes is the same as a PA projection because the x-rays enter at the plantar (posterior) surface and exit at the dorsum (anterior) surface *(Fig. 1-70).*

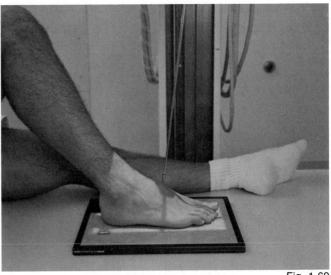

Dorsoplanter (AP) Projection   Fig. 1-69

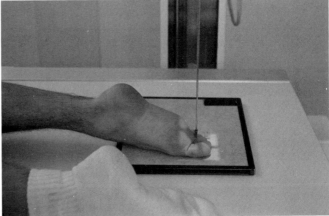

Plantodorsal (PA) Projection   Fig. 1-70

47. Palmar *(pal'mar)* (Volar)
- Refers to the **palm of the hand.**
  In the anatomical position this would be the same as the **anterior** surface of the hand.

NOTE: The term **volar** is more often used to refer to the palm of the hand, the palmar surface. However, volar may also be used to refer to the sole of the foot. ("Vola" literally means the hollow of the hand or foot.)

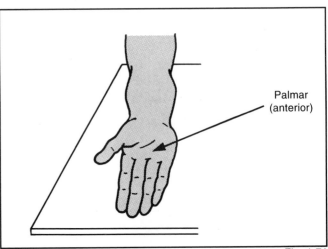

Palmar (Volar) Surface   Fig. 1-71

Terms Related to Movements

The final group of positioning and related terms that every radiographer should know are those relating to various movements. Many of these are listed as paired terms describing movements in opposite directions.

48. Flexion
- In flexing or bending a joint, **the angle** between parts **is decreased.**

 vs.

49. Extension
- In extending or straightening a joint, **the angle between parts is increased.**

 Extension is moving from a flexed to a straightened position. Going beyond this straightened position is termed **hyperextension.**

50. Hyperextension
- Extending a joint **beyond the straight or neutral position.**

Example: A hyperextended elbow or knee results when the joint is extended beyond the straightened or neutral position. This is not a natural movement for these two joints and results in injury or trauma.

NOTE: A special use of flexion and extension involves the spine. Flexion is bending forward and extension is returning to the neutral position. A backward bending beyond the neutral position is hyperextension.

 A second example of a special use of the term hyperextension is that of the wrist wherein the carpal canal or carpal tunnel view of the carpals is visualized by a special hyperextended wrist movement, also called dorsiflexion. (See Chapter 4 for the carpal canal projections.)

51. Ulnar Flexion (Radial Deviation) of Wrist
- To **decrease** the angle (flex) **between the hand and the ulnar side** of the forearm.

 vs.

52. Radial Flexion (Ulnar Deviation) of Wrist
- To **decrease** the angle (flex) **between the hand and the radial side** of the distal forearm (flex toward thumb side).

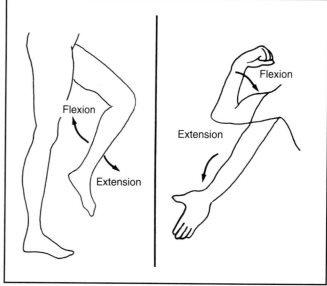

Flexion - Extension   Fig. 1-72

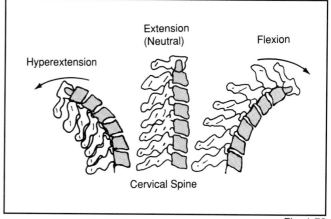

Fig. 1-73
Flexion, Extension and Hyperextension of Spine

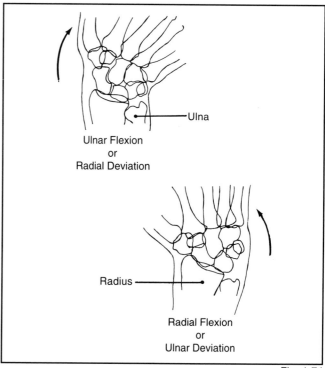

Movements of Wrist Joint   Fig. 1-74

Terms Related to Movements continued

53. Dorsiflexion *(dor″si-flek′shun)* **of Ankle**
- To **decrease the angle** (flex) between the dorsum pedis and the lower leg, moving foot and toes upward.

vs.

54. Plantar Flexion of Ankle
- **Extending the ankle joint,** moving foot and toes downward from the normal position.

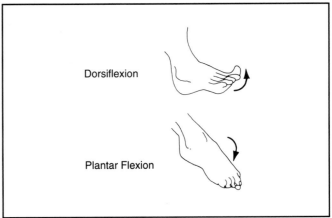

Movements of Ankle Joint   Fig. 1-75

55. Eversion *(ē-ver′zhun)*
- An **outward stress movement** of the foot at the ankle joint without rotation of the leg.
  The plantar surface (sole) of the foot is turned away from the median plane of the body (sole faces more laterally).
  The leg does **not** rotate, and stress is applied to the medial aspect of the ankle joint.

vs.

56. Inversion *(in-ver′zhun)*
- An **inward stress movement** of the foot at the ankle joint without rotation of the leg.
  The plantar surface of foot (sole) is turned more medially.
  The leg does **not** rotate, and stress is applied to the lateral aspect of the ankle joint.

NOTE: Correctly used, these terms refer to stress movements as described, and **not** to the usual medial and lateral rotational movements used for oblique positioning of the ankle joint.

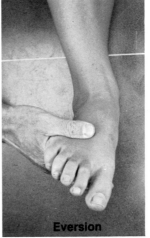 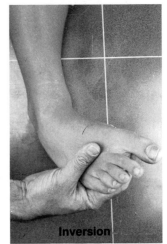

Fig. 1-76   Movements of Ankle Joint   Fig. 1-77

57. Medial Rotation (Internal Rotation)
- A rotation or turning of a body part, moving the **anterior** aspect of the part **toward the inside or median plane.**

vs.

58. Lateral Rotation (External Rotation)
- A rotation of an **anterior** body part **toward the outside or away from the median plane.**

NOTE: Remember that these terms describe the movement of the **anterior** aspect of the part being rotated. Thus in the forearm movements *(Fig. 1-78)* the anterior aspect of the forearm moves medially or internally on the medial rotation, and laterally or externally on the lateral rotation.

Another example is the medial and lateral obliques of the knee in which the **anterior** part of the knee is rotated medially and laterally respectively (Chapter 6).

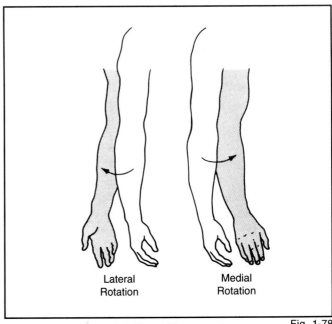

Rotational Movements   Fig. 1-78

Terms Related to Movements continued

59. Abduction *(ab-duk'shun)*
- A movement of arm or leg **away** from body, a lateral movement (to draw away from).

  Another application of this term is the abduction of the fingers or toes, which means spreading them apart.

vs.

60. Adduction *(ah-duk'shun)*
- A movement of arm or leg **toward** the body, to draw toward a center or medial line.

  Adduction of the fingers or toes means moving them together or toward each other.

NOTE: A memory aid is to associate the d in towar<u>d</u> with the d in a<u>d</u>duction.

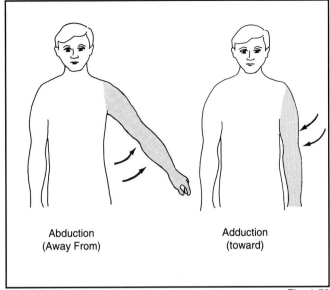

Abduction
(Away From)   Adduction
                     (toward)

Movements of Extremities   Fig. 1-79

61. Supination *(su″pi-na'shun)*
- A rotational movement of the hand into the anatomical position (palm up in supine position or forward in erect position).

  This movement rotates the radius of the forearm laterally along its long axis.

vs.

62. Pronation *(pro-na'shun)*
- A rotation of hand into the opposite of the anatomical position (palm down or back).

NOTE: To help remember these terms, relate them to the body positions of supine and prone. Supine or supination means face up or palm up, and prone or pronation means face down or palm down.

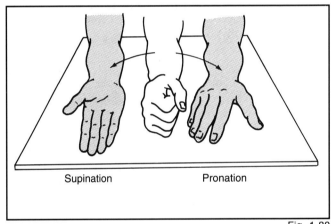

Supination   Pronation

Movements of Hand   Fig. 1-80

63. Protraction *(pro-trak'shun)*
- A **movement forward** from a normal position.

vs.

64. Retraction *(re-trak'shun)*
- A **movement backward,** or the condition of being drawn back.

Example: Protraction is moving the jaw forward (sticking the chin out) or drawing the shoulders forward. Retraction is the opposite of this, moving the jaw backward or squaring the shoulders, as in a military stance.

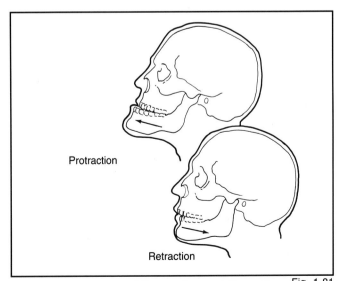

Protraction

Retraction

Movements of Protraction and Retraction   Fig. 1-81

Terms Related to Movements continued

65. Elevation
- **A lifting, raising** or **moving of a part superiorly.**

vs.

66. Depression
- **A letting down, lowering** or **moving of a part infe-riorly.**

Example: Shoulders are elevated when raising them, as occurs when shrugging the shoulders. Depressing the shoulders is lowering them, as in positioning them for a lateral cervical spine.

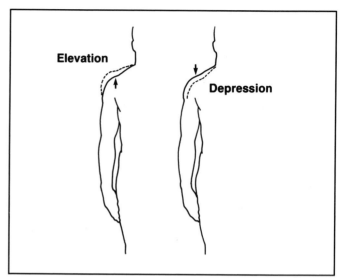
Fig. 1-82
Elevation and Depression Movements of Shoulders

67. Circumduction *(ser″kum-duk′shun)*
- To **move around in the form of a circle.**
  These involve sequential movements of flexion, abduction, extension and adduction, resulting in a cone type movement at any joint with the four movements possible (e.g., fingers, wrist, arm or leg).

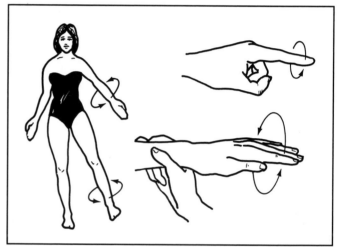
Circumduction Movements   Fig. 1-83

68. Tilt
- **A slanting or tilting movement.**
- To move into a **slanting position with respect to the long axis.**
  The body part is slanted or **tilted** 15° in the example in *Fig. 1-84* such that the CR is **not** aligned with or parallel to the long axis, and the long axis of the head is **not** aligned with the long axis of the body. (Observe that no rotation has occurred in relation to the long axis; however the long axis of the head would **not** be parallel to the long axis of the body, even if the chin were pulled down as for an AP projection, thus the 15° tilt.)

vs.

69. Rotation
- To **turn or rotate a body part on its axis.**
- A **rotational movement.**
  The body part is **rotated** 37° from a PA projection in the example in *Fig. 1-85*. (Observe that no tilting has occurred in that the long axis of the head is still aligned with or parallel to the long axis of the body.)

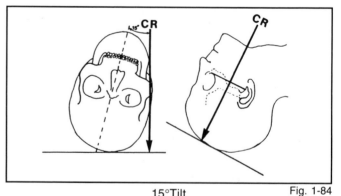
15°Tilt   Fig. 1-84
(Tangential Projection for Zygomatic Arch)

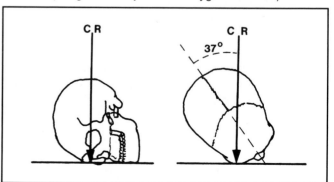
37° Rotation from PA   Fig. 1-85
(Parieto-orbital Projection for Optic Foramen)

Summary of Potentially Misused Terms

The following three terms, **position, projection, and view,** are often used incorrectly in practice, resulting in confusion and error. It is essential that these terms be understood and used correctly.

Position

- A correct positioning term describing positions used in reference to the **body part closest to film,** or by the surface on which the patient is lying (decubitus). Therefore, the term position as used in this text describes specific **lateral, oblique,** and **decubitus** positions, (such as left lateral, left posterior oblique or a lateral decubitus position as illustrated).

Following are examples of the correct use of the term **position** as used in this textbook:
- **Right or left lateral position**
- **Anterior or posterior oblique position**
- **Medial or lateral oblique position** (upper or lower limbs)
- **Right or left lateral decubitus position** (chest or abdomen)
- **Ventral or dorsal decubitus position** (chest or abdomen)

As noted previously, this term is also used to describe a **general body position** such as **supine, prone, recumbent or erect.**

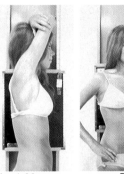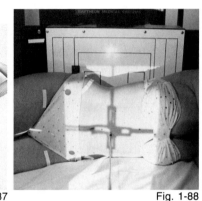

Fig. 1-86
L Lat. Position

Fig. 1-87
LPO Position

Fig. 1-88
L Lat. Decub. Position (AP)

Projection

- **A correct positioning term describing or referring to the path of the x-ray beam,** projecting an image on radiographic film or other image receptor.

Following is a list of examples of the correct use of the term **projection** as used in this text, which in most cases is preceded by a specific description of the points of entrance and exit.
- **AP or PA projection** (as illustrated)
- **Submentovertex (SMV) projection** (as illustrated)
- **Parietoacanthial projection** (special skull projection)
- **AP lordotic projection** (special chest projection)
- **Inferosuperior axial projection** (special shoulder and hip projections)
- **Dorsoplantar projection** (AP projection of the foot)
- **Mediolateral or lateromedial projections** (used to indicate specific lateral projections such as for the foot or ankle, or to describe specific projections for mammography.)
- **Axial** and **tangential projections** (terms 8 & 9) These two terms refer to, or describe the path of the x-ray beam in general rather than specifically indicating the points of entrance and exit. Therefore, these terms are used with projection rather than position. (They would not be used as positions because they do not refer to, or describe a specific body position in reference to the film or on which surface they are lying.)

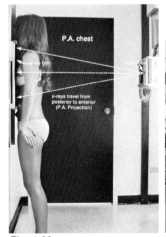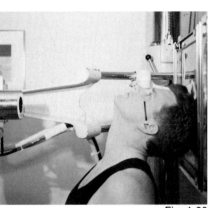

Fig. 1-89
PA Projection

Fig. 1-90
Submentovertex (SMV) Projection

View

- Is **not** a positioning term.
- Should **only** be used in discussing the radiograph or image.
- Represents the **radiographic image** as seen from the vantage of the film or other image receptor such as a fluoroscopic screen.

Summary: View is the exact opposite of projection and should **not** be used as a positioning term.

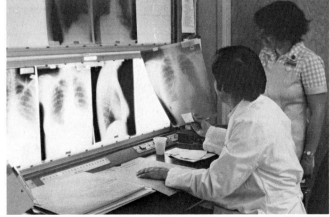

Viewing Radiographs

Fig. 1-91

Part III Basic Imaging Principles

Evaluation Criteria

The goal of every radiographer should not be just to take a "passable" or merely a "diagnostic" radiograph wherein only obvious pathological changes are evident, but the goal should be an **optimum image** which can be **evaluated by a definable standard,** as described under evaluation criteria. The less than optimal radiograph may be considered passable if exposure factors are sufficient to result in a merely diagnostic image, but it may demonstrate sloppy and careless technique; the markers may not be placed correctly, or the centering or collimation may be off. Other carelessness may also be evident such as not being aligned to the long axis of the film, or unnecessary magnification or distortion may be evident by improper tube-part-film placement or alignment.

Therefore, it is imperative that the goal for every radiograph taken should be that optimal image as evaluated against the definable standard described under evaluation criteria. An example of evaluation criteria as used in this text for a lateral forearm is given in *Fig. 1-92.*

Positioning Accuracy

Part Placement on Film holder

Positioning accuracy first includes **correct placement of the part to be demonstrated on the cassette so that all of the anatomy to be visualized is within the collimated borders,** but no unnecessary anatomy is irradiated. This means a large enough cassette must be selected and the collimation field be opened large enough to include all of the body part being radiographed, but not so large as to expose body parts not required for diagnosis.

Part-Film Alignment

The film holder should also be placed in correct alignment to the part. For example, a radiographic examination of an average forearm requires an 11 x 14 in. (28 x 35 cm) cassette placed so that the long axis of the forearm is aligned to the long axis of the film and the collimation field is restricted just to the area of the forearm *(Fig.1-93)*.

A general rule states that the **long axis of the body part should be aligned with the long axis of the film** as shown in *Fig. 1-93*. The exception to this general rule is in those cases where the body part needs to be angled on the cassette from corner to corner to insure that both joints of the body part are included on the film. An example is the femur or leg on a large adult which may need to be placed diagonally (corner to corner) on the 14 x 17 in. (35 x 43 cm) cassette to insure that the joints at both ends are well visualized. When this is done the collimation field must then also be rotated and aligned to the body part.

Also when two or more projections are taken on the same film, such as an AP and lateral forearm taken on one 11 x 14 in. (28 x 35 cm), the long axis of the body part should always be aligned the same way with the parts running in the same direction.

Rotation

Positioning accuracy also requires that the part being radiographed be correctly positioned so that the specific projection or position being taken **will visualize the body part precisely as planned.** For example the lateral forearm correctly positioned with **no rotation** will result in the ulnar head being directly superimposed and centered through the distal radius. (See evaluation criteria, *Fig. 1-92* and radiograph, *Fig. 1-94*).

Evaluation Criteria:
- The elbow should be flexed 90° and the forearm should be aligned to the long axis of the half of exposed film.
- The carpals should be visible distally, and the distal humerus proximally.
- No rotation: Ulnar head of distal ulna should be directly superimposed and centered over radius; humeral epicondyles should be directly superimposed.
- Radial head should superimpose coronoid process; radial tuberosity should not be seen in profile.
- Wrist and elbow joints will be only partially open due to beam divergence.
- Lateral collimation borders should be visible but borders at both ends should be minimal so as not to cut off essential anatomy of joints.
- Optimum exposure with no motion should visualize sharp bone margins and clear trabecular markings throughout. Densities should be similar at distal and proximal ends of forearm.
- Patient ID should be clear and legible and R or L marker visible on lateral border without superimposing anatomy.

Lateral Forearm Criteria   Fig 1-92

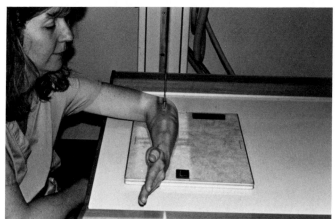

Lateral Forearm   Fig 1-93

11

14

Lateral Forearm   Fig 1-94

Film Markers and Patient Identification

A **minimum** of two types of markers should be imprinted in the emulsion of **every** radiograph. These are **patient identification and date,** and **anatomical side markers.**

Patient identification and date

Generally this patient information which includes data such as name, date, case number, and institution is provided on an index card, then photoflashed on the film in the space provided by a lead block in the film holder *(Fig. 1-95)*. Each film holder should have a marker on the exterior indicating this area where the patient ID, including the date, will be flashed. Care must be taken so this area does not superimpose the essential anatomy being demonstrated. Figure 1-96 demonstrates a wrist with the patient information visible, along with an "R" (right) marker.

Throughout this text the preferred location of this patient ID marker in relationship to the body part is shown, as well as the preferred place for the Right or Left marker. These are shown on each positioning page in the small box drawing indicating the correct film size and the film position orientation, lengthwise or crosswise.

A general rule is to place the patient ID information at the top margin of the film on chests, and on the lower margin on abdomens *(Figs. 1-97 and 98)*. This marker should always be placed where it is the least likely to superimpose essential anatomy.

Anatomical Side Marker

In addition to the patient ID information, a right or left radiopaque marker must also appear on every radiograph correctly indicating the patient's right or left side, or to indicate which limb is being radiographed, the right or left. These may be either the word "Right" or "Left" or just the initials "R" or "L". This side marker should preferably be placed directly on the film holder alongside the collimated border of the side being identified with the placement such that the marker will not "cover up" or superimpose essential anatomy.

Remember however these are radiopaque markers and thus must be placed just within the collimation field so they will be exposed by the x-ray beam and imprinted in the film emulsion.

The two markers, the Patient ID and anatomical side marker, must be correctly placed on **ALL** radiographs. Generally it is **not** an acceptable practice to write this information on the film after it is processed because of legal and liability problems from potential mismarkings. A **radiograph taken without these two markers should be repeated,** which obviously results in unnecessary radiation to the patient making this a serious error.

Additional markers or identification

Certain other markers or identifiers may also be used such as **radiographer initials**, which are generally placed on the R or L marker to identify the specific radiographer responsible for that exam. Sometimes the exam room number is also included. **Time indicators** are also commonly used noting the minutes of elapsed time in a series such as the 1 min, 5 min, 15 min and 20 min series of radiographs taken in an intravenous urogram (IVU) procedure.

Another important marker on all decubitus positions is a **decub** marker or some type of indicator such as an **arrow identifying which side is up.** A special type of R or L marker such as a

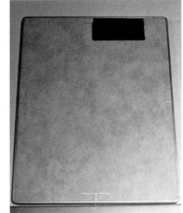
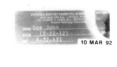

Fig 1-95   Patient ID Info.   Fig 1-96

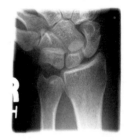

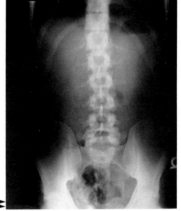
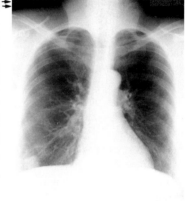

Fig 1-97   Correctly placed side markers and patient ID info.   Fig 1-98

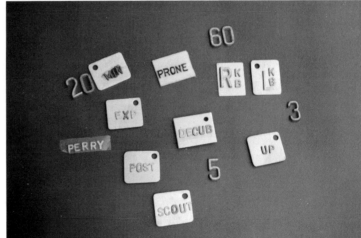

Sample Markers   Fig 1-99

mercury ball marker wherein the mercury ball drops to the down side of the marker may also be used to indicate erect or decub positions. If this type of R or L mercury ball marker is not used when the film is placed vertically, then an **"upright"** or **"erect"** marker and/or an arrow must be used to identify erect chest or abdomen positions compared to recumbent, and to indicate which side is up.

Inspiration (INSP) and **expiration** (EXP) markers are used for special comparison PA projections of the chest. **Internal** (INT) and **external** (EXT) markers are also used for rotation projections such as for the proximal humerus and shoulder. Sample markers are shown in *Fig. 1-99*.

Radiographic Quality

A study of radiographic quality or radiographic technique includes all those factors or variables which relate to the precision or accuracy with which the structures and tissues being radiographed are reproduced on radiographic film or other image receptors. Certain of these factors or variables relate more directly to radiographic positioning and a discussion of the applied aspects of these factors follow.

Exposure Factors

The three exposure factors, kilovoltage (kVp), milliamperage (mA) and exposure time (seconds, s) are the primary controlling factors for contrast, density and definition or unsharpness respectively.

Kilovoltage (kVp) primarily controls the **quality** or penetrating ability of the x-ray beam and as such controls the **contrast** scale of a radiograph.

Milliamperage (mA) and **Time** (s) are usually combined into milliampere seconds (mAs) as the primary factor controlling the **quantity** of the x-ray beam. Therefore, mAs is the primary controlling factor of the density of a radiograph. Time or length of exposure in seconds (s) or milliseconds (ms) can be changed in combination with mA to control motion during the exposure resulting in loss of definition or image unsharpness. Therefore, to obtain that optimum exposure as described for each projection or position under evaluation criteria requires a good understanding of these exposure variables which are set on the control panel by the radiographer for each exposure *(Fig. 1-100)*.

Image Quality Factors

Certain factors by which one evaluates the quality of a radiographic image are termed image quality factors. Every radiographer must understand these factors as described in this chapter so that they may be evaluated, described and used to produce that optimum quality radiograph which is the goal for every radiographic examination. These four image quality factors are **density, contrast, detail, and distortion.**

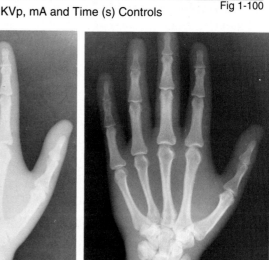
KVp, mA and Time (s) Controls   Fig 1-100

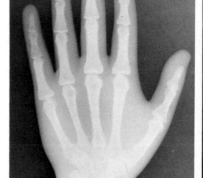
Fig 1-101   Fig 1-102
2.5 mAs (60 kVp)   5 mAs (60 kVp)

1. Density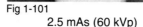

Definition

Radiographic density can be described as **the amount of blackening of the finished radiograph**. The higher the amount of blackening the greater the density and the less the amount of light which will pass through the radiograph when placed in front of an illuminator or light source.

Controlling Factors

The **primary controlling factor of density is mAs** which controls density by directly controlling the quantity or amount of x-rays emitted from the x-ray tube during an exposure. Thus twice the mAs will double the quantity of x-rays emitted and double the density.

In addition to mAs, **distance** is also a controlling factor for radiographic density. Distance affects density according to the inverse square law. For example, twice the distance will reduce density by one-fourth. Distance then has a significant effect on density but since a standard distance is generally used, mAs becomes the variable used to either increase or decrease radiographic density.

Density Change Rule

A general rule states that mAs must be changed at least 30 per cent to make a noticeable change in radiographic density. Therefore if a radiograph is underexposed enough to be unacceptable, a 30 per cent increase would make a noticeable change but would not be enough to correct the radiograph. A good general rule suggests **a doubling is generally the minimal change in mAs required to correct such an underexposed radiograph.**

For example if a hand taken with 2.5 mAs was too light or underexposed to a degree which warranted a repeat, *(Fig. 1-101)*, then the mAs should be increased to 5 mAs if kVp and other factors were not changed *(Fig. 1-102)*. In the same way, an overexposed or too dark radiograph that warrants repeating, generally requires cutting the mAs in half if other factors are not changed.

Summary: Adequate density must be present on the finished radiograph to accurately visualize those tissues or organs being radiographed. Too little density (underexposed) or too much density (overexposed) will not accurately visualize these tissues or structures.

2. Contrast

Definition

Radiographic contrast is defined as **the difference in density on adjacent areas of a radiograph or other image receptor.** This can also be defined as the **variation in density.** The greater this variation, the higher the contrast. The less this variation or the less difference between density on adjacent areas, the lower the contrast. This is demonstrated by the step wedge in *Fig. 1-103* which shows greater differences in densities between adjacent areas, thus **high** contrast.

Contrast can also be described as long scale or short scale contrast referring to the range of all optical densities from the lightest to the blackest parts of the radiograph. This is again demonstrated in *Figs. 1-103* and *104* showing **high contrast** with greater differences in adjacent densities, and a **short scale contrast** because there are fewer different density steps.

Purpose or Function

The purpose or function of contrast is to **make the anatomical detail of a radiograph more visible.** Therefore, optimum radiographic contrast is important and an understanding of contrast is essential in evaluating radiographic quality. Lower or higher contrast is not necessarily good or bad by itself. For example, lower contrast with less difference between adjacent densities (long scale contrast) is more desirable on certain exams such as on chest radiographs where the many different shades of gray are needed to visualize the very fine lung markings. This is demonstrated by comparing the two chest radiographs in *Figs. 1-104* and *105*. The low contrast (long scale) chest in *Fig. 1-105* demonstrates more shades of gray as evident by the faint outlines of the ribs and vertebrae visible through the heart and mediastinal structures. These shades of gray outlining the ribs and vertebrae are less visible through the mediastinum on the high contrast chest radiograph in *Fig. 1-104.*

A higher contrast (short scale) may be more desirable for demonstrating certain skeletal structures where more difference in adjacent densities is needed to clearly visualize outlines or borders, such as for the upper or lower limbs. In general however, radiographs with very high contrast (short scale) often lack information and a lower or long scale contrast radiograph demonstrating a greater number of different densities may result in more diagnostic information and thus, in general, be more desirable.

Controlling Factors

The primary controlling factor for contrast is **kVp.** Kilovoltge controls the energy or penetrating power of the primary beam. The higher the kVp, the greater the energy and the more uniformly the x-ray beam penetrates the various mass densities of all tissues. Thus higher kVp produces less variation in attenuation (differential absorption), resulting in lower contrast.

Kilovoltage (kVp) is also a secondary controlling factor of density. Higher kVp, resulting in both more x-rays and greater energy x-rays, will cause more x-ray energy to reach the film with a corresponding increase in overall density. A general rule of thumb states that a **15% increase in kVp will increase density the same as doubling the mAs.** Thus in the lower kVp range such as at 50-70 kVp, an 8-10 kVp increase will double the density (equivalent to doubling the mAs). In the 80 to 100 kVp range, it requires a 12 to 15 kVp increase to double the density.

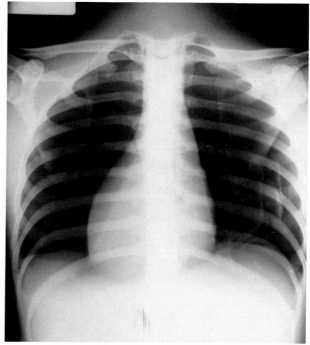

Fig 1-103   Fig 1-104

High Contrast, **Short** Scale 50 kVp, 800 mAs

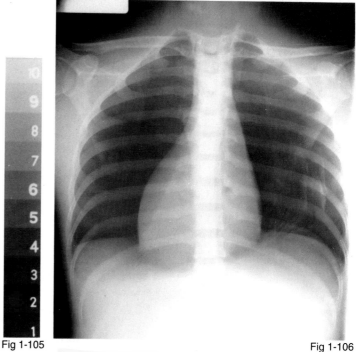

Fig 1-105   Fig 1-106

Low Contrast, **Long** Scale 110 kVp, 10mAs

The importance of this relates to radiation protection because as kVp is increased, mAs can be significantly reduced resulting in less radiation to the patient.

Summary: A general rule states that the **highest kVp and lowest mAs which yields sufficient diagnostic information should be used on each radiographic examination.** This will both reduce patient exposure and in general result in radiographs with good diagnostic information.[1]

---

[1] Statkiewiez, M.L. and Ritenour, E.R.: **Radiation Protection for Student Radiographers.** Denver; Multi-Media Publishing Inc. 1983.

3. Detail

Definition

Recorded detail (sometimes referred to as definition) can be defined as **the sharpness of structures on the radiograph.** This sharpness of image detail is demonstrated by the clarity of sharpness of fine structural lines and by the borders of tissues or structures as visible on the radiographic image. Lack of detail or definition is known as blur or unsharpness.

Controlling Factors

The optimum radiograph will display good image sharpness as described for each exam in this text under evaluation criteria. The greatest deterrent to image sharpness as related to positioning is **motion**.

Additional factors which control or influence detail are **focal spot size**, **SID** (Source Image receptor Distance) and **OID** (Object Image receptor Distance). The use of the smaller focal spot results in less geometric unsharpness, thus a sharper image or better detail. (See page 36.) Therefore, the small focal spot as selected on the control panel should be used whenever possible.

Combined with a small focal spot, an **increase in SID** and a **decrease in OID** will result in less geometric unsharpness, which will **increase** detail, as described in the section which follows on distortion.

Two Types of Motion

There are two types of motion which influence radiographic detail. These are voluntary and involuntary motion.

Voluntary motion, from breathing or movement of body part during exposure, can be avoided or at least minimized by certain factors during positioning. The use of support blocks, sandbags or other immobilization devices can be used effectively to reduce motion. These are most effective for exams of upper or lower limbs as will be demonstrated throughout this text. Retention bands to support patients for exams of the chest or abdomen will also be demonstrated for weak or unsteady patients as a way to prevent patient movement during the exposure.

Involuntary motion such as from peristaltic action of abdominal organs is more difficult if not impossible to control completely. If image unsharpness is present due to motion, it is important to be able to determine from the radiograph if this blurring or unsharpness is due to voluntary or involuntary motion because there are different ways to control these two types of motion.

Difference between voluntary and involuntary motion.

Voluntary motion, which is much easier to prevent, is characterized by **generalized blurring of linked structures,** such as is evident in *Fig. 1-107.*

Involuntary motion such as from peristalsis, is more difficult to control and can be identified by **localized unsharpness** or blurring as demonstrated by the small arrows in the upper left abdomen *(Fig. 1-108).* Sometimes certain relaxing techniques, or in some cases careful breathing instructions may help in reducing involuntary motion. **Short exposure time** however is the best and sometimes the only way to minimize image unsharpness due to involuntary motion.

A general rule to minimize image unsharpness due to voluntary motion is to **always use support devices when needed**; and for minimizing both kinds of motion use **a faster film-screen combination** and as **short exposure time as possible**. Since mA x

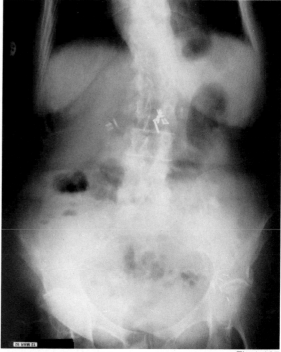

Voluntary Motion (Breathing Motion) Fig 1-107

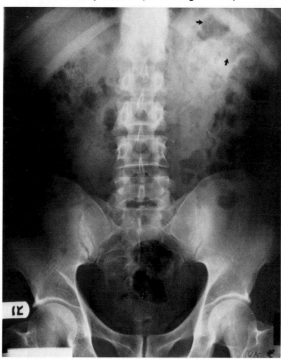

Involuntary Motion   Fig 1-108
(From peristaltic action in upper left abdomen)

s = mAs, mA and time (in seconds, s, or milliseconds, ms) are inversely proportioned. If one doubles the mA, the time can be cut in half. In general, one should use as high mA and as short exposure time as possible within the limits of the specific equipment being used.

Summary: Loss of detail is most often caused by **motion**, either voluntary or involuntary, which is primarily **controlled by use of immobilization devices and short exposure times.**

The use of the **small focal spot**, the **least possible OID** and a **greater SID**, also improve the recorded detail or definition on the radiograph as described and illustrated on a following page.

4. Distortion

Definition

The fourth image quality factor by which one evaluates and describes radiographic quality is **distortion,** which can be defined as **the misrepresentation of object size or shape as projected onto radiographic recording medium.** Magnification sometimes is listed as a separate factor but since it is a size distortion, it can be included along with shape distortion. Therefore, distortion, whether it is shape or size distortion, is a misrepresentation of the actual object and as such is undesirable.

However, **no radiograph is an exact image of the body part being radiographed. This is impossible because there is always some magnification and/or distortion due to OID** (Object Image receptor Distance) **and the divergence of the x-ray beam.** Therefore, distortion must be minimized and controlled.

X-ray Beam Divergence

This is a basic but important concept to understand in a study of radiographic positioning. X-ray beam divergence occurs because x-rays originate from a narrow source in the x-ray tube and diverge or spread out to cover the entire film or image receptor *(Fig. 1-109).*

The size of the x-ray beam (collimation field size) is limited by adjustable collimators which absorb periphery x-rays on four sides thereby controlling the size of the collimation field. The larger the collimation field and the shorter the SID, the greater the angle of divergence at the outer margins. This increases the potential for distortion at these outer margins. In general, only the exact center point of the x-ray beam, the central ray (CR), has no divergence as it penetrates the body part and strikes the film at exactly **90°** or **perpendicular** to the plane of the x-ray film. This results in the least possible distortion at this point. All other aspects of the x-ray beam strike the film at some angle other than 90° with the angle of divergence increasing to the outermost portions of the x-ray beam.

The drawing in *Fig. 1-109* demonstrates three points on the body part (marked A, B, and C) projected onto the film. The amount of magnification (increase in image size) in this example is the distance between A_1 and A_2, or between B_1 and B_2. (C indicates the point of the CR.) Therefore, due to the effect of the divergent x-ray beam, combined with at least some OID, this type of size distortion is inevitable and its effect as well as other types of shape distortion must be controlled.

The x-ray beam divergence combined with the size of the focal spot also creates geometric unsharpness due to the penumbra effect as described on the following page.

Controlling Factors

Four primary controlling factors of distortion are (1) **SID,** (2) **OID, (3) Object alignment** and (4) **CR** (Central ray).

1. SID: The effect of SID (Source Image receptor Distance) on size distortion is demonstrated in *Fig. 1-110.* Note that at **a greater SID there is less magnification** than at a shorter SID. This is the primary reason chest radiographs are taken at 72 in. (183 cm) rather than at the more common minimum 40 in. (102 cm). The size of the heart is an important consideration in chest radiography and a 72 in. (183 cm) SID results in less magnification of the heart and other structures within the thorax.

Minimum 40 in. (102 cm) SID: For many years it has been common practice to use 40 inches (102 cm) as the standard SID for most radiographic exams. However, in the interest of **decreasing patient exposure** and **improving recorded detail or definition,** it is becoming more common to increase the standard SID to 42, 44 or 48 inches (107, 112 or 122 cm). Studies have shown for example, that increasing the SID from 40 to 48 inches will reduce the entrance dose to the patient by

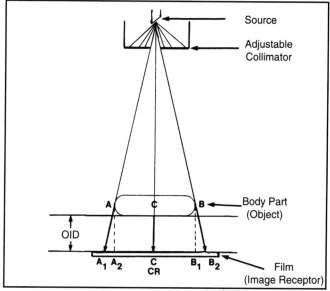

X-Ray Beam Divergence   Fig. 1-109

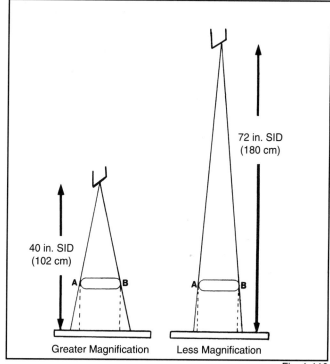

Effect of SID   Fig. 1-110

12.5%, with an integral dose (total tissue volume irradiated) reduction of 11%.[1]

Also due to the x-ray beam divergence principle described above, this increase in SID has the added benefit of **decreasing** magnification and distortion, thus decreasing geometric unsharpness which **increases** the recorded detail or definition.

Due to problems of shorter technologists not being able to reach the tube at the greater SID distances, and the increase in mA required (50% increase in changing from 40 to 48 inches), many departments still use the standard 40 in. (102 cm) SID. Also some departments use a 44 in. (112 cm) SID for Bucky tray procedures and 40 in. (102 cm) for table-top exams because the distance between the table top and Bucky tray is 3 to 4 inches on most floating type table tops. In addition some of the newer x-ray tubes with steep anode angles require a greater than 40 in. (102 cm) SID for sufficient field coverage for the larger films. Therefore, throughout this text the suggested SID as listed on each positioning page is a **minimum** of 40 in. (102 cm). Departmental protocol concerning this will need to be determined by each radiographer.

[1] Kebart, R.C. and Jame, C.C., Benefits of Increasing Focal Film Distance. Radiologic Technology **62-6**:434-441, 1991.

Distortion: Controlling Factors continued

2. OID: The effect of OID (Object Image receptor Distance) on magnification or size distortion is clearly illustrated in *Fig. 1-111*. **The closer the object being radiographed is to the image receptor, the less the magnification and the better the detail or definition.**

This is one advantage for taking radiographs of the upper and lower limbs table top rather than Bucky. (Film in cassette is placed under the patient on the table top rather than in the Bucky tray.) The Bucky tray in most floating type table tops is from 3 to 4 in. (8-10 cm) below the table top which increases the OID. This not only increases magnification but also **decreases image sharpness** (definition).

Focal Spot Size and Image Unsharpness: For purposes of describing the principle of x-ray beam divergence and the controlling factors of distortion, a point source has been used in the illustrations for the source of x-rays at the x-ray tube. In actuality the source of x-rays is from an **area** on the anode known as the **focal spot.** The size of the focal spot is determined by the **size of filament at the cathode,** and by the **angle of the target area** on the anode. The selection of the small focal spot on a dual-focus x-ray tube, or the use of a smaller angle anode x-ray tube will result in **less blurring or unsharpness of the image** due to the penumbra effect of geometric unsharpness *(Fig. 1-112).* The penumbra is shown to be greater on the cathode side.

The anode angle is determined by the equipment manufacturer and thus is not a variable controlled by the technologist. The selection of the smaller focal spot on a dual-focus x-ray tube is a variable controlled by the technologist. However even with the smallest focal spot possible, some penumbra is present. The **effect of this geometric unsharpness is greatly increased or magnified when the OID is increased or the SID decreased.** Therefore, not only does an increase in OID and a decrease in SID result in an increase in size distortion or magnification of the image, but this also increases the overall blurring or unsharpness of the radiographic image.

3. Object Alignment: The third important controlling factor of distortion as related to positioning is object alignment. This refers to the **alignment or plane of the object being radiographed in relationship to the plane of the x-ray film** or other image receptor. If the object plane is not parallel to the plane of the film, distortion occurs as shown on the left in *Fig. 1-113.* Two effects are demonstrated when the object is not aligned correctly or is not parallel to the film. First is distortion by way of **foreshortening** or **reduction in image size** compared to object size; or **elongation** which is an **increase in image size** compared to object size. The greater the angle of inclination of the object, the greater the amount of distortion.

A second effect of improper object alignment is **distortion of the joints or ends of bony structures.** This is best demonstrated on joints involving the upper and lower limbs. For example if a finger being radiographed is not parallel to the film, the joint spaces between the phalanges would not be visualized as being open because of the overlapping of the ends of the bones as demonstrated on this drawing. This demonstrates an important positioning principle. **Correct object alignment** (wherein the plane of the body part being x-rayed is as near parallel as possible to the plane of the film) **results in less distortion and more open joint spaces.**

4. Central Ray (CR): Another important principle in positioning and the fourth controlling factor of distortion is **correct use of the CR.** As described previously under the x-ray beam divergence principle, in general only the exact center of the x-ray beam, the CR, has no divergence as it projects that part of the object at 90° or perpendicular to the plane of the film. Therefore, **there is the least possible distortion at the CR,** as x-rays can travel through a joint space at this point unimpeded.

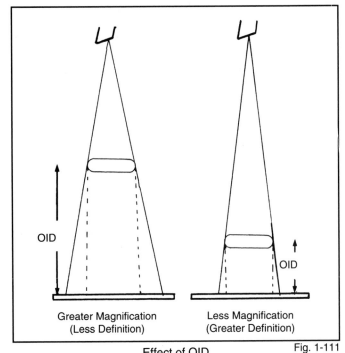

Greater Magnification   Less Magnification
(Less Definition)   (Greater Definition)

Effect of OID   Fig. 1-111

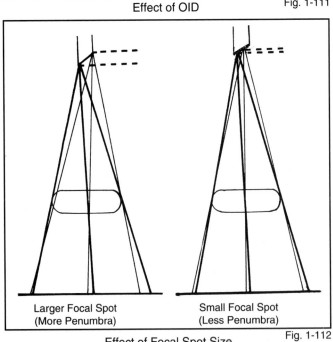

Larger Focal Spot   Small Focal Spot
(More Penumbra)   (Less Penumbra)

Effect of Focal Spot Size   Fig. 1-112

"Closed" Joint Spaces   "Open" Joint Spaces

Fig. 1-113

Object Alignment and Distortion

Central Ray continued

Distortion increases as the angle of divergence increases from the center of the x-ray beam to the outer edges. Therefore **the closer to the point of the CR, the less the distortion**. This is why correct centering or correct CR placement is important in minimizing image distortion.

An example of correct CR placement for an AP knee is shown in *Fig. 1-114a*. The CR will pass through the knee joint space with minimal distortion and the joint space should appear open.

Figure 1-114b demonstrates correct centering for an AP femur wherein the CR is directed to the area of the mid-femur. The knee joint, however, is now exposed by divergent rays (as shown by arrow) which will create distortion of knee joint structures. The knee joint space will therefore **not** appear open on this projection.

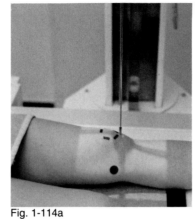
Fig. 1-114a
Correct CR for AP knee

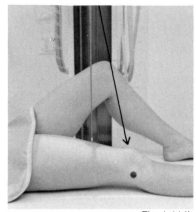
Fig. 1-114b
Correct CR for femur, but not for knee
(distortion occurs at knee)

Summary: Distortion, which is a misrepresentation of size and shape on the radiographic image, can be minimized by four controlling factors:

1. **SID** - Increase in SID decreases distortion (also increases definition).
2. **OID -** Decrease in OID decreases distortion (combined with small focal spot, decrease in OID also increases definition).
3. **Object Alignment** - Distortion is decreased with correct object alignment (plane of object is parallel to plane of film).
4. **CR** - Correct CR placement decreases distortion in that the center-most portion of the x-ray beam with the least divergence is used to the best advantage.

Anode Heel Effect

The anode heel effect describes a phenomenon wherein **the intensity of the radiation emitted from the cathode end of the x-ray field is greater than that at the anode end.** This is due to the angled design of the anode face such that there is greater attenuation or absorption of the x-rays at the anode end. The reason for this is those x-rays emitted from deeper within the anode must travel through more anode material before exiting at the anode end than those emitted in the direction of the cathode.

Studies show that the difference in intensity from the cathode to anode end of the x-ray beam can vary from 30% to 50% depending on the target angle using a 17 in. (43 cm) film at 40" (102 cm) SID *(Fig. 1-115).*[1] In general the smaller the focal spot, the greater the heel effect.

This effect is most pronounced at shorter SID because as the SID is decreased the angle or spread of beam that must be used to cover a given field size is increased as demonstrated in *Fig. 1-115*. Thus the **anode heel effect is most pronounced with a larger film using a smaller focal spot, at a shorter SID.**

Positioning Considerations

Obtaining optimum exposures of certain body parts which have a significant variation in thickness along the axis of the x-ray beam should include correct use of this anode heel effect by **placing the thicker body part at the cathode end of the x-ray table**. (The cathode and anode ends of the x-ray tube are usually marked on the protective housing near the cable connections.)

The abdomen, spine and long bone extremities are common examples of anatomic structures that vary enough in thickness or density that correct use of the anode heel effect is recommended for optimum radiographic images.

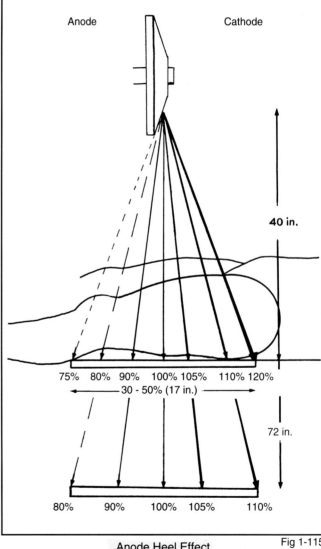
Anode Heel Effect
Fig 1-115

Exception: It should be noted that it is not always practical or even possible to take advantage of the anode heel effect (depending on the patient's condition or the arrangement in a room of specific x-ray equipment).

[1] Gratale, P, Wright, D. L., and Daughtry, L., Using the Anode Heel Effect for Extremity Radiography. Radiologic Technology **61-3** ; 1990; pp 195-198.

Part IV Principles of Radiation Protection

As a professional fully responsible for one's actions, the responsibility of **radiation protection** for both the patient and fellow workers is especially important for radiologic technologists. A complete study and understanding of radiation protection is essential for every radiographer but is beyond the scope of this anatomy and positioning text. However, the application or applied principles of radiation protection is very much an essential part of a course in radiographic anatomy and positioning because it is the responsibility of every radiographer to **always assure that the radiation dose to both the patient and the radiographer be kept as low as possible.**

Radiographer Protection

Radiographers must always remember that by the very nature of their work they are occupationally exposed to radiation and therefore, need to follow all safety practices possible to limit exposure.

Federal standards allow radiographers to receive up to 5 rem per year, a maximum permissible dose (MPD) which is ten times larger than the dose limit for the general population. However, because of the small risk of long-term effects of low level radiation, it is important that radiographers limit their exposure as much as possible. There is a protection principle called **ALARA** that goes much further in protecting the worker than the MPD level. This principle states that occupational exposure should be kept "**As Low As Reasonably Achievable**". This is an important principle that all radiographers should strive for and following is a summary of four important ways this can be achieved:

1. **Always** wear a film badge or other monitoring device. Although the badge doesn't lower exposure of the wearer, the existence of long term accurate records of badge readings aids in the evaluation of a radiation safety program.
2. If restraining patients is necessary, the person assisting with the restraining should **NEVER** stand in the primary or useful beam and should **ALWAYS** wear protective aprons and gloves. Use restraint devices or retention bands whenever possible and only as a last resort should anyone stay in the room to restrain patients, this should **never** be radiology personnel.
3. For portables or other trauma patient exams and fluoroscopy procedures, **ALWAYS** wear lead aprons and stand as far away as possible (inverse square law principle) from the x-ray source for protection against exposure by scatter radiation.
4. Practice the use of close collimation, filtration of primary beam, higher kVp techniques, high speed screens and minimum repeat exams. Exposure of the radiographer is due primarily to scattered radiation from the patient. Therefore, reduction in patient exposure results in reduction in exposure of the radiographer as well.

Patient Protection

Each professional radiographer subscribes to a code of ethics which includes responsibility for controlling and limiting the radiation exposure to patients under their care. This is a serious responsibility and each of the following six specific ways of reducing patient exposure needs to be understood and consistently put into practice as described on the following pages. They are as follows:

1. **Minimum repeat radiographs**
2. **Correct filtration**
3. **Accurate collimation**
4. **Specific area shielding** (gonadal shielding)
5. **Protection for pregnancies**
6. **Use of optimum exposure factors and high speed screen-film combinations.**

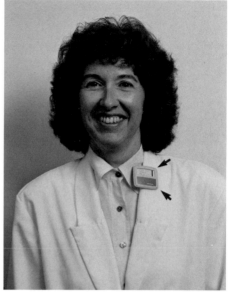

Fig 1-116

Radiographer wearing a film badge to monitor individual occupational radiation exposure. (Should be worn near the neck area **not** covered by the lead apron if such is worn.)

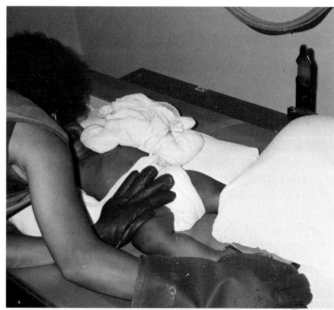

Wearing lead apron and gloves if restraining patient is necessary.   Fig 1-117

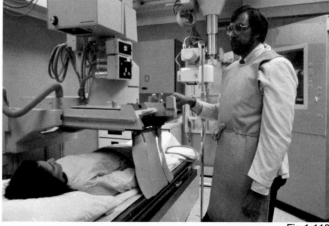

Radiographer protection in flouroscopy   Fig 1-118

Patient Protection continued

1. Minimum Repeat Radiographs

The first and most basic way to prevent unnecessary radiation is to **avoid unnecessary repeat radiographs**. One of the causes for repeat radiographs is **poor communication** between the radiographer and the patient. Breathing instructions which are unclear and not understood are one of the common causes of motion and the need to repeat radiographs. When procedures are not clearly explained, the patient can have added anxiety and nervousness because of the fear of the unknown. This stress from uncertainty and fear often increases the patient's state of mental confusion and ability to cooperate fully. To prevent this the radiographer must take the necessary time, even with heavy schedules and full work loads, to **carefully and fully explain the breathing instructions as well as the procedure in general in simple terms that the patient can understand.**

Patients need to be forewarned of any movements or strange noises by the equipment during the exposure. Also any burning sensation or other possible effects from injections during exposures should be explained to the patient.

Carelessness in positioning or **selection of incorrect exposure factors** are also common causes for repeats and should be avoided.

Correct and accurate positioning requires a good knowledge and understanding of anatomy because this allows the radiographer to visualize the size, shapes and locations of structures being radiographed. This is the reason for combining the anatomy with positioning in every chapter of this text.

2. Correct Filtration

Filtration of the primary x-ray beam reduces exposure to the patient by absorbing most of those lower energy "unuseful" x-rays which primarily expose the patient's skin and superficial tissue. The net effect of filtration is a "hardening" of the x-ray beam resulting in an increase in the effective energy or penetrability of the x-ray beam.

Filtration is described in two ways. First is **inherent** or built-in filtration from the structures making up the x-ray tube itself. For most x-ray tubes this is approximately .5 mm aluminum (Al) equivalent. Second and more important to radiographers is **added filtration**, which is the amount of filtration added between the x-ray tube and the collimator.

Aluminum (Al) is the metal most commonly used for filters in diagnostic radiology, with Molybdenum (Mo) often used in mammography. The amount of required added filtration as established by federal laws is dependent on the operating kVp range of the equipment. The manufacturers of x-ray equipment are required to meet these standards. The filtration of diagnostic imaging equipment is checked yearly (and after a major equipment service such as replacement of the tube or collimator) by qualified personnel such as a medical physicist. The responsibility of the radiographer is to check to see that the proper filter material for each tube is in place.

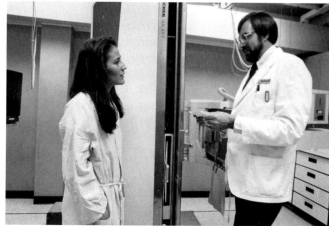
Fig 1-119
Clear precise instructions help relieve patient anxieties

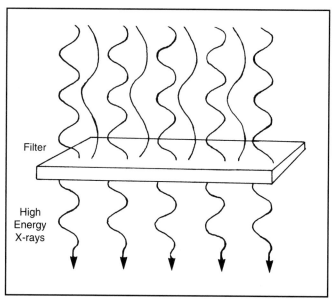
Fig 1-120
Filtration removes low energy X-rays (which are not useful) from the beam by absorbing them while permitting higher energy X-rays to pass through.

Patient Protection continued

3. Collimation

Accurate collimation is another important way to reduce patient exposure by limiting the size and shape of the x-ray beam to only the area of clinical interest, or that area required to be visualized on the film or other image receptor. Careful and accurate collimation is stressed and demonstrated throughout this text.

The variable rectangular collimator is commonly used for general purpose diagnostic radiographic equipment. The illuminated light field carefully defines the x-ray beam field on accurately calibrated equipment and can be used effectively to determine tissue area being irradiated.

The concept of divergence of the x-ray beam must be considered in accurate collimation. Therefore, the illuminated field size as it appears on the skin surface of the patient will appear smaller than the actual size of the anatomical area to which one is collimating. This is most evident on an exam such as a lateral thoracic or lumbar spine *(Fig. 1-121)* wherein there is considerable distance from the skin surface of the light field to the film in the Bucky tray. In such cases the light field when collimated correctly to the area of interest will appear much too small unless one considers the divergence of the x-ray beam.

Automatic Positive Beam Limitation (PBL): All general purpose x-ray equipment in the United States require collimators with PBL features which automatically collimate the useful x-ray beam to the film size. This PBL feature consists of sensors in the film cassette holder which when activated by placing a cassette in the cassette holder (Bucky tray) automatically signals the collimator to adjust the x-ray beam to that size film.

The PBL device can be deactivated or overridden with a key but this should only be done under special conditions where larger collimation by manual control is needed. A red warning light automatically comes on as a reminder that the PBL system has been deactivated and regulations require that the key cannot be removed while the system is being overridden *(Fig. 1-122)*.

Manual Collimation: Even with automatic collimation, PBL, the operator can also manually reduce the collimation field size from that which is set automatically. This should be done for all exams where the film size is larger than the critical area being radiographed. Accurate manual collimation also is required for exams of the upper and lower limbs taken table top wherein the PBL device is not activated. Throughout the positioning pages of this text, collimation guidelines are provided to maximize patient protection by careful and accurate collimation.

This practice of close collimation to only the area of interest reduces patient exposure **two ways.** First it **reduces the volume of tissue directly irradiated,** and second it **reduces the accompanying scatter radiation.** This scatter radiation resulting from lack of accurate collimation or other shielding not only adds unnecessary increased patient exposure but also results in a decrease in image quality by the "fogging" effect of scatter radiation. (This is especially true in high volume tissue areas such as the abdomen or chest.)

Reasons for Four-sided Collimation if Possible: In addition to reducing patient exposure and improving image quality, another reason for this general rule of at least some visible collimation on all four sides is a check system insuring that maximum collimation did occur. If there is no collimation border visible on the radiograph on any one or more sides on exams taken table top where there is no automatic collimation, then of course there is no evidence that the primary beam was restricted at all on that portion.

An added benefit for at least some collimation on all four sides if

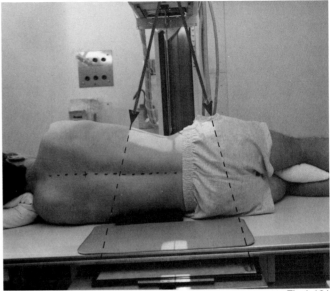

Close Four Sided Collimation (Collimation field may appear too small due to divergence of x-rays)   Fig 1-121

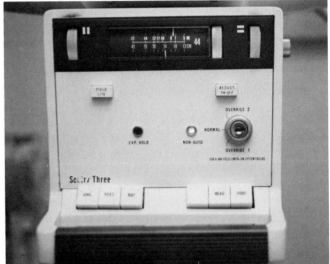

Automatic Collimation (PBL)   Fig 1-122

possible is to be able to check the final radiograph for **correct central ray location**. This is done by placing a large imaginary X from the four corners of the collimation field as seen on the resultant radiograph. The exact center of this X indicates where the CR was located.

Summary: The practice of close collimation to the area of clinical interest results in a significant **decrease in patient exposure** and **increases image quality** through decreased scatter.

Collimation Rule: A general rule followed throughout this text indicates that **collimation borders should be visible on the film on all four sides if the film size is large enough to allow this without "cutting off" essential anatomy.** For some body parts such as a large adult abdomen, extra side collimation as visible on the radiograph may not be possible. For most exams however such as for the upper and lower limbs, spine and skull, four-sided collimation as visible on the radiograph is possible without cutting off essential anatomy.

Patient Protection continued

4. Specific Area Shielding

Specific area shielding is required when especially sensitive tissue or organs such as the lens of the eye, breasts and gonads are in or near the useful beam. Examples of this type of area shielding are **breast** and **gonadal** shields which can be used over juvenile breasts and gonads for certain examinations such as a scoliosis spine series *(Figs. 1-123 and 124)*. Another example is a type of eye shield which can be used when radiographing parts of the skull if such do not obscure essential anatomy.

The most common area shielding is **gonadal shielding**, used to protect the reproductive organs from irradiation when they are in or near the primary beam. There are two general types of specific area shielding available as follows:

1. **Shadow Shields:** As the name implies shadow shields, which are attached to the tube head, are devices placed between the x-ray tube and the patient thus casting a shadow of the shield over the specific areas being shielded. One such type of shield is shown in *Fig. 1-123* wherein the shield is attached to a flexible arm which can be adjusted to cast a shadow from the collimator light over the gonads or other areas being shielded.

   Another newer type is shown in *Fig. 1-124* wherein certain individual radiopaque breast and gonad shields are attached with magnets directly to the bottom of the collimator. These are frequently combined with clear lead compensating filters used to provide a more uniform exposure over parts of the body that are not uniform in thickness or density, such as used on the thoracic and lumbar spine scoliosis radiograph of *Fig. 1-125*.

2. **Flat Contact Shields**: Flat contact gonadal shields are most commonly used for patients in recumbent positions. Contact shields may be larger vinyl-covered lead shields placed over the gonadal area in general. This is demonstrated in *Fig. 1-126,* showing shielding for a lateral femur. These shields are generally from the same lead-impregnated vinyl materials used for lead aprons of sufficient thickness to shield primary radiation.

   Contact shields specifically for gonads, such as for the testes on the male or ovaries on female patients, may be smaller vinyl covered lead material of appropriate lead thickness cut into various shapes to be placed directly over the reproductive organs *(Figs. 1-127 and 128)*.

   Gonadal shields for males should be placed distally to the lower margin of the pubic symphysis covering the area of the testes or scrotum. Gonadal shielding on females to cover the area of the ovaries, fallopian tubes and uterus is a little more difficult to determine. A general guideline for female adults is to shield an area 3-4 in. (8-10 cm) superior to the pubic symphysis, and 1.5 - 2 in. (4-5 cm) each way from the pelvic midline. Various shaped shields may be used such as oval, round, heart-shaped, V or U shaped and triangular. The shielded area would be proportionally smaller on youth. A one year old female would require an oval shield only about 1 in. (2.5 cm) wide and 1.5 in. (4 cm) long placed directly superior to the pubic symphysis.

   For females such flat contact shields placed correctly over the gonads can reduce exposure by approximately 50%. The reduction in exposure to the gonads for male patients is greater, up to 90-95% when contact shields are used correctly.[1]

---

[1] Statkiewiez, M.L. and Ritenour, E.R.: **Radiation Protection for Student Radiographers.** Denver; Multi-Media Publishing Inc. 1983.

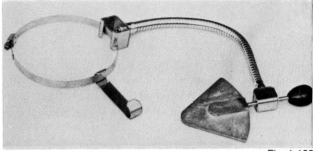

Shadow Shield on Flexible Arm Fig. 1-123
(Courtesy of Nuclear Associates, Carle, NY)

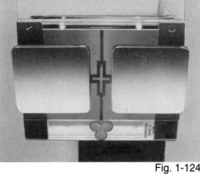

Fig. 1-124
Clear pb Filter with Breast and Gonad Shadow Shields in Place.
(Courtesy of Nuclear Associates)

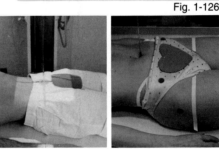

Fig. 1-126

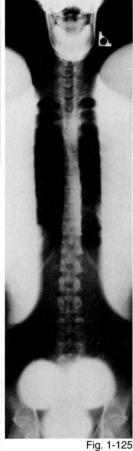

Fig. 1-125
AP Spine for Scoliosis with Compensating Filter and Breast and Gonad Shields in Place.
(Courtesy of Nuclear Asso.)

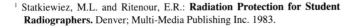

Fig. 1-127   Fig. 1-128
Flat Contact Shields

Summary Rules for Specific Area Shielding

Consistent and correct use of specific area shielding is a challenge for each radiographer because of the added time and equipment required. The importance, however, of protecting radiation sensitive organs of children and adults of reproductive age from unnecessary radiation exposure should be sufficient motivation to consistently practice the following three rules:

1. **Should be used on all potentially reproductive patients.** A common departmental policy is to include specific area shielding for all children and those adults of reproductive age.

2. **Should be used when the radiation sensitive areas lie within or near (2 in. or 5 cm) the primary beam unless such shielding obscures essential diagnostic information.**

3. **Accurate beam collimation** and **careful positioning must accompany the use of such shielding.** Specific area shielding is important, but this should always be a **secondary** protective measure and **not** a substitute for accurate collimation.

Patient Protection continued

5. Protection for Pregnancies

Pregnancies and potential pregnancies require special consideration for all women of child bearing age because of the evidence that the developing embryo is especially sensitive to radiation. This concern is particularly critical during the first two months of pregnancy when the fetus is most sensitive to radiation exposure and the mother is usually not yet aware of the pregnancy. Therefore, because of the concern for **potential pregnancies** of women of childbearing age, the ten-day rule has been recommended by the ICRP (International Commission on Radiation Protection).

Ten-day Rule: The ten-day rule states that **all radiologic examinations involving the pelvis and lower abdomen should be scheduled during the first ten days following the onset of menstruation.** This is the time when it is most certain that there is no pregnancy. The exception to this rule would be if the attending physician believes it is in the best interest of the patient to have the exam even after this ten day period with the potential hazards.

In large departments it is impractical if not impossible to insure that all such examinations be scheduled following this ten-day rule. However, posters or signs *(Fig. 1-129)* should be posted in examination rooms and waiting room areas reminding the patient to inform someone of their known pregnancy or potential pregnancy.

If the ten-day rule cannot always be followed for potential pregnancies, it is important to use all those radiation protection practices already described, especially careful collimation and gonadal shielding.

For **known pregnancies**, the following exams result in higher doses to the fetus and may require confirmation from the referring physician and the radiologist that the exam is indicated:

• Lumbar spine
• Pelvis
• Sacrum and coccyx
• Proximal femur and hip
• Intravenous Urogram. (IVU)
• Gallbladder
• Fluoroscopic procedures (abdomen)
• Computed tomography (abdomen)

6. Optimum Exposure Factors and High Speed Screen-Film Combinations

Another final important radiation protection practice involves the use of those optimum exposure factors and high speed screen-film combinations which reduce patient exposure.

The selection of optimum exposure factors should not only result in the highest quality radiograph possible yielding maximum diagnostic information but should also result in the least possible patient dose. The use of high kVp techniques with lower mAs significantly reduces patient dose as already described in this chapter under the discussion of contrast and density. A general rule was given which states that **the highest kVp and the lowest mAs possible should be selected which results in a diagnostically acceptable radiograph.**

The use of optimum screen-film combinations also reduces patient dose dramatically. For average speed screens about 95% of the radiographic exposure results from light emitted by

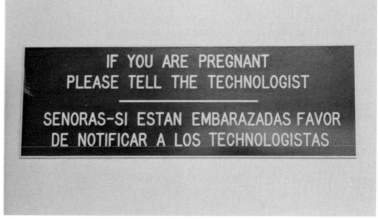

Warning Sign   Fig. 1-129a
(Courtesy of St. Joseph's Hospital, Phoenix, AZ)

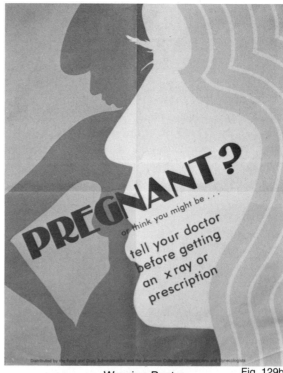

Warning Poster   Fig. 129b

the intensifying screens and only 5% from the primary rays. This per cent is even higher with high speed screens commonly used today such as rare earth screens, thus reducing patient dose even more.

Certain films with thicker emulsion or with different chemical dyes are faster or more sensitive thus reducing the amount of exposure required. The use of higher speed screens and films however, does reduce image definition or sharpness of detail. Therefore it is common practice to use detail screens with table top exams, such as upper and lower limbs, when a grid is not used. A general rule similar to the kVp-mAs rule states "**Use the highest speed screen-film combination which results in diagnostically acceptable radiographs**".

Part V Basic Principles of Radiographic Positioning

Professional Ethics and Patient Care

The medical radiographer (radiologic technologist) is a medical professional and an important member of the health care team responsible in general for radiologic examination of patients. This requires not only a broad understanding of anatomy terminology used in this profession, an understanding of the basic imaging principles and radiation protection as covered in the first part of this chapter, but also an understanding of what it means to be a professional responsible for the patients under their care. This includes being responsible for ones actions under a specific code of ethics.

The term ethics in general refers to the moral principles of behavior of individuals. More specifically a **Code of Ethics** describes the **rules of acceptable conduct toward others,** as defined within certain professions.

As a medical professional responsible for the welfare of patients in their care, radiologic technologists must adhere to a strict code of conduct with absolute honesty in carrying out their tasks and responsibilities in a professional manner. They must also remember that they are a supporting member of the medical team which includes radiologists and referring physicians.

The current code of ethics as printed on this page reflects the recognition of the radiologic technologist as a professional who "**practices ethical conduct appropriate to the profession, and protects the patient's right to quality radiologic technology care**" (principle 8). Principle 7 also emphasizes the added responsibilities as a professional who "**performs services in accordance with an accepted standard of practice, and demonstrates expertise in limiting the radiation exposure . . .**"

This code of ethics and the increased recognition of radiologic technology as a profession indicating responsibility for their actions and behavior, places additional responsibility on technologists in the areas of radiation protection and optimum quality radiographs. Throughout this text emphasis has been given to radiation protection for the patient in that gonadal shielding and collimation notations are included on each positioning page for all projections or positions.

Responsibility by the technologist for "**quality radiologic technology care**" (principle 8) has also been recognized in this text in that evaluation criteria sections are included with each projection or position which identifies a definable standard for each radiographic image described and illustrated.

Code of Ethics

1. *The Radiologic Technologist conducts himself/herself in a professional manner, responds to patient needs and supports colleagues and associates in providing quality patient care.*

2. *The Radiologic Technologist acts to advance the principle objective of the profession to provide services to humanity with full respect for the dignity of mankind.*

3. *The Radiologic Technologist delivers patient care and service unrestricted by concerns of personal attributes or the nature of the disease or illness, and without discrimination, regardless of sex, race, creed, religion, or socioeconomic status.*

4. *The Radiologic Technologist practices technology founded upon theoretical knowledge and concepts, utilizes equipment and accessories consistent with the purpose for which it has been designed, and employs procedures and techniques appropriately.*

5. *The Radiologic Technologist assesses situations, exercises care, discretion and judgment, assumes responsibility for professional decisions, and acts in the best interest of the patient.*

6. *The Radiologic Technologist acts as an agent through observation and communication to obtain pertinent information for the physician to aid in the diagnosis and treatment management of the patient, and recognizes that interpretation and diagnosis are outside the scope of practice for the profession.*

7. *The Radiologic Technologist utilizes equipment and accessories, employs techniques and procedures, performs services in accordance with an accepted standard of practice, and demonstrates expertise in limiting the radiation exposure to the patient, self and other members of the health care team.*

8. *The Radiologic Technologist practices ethical conduct appropriate to the profession, and protects the patient's right to quality radiologic technology care.*

9. *The Radiologic Technologist respects confidences entrusted in the course of professional practice, protects the patient's right to privacy, and reveals confidential information only as required by law or to protect the welfare of the individual or the community.*

10. *The Radiologic Technologist continually strives to improve knowledge and skills by participating in educational and professional activities, sharing knowledge with colleagues and investigating new and innovative aspects of professional practice. One means available to improve knowledge and skills is through professional continuing education*

ADOPTED BY:
THE AMERICAN SOCIETY OF RADIOLOGIC TECHNOLOGISTS
THE AMERICAN REGISTRY OF RADIOLOGIC TECHNOLOGISTS
as revised in September, 1989

Positioning Method Sequence
(Fixed table top and floating table top
with film in Bucky tray under table)

The positioning pages which follow in this text describe the positioning of each body part using a standard step by step positioning sequence. The differences in the specific types of equipment being used will require some adaptation and adjustments.

Improvements and changes in x-ray equipment are continually being made. One example is the floating table top equipment now in common use. This allows the radiographer to easily move the entire patient and table top together as described below in a step by step sequence. However, fixed table top equipment is also in use and radiographers need to adapt positioning methods and procedures based on the available equipment.

In general the part-film-tube centering method and sequence as described in this text can be used with either a fixed table top Bucky tray combination or a floating table top Bucky tray system.

Floating Table Top Equipment:
(Part positioned to CR)
With a floating table top and independent Bucky tray system the patient does not need to be moved or slid around on the table top in that the patient and table top can be moved together. With this system the positioning method and sequence is described as a three-step method.

1. Patient and Part Positioning: The patient is first assisted onto the table (with table top in a locked position to prevent patient from falling). The patient is then positioned into a specific supine, prone, oblique or lateral body position as needed.

2. CR-film Alignment: After the patient is on the table, the CR (x-ray tube) is then aligned and centered to the film (cassette) as correctly placed in the Bucky tray, lengthwise or crosswise. This includes setting the correct SID (Source Image receptor Distance), and angling the CR if this is required.

3. Patient-CR Alignment: After the CR and film are aligned and the patient and/or body part is positioned correctly on the table, then the table top is unlocked and the patient and table top together are moved as needed to align the CR to the correct centering point on the patient as indicated by the CR indicator in the lighted exposure field.

The exact sequence of positioning is of course not as important as understanding the principles of positioning. However, every radiographer should learn a positioning sequence that can be used with different types of equipment and that is efficient and also easiest for them and for the patient. This text describes certain suggested positioning steps and sequences on each positioning page to guide student radiographers through this learning process.

Floating Table Top Positioning Sequence
3-step method

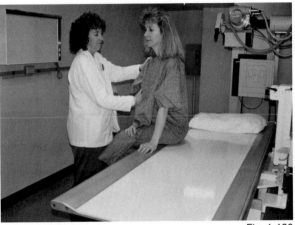

Step 1. Patient and Part Positioning   Fig. 1-130

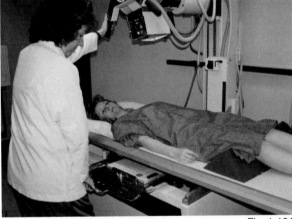

Step 2. CR-Film Alignment   Fig. 1-131

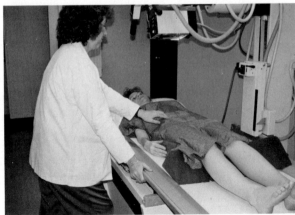

Step 3. Patient - CR Alignment   Fig. 1-132

Positioning Method Sequence continued

Fixed Table top Equipment: (Part positioned and centered to table and/or film)

The following four-step positioning sequence is generally followed when using fixed table top, Bucky tray equipment:

1. Patient Position: Patient is assisted onto the x-ray table and placed into a specific supine, prone, oblique or lateral body position.

2. Part Position: Using topographical landmarks the patient is then moved or slid on the table top as required to align or center the part being radiographed to the center line or to parallel longitudinal lines on the table top.

3. Film Centered: The film in the Bucky tray is then moved along the length of the table as needed to center the film to the part being radiographed, again using topographical landmarks on patient.

4. CR Centered: The x-ray tube (at correct SID) is moved into position by aligning the CR (central ray) to the center of the film. If the CR requires angling, the CR and film are then aligned and moved as needed to correctly center and project the part to the center of the film.

At this time a final check for correct centering can be made by observing the correct CR location on the body part and making adjustments of tube, film, or part as needed.

Table Top and/or Portable Procedures

Certain exams of the upper and lower limbs are taken non-grid wherein the film is not placed in the moving grid Bucky tray under the table top but rather the film (cassette) is placed directly **on** the table top under the patient. This is also true for certain emergency type procedures taken directly on the stretcher or cart; or for portables taken in patient's rooms. The above positioning steps in general however can still be followed.

Fixed Table top Positioning Sequence
(4-step method)

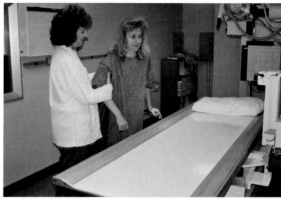

Step 1. Patient Position   Fig. 1-134

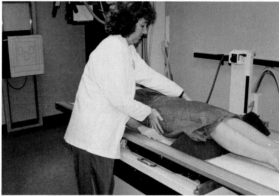

Step 2. Part Position   Fig. 1-135

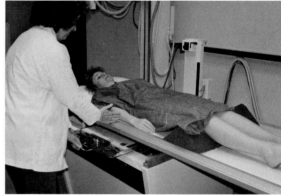

Step 3. Film Centered   Fig. 1-136

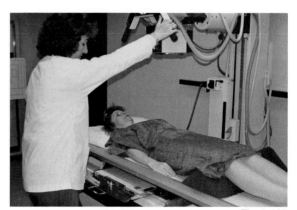

Step 4. CR Centered   Fig. 1-137

General Protocol and Order for General Diagnostic Radiographic Procedures

Each radiology department should establish an agreed on protocol and order by which all general diagnostic radiographic procedures are performed. This is necessary for an orderly and effective working system whereby all radiographers (students or graduate technologists) follow the same order and procedure. The specific items included as well as the order of these various steps of procedure will vary depending on the location, type and size of department. Following is a sample of such a protocol as established and used by a U.S. mid-western university hospital.[1]

GENERAL PROTOCOL FOR RADIOGRAPHERS DURING RADIOGRAPHY OF PATIENTS

1. Read and assess requisition completely.
2. Determine which screen-film combination you will need.
3. Determine what size and number of cassettes you will need.
4. Stock passbox/cassette cabinet with proper amount and type of cassettes.
5. Prepare radiographic room.
6. Correctly identify the patient. (Check arm band or have patient repeat full name.)
7. Dress patient correctly. (Sometimes done by nurse or transaide.)
8. Explain to the patient what you will be doing and what is expected of them.
9. ASSIST the patient to position and place you want them for the first film.
10. Measure the part to be radiographed.
11. Determine the radiographic technique to be used and set on the machine.
12. Position the patient accurately.
13. Collimate the beam so that only the area of interest is included.
14. Identify right and left side of patient with the proper lead marker.
15. Restrain the patient if needed.
16. Use lead gonadal shielding on anyone under 50 years of age.
17. Provide lead aprons and lead gloves, if necessary, for EVERYONE assisting with restraint in the room.
18. Take exposure, while watching patient through window.
19. Repeat steps 8 through 18 for each radiographic view needed.
20. Patient is not to be left alone in the radiographic room unless restrained and holding a pull cord.
21. Explain that you are going to develop and view the films you have taken to determine if adequate radiographs have been taken.
22. Fog each exposed cassette with the patient's identification card.
23. Place exposed cassettes in a pass box to the darkroom.
24. Record the date, time, number of films, name, room number, technique used, and patient history on the requisition.
25. Properly critique radiographs. If no radiograph needs to be repeated, place in proper slot or send with patient if indicated.
26. Place a corrected patient exam card in the designated computer terminal completed box, including the time, room number, number of films and rejects.
27. Assist the patient from table to wheel chair, cart or walking position.
28. Open door for the patient.
29. Explain to out-patients where they are to go next. Take in-patients to the proper holding area and place a TO GO card in the transaide area.
30. Straighten up the radiographic room, change linens and clean off table with alcohol so room will be ready for the next patient.
31. Wash your hands.

---

[1]Submitted by Kathy Martensen, BS, RT(R), University of Iowa Hospitals and Clinics, Iowa City, Iowa

Basic and Optional Projections/Positions

Certain **basic** and **optional** projections or positions are demonstrated and described in this text for each radiographic examination or procedure commonly done in radiology departments throughout the United States. This national standard or norm of basic and optional projections/positions was determined by a national survey and questionnaire as described in the front pages of this text.

Optional Projections/Positions

In addition to the basic or routine projections/positions, there are certain optional or extra projections/positions also included for each examination or procedure described in this text. The national survey helped determine these which are defined as those **projections/ positions most commonly taken to better demonstrate specific anatomical parts,** or **for certain pathological conditions** or **which may be necessary for patients who cannot cooperate fully.** (They are **not** optional as to whether or not they need to be learned and mastered.)

Principles for Determining Positioning Routines

There are two general rules or principles which if understood will help one remember and understand why certain minimum projections are taken as routine or as basic projections/positions for various radiographic examinations or procedures.

1. **Need for a minimum of <u>two</u> projections/positions**

   A general rule in diagnostic radiology suggests that a minimum of two projections taken as near 90° from each other as possible are required in most radiographic procedures. Exceptions include mass chest screening which may include only a single PA projection. The KUB (kidneys, ureter, and bladder) of the abdomen or other cases where only one projection provides ample information are also exceptions.

   There are three reasons for this general rule of a minimum of two projections taken as near 90° from each other as possible.

   a. Problem of anatomical structures being superimposed: In general, a single projection should never be taken for any routine radiographic examination because of the superimposition of body parts. Certain pathological conditions such as some fractures, small tumors, etc., may not be visualized on one projection only.

   Example: A small chest lesion is shown posteriorly on the lateral chest radiograph in *Fig. 1-139.* This lesion is not visible on the PA projection in *Fig. 1-138,* because it is superimposed by the dense heart shadow.

   b. Localization of lesions or foreign bodies: A minimum of two projections, taken at 90° or as near right angles from each other as possible, are essential in determining the location of any lesion or foreign body *(Fig. 1-140).*

   Example: Foreign bodies (the white densities are metallic fragments) embedded in tissues of the hand. Note that both the PA and lateral projections are necessary to determine the exact location of these metallic fragments.

   c. Determination of alignment of fractures: Any fracture requires a minimum of two projections, taken at 90° or as near right angles as possible, both to visualize fully the fracture site and to determine alignment of the fractured parts.

   Example: Two positions or projections of the fractured lower leg, 90° from each other, are required to allow the physician to determine alignment of the fractured tibia and fibula *(Figs. 1-141 and 142).*

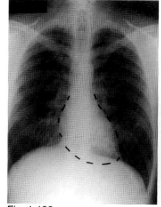

Fig. 1-138
PA Radiograph   Fig. 1-139
Lateral Radiograph

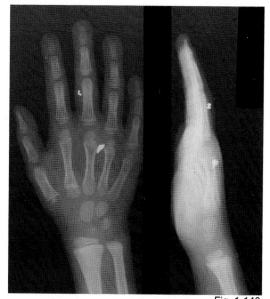

Foreign Bodies   Fig. 1-140

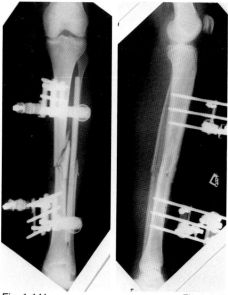

Fig. 1-141   For Fracture Alignment   Fig. 1-142

2. **A minimum of <u>three</u> projections/positions when joints are in prime interest area**

This general rule or principle suggests that all radiographic procedures of the skeletal system involving joints require a minimum of **three** projections/ positions rather than only two. These are **AP or PA, lateral and oblique.**

The reason for this is more information is needed than can be provided on only two projections. For example with the multiple surfaces and angles of the bones making up the joint, a small oblique chip fracture or other abnormality within the joint space may not be visualized on either the frontal or the lateral views but may be well demonstrated in the oblique position.

Examples of exams requiring **three** positions or projections (joint is in prime interest area):

- fingers
- toes
- hand
- wrist
- elbow
- ankle
- foot
- knee

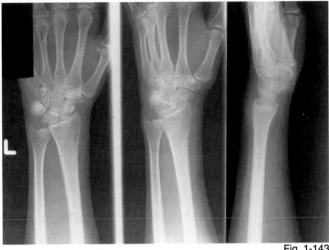

Wrist (Requires three projections/positions) Fig. 1-143

Examples of exams requiring **two** positions or projections (long bones and chest):

- forearm
- humerus
- femur
- tibia-fibula
- chest

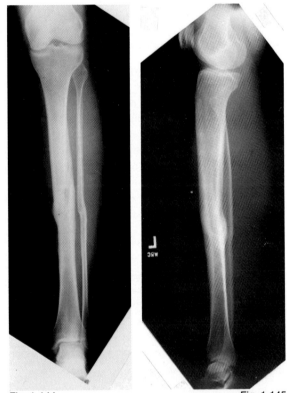

Fig. 1-144   Fig. 1-145

Lower Leg (Requires two projections/positions)
(This is the same patient as Figs. 1-141 and 142 on preceding page)

Chapter 2

Radiographic Anatomy and Positioning of the Chest

Contributions by: Karen Brown, RT (R)

Kathy Martensen, BS, RT (R)

Contents

Chest

Part I Radiographic Anatomy

Chest radiographic examinations are the most common of all radiographic procedures. It is common for student radiographers to begin their clinical experience taking chest radiographs. Before beginning such clinical experience however, it is important to learn and understand chest anatomy well, including relative relationships of all anatomy within the chest cavity.

CHEST

The chest or thorax is the upper part of the trunk between the neck and the abdomen. Radiographic anatomy of the chest is divided into three sections; the **bony thorax**, the **respiratory system proper**, and the **mediastinum**.

Bony Thorax

The **bony thorax** is that part of the skeletal system providing a protective framework for the parts of the chest involved with breathing and blood circulation. **Thoracic viscera** is the term used to describe these parts of the chest consisting of the lungs and the remaining thoracic organs contained in the mediastinum.

The bony thorax consists of the **sternum** (breastbone) anteriorly, the **two clavicles** (collarbones) connecting the sternum to the two **scapulae** (shoulder blades), the **twelve pairs of ribs** circling the bony thorax and the **twelve thoracic vertebrae** posteriorly. A detailed description of the parts of the bony thorax is presented in chapter 10.

Topographic Positioning Landmarks
Accurate and consistent radiographic positioning requires certain landmarks or reference points which one can use to center the film correctly to insure that all essential anatomy is included on that specific projection. These topographic landmarks need to be parts of the body that are easily and consistently located on patients, such as parts of the bony thorax. For chest positioning two of these landmarks are the vertebra prominens and the jugular notch.

1. Vertebra Prominens (7th cervical vertebra)
This can be an important landmark for locating the central ray location on a PA chest projection. It can be readily palpated on most patients by applying light pressure with the finger tips at the base of the neck. The vertebra prominens is the first prominent process felt as you gently but firmly palpate down the back of the neck with the head dropped forward. With a little practice this landmark can be readily located on most patients, especially if the head and neck is flexed forward.

2. Jugular notch (manubrial or suprasternal notch)
The jugular notch is an important landmark for locating the central ray location on AP chest projections. This is easily palpated as a deep notch or depression on the superior portion of the sternum below the thyroid cartilage (commonly known as Adam's apple).

The mid-thorax, at the level of T7 (7th thoracic vertebra), can easily be located from these two landmarks as will be described later in this chapter.

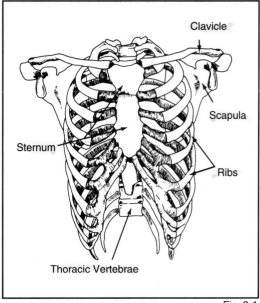

Bony Thorax   Fig. 2-1

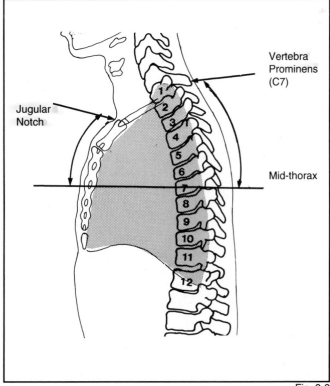

Topographic Landmarks   Fig. 2-2

Chest

Respiratory System

Respiration is the exchange of gaseous substances between the air we breathe and the blood stream. This is brought about by the respiratory system which consists of those parts of the body through which air passes as it travels from the nose and mouth into the lungs. The four parts of the respiratory system are the **pharynx**, **trachea**, **bronchi** and **lungs** as illustrated and described in detail on the following pages.

Diaphragm

An important structure of the respiratory system is the dome-shaped **diaphragm** which is the chief muscle of inspiration. As the dome of the diaphragm moves downward, it **increases** the volume of the thoracic cavity. This, along with certain other dimensional movements of the thorax described later in this chapter, **decreases** the intrathoracic pressure, resulting in air being drawn into the lungs through the nose and mouth, pharynx, larynx, trachea, and bronchi.

Pharynx *(far'inks)* (upper air way)

The pharynx is a structure or passageway important to the respiratory system because air must pass through it prior to entering the respiratory system proper, which begins with the larynx or voice box. The pharynx, also referred to as the upper airway or the upper respiratory tract, is that posterior area between the nose and mouth above and the larynx or voice box and the esophagus below. This is the area that serves as a passageway for both food and fluids as well as air, thus making it common to both the digestive and respiratory systems. For this reason it is not considered part of the respiratory system proper.

The pharynx has three divisions as shown in *Fig. 2-4,* the **naso-pharynx** *(na"zo-far'inks)*, **oropharynx** *(o"ro-far'inks)* and **laryngopharynx** *(lah-ring"go-far'inks)*. The interior of the pharynx communicates posteriorly with the cavities, the nose above (nasopharynx), the mouth (oropharynx), and the larynx below (laryngopharynx), as well as the esophagus. The **soft palate**, the back portion of which is called the **uvula** *(ū'vu-lah)*, is the point of separation of the nasopharynx from the oropharynx. The laryngopharynx lies above and posterior to the larynx and extends from the upper border of the **epiglottis** *(ĕp"ĭ-glot'is)* to where the laryngopharynx narrows to join the esophagus.

The dotted black lines indicate the pathway which air may take from the external environment to the trachea and eventually to the lungs. Note that air passing through either the nose or mouth must pass through at least some portion of the pharynx.

Two additional structures shown on this sectional lateral drawing are the **hyoid bone** and the **thyroid cartilage** (Adam's Apple), which are described in more detail in the next section on the larynx.

Esophagus

The esophagus is part of the digestive system which connects the pharynx with the stomach. Note the relationship of the esophagus to both the pharynx and the larynx. It is continuous with the pharynx at its origin at the approximate level of **C5** (fifth cervical vertebra) which is also the level of the thyroid cartilage anteriorly. The esophagus continues downward to the stomach, posterior to the larynx and trachea. (Chapter 14 describes the esophagus in detail along with the upper digestive system.)

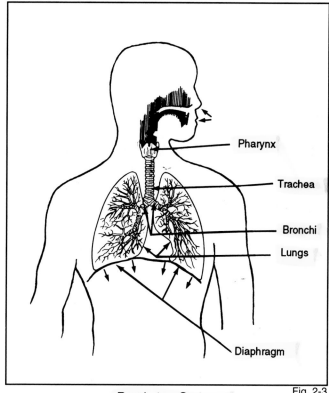

Respiratory System　　　Fig. 2-3

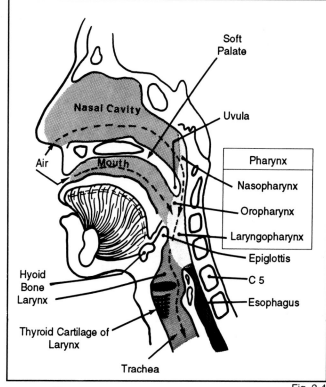

Pharynx, Upper Airway (Midsagittal Section)　Fig. 2-4

Respiratory System continued

The four parts of the respiratory system important in chest radiography are as follows:

1. **Larynx** *(lar'inks)* (voice box)
2. **Trachea** *(tra'ke-ah)*
3. **Right and left bronchi** *(bron'chi)*
4. **Lungs**

The larynx, trachea and bronchi form a continuous, tubular structure through which air can pass from the nose and mouth into the lungs as shown in *Fig. 2-3* and *4* on the preceding page.

1. Larynx (voice box)

The **larynx** or voice box, is a cagelike, cartilaginous structure approximately 5 centimeters in length in an adult. The larynx is in the anterior portion of the neck, suspended from a small bone called the **hyoid**. The hyoid bone is found in the upper neck just below the tongue or floor of the mouth. The hyoid bone is **not** part of the larynx.

The larynx serves as the organ of voice. Sounds are made as air passes between the vocal cords located within the larynx. The upper margin of the larynx is at the approximate level of **C3** (third cervical vertebra). Its lower margin, where the larynx junctions with the trachea, is at the level of **C6** (sixth cervical vertebra).

The framework of the larynx consists of nine cartilages, the largest of which is called the **thyroid cartilage** (Adam's apple), as shown in *Fig. 2-5*. This cartilage is a prominent structure that is easy to locate; therefore, it becomes an important positioning landmark. As noted on the preceding page, the laryngeal prominence of the thyroid cartilage is located at approximately the level of **C5** (fifth cervical vertebra) and is an excellent topographical reference for locating specific skeletal structures in this region.

A small structure known as the **epiglottis**, located at the upper margin of the larynx, acts as a lid for the slanted opening of the larynx, as shown in *Fig. 2-6*. During the act of swallowing, the epiglottis flips down and covers the laryngeal opening and prevents food and fluid from entering the larynx, and bronchi. This anatomical relationship is demonstrated in *Fig. 2-6*, as well as *Fig. 2-4* on the preceding page.

Cross Section of Larynx

Due to the wide acceptance of CT (computed tomography) and ultrasonography, it is important for the radiographer to recognize anatomical structures in cross section. Figure 2-7 shows a computed tomogram through the mid-portion of the larynx at the level of C5. Only major structures are labeled on this radiograph. A more detailed study of the cross sectional anatomy of the chest is found in Chapter 21 on thoracic computed tomography.

Note: Conventional CT images such as seen here are viewed as though one were at the patient's feet looking up toward the head.

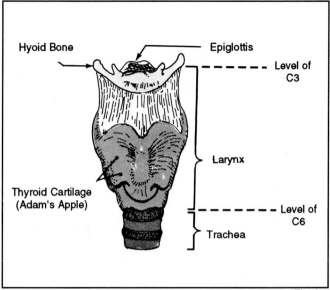

Larynx (Frontal View)   Fig. 2-5

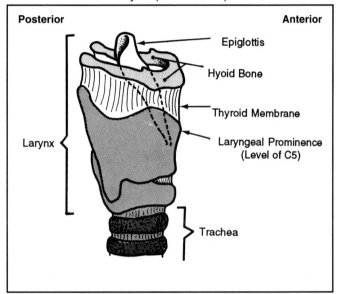

Larynx (Lateral View)   Fig. 2-6

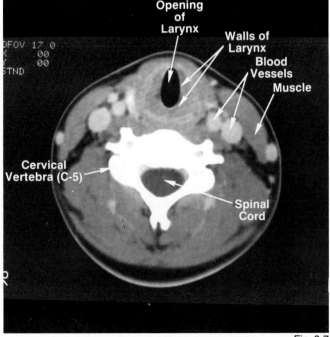

CT Image of Neck through Larynx
(cross section at level of C5)   Fig. 2-7

2. Trachea

Continuing from the larynx downward, the second division of the respiratory system proper is the **trachea** or windpipe. It is a fibrous muscular tube about 3/4 in. (2 cm) in diameter and 4.5 in. (11 cm) long. Approximately twenty C-shaped rings of cartilage are embedded in its walls. These provide rigidity to keep the airway open by preventing the trachea from collapsing during inspiration.

The trachea, located just anteriorly to the esophagus, extends from its junction with the larynx at the level of **C6** (6th cervical vertebra) downward to the level of **T4** or **T5** (4th or 5th thoracic vertebra) where it divides into right and left primary bronchi.

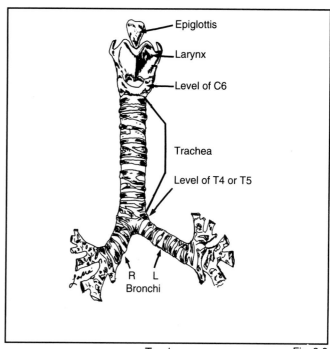

Trachea   Fig. 2-8

Radiographs

The AP and lateral radiographs of the upper airway visualize both the air-filled trachea and the esophagus also containing some air. Certain enlargements or other abnormalities of the thymus or thyroid glands may be demonstrated on such radiographs, as well as pathology within the airway system itself.

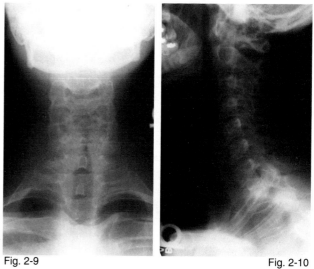

Fig. 2-9   Fig. 2-10
AP Upper Airway   Lateral Upper Airway

Cross Section of Trachea

Figure 2-11 is a CT image through the upper chest at the approximate level of T3. Observe again that the trachea is located anteriorly to the esophagus, both of which are anterior to the thoracic vertebrae. The upper lungs are located to each side of the trachea and the thoracic vertebrae.

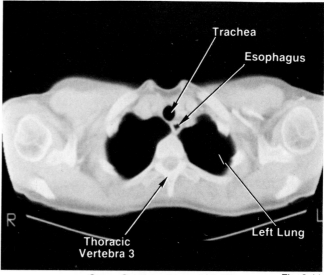

Cross Section at Level of T3   Fig. 2-11

3. Right and Left Bronchi

The third part of the respiratory system consists of the **right** and **left bronchi,** also known as the right and left primary or main stem bronchi.

The right bronchus is wider but shorter than the left bronchus. The angle of divergence from the distal trachea is also less abrupt for the right bronchus than for the left. This **difference in size and shape** between the two primary bronchi is important in radiology because food particles or other foreign matter which happens to enter the respiratory system is more likely to enter and lodge in the **right** bronchus.

The **right bronchus** is about 1 in. or 2.5 cm long and 1.3 cm in diameter. The angle of divergence of the right bronchus is only about 25°.

The **left bronchus** is smaller in diameter (1.1 cm) than the right but about twice as long (2 in. or 5 cm). The divergent angle of the left bronchus is approximately 37°. This increased angle and the smaller diameter make food particles or other foreign matter **less** likely to enter the left bronchus compared to the right.

The **carina** (kah-ri′nah) is a specific prominence or ridge of the lowest tracheal cartilage as seen at the bottom of the trachea where it divides into right and left bronchi. As viewed from above through a bronchoscope, the carina is to the left of the midline, and the right bronchus appears more open than the left, which clearly demonstrates why particles coming down the trachea are more likely to enter the right bronchus.

The position of the carina, as shown in *Fig. 2-12,* is at the lower level of the division into the right and left primary bronchi, This is used as a specific reference point or level for computed tomography (CT) of the thorax as described in Chapter 22.

Secondary Bronchi, Lobes and Alveoli

In addition to the difference in size and shape between the right and left bronchi, another important difference is that the **right** bronchus divides into **three** secondary bronchi, but the **left** divides into only **two** with each entering individual lobes of the lungs. Thus the **right lung** contains **three lobes** and the **left** contains **two lobes**, as demonstrated in both *Figs. 2-12* and *13*. These secondary bronchi continue to subdivide into smaller branches termed **bronchioles** that spread to all parts of each lobe.

Each of these small **terminal bronchioles** terminates or ends in very small air sacs or air spaces called **alveoli.** There are from 500 to 700 million of alveoli within the two lungs. It is here that oxygen and carbon dioxide are exchanged with the blood through the thin walls of the alveoli.

Cross Section of Bronchi and Lungs

Figure 2-14 demonstrates a CT image through the right and left primary or main stem bronchi at the approximate level of T7. This section is just below the termination of the trachea, thus the trachea is not shown but the air-filled right and left bronchi are visualized. Note that the left bronchus is longer but is smaller in diameter at its distal end than the right bronchus, as indicated by the arrows.

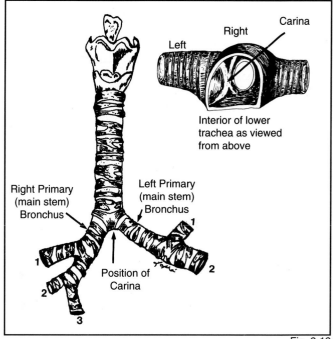

Bronchi   Fig. 2-12

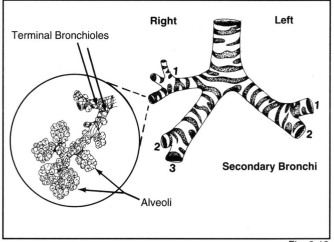

Secondary Bronchi and Alveoli   Fig. 2-13

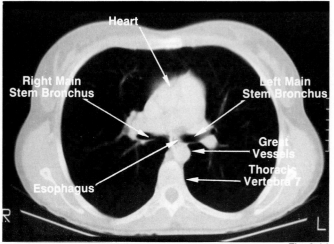

CT Image of Lungs and Heart   Fig. 2-14
(cross section at level of T7)

4. Lungs

The fourth and last division of the respiratory system is made up of the two large, spongy **lungs**, located on each side of the thoracic cavity. The lungs fill all of the space not occupied by other structures. It is important to remember that the right lung is made up of **three** lobes, the **upper** or **superior**, **middle**, and **lower** or **inferior** lobes, divided by **two deep fissures**. The left lung has only **two** lobes, the **upper** or **superior**, and **lower** or **inferior**, separated by a **single deep oblique fissure**.

The lungs are made up of a light spongy but highly elastic substance called **parenchyma**. This allows for the breathing mechanism which includes expansion and contraction of the lungs which brings oxygen in and removes the carbon dioxide from the blood through the thin walls of the alveoli.

Each lung is contained in a delicate double walled sac or membrane called the **pleura**. The double walled pleura completely surrounding the lung is visualized in both the frontal view drawing in *Fig. 2-15* and the cross-sectional drawing in *Fig. 2-16*. The outer layer of this pleural sac lines the inner surface of the chest wall and diaphragm and is called the **parietal pleura**. The inner layer covering the surface of the lungs, including dipping into the fissures between the lobes is called the **pulmonary** or **visceral pleura** (*Fig. 2-16*).

The potential space between the double walled pleura is called the **pleural cavity**. When a lung collapses or when air or fluid collects between these two layers then this space may be visualized radiographically. Air or gas present in this pleural cavity results in a condition called a **pneumothorax** wherein the air or gas pressure in the pleural cavity may cause the lung to collapse.

Cross Section of Lungs and Heart

The drawing in *Fig. 2-16* demonstrates a cross-sectional view through the lower third of the mediastinum and lungs (as viewed from the head, or top down). Clearly demonstrated is the double walled membrane, the **pleura** which completely encloses the lungs including around the heart. The outer membrane, the **parietal pleura** and the inner membrane, the **pulmonary** or **visceral pleura** are clearly visible as is the potential space between them, the **pleural cavity**.

The double walled **pericardial sac** which surrounds the heart is also identified. This drawing demonstrates the relationship of the pericardial sac surrounding the heart with the pleural sac surrounding the lungs. The pleural and pericardial spaces or cavities are exaggerated on this drawing to better demonstrate these parts. Normally there is no space between the double walls of the pericardial sac or between the parietal and visceral pleura unless pathology is present.

CT Cross Sectional Image

The CT image in *Fig. 2-17* also illustrates a sectional view of the lower thoracic cavity as viewed from the standard feet position, or bottom-up view. This level (9th thoracic vertebra) shows the relationship and relative size of the heart, descending aorta and lungs. The heart is located slightly more to the **left** as can also be seen on a PA chest radiograph. The heart is shown to be located in the very **anterior** portion of the chest cavity directly behind the sternum. The esophagus is directly posterior to the heart, with the descending aorta between the esophagus and the thoracic vertebrae.

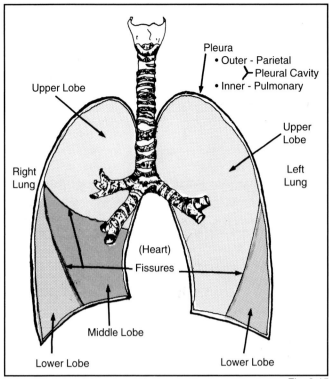

Lungs   Fig. 2-15

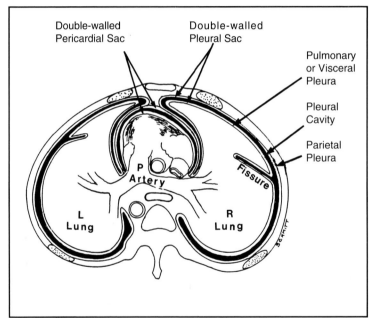

Cross Section of Lower Mediastinum and Lungs   Fig. 2-16

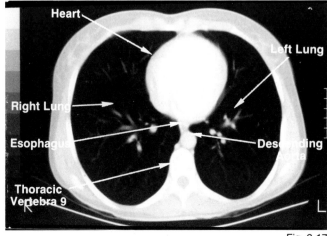

CT Image of Lower Thorax   Fig. 2-17
(level of T9)

Chest Radiograph

Enormous amounts of medical information can be obtained from a properly exposed and carefully positioned PA chest radiograph. Although the technical factors are designed to optimally visualize the lungs and other soft tissues, the bony thorax can also be seen. The clavicles, scapulae and ribs can be identified by carefully studying the chest radiograph in *Fig. 2-18*. The sternum and thoracic vertebrae are superimposed along with mediastinal structures such as the heart and great vessels; therefore, the sternum and vertebrae are not well visualized on a PA chest radiograph.

The lungs and trachea (enhanced by a dotted outline) of the respiratory system are well shown, although usually the bronchi are not easily seen. The first portion of the respiratory system, the larynx, is usually above the top border of the radiograph and cannot be seen. The heart, the large blood vessels and the diaphragm are also well visualized.

The parts labelled A-F on the radiograph are also demonstrated on the drawing in *Fig. 2-19*.

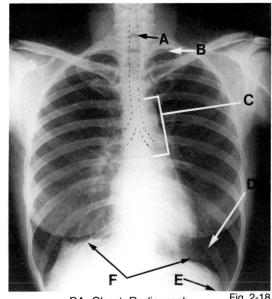

PA Chest Radiograph — Fig. 2-18

Parts of Lungs

Other parts of the lungs important radiographically are as follows:

The **hilum** (hilus) which is the central, wedge-shaped area of each lung where the bronchi, blood vessels, lymph vessels and nerves enter and leave the lungs.

The **apex** of each lung is that **rounded upper area above the level of the clavicles**. As can be seen in *Figs. 2-18* and *20*, the apices of the lungs extend well up into the lower neck area to the level of T1 (first thoracic vertebra). This important part of the lungs must be included on chest radiographs. The **base** of each lung is the lower concave area of each lung that rests on the **diaphragm**. The diaphragm is a muscular partition separating the thoracic and abdominal cavities.

The **costophrenic angle** refers to the extreme outermost corner of each lung where the diaphragm meets the ribs. In positioning for chest radiographs it is especially important to know the relative locations of the uppermost and lowermost parts of the lungs, namely the apices and the costophrenic angles respectively.

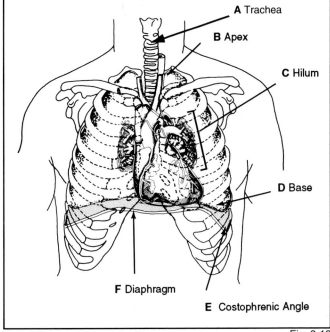

A Trachea
B Apex
C Hilum
D Base
E Costophrenic Angle
F Diaphragm

Lungs — Fig. 2-19

Lateral Chest View

The lateral chest radiograph in *Fig. 2-20* is marked to demonstrate the same parts as labelled in the adjoining drawing, *Fig. 2-21*. This drawing shows the left lung as seen from the medial aspect. Since this is the left lung, only two lobes are seen. Note that some of the lower lobe extends above the level of the hilum posteriorly, while some of the upper lobe extends below the hilum anteriorly. The posterior part of the diaphragm is the most inferior part of the diaphragm. The single deep **oblique fissure** dividing the two lobes of the left lung is again shown on this lateral view.

It is of significance, radiographically, to know that the right lung is usually about one inch shorter than the left lung. The reason for this difference is the large space-occupying liver located in the right upper abdomen which pushes up on the right **hemidiaphragm**. (The right half of the diaphragm is termed the right hemidiaphragm.) The right and left hemidiaphragms are seen on the lateral chest radiograph in *Fig. 2-20*. The more superior of the two is the right hemidiaphragm.

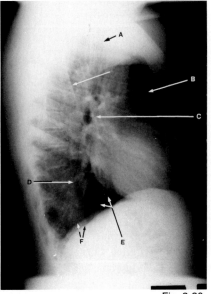

Fig. 2-20
Lateral Chest Radiograph

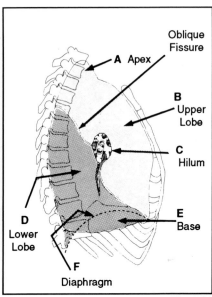

A Apex
Oblique Fissure
B Upper Lobe
C Hilum
D Lower Lobe
E Base
F Diaphragm

Fig. 2-21
Medial Left Lung

Chest

Mediastinum

The medial portion of the thoracic cavity between the lungs is called the **mediastinum**. Four structures that are radiographically important are located in the mediastinum: the **heart and great vessels**, the **trachea**, the **esophagus**, and the **thymus gland**.

Thymus Gland

The thymus gland, located behind the upper sternum, is said to be a temporary organ because it reaches its maximum size at puberty, then gradually decreases until it almost disappears in the adult. It may be visualized on chest radiographs of children but generally not for adults where the denser lymphatic tissue has been replaced by fat. At its maximum development the thymus gland lies above and anterior to the heart and pericardium.

Heart

The heart and the roots of the great vessels are enclosed in a double-walled sac called the **pericardial sac**. The heart is located posterior to the body of the sternum and anterior to the 5th to 8th thoracic vertebrae. It lies obliquely in the mediastinal space and approximately two-thirds of the heart lies to the left of the median plane.

Great Vessels

The great vessels in the mediastinum are the inferior and superior vena cava, aorta, and large pulmonary arteries and veins. The **superior vena cava** is a large vein which returns blood to the heart from the upper half of the body, as shown in *Figs. 2-22* and *23*. The **inferior vena cava**, also shown in *Fig. 2-23* is a large vein returning blood from the lower half of the body.

The **aorta** is the largest artery in the body, being about one inch in diameter in an average adult. It carries blood to all parts of the body through its various branches. The aorta is divided into three parts: the **ascending aorta**, coming up out of the heart, the **arch of the aorta**, and the **descending aorta**, which passes down through the diaphragm into the abdomen.

Various **pulmonary arteries and veins** which are present in the mediastinum are shown in *Figs. 2-23* and *24*. These supply blood and return blood to and from all segments of the lungs. The arterial network surrounds the small air sacs or alveoli, where oxygen and carbon dioxide are exchanged with the blood.

See **Chapter 23** Part I, Anatomy for Angiography, for more complete drawings of the heart and great vessels as part of the total body circulatory system including total body drawings of major arteries and veins.

Trachea and Esophagus

The trachea, within the mediastinum, separates into the **right and left primary and secondary bronchi**, as shown in *Fig. 2-23*.

The proximal esophagus is located **posterior to the trachea**, as shown in *Fig. 2-22*. The esophagus continues down through the mediastinum **anterior to the descending aorta** until it passes through the diaphragm into the stomach.

Note also in *Fig. 2-24* that the heart is located in the very **anterior** aspect of the thoracic cavity, directly behind the sternum.

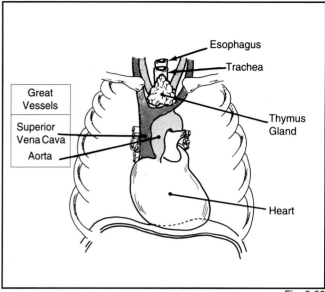

Structures within Mediastinum
(Anterior View)

Fig. 2-22

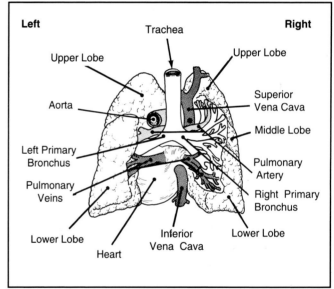

Lungs and Structure within Mediastinum
(Posterior View)

Fig. 2-23

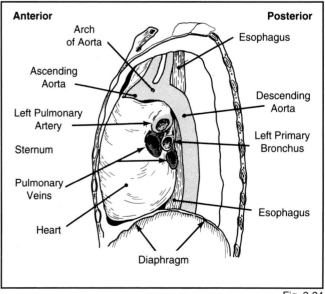

Mediastinal Relationships on
Left Side with Lung Removed

Fig. 2-24

2 Chest

Part II Radiographic Positioning

Body Habitus

The general form or shape of the body is termed **body habitus**. The four common body types are illustrated in *Fig. 2-25*. These different body shapes require special consideration in chest radiography. For example the massive built **hypersthenic**, representing only about 5% of the population, have a thorax which is very **broad** and very **deep** from front to back, but is **shallow** in vertical dimension as shown in *Figs. 2-26* and *27*. Therefore, care must be taken that the sides or the costophrenic angles are not cut off on a PA chest which must be taken with the film placed crosswise. Insure that the anterior or posterior margins are included on the lateral.

The other extreme is the very slender **asthenic** representing only about 10% of the population. Their thorax is **narrow** in width and **shallow** from front to back, but is very **long** in its vertical dimension. Therefore, in positioning for such a chest one must insure that the film is long enough to include both the upper apex areas which extend well above the clavicles, as well as the lower costophrenic angles. A thinner, hyposthenic type chest is shown in *Figs. 2-28* and *29*. Care in collimation for such patients must also be exercised so the costophrenic angles are not cut off on the lower margin.

Breathing Movements

Movements of the bony thorax during inspiration (taking air in) and expiration (expelling air) greatly change the dimensions of the thorax, and thus the thoracic volume. To increase the volume of the chest during inspiration, the thoracic cavity increases in diameter in **three dimensions**.

The first of these is the **vertical diameter**, which is increased primarily by the diaphragm contracting and lowering, thereby increasing the thoracic volume.

The **transverse diameter** is the second dimension increased during inspiration, occurring when the ribs swing outward and upward. This lateral movement increases the transverse diameter of the thorax.

The third dimension to be increased is the **anteroposterior diameter**, also increased during inspiration by the raising of the ribs, especially the second through the sixth ribs. During expiration the elastic recoil of the lungs, along with the weight of the thoracic walls, causes the three diameters of the thorax to return to normal.

Degree of Inspiration

To determine the degree of inspiration in chest radiography, one should be able to identify and count all twelve pairs of ribs on a chest radiograph. The first and second pairs are the most difficult to locate. When a chest radiograph is taken, it is important that the patient take as deep a breath as possible and then hold it to fully aerate the lungs.

The best way to determine the degree of inspiration is to observe how far down the diaphragm has moved by counting the pairs of ribs in the lung area above the diaphragm. A general rule for average adult patients is to "show" a **minimum** of ten ribs on a good PA chest radiograph. To determine this, start at the top with rib number one and count down to the tenth rib posteriorly. The posterior part of each rib, where it joins a thoracic vertebra, is the most superior part of the rib. The diaphragm should always be checked to see that it is below the level of the tenth rib, as shown on the radiograph in *Fig. 2-30*. (On this example, eleven posterior ribs are shown, which is what can be expected on most healthy patients.)

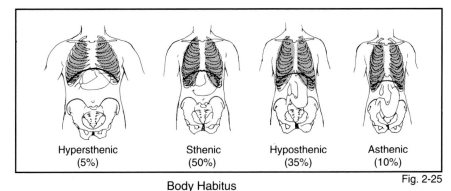

Body Habitus

| Hypersthenic (5%) | Sthenic (50%) | Hyposthenic (35%) | Asthenic (10%) |

Fig. 2-25

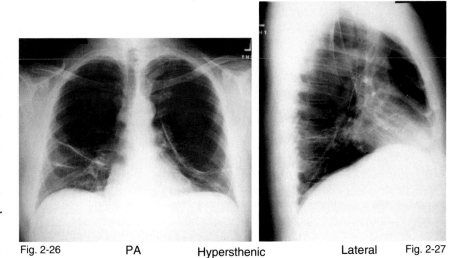

Fig. 2-26   PA   Hypersthenic   Lateral   Fig. 2-27

Fig. 2-28   PA   Hyposthenic   Lateral   Fig. 2-29

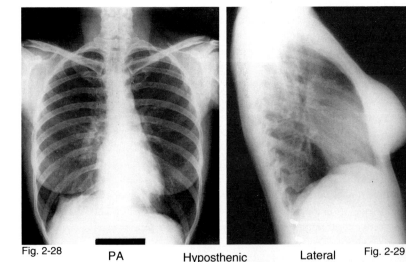

Posterior Ribs   Fig. 2-30

Patient Preparation

Patient preparation for chest radiography includes the removal of all opaque objects from the chest and neck regions, including clothes with buttons, snaps, hooks or any objects that would be visualized on the radiograph as a shadow. To insure that all such objects are removed from the chest region, the usual procedure is to ask the patient to remove all clothing, including bras, along with necklaces or other objects around the neck. The patient then puts on a hospital gown with the opening in the back.

Long hair braided or tied together in bunches with rubber bands or other fasteners may cause suspicious shadows on the radiograph if it is left superimposing the chest area. Oxygen lines or pacemaker wires should be carefully moved to the side of the chest if possible.

Radiation Protection

Patients should be protected from unnecessary radiation for all diagnostic radiographic examinations. This is especially true for chest radiography because these are the most common of all radiographic examinations and are done repeatedly on persons throughout their lifetime.

Repeat Exposures: Even though chest radiographic exams are often considered the simplest of all radiographic procedures, they are also the exam with the highest number of repeats in many radiology departments. Therefore, it is important to minimize unnecessary radiation exposure from repeat exposures by taking extra care in positioning and in the selection of correct exposure factors. It is also important to reduce patient dose as much as possible through the use of correct radiation protection practices by way of close collimation and gonadal shielding.

Collimation: Careful collimation is important in chest radiography. Restricting the primary x-ray beam by collimation not only reduces patient dose by reducing the volume of tissue irradiated, but also reduces patient exposure by the accompanying reduction in scatter radiation.

Utilizing the collimation guidelines as described on the following positioning pages will allow for consistent optimum chest collimation.

Gonadal Shielding: In addition to careful collimation, a leaded gonadal shield should be used for the abdominal area below the lungs. This is especially important for children, pregnant women and for all those of child-bearing age. A minimal rule is that **gonadal shielding should be used on all patients of reproductive age.** Many departments however, have a general policy of gonadal shielding for all patients in chest radiography.

A common type of gonadal shield for chest radiography is the apron type vinyl-covered lead shield with ties by which the shield can be tied around the waist. This should provide shielding from the level of the iliac crests or slightly higher, to the mid-thigh area.

Other types of free standing adjustable mobile shields may also be used for this purpose.

Back Scatter Protection: To protect the gonads from scatter and secondary radiation from the chest film holder device and the wall behind it, some references suggest a free standing shield or a wrap around shield also be placed **between the patient and the chest board and wall.**

Technical Factors

Kilovoltage (kVp): Generally kVp should be high enough to result in sufficient contrast to demonstrate the many shades of gray needed to visualize the finer lung markings. Thus in general, chest radiography uses **low contrast**, described as a **long scale contrast** with more shades of gray. This requires high kVp of 100 to 125.

Lower kVp, yielding high contrast, will not provide sufficient penetration to visualize well the fine lung markings in the areas behind the heart and at the lung bases. Too high contrast is evident when the heart and other mediastinal structures appear underexposed even though the lung fields are sufficiently penetrated.

Patients with less dense, expanded lungs such as with emphysema or hyper expanded lungs will require a decrease in kVp or other exposure factors.

As a general rule in chest radiography, the use of high kVp (above 100) requires the use of grids. Either moving grids or fine line focused fixed grids can be used.

Exceptions to this are some portable chests taken with equipment that is limited to 80-90 kVp, where screens may be used rather than grids.

Exposure Time and Milliamperage (mAs - milliampere seconds): Generally chest radiography requires the use of high mA and short exposure times to minimize the chance of motion and resultant loss of sharpness.

Sufficient mAs should be used to provide for optimum density of lungs and mediastinal structures. A determining factor for this on PA chest radiographs is to be able to **see faint outlines of at least the mid and upper vertebrae and posterior ribs through the heart and other mediastinal structure shadows.**

Placement of Film Markers: Throughout the positioning sections of this text, the correct or best placement of patient ID information and film markers is indicated. The top portion of each positioning page includes a box drawing demonstrating the correct film holder size and placement (lengthwise or crosswise), and indicates the best location for patient ID, as well as the location and type of film marker used for that specific projection or position. The use of a grid or screen film holder is indicated along with a suggested kVp range.

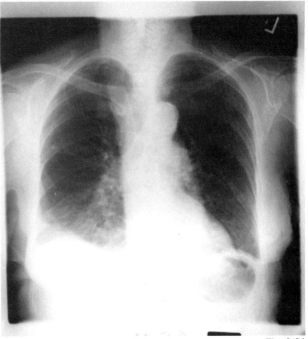

PA Chest
(with correct collimation, exposure and film markers)

Fig. 2-31

Breathing Instructions

Breathing instructions are very important in chest radiography because any chest or lung movement occurring during the exposure will result in "blurring" of the radiographic image. It is also imperative that chest radiographs be taken on **full** inspiration to demonstrate the lungs as they appear fully expanded. However, the full inspiration should not be forced to the point of strain, causing unsteadiness. This needs to be explained to the patient prior to the exposure as the patient is being positioned.

Also, more air can be inhaled without too much strain on the **second** breath compared to the first. Therefore, the patient should be asked to **hold the second full breath** rather than the first. It may be necessary to practice this breathing procedure with the patient before actually making the exposure.

Inspiration and Expiration

Occasionally there are exceptions to taking chest radiographs on full inspiration only. For certain conditions comparison radiographs are taken on both full inspiration and full expiration. Indications for this are a possible small pneumothorax (air or gas in the pleural cavity), fixation or lack of normal movement of the diaphragm, the presence of a foreign body, or to distinguish between an opacity in the rib or in the lung. When such comparison radiographs are taken, they should be labelled "inspiration" and "expiration". Note the pnuemothorax of the upper right lung demonstrated in the chest radiograph in *Fig. 2-33* (see arrows). This is not evident on the inspiration radiograph of the same patient taken at the same time in *Fig. 2-32*.

Erect Chest Radiographs

All chest radiographs should be taken in an erect position if the patient's condition allows. Three reasons for this are as follows:

1. To allow the diaphragm to move down farther.
   An erect position causes the liver and other abdominal organs to drop, allowing the diaphragm to move farther down on full inspiration, thus allowing the lungs to fully aerate.

2. To show possible air and fluid levels in the chest.
   If both air and fluid are present within a lung or within the pleural space, the heavier fluid, such as blood or serum, will gravitate to the lowest position, while the air will rise. In the recumbent position, a pleural effusion will spread out over the posterior surface of the lung, resulting in a hazy appearance of the entire lung. In the upright position, fluid will locate near the base of the lung. The erect chest radiograph (Fig. 2-34) shows excess fluid in the left lower thoracic cavity. The supine radiograph (Fig. 2-35) shows a generalized hazy appearance of the entire right lung.

3. To prevent engorgement and hyperemia of pulmonary vessels.
   The term engorgement literally means "distended or swollen with fluid".[1] Hyperemia refers to an excess of blood in a part due to a relaxation of the distal small blood vessels or arterioles.

   An erect position in general, tends to minimize engorgement and hyperemia of pulmonary vessels which can change the appearance of these vessels.

Seventy-Two inch (180 cm) SID

Chest radiographs taken at a minimum 40 in. (102 cm) rather than 72 in. (180 cm) will cause increased magnification of the heart shadow which

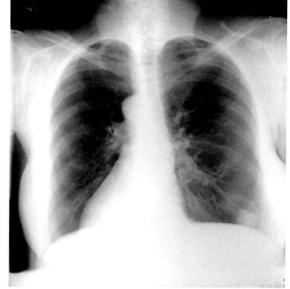

Inspiration   Fig. 2-32
(Courtesy of Llori Lundh)

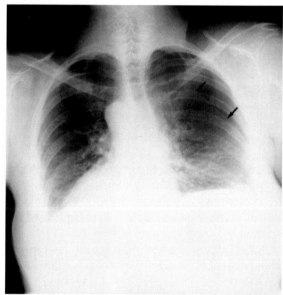

Expiration   Fig. 2-33
(Courtesy of Llori Lundh)

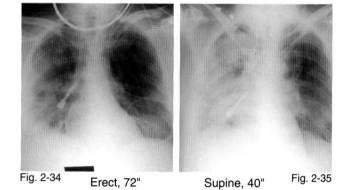

Fig. 2-34   Erect, 72"   Supine, 40"   Fig. 2-35

complicates the diagnosis of possible cardiac enlargement. The reason for this is greater magnification due to increased divergence or angle of the x-ray beam at a shorter SID as described in Chapter One. A longer SID, such as 72 in. or 180 cm, results in the use of a straighter or less divergent x-ray beam resulting in less magnification.

---

[1] Dorland's Medical Dictionary, 24th edition.

Evaluation Criteria

The description for each chest projection or position in this chapter includes an evaluation criteria section. In this section specific criteria are listed and described by which one can evaluate the resultant radiograph. The goal of every radiographer should be to take the "optimal" radiograph. These evaluation criteria provide **a definable standard** by which every chest radiograph can be evaluated to determine where improvements can be made.

Certain important evaluation criteria related to positioning which are common to all routine PA and lateral chest radiographs are as follows:

PA Chest Positioning

1. True PA, no rotation: Even a slight amount of rotation on a PA chest projection will result in distortion of size and shape of the heart shadow since the heart is located anteriorly in the thorax. Therefore, it is important that there be **NO** rotation. To prevent rotation insure that the patient is standing evenly on both feet with both shoulders rolled forward and downward. Also, check the posterior aspect of the shoulders, as well as the lower posterior rib cage and the pelvis to insure no rotation. Scoliosis or curvature of the thoracic spine makes it more difficult to prevent rotation and extra care is required to avoid rotation for such patients.

Rotation on chest radiographs can be determined two ways. First, by the overall symmetrical appearance of the thorax as determined by **the distance from the mid-vertebral column to the lateral borders of the ribs** on each side. (See *Figs. 2-36* and *37*.)

A second method of determining rotation is by carefully examining both sternoclavicular joints for symmetrical appearance in relationship to the spine. On a true PA chest without any rotation, both the **right and left sternoclavicular joints will be the same distance from the spine.** (Note the rotation as evident by distance between the sternoclavicular joint spaces and the center of the spinal column.) This becomes more obvious on the enlargement of the sternoclavicular area in *Fig. 2-38*.

2. Extending the chin: Sufficiently extending the patient's chin will insure that the chin and neck are not covering up or superimposing the uppermost lung regions, the apices of the lungs. This is demonstrated by the two radiographs in *Figs. 2-39* and *40*. Also, be sure the upper collimation border is high enough so the apices are not cut off.

3. Minimizing breast shadows: For those patients with large pendulous breasts, the patient should be asked to lift them up and outward, then remove hands as they lean against the film holder to keep them in this position. This will lessen the effect of breast shadows over the lower lung fields. Remember, however, that depending on the size and density of the breasts, breast shadows over the lung fields cannot be totally eliminated *(Fig. 2-41)*.

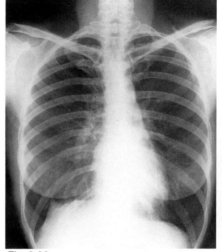
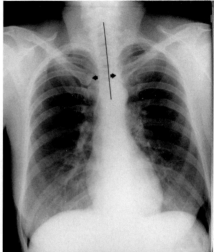

Fig. 2-36   Without Rotation   With Rotation   Fig. 2-37

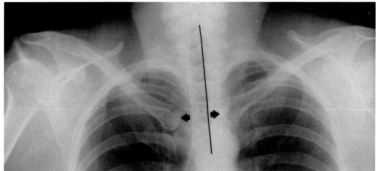

Closeup, With Rotation   Fig. 2-38

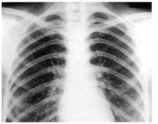

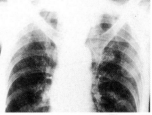

Fig. 2-39   Chin Up   Chin Down   Fig. 2-40

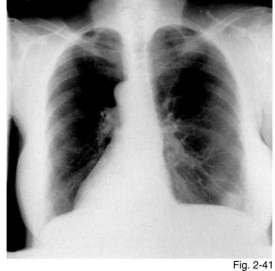

Fig. 2-41

Breast Shadows Evident

Radiographic Positioning continued

Lateral Chest Positioning

1. Side closest to the film: The patient's side closest to the film is best demonstrated on the finished radiograph. A left lateral should be done unless departmental protocol indicates otherwise. A left lateral will better demonstrate the heart region because the heart is located primarily in the left thoracic cavity.

2. True lateral, NO rotation or tilt: Insure that the patient is standing straight with weight evenly distributed on both feet with arms raised. As a check against rotation, confirm that the posterior surfaces of the thorax are directly superimposed as viewed from the position of the x-ray tube. Due to the divergent x-ray beam, this requires that the side farthest from the film needs to be **rotated slightly anteriorly**, especially on wide, broad-shouldered patients. This is necessary so that the posterior surfaces of the right and left aspects of the thorax are **directly superimposed, as viewed from the x-ray tube**, considering the divergent x-ray beam. An accurate collimation light skimming the posterior surfaces of both the right and left halves of the thorax can also be used to determine the amount of anterior rotation needed.

Possible rotation on a lateral chest radiograph can then be determined by viewing the posterior ribs. The right and left ribs will be directly superimposed on a true lateral as demonstrated in *Fig. 2-42*, compared to *Fig. 2-43* with rotation.

A second way to detect rotation is to determine how nearly the hemidiaphragms and costophrenic angles are superimposed. On a true lateral with no rotation the costophrenic angles will be directly superimposed and appear as one *(Fig. 2-42)*.

There should also be **no tilt. The midsagittal plane must be parallel to the film.** This means that if the patient's shoulders are firmly against the film holder, the lower lateral thorax and/or hips may be an inch or two away. This is especially true on broad shouldered patients.

Tilt is also detected on the radiograph by lack of superimposition of costrophrenic angles.

3. Arms raised high: Insure that the patient raises both arms sufficiently high to prevent superimposition on the chest field. Patients who are weak or unstable may need to grasp a support *(Fig. 2-44)*.

When the patient's arms are not raised sufficiently, the soft tissues of the upper arm will superimpose portions of the lung field as demonstrated in *Fig. 2-45*. (Arrows demonstrate margins of soft tissues of the arms overlying upper lung fields.)

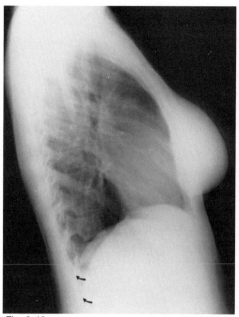

Fig. 2-42   Without Rotation

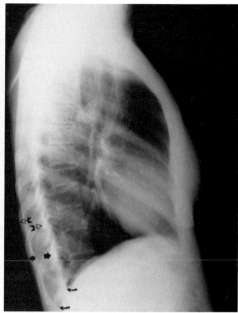

With Rotation   Fig. 2-43

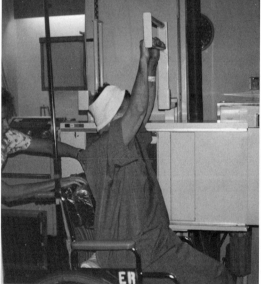

Arms Raised High   Fig. 2-44

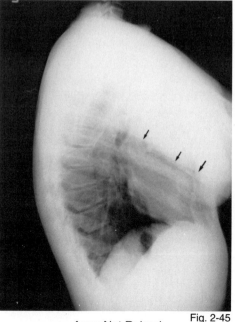

Arms Not Raised   Fig. 2-45

Central Ray Location

Traditional Top-of-Shoulder, CR to Center of Film Method (Not recommended)

Traditionally the top of the shoulder and the exterior borders of the thorax have been used as positioning landmarks for chest radiography. This method which usually includes placing the top of the cassette about 2 in. above the shoulder and centering the CR to the center of the film may be a good method for centering the lungs to a full 14 x 17 in. (35 x 43 cm) film on an average male adult with a typical sthenic body habitus *(Fig. 2-46)*. However, this positioning method is inconsistent considering variations in lung field dimensions due to differences in body habitus, as well as differences in overall size of patients as demonstrated by comparing *Figs. 2-46* and *47*. The center of the lungs is shown to be near the center of the film for this male, but is near the upper third of the film on this older female. Therefore the CR obviously was **not** centered to the lungs in *Fig. 2-47*, which also resulted in inaccurate collimation. Variables such as spinal curvature (kyphosis) on older patients, obesity, and muscular build all indicate the need for a chest positioning method which **consistently centers the central ray to the center of the lung fields with accurate collimation on both top and bottom.**

Central Ray Location Method (Recommended)

As described in Chapter 1, accurate central ray location to the center of the anatomical part being radiographed is important to prevent distortion of anatomical parts and for consistent exposures by phototiming devices. This is especially true for chest radiographs.

Bony topographical landmarks are consistent and reliable as a means of determining CR locations. Two such specific landmarks for locating the center of the lung fields are as follows:

1. Vertebra Prominens (PA Chest): The vertebra prominens is the long sloping spinous process of C7 which corresponds to the level of the first thoracic vertebra and to the uppermost margin of the apex of the lungs. This topographical landmark, which can be readily palpated on most patients at the base of the neck, is the preferred landmark for location of the CR

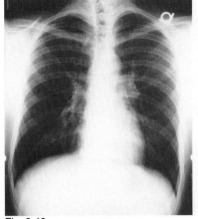
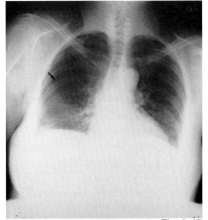

Fig. 2-46   Average Male   **PA Chest**   Small Female   Fig. 2-47
(Correct CR and Collimation)   **(Incorrect** CR and Collimation)

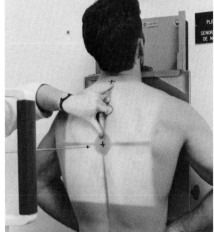
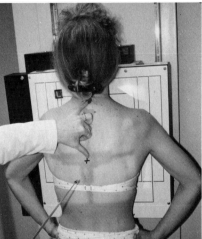

Fig. 2-48   Correct CR Utilizing Vertebra Prominens   Fig. 2-49

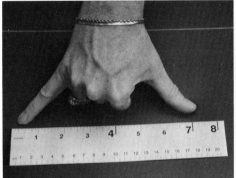
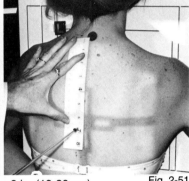

Fig. 2-50   Hand Spread Method - 7 or 8 in. (18-20 cm)   Fig. 2-51

on a PA chest as shown in *Fig. 2-48* and *2-49*. For the average female this is down about 7 in. (18 cm), and for the male is about 8 in. (20 cm).

One way of determining this distance is by an average hand spread as shown. Most hands can reach the 7 inches, and the 8 inches can be determined by estimating an additional inch. If the hand spread method is used, one should practice with a ruler to **consistently determine these distances** (see *Fig. 2-50*).

Another preferred method is to use a cardboard guide or other simple ruler type device placed against the patient's back that is readily available and easy to use as shown in *Fig. 2-51*.

These variations between male and female are true for the general population with crossover exceptions wherein certain larger athletic type females may also have larger lung fields and some males smaller lungs. However, for purposes of chest positioning for the general population, these average measurements of **7 inches for a female** and **8 inches for a male** can be used as reliable guidelines.

NOTE: Appendix A at the end of this chapter describes a study which determined that the center of the lung field on **80 - 85 %** of adults is at the **mid 7th** thoracic vertebra. For **15 - 20 %** of larger athletic types the central point of the lungs are at the **T7- T8 interspace**, and on a few at the **mid 8th** thoracic vertebra.

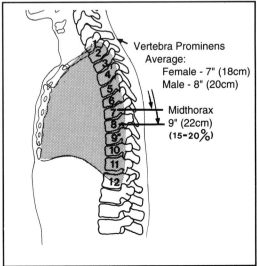

Vertebra Prominens
Average:
    Female - 7" (18cm)
    Male - 8" (20cm)

Midthorax
9" (22cm)
(15-20%)

Fig 2-52
Topographical Landmarks for PA Chest

Central Ray Location continued

2. Jugular Notch (AP Chest): The easily palpated jugular notch anteriorly is the recommended landmark for location of the CR for AP chest radiographs. The level of T 7 on an average adult is 3 to 4 in. (8-10 cm) below the jugular notch. For most older patients this will be approximately **3 in. (8 cm)**. For younger and/or athletic types this will be nearer **4, or even 5 in. (10-12 cm)**.

This distance can also be determined by the radiographer's hand spread. The average sized hand placed flat with the fingers together is approximately 3 in. (8 cm). See *Fig. 2-54*.

Lung Dimensions and Film Holder Placement

PA or AP chest radiographs are most commonly taken with the cassette film holder placed lengthwise. However, contrary to common belief, **the width or horizontal dimension of the average PA or AP chest is greater than the vertical dimension.** (See Appendix A at the end of this chapter.)

The study described in appendix A also shows that the width or horizontal dimension on a PA or AP chest is **greater than 13 in.** (33 cm) on **15 to 20%** of patients. This requires that the 14 x 17 in. (35x43 cm) film holder be placed **crosswise** so as not to cut off lateral lung margins on these patients.

PA Chest: Most erect PA chests are done with dedicated chest units which may not allow for this crosswise placement of the film. However, cassettes with portable stationary grids can be used (placed crosswise) for this purpose.

As the patient faces the chest film holder, one can determine the potential need to place the film crosswise on larger patients by standing behind the patient and placing your hands squarely on each side of the chest. **If there is any doubt that both sides of the chest can be included, the film holder should be placed crosswise remembering that the height of the average lungs is less than the width.**

AP Chest: For AP chest radiographs (usually taken at less than 72 in. or 180 cm with an accompanying increase in divergence of the x-ray beam) the chance of the side borders of the lungs being cut off increases if the film is placed lengthwise. Therefore, **it is recommended that for AP chest radiographs the 14 x 17 in. (35x43 cm) film be placed crosswise,** with the **film and CR centered to a point 3 to 4 in. (8-10 cm) below the jugular notch** *(Fig. 2-54)*.

Collimation Guidelines

First center the CR to the level of T7, then adjust the collimation borders. **Side collimation borders** can easily be determined by **adjusting the illuminated field margins to the outer skin margins** on each side of the posterior chest surface (remembering that lungs expand during deep inspiration). The upper and lower collimation borders, however, are more difficult to determine because these lung margins are not visible externally.

A reliable method for upper and lower chest collimation is to **adjust the upper border of the illuminated light field to the vertebra prominens,** which with the divergent rays will result in an upper collimation margin on the film of about 1.5 in. or 4 cm above the vertebra prominens *(Figs. 2-55 and 56)*. This will then also result in a lower collimation border of 1.5 in. (4 cm) below the costophrenic angles, if the CR was correctly centered. The 1.5 in. or 4 cm allowance above and below the lungs allows for some margin of error in CR placement without cutting off upper or lower lungs.

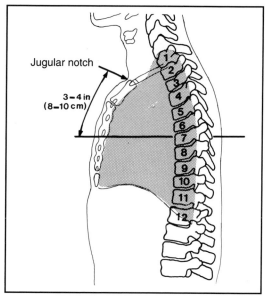

Topographical Landmark for AP Chest   Fig. 2-53

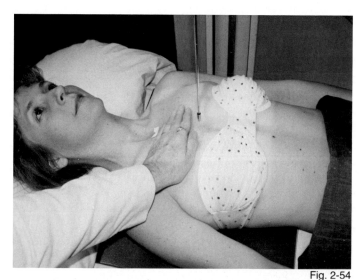

Fig. 2-54
Film Crosswise, CR 3-4 in. (8-11cm) Below Jugular Notch

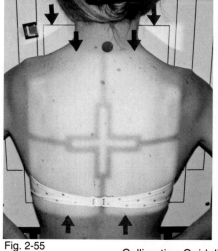
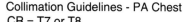

Fig. 2-55

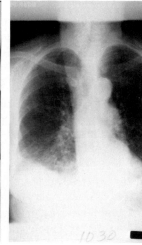

Fig. 2-56

Collimation Guidelines - PA Chest
CR = T7 or T8
Sides = outer skin margins
Upper = level of vertebra prominens

Standard and Optional Operating Procedures

Certain basic and optional projections or positions for the chest are demonstrated and described on the following pages as suggested standard and optional departmental procedures.

Basic Projections

Standard or basic projections, also sometimes referred to as routine projections or departmental routines are **those projections or positions commonly taken on average patients who are helpful and can cooperate in performing the procedure.**

Optional Projections

Optional projections are **those more common projections or positions taken as extra or additional projections to better demonstrate certain pathologic conditions or specific body parts.** (This does not mean they are optional as to whether or not they are important, or whether or not they need to be learned and mastered.)

National Survey

Departmental standard and optional operating procedures (departmental routines) for the chest are very consistent throughout the United States. This was determined by the results of a national survey completed to determine national norms for standard and optional radiographic operating procedures for the chest and upper airway.

Chest Routine

Chest	U.S. Average (538)	
	Basic	Optional
PA	99%	
Lateral	99%	
AP supine		82%
Decub		70%
AP lordotic		38%
Obliques		30%

Upper Airway Routine

Upper Airway	U.S. Average (485)	
	Basic	Optional
Lateral	99%	
AP	75%	

Summary

Chest: These results indicate that **99%** of all departments throughout the United States responding to the survey for radiographic procedures of the chest include the **PA** projection and the **lateral** position as standard or routine.

This survey also indicates that according to the frequency indicated in the survey for optional projections or positions, **82%** do the **AP supine, 70%** the **decubitus, 38%** the **AP lordotic** and **30%** the **obliques**. Therefore, each of these are described and demonstrated in this chapter.

Upper Airway: For the upper airway to demonstrate the air-filled larynx and trachea as well as the region of the thyroid and thymus glands, the survey results indicate that 95% of all departments include the lateral position as routine or standard and 75% include the AP projection. No common optional projections for this procedure were indicated.

Basic and Optional Routines

| Chest
Basic
• PA
• Lateral |

| Chest (Optional)
• AP supine or semi-erect
• Lateral decubitus
• AP lordotic
• Obliques |

| Upper Airway
Basic
• Lateral
• AP |

Chest

• PA Projection
(Ambulatory patient)

Chest
Basic
• **PA**
• Lateral

Structures Best Shown:
Lungs, including both apices, air-filled trachea, bronchi, heart and great vessels, diaphragm to include costophrenic angles, and bony thorax.

Technical Factors:
• Film Size - 14 x 17 in. (35 x 43 cm), lengthwise or crosswise (see NOTE).
• Moving or stationary grid.
• 110-125 kVp range.

Shielding: Secure lead shield around waist or use an adjustable mobile shield to protect gonads.

Patient Position:
• Patient erect, feet spread slightly, weight equally distributed on both feet.
• Chin raised, resting against film holder.
• Hands on lower hips, palms out, elbows partially flexed.
• Shoulders rotated forward against film holder to allow scapulae to move laterally clear of lung fields. Also depress shoulders downward to move clavicles below the apices.
• See page 61 for positioning women with large pendulous breasts.

Part Position:
• Align midsagittal plane to midline of film holder with equal margins between lateral thorax and sides of film holder.
• Insure **no rotation** of thorax.

Central Ray:
• CR **perpendicular** to the film and centered to the **midsagittal plane at the level of T7** (7-8 in. or 18-20 cm below vertebra prominens).
• Center cassette to CR.
• 72 in. (180 cm) SID.

Collimation: Collimate on four sides to area of lung fields. (Top border of illuminated field should be to level of vertebra prominens, and lateral borders to outer skin margins.)

Respiration: Exposure made at end of 2nd full inspiration.

NOTE: Place cassette crosswise for larger or hypersthenic type patients. See page 64 for further explanations.

Evaluation Criteria:
• **No rotation**, both sternoclavicular joints should be the same distance from the vertebral column; the distance from the lateral borders of the ribs to the vertebral column should be the same on each side, from the upper to the lower rib cage.
• Scapulae should not superimpose the lungs if shoulders are rotated forward sufficiently.
• Collimation margins should appear on four sides on smaller patients. The center of the collimation field should be to area of T7 on average patients.
• Entire lungs should be included on film, superior apices to the lower costophrenic angles.
• Larger breast shadows should primarily be lateral to lung fields, with correct placement during positioning.
• **Full inspiration** should result in a minimum of 10 posterior ribs visualized above diaphragm.
• **No motion** should result in sharp outlines of diaphragm and heart borders.

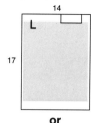
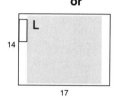

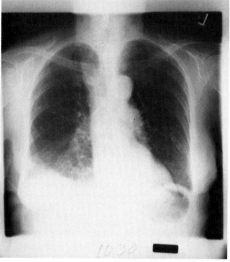

PA Chest   Fig. 2-57

PA Chest   Fig. 2-58

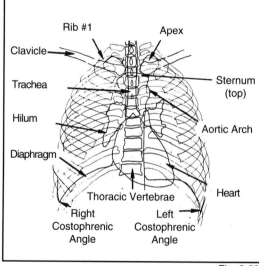

PA Chest   Fig. 2-59

• Optimum exposure and sufficient long contrast scale should visualize the fine vascular lung markings throughout lungs. **Faint outlines should be visible of at least the mid and upper thoracic vertebrae and posterior ribs through the heart and mediastinal structure shadows.**
• Patient ID should be clear and legible; and correctly placed R or L marker should be visible without superimposing lung area.

• PA Projection
(with cart or stretcher if patient cannot stand)

<table>
<tr><td>

Chest
Basic
• **PA**
• Lateral

</td></tr>
</table>

Structures Best Shown:
Lungs, including both apices, air-filled trachea, heart and great vessels, diaphragm to include costophrenic angles, and bony thorax.

Technical Factors:
• Film Size - 14 x 17 in. (35 x 43 cm) lengthwise or crosswise.
• Moving or stationary grid.
• 110 - 125 kVp range.

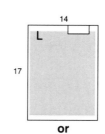

or

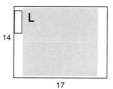

Shielding: Secure lead shield around waist to shield gonads.

Patient Position:
• Patient erect, seated on cart, legs over the edge.
• Arms around cassette unless a chest film holder is used, then position as for an ambulatory patient.
• Shoulders rotated forward and downward.
• **No** rotation of thorax.

Part Position:
• Adjust the height of film holder so top of cassette is about 2 in. (5 cm) above top of shoulders.
• If portable cassette is used because patient cannot be placed up against chest board, place pillow or padding on lap to raise and support cassette as shown, but keep cassette against chest for minimum OID *(Fig. 2-61)*.

Central Ray:
• CR **perpendicular** to the film and centered to the **midsagittal plane at the level of T7**, (7-8 in. or 18-20 cm below vertebra prominens).
• Center cassette to level of CR.
• 72 in. (180 cm) SID.

Collimation: Collimate to area of lung fields. (Upper border of illuminated field should be to level of vertebra prominens, which with divergent rays will result in upper collimation border on film of about 1.5 in. or 4 cm above apex of lungs.)

Respiration: Make exposure upon **2ⁿᵈ full inspiration.**

NOTE: Insure that patient is stable and will not waver or move during exposure.

Evaluation Criteria:
• Radiograph should appear similar to ambulatory PA chest as described on preceding page.

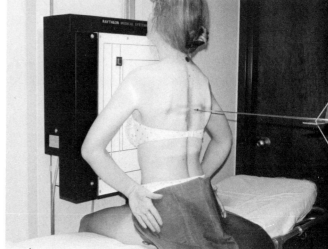

PA Chest
(Patient Against Chestboard)   Fig. 2-60

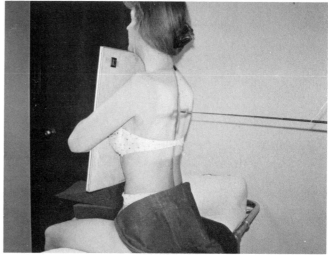

PA Chest
(Patient Holding Cassette)   Fig. 2-61

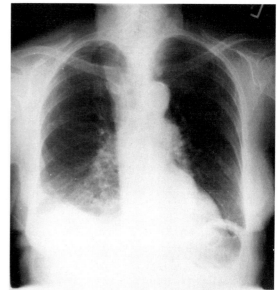

PA Chest   Fig. 2-62

Chest
Basic
• PA
• **Lateral**

• Lateral Position
(Ambulatory patient)

Structures Best Shown:
Lungs, trachea, heart and great vessels, diaphragm to include posterior costophrenic angles, and bony thorax.

Technical Factors:
• Film Size - 14 x 17 in. (35 x 43 cm), lengthwise.
• Moving or stationary grid.
• 110 - 125 kVp.

Shielding: Secure lead shield around waist or use mobile lead shield to protect gonads.

Patient Position:
• Patient erect, left side against film (unless patient's complaint is on right side, then do a right lateral if departmental protocol includes this option).
• Weight evenly distributed on both feet.
• Raise arms above head.
• Keep chin up.

Part Position:
• Center patient to film by checking anterior and posterior aspects of thorax.
• Position in a **true lateral** position (check posterior thorax from position of x-ray tube to determine the amount of **anterior rotation** needed, due to the divergent CR (see pg.62).

Central Ray:
• CR **perpendicular** to and directed to level of **T 7** (3-4 in. or 8-10 cm below level of jugular notch). Top of cassette should be about 1 in. or 2.5 cm above level of shoulders.
• 72 in. (180 cm) SID.

Collimation: Collimate on four sides to area of lung fields (top border of light field to level of vertebra prominens).

Respiration: Exposure made at end of **2ⁿᵈ full inspiration**.

NOTE: • Insure that midsagittal plane is **parallel to film**, which for slender but broader shouldered patients will result in hips and lower thorax **not** being against film holder. This increase in OID of the lower chest will result in the costophrenic angles of the lungs being projected lower due to the divergence of the x-ray beam. Therefore, the film holder needs to be lowered a **minimum** of 1 in. or 2 cm on this type of patient with this increase in OID of the lower chest to prevent cut-off of costophrenic angles.
• If patient is weak and unsteady, take lateral on cart or in wheel chair as shown on following page.

Evaluation Criteria:
• **No rotation**, ribs posterior to vertebral column should be directly superimposed; costophrenic angles should be aligned and superimposed.
• Chin and arms should be elevated sufficiently to prevent excessive soft tissues from superimposing apices.
• Image should include lung apices at the top and costophrenic angles on the lower margin of the film.
• Collimation margins should appear on all four sides, on smaller patients. The center of the collimation field should be at the level of T 7 on average patients.
• The hilum region should be in the approximate center of the film.
• **NO motion**, should be evidenced by sharp outlines of the diaphragm and lung markings.
• Should have sufficient exposure and long scale contrast to **visualize lung markings through the heart shadow and upper lung areas**, without over-exposing other regions of the lungs.

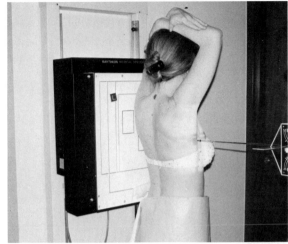
Lateral Chest   Fig. 2-63

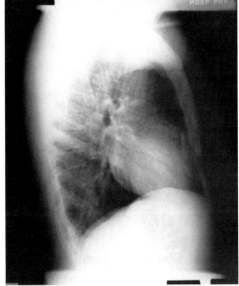
Lateral Chest   Fig. 2-64

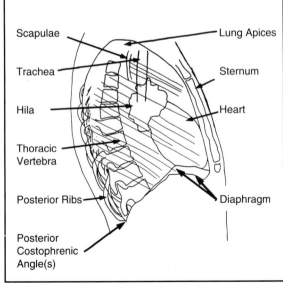
Lateral Chest   Fig. 2-65

Labels: Scapulae, Trachea, Hila, Thoracic Vertebra, Posterior Ribs, Posterior Costophrenic Angle(s), Lung Apices, Sternum, Heart, Diaphragm

• Patient ID should be clear and legible, with correctly placed R or L marker visible without superimposing lung area.

• Lateral Position
(with a wheel chair or cart, if patient cannot stand)

Chest
Basic
• PA
• **Lateral**

Structures Best Shown:
Lungs, trachea, heart and great vessels, diaphragm including posterior costophrenic angles, and bony thorax.

Technical Factors:
• Film Size - 14 x 17 in. (35 x 43 cm), lengthwise.
• Moving or stationary grid.
• 110 - 125 kVp.

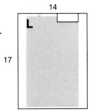

Shielding: Secure lead shielding around waist to protect gonads.

Patient Position on Cart:
• Patient seated on cart; legs over the edge if this is easier for patient (insure that cart does not move).
• Arms crossed above head, or hold on to arm support as shown.
• Keep chin up.

Patient Position in Wheelchair:
• Place pillow or other support under smaller patients so arm rests of wheel chair do not superimpose lungs.
• Turn patient in wheel chair to lateral position as close to film holder as possible.
• Have patient lean forward and place support blocks behind back; raise arms above head and hold on to support bar - **keep arms high.**
• Keep chin up.

Part Position:
• Center patient to film by checking anterior and posterior aspects of thorax.
• Insure **NO** rotation by viewing patient from tube position.

Central Ray:
• CR **perpendicular** to and directed to level of **T7**. (3-4 in. or 8-10 cm below to level of jugular notch.)
• 72 in. (180 cm) SID.
• Center cassette to level of CR. (Top of cassette should be about 1 in. (2.5 cm) above shoulders.)

Collimation: Collimate on four sides to area of lung fields.

Respiration: Exposure made at end of **2nd full inspiration.**

NOTE: • If patient comes to the department in a wheel chair but is too weak or unsteady to stand erect, then take lateral with patient remaining seated in wheel chair. Place support behind back with arms raised and holding onto support bar as shown in *Fig. 2-67.*
• Always attempt to have patient sit completely erect on cart if possible *(Fig. 2-66)*. However, if patient is in a condition that does not allow this, the head end of the cart can be raised to as near an erect position as possible using a radiolucent support behind back *(Fig. 2-68)*. Attempts should be made however, to get patient in as near an erect position as possible.

Evaluation Criteria:
Radiograph should appear similar to ambulatory lateral position as described under evaluation criteria on preceding page.

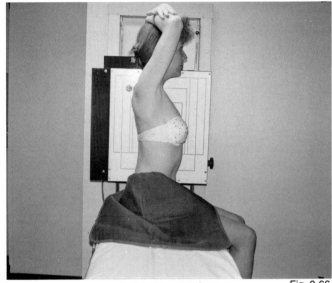

Left Lateral on Cart   Fig. 2-66

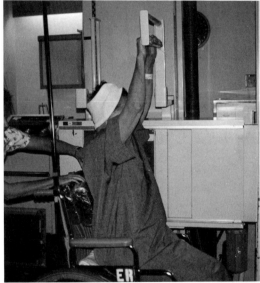

Left Lateral in Wheel Chair   Fig. 2-67

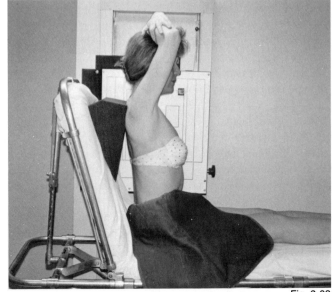

Erect, Supported Left Lateral   Fig. 2-68

• AP Projection
Supine or Semi-Erect (in department or as bedside portable)

Chest
Optional
• **AP Supine or Semi-erect**
• Lateral Decubitus (AP)
• AP Lordotic
• Obliques

Structures Best Shown:
Lungs, air-filled trachea, bony thorax, diaphragm including costophrenic angles, and heart and great vessels. Heart shadow will be magnified due to shorter SID and AP projection.

Technical Factors:
• Film Size - 14 x 17 in. (35 x 43 cm) crosswise.
• Stationary grid or screens. (Screens commonly used with portables at 80-90 kVp.)
• 100 - 120 kVp range with grid.

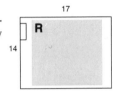

Shielding: Place lead shield to shield gonads.

Patient Position:
• Patient supine on cart; if possible, the head end of the cart or bed should be raised into a semierect position (see NOTE below).
• Roll shoulders forward as much as possible by rotating arms medially.

Part Position:
• Place film holder under or behind patient, align top of film 4 in. (10 cm) above level of jugular notch (2 in. or 5 cm above shoulders).
• Center patient to film holder; check by viewing patient from the top or tube position.

Central Ray:
• CR **perpendicular** to the **sternum** (see note). CR to area of **T7**, 3-4 in. or 8-10 cm below jugular notch (can be determined by hand method as shown in *Fig 2-69*).
• For supine position, raise tube to at least a 40 in. (102 cm) SID, although more distance is preferred. (See NOTE).

Collimation: Collimate to area of lung fields.

Respiration: Exposure made at end of 2nd full inspiration.

NOTE: •Crosswise film placement is recommended to minimize chance of lateral cut-off. This requires **accurate CR alignment to center of film** to prevent grid cut-off if grid is used.
• For semi-erect position, use 60 in. (150 cm) or even 72 in. (180 cm) SID if this is possible to obtain. Always indicate the SID used; also indicate those projections obtained, such as AP supine or AP semi-erect.
• Placing the CR perpendicular to the sternum rather than the film prevents the clavicles from obscuring the apices.

Evaluation Criteria:
• Evaluation criteria for those taken in supine or semi-erect positions should be similar to those for a PA projection described on a preceding page, with three exceptions. They are as follows:
(1) The heart will appear larger due to increased magnification from a shorter SID.
(2) Possible chest effusion and other potential pathologies for this type of patient will often obscure vascular lung markings when compared to a fully erect PA chest projection.
(3) Usually there will not be as full an inspiration, with only 8 or 9 posterior ribs visualized above diaphragm. Thus the lungs will appear more dense because the lungs are not fully aerated.

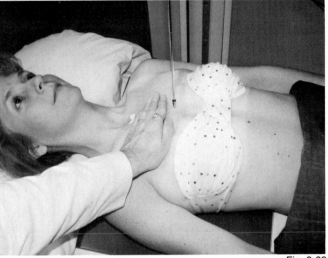

AP Supine   Fig. 2-69

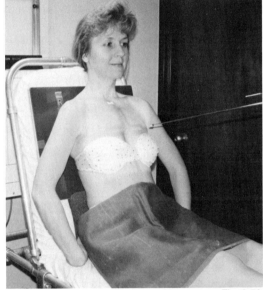

AP Semi-erect   Fig. 2-70

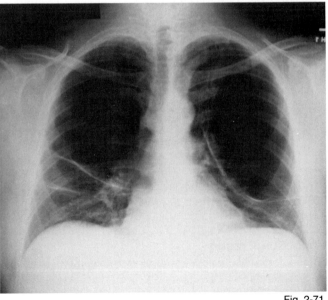

AP   Fig. 2-71

Lateral Decubitus Position

Chest
Optional
- AP Supine or Semierect
- **Lateral Decubitus** (AP)
- AP Lordotic
- Obliques

Structures Best Shown:
Small pleural effusions by demonstrating air-fluid levels in pleural space, or small amounts of air in pleural cavity for possible pneumothorax. (See NOTE.)

Technical Factors:
- Film Size - 14 x 17 in. (35 x 43 cm.), **crosswise**. (Crosswise with respect to patient.)
- Moving or stationary grid.
- 110 - 125 kVp range.

Shielding: Place lead shield to shield gonads.

Patient Position:
- Use a cardiac board on the cart or place a radiolucent pad under patient as shown.
- Place pillow under head.
- Patient lying on right side for right lateral decubitus and on left side for left lateral decubitus. (See NOTE below.)
- Raise both arms above head to clear lung field; place back of patient firmly against film holder. Secure stretcher to prevent forward movement and resultant falling of patient.
- Flex knees slightly and insure that pelvis and shoulders are parallel to film with **no** body rotation.

Part Position:
- Adjust height of film holder to center thorax to film (see NOTE).
- Adjust patient and cart so top of film is about 4 in. (10 cm) above level of jugular notch (2 in. or 5 cm above shoulders).

Central Ray:
- CR **horizontal** to and directed to center of film, to the area of **T7**, 3-4 in. (8-10 cm) inferior to level of jugular notch. (A **horizontal** beam **must** be used to show air-fluid level or pneumothorax.)
- 72 in. (180 cm) SID.

Collimation: Collimate to area of lung fields. (See NOTE.)

Respiration: Exposure made at end of 2nd full inspiration.

Alternate Positioning Routine: Some departmental routines place the head 10° lower than the hips to reduce the apical lift caused by the shoulder, thereby allowing the entire chest to remain horizontal.

NOTE: • Place appropriate marker to indicate which side of chest is up.
- May be taken as a right or left lateral decubitus. For **possible fluid** in pleural cavity (pleural effusion) the suspected side should be **down**. Insure that the side of the chest that is down is **not** cut off.
- For possible small amounts of **air** in pleural cavity (pneumothorax) the affected side should be **up** and care must be taken to **not** cut off this side of the chest.

Evaluation Criteria:
- **No rotation**, should have equal distance from vertebral column to the lateral borders of ribs on both sides; and sternoclavicular joints should be same distance from the vertebral column.
- Entire lungs including apices and both lateral borders should be included.

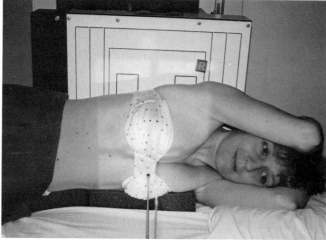

Left Lateral Decubitus Position   Fig. 2-72
(AP Projection)

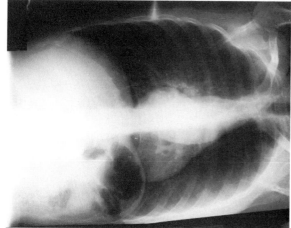

Left Lateral Decubitus   Fig. 2-73

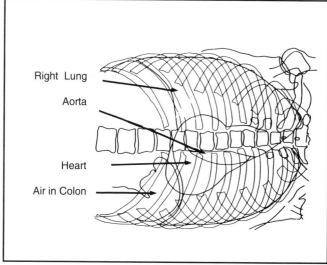

Right Lung
Aorta
Heart
Air in Colon

Left Lateral Decubitus   Fig. 2-74

- Center of collimation field should be to area of T7 on average size patients.
- Arms should not superimpose upper lungs.
- **No motion**, diaphragm and heart borders should appear sharp.
- Optimum contrast scale and exposure should result in **faint visualization of vertebrae and ribs through heart shadow.**
- Patient ID with appropriate marker indicating which side is up should be visible without superimposing lung area.

AP Lordotic Projection

Chest
Optional
• AP supine or semierect
• Lateral Decubitus (AP)
• **AP Lordotic**
• Obliques

Structures Best Shown:
Apices without clavicular superimposition and interlobar effusions.

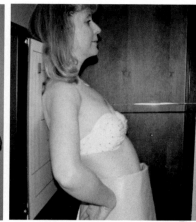

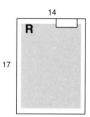

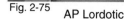

Technical Factors:
• Film Size - 14 x 17 in. (35 x 43 cm), lengthwise.
• Moving or stationary grid.
• 110 - 125 kVp range.

Shielding: Secure lead shield around waist to shield gonads.

Fig. 2-75   AP Lordotic   AP Lordotic   Fig. 2-76

Patient Position:
• Have patient stand about one foot away from film holder and lean back with shoulders, neck and back of head against film holder.
• Rest both hands on hips, palms out; roll shoulders forward.

Part Position:
• Center midsagittal plane to center of film.

Central Ray:
• CR **perpendicular** to film, centered to **mid-sternum** (3-4 in. or 9 cm below jugular notch).
• Center cassette to CR. (Top of film should be about 3 or 4 in. (8-10 cm) above shoulders on average patient.)
• 72 in. (180 cm) SID.

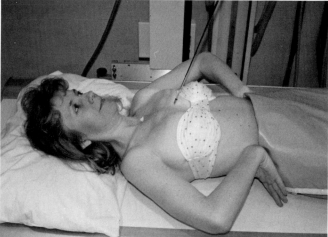

Exception: Semi-axial AP   Fig. 2-77

Collimation: Collimate to area of lungs of interest.

Respiration: Exposure made at end of **2ⁿᵈ full inspiration.**

Exception: (*Fig. 2-77*)
• If patient is weak and unstable and/or is not able to assume the lordotic position, an **AP semi-axial projection** may be taken with the patient in an erect or supine position with back against table or film holder. Shoulders are rolled forward and arms positioned as for lordotic position.
   The **CR** is directed **15 to 20° cephalad** to the area of the mid-sternum.

Evaluation Criteria:
• Clavicles should appear nearly horizontal and above or superior to apices.
• **No rotation**, sternal ends of the clavicles should be the same distance from vertebral column on each side. The lateral borders of the ribs on both sides should appear to be near equal distances from the vertebral column.
• Center of collimation field should be mid-sternum with more collimation visible on the bottom.
• Ribs appear distorted with posterior ribs appearing nearly horizontal.
• **No motion**, diaphragm, heart and rib outlines should appear sharp.

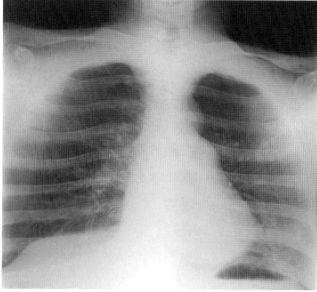

AP Lordotic   Fig. 2-78

• Optimum contrast scale and exposure should **visualize the faint vascular markings of lungs, especially in area of apices and upper lungs.**
• Patient ID with correct R or L marker should be visualized without superimposing lung area.

• Anterior Obliques (RAO & LAO)

<table>
<tr><td>

Chest
Optional
• AP
• Lateral Decubitus
• AP Lordotic
• **Obliques**

</td></tr>
</table>

Technical Factors:
• 14 x 17 in. (35 x 43 cm), lengthwise.
• Moving or stationary grid.
• 110 - 125 kVp range

Shielding: Secure lead shield around waist to shield gonads.

Structures Best Shown:

LAO • Right lung, trachea, bony thorax with heart and aorta in front of vertebral column.

RAO • Left lung, trachea, bony thorax, with heart and aorta in front of vertebral column.

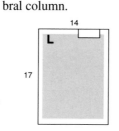

Patient Position:
• Patient erect, rotated 45° with left anterior shoulder against film holder for the LAO, and 45° with right anterior shoulder against film holder for the RAO. (See NOTE for 60° LAO.)
• Flex the arm nearest film holder and place hand on hip, palm out.
• Raise opposite arm to clear lung field and rest hand on chest film holder for support, keeping arm raised as high as possible.
• Have patient look straight ahead; keep chin raised.

Part Position:
• As viewed from the position of the x-ray tube, center the patient to the film.

Central Ray:
• CR **perpendicular** to and directed to level **of T7**. (7-8 in. or 8-10 cm below level of vertebra prominens.)
• 72 in. (180 cm) SID.

Collimation: Collimate to area of lungs.

Respiration: Exposure made at end of **2ⁿᵈ full inspiration**.

NOTE: • For **anterior** obliques, the side of interest is generally the side **farthest** from the film. Thus the **RAO** will best visualize the **left** lung.
• Certain positions for studies of the **heart** require an **LAO** with more rotation, **60°**.
• Less rotation (15-20°) may be of value for better visualization of the various areas of the lungs for possible pulmonary diseases.

Evaluation Criteria:
• To evaluate a 45° rotation, the distance from the outer margin of the ribs to the vertebral column on the side farthest from the film should be approximately twice the distance as the side closest to the film.
• Both lungs from the apices to the costophrenic angles should be included.
• Center of collimation field should be to the mid-lung area at the level of T7.
• The air-filled trachea, great vessels and heart outlines are best visualized on a 60° LAO. (A 45° RAO will also visualize these structures.)

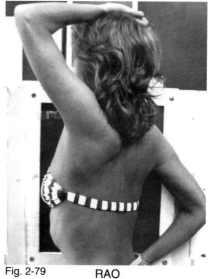
Fig. 2-79   RAO

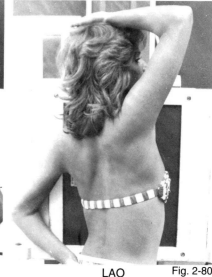
LAO   Fig. 2-80

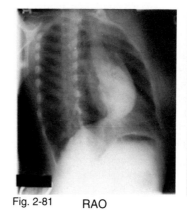
Fig. 2-81   RAO

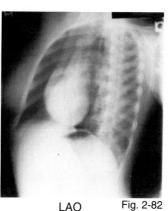
LAO   Fig. 2-82

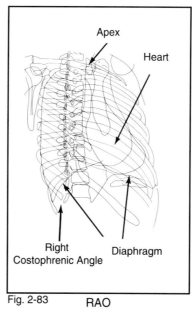
Fig. 2-83   RAO

Apex   Heart   Right Costophrenic Angle   Diaphragm

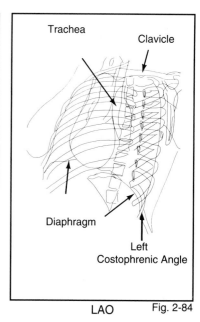
LAO   Fig. 2-84

Trachea   Clavicle   Diaphragm   Left Costophrenic Angle

• **No motion:** The outline of the diaphragm and heart should appear sharp.
• Optimum exposure and sufficient, long contrast scale will result in **visualization of general vascular markings of the lungs and faint rib outlines throughout lungs, except through the most dense part of the heart shadow.**
• Patient ID and correctly placed R or L marker should be visible without superimposing lung area.

• Posterior Obliques (RPO & LPO)

Chest
Optional
• AP
• Lateral Decubitus
• AP Lordotic
• **Obliques**

Exception: Posterior obliques can be taken if patient cannot assume an erect position for anterior obliques or if supplementary projections are required.

Structures Best Shown:

LPO • Left lung, trachea, bony thorax, with heart and aorta in front of vertebral column.

RPO • Right lung, trachea, bony thorax, with heart and aorta in front of vertebral column.

Technical Factors:

• Film Size - 14 x 17 in. (35 x 43 cm), lengthwise.
• Moving or stationary grid.
• 110 - 125 kVp range.

Shielding: Secure lead shield around waist to shield gonads.

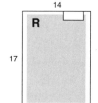

Patient Position: (Erect)

• Patient erect, rotated 45° with right posterior shoulder against film holder for RPO, and 45° with left posterior shoulder against film holder for LPO.
• Raise the arm closest to the film and support behind head. Place other arm on hip with palm out, or place both hands on hips with palms out as shown.
• Have patient look straight ahead.

Recumbent Position:

• If patient cannot stand or sit, posterior obliques on table can be taken.
• Place supports under head and under elevated hip and shoulder.

Part Position:

• Top of film holder about 1 in. (2 cm) above vertebra prominens, or about 5 in. (12 cm) above level of jugular notch (2 in. or 5 cm above shoulders).
• Center thorax to film.

Central Ray:

• CR **perpendicular** to the level of **T7**.
• 72 in. (180 cm) SID.

Collimation: Collimate to area of lungs.

Respiration: Exposure made at end of **2nd full inspiration.**

NOTE: • **Posterior** obliques best visualize the side **closest** to the film.
• Posterior positions show the same anatomy as the opposite anterior oblique. Thus the LPO position corresponds to the RAO, and the RPO to the LAO.

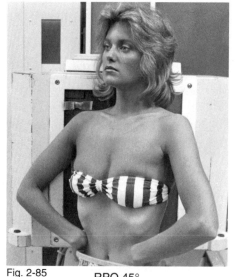

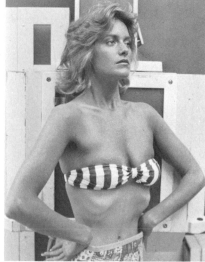

Fig. 2-85   RPO 45°   LPO 45°   Fig. 2-86

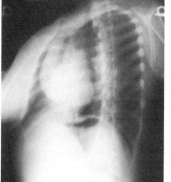

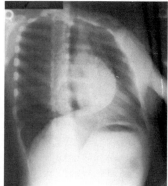

Fig. 2-87   RPO   LPO   Fig. 2-88

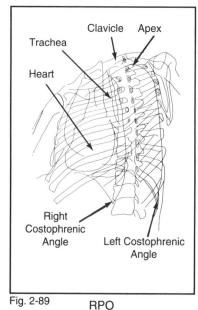

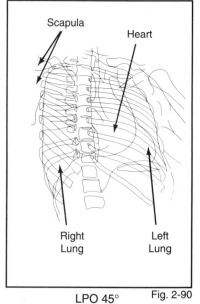

Fig. 2-89   RPO   LPO 45°   Fig. 2-90

Evaluation Criteria:

Positioning criteria are similar to that of anterior obliques described on previous page. However, due to increased magnification of anterior diaphragm, lung fields usually appear shorter on posterior obliques compared to anterior obliques. The heart and great vessels also appear larger on posterior obliques because they are farther from the film.

• Lateral Position

Upper Airway
Basic
• **Lateral**
• AP

Structures Best Shown:
Air-filled larynx and trachea, the region of thyroid and thymus glands and upper esophagus if opacified.

Technical Factors:
• Film Size - 10 x 12 in. (24 x 30 cm), lengthwise.
• Moving or stationary grid.
• 80 ± 6 kVp range. (See NOTE below.)

Shielding: Secure lead shield around waist to shield gonads.

Patient Position:
• Upright if possible, seated or standing in a lateral position (may be taken in R or L lateral, and may be taken recumbent tabletop if necessary).

Part Position:
• Position patient to center upper airway to center of film (larynx and trachea lie anterior to cervical and thoracic vertebrae).
• Rotate shoulders posteriorly with arms hanging down clasping hands behind back.
• Raise chin slightly and have patient look directly ahead.
• Adjust film height to place top of film at level of EAM, (external auditory meatus) which is the opening of the external ear canal. (See NOTE if area of primary interest is the trachea rather than the larynx.)

Central Ray:
• CR **perpendicular** to film at level of **C6 or 7**, midway between the laryngeal prominence of the thyroid cartilage and the jugular notch. (See NOTE for lower centering if trachea is area of primary interest.)
• 72 in. (180 cm) SID if possible to minimize magnification.

Collimation: Collimate to area of interest.

Respiration:
• Exposure should be made **during a slow deep inspiration** to insure filling trachea and upper airway with air.

NOTE:
• **Exposure:** Exposure for the lateral of the upper airway in the neck region should be that of a soft tissue lateral. If the trachea is the primary area of interest, the exposure should be approximately that of a lateral chest.
• **Centering for trachea area:** If the primary interest area is the trachea, the film and CR should be lowered about 1.5 to 2 in. (4-5 cm) to center the entire trachea (level of C6 to T4 or 5) to the film, which places the CR at the jugular notch.

Evaluation Criteria:
• The larynx and trachea should be filled with air and well visualized. Centering for the **upper airway** (larynx and proximal trachea) should include the EAM at the upper border of the film and T3 or 4 on the lower border. If the **trachea** is the primary area of interest, the centering should be lower to center the area of the trachea (C6 to T4 or 5) to the film.
• The shadows of the shoulders should primarily be posterior to and not superimpose the area of the trachea.
• Collimation borders should appear on both sides with ideally only minimal (1/8 in. or less) borders on top and bottom. The center of the collimation field should be to the CR location as described above.
• Optimum exposure includes a soft-tissue technique wherein the air-filled larynx and upper trachea are not overexposed. The cervical vertebrae will appear underexposed.
• Patient ID and correctly placed R or L marker should be visible without superimposing essential anatomy.

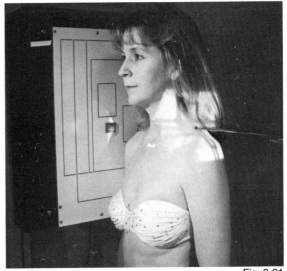

Lateral — Fig. 2-91

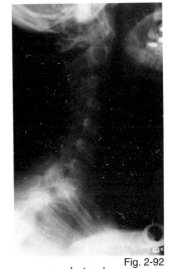

Lateral — Fig. 2-92

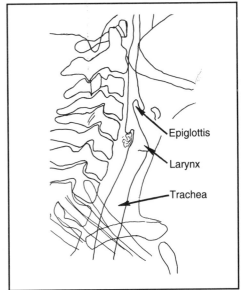

Epiglottis

Larynx

Trachea

Lateral — Fig. 2-93

Chest - Upper Airway

• AP Projection

Upper Airway
Basic
• Lateral
• AP

Structures Best Shown:
Air-filled larynx and trachea, the region of thyroid and thymus glands and upper esophagus if opacified.

Technical Factors:
• Film Size - 10 x 12 in. (24 x 30 cm), lengthwise.
• Moving or stationary grid.
• 80 ± 6 kVp range.

Shielding: Secure lead shield around waist to protect gonads.

Patient Position:
• Upright if possible, seated or standing with back of head and shoulders against film holder. (May be taken recumbent table top if necessary.)

Part Position:
• Align midsagittal plane to midline of grid or table.
• Raise chin so that **acathiomeatal line is perpendicular to the film**; have patient look directly ahead.
• Adjust the film height to place top of film about 1 or 1.5 in. (3-4 cm) below EAM. (See NOTE for explanation of centering.)

Central Ray:
• CR **perpendicular** to film at level of T1-2, about 1 in. (2.5 cm) above the jugular notch.
• Minimum 40 in. (102 cm) SID.

Collimation: Collimate to area of interest.

Respiration:
• Exposure should be made **during a slow deep inspiration** to insure filling trachea and upper airway with air.

NOTE:
• **Exposure:** Exposure for this AP projection should be approximately that of an AP of the cervical and/or thoracic spine.
• **Centering for upper airway and trachea:** Centering for this AP projection is slightly lower than for the lateral position described on the previous page because the most proximal larynx area is not visualized on the AP due to the superimposed base of skull and mandible. Therefore, more of the trachea can be visualized.

Evaluation Criteria:
• The larynx and trachea should be filled with air and well visualized. (See NOTE for centering explanation.) The area of the proximal cervical vertebrae (the lower margin of the shadow of the superimposed mandible and base of skull) to the mid-thoracic region should be included.
• There should be no rotation as evidenced by the symmetrical appearance of the sternoclavicular joints.
• Collimation borders should appear on both sides with ideally only minimal (1/8 in. or less) borders on top and bottom. The center of the collimation field should be to area of T1-2.
• Optimum exposure should be dark enough to visualize the air-filled trachea through the cervical and thoracic vertebrae.
• Patient ID and correctly placed R or L marker should be visible without superimposing essential anatomy.

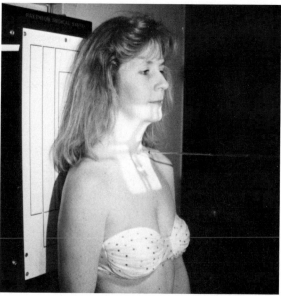
AP   Fig. 2-94

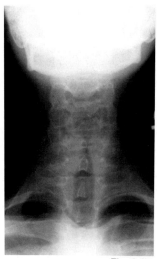
AP   Fig. 2-95

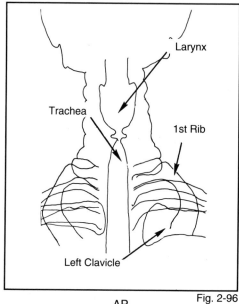
Larynx
Trachea
1st Rib
Left Clavicle
AP   Fig. 2-96

Appendix A

CR Location Chest Positioning Method [1]

Following is a sample of the data sheet used to determine accurate CR locations for chest positioning with corresponding accurate collimation. Included are actual lung measurements from radiographs which are compared with the centering estimates used in positioning for the chest radiographs using the hand spread method. (The printed ruler on this page can be used to determine hand spread measurements.)

It should be noted that measurements "C" and "A" are greater than the corresponding measurements "D" or "B" on the radiograph because of the curvature of the thorax. This difference will be greater on older patients with spinal curvature (kyphosis) and for those with more of a barrel shaped chest.

Note also in the total sample of 130 patients, the average height of the lungs was **10.4 in.** and the average width was **11.7 in.** (average width is 1.3 in. greater than height). It is also interesting to note that only 13 patients had lung height measurements greater than the width, and these were smaller patients weighing only an average of 131 lbs.

The 30 patients in this sample, however, who weighed over 200 lbs. had an average lung width of **13 in.** Therefore for most of these patients the film should be placed crosswise to prevent side cut off. The average lung height on these larger patients was only **10.7 in.** indicating that a 14 x 17 in. film can safely be placed crosswise without danger of lung cut-off on top or bottom.

It should be remembered, however, that these are averages and there are exceptions such as larger well developed athletic type patients, for which the height may be greater than the width.

Chest CR and Lung Measurement Study

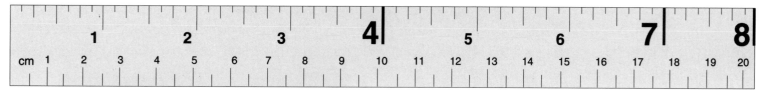

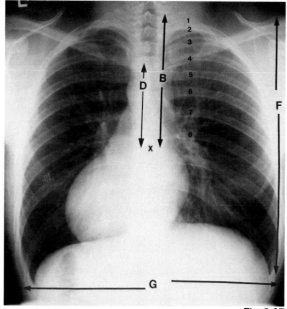

Larger than Average Male, CR=T8   Fig. 2-97
Actual Lung Measurements: width(G)=13in., height(F)=12.5in.

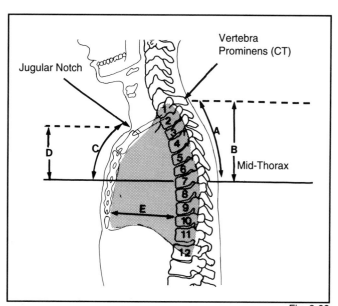

CR and Landmarks
(Average Patient)   Fig. 2-98

Patient Data					Centering Est. (Hand Spread Method)		Measurements of Lung Dimensions (from film)					Upper Collimation (from film)	Critique Remarks
					AP & Lat.	PA			Height	Depth	Width		
Case Number	Height	Weight	Age	M/F	C	A	D	B	F	E	G	H	
*Averages:	5'8"	162 lbs.	48	±50/50	3-4"	M =8" F=7"	2.7"	4.8"	10.4"	8.5"	11.7"	.98"	
(30 patients +200 lbs)		+200 lbs.							10.7"		13"		requires film crosswise
(13 patients F>G)		131 lbs.							11.4"		10.5"		height greater than width

* total sample 130 adult patients

[1]NOTE: This CR location chest positioning method and the chest measurements quoted in this chapter were determined by the author in cooperation with Kathy Martensen, R.T., University of Iowa and Karen Brown, R.T., William Gize and Tonya Morisette, St. Joseph's Hospital, Phoenix, AZ.

Chapter 3

Radiographic Anatomy and Positioning
of the
Abdomen

Contributions by: John P. Lampignano, M Ed, RT (R)
Kathy Martensen, BS, RT (R)
Barry T. Anthony, RT (R)

Contents

3 Abdomen

Part I Radiographic Anatomy

Abdominal Radiography

This chapter covers the anatomy and positioning for what is often called "plain" films of the abdomen. The most common is an AP supine abdomen, also sometimes called a KUB (**K**idneys, **U**reters and **B**ladder). These are taken without injection of contrast media. (The abdominal studies utilizing contrast media are described in later chapters.) Plain radiographs of the abdomen (KUB) are commonly taken prior to scheduling abdominal examinations utilizing contrast media to rule out certain pathologies.

Acute Abdominal Series: Certain acute or emergency conditions of the abdomen may develop from conditions such as bowel obstruction, perforations involving free air or fluid in the abdomen, or a possible intra-abdominal mass. These acute or emergency conditions require what is commonly called an "acute abdominal series", or a "3-way abdomen" series wherein several abdominal radiographs are taken in different positions to demonstrate air fluid levels and/or free air. Accurate positioning for all of these abdominal radiographs requires a good understanding of anatomy and relationships of the organs and structures within the abdominopelvic cavity.

Topographic Landmarks

One must be able to locate certain bony landmarks on the patient and to use these landmarks to position the patient in relationship to the film for abdominal radiographs. These landmarks are called topographic landmarks and can be located on the patient by careful palpation (light pressure applied by the hand).

The following five palpable landmarks are important in positioning the abdomen. Each of these landmarks is marked on the model, drawings and radiograph on this page. One may wish to practice finding these bony landmarks on oneself before attempting to locate them on a patient the first time. Positioning for abdominal radiographs in either AP or PA projections requires a quick but accurate location of these landmarks on all types of patients, the thin as well as the heavy set or muscular patients.

A. Iliac Crest: The crest of ilium (iliac crest) is the upper, curved border of the ilium. The ilium is the large wing-like portion of each half of the pelvis. The crest can be felt along its entire length through the lateral wall of the abdomen.

B. Anterior Superior Iliac Spine (ASIS): The second important landmark is the prominent anterior end of the iliac crest, known as the anterior superior iliac spine, or ASIS. The ASIS can be found by locating the iliac crest, then palpating anteriorly until a prominent projection or bump is felt.

C. Greater Trochanter of Femur: The next important palpable area is the greater trochanter of the femur. The most superior portion of this large prominence lies about 1 or 1.5 in. (3 or 4 cm) above the level of the symphysis pubis. (See radiograph, *Fig. 3-4.*)

D. Ischial Tuberosity: A fourth topographic landmark is the ischial tuberosity. These two bony prominences bear most of the weight of the trunk when a person is seated. Each ischial tuberosity is about 1.5 in. or nearly 4 cm below the level of the symphysis pubis.

Palpating this landmark may be embarrassing as well as uncomfortable for the patient. Therefore, the iliac crest and/or the greater trochanter can be used instead for positioning a PA abdomen in the prone position.

E. Symphysis Pubis: A fifth topographic landmark is the symphysis pubis, the anterior junction of the two pubic bones. The symphy-

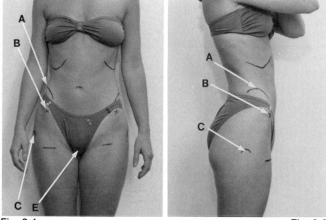
Fig. 3-1   Topographic Landmarks   Fig. 3-2

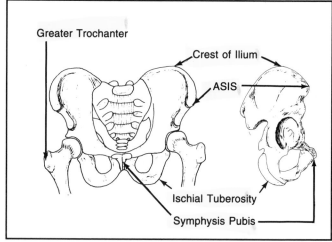
Topographic Landmarks   Fig. 3-3

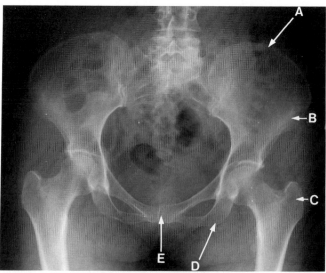
Topographic Landmarks (AP Pelvis)   Fig. 3-4

sis pubis itself is a vertical midline structure. The most anterior part of the pubis, however, is the structure which can be palpated with the patient in the supine position.

Palpating this landmark may also be embarrassing to the patient and with some practice one can also determine the level of the pubic symphysis by palpating the greater trochanter and the ASIS, and/or the iliac crest.

Vertebral Column

The lower vertebral column, which forms the posterior portion of the abdominopelvic cavity, is composed of the lumbar spine, sacrum *(sa'krum)* and coccyx *(kok'siks)*.

The **lumbar spine** consists of five large vertebrae. The **sacrum** is made up of five bony segments fused into one bone articulating on either side with the two ilia of the pelvis. Three to five incompletely developed vertebrae fuse in the adult to form the small **coccyx.**

Note that the **crest of the ilium is at the same level as the disc space between the fourth and fifth lumbar vertebrae.**

Abdominal Muscles

There are many muscles associated with the abdominopelvic cavity; however, the following three are the most important in abdominal radiography:

1. **Diaphragm**
2. **Left psoas** *(sō'es)* **major**
3. **Right psoas major**

The **diaphragm** is an umbrella-shaped muscle separating the abdominal cavity from the thoracic cavity. The diaphragm must be perfectly motionless during radiography of either the abdomen or the chest. Motion of the patient's diaphragm can be stopped by providing appropriate breathing instructions.

The two **psoas major** muscles are located on either side of the lumbar vertebral column. The lateral borders of these two muscles should be visible on a diagnostic abdominal radiograph.

Cross Section of Abdomen

Computed tomographic (CT) images of the abdominal cavity result in excellent visualization of bony and soft tissue structures. CT sections are viewed as though one were at the patient's feet looking up toward the head. Structures on the viewer's left are actually right side structures. The CT image shown in *Fig. 3-7* is through the level of the **fourth lumbar vertebra.** Note that bony anatomy with high density, such as the body of L4, appear white; while soft tissue structures, such as the **psoas major muscles,** appear gray. The white irregular shaped structure visualized in the abdominal cavity is barium-filled small intestine.

Abdominal Cavity

The abdominopelvic cavity is lined with a double-walled, saclike membrane called the **peritoneum** *(per"i-to-ne'um)*. The outer layer adhering to the abdominal and pelvic cavities is the **parietal** *(pah-ri'e-tal)* peritoneum, and the inner portion covering certain organs is the **visceral** *(vis'er-al)* peritoneum. The **peritoneal cavity** is the space inside the peritoneal lining.

Certain portions of the inner visceral peritoneum completely enclose some organs such as the small intestine to form a double fold called the **mesentery** *(mes'en-ter"e)* or **omentum** *(o-men'tum)*, which stabilize and support these structures.

Some structures are only partially covered by the visceral mesentery such as the ascending and descending colon. Certain other structures within the abdomen are completely behind or posterior to the parietal peritoneum, such as the kidneys, ureters and large blood vessels like the aorta and inferior vena cava. These are called **retroperitoneal** structures. More detail of the abdominal cavity and associated abdominal organs is included in Chapter 15 of the lower gastrointestinal system. (Pages 451 and 452.)

Note: The cross sectional drawing in *Fig. 3-8* is simplified to demonstrate peritoneum and mesentery. If all loops of bowel and other organs of the abdominal cavity were drawn in, there would be very little actual space left in the peritoneal cavity, as evident by comparing this drawing to the C.T. image in *Fig. 3-7.*

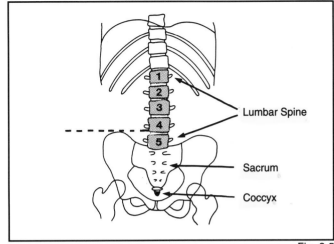

Lower Vertebral Column   Fig. 3-5

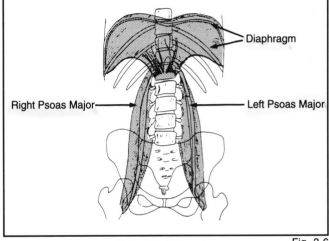

Abdominal Muscles   Fig. 3-6

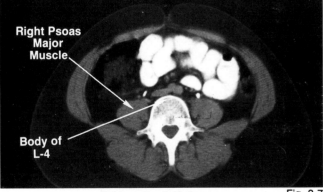

CT Image of Abdomen   Fig. 3-7
(Level of L4)

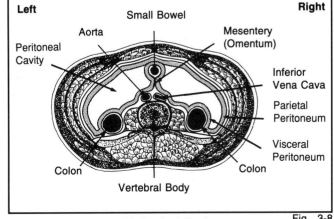

Abdominal Cavity   Fig. 3-8
(Cross Section)

Abdomen

Abdominal Organ Systems

The various organ systems found within the abdominopelvic cavity are presented only briefly in this chapter. Each of these systems is described in greater detail in later chapters devoted to those specific systems.

The digestive system along with its accessory organs (the liver, gallbladder and pancreas) fills much of the abdominal cavity. The organs of the digestive system are listed as follows:

- Mouth
- Pharynx
- Esophagus
- **Stomach**
- **Small intestine** } In abdominal cavity
- **Large intestine**

Mouth, Pharynx and Esophagus: The digestive system begins at the **mouth** and continues as the **pharynx and esophagus.** The esophagus is located in the mediastinum of the thoracic cavity.

Stomach

The stomach is the first organ of the digestive system found in the abdominal cavity. The stomach is an expandable reservoir for swallowed food and fluids. The three main subdivisions of the stomach are the **fundus, body and pyloric antrum.** The fundus is the proximal portion superior to the esophageal opening. The distal portion, which continues as the small intestine, is the pyloric antrum. The major part of the stomach between the fundus and the pyloric antrum is termed the body. The radiographic and anatomical position of the stomach is highly variable depending on body build, posture and stomach contents.

The **greater curvature** is four to five times longer than the **lesser curvature** and is convex rather than concave.

Openings of Stomach: The two openings of the stomach are guarded by circular sphincter muscles. Between the esophagus and stomach is the **esophagogastric junction** (cardiac orifice), while the **pyloric** orifice, or **pylorus,** is located between the stomach and small intestine. When the stomach is empty it tends to collapse, except for the upper portion or fundus. A gas bubble is usually seen in the fundus, just below the left hemidiaphragm, on a radiograph of an upright person. The empty stomach lining forms longitudinal folds termed **rugae** *(roo'je),* which mostly disappear when the stomach is full.

Gas Bubble in Fundus of Stomach: Due to the gas bubble that rises to the top of the stomach, the fundus is all that is visible on a plain abdominal radiograph in the upright position (see small arrows *Fig. 3-12*). Note that the fundus of the stomach lies just below the left hemidiaphragm. The rest of the stomach blends in with other abdominal structures and is not readily visible.

Barium Sulfate in Stomach: A dense suspension of barium sulfate and water has been ingested by the patient in *Fig. 3-13,* resulting in the entire stomach being visualized. The parts of the stomach as labeled on the radiograph are: (A) fundus, (B) body, (C) pyloric antrum, (D) pyloric orifice or pylorus, and (E) esophagogastric junction (cardiac orifice).

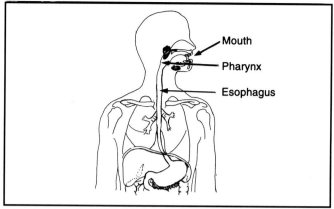

Upper Digestive Tract   Fig. 3-9

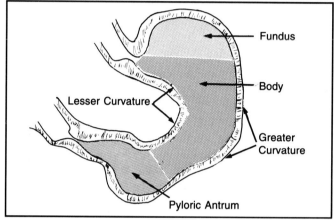

Stomach   Fig. 3-10

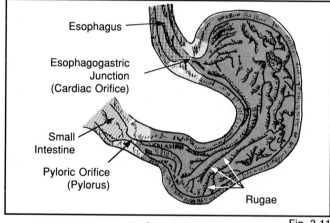

Stomach   Fig. 3-11

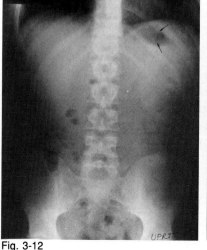

Fig. 3-12
Upright Abdominal

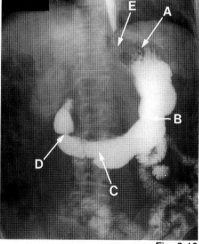

Fig. 3-13
Radiograph of Stomach

Small Intestine

The next portion of the digestive tract, the small intestine, consists of three parts:
  A. **Duodenum** *(du"o-de'num)*
  B. **Jejunum** *(je-joo'num)*
  C. **Ileum** *(il'e-um)*

The small intestine begins at the **pyloric orifice** and extends 15 to 18 feet (4.5 to 5.5 meters), then joins the large intestine at the (D) **ileocecal valve.**

Duodenum: The first portion of the small intestine, the **duodenum,** is the shortest, but the widest in diameter of the three segments. It is about 10 in., or 25 cm, in length. When filled with contrast medium, the duodenum looks like the letter C. The proximal portion of the duodenum is called the duodenal bulb or cap. It has a certain characteristic shape, usually well seen on barium studies of the upper gastrointestinal tract. Ducts from the liver, gallbladder and pancreas drain into the duodenum.

Jejunum and Ileum: The remainder of the small bowel lies in the central and lower abdomen. The first two-fifths following the duodenum is termed the **jejunum,** while the distal three-fifths is called the **ileum.** (Note the spelling of il<u>e</u>um as compared to the superior portion of the hip bone, which is spelled i-l-<u>i</u>-u-m.)

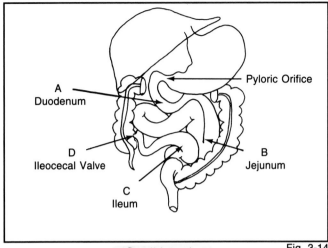

Small Intestine   Fig. 3-14

Radiograph of Small Intestine

Air is seldom seen within the entire small intestine on a plain abdominal radiograph of a healthy, ambulatory adult. The radiograph in *Fig. 3-15* visualizes the stomach, small intestine and proximal large intestine because they are filled with radiopaque barium sulfate. The identified general areas are: (A) the duodenum, (B) the jejunum, (C) the ileum, and (D) the ileocecal valve.

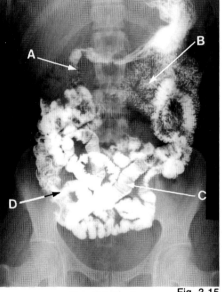

Small Intestine   Fig. 3-15
Radiograph

Cross Section of Abdomen

Computed tomography of the abdomen utilizes barium or iodine-containing compounds to outline the gastrointestinal tract. Figure *3-16* is a CT image through the distal stomach and duodenum. The **distal stomach** is shown partially filled with a barium mixture and partially filled with air. Some of the barium mixture has passed into the **small intestine** to outline the proximal duodenum.

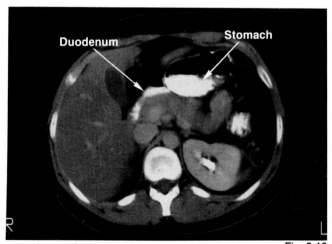

CT Image of Abdomen   Fig. 3-16
(level of distal stomach and duodenum)

Large Intestine

The last of the digestive system organs is the large intestine. The large intestine begins in the lower right quadrant at the junction with the small intestine. That portion of the large intestine below the **ileocecal valve** is a saclike area termed the **cecum.** The **appendix** is attached to the posteromedial aspect of the cecum. The vertical portion of the large bowel above the cecum is the **ascending colon,** which joins the **transverse colon** at the **right colic** (*kol´ik,* referring to colon) **flexure** (hepatic flexure). The transverse colon joins the **descending colon** at the **left colic flexure** (splenic flexure). The descending colon continues as the S-shaped **sigmoid colon** in the lower left abdomen. The **rectum** is the final 6 in., or 15 cm, of the large intestine. The rectum ends at the **anus,** the sphincter muscle at the terminal opening of the large intestine.

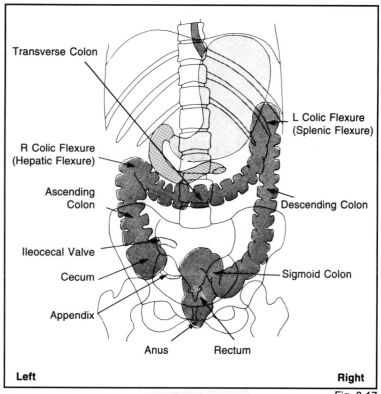

Large Intestine   Fig. 3-17

Radiograph of Large Intestine

Portions of the large intestine can usually be seen on a plain abdominal radiograph due to contained fecal matter and varying amounts of gas. In addition, the muscles of the large bowel cause the formation of large saclike divisions termed **haustra,** which give the large bowel a different internal appearance than the small bowel. Radiopaque contrast medium must be added to the clean large bowel during the radiographic examination, termed a barium enema, in order to visualize all of the large intestine. A barium enema radiograph *(Fig. 3-18)* shows the following labeled anatomy: (A) anus, (B) rectum, (C) sigmoid colon, (D) descending colon, (E) left colic (splenic) flexure, (F) transverse colon, (G) right colic (hepatic) flexure, (H) ascending colon, and (I) cecum.

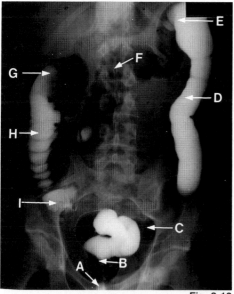

Large Intestine
Radiograph   Fig. 3-18

Cross Section of Abdomen

The computed tomographic image shown in *Fig. 3-19* is through the lower abdomen and shows primarily intestinal structures within the abdominal cavity. The loops of **small intestine** are well shown due to the contained barium mixture. The portion of **large intestine** best seen is filled with air and fecal matter. Since the labeled portion is in the lower right quadrant, it is the cecum part of the large intestine.

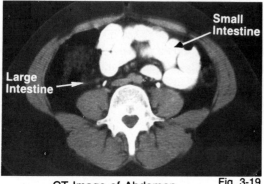

CT Image of Abdomen   Fig. 3-19

Accessory Digestive Organs

Certain accessory organs of digestion also located in the abdominal cavity are:

- **Pancreas**
- **Liver**
- **Gallbladder**

Pancreas: The pancreas is an elongated gland located posterior to the stomach and near the posterior abdominal wall, between the duodenum and the spleen. The head of the pancreas is nestled in the C-loop of the duodenum. The body and tail of the pancreas extend toward the upper left abdomen.

The pancreas which is not seen on a plain abdominal radiograph, manufactures several digestive juices that move to the duodenum via a main pancreatic duct, as needed, for digestion. In addition, the pancreas produces certain hormones, such as insulin, that are necessary to normal well-being.

Liver: The liver is the largest solid organ in the body, occupying most of the upper right quadrant. One of its numerous functions is the production of bile, which assists in the digestion of fats. If bile is not needed for digestion, it is stored and concentrated for future use in the gallbladder.

Gallbladder: The gallbladder is a pear-shaped sac located beneath the liver. The primary functions of the gallbladder are to store and concentrate bile, and to contract and release bile when stimulated by an appropriate hormone.

Radiograph of Gallbladder

The gall bladder in most cases cannot be visualized on a radiograph without contrast media. Only about 15% of all gallstones contain enough calcium to be visualized on a plain abdominal radiograph. Figure 3-21 demonstrates the gallbladder following oral ingestion of contrast media. The average size, location and saclike appearance of the gallbladder is well demonstrated on this radiograph.

Cross Section of Abdomen

A CT image through the lower liver, as shown in *Fig. 3-22* visualizes numerous soft tissue structures. The **liver** is shown with multiple white densities throughout its substance. These are blood vessels in the liver since this examination was done following the venous injection of an iodinated contrast medium. The **gallbladder** appears as a lower density darker structure as compared to the surrounding liver. The head of the **pancreas** is well shown near the duodenum.

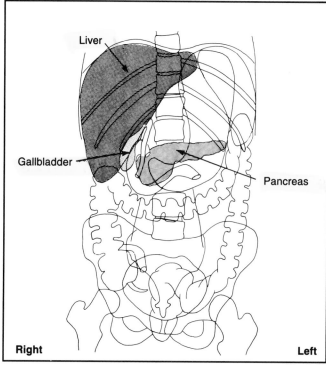

Right   **Left**

Accessory Organs of Digestion   Fig. 3-20

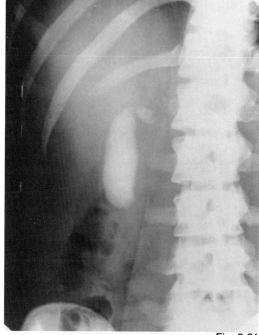

Radiograph of Gallbladder   Fig. 3-21

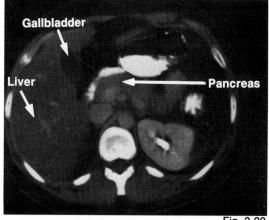

CT Image of Abdomen   Fig. 3-22
(level of lower liver, gallbladder, and pancreas)

Bile Ducts

Bile formed in the liver travels through either the **right** or **left hepatic ducts** and, finally, into the **common hepatic duct.** Bile then travels to the gallbladder to be stored via the **cystic duct.** When needed for digestion, concentrated bile from the gallbladder travels back through the cystic duct to the **common bile duct** and finally into the duodenum. The common bile duct may join the main pancreatic duct before emptying into the duodenum. Near the terminal opening, the duct walls contain circular muscle fiber called the **sphincter of Oddi** which controls bile flow into the duodenum.

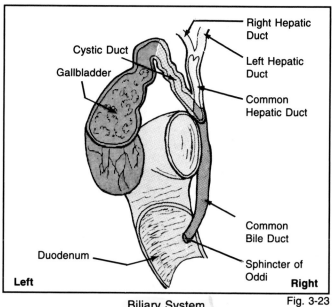

Biliary System   Fig. 3-23

(Spleen)

The spleen is not directly associated with the digestive system since it is considered part of the circulatory system which includes the lymphatic organs, however, it is an important abdominal organ and does occupy a space to the left of the stomach in the upper left quadrant. The spleen is often visualized on plain abdominal radiographs, particularly if the organ is enlarged. It is a very fragile organ and is sometimes lacerated during trauma to the lower left rib cage.

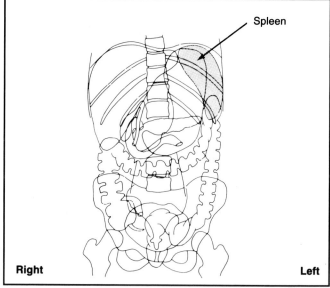

Spleen   Fig. 3-24

Cross Section of Abdomen

A CT image through the upper abdomen clearly visualizes the liver, stomach, and spleen. The large **liver** occupies the entire upper right side and some of the upper left side as well. The contrast-filled stomach is clearly differentiated from the **spleen,** which is located high and posterior in the upper left abdominal cavity. Blood vessels show well on this contrast-enhanced scan, including the large abdominal **aorta** and the **inferior vena cava.**

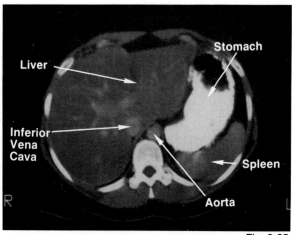

CT Image of Abdomen   Fig. 3-25
(level of upper abdomen, liver,
stomach and spleen)

Urinary System

In addition to the digestive system with its accessory organs, the urinary system is also an important abdominal system and will be introduced in this chapter.

The urinary system is composed of:

- two **kidneys**
- two **ureters** *(u-re'ter)[1]* or *(yoo-re'ter)[2]*
- one **urinary bladder**
- one **urethra** *(u-re'thrah)[1]* or *(yoo-re'thra)[2]*

Each **kidney** drains by way of its own **ureter** to the single **urinary bladder.** The bladder, situated above and behind the symphysis pubis, serves to store urine. Under voluntary control, the stored urine passes to the exterior via the **urethra.** The two **adrenal** *(ad-re'nal)* **glands** of the endocrine system are located at the superomedial portion of each kidney. The bean-shaped kidneys are located on either side of the lumbar vertebral column. The right kidney is usually situated a little lower than the left one, due to the presence of the large liver on the right. Waste materials and excess water are eliminated from the blood by the kidneys and are transported through the ureters to the urinary bladder.

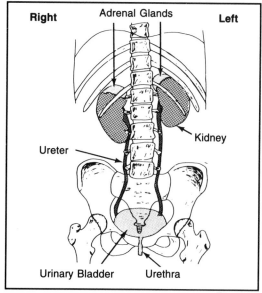

Urinary System   Fig. 3-26

Excretory Urogram (Intravenous Urogram, IVU)

The kidneys are usually faintly seen on a plain abdominal radiograph due to a fatty capsule that surrounds each kidney. The contrast medium examination shown in *Fig. 3-27* is termed an **excretory urogram,** *(eks'kre-to-re u'ro-gram)* also correctly termed an **intravenous urogram** (IVU), which is a radiographic examination of the urinary system wherein the contrast media is injected intravenously. During this examination the hollow organs of this system are visualized. The organs as labeled are: (A) left kidney, (B) left ureter, (C) urinary bladder, and (D) the area of the right adrenal gland. (Additional anatomy and positioning for the urinary system will be covered in Chapter 17.)

Note: Another term, **Intravenous Pyleogram (IVP)** has often been used for this examination. However, this is **not** an accurate term for this exam because "pyelo" refers to the renal pelvis of the kidney and the excretory urogram includes a study of the entire urinary tract, which includes the total collecting system. Therefore, throughout this textbook the term excretory urogram or intravenous urogram (IVU) will be used.

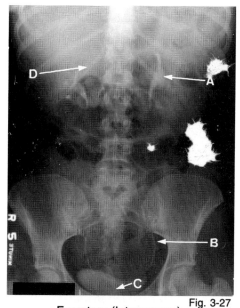

Fig. 3-27
Excretory (Intravenous) Urogram, IVU

Cross Section of Abdomen

The paired **kidneys** of the urinary system are also well visualized on the CT image in *Fig. 3-28,* taken during an IVU examination. The intravenous contrast material is being excreted by the kidneys in preparation for elimination from the body via the urinary bladder and urethra.

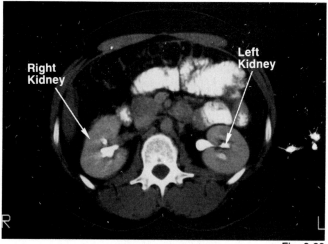

Fig. 3-28
CT Image of Abdomen (level of kidneys)

---

[1] Dorland Illustrated Medical Dictionary, 24th Edition
[2] New World Dictionary, Second College Edition

Quadrants and Regions

To help describe the locations of various organs or other structures within the abdominopelvic cavity, the abdomen may be divided into either four quadrants or into nine regions.

Four Abdominal Quadrants

If two imaginary perpendicular planes were passed through the abdomen at the unbilicus or navel, they would divide the abdomen into four quadrants. One plane would be transverse through the abdomen at the level of the umbilicus, while the second plane would coincide with the midsagittal plane and would pass through both the umbilicus and the symphysis pubis. These two planes would divide the abdominopelvic cavity into four quadrants: the **right upper quadrant** (RUP), the **left upper quadrant** (LUQ), the **right lower quadrant** (RLQ), and the **left lower quadrant** (LLQ).

Note: The four-quadrant system is generally adequate for use in radiographically localizing any particular organ, but the nine regions also need to be known and understood.

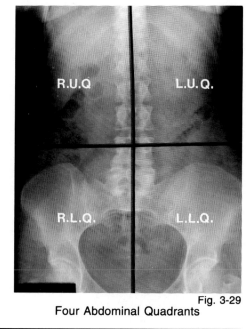

Fig. 3-29
Four Abdominal Quadrants

Nine Abdominal Regions

The abdominopelvic cavity can be further divided into nine regions by using two horizontal (or transverse) and two vertical imaginary planes. The two vertical planes would be parallel to the midsagittal plane, and midway between it and each anterior superior iliac spine. One transverse plane would be located at the lower border of the first lumbar vertebra and the second at the level of the body of the fifth lumbar vertebra. These four imaginary planes divide the abdominopelvic cavity into the nine regions.

Names of Regions: The names of these nine regions are listed in *Fig. 3-31*. The upper three regions are the **right and left hypochondriac regions** and the **epigastric region**. The middle three are the **right and left lateral regions** (formerly known as lumbar regions) and the **umbilical region**. The bottom three are the **right and left inguinal regions** (formerly known as iliac regions) and the **pubic** (formerly known as the hypogastric region).

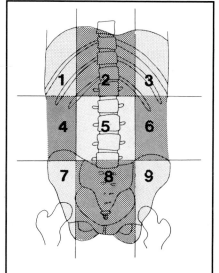

Fig. 3-30

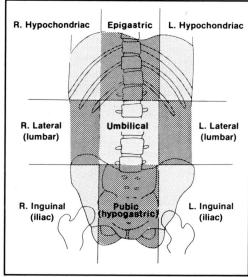

R. Hypochondriac	Epigastric	L. Hypochondriac
R. Lateral (lumbar)	Umbilical	L. Lateral (lumbar)
R. Inguinal (iliac)	Pubic (hypogastric)	L. Inguinal (iliac)

Fig. 3-31

Nine Abdominal Regions

Body Habitus

Positioning for the abdomen requires an understanding of the common variations in body habitus and how these variations determine dimensions of the abdomen. For example the sthenic-hypersthenic type patient is very broad and a 14 x 17 in. (35 x 43 cm) film holder placed lengthwise as done for the average size patient may not be wide enough. Therefore, two films placed crosswise may need to be used as indicated in the positioning pages of this chapter.

Another exception is the asthenic type which has a very long trunk but not wide. The usual 14 x 17 in. (35 x 43 cm) film holder placed lengthwise may be wide enough but may not be long enough to include

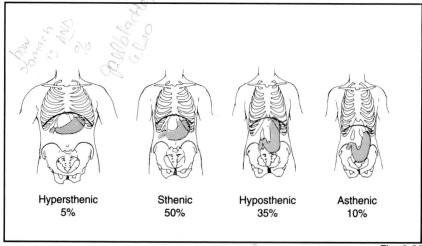

| Hypersthenic 5% | Sthenic 50% | Hyposthenic 35% | Asthenic 10% |

Body Habitus

Fig. 3-32

both the upper and lower abdominal regions. For this type of patient two films may be required, one centered high enough to include the diaphragm and the second centered lower to include the symphysis pubis.

Note also, the difference in the shape and location of the stomach within the abdominal cavity. This will be discussed further in chapter 14 (the upper GI tract).

Part II Radiographic Positioning

Patient Preparation

Patient preparation for abdominal radiography includes removal of all clothing and any opaque objects in the area to be radiographed. A hospital gown should be put on with the opening and ties in the back. Shoes and socks may remain on the feet.

Some abdominal radiographs, particularly those requiring contrast media, necessitate special instructions to the patient prior to the examination. Instructions may include such things as fasting or a laxative the night before, but the "plain" abdominal radiograph (KUB) or the acute abdominal series are usually taken "as is".

General Positioning Considerations

Make the patient as comfortable as possible on the radiographic table. A pillow under the head and support under the knees will enhance the patient's comfort. Place clean linen on table and cover patient's legs to keep them warm and to protect their modesty. Adjust the midsagittal plane to coincide with the midline of the table or the midline of the film holder. Be sure that the pelvis is not rotated, and adjust the arms at the patient's sides, away from the abdomen.

Breathing Instructions

One of the key factors in good abdominal radiography is the prevention of motion. This may be due to either **voluntary** movements from breathing or from **involuntary** movements such as peristaltic action of the bowel. The difference between these two types of motion is clearly illustrated in Chapter 1. However, what is important to remember in preventing motion in abdominal radiography is to use **as short exposure times as possible,** to prevent or minimize the effects of involuntary motion.

A second way to prevent voluntary motion is by careful breathing instructions to the patient. Most abdominal radiographs are taken on expiration, the patient is instructed to "take in a deep breath . . . let it all out and hold it — don't breathe". Before making the exposure, it is important to observe the patients to insure they are following instructions; and, that sufficient time has been allowed for all breathing movements to cease.

Film Markers

Film markers such as patient ID information should be clear and legible. Correctly placed R and L markers and "up side" markers on erect and decubitus projections should be visible without superimposing abdominal structures. On the positioning pages for the abdomen which follow in this chapter, are suggested locations for all film markers. These are indicated in the small box drawings at the top of the page indicating film size for each projection.

Radiation Protection

Patients must be protected from unnecessary radiation for all radiographic examinations. Good radiation protection practices are especially important in abdominal radiography due to the proximity of the radiation sensitive gonadal organs.

Repeat Exposures: Careful positioning and selection of correct exposure factors are ways of reducing unnecessary exposures from repeat examinations. Following breathing instructions carefully also assists in eliminating repeats due to motion caused by breathing during the exposure.

Collimation: Chapter one states a general collimation rule that **collimation borders should be visible on all four sides if the film is large enough to allow this without "cutting off" essential anatomy.** For abdominal radiographs of average to small patients, side collimation smaller than the film size is possible and should be practiced if it does not cut off abdominal anatomy. Extra side collimation can be adjusted manually so the lateral margins of the light field are visible on the outer edges of the patient's abdomen, *(Figs. 3-33 and 34).* Considering the divergent rays this will avoid cutting off abdominal anatomy and still show side collimation margins on the radiograph. However, if the patient is too broad, extra side collimation inside film borders may not be possible.

Collimation on the top and bottom should be adjusted directly to the margins of the film holder allowing for divergence of the x-ray beam. Essential anatomy will be cut off on full size adults if extra collimation margins are shown on the top and bottom borders of the radiograph.

Gonadal Shielding: Chapter one states an important rule that for **all patients of reproductive age gonadal shielding is needed if the gonads lie within or close to** (2 in. or 5 cm) **the primary field, unless such shielding covers an area of primary interest on the image receptor.** Applying this to abdominal radiographs, **gonad shields should be used** (as shown in *Fig. 3-33*) **for males** with the upper edge of the shield carefully placed at the pubic symphysis. For females, *(Fig. 3-34)* gonadal shields may be used when such shields do not obscure essential anatomy in the lower abdominopelvic region. Generally, this decision to shield female gonads on abdomen radiographs should be made by a physician to determine if essential anatomy will be obscured.

Exposure Factors

The principal exposure factors for abdominal radiographs are:
1. Medium kVp (70-80)
2. Short exposure time
3. Adequate mAs for sufficient density

Correctly exposed abdominal radiographs on an average sized patient should visualize the lateral borders of the psoas muscles, lower liver margin, kidney outlines and lumbar vertebrae transverse processes. This requires moderate contrast using medium kVp exposure to allow for visualization of various abdominal structures, including possible small semi-opaque stones in the gall bladder or kidneys.

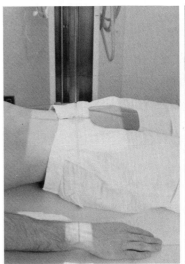 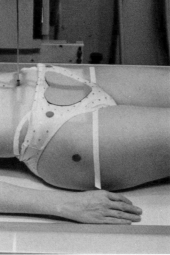

Fig. 3-33   Collimation and Gonadal Shielding   Fig. 3-34

Abdomen

Standard and Optional Operating Procedures

Certain basic and optional projections or positions for the abdomen are demonstrated and described on the following pages as suggested standard and optional departmental procedures.

Standard or Basic projections, also sometimes referred to as **routine projections** or **departmental routines** are those projections commonly taken on average patients who are helpful and can cooperate in performing the procedure.

Optional projections are those more common projections or positions taken as extra or additional projections to better demonstrate certain pathological conditions or specific body parts.

Abdominal Radiographic Routines

Radiographic examinations of the abdomen are done for a wide variety of symptoms and for various purposes as described at the beginning of this chapter. The most common radiographic exam of the abdomen is the "plain" abdomen often called a KUB. More acute conditions require what is termed an acute abdomen series, requiring abdominal radiographs taken in various patient positions, such as erect or lateral decubitus using a horizontal x-ray beam. The routines for the acute abdomen series may vary depending on physician preference and what is customary or common in different institutions or different parts of the country as shown in the following survey results.

National Survey:

Departmental basic and optional operating procedures for the abdomen are fairly consistent throughout the United States as shown on the following chart. (The number in each region box indicates the number of responding institutions to the survey in that region.)

Abdomen (KUB)	U. S. Average (529)		East (198)		Midwest (244)		West (77)	
	Basic	Optional	Basic	Optional	Basic	Optional	Basic	Optional
AP Supine	98%		98%		98%		96%	
Lat. Decub.		30%		—		—		—
AP Erect		21%		24%				12%
PA Prone		19%		22%		17%		12%
Dorsal Decub.		5%						
Acute Abdomen								
AP Supine	98%		98%		98%		96%	
AP Erect	92%		92%		92%		91%	
PA Chest	60%		61%		61%		62%	
Lat. Decub.	(23%)	58%	(22%)	60%	(24%)	62%	(26%)	44%

Explanations

Abdomen (KUB): The above results demonstrate that for the KUB abdomen examination, the **AP supine** is overwhelmingly the basic projection, with the **lateral decubitus, AP erect, PA prone** and **dorsal decub lateral** as optional projections in this order. The regional differences were primarily in the western states where fewer routines include the AP erect and the PA prone as optional.

Acute Abdomen: The acute abdomen series results demonstrate that the **AP supine** and **AP erect** are by far the most frequent basic routines, followed by the **PA chest** also listed as basic in the acute abdomen series by the majority of respondents. This is very consistent throughout the U.S. The primary regional difference is the **lateral decubitus** which is less frequently included in the western states as optional, but more frequently as a basic projection.

Because of these differences this text will list and demonstrate two possible routines for the acute abdomen series. First will be the "three-way" acute abdomen routine, with the "two-way" routine also presented as an alternative.

The erect PA chest is included in the recommended three-way acute abdomen routine. One reason is that the erect chest best visualizes free air under the diaphragm. The erect abdomen will of course also visualize free air if the film holder is positioned high enough to include the diaphragm, however, the exposure technique for the chest best visualizes this air if it is present. Also, certain chest diseases such as basal pneumonia are frequently associated with abdominal pain suggesting the need for a PA chest as part of the acute abdomen routine.

Basic and Optional Routines as presented in positioning pages of this chapter which follow

Abdomen (KUB)
Basic
• AP Supine
Optional
• Lat. Decub. (AP)
• AP Erect
• PA Prone
• Dorsal Decub. (Lat)

Acute Abdomen
(Three-way)
Basic
• AP Recumbent
• AP Erect
• PA Chest Erect
Optional
• Left Lat. Decub. (AP)

Acute Abdomen
(Two-way)
Basic
• AP Supine
• AP Erect

• AP Projection, Supine
(KUB)

Abdomen
Basic
• AP Supine (KUB)

Structures Best Shown:
Liver, spleen, kidneys, abnormal masses, calcifications or accumulations of gas. Pelvis, lumbar spine and lower ribs are also well shown.

Technical Factors:
• Film Size - 14 x 17 in. (35 x 43 cm), lengthwise.
• Moving or stationary grid.
• 70-80 kVp range.

Patient Position:
• Provide clean pillow for head. Place arms at patient's sides, away from body.
• Supine with midsagittal plane centered to midline of table and/or cassette.
• Legs extended (not crossed) with support under knees.

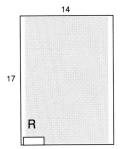

Shielding:
• Use gonadal shields on males (also on females of reproductive age if such shielding does not obscure essential anatomy as determined by a physician).
• **NO** x-rays of pregnancies (unless contraindicated), apply 10 day rule. (Do not take abdominal x-rays except during the first 10 days following menstruation to best insure no pregnancy.)

Part Position:
• Center of cassette to **level of iliac crests**, with bottom margin at pubic symphysis. (See NOTE.)
• **No rotation** of pelvis or shoulders. (Check that both ASIS, anterior superior iliac spine, are the same distance from table or film holder.)

Central Ray:
• CR **perpendicular** to and directed to **center of film.**
• Minimum 40 in. (102 cm) SID.

Collimation: Collimate closely on all four sides.

Respiration: Exposure made at end of **expiration**.

NOTE: •A tall asthenic type patient may require **two radiographs** lengthwise, one centered lower to include the symphysis pubis and the second, centered high enough to include the upper abdomen and diaphragm.
• A broad hypersthenic type patient may also require two 14 x 17 films placed **crosswise**, one centered lower to include the symphysis pubis and the second for the upper abdomen, with a minimum of 1 to 2 in. (3-5 cm) overlap.

Evaluation Criteria:
• Lower margin of radiograph should include at least the superior portion of the arch of the symphysis pubis.
• Upper abdomen should be included visualizing the upper margins of the kidneys as well as the lower portion of the dense liver and the area of the spleen. (See NOTE for possible two radiographs.)
• Vertebral column should be aligned to center of radiograph.
• **No rotation:** Pelvis and lumbar vertebrae should appear symmetrical. (R and L iliac wings appear equal in size, and shape and spinous processes should appear in center of vertebrae.)
• Lateral collimation margins should be visible for most patients unless such would cut off essential abdominal anatomy.

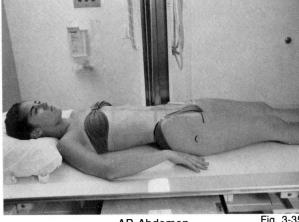

AP Abdomen   Fig. 3-35

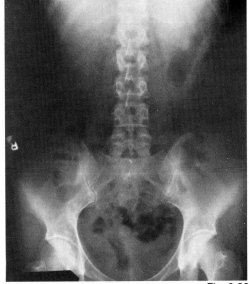

AP Abdomen   Fig. 3-36

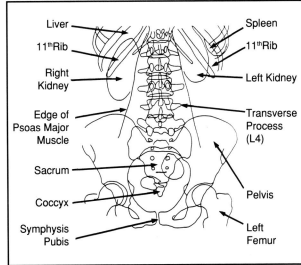

AP Abdomen   Fig. 3-37

• **No motion**: ribs and gas bubble margins appear sharp.
• Should have sufficient exposure (mAs) and long scale contrast (kVp) to visualize psoas muscle outlines, lumbar transverse processes and ribs. Margins of liver and kidneys should be visible on smaller to average size patients.
• Patient ID and R or L marker are correctly placed.

• PA Projection, Prone

Abdomen
Optional
• **PA Prone**
• Lat. Decub. (AP)
• AP Erect
• Dorsal Decub. (Lat.)

Structures Best Shown:
Liver, spleen, kidneys, abnormal masses, calcifications or accumulations of gas. Pelvis, lumbar spine and lower ribs are also shown.

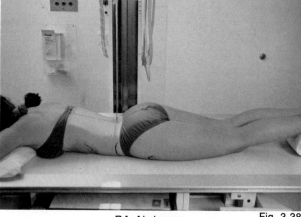

PA Abdomen   Fig. 3-38

NOTE: This PA projection should be considered when kidneys are not of primary interest because of the greatly reduced gonadal dose on females compared to the AP projection.

Technical Factors:
- Film Size - 14 x 17 in. (35 x 43 cm), lengthwise.
- Moving or stationary grid.
- 70-80 kVp range.

Patient Position:
- Prone with midsagittal plane of body centered to midline of table and/or film holder.
- Legs extended with support under ankles.
- Arms up beside head, provide clean pillow.

Shielding:
- Use gonadal shields on males.
- **NO** x-rays of pregnancies (unless contraindicated) apply 10 day rule if possible.

Part Position:
- No rotation of pelvis or shoulders and chest.
- Center of cassette to **iliac crest** (see NOTE).

Central Ray:
- CR **perpendicular** to and directed to **center of film.**
- Minimum 40 in. (102 cm) SID.

Collimation: Collimate closely on all four sides.

Respiration: Exposure made at end of **expiration.**

NOTE: Tall asthenic type patients may require two films lengthwise; broad hypersthenic types may also require two films but placed crosswise.

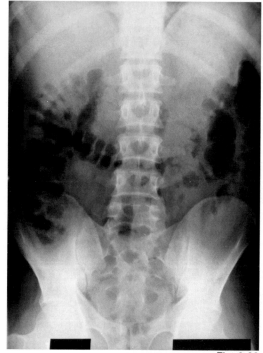

PA Abdomen   Fig. 3-39

Evaluation Criteria:
- Lower margin of radiograph should include at least the superior portion of the arch of the symphysis pubis.
- Upper abdomen should be included visualizing the upper margins of the kidneys as well as the lower portion of the dense liver and the area of the spleen. (See NOTE for possible two radiographs.)
- Vertebral column should be aligned to center of radiograph.
- **No rotation:** Pelvis and lumbar vertebrae should appear symmetrical (R and L iliac wings appear equal in size and shape and spinous processes should appear in center of vertebrae).
- Lateral collimation margins should be visible for most patients unless such would cut off essential abdominal anatomy.
- **No motion**: Ribs and gas bubble margins should appear sharp and clear.
- Should have sufficient exposure (mAs) and long scale contrast (kVp) to visualize psoas muscle outlines, lumbar transverse processes and ribs. Margins of liver and kidneys should be visible on smaller to average size patients.

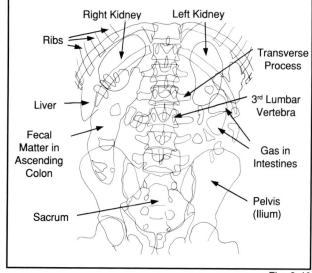

PA Abdomen   Fig. 3-40

- Patient ID should be clear and legible and correctly placed R or L marker should be visible without superimposing abdominal structures.

• Lateral Decubitus Position
AP Projection

Abdomen
Optional
• PA Prone
• **Lat. Decub. (AP)**
• AP Erect
• Dorsal Decub. (Lat.)

Structures Best Shown:
Liver, spleen, kidneys, abdominal masses, air-fluid levels and accumulations of gas or free intra-abdominal air. (Free intra-abdominal air, however, is best demonstrated with chest technique on erect PA chest in three-way acute abdominal series.)

Technical Factors:
• Film Size - 14 x 17 in.(35 x 43 cm), crosswise.
• Moving or stationary grid.
• 70-80 kVp range.

Patient Position:
• Lateral recumbent on radiolucent pad, back firmly against table or vertical grid device. (Lock wheels on cart so as not to move away from table or grid.)
• Knees partially flexed, one on top of the other to stabilize patient.
• Arms up near head, provide clean pillow.

Shielding:
• Use gonadal shield on males.
• No x-rays of pregnancies (unless contraindicated), apply 10 day rule if possible.

Part Position:
• Adjust patient and cart so center of film and CR is about **2 in. or 5 cm above level of iliac crests** (to include diaphragm), with **top of film approximately under the axilla.**
• Insure **no rotation** of pelvis or shoulders.
• Adjust height of cassette to center midsagittal plane of patient to center of film but insure that **up side of abdomen is clearly included on the film.**

Central Ray:
• CR **horizontal**, directed to **center of film**. (A **horizontal** beam **must** be used to show air-fluid levels and free intra-abdominal air.)
• Minimum 40 in. (102 cm) SID.

Collimation: Collimate on four sides.

Respiration: Exposure made at end of **expiration.**

NOTE: • Patient should be on side a minimum of **5 minutes** before exposure (to allow possible free intra-abdominal air to rise).
• **Left lateral decubitus** best demonstrates free air within abdominal cavity in the area of the liver in the right upper abdomen.
• Place arrow or other appropriate marker to indicate which side is up.

Evaluation Criteria:
• Upper margin of radiograph should include the diaphragm.
• **No rotation**: Pelvis should appear symmetrical with right and left iliac wings appearing equal in size and shape, and the outer margins of the ribs should be the same distance from the vertebral column.
• If both sides cannot be included, **the upper side must be included.**
• **No motion**: Diaphragm, ribs and gas shadow margins appear sharp.
• Overall exposure and density should appear slightly less than supine abdomen to better visualize air-fluid levels and free intra-abdominal air if present.

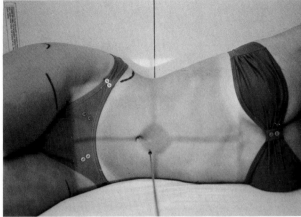
L Lat. Decub. (AP) Fig. 3-41

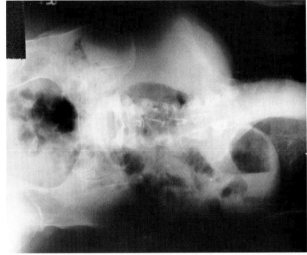
L Lat. Decub. (AP) Fig. 3-42

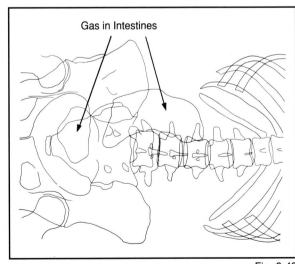
Gas in Intestines
L Lat. Decub. (AP) Fig. 3-43

• Patient ID should be clear and legible. R or L marker and arrow or other marker indicating up side, should be visible in pelvic area or where least likely to superimpose abdominal contents.

Abdomen

•Erect AP Projection

Structures Best Shown:
Liver, spleen, kidneys, abnormal masses, air-fluid levels, accumulations of gas or free intra-abdominal air. (Free intra-abdominal air, however, is best demonstrated with chest technique on erect PA chest as part of three-way acute abdominal series.)

Technical Factors:
• Film Size - 14 x 17 in. (35 x 43 cm) lengthwise.
• Moving or stationary grid.
• 70-80 kVp range.

Patient Position:
• Upright, legs slightly spread, back against table or grid device. (See NOTE for weak or unsteady patients.)
• Arms at sides away from body.
• Midsagittal plane of body centered to midline of table. Generally, the center of film is 2 in. (5 cm) above the iliac crest to include diaphragm (see NOTE).

Shielding:
• Use gonadal shields on males (use shaped contact shield or adjustable mobile shield as used in chest radiography).
• No pregnancies (unless contraindicated), use 10 day rule if possible.

Part Position:
• No rotation **of pelvis or shoulders.**
• Adjust height of film holder so center of film is **about 2 inches above iliac crest,** (to include diaphragm), with **top of film directly under the axilla.**

Central Ray:
• CR **perpendicular** to film holder but **horizontal** if table is tilted. (See NOTE).
• Minimum 40 in. (102 cm) SID.

Collimation: Collimate closely on all four sides. (Do **NOT** cut off upper abdomen.)

Respiration: Exposure made at end of **expiration.**

NOTE: • For weak or unsteady patients a compression band may be placed across chest and knees as table with footboard is raised from horizontal to vertical. Table may be left at a slight tilt **if horizontal x-ray beam is used.**
• Generally, centering should be high enough to include diaphragm, however, some routines include centering to the iliac crests to include all of the lower abdomen **if** an erect PA chest is also taken (see 3-way abdomen series); or two radiographs may be taken especially on a tall asthenic type patient. One is centered high to include the diaphragm, and, the second is centered lower to include the pubic symphysis. Broad hypersthenic type patients may also require two films placed crosswise.
• Patient should be upright a minimum of **5 minutes** before exposure. (If a patient cannot maintain an erect position, a lateral decubitus (AP) may be taken.)

Evaluation Criteria :
• Vertebral column should be aligned to center of radiograph.
• **No rotation:** pelvis and lumbar vertebrae should appear symmetrical (R and L iliac wings appear equal in size and shape and spinous processes should appear in center of vertebrae).
• Lateral collimation margins should be visible for most patients unless such would cut off essential abdominal anatomy.
• **No motion:** ribs, diaphragm and gas bubble margins should appear sharp.
• Should have sufficient exposure (mAs) and long scale contrast (kVp) to visualize margins of liver and kidneys as well as psoas muscle outline, lumbar transverse processes and ribs on small to average sized patients, unless these areas are obscured by gas in bowel.
• Free intra-abdominal air should be seen under diaphragm if present.
• Patient ID should be clear and legible.

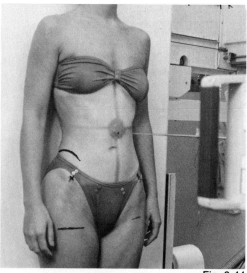

Erect AP   Fig. 3-44

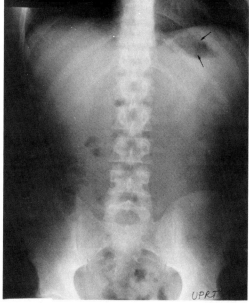

Erect AP   Fig. 3-45

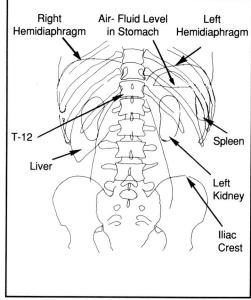

Erect AP   Fig. 3-46

• R or L marker and erect marker should be visible without superimposing essential anatomy

• Dorsal Decubitus (Lateral) Position

Abdomen
Optional
• PA Prone
• Lat. Decub. (AP)
• AP Erect
• **Dorsal Decub.(Lat.)**

Structures Best Shown:
Abnormal masses, accumulations of gas, air-fluid levels, aneurysms, calcification of aorta or other vessels and umbilical hernias.

Technical Factors:
- Film Size - 14 x 17 in. (35 x 43 cm) crosswise.
- Moving or stationary grid.
- 70-80 kVp range.

Patient Position:
- Supine on radiolucent pad, side against table or vertical grid device. (Secure cart so as not to move away from table or grid device.)
- Pillow under head, arms up beside head, provide support under partially flexed knees.

Shielding:
- Use gonadal shields on males.
- No pregnancies (unless contraindicated, use 10 day rule if possible).

Part Position:
- Adjust patient and cart so center of film and CR is **about 2 in. or 5 cm above level of iliac crest** (to include diaphragm).
- Insure **no rotation** of pelvis or shoulders. (Check that line between two ASIS is perpendicular to film.)
- Adjust height of film holder to align mid-axillary line to center line of film holder.

Central Ray:
- CR **horizontal,** to **center of film** (approximately 2 in. or 5 cm above iliac crest and about 1.5 in. or 4 cm posterior to level of ASIS).
- Minimum 40 (102 cm) SID.

Collimation: Collimate closely to abdomen soft tissue borders, especially upper and lower margins.

Respiration: Exposure made at end of **expiration**.

NOTE: May be taken as a right or left lateral; appropriate R or L lateral marker should be used indicating which side is against film. An arrow or other marker indicating up side should also be used.

Evaluation Criteria:
- Diaphragm should be well visualized.
- Collimation borders should be seen on long sides of radiograph on average or small patients without cutting off anterior or posterior aspects of abdomen.
- **No rotation**: Posterior ribs should be superimposed as well as R and L iliac wings and ASIS of pelvis.
- **No motion**: Diaphragm and gas bubble margins should appear sharp.
- Overall density and contrast scale should visualize soft tissue structures within abdomen, especially the ante-vertebral space for possible calcification of aorta and other vessels. Vertebral outlines should be clearly visible below diaphragm.
- Patient ID should be clear and legible and an arrow or other marker indicating the up side and a R or L lateral marker should be visible.

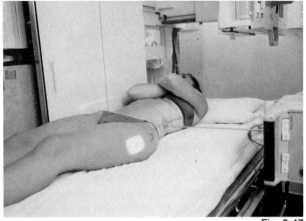

Dorsal Decub. (R Lat.)   Fig. 3-47

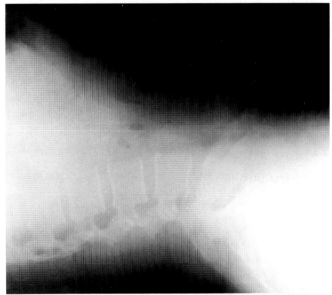

Dorsal Decub. (L Lat.)   Fig. 3-48

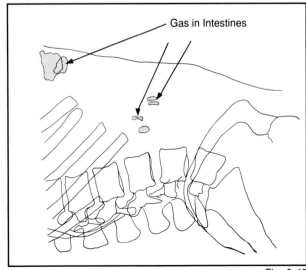

Gas in Intestines

Dorsal Decub. (L Lat.)   Fig. 3-49

Acute Abdominal Series
Three-way Abdomen

Acute Abdomen
(Three-way)
Basic
• **AP Recumbent**
• **AP Erect**
• **PA Chest**
Optional
• **Left Lat. Decub.**

Common Reasons for Acute Abdominal Series:
1. Perforated hollow viscus
2. Obstruction
3. Infection
4. Intra-abdominal mass
5. Post-op (abdominal surgery)

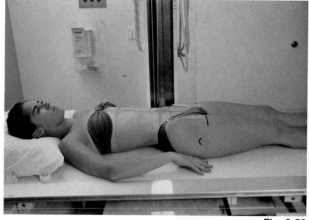

AP Supine   Fig. 3-50

Remember to take erect radiographs first if patient comes to the department in an erect position.

Film Holder, Collimation and Shielding:
• 14 x 17 in. (35 x 43 cm), moving or stationary grids. Collimation and shielding the same as described on preceding pages.

Patient and Part Positioning:
• Note that on the AP erect abdomen as described on a previous page, some routines include centering to the iliac crest to include the lower abdomen, **if** the erect PA chest is included to demonstrate possible free intra-abdominal air under the diaphragm.
• Other departmental routines include centering higher to include the diaphragm on erect abdomen radiographs even if a PA chest is included in the series. Some departments routinely include two erect abdomen films, one centered high for the diaphragm and a second centered lower to include the pubic symphysis. Each radiographer should know the preferred routine in his/her department.

Breathing Instructions:
• Chest taken on full inspiration, and abdomen on expiration.

Central Ray:
• Same as described on preceding pages.

NOTE: • Left lateral decubitus replaces erect position, if the patient is too ill to stand.
• **Horizontal beam** is necessary to visualize air-fluid levels.
• **Upright chest** best visualizes free air under diaphragm.
• Patient should be upright or on the side for decubitus for a minimum of **five minutes** before exposure.

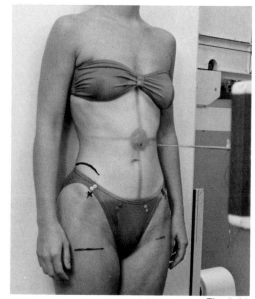

AP Erect   Fig. 3-51

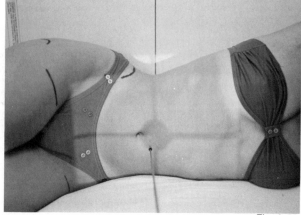

L Lat. Decub. (Optional)   Fig. 3-52

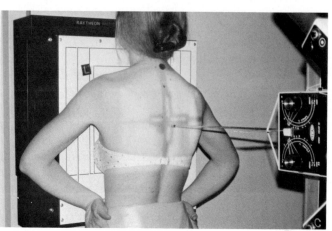

PA Chest Erect   Fig. 3-53

Acute Abdominal Series
Two-way Abdomen

Acute Abdomen
(Two-way)
Basic
• **AP Recumbent**
• **AP Erect**
(to include diaphragm)

Common Reasons for Acute Abdominal Series:
1. Perforated hollow viscus
2. Obstruction
3. Infection
4. Intra-abdominal mass
5. Post-op (abdominal surgery)

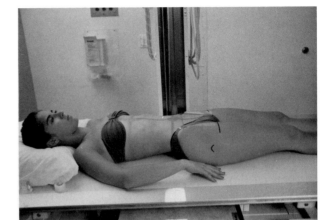

AP Supine   Fig. 3-54

Remember to take erect radiograph first if patient comes to the department in an erect position.

Technical Factors:
• Film Size - 14 x 17 in. (35 x 43 cm), moving or stationary grids.
• 70-80 kVp range.

Collimation and Shielding:
Collimation and shielding the same as described on preceding pages.

Patient and Part Positioning:
• Patient positioning and centering the same as described on preceding pages. For **AP supine, film holder should be centered to iliac crest,** and for **AP erect, 2 inches or more above crest to include diaphragm.**

Central Ray:
• Same as on preceding pages; **horizontal** CR must be used with erect abdomen.

Breathing Instructions:
• Exposures taken on **expiration**. Remember to insure that all breathing movements have stopped prior to making exposure.

NOTE: • The two-way abdomen may be taken as an alternative routine rather than the three-way abdomen for an acute abdominal series with above noted possible symptoms.
• With this two-way abdomen routine it is essential that the **diaphragm be included** on the erect abdomen radiograph. Some departments routinely also take a second erect abdomen centered lower to include the pubic symphysis.

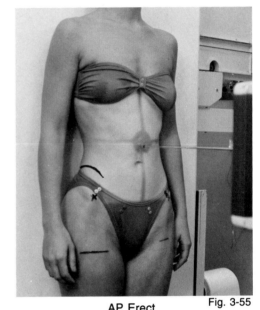

AP Erect   Fig. 3-55
(to include diaphragm)

Evaluation Criteria:
See previous pages for correct evaluation of these radiographs.

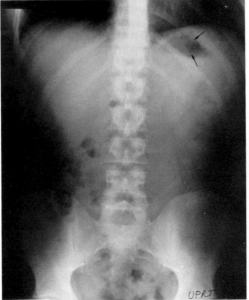

Fig. 3-56
AP Erect

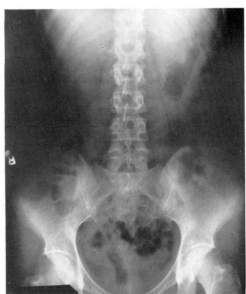

Fig. 3-57
AP Supine

Chapter 4
Radiographic Anatomy and Positioning of the Upper Limb

Contributions by: John Lampignano, MA, RT (R)
Kathy Martensen, RT (R)

Contents

Part I Radiographic Anatomy

Upper Limb (Extremity)

The bones of the upper limb are divided into four main groups; hand and wrist, forearm, humerus, and shoulder girdle. The first group; the hand and wrist, and the second group; the forearm and the elbow including the distal humerus, are described and illustrated on drawings and radiographs in this chapter. Each of the bones, their shape and structure, as well as the articulates or joints of the upper limb must be thoroughly understood by radiographers to be able to identify and demonstrate each part on radiographs.

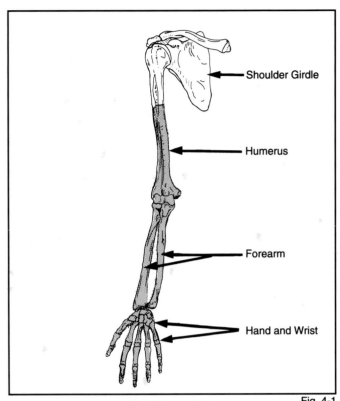

Right Upper Limb
(Anterior View)
Fig. 4-1

Hand and Wrist

The 27 bones on one hand and wrist are divided into three groups:

1. Phalanges (fingers and thumb)	14
2. Metacarpals (palm)	5
3. Carpals (wrist)	8
Total	27

The most distal bones of the hand are the **phalanges**, *(fa-lan´jez)* which make up the digits (fingers and thumb). The second group of bones are the **metacarpals,** *(met´ah-kar´pals)* which make up the palm of each hand. The third group of bones, the **carpals,** *(kar'pals)* compose the bones of the wrist.

Phalanges - Fingers and Thumb (digits)

Each finger and thumb is called a digit, and each digit consists of two or three separate small bones called phalanges [singular is **phalanx** *(fa´lanks)*]. The digits are numbered starting with the thumb as number one and ending with the little finger as digit number five.

Each of the four fingers (digits two, three, four and five) are made up of three phalanges: the **proximal, middle and distal.** The thumb, or first digit, has just two phalanges, the **proximal and distal**.

Metacarpals (palm)

The second group of bones of the hand, making up the palm, are the five metacarpals. These bones are numbered in the same way the digits are numbered, with the first metacarpal being on the thumb or lateral side when the hand is in the anatomical position.

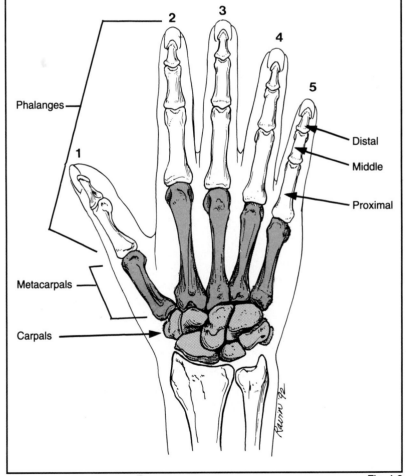

Left Hand & Wrist (Posterior View)   Fig. 4-2

Joints of the Hand

The joints or articulations between the individual bones of the upper limb are important in radiology because small chip fractures may occur near the joint spaces. Therefore, accurate identification of all joints of the phalanges and metacarpals of the hand is required.

Thumb (first digit): The thumb has only two phalanges, so the joint between them is called the **interphalangeal** or **IP joint**. The joint between the first metacarpal and the proximal phalanx of the thumb is called the **first metacarpophalangeal** or **MP joint**. Note that the name of this joint consists of the names of the two bones making up this joint. The proximal bone is named first, followed by the name of the distal bone.

Fingers (second through fifth digits): The second through fifth digits have three phalanges, therefore they would also have three joints each. Starting from the most distal portion of each digit, the joints are the **distal interphalangeal** or **DIP joint,** then the **proximal interphalangeal** or **PIP joint** and, most proximally, the **metacarpophalangeal** or **MP joint.**

Metacarpals. The metacarpals articulate with the phalanges at their distal ends and are called **metacarpophalangeal** or **MP joints.** At the proximal end, the metacarpals articulate with the respective carpals and are called **carpometacarpal** or **CM joints.**

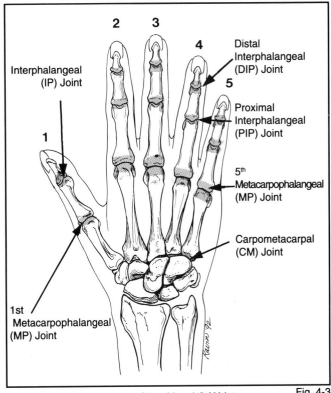

Joints of the Hand & Wrist   Fig. 4-3

Review Exercise with Radiograph

In identifying joints and phalanges of the hand, it is important to remember that the specific digit and hand must be included in descriptions. A radiograph of a hand *(Fig. 4-4)* demonstrates the phalanges and metacarpals as well as the joints that have been described above. A good review exercise includes covering up the answers below while identifying each part labelled A-R on this radiograph.

A. Carpometacarpal joint of first digit of right hand
B. First metacarpal of right hand
C. Metacarpophalangeal joint of first digit of right hand
D. Proximal phalanx of the first digit (or thumb) of right hand
E. Interphalangeal joint of first digit (or thumb) of right hand
F. Distal phalanx of first digit (or thumb) of right hand
G. Second metacarpophalangeal joint of right hand
H. Proximal phalanx of second digit of right hand
I. Proximal interphalangeal joint of second digit of right hand
J. Middle phalanx of second digit of right hand
K. Distal interphalangeal joint of second digit of right hand
L. Distal phalanx of third digit of right hand
M. Middle phalanx of fourth digit of right hand
N. Distal interphalangeal joint of fifth digit of right hand
O. Proximal phalanx of third digit of right hand
P. Fifth metacarpophalangeal joint of right hand
Q. Fourth metacarpal of right hand
R. Fifth carpometacarpal joint of right hand

NOTE: Radiographs of the limbs such as the hands or feet are generally placed on an illuminator with the fingers or toes up, as in *Fig. 4-4* and on succeeding pages.

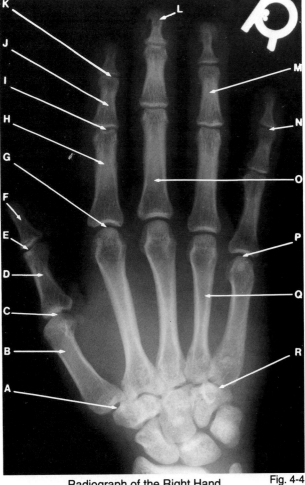

Radiograph of the Right Hand   Fig. 4-4

Carpals (wrist)

Following the phalanges (digits-fingers and thumbs), and the metacarpals (palm), are the third group of bones of the hand and wrist, the **carpals** or bones of the wrist. It is easiest to learn the names of the eight carpals by dividing them into two rows of four each.

Proximal row: Beginning on the lateral or thumb side is the **scaphoid,** *(skaf´oid)* sometimes referred to as the navicular. It should be noted that one of the tarsal bones of the foot is also sometimes called the navicular or scaphoid. However, correct terminology for the tarsal bone of the **foot** is **navicular** and the carpal bone of the **wrist** is **scaphoid.**

The **scaphoid,** a boat shaped bone, is the largest bone in the proximal row and **articulates with the radius proximally.** Its location and articulation with the forearm make it important radiographically because it is one of the most frequently fractured carpal bones.

The **lunate** (moon shaped) is the second carpal in the proximal row and **also articulates with the radius.** It is distinguished by its deep concavity on its distal surface where it articulates with the capitate of the distal row of carpals.

The **third** carpal is the **triquetrum** *(tri-kwe´trum)* which is distinguished by its pyramidal shape and its articulation with the small pisiform anteriorly.

The **pisiform** *(pi´si-form)* (pea shaped) is the smallest of the carpal bones and is located anteriorly to the triquetrum as most evident in the anterior view *(Fig. 4-6)* and the carpal canal view in *Fig. 4-7.*

Distal Row: The second more distal row of four carpals articulate with the five metacarpal bones distally. Starting again on the lateral or thumb side is the **trapezium,** *(trah-pe´ze-um)* a somewhat irregularly shaped bone located between the scaphoid medially and the first metacarpal distally. Next is the wedge shaped **trapezoid,** *(trap´e-zoid)* the smallest bone in the distal row. This is followed by the largest of the carpal bones, the **capitate,** *(kap´i-tat)* or Os Magnum meaning large bone. It can also be remembered by its large rounded head which proximally fits into a concavity formed by the scaphoid and lunate bones.

The last carpal in the distal row is the **hamate** *(ham´ate)* which is easily distinguished by the hook-like process called the **hamulus** *(ham´u-lus)* or hamular process projecting from its palmar surface which can readily be palpated. *(See Fig. 4-7.)*

Carpal Canal

Figure 4-7 is a drawing of the carpals as they would appear looking tangentially down the wrist and arm from the palm or volar side of a hyperextended wrist. This drawing demonstrates the carpal canal formed by the concave anterior or palmar aspect of the carpals. The anteriorly located pisiform and the hamulus process of the hamate are best visualized on this view. The term hamate means hooked, describing the shape of the hamate as seen in the drawing. The trapezium and its relationship to the thumb and trapezoid is well demonstrated.

Summary Chart of Carpal Terminology

The preferred terms as listed will be used throughout this text. Secondary terms listed as synonyms in this chart are terms commonly used in earlier literature.

The names of these eight carpals may be more easily remembered by utilizing the mnemonic on the right.

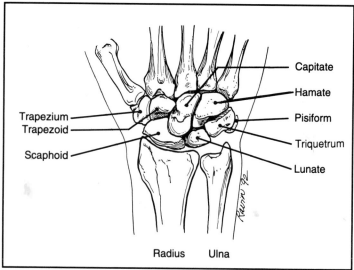

Right Carpals (Dorsal or Posterior View)   Fig. 4-5

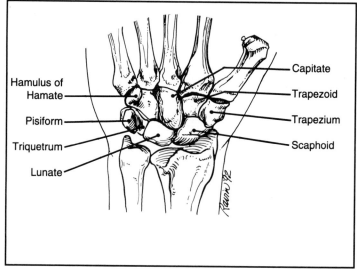

Right Carpals (Palmar or Anterior View)   Fig. 4-6

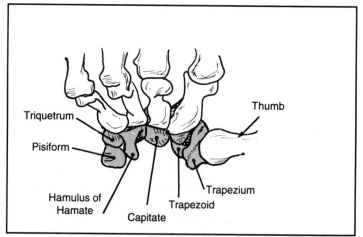

Carpal Canal   Fig. 4-7

Mnenonic	Preferred Term	Synonyms
Send	Scaphoid	(Navicular)
Letter	Lunate	(Semilunar)
To	Triquetrum	(Triangular or Cuneiform)
Peter	Pisiform	
To	Trapezium	(Greater Multangular)
Tell (him to)	Trapezoid	(Lesser Multangular)
Come	Capitate	(Os Magnum)
Home	Hamate	(Unciform)

Carpals continued

Review Exercise with Radiographs

Five projections for the wrist are shown in *Fig. 4-8* through *4-12*. A good review exercise is to cover up the answers below and identify each of the carpal bones as labeled. Then check your answers with those listed below.

Note in the lateral position *(Fig. 4-12)* that the trapezium and the scaphoid are located more anteriorly. Note also that the ulnar flexion best demonstrates the scaphoid without the foreshortening and overlapping as seen on the PA. The radial flexion best demonstrates the interspaces and the carpals on the ulnar (lateral) side of the wrist, namely (H) the hamate, (C) and (D) the triquetrum and pisiform respectively, and (B) the lunate. The outline of the end-on view of the hamulus process of the hamate (h) can also be seen on this radial flexion radiograph. This hamulus process is also demonstrated well on the carpal canal projection of *Fig. 4-11,* as is the hook-like process of (D) the pisiform.

A. Scaphoid
B. Lunate
C. Triquetrum
D. Pisiform
E. Trapezium
F. Trapezoid
G. Capitate
H. Hamate
h. Hamulus (hamular process) of hamate

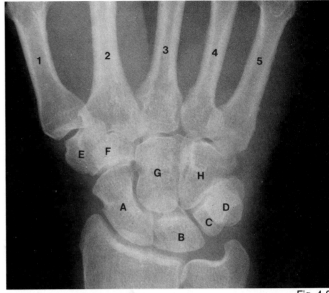

PA Wrist   Fig. 4-8

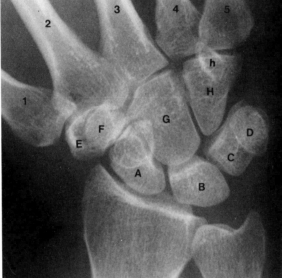
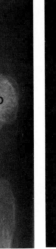

Radial Flexion   Fig. 4-9

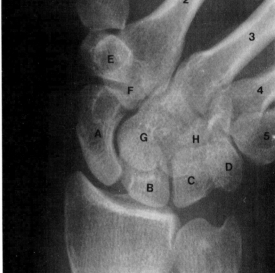

Ulnar Flexion   Fig. 4-10

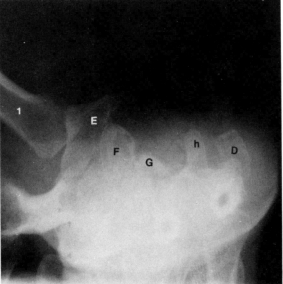

Carpal Canal   Fig. 4-11

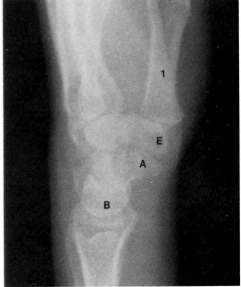

Lateral   Fig. 4-12

Forearm - Radius and Ulna

The second group of upper limb bones are those of the forearm, namely the **radius** on the lateral or thumb side and the **ulna** on the medial side.

Starting at the distal forearm or wrist joint are small conical projections termed **styloid processes**, located at the extreme distal end of both the radius and the ulna *(Fig.4-14)*. The radial styloid process can be palpated on the thumb side of the wrist joint. The radial styloid process extends more distally than does the ulnar styloid process.

The **ulnar notch** is a small depression on the medial aspect of the distal radius. The head of the ulna fits into the ulnar notch.

The **head of the ulna** is located near the wrist at the **distal** end of the ulna. When the hand is pronated, the ulnar head and styloid process are easily felt and seen on the little finger side of the distal forearm.

The **head of the radius** is located at the **proximal** end of the radius near the elbow joint. The long midportion of both the radius and the ulna is termed the **shaft** or **body**.

The radius is the shorter of the two bones of the forearm and is the only one of the two directly involved in the wrist joint. During the act of pronation, the radius is the bone that rotates around the more stationary ulna.

The proximal radius demonstrates the round disc-like **head**, and the **neck** of the radius, a tapered constricted area directly below the head. The rough oval process on the medial and anterior side of the radius, just distal to the neck, is the **radial tuberosity**.

Proximal Ulna *(Fig. 4-15)*

The ulna is the longer of the two bones of the forearm and is primarily involved in the formation of the elbow joint. The two beak-like processes of the proximal ulna are termed the **olecranon** and **coronoid processes**. The olecranon process can be easily palpated on the posterior aspect of the elbow joint.

The medial margin of the coronoid process opposite the radial notch is commonly referred to as the **coronoid tubercle**. (See AP elbow radiograph in *Fig 4-19*).

The large, concave depression or notch articulating with the distal humerus is the **trochlear** *(trok´le-ar)* **notch** (semilunar notch). The small, shallow depression located on the lateral aspect of the proximal ulna is the **radial** *(ra´de-al)* **notch.** The head of the radius articulates with the ulna at the radial notch. This joint or articulation is the proximal radio-ulnar joint that combines with the distal radio-ulnar joint to allow rotation of the forearm during pronation. During the act of pronation the radius crosses over the ulna near the upper third of the forearm (see page 108).

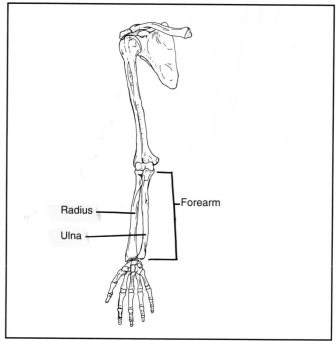

Right Upper Limb (Anterior View)   Fig. 4-13

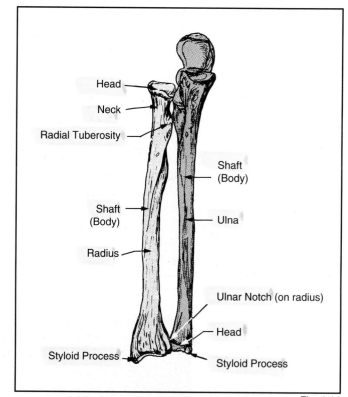

Right - Radius and Ulna (Anterior View)   Fig. 4-14

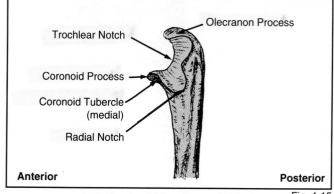

Left Proximal Ulna (Lateral View)   Fig. 4-15

Distal Humerus

The parts of the proximal humerus are covered in chapter five with the shoulder girdle. The mid and distal humerus however, are included in this chapter as part of the elbow joint.

The **shaft** or body of the humerus is the long center section, and the expanded distal end of the humerus is the **humeral condyle**. The articular portion of the humeral condyle is divided into two parts, the **trochlea** *(trok'le-ah)* and the **capitulum** *(kah-pit'u-lum)*.

The **trochlea** (meaning pulley) is shaped like a pulley or spool with two rim-like outer margins, and a depressed center portion called the **trochlear sulcus** or groove. This depression of the trochlea appears circular on a lateral end-on view, and on a lateral elbow radiograph appears as a less dense (more radiolucent) area as seen in *Figs. 4-17* and *4-20*. The trochlea is located more medially and articulates with the **ulna**.

The **capitulum**, meaning "little head," which in earlier literature was called **capitellum**, *(kap"i-tel'um)* is located on the lateral aspect articulating with the head of the **radius**. (A memory aid is to associate the **cap**itulum, "cap" with the "head" of the radius.)

The articular surface making up the rounded articular margin of the capitulum is smaller than that of the trochlea as seen in *Fig. 4-18*. This becomes significant in evaluating for a true lateral position of the elbow, as does also the direct superimposition of the two **epicondyles** *(ep"e-kon'dils)*.

The **lateral epicondyle** is that small projection on the lateral aspect of the distal humerus above the capitulum. The medial epicondyle is larger and more prominent than the lateral and is located on the medial edge of the distal humerus proximal to the trochlea. In a true lateral position, the directly superimposed epicondyles (which are difficult to recognize) are seen to be just proximal to the circular appearance of the trochlear sulcus *(Figs. 4-17* and *4-20)*.

The distal humerus has specific **depressions** on both the anterior and posterior surfaces. The two shallow **anterior depressions** are the **coronoid fossa** and the **radial fossa** *(Figs. 4-16 and 17)*. As the elbow is completely flexed, the coronoid process and the radial head are received by these respective fossa, as the names indicate.

The deep **posterior depression** is the **olecranon fossa**. The olecranon process of the ulna fits into this depression when the arm is fully extended. Soft tissue detail by way of specific fat pads located within the deep olecranon fossa is important in trauma diagnosis of the elbow joint.

The lateral view of the elbow clearly demonstrates specific parts of the proximal radius and ulna. The **head** and **neck** of the radius are well demonstrated, as are the **radial tuberosity** (partially seen on the anterior aspect of the proximal radius) and the large concave **trochlear (semilunar) notch.**

True Lateral Elbow: Specific positions such as an accurate lateral with **90° flexion** with possible associated visualization of fat pads are essential for evaluation of joint pathology for the elbow. A good criteria or a good means of evaluating for a true lateral position of the elbow when flexed 90° is the appearance of the three concentric arcs, as labeled in *Fig. 4-18*. The first and smallest arc is the **trochlear sulcus**. The second intermediate arc appears double-lined as the outer ridges or rounded edges of the **capitulum** and **trochlea**.[1] The **trochlear notch of the ulna** appears as a third arc of a true lateral elbow. If the elbow is even slightly rotated from a **true** lateral, these arcs will not appear aligned in this way and the elbow joint space will not be as completely open.

---

[1] Berquist, TH; **Imaging of Orthopedic Trauma and Surgery**; W. B. Saunders; 1986; pp 583-584.

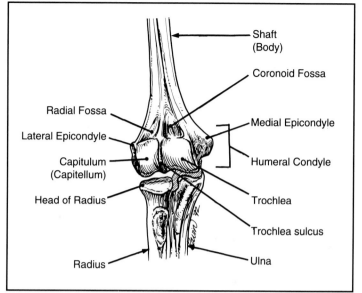

Distal Humerus (Anterior View)   Fig. 4-16

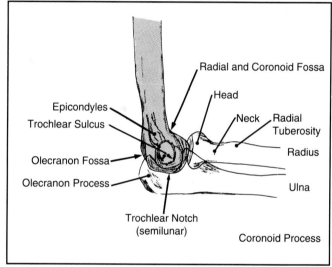

Lateral Elbow   Fig. 4-17

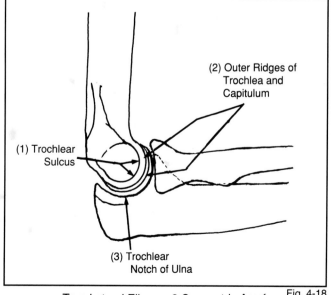

True Lateral Elbow – 3 Concentric Arcs[1]   Fig. 4-18

Radiographs of Elbow

These AP and lateral radiographs of the elbow provide a review of anatomy and demonstrate the three concentric arcs as evidence of a true lateral position.

A. Medial epicondyle   E. Capitulum
B. Trochlea   F. Lateral epicondyle
C. Coronoid tubercle
D. Radial head

H. Superimposed epicondyles of humerus
I. Trochlear sulcus (1st or smallest arc)
J. Trochlear notch (3rd arc)
K. Olecranon process
L. Outer ridge of trochlea (which along with outer ridge of capitulum appears as a second double-lined arc)
M. Coronoid process   O. Radial Neck
N. Radial head   P. Radial tuberosity

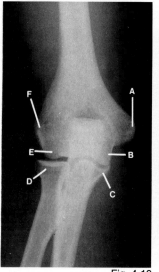
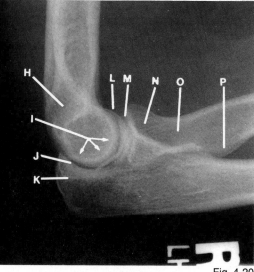

AP   **Fig. 4-19**   Lateral   **Fig. 4-20**

Classification of Joints

A general description of joints or articulations with the various classifications and movement types is described in Chapter one. These will be reviewed and described more specifically for each joint of the hand, wrist, forearm and elbow.

Classification and Movement Types

All joints of the human body are divided into three possible classifications according to the type of tissue which separates the ends of bones of these joints. These three classifications are **fibrous joints, cartilaginous joints** and **synovial joints.** All joints of the hand, wrist, forearm and elbow are classified as **synovial joints,** characterized by a fibrous capsule containing synovial fluid.

Joints are also described and classified according to their mobility or lack of mobility. The three mobility types are **synarthrosis** (immovable), **amphiarthrosis** (limited movement) and **diarthrosis** (freely movable). All synovial type joints enclosed by a fibrous capsule containing synovial fluid are by the nature of their structure **freely movable** or **diarthrodial**.

Joints are further divided into various sub groups according to descriptions of their movement types. These possible six movement types are **gliding, hinge, pivot, condyloid, saddle** and **ball and socket joints.** Since all joints to be described in this chapter are classified as synovial and freely movable or diarthrodial type, only the movement types differ.

Hand and Wrist

Interphalangeal (IP) Joints: Beginning distally with the phalanges, all interphalangeal joints are **hinge type** joints with movements in two directions only, **flexion** and **extension**. This movement is in one plane only, around the **transverse axis**. This includes the single interphalangeal joint of the thumb (1st digit), and the distal and proximal interphalangeal joints of the fingers (2nd-5th digits).

Metacarpophalangeal (MP) Joints: The second through fifth metacarpophalangeal joints (the base of the fingers) are **condyloid type** joints that allow movement in four directions, **flexion, extension, abduction** and **adduction. Circumduction** movement also occurs at these joints which is a cone-like sequential movement of these four directions. Both the first metacarpophalangeal and the first carpometacarpal (MP) joints of the thumb are **saddle type** joints. The best example of the saddle joint is the first carpometacarpal joint as this best demonstrates the shape and the movements of a saddle joint. The first metacarpopha-

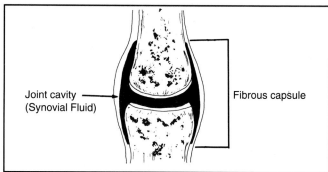

Joint cavity (Synovial Fluid)   Fibrous capsule

Synovial Joints (Diarthrodial - Freely Moveable)   **Fig. 4-21**

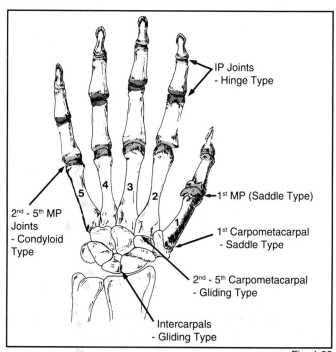

IP Joints - Hinge Type

2nd - 5th MP Joints - Condyloid Type

1st MP (Saddle Type)

1st Carpometacarpal - Saddle Type

2nd - 5th Carpometacarpal - Gliding Type

Intercarpals - Gliding Type

Joints of the Hand & Wrist (Posterior view)   **Fig. 4-22**

langeal joint is also classified as a saddle joint although it is not as good an example.

The second through fifth carpometacarpal joints are **gliding type** or plane joints, which allow the least amount of movement of the synovial class joints. The joint surfaces are flat or slightly curved with movement limited by a tight fibrous capsule. The intercarpal joints between the various carpals also only have a **gliding type** movement.

Classification of Joints continued

Wrist Joint

The wrist joint is a **condyloid-type** joint. Of the two bones of the forearm, only the radius articulates directly with carpal bones. This articulation is therefore called the **radiocarpal** joint. The two carpals directly involved in the radiocarpal joint are the **scaphoid** and the **lunate**. The **triquetral** bone, however, is also part of the wrist joint in that it is opposite the **articular disk**. The articular disk is part of the articulation or joint between the distal radius and ulna of the forearm, called the **distal radio-ulnar joint**. The wrist joint proper therefore includes both the articulation between the radius and the carpal bones (radiocarpal joint) as well as the distal radio-ulnar articulation which also involves the articular disk and the triquetrum.

The total wrist joint is enclosed by an articular capsule strengthened by numerous radiocarpal ligaments which allow movements in four directions plus circumduction.

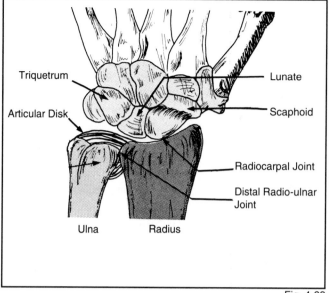

Left Wrist Joint (Posterior View)   Fig. 4-23

Elbow Joint

The elbow joint is generally considered a **hinge type** (ginglymus) joint with flexion and extension movements between the humerus, and the ulna and radius. The complete elbow joint, however, includes three joints enclosed in one articular capsule. In addition to the hinge joints between the humerus and ulna and the humerus and radius, the proximal radio-ulnar joint (pivot type) is also considered part of the elbow joint.

Summary of Hand, Wrist, Forearm and Elbow Joints

Classification: *Synovial* (Articular capsule containing synovial fluid)

Mobility Type: *Diarthrodial* (freely movable)

Movement Type:

1. Interphalangeal joints   - **Hinge** (ginglymus)

2. Metacarpophalangeal joints
    First digit (thumb)   - **Saddle** (sellar)
    Second-fifth digits   - **Condyloid**

3. Carpometacarpal joints
    First digit (thumb)   - **Saddle** (sellar)
    Second-fifth digits   - **Gliding** (plane)

4. Intercarpal joints   - **Gliding** (plane)

5. Radiocarpal joint   - **Condyloid**

6. Proximal and Distal
    Radio-ulnar joints   - **Pivot** (Trochoidal)

7. Elbow joint
    Humero-ulnar
       and   }   - **Hinge** (ginglymus)
    Humeroradial
    Proximal radio-ulnar   - **Pivot**

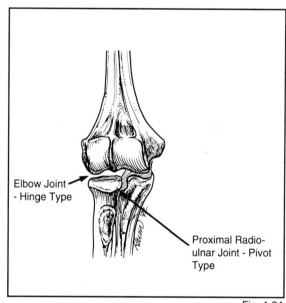

Elbow Joint   Fig. 4-24

Wrist Joint Movement Terminology

Certain terminology involving movements of the wrist joint may be confusing but need to be understood by radiographers because special projections of the wrist are described by these movements. These terms are **ulnar flexion** or **radial deviation** and **radial flexion** or **ulnar deviation**.

The term flexion is described in Chapter One under Terminology as a "bending of a joint wherein the angle between the parts is decreased". Usual flexion of the wrist joint involves the anterior surface of the wrist and is a forward bending wherein the angle between the anterior hand and forearm is decreased.

Ulnar or radial flexion involves a **lateral bending** at the wrist joint. If the hand is forced toward the ulnar side of the forearm with the hand pronated, the wrist joint near the distal ulna will be flexed wherein the angle between the lateral aspect of the hand and forearm is decreased. This motion, termed **ulnar flexion** or **radial deviation**, serves to open up the carpal joints on the opposite side of the wrist. The carpals best demonstrated in this position are those located most medially when the hand is pronated, namely the scaphoid, trapezium and trapezoid. This motion is most often used to obtain a better view of the **scaphoid**.

If the hand is forced toward the radial or thumb side of the forearm with the hand pronated, the wrist joint near the distal radius will be flexed laterally. This motion, termed **radial flexion** or **ulnar deviation**, serves to open up the carpal joints on the lateral or little finger side of the wrist. The carpals best demonstrated are the lunate, triquetrum, pisiform and hamate. This motion is used most often to better demonstrate the **lunate**.

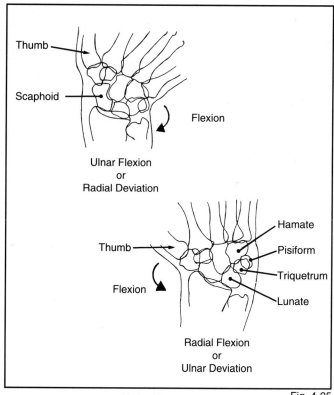

Wrist Movements   Fig. 4-25

Forearm Rotational Movements

The radio-ulnar joints of the forearm also involve some special rotational movements which need to be understood in radiographing the forearm. For example the **forearm generally should not be radiographed in a pronated position (a PA projection)** which may appear to be the most natural position for the forearm and hand. The forearm is rather routinely radiographed in an **AP projection** with the hand **supinated**, or palm up. The reason becomes clear in studying the "cross over" position of the radius and ulna when the hand is pronated. This results from the unique pivot-type rotational movements of the forearm involving both the proximal and distal radio-ulnar joints.

Therefore, to prevent superimposition of the radius and ulna resulting from these pivot-type rotational movements, the forearm is radiographed with the hand supinated for an AP projection.

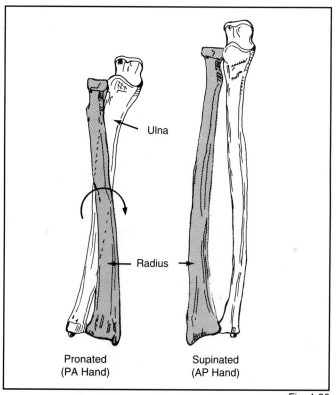

Forearm Rotational Movements   Fig. 4-26

Part II Radiographic Positioning

General Positioning Considerations

Radiographic examinations involving the upper limb are generally done with the patient seated sideways at the end of the table in a position that is not strained or uncomfortable. An extended table top as is shown in *Fig. 4-27* may make this a little more comfortable, especially if the patient is in a wheelchair. The patient should also be turned away from the x-ray beam and the body positioned out of the region of scatter radiation as much as possible. The height of the table top should be near shoulder height so the arm can be fully supported as shown.

Trauma Patients: Trauma patients can be radiographed on the table or taken directly on the cart as shown in *Fig. 4-28*. The patient should be moved to one side to provide the necessary space on the cart for the cassette. Sand bags, radiolucent blocks and/or other support devices may be used to provide support and prevent motion.

Distance

A common minimum SID (source-image receptor distance) is 40 in. or 102 cm. When radiographing with cassettes directly on the table top, to maintain a constant SID the tube height must be increased as compared to radiographs taken with the cassette in the Bucky tray. This difference is generally 3-4 in. (8-10 cm) for floating type table tops. The same minimum 40 in. (102 cm) SID should also be used when radiographing directly on the cart, unless exposure factors are adjusted to compensate for a change in SID.

NOTE: See page 35 for a discussion on the minimal 40 in. (102 cm) SID.

Gonadal Shielding

Gonadal shielding is important for exams of the upper limb because of the proximity of the gonads to the divergent x-ray beam as well as scatter radiation. This is true for those patients seated at the end of the table as well as those trauma patients taken on the cart. Therefore a lead vinyl covered shield should be draped over the patient's lap or gonadal area as shown in *Figs. 4-27* and *28*. Even though the gonadal rule states this should be done on patients of reproductive age (50 or younger) when the gonads lie within or close to the primary field, it is a good practice to provide gonadal shielding for all patients.

Collimation, General Positioning and Markers

The collimation rule should again be followed, namely that **collimation borders should be visible on all four sides if the film is large enough to allow this without cutting off essential anatomy**. A general rule however, concerning film size is to **use the smallest film size possible for the specific part being radiographed.** Four-sided collimation is generally possible however, even with a minimal size film for most if not all radiographic exams of the upper limb.

Two or more projections may be taken on one film. This requires close collimation.

A general positioning rule especially applicable to the upper limbs is to **always place the long axis of the part being radiographed parallel to the long axis of the film.** If more than one projection is taken on the same film, the part should be parallel to the long axis of the part of the film being used. Also, **all body parts should be oriented in the same direction** when two or more projections are taken on the same film.

Correct placement of patient ID information and side markers within the collimation borders must be demonstrated on each radiograph.

Correct Centering

Accurate centering and alignment of the body part to the film and correct central ray location is especially important for exams of the upper limb where shape and size distortion must be avoided and the narrow joint spaces clearly demonstrated. Therefore the part being radiographed should be **parallel to the plane of the cassette, the central ray should be 90° or perpendicular** and should be **directed to the correct centering point** as indicated on each positioning page. (There are exceptions to the 90° perpendicular rule as indicated in the specific positioning pages which follow.)

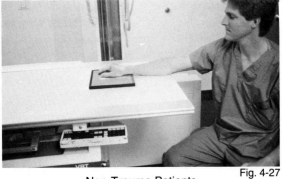

Non-Trauma Patients   Fig. 4-27

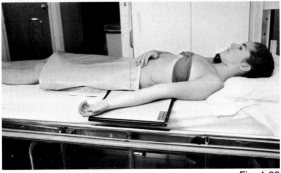

Trauma Patients   Fig. 4-28

Exposure Factors

The principal exposure factors for radiographs of the upper limbs are:
1. Lower to medium kVp (50-70)
2. Short exposure time
3. Small focal spot
4. Adequate mAs for sufficient density

Correctly exposed radiographs of the upper limbs should visualize soft tissue margins and fine trabecular markings of all bones being radiographed.

Cassettes

Cassettes with intensifying screens are used. Single screen and single emulsion film are common and used for adult extremities to achieve better recorded detail. Grids are not generally used for the upper limbs unless the body part, (such as the shoulder) measures more than 10 cm. (Some references suggest a grid for over 13 cm.)

Increase Exposure with Cast:

An upper limb with a cast will require an increase in exposure. The thickness of the cast and the body part will affect the increase in exposure required. A recommended general conversion guide for casts is as follows:

• Small to medium dry plaster cast:	- increase 5-7 kVp.

• Large or wet
   plaster cast:
	- double mAs **or**
	   increase 8-10 kVp.

• Fiberglass cast:	- increase 3-4 kVp.

National Survey

Departmental standard and optional operating procedures (departmental routines) for exams of the upper limb were very consistent throughout the United States. This was determined by the results of a survey completed to determine national norms for such standard and optional operating procedures.

Hand Routine

Hand	U.S. Average	
	Basic	Optional
• PA	90%	
• Obl.¹ without block (digits not parallel)	68%	
or Obl. with block (digits parallel)	35%	(7%)
• Lateral (fan lat.)	62%	(11%)
or Lateral (fingers superimposed)	29%	(20%)

¹ Not recommended or demonstrated in this text for a routine oblique hand position.

Wrist Routine

Wrist	U.S. Average	
	Basic	Optional
• PA	96%	
• Oblique (45°)	94%	
• Lateral	98%	
• Ulnar Flex.	24%	(47%)
• Carpal Canal		(20%)
• Radial Flex.		(19%)
• Carpal Bridge		(15%)
• Stecher		(5%)

Finger Routine

Fingers	U.S. Average	
	Basic	Optional
• PA¹ (finger only)	57%	(5%)
or PA¹ (entire hand)	43%	(11%)
• Lateral	94%	
• Oblique	87%	
Thumb		
• AP	93%	
• Lateral	94%	
• Obl.¹ (thumb only)	58%	(5%)
or Obl.¹ (include PA hand)	35%	(8%)

¹ Both options covered in this text.

Forearm Routine

Forearm	U.S. Average	
	Basic	Optional
• AP	99%	
• Lateral	99%	
• Oblique		(5%)

Elbow Routine

Elbow	U.S. Average	
	Basic	Optional
• AP	99%	
• Lateral	98%	
• Oblique	72%	
• Coyle Trauma Method	8%	(20%)
• Jones Method		(3%)

Summary

One revealing and unexpected result of this survey was the indicated routine for the **oblique hand**. Sixty-eight percent indicated their routine to be without the use of a block or support for the thumb and fingers wherein the digits are not parallel to the film. However, this is not the recommended method as described in this text for a routine oblique hand. Rather, the routine oblique hand in this chapter includes the use of a radiolucent step block or wedge block supporting the digits in a 45° oblique position **parallel to the film** to better demonstrate the phalanges.

For the wrist and elbow, the results for routine and most common optional projections/positions were consistent throughout the U.S.

Survey Questions on Long Bone Exams

One of the questions on the survey asked for the department routine when radiographing long bones such as the forearm, humerus, leg or femur. The results were as follows:

_84%_ a. **Both** joints of the long bone in question are to be included and clearly visible on the film.

_12%_ b. Only **one joint nearest the injury** is to be well visualized on film (joint to be 1.5 to 2 in. from any end of film).

_4%_ c. Other _(write-ins)_

There was a significant difference in the percentage selecting **b** rather than **a** between various regions of the U.S. Twenty percent (20%) of western states selected **b**, but only 10% of eastern and midwestern states for a total average of 12%. This indicates that twice as many departments in the west include only one joint as routine compared to the east and midwest. However, since the majority of departments throughout the U.S. routinely include both joints, this will be the recommended routine in this text. An alternate routine including only one joint will also be described.

Humerus Routine

Humerus	U.S. Average	
(Non-Trauma Routine)	Basic	Optional
• AP	99%	
• Rotational Lateral	98%	
Humerus (Trauma Routine - possible fracture or dislocation)		
• AP (Neutral Rotation)	98%	
• Lateral (Mid & Distal)	59%	
• Transthoracic Lat. (proximal)	60%	(23%)
Chapter 5		
• Scapular Y (proximal)	17%	(21%)

Summary
The routines for the **non-trauma humerus** were very consistent with a non-trauma routine of an **AP** and a **rotational lateral**.

The trauma routine for the mid and proximal humerus is not as clear. The projections for the proximal humerus are related more to shoulder projections and routines and in this text these are included in Chapter 5 with the proximal humerus and shoulder girdle.

Standard and Optional Operating Procedures

Certain basic and optional projections or positions for the hand, wrist, forearm and elbow are demonstrated and described on the following pages as suggested standard and optional departmental procedures.

Basic Projections
Standard or basic projections, also sometimes referred to as routine projections or departmental routines are **those projections or positions commonly taken on average patients who are helpful and can cooperate in performing the procedure**.

Optional Projections
Optional projections are those **more common projections or positions taken as extra or additional projections to better demonstrate certain pathologic conditions or specific body parts**. (This does not mean they are optional as to whether or not they are important, or whether or not they need to be learned and mastered.)

Basic and Optional Projections

Fingers
Basic
• PA
• Oblique
• Lateral

Thumb
Basic
• AP
• Lateral
• Oblique

Hand
Basic
• PA
• Oblique
• Lateral

Wrist
Basic
• PA
• Oblique
• Lateral

Wrist
Optional
• Ulnar Flex.
• Radial Flex.
• Carpal Canal
• Carpal Bridge

Forearm
Basic
• AP
• Lateral

Wrist & Forearm
(Post Reduction in Cast)
• PA
• Lateral

Elbow
Basic
• AP
• Oblique
• Lateral

Elbow
Optional
• Acute Flexion
(Jones Position)
• Coyle Trauma Method
• Radial Head Projections

Humerus
Basic
• AP
• Rotational Lateral

Humerus
(Trauma Routine)
Basic
• AP Neutral Rotation
• Lateral (Mid or Distal)
(Proximal Humerus - Ch. 5)

• PA Projection

Fingers
Basic
• **PA**
• Oblique
• Lateral

Structures Best Shown:
Distal, middle and proximal phalanges, distal metacarpal and associated joints.

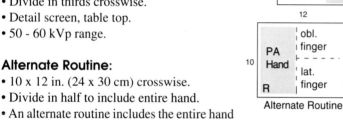

Technical Factors:
• Film Size - 8 x 10 in. (18 x 24 cm).
• Divide in thirds crosswise.
• Detail screen, table top.
• 50 - 60 kVp range.

Alternate Routine:
• 10 x 12 in. (24 x 30 cm) crosswise.
• Divide in half to include entire hand.
• An alternate routine includes the entire hand for the PA projection of the finger for possible secondary trauma or pathology to other aspects of the hand and wrist. Oblique and lateral projections would be of affected finger only.

Patient Position:
• Patient seated at end of table with elbow flexed about 90° with hand and forearm resting on table.

Shielding:
Place lead shield over patient's lap.

Part Position:
• Pronate hand with fingers extended.
• Center and align long axis of affected finger to long axis of unmasked portion of cassette.
• Separate adjoining fingers from affected finger.

Central Ray:
• CR **perpendicular** to film, directed to **proximal interphalangeal (PIP) joint.**
• Minimum 40 in. (102 cm) SID.

Collimation:
Collimate on four sides to area of affected finger.

Evaluation Criteria:
• Entire finger in question (distal, middle and proximal phalanges) and approximately the distal one-third of metacarpal should be included, with collimation visible on all four sides.
• The center of the collimation field should be at the PIP joint.
• Long axis of finger should be aligned to long axis of portion of film being used.
• No rotation of fingers as evidenced by:
  - The symmetrical appearance of both sides or concavities of the shafts of phalanges and distal metacarpals.
  - The amount of tissue on each side of the phalanges should appear equal.
• Fingers should be separated from both sides of finger being examined so there is no overlapping of soft tissues.
• Interphalangeal joints should appear open indicating hand was fully pronated and correct CR location.
• Optimum exposure and contrast scale with no motion will demonstrate soft tissue margins and clear, sharp bony trabecular markings.
• Patient ID information should be clear and legible with R or L markers visible on a lateral margin without superimposing anatomy.
• **Alternate Routine** - see PA hand.

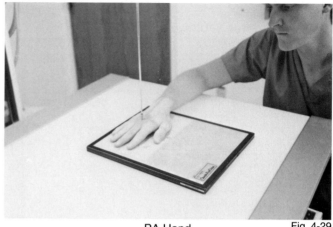

PA Hand
(Alternate Routine)   Fig. 4-29

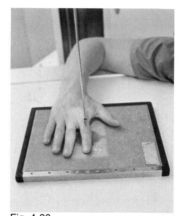

Fig. 4-30
PA, 2nd Digit   Fig. 4-31
                                     PA, 4th Digit

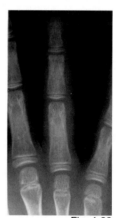

Fig. 4-32
PA, 4th Digit

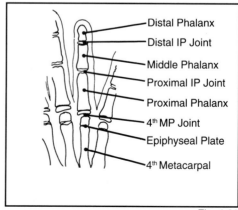

- Distal Phalanx
- Distal IP Joint
- Middle Phalanx
- Proximal IP Joint
- Proximal Phalanx
- 4th MP Joint
- Epiphyseal Plate
- 4th Metacarpal

PA, 4th Digit   Fig. 4-33

• Oblique Position

Fingers
Basic
• PA
• **Oblique**
• Lateral

Structures Best Shown:

Phalanges, interphalangeal and metacarpophalangeal joints in oblique position.

Technical Factors:

- Film Size - 8 x 10 in. (18 x 24 cm).
- Divide in thirds crosswise.
- Detail screen, table top.
- 50 - 60 kVp range.
- Accessories: 45° foam wedge block or step wedge.

Patient Position:

- Patient seated at end of table with elbow flexed about 90° with hand and wrist resting on cassette with fingers extended.

Shielding: Place lead shield over patient's lap to shield gonads.

Part Position:

- Place hand with fingers fully extended against 45° foam wedge block placing hand in a 45° lateral oblique (thumb side up).
- Position hand on cassette so the long axis of finger is aligned with long axis of unmasked 1/3 of film.
- Separate fingers and carefully place finger being examined against block so it is supported in a 45° oblique and is **parallel to film.**

Central Ray:

- CR **perpendicular** to film, directed to **proximal interphalangeal** (PIP) joint.
- Minimum 40 in. (102 cm) SID.

Collimation: Collimate on four sides to finger being examined.

Optional Medial Oblique: 2nd digit may also be taken in a 45° medial oblique (thumb side down) with thumb and other fingers flexed to prevent superimposition. This places part closer to film for improved definition but may also be more painful for patient.

Evaluation Criteria:

- Entire finger in question (distal, medial and proximal phalanges) and the metacarpophalangeal joint should be included positioned in a 45° oblique with collimation on all four sides.
- Long axis of finger should be aligned to long axis of portion of film being used.
- Center of collimation field should be to the PIP joint.
- Interphalangeal and metacarpophalangeal joint spaces should be open indicating correct central ray location and that the phalanges are parallel to the film.
- Optimum exposure and contrast scale with no motion will demonstrate soft tissue margins and clear, sharp bony trabecular markings.
- Patient ID information should be clear and legible with R or L marker visible on a lateral margin without superimposing anatomy.

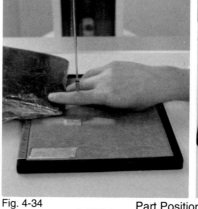

Fig. 4-34   Part Position   Fig. 4-35

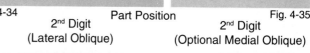

2nd Digit (Lateral Oblique)   2nd Digit (Optional Medial Oblique)

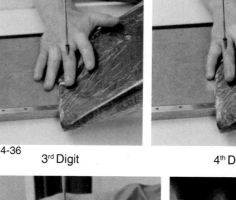
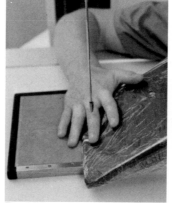
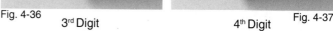

Fig. 4-36   3rd Digit   4th Digit   Fig. 4-37

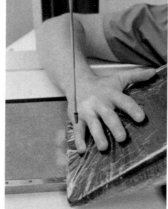

Fig. 4-38   5th Digit   4th Digit   Fig. 4-39

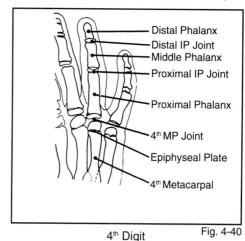

- Distal Phalanx
- Distal IP Joint
- Middle Phalanx
- Proximal IP Joint
- Proximal Phalanx
- 4th MP Joint
- Epiphyseal Plate
- 4th Metacarpal

4th Digit   Fig. 4-40

• Lateral Position

Fingers
Basic
• PA
• Oblique
• **Lateral**

Structures Best Shown:
Phalanges, interphalangeal and metacarpo-phalangeal joints in lateral position.

Technical Factors:
• Film Size - 8 x 10 in. (18 x 24 cm).
• Divide in thirds crosswise.
• Detail screen, table top.
• 50 - 60 kVp range.
• Accessories: Sponge support block.

Patient Position:
• Patient seated at end of table with elbow flexed about 90° with hand and wrist resting on cassette with fingers extended.

Shielding: Place lead shield over patient's lap to shield gonads.

Part Position:
• Place hand in lateral position (thumb side up) with finger to be examined fully extended centered to unmasked portion of film. (See NOTE for 2nd digit lateral.)
• Flex unaffected fingers.
• Align finger to long axis of unmasked film.
• Use sponge block or other radiolucent device to support finger and prevent motion. (Have patient hold support block with other hand or use sand bags.)
• Insure that long axis of finger is **parallel to film**.

Central Ray:
• CR **perpendicular** to film, to **proximal interphalangeal (PIP) joint.**
• Minimum 40 in. (102 cm) SID.

Collimation: Collimate on four sides to finger being examined.

NOTE: For second digit, a thumb side down lateral is advised if patient can assume this position, placing the second digit in contact with cassette. (Definition is improved with less object-image receptor distance.)

Evaluation Criteria:
• Entire finger in question (distal, middle and proximal phalanges) and the metacarpophalangeal joint should be included with collimation on all four sides.
• The center of the collimation field should be at the PIP joint.
• Long axis of finger should be aligned to long axis of portion of film being used.
• Interphalangeal joint spaces should be open indicating correct central ray location and that the phalanges are parallel to film.
• Finger should be in true lateral position as indicated by the concave appearance of anterior surface of the shaft of phalanges and by the anterior projecting rounded ends of proximal and middle phalanges.
• Metacarpophalangeal joints of 2nd and 3rd fingers should appear somewhat open with minimal superimposition, but 4th and 5th metacarpophalangeal joints will be obscured by overlapping structures.
• Optimum exposure and contrast scale with no motion will demonstrate soft tissue margins and clear sharp bony trabecular markings.
• Patient ID information with R or L marker is visible on lateral margin of collimated field without superimposing anatomy.

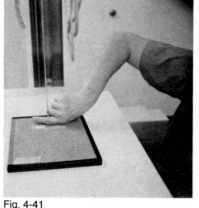
Fig. 4-41   2nd Digit

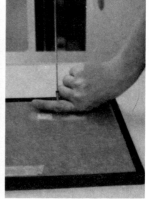
2nd Digit   Fig. 4-42

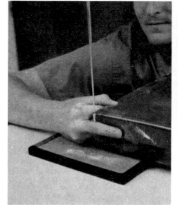
Fig. 4-43   3rd Digit

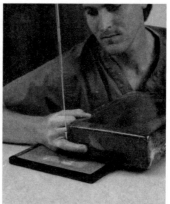
4th Digit   Fig. 4-44

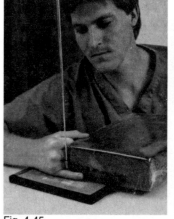
Fig. 4-45   5th Digit

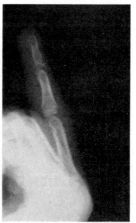
4th Digit   Fig. 4-46

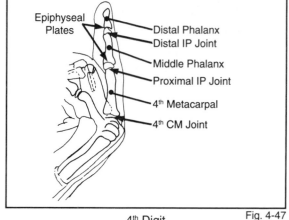
Epiphyseal Plates
Distal Phalanx
Distal IP Joint
Middle Phalanx
Proximal IP Joint
4th Metacarpal
4th CM Joint

4th Digit   Fig. 4-47

• AP Projection

Thumb
Basic
• **AP**
• Lateral
• Oblique

Structures Best Shown:
Distal and proximal phalanges, first meta-carpal and associated joints.

Technical Factors:
• Film Size - 8 x 10 in. (18 x 24 cm).
• Divide in thirds crosswise.
• Detail screen, table top.
• 50 - 60 kVp range.

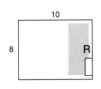

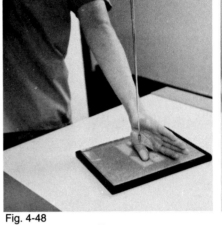

Fig. 4-48
AP

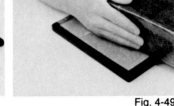

Fig. 4-49
PA (exception)

Patient Position – AP:
• Patient standing with arm behind back, hand supinated.
  or
  May be taken with patient seated facing table, arms extended in front with hand rotated internally to supinate thumb for AP projection.

Shielding: Place lead shield over patient's lap to shield gonads.

Part Position – AP:
(It is suggested you first demonstrate this awkward position on yourself for better cooperation and understanding by the patient.)
• Internally rotate hand with fingers extended until posterior surface of thumb is in contact with film.
• Center **1st MP joint** to center of unmasked portion of film. (Remember 1st metacarpal is considered part of thumb.)
• Align thumb to long axis of unmasked third of film.

Exception - PA: (Only if patient cannot position for above AP)
• Place hand in a near lateral position and rest thumb on a sponge support block which is high enough so thumb is not obliqued but in position for a **true PA** projection **parallel** to the cassette.
• Align thumb and support block to long axis of unmasked third of film.
• (The PA is not advisable as a routine because of loss of definition due to increased object-image receptor distance.)

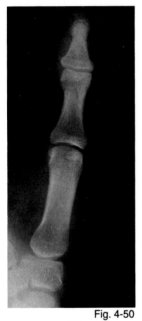

Fig. 4-50
AP

Central Ray:
• CR **perpendicular** to film, to **1st metacarpophalangeal (MP) joint.**
• Minimum 40 in. (102 cm) SID.

Collimation: Collimate on four sides to area of thumb remembering the **thumb includes the entire 1st metacarpal.**

Evaluation Criteria:
• Entire thumb (from distal tip of thumb to 1st carpometacarpal joint) and the carpal, trapezium, should be visualized and centered to the film.
• Collimation on all four sides.
• Long axis of thumb should be aligned to long axis of portion of film being used.
• The center of the collimation field should be at the 1st MP joint.
• No rotation as evidenced by symmetrical appearance of both concave sides of phalanges and by the equal amounts of soft tissue appearing on each side of phalanges.
• Interphalangeal and metacarpophalangeal joints should appear open.
• Optimum exposure and penetration with no motion will demonstrate soft tissue margins and clear sharp bony trabecular markings for the 1st metacarpal and the phalanges.
• Patient ID information should be clear and legible and R or L markers should be visible on lateral margin of the collimated field without superimposing anatomy.

Distal Phalanx
IP Joint
Proximal Phalanx
MP Joint
Sesamoid Bones
1st Metacarpal
1st CM Joint
Trapezium

AP   Fig. 4-51

• Lateral Position

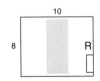

Thumb
Basic
• AP
• Lateral
• Oblique

Structures Best Shown:
Distal and proximal phalanges and metacarpal of 1st digit in lateral position along with associated opened joints and sesamoid bones if present.

Technical Factors:
- **Film Size** - 8 x 10 in. (18 x 24 cm).
- Divide in thirds crosswise.
- Detail screen, table top.
- 50 - 60 kVp range.

Patient Position:
- Patient seated at end of table with elbow flexed about 90° with hand resting on cassette, palm down.

Shielding: Place lead shield over patient's lap to shield gonads.

Part Position:
- Start with hand pronated and thumb abducted, with fingers and hand slightly arched, then rotate hand medially until thumb is in a true lateral position. (May need to provide sponge or other support under lateral portion of hand.)
- Align long axis of thumb to long axis of unmasked portion of film.
- Center **1st MP joint** to center of unmasked portion of film.
- Entire lateral aspect of thumb should be in direct contact with cassette.

Central Ray:
- CR **perpendicular** to film, directed to **first metacarpophalangeal (MP) joint.**
- Minimum 40 in. (102 cm) SID.

Collimation: Collimate on four sides to thumb area. (Remember the thumb includes the **entire first metacarpal.**)

Evaluation Criteria:
- Entire thumb (from distal tip of thumb to 1st carpometacarpal joint) and the carpal, trapezium, should be visualized and centered to the film.
- Collimation on all four sides.
- The center of the collimation field should be at the 1st MP joint.
- Thumb should be in true lateral position evidenced by the concave shaped anterior surface of proximal phalange and 1st metacarpal, and the relatively straight posterior surfaces.
- Interphalangeal and metacarpophalangeal joints should appear open.
- Optimum exposure and penetration with no motion will demonstrate soft tissue margins and clear sharp bony trabecular markings for the 1st metacarpal and the phalanges.
- Patient ID information should be clear and legible and R or L markers should be visible on lateral margin of the collimated field without superimposing anatomy.

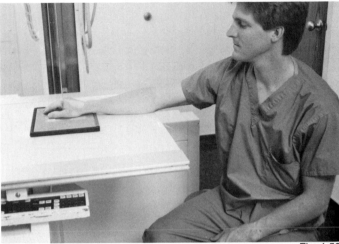

Patient Position - Lateral Thumb — Fig. 4-52

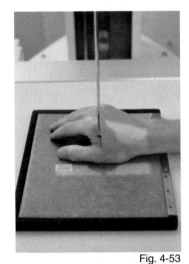

Fig. 4-53
Part Position

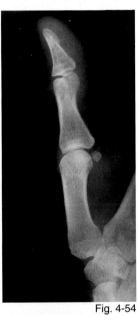

Fig. 4-54
Lateral Thumb

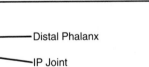

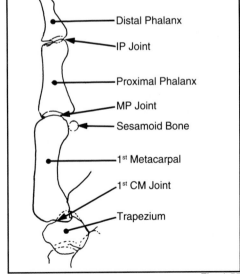

- Distal Phalanx
- IP Joint
- Proximal Phalanx
- MP Joint
- Sesamoid Bone
- 1st Metacarpal
- 1st CM Joint
- Trapezium

Lateral Thumb — Fig. 4-55

• Oblique Position

Thumb
Basic
• AP
• Lateral
• **Oblique**

Structures Best Shown:
Distal and proximal phalanges and metacarpal of 1st digit and associated joints all in oblique position and sesamoid bones if present.

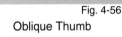

Technical Factors:
• Film Size - 8 x 10 in. (18 x 24 cm).
• Divide in thirds crosswise.
• Detail screen, table top.
• 50 - 60 kVp range.

Alternate Routine:
• 10 x 12 in. (24 x 30 cm) crosswise.
• Divide in half to include entire hand.
• An alternate routine includes the entire hand for the oblique thumb for possible secondary trauma or pathology on other aspects of hand. AP and lateral would be of thumb only.

Alternate Routine

Patient Position:
• Patient seated at end of table with elbow flexed about 90° with hand resting on cassette.

Shielding:
Place lead shield over patient's lap to shield gonads.

Part Position:
• **Abduct thumb** slightly with palmar surface of hand in contact with cassette. (This will naturally place thumb into a 45° oblique position.)
• Align long axis of thumb to long axis of unmasked third of cassette.
• Center **1st MP joint** to center of unmasked portion of film.

Central Ray:
• CR **perpendicular** to film, directed to **first metacarpophalangeal (MP) joint.**
• Minimum 40 in. (102 cm) SID.

Collimation:
Collimate on four sides to thumb, insure that **all of first metacarpal is included.**

Evaluation Criteria: (Oblique thumb only)
• Entire thumb (from distal tip of thumb to 1st carpometacarpal joint) and the carpal bone, trapezium, should be visualized in a 45° oblique position and be centered to portion of film being used with collimation on all four sides.
• The center of the collimation field should be at the 1st MP joint.
• Long axis of thumb should be aligned to long axis of portion of film being used.
• Interphalangeal and metacarpophalangeal joints should appear open.
• Optimum exposure and contrast scale with no motion will demonstrate soft tissue margins and clear sharp bony trabecular markings for the 1st metacarpal and the phalanges.
• Patient ID information should be clear and legible and R or L markers should be visible on lateral margin of the collimated field without superimposing anatomy.
• **Alternate Routine** - see PA hand.

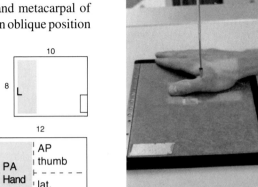

Fig. 4-56
Oblique Thumb

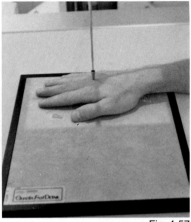

Fig. 4-57
Oblique Thumb with PA Hand
(Alternate Routine)

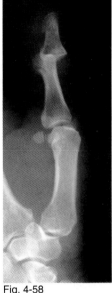

Fig. 4-58
Oblique Thumb

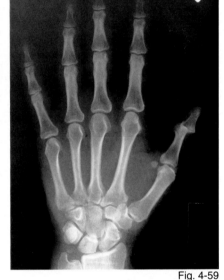

Fig. 4-59
Oblique Thumb with PA Hand
(Note dislocated distal phalanx of thumb)

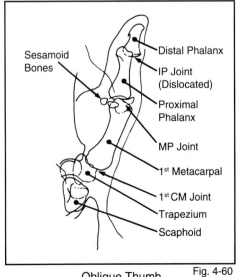

Oblique Thumb

Fig. 4-60

Sesamoid Bones

Distal Phalanx
IP Joint (Dislocated)
Proximal Phalanx
MP Joint
1st Metacarpal
1st CM Joint
Trapezium
Scaphoid

• PA Projection

Hand
Basic
• **PA**
• Oblique
• Lateral

Structures Best Shown:
Phalanges, metacarpals, carpals and all joints of hand. Results in an oblique view of thumb.

Technical Factors:
- Film Size - 10 x 12 in. (24 x 30 cm).
- Divide film in half crosswise.
  or (for large hand)
  - 8 x 10 in. (18 x 24 cm) lengthwise.
- Detail screen, table top.
- 50 - 60 kVp range.

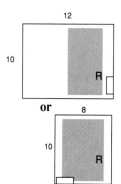

Patient Position:
- Patient seated at end of table with elbow flexed about 90° with hand and forearm resting on table.

Shielding: Place lead shield over patient's lap to shield gonads.

Part Position:
- Pronate hand with palmar surface in contact with cassette.
- Center hand and wrist to unmasked half of film.
- Align long axis of hand and forearm with long axis of portion of film being exposed.
- Spread fingers slightly.

Central Ray:
- CR **perpendicular** to film, directed to the **third metacarpophalangeal (MP) joint.**
- Minimum 40 in. (102 cm) SID.

Collimation: Collimate on four sides to outer margins of hand and wrist.

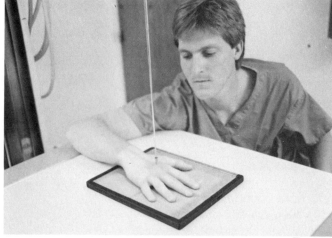

Patient Position - PA Hand   Fig. 4-61

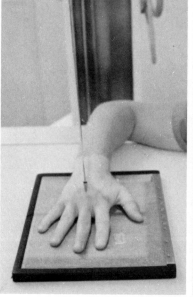

Part Position   Fig. 4-62

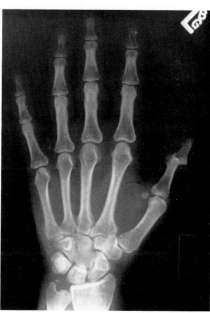

PA Hand   Fig. 4-63

NOTE: If exams of both hands and/or wrists are requested, they should be positioned and exposed separately for correct CR placement.

Evaluation Criteria:
- Entire hand, wrist and distal forearm should be included with collimation margins visible on all four sides.
- Center of collimation field should be to 3rd MP joint indicating correct CR placement.
- Long axis of hand and wrist should be aligned to long axis of film.
- **No rotation** of hand as evidenced by:
  - the symmetrical appearance of both sides or concavities of the shafts of the metacarpals and phalanges (except for the 1st metacarpal - phalanges of the obliqued thumb).
  - the amount of soft tissue on each side of the phalanges should appear equal.
- Digits should be slightly separated with soft tissues not overlapping.
- Metacarpophalangeal and interphalangeal joints should appear open indicating correct CR location and that hand was fully pronated.
- Optimum exposure and penetration with no motion will be evidenced by soft tissue margins and fine trabecular markings of the bones appearing clear and sharp.
- Patient ID should be clear and legible and R or L markers visible on lateral border of the collimated field without superimposing anatomy.

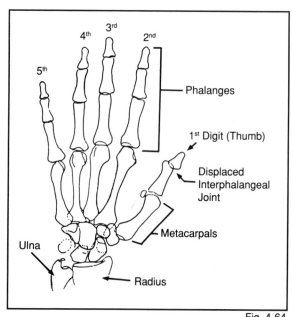

PA Hand   Fig. 4-64

• Oblique Position

Hand
Basic
• PA
• **Oblique**
• Lateral

Structures Best Shown:
Phalanges, metacarpals, carpals and all joints in oblique position.

Technical Factors:
• Film Size - 10 x 12 in. (24 x 30 cm).
• Divide film in half crosswise.
    or (for large hand)
    - 8 x 10 in. (18 x 24 cm), lengthwise.
• Detail screen, table top.
• 50 - 60 kVp range.

Patient Position:
• Patient seated at end of table with elbow flexed about 90° with hand and forearm resting on table.

Shielding: Place lead shield over patient's lap to shield gonads.

Part Position:
• Pronate hand on cassette and align long axis of hand and forearm to long axis of portion of film being exposed.
• Center hand and wrist to unmasked half of film.
• Rotate entire hand and wrist laterally 45° and support with radiolucent wedge or step block as shown so all digits are separated and **parallel to film.** (See exception below.)

Central Ray:
• CR **perpendicular** to film, directed to the **third metacarpophalangeal (MP) joint.**
• Minimum 40 in. (102 cm) SID.

Collimation: Collimate on four sides to outer margins of hand and wrist.

Exception: It is advisable for a routine oblique hand to use a support block as shown to place digits parallel to film. This prevents foreshortening of phalanges and obscuring of interphalangeal joints. Only if the phalanges are not in the area of interest, should the oblique position for metacarpals be taken with thumb and finger tips touching cassette.

Evaluation Criteria:
• Entire hand, wrist and about 1 inch (2.5 cm) of distal forearm should be visualized with collimation margins on all four sides.
• The center of the collimation field should be at the 3rd MP joint.
• Long axis of hand and wrist should be aligned to long axis of film.
• 45° oblique is evidenced by:
  - Mid-shafts of 3rd, 4th and 5th metacarpals should not overlap.
  - Some overlap of distal heads of 3rd, 4th and 5th metacarpals but no overlap of distal 2nd and 3rd metacarpals.
• Metacarpophalangeal and interphalangeal joints should be open without foreshortening of mid and distal phalanges indicating fingers were parallel to film.
• Optimum exposure and penetration with no motion will be evidenced by clear and sharp fine trabecular markings of the bones. Soft tissue margins will also be visualized.
• Patient ID should be clear and legible and R or L markers visible on lateral border of the collimated field without superimposing anatomy.

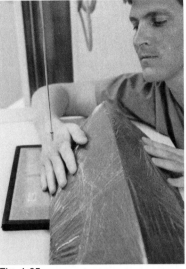

Fig. 4-65
Routine Oblique Hand
(Digits parallel)

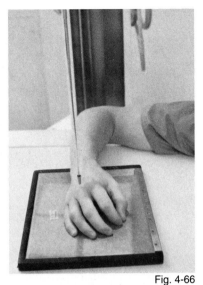

Fig. 4-66
Exception: Oblique Hand for Metacarpals
(Digits not parallel)

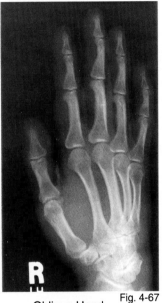

Fig. 4-67
Oblique Hand
(Digits parallel)

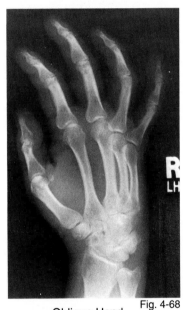

Fig. 4-68
Oblique Hand
(Digits not parallel)

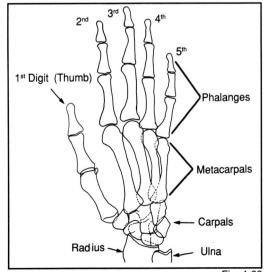

Fig. 4-69
Oblique Hand
(Digits parallel)

• Lateral "Fan" Position

Hand
Basic
• PA
• Oblique
• **Lateral**

Structures Best Shown:
Phalanges, metacarpals and carpals superimposed in a lateral position, except for thumb which is shown in a true PA projection. (With some magnification.)

Technical Factors:
• Film Size - 8 x 10 in. (18 x 24 cm) lengthwise.
• Detail screen, table top.
• 54 - 64 kVp range. (Increase 4 or 5 kVp from PA and oblique.)

Patient Position:
• Patient seated at end of table with elbow flexed about 90° with hand and forearm resting on table.

Shielding:
Place lead shield over patient's lap to shield gonads.

Part Position:
• Align long axis of hand and forearm to long axis of film with center of film to metacarpophalangeal joints.
• Rotate hand and wrist into a lateral position with thumb side up.
• Spread fingers and thumb into a "fan" position and support each digit on radiolucent step block as shown. Insure that all digits including the thumb are parallel to film and that the metacarpals are **not** obliqued but remain in a true lateral position.

Central Ray:
• CR **perpendicular** to film, directed to **1st metacarpophalangeal (MP) joint.**
• Minimum 40 in. (102 cm) SID.

Collimation:
Collimate on four sides to outer margins of hand and wrist.

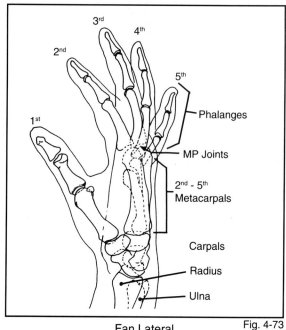

Patient Position - Fan Lateral   Fig. 4-70

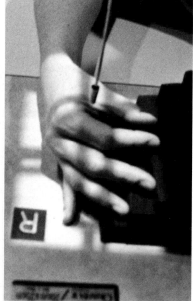

Fig. 4-71
Part Position - Fan Lateral

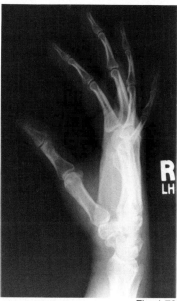

Fig. 4-72
Fan Lateral

Evaluation Criteria:
• Entire hand, wrist and about 1 inch (3-5 cm) of the distal forearm should be included with collimation margins visible on all four sides.
• The center of the collimation field should be to 1st MP joint.
• Long axis of hand and wrist should be aligned to long axis of film.
• Hand and wrist should be in a true lateral position evidenced by:
 - Distal radius and ulna directly superimposed.
 - Metacarpals are directly superimposed.
• Fingers should appear equally separated with phalanges in lateral position with joint spaces open indicating fingers were parallel to film.
• Thumb should appear as in a PA projection completely free of superimposition with joint spaces open.
• Optimum exposure and contrast scale with no motion will demonstrate outlines of individual metacarpals through shadows of superimposing metacarpals. Mid and distal phalanges of both thumb and fingers should appear sharp and be visible but will appear slightly overexposed.
• Patient ID should be clear and legible and R or L markers visible on lateral margin without superimposing anatomy.

Fan Lateral   Fig. 4-73

• Lateral in Extension and Flexion
(Alternates to Fan Lateral position - see NOTE)

Hand
Basic
• PA
• Oblique
• **Lateral**

Structures Best Shown:
Phalanges, metacarpals and carpals superimposed in a lateral position, except for thumb which is shown in a true PA projection. (With some magnification.)

Technical Factors:
• Film Size - 8 x 10 in. (18 x 24 cm) lengthwise.
• Detail screen, table top.
• 54 - 64 kVp range. (Increase 4 kVp from PA and oblique.)

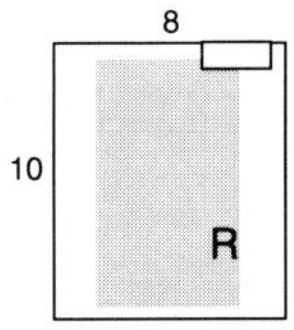

Patient Position:
• Patient seated at end of table with elbow flexed about 90° with hand and forearm resting on table.

Shielding: Place lead shield over patient's lap to shield gonads.

Part Position:
• Rotate hand and wrist 90° to cassette, thumb side up, into a true lateral position.

Lateral in Extension:
• Extend fingers and thumb and support against a radiolucent support block. Insure that all fingers are directly superimposed for a true lateral position.

Lateral in Flexion:
• Flex finger into a natural flexed position with thumb lightly touching the first finger.
• Thumb should be parallel to film.
• Insure that fingers are directly superimposed with the entire hand in a true lateral position.

Central Ray:
• CR **perpendicular** to film directed to the **MP joints.**
• Minimum 40 in. (102 cm) SID.

Collimation: Collimate on four sides to outer margins of hand and wrist.

NOTE: These two positions are alternate positions for the recommended fan lateral. • The lateral position in extension may be taken for localization of foreign bodies and fractures of metacarpals.

Evaluation Criteria:
• Entire hand, wrist and about 1 inch (2.5 cm) of the distal forearm should be included with collimation margins visible on all four sides.
• The center of the collimation field should be at the MP joints.
• Long axis of hand and wrist should be aligned to long axis of film.
• Hand and wrist should be in a true lateral position evidenced by:
  - Distal radius and ulna are directly superimposed.
  - Metacarpals and phalanges are directly superimposed.
• Thumb should appear as in a PA projection free of superimposition with joint spaces open.
• Optimum exposure and penetration without motion will visualize outlines of individual metacarpals and phalanges through shadows of superimposing structures. Trabecular markings of thumb should appear clear and sharp.
• Patient ID should be clear and legible and R or L markers visible on lateral margin without superimposing anatomy.

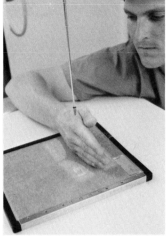
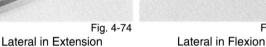

Fig. 4-74
Lateral in Extension

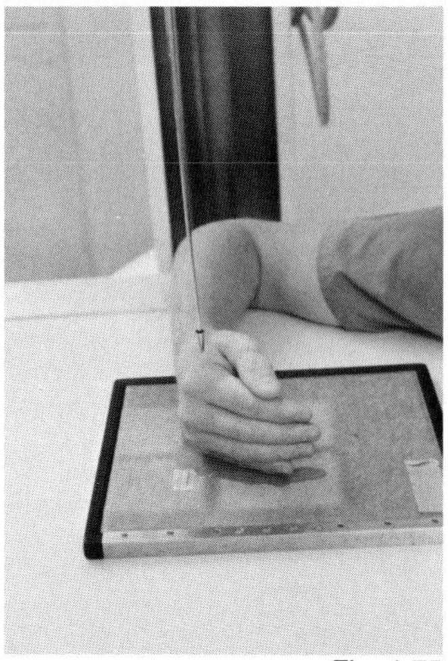

Fig. 4-75
Lateral in Flexion

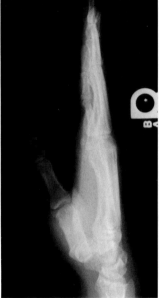
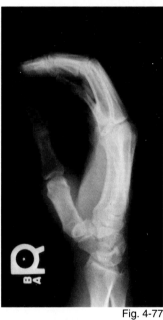
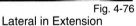

Fig. 4-76
Lateral in Extension

Fig. 4-77
Lateral in Flexion

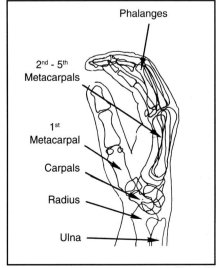

Fig. 4-78
Lateral in Flexion

Wrist

• PA Projection

Structures Best Shown:
Mid and proximal metacarpals, carpals, distal radius and ulna and associated joints.

Technical Factors:
• Film Size - 8 x 10 in. (18 x 24 cm).
• Divide in half, crosswise.
• Detail screen, table top.
• 60 ± 6 kVp range.

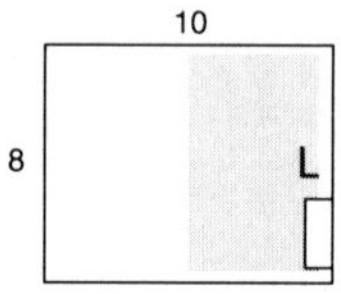

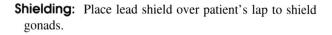

Patient Position:
• Patient seated at end of table with elbow flexed about 90° with hand and wrist resting on cassette, palm down.
• Drop shoulder or raise table height so shoulder, elbow and wrist are on same horizontal plane.

Shielding: Place lead shield over patient's lap to shield gonads.

Part Position:
• Align long axis of hand and forearm to center of the long axis of the unmasked half of cassette, with carpal area to center of unmasked film.
• With hand pronated, arch hand only slightly **to place wrist and carpal area in close contact with cassette.**

Central Ray:
• CR **perpendicular** to film, directed to **mid-carpal area**.
• Minimum 40 in. (102 cm) SID.

Collimation: Collimate to wrist on all four sides, include distal radius and ulna and mid-metacarpal area.

Alternate AP: To better demonstrate intercarpal spaces and distal radius and ulna, an AP wrist may be taken with hand slightly arched to place **wrist and carpals in close contact with cassette** (*Fig. 4-80*).

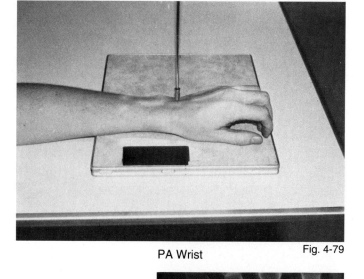

PA Wrist   Fig. 4-79

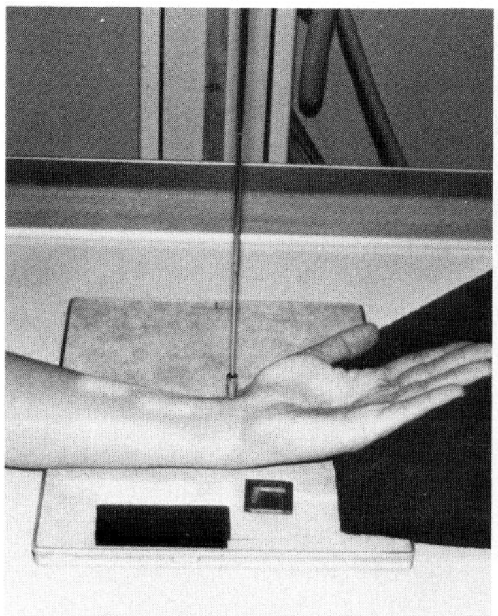

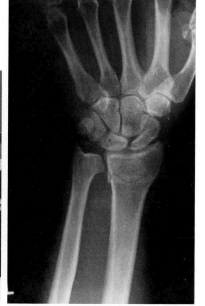

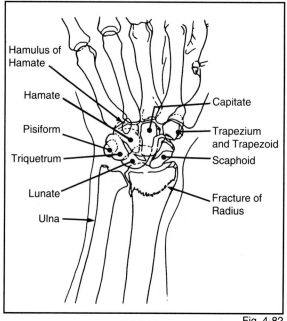

Alternate AP Wrist Fig. 4-80   PA Wrist   Fig. 4-81

Evaluation Criteria:
• Distal radius, ulna, and all carpals at least to mid-metacarpal area should be visualized, centered to the mid portion and to the long axis of that part of film being used with collimation margins on all four sides.
• The center of collimation field should be to mid-carpal area.
• **True PA** as evidenced by:
 - equal concavity shapes on each side of shafts of proximal metacarpals.
 - near equal distances between proximal metacarpals; and separation of distal radius and ulna except for **minimal** superimposition at distal radio-ulnar joint.
• Optimum exposure and contrast with no motion should visualize soft tissues such as pertinent fat pads, as well as the bony margins of the carpals with sharp borders and clear trabecular markings. (The intercarpal spaces will not all appear open because of irregular shapes and resultant overlapping).
• Patient ID should be clear and legible and R and L markers visible on a lateral margin of the film within the collimation field without superimposing anatomy.

PA Wrist   Fig. 4-82

Labels in figure:
Hamulus of Hamate
Hamate
Pisiform
Triquetrum
Lunate
Ulna
Capitate
Trapezium and Trapezoid
Scaphoid
Fracture of Radius

• Oblique Position

Wrist
Basic
• PA
• **Oblique**
• Lateral

Structures Best Shown:
Mid and distal metacarpals, carpals (especially trapezium and scaphoid), distal radius and ulna and associated joints.

Technical Factors:
• Film Size - 8 x 10 in. (18 x 24 cm).
• Divide in half, crosswise.
• Detail screen, table top.
• 60 ± 6 kVp range.

Patient Position:
• Patient seated at end of table with elbow flexed about 90° with hand and wrist resting on cassette, palm down.
• Drop shoulder or raise table height so shoulder, elbow and wrist are on same horizontal plane.

Shielding: Place lead shield over patient's lap to shield gonads.

Part Position:
• Align hand and wrist to the center of, and to the long axis of the unmasked half of cassette.
• From pronated position, rotate wrist and hand laterally 45°.
• For stability place a 45° support under thumb side of hand to support hand and wrist in a 45° oblique position, *(Fg. 4- 84)* or partially flex fingers to arch hand to lightly rest finger tips on cassette.

Central Ray:
• CR **perpendicular** to film, directed to the **mid-carpal area.**
• Minimum 40 in. (102 cm) SID.

Collimation: Collimate to wrist on all four sides, include distal radius and ulna and at least to the mid-metacarpal area.

Evaluation Criteria:
• Distal radius, ulna, carpals and at least to mid-metacarpal area should be visualized, centered to the mid portion and to the long axis of that part of film being used with collimation margins on all four sides.
• The center of collimation field should be to mid-carpal area.
• The trapezium in its entirety should be well visualized as well as the scaphoid which has only slight superimposition of other carpals on its medial aspects.
• The proximal 3rd, 4th, 5th metacarpals as well as the distal radius and ulna should appear with some superimposition.
• Correct exposure with adequate penetration with no motion will demonstrate the carpals and their overlapping borders. The trabecular markings of all bones visualized will be sharp and clear. Soft tissue margins such as pertinent fat pads should be visible.
• Patient ID should be clear and legible and R and L markers visible on a lateral margin of the film within the collimation field without superimposing anatomy.

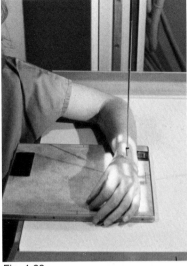

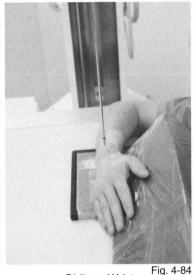

Fig. 4-83 Oblique Wrist

Oblique Wrist
(with 45° support)

Fig. 4-84

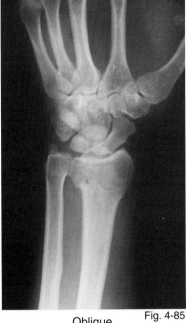

Oblique   Fig. 4-85

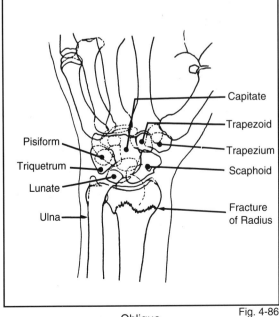

Pisiform
Triquetrum
Lunate
Ulna

Capitate
Trapezoid
Trapezium
Scaphoid
Fracture of Radius

Oblique   Fig. 4-86

• Lateral Position

Wrist
Basic
• PA
• Oblique
• **Lateral**

Structures Best Shown:
Superimposed proximal metacarpals, carpals, distal radius and ulna and wrist joint.

Technical Factors:

- Film Size - 8 x 10 in. (18 x 24 cm), lengthwise.
- Detail screen, table top.
- 64 ± 6 kVp range. (Increase 4 kVp from PA and oblique)

Patient Position:
- Patient seated at end of table with both arm and forearm resting on the table with elbow flexed about 90° and wrist and hand on cassette in thumb up lateral position. Shoulder, elbow and wrist should be on same horizontal plane.

Shielding: Place lead shield over patient's lap to shield gonads.

Part Position:
- Align hand and forearm to the center of and to the long axis of the cassette.
- Adjust the hand and wrist into a **true lateral** position with fingers comfortably flexed (*Fig. 4-87*); or if support is needed to prevent motion, use a radiolucent support block and sandbag and place block against extended hand and fingers (*Fig. 4-88*).

Central Ray:
- CR **perpendicular** to film, directed to **mid-wrist joint.**
- Minimum 40 in. (102 cm) SID.

Collimation: Collimate on all four sides, including distal radius and ulna and at least to mid-metacarpal area.

Evaluation Criteria:
- Distal radius and ulna, carpals and at least to mid-metacarpal area should be visualized, centered to the mid portion and to the long axis of that part of film being used.
- Collimation margins should be visible on all four sides.
- The center of the collimation field should be to the wrist joint.
- **True lateral** position as evidenced by:
  - Ulnar head of distal ulna should be centered and directly superimposed over radius.
  - Proximal metacarpals should all appear aligned and superimposed.
- Optimum exposure and adequate penetration with no motion will visualize soft tissue such as margins of pertinent fat pads, as well as the borders of the distal ulna through the superimposed radius. The fine trabecular markings of all bones should appear clear and sharp.
- Patient ID should be clear and legible and R or L marker be visible on a lateral margin of the film without superimposing anatomy.

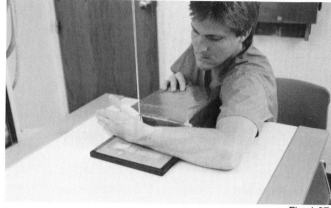

Lateral Wrist   Fig. 4-87

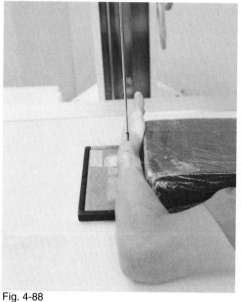

Fig. 4-88
Lateral Wrist

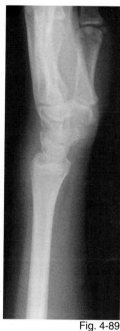

Fig. 4-89
Lateral Wrist

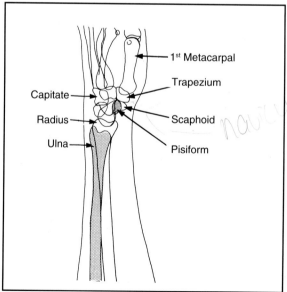

Lateral Wrist   Fig. 4-90

• Ulnar Flexion, PA Projection

Warning: Do **not** attempt this position with possible wrist trauma before routine series has been completed to evaluate for possible fractures of distal forearm and/or wrist.

Structures Best Shown:
Scaphoid without foreshortening with opened spaces between adjacent carpals. Also, to a lesser degree visualizes the trapezium and trapezoid.

Technical Factors:
• Film Size - 8 x 10 in. (18 x 24 cm).
• Divide in half, crosswise (if combined with other projections).
• Detail screen, table top.
• 60 ± 6 kVp range.

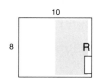

Patient Position:
• Patient seated at end of table with elbow flexed at 90° resting on table with wrist and hand on cassette, palm down with shoulder, elbow and wrist on same horizontal plane.

Shielding: Place lead shield over patient's lap to shield gonads.

Part Position:
• Position wrist as for a PA projection, palm down with arm and hand aligned to center of long axis of unmasked portion of film.
• Without moving forearm, gently evert (move toward ulnar side) as far as patient can tolerate without lifting or obliquing distal forearm.

Central Ray:
• Angle CR **15-20° proximally** (along long axis of forearm, toward elbow) to direct the **CR perpendicular to the scaphoid**.
• Center CR to **scaphoid** (Locate scaphoid at a point 3/4 in. or 2 cm proximal to, and 3/4 in. or 2 cm lateral to the 1st MP joint.)
• Minimum 40 in. (102 cm) SID.

Collimation: Collimate on all four sides to area of interest.

NOTE: The purpose of the 15-20° angle toward the elbow is to direct the CR **perpendicular** to the scaphoid to prevent foreshortening. An increased angle over 15° may be necessary to elongate the scaphoid to demonstrate fracture lines more clearly. (See 25° Angle, *Fig. 4-93*.)

Evaluation Criteria:
• Scaphoid should be clearly demonstrated without distortion (foreshortening), with adjacent carpal interspaces open.
• The distal radius and ulna, the carpals and proximal metacarpals should be visualized. The long axis of forearm should be aligned to long axis of the portion of exposed film with collimation margins on all four sides.
• The center of collimation field (CR location) should be to the scaphoid.
• No rotation of wrist as evidenced by appearance of distal radius and ulna with only **minimal** superimposition of distal radio-ulnar joint.
• Extreme ulnar flexion should be evident by the angle of the long axis of the metacarpals to that of the radius and ulna.

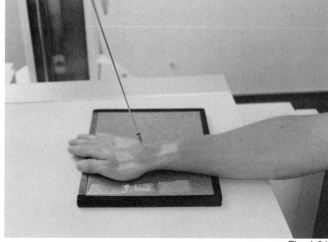

PA Wrist - Ulnar Flexion (15° Angle)   Fig. 4-91

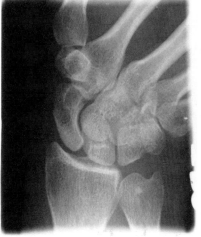 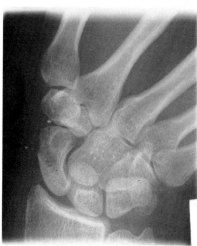

15° Angle   Fig. 4-92   25° Angle   Fig. 4-93

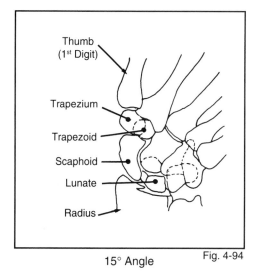

15° Angle   Fig. 4-94

• Correct exposure and adequate penetration with no motion will visualize the scaphoid borders and trabecular markings clearly and sharply.
• Patient ID marker should be clear and legible and R or L marker visible within the collimation field without superimposing anatomy.

Wrist

• Radial Flexion, PA Projection

Warning: Do **not** attempt this position with possible wrist trauma before routine series has been completed to evaluate for possible fractures of distal forearm and/or wrist.

Wrist
Optional
• Ulnar Flexion
• **Radial Flexion**
• Carpal Canal
• Carpal Bridge

Structures Best Shown:
Carpals with more opened interspaces on ulnar (lateral) side of wrist, especially the lunate, triquetrum, pisiform and hamate.

Technical Factors:
• Film Size - 8 x 10 in. (18 x 24 cm).
• Divide in half, crosswise.
• Detail screen, table top.
• 64 ± 6 kVp range.

Patient Position:
• Patient seated at end of table with elbow flexed at 90° resting on table with wrist and hand on cassette, palm down with shoulder, elbow and wrist on same horizontal plane.

Shielding: Place lead shield over patient's lap to shield gonads.

Part Position:
• Position wrist as for a PA projection, palm down with arm and hand aligned to center of long axis of unmasked portion of film.
• Without moving forearm, gently invert (move medially toward thumb side) as far as patient can tolerate without lifting or obliquing distal forearm.

Central Ray:
• CR **perpendicular** to film, directed to **mid-carpal area.**
• Minimum 40 in. (102 cm) SID.

Collimation: Collimate on all four sides to area of interest.

Evaluation Criteria:
• The carpals with adjacent interspaces more open should be best visualized on the medial (radius) side of the wrist.
• The distal radius and ulna, the carpals and proximal metacarpals should be visualized. The long axis of forearm should be aligned to long axis of the portion of exposed film with collimation margins on all four sides.
• The center of collimation field should be to the mid-carpal area.
• No rotation of wrist as evidenced by appearance of distal radius and ulna (should be similar to a PA wrist projection).
• Extreme radial flexion should be evident by the angle of the long axis of the metacarpals to that of the radius and ulna.
• Correct exposure and adequate penetration with no motion will visualize the scaphoid borders and trabecular markings clearly and sharply.
• Patient ID marker should be clear and legible and R or L marker visible within the collimation field without superimposing anatomy.

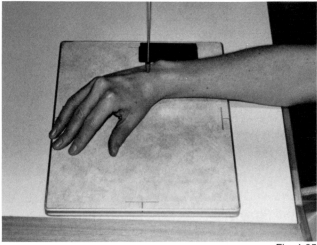

PA Wrist - Radial Flexion   Fig. 4-95

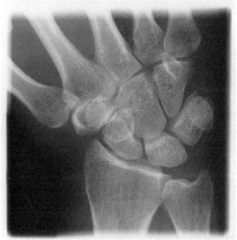

Radial Flexion   Fig. 4-96

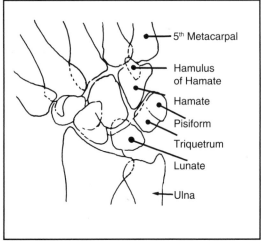

- 5th Metacarpal
- Hamulus of Hamate
- Hamate
- Pisiform
- Triquetrum
- Lunate
- Ulna

Radial Flexion   Fig. 4-97

• Carpal Canal - Tangential, Inferosuperior Projection
(Gaynor - Hart Method)

Warning: Do **not** attempt this position with possible wrist trauma before routine series has been completed to evaluate for possible fractures of distal forearm and/or wrist.

Wrist
Optional
• Ulnar Flexion
• Radial Flexion
• **Carpal Canal**
• Carpal Bridge

Structures Best Shown:
Carpal tunnel or canal made up of the palmar aspect of the trapezium, tuberosity of scaphoid, palmar aspects of trapezoid and capitate, the hamulus process of the hamate, the triquetrum (which is mostly superimposed), and the pisiform.

Technical Factors:
• Film Size - 8 x 10 in. (18 x 24 cm).
• Divide in half, crosswise.
• Detail screen, table top.
• 64 ± 6 kVp range.

Patient Position:
• Patient seated at end of table with elbow flexed at 90° resting on table with wrist and hand on cassette, palm down, (pronated).

Shielding: Place lead shield over patient's lap to shield gonads.

Part Position:
• Align forearm and wrist to long axis of unmasked portion of film.
• Ask patient to hyperextend wrist (dorsiflex) as far as possible by grasping the fingers with other hand and gently but firmly hyperextending the wrist until the long axis of the metacarpals and fingers are as near vertical as possible (without lifting the wrist and forearm from the cassette). May also use gauze to have patient pull fingers back.
• Rotate entire hand and wrist about **10° internally** (toward radial side) to prevent superimposition of pisiform and hamate.

Central Ray:
• Angle CR **25-30° to the long axis of the hand**. (The total CR angle in relationship to the film will have to be increased if patient cannot hyperextend wrist as far as indicated above.)
• Direct CR to a point **1 inch distal to the base of the 3rd metacarpal**.
• Minimum 40 in. (102 cm) SID.

Collimation: Collimate on four sides to area of interest.

NOTE: If patient cannot assume this hyperextended position, see alternate supero-inferior projection on following page.

Evaluation Criteria:
• The carpals should be demonstrated in a tunnel-like "arched" arrangement on the inferosuperior projection.
• The center of the collimation field should be to the mid point of the carpal canal.
• The pisiform and the hamulus process should be clearly visualized in profile without superimposition.
• The rounded palmar aspect of the trapezoid, and the adjacent and overlaying tubercle of the scaphoid should be visualized in profile; as well as that aspect of the trapezoid articulating with the 1st metacarpals.
• Correct exposure and adequate penetration without motion should visualize the carpals in profile with trabecular markings appearing clear and sharp.
• Patient ID marker should be clear and legible and R or L marker visible without superimposing anatomy.

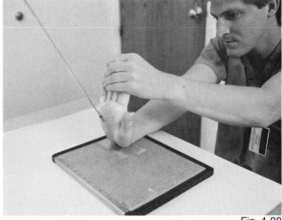

Tangential Projection   Fig. 4-98

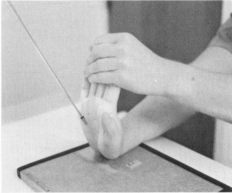

Tangential Projection   Fig. 4-99

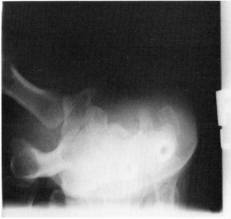

Tangential Projection   Fig. 4-100

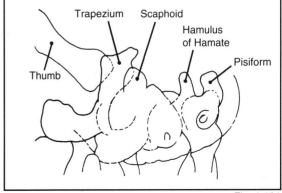

Tangential Projection   Fig. 4-101

• Carpal Canal - Alternate Supero-inferior Projection

Warning: Do **not** attempt this position with possible wrist trauma before routine series has been completed to evaluate for possible fractures of distal forearm and/or wrist.

Wrist
Optional
• Ulnar Flexion
• Radial Flexion
• **Carpal Canal**
• Carpal Bridge

Structures Best Shown:
Carpal tunnel or canal made up of the palmar aspect of the trapezium, tuberosity of scaphoid, palmar aspects of trapezoid and capitate, the hamulus process of the hamate, the triquetrum (which is mostly superimposed), and the pisiform.

Technical Factors:
• Film Size - 8 x 10 in. (18 x 24 cm).
• Divide in half, crosswise.
• Detail screen, table top.
• 64 ± 6 kVp range.

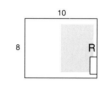

Alternate Projection:
If patient cannot hyperflex wrist sufficiently as shown on preceding page, then this alternate supero-inferior projection may be taken. This however, will not result in the same tunnel view of the arched carpals and the carpals will not be as well visualized in profile. Therefore this should only be taken as an alternate projection when the hyperflex wrist is not possible.

Shielding:
Secure a lead shield around patient's waist to shield gonads.

Patient and Part Position:
• Have patient stand at end of the table and place the palmar surface of the hand flat on the cassette. Then hyperextend the wrist by slowly leaning forward as far as can be tolerated, allowing the palmar surface of the hand to raise off the cassette 1 to 1.5 inches (3-4 cm) as shown.
• The long axis of the forearm should be about 25-35° from the perpendicular CR.

Central Ray:
• Direct CR **tangentially** to the **mid-carpal canal, perpendicular** to the film.
• Minimum 40 in. (102 cm) SID.

Collimation:
Collimate on four sides to area of interest.

Evaluation Criteria:
• The carpals should be demonstrated in a tunnel-like "arched" arrangement on the inferosuperior projection. (The supero-inferior projection will not demonstrate the tunnel-like arrangement.)
• The center of the collimation field should be to the midpoint of the carpal canal.
• The pisiform and the hamulus process should be clearly visualized in profile without superimposition.
• The rounded palmar aspect of the trapezoid, and the adjacent and overlaying tubercle of the scaphoid should be visualized in profile; as well as that aspect of the trapezoid articulating with the 1st metacarpal.
• Correct exposure and adequate penetration without motion should visualize the carpals in profile with trabecular markings appearing clear and sharp.
• Patient ID marker should be clear and legible and R or L marker visible without superimposing anatomy.

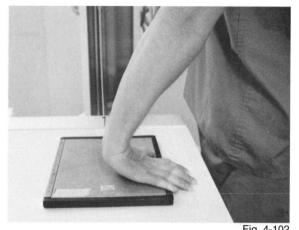

Fig. 4-102
Tangential Supero-inferior Projection

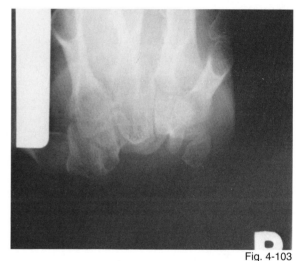

Fig. 4-103
Tangential Supero-inferior Projection

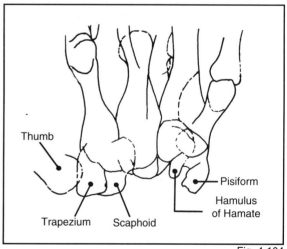

Fig. 4-104
Tangential Supero-inferior Projection

• Carpal Bridge - Tangential Projection

Warning: Do **not** attempt this position with possible wrist trauma before routine series has been completed to evaluate for possible fractures of distal forearm and/or wrist.

<table>
<tr><td>

Wrist

Optional
• Ulnar Flexion
• Radial Flexion
• Carpal Canal
• **Carpal Bridge**

</td></tr>
</table>

Structures Best Shown:

Tangential view of carpals, especially for demonstration of possible calcifications or chip fractures of the dorsal aspect of the carpals.

Technical Factors:

• Film Size - 8 x 10 in. (18 x 24 cm).
• Divide in half, crosswise.
• Detail screen, table top.
• 64 ± 6 kVp range.

Shielding: Secure lead shield around waist to shield gonads.

Patient Position:

• With patient standing or seated at end of the table, ask them to lean over and place dorsal surface of hand, **palm upward,** on cassette.

Part Position:

• Flex wrist gently as far as can be tolerated or until the hand and forearm form a right angle.

Central Ray:

• Angle the CR **45°** to the large axis of the forearm.
• Direct the CR to a **mid point of the distal forearm about 1.5 inches proximal to the wrist joint.**
• Minimum 40 in. (102 cm) SID.

Collimation: Collimate on all four sides to area of interest.

Evaluation Criteria:

• Should demonstrate a tangential view of the dorsal aspect of the scaphoid, lunate and triquetrium. An outline of the superimposed capitate and trapezium should also be visible.
• The center of the collimation field should be to the area of the proximal 3rd metacarpal.
• Correct exposure with adequate penetration without motion should visualize sharp borders and trabecular markings of the more posterior carpals as described above. Outlines of the proximal metacarpals should be visualized through other superimposed structures.
• Patient ID marker should be clear and legible with R or L marker visible without superimposing anatomy.

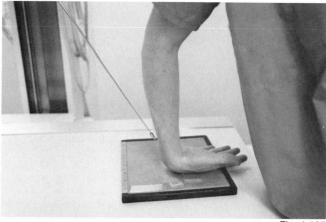

Carpal Bridge   Fig. 4-105

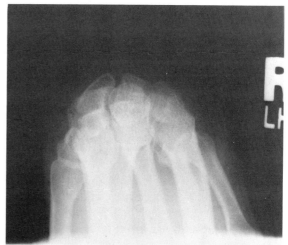

Carpal Bridge   Fig. 4-106

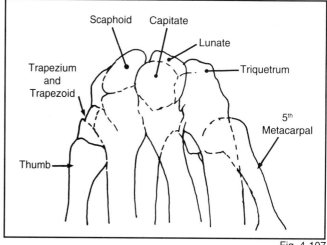

Carpal Bridge   Fig. 4-107

• AP Projection

Forearm
Basic
• **AP**
• Lateral

Structures Best Shown:
Entire radius and ulna, proximal row of carpals, elbow and distal end of humerus.

Technical Factors:
- Film Size - 11 x 14 in. (30 x 35 cm) or
  - 14 x 17 in. (35 x 43 cm).
- Divide in half, lengthwise.
- Detail screen, table top.
- 64 ± 6 kVp range.
- To make best use of the Anode-Heel Effect, place elbow at cathode end of x-ray beam.

11 (14)

14 (17)

L

Patient Position:
- Patient seated at end of table with hand and arm fully extended **palm up (supinated).**

Shielding: Place lead shield over patient's lap to shield gonads.

Part Position:
- Drop shoulder to place entire upper limb on same horizontal plane.
- Align and center forearm to the long axis of unmasked portion of film.
- Have patient lean laterally as necessary to place entire wrist, forearm and elbow in as near a true frontal position as possible. (Medial and lateral epicondyles the same distance from film.)

Central Ray:
- CR **perpendicular** to film, directed to **mid-forearm.**
- Minimum 40 in. (102 cm) SID.

Collimation: Collimate both lateral borders to the actual forearm area; and at both ends collimate to avoid cutting off anatomy at either joint. Considering divergence of the x-ray beam, insure that a **minimum** of 1 in. or 2.5 cm distal to wrist joint, and 1 in. or 2.5 cm proximal to elbow joint is included on the film.

Alternate Routine:
The routine for long bones in some departments is to only include the one joint nearest the site of injury. This then includes only about 3/4 of the forearm but places the one joint of interest about 2 inches (5 cm) from the end of the film with better demonstration of this joint because of less divergence of the x-ray beam in joint area. A smaller 10 x 12 in. (24 x 30 cm) film divided lengthwise may best be used for this routine.

Evaluation Criteria:
- The long axis of the forearm should be aligned to the long axis of the half of exposed film.
- The carpals should be included distally, and the distal humerus proximally.
- Humeral epicondyles should be visible in profile with radial head, neck and tuberosity slightly superimposed by ulna. There should only be slight superimposition at the distal radioulnar joint.
- Wrist and elbow joint spaces will be only partially opened because of beam divergence. (See alternate routine above.)
- Lateral collimation borders should be visible on each side of forearm and borders at both ends should include essential anatomy of joints.
- Optimum exposure with no motion should visualize sharp bone margins and clear trabecular markings throughout. Densities should be similar at distal and proximal ends of forearm.
- Patient ID should be clear and legible and R or L markers visible on lateral border without superimposing anatomy.

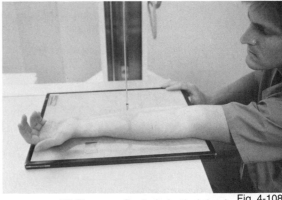
AP Forearm (include both Joints) Fig. 4-108

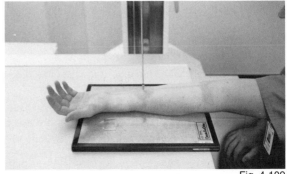
Alternate Routine (include only joint nearest injury) Fig. 4-109

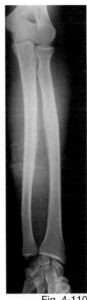
Fig. 4-110
AP (both joints)

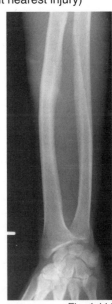
Fig. 4-111
AP (wrist joint)

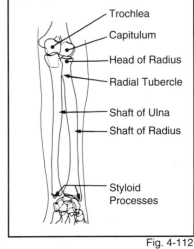
Trochlea
Capitulum
Head of Radius
Radial Tubercle
Shaft of Ulna
Shaft of Radius
Styloid Processes
Fig. 4-112
AP (both joints)

• Lateral Positon

Forearm
Basic
• AP
• **Lateral**

Structures Best Shown:
Entire radius and ulna, proximal row of carpals, elbow and distal end of humerus.

Technical Factors:
• Film Size - 11 x 14 in. (30 x 35 cm) or
        - 14 x 17 in. (35 x 43 cm).
• Divide in half, lengthwise.
• Detail screen, table top.
• 64 ± 6 kVp range.
• To make best use of the Anode-Heel Effect, place elbow at cathode end of x-ray beam.

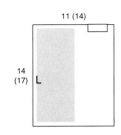

Patient Position:
• Patient seated at end of table with elbow flexed 90°.
• Drop shoulder to place entire upper limb on same horizontal plane.

Shielding:
Place lead shield over patient's lap to shield gonads.

Part Position:
• Align and center forearm to the long axis of unmasked portion of film.
• Rotate hand and wrist into **true lateral** (thumb up) **position** and support hand to prevent motion. (Insure that distal radius and ulna are directly superimposed.)

Central Ray:
• CR **perpendicular** to film, directed to **mid-forearm**.
• Minimum 40 in. (102 cm) SID.

Collimation:
Collimate both lateral borders to the actual forearm area; and at both ends collimate to avoid cutting off anatomy at the joints. Considering divergence of the x-ray beam, insure that a **minimum** of 1 in. or 2.5 cm distal to wrist joint, and 1 in. or 2.5 cm proximal to elbow joint is included on the film.

Alternate Routine:
The routine for long bones in some departments is to only include the one joint nearest the site of injury. This then includes only about 3/4 of the forearm but places the one joint of interest about 2 inches from the end of the film with better demonstration of this joint because of less divergence of the x-ray beam in joint area. A smaller 10 x 12 in. (24 x 30 cm) film divided lengthwise may best be used for this routine.

Evaluation Criteria:
• The elbow should be flexed 90° and the forearm should be aligned to the long axis of the half of exposed film.
• A minimum of the distal row of carpals should be visible distally, and the distal humerus proximally.
• **No Rotation:** Head of distal ulna should be directly superimposed and centered over radius; humeral epicondyles should be directly superimposed.
• Radial head should superimpose coronoid process; radial tuberosity should not be seen in profile.
• Wrist and elbow joints will be only partially open due to beam divergence. (See alternate routine above.)
• Lateral collimation borders should be visible but borders at both ends should be minimal so as not to cut off essential anatomy of joints.
• Optimum exposure with no motion should visualize sharp bone margins and clear trabecular markings throughout. Densities should be similar at distal and proximal ends of forearm.
• Patient ID should be clear and legible and R or L markers visible on lateral border without superimposing anatomy.

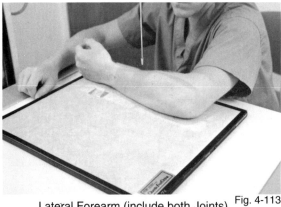

Lateral Forearm (include both Joints)   Fig. 4-113

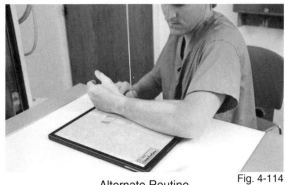

Alternate Routine   Fig. 4-114
(include only joint nearest injury)

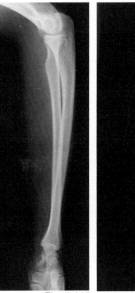

Fig. 4-115   Fig. 4-116
Lat. (both joints)   Lat. (wrist joint)

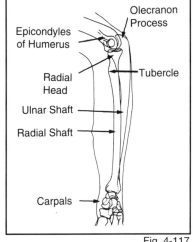

Fig. 4-117
Lateral (both joints)

Wrist and Forearm

• PA Projection

(Post Reduction, in Cast)

Wrist & Distal Forearm
(Post reduction)
• **PA**
• Lateral

Structures Best Shown:

Forearm and wrist to check for alignment and/or healing of fracture fragments.

Technical Factors:

- Film Size: Wrist - 10 x 12 in. (24 x 30 cm).
  Forearm - 11 x 14 in. (30 x 35 cm).
- Divide in half, lengthwise.
- Detail screen, table top.
- 65-75 kVp range.
- mAs increase - see NOTE below.

10 (11)

12
(14)

R

Patient Position:

- Ambulatory patient - seat at end of table with hand and forearm resting on cassette on table top, palm down (pronate).
- Stretcher patient - move patient to one side of stretcher and place hand and forearm on cassette, palm down.

Shielding: Place lead shield over patient's lap or gonadal area.

Part Position:

- Align hand and forearm to long axis of portion of unmasked film.
  Wrist - Center the wrist and forearm to include the metacarpals of the hand on the end of the film.
  Forearm - Center the entire forearm to film, including **both** wrist and elbow joints on the film.

Central Ray:

- CR **perpendicular** to film, directed to the **mid point of the film.**
- Minimum 40 in. (102 SID).

Collimation:
Collimate to four sides with only minimal collimation at both ends to not cut off essential anatomy.

NOTE: • Because of added cast density, increase 5-7 kVp from forearm technique for small to average dry casts. Double mAs **or** increase 8-10 kVp for wet or large casts. For fiberglass cast, increase only 3-4 kVp.
- Forearm post reduction in cast is usually taken PA rather than AP as for routine forearm because the cast prevents or makes very difficult rotating the forearm into position for a true AP.
- Post reduction films always include two projections taken 90° from each other to check for correct alignment in both dimensions.

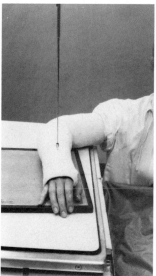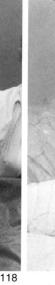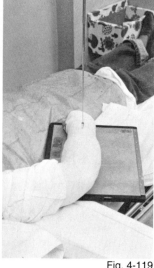

Fig. 4-118
PA Wrist (Erect)

Fig. 4-119
PA Wrist (Supine)

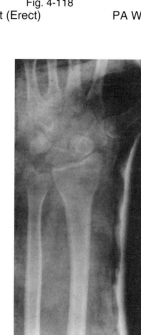

Fig. 4-120
PA Wrist

Evaluation Criteria:

Wrist:

- Should demonstrate distal two-thirds of forearm, carpals and metacarpals through cast, aligned to long axis of film with collimation borders visible on four sides, (only minimal borders at both ends to avoid cutting off essential anatomy).

Forearm:

- Should include both elbow and wrist joints on film. (Forearm should be aligned to long axis of film with collimation borders on both lateral margins, but only minimal at end to avoid cutting off either joint.

- **True PA projection** as evidenced by near equal distance between proximal metacarpals and only minimal superimposition at distal radio-ulnar joint.
- Correct exposure and adequate penetration without motion should clearly visualize outlines of distal radius and ulna and the metacarpals. The carpals in general and trabecular markings of all bones however, will appear unclear and hazy because of the semi-opaque cast material.
- Patient ID marker should be clear and legible with R or L marker visible on lateral border without superimposing anatomy.

• Lateral Position
(Post Reduction, in Cast)

> **Wrist & Distal Forearm**
> (Post reduction)
> • PA
> • **Lateral**

Structures Best Shown:
Forearm and wrist to check for alignment and/or healing of fracture fragments.

Technical Factors:
- Film Size: Wrist - 10 x 12 in. (24 x 30 cm).
  Forearm - 11 x 14 in. (30 x 35 cm).
- Divide in half, lengthwise.
- Detail screen, table top.
- 65-75 kVp range.
- mAs or kVp increase - see NOTE below.

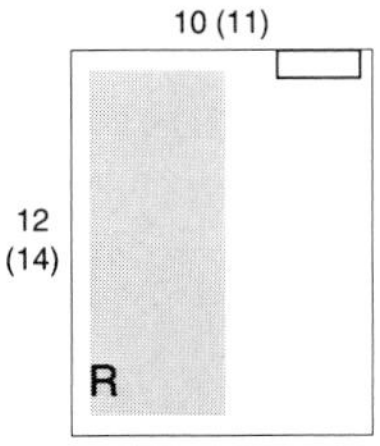

Patient Position:
- Ambulatory patient - seat at end of table with hand and forearm resting on cassette on table top in lateral position.
- Stretcher patient - move patient to one side of stretcher and place hand and forearm on cassette in lateral position.

Shielding:
Place lead shield over patient's lap or gonadal area.

Part Position:
- Align forearm and wrist to long axis of film.
- Rotate hand and wrist into a true lateral position.
  Elbow - Include at least the metacarpals at the end of film.
  Forearm - Center entire forearm to film including both wrist and elbow joints.

Central Ray:
- CR **perpendicular** to film, directed to the **mid point of the film.**
- Minimum 40 in. (102 cm SID).

Collimation:
Collimate to four sides with only minimal collimation at both ends to avoid cutting off essential anatomy.

NOTE: • Because of added cast density, for small to average plaster casts increase 5-7 kVp from forearm technique. Double mAs **or** increase 8-10 kVp for wet or large casts. For fiberglass cast, increase only 3-4 kVp.
• Post reduction films always include two projections taken 90° from each other to check for correct alignment in both dimensions.

Evaluation Criteria:
Wrist:
- Should demonstrate distal two-thirds of forearm, carpals and metacarpals through cast, aligned to long axis of film with collimation borders visible on four sides, (only minimal borders at both ends to avoid cutting off essential anatomy).

Forearm:
- Should include both elbow and wrist joints on film. (Forearm should be aligned to long axis of film with collimation borders on both lateral margins, but only minimal at end to avoid cutting off either joint.
- True lateral as evidenced by direct superimposition of distal radius and ulna.
- Correct exposure and adequate penetration without motion should visualize at least faint outlines of carpals as well as faint outlines of the superimposed proximal 2nd-5th metacarpals and distal radius and ulna.
- Patient ID should be clear and legible with R or L marker visible on lateral border without superimposing anatomy.

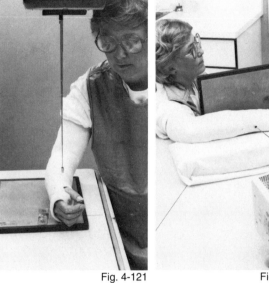

Fig. 4-121
Lateral (Erect)

Fig. 4-122
Lateral (Crosstable)

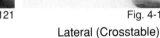

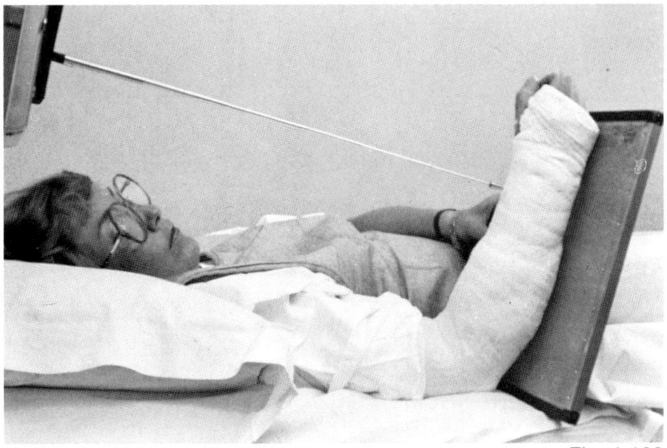

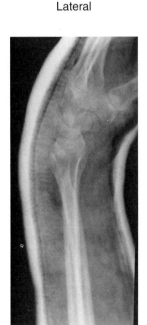

Lateral
Fig. 4-123

Fig. 4-124
Lateral

• AP Projection

Elbow
Basic
• **AP**
• Oblique
• Lateral

Structures Best Shown:
Distal humerus, elbow joint space and proximal radius and ulna.

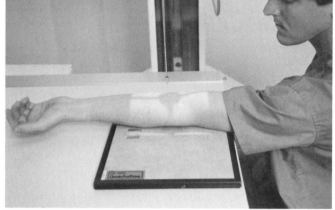

AP (Fully Extended)   Fig. 4-125

Technical Factors:
• Film Size - 10 x 12 in. (24 x 30 cm).
• Divide in half, crosswise
• Detail screen, table top.
• 66 ± 6 kVp range.

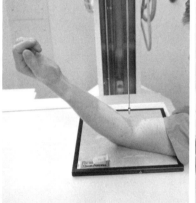

Patient Position:
• Patient seated at end of table with elbow fully extended if possible.

Shielding: Place or secure lead shield over pelvic area to protect gonads.

Part Position:
Fully Extended:
• Extend elbow, supinate hand and align arm and forearm to long axis of unmasked portion of film, with elbow joint to the center of unmasked film.
• Have patient lean laterally as necessary for **true AP projection**. (Palpate epicondyles to insure equal distance from the film.)
• Support hand as needed to prevent motion.

Partially Flexed: (If patient cannot fully extend elbow.)
• **Two** AP projections required; one with **forearm parallel** to film, and one with **humerus parallel** to film.
• Place support under wrist and forearm for projection with humerus parallel to film.
• Increase exposure 4-6 kVp, because of increased part thickness due to partial flexion.

Fig. 4-126   AP (Partially Flexed)   Fig. 4-127

Central Ray:
• CR **perpendicular** to film, directed to **mid-elbow joint,** which is approximately 3/4 in. (2 cm) distal to mid point of a line between epicondyles.
• Minimum 40 in. (102 cm) SID.

Collimation: Collimate on four sides to area of interest.

NOTE: If patient cannot even partially extend elbow, and elbow remains **flexed near 90°**, take the two AP projections as described above under Partially Flexed but **angle the CR 10-15°** into elbow joint.

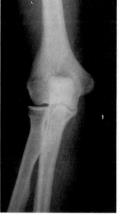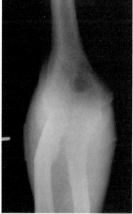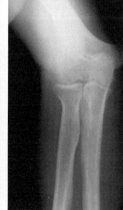

Fig. 4 -128   Fig. 4 -129   Fig. 4 -130
AP (Extended)   Humerus Parallel   Forearm Parallel
                    AP (Partially Flexed)

Evaluation Criteria:
• Long axis of arm should be aligned to long axis of the half of exposed film.
• Elbow joint space should be open and centered to exposed area of film.
• Collimation borders should be visible on all four sides with mid-elbow joint to center of collimation field.
• Epicondyles should both be in profile with medial most prominent.
• A portion of the radial head and about 1/2 of neck should be superimposed by ulna.
• Optimum exposure and penetration with no motion should visualize sharp bone margins. Trabecular marking should appear clear and sharp.
• Patient ID should be clear and legible and R or L marker visible on lateral border without superimposing anatomy.

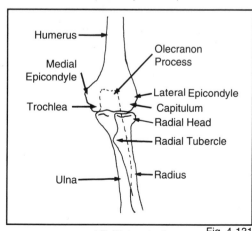

AP (Extended)   Fig. 4-131

• Oblique Position (Medial, Internal Oblique)

Elbow
Basic
• AP
• **Oblique**
• Lateral

Structures Best Shown:
Oblique view of distal humerus and proximal radius and ulna.
Internal Oblique - Coronoid process of ulna in profile.

NOTE: Choice of internal and/or external oblique is determined by departmental routines or by area of interest, either the coronoid process or the radial head and neck.

Technical Factors:
• Film Size - 10 x 12 in. (24 x 30 cm).
• Divide in half, crosswise.
• Detail screen, table top.
• 66 ± 6 kVp range.

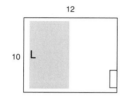

Patient Position:
• Patient seated at end of table with arm fully extended with shoulder and elbow on same horizontal plane (lower shoulder as needed).

Shielding: Place lead shield over patient's lap to protect gonads.

Part Position:
• Align arm and forearm to long axis of unmasked portion of film. Center elbow joint to center of unmasked film.
• Pronate hand into a natural palm down position and rotate arm as needed until distal humerus and anterior surface of elbow is rotated **45°**. (Palpate epicondyles to determine a 45° rotation of distal humerus.)

Central Ray:
• CR **perpendicular** to film, directed to **mid-elbow joint** (approximately 3/4 in. or 2 cm distal to mid point of line between epicondyles as viewed from the x-ray tube).
• Minimum 40 in. (102 cm) SID.

Collimation: Collimate on four sides to area of interest.

Evaluation Criteria:
• Long axis of arm should be aligned to long axis of the half of exposed film with elbow joint centered to center of four-sided collimation.
• The medial epicondyle and the trochlea should appear elongated and in partial profile.
• Olecranon process of ulna should appear seated in olecranon fossa and trochlear notch should be visible in obliqued position.
• **Coronoid process** should be well demonstrated in profile with associated joint space open.
• Radial head and neck should be superimposed and near centered on proximal ulna.
• Optimum exposure and penetration with no motion should visualize sharp bone margins. Trabecular markings should be visible and appear sharp on those parts of humerus, radius and ulna that are not superimposed.
• Patient ID should be clear and legible and R or L markers visible on lateral border without superimposing anatomy.

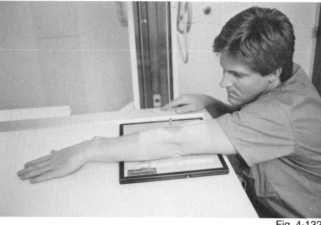

Medial, Internal Oblique   Fig. 4-132

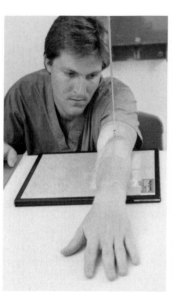

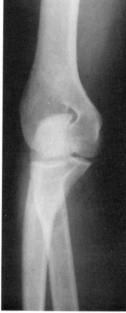

Fig. 4 -133   Fig. 4 -134
Close-up, Showing   Medial, Internal
45° Oblique   Oblique

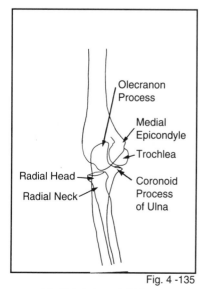

Fig. 4 -135
Medial, Internal Oblique

• Oblique Position (Lateral, External Oblique)

Elbow
Basic
• AP
• **Oblique**
• Lateral

Structures Best Shown:
Oblique view of distal humerus and proximal radius and ulna.
External Oblique - radial head and neck

NOTE: Choice of internal and/or external oblique should be determined by departmental routines or by area of interest, coronoid process or radial head and neck.

Technical Factors:
- Film Size - 10 x 12 in. (24 x 30 cm).
- Divide in half, crosswise
- Detail screen, table top.
- 66 ± 6 kVp range.

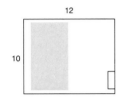

Patient Position:
- Patient seated at end of table with arm fully extended with shoulder and elbow on same horizontal plane (lower shoulder as needed).

Shielding: Place lead shield over patient's lap to protect gonads.

Part Position:
- Align arm and forearm to long axis of unmasked portion of film. Center elbow joint to center of unmasked film.
- Supinate hand and rotate laterally the entire arm so the distal humerus and the anterior surface of elbow joint is 45° to cassette.
  (Will need to lean laterally for sufficient lateral rotation). Palpate epicondyles to determine a 45° rotation of distal humerus.

Central Ray:
- CR **perpendicular** to film, directed to **mid-elbow joint,** (a point approximately 3/4 in. (2 cm) distal to midpoint of line between epicondyles as viewed from the x-ray tube).
- Minimum 40 in. (102 cm) SID.

Collimation: Collimate on four sides to area of interest.

Evaluation Criteria:
- Long axis of arm should be aligned to long axis of the half of exposed film with elbow joint centered to center of four-sided collimation.
- The lateral epicondyle and the capitulum should appear elongated and in profile.
- **Radial head, neck and tuberosity** should be visualized entirely free of superimposition.
- Elbow joint space should appear open.
- Optimum exposure and penetration with no motion should visualize sharp bone margins. Trabecular markings should be visible and appear sharp on those parts of humerus, radius and ulna that are not superimposed.
- Patient ID should be clear and legible and R or L markers visible on lateral border without superimposing anatomy.

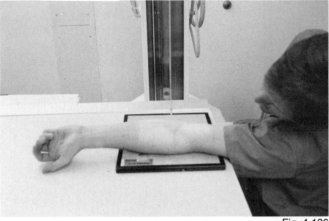
Lateral, External Oblique   Fig. 4-136

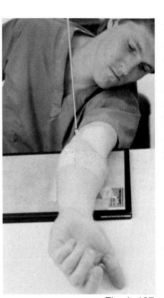
Fig. 4 -137
Close-up, Showing
45° Lateral Rotation

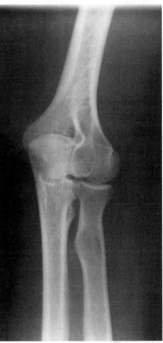
Fig. 4 -138
Lateral, External Oblique

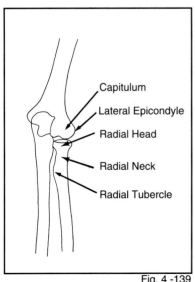

- Capitulum
- Lateral Epicondyle
- Radial Head
- Radial Neck
- Radial Tubercle

Fig. 4 -139
Lateral, External Oblique

Elbow

• Lateral Position

Elbow
Basic
• AP
• Oblique
• **Lateral**

Structures Best Shown:

Lateral view of distal humerus and proximal forearm. Clearly visualizes olecranon process with epicondyles superimposed.

Technical Factors:

• Film size - 8 x 10 in. (18 x 24 cm), crosswise.
• Detail screen, table top.
• 66 ± 6 kVp range.

Patient Position:

• Patient seated at end of table with elbow **flexed 90°**. (See NOTE.)

Shielding: Place lead shield over patient's lap to protect gonads.

Part Position:

• Align long axis of forearm to long axis of cassette and center elbow joint to center of film.
• Drop shoulder so humerus and forearm are on same horizontal plane.
• Rotate hand and wrist into true lateral position, thumb side up.
• Place support under hand and wrist to elevate hand and distal forearm slightly as needed for true lateral elbow (epicondyles superimposed).

Central Ray:

• CR **perpendicular** to film, directed to **mid elbow joint** (a point approximately 1.5 in. or 4 cm medial to easily palpated posterior surface of olecranon process).
• Minimum 40 in. (102 cm) SID.

Collimation: Collimate on four sides to area of interest.

NOTE: Diagnosis of certain important joint pathology is dependent on 90° flexion of the elbow joint. Therefore, unless there are counter indications such as severe trauma and/or dislocation, the lower arm should be flexed **90°** or at **a right angle** to the humerus. Also, a second reason for the full 90° flexion is that the olecranon process will not be fully seen in profile with less than 90°.

• **Exception:** Certain soft tissue diagnoses require less flexion of only 30 to 35°, but these should be taken only when specifically indicated.

Evaluation Criteria:

• Long axis of arm should be aligned to long axis of film with elbow joint flexed 90° and centered to center of film and centered to four-sided collimation field.
• **True lateral**, best indicated by the three concentric arcs of (1) the trochlear sulcus, (2) ridge of capitulum and trochlea and (3) trochlear notch of ulna. (See *Figs. 4-141* and *142* and page 105.) Also the humeral epicondyles should be superimposed.
• Olecranon process should be visualized in profile.
• Part of the radial head will be superimposed by the coronoid process.
• Optimum exposure with no motion should visualize sharp bone margins and clear trabecular markings throughout. Densities should be similar at distal and proximal ends of forearm.
• Patient ID should be clear and legible and R or L markers visible on lateral border without superimposing anatomy.

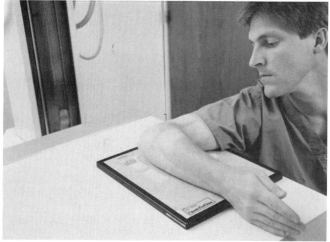

Lateral

Fig. 4-140

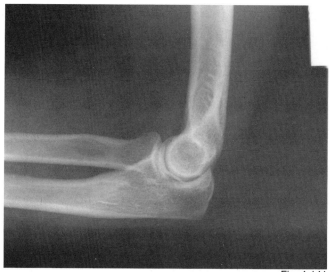

Lateral

Fig. 4-141

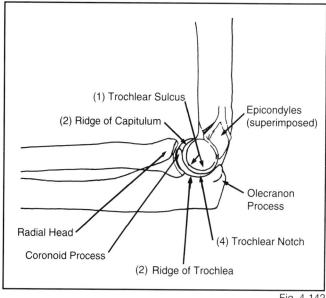

(1) Trochlear Sulcus
(2) Ridge of Capitulum
Epicondyles (superimposed)
Radial Head
Coronoid Process
Olecranon Process
(4) Trochlear Notch
(2) Ridge of Trochlea

Lateral

Fig. 4-142

• Acute Flexion "Jones" Position

Elbow
Optional
• **Acute Flexion**
   (Jones Position)
• Coyle Trauma Methods
• Radial Head Projections

Structures Best Shown:
Olecranon process in profile, and superimposed outlines of bones of forearm and arm.

NOTE: Two projections are required, one with **CR perpendicular to humerus** and one with CR angled to be **perpendicular to forearm.**

Technical Factors:
• Film Size - 8 x 10 in. (18 x 24 cm) lengthwise (or divide in half, crosswise for two projections)
• Detail screen, table top.
• 66 ± 6 kVp range.
   (Increase 4-6 kVp for proximal forearm.)

Patient Position:
• Patient seated at end of table with acutely flexed arm resting on cassette.

Shielding: Place lead shield over patient's lap.

Part Position:
• Align and center humerus to long axis of film with forearm acutely flexed, with fingertips resting on shoulder.
• Adjust cassette to center elbow joint region to center of film.
• Palpate epicondyles and insure they are the same distances from cassette for **no rotation.**

Central Ray:
Distal Humerus: (Tangential projection of olecranon process)
• CR **perpendicular to film, and humerus**, directed to **a point midway between epicondyles.**
• Minimum 40 in. (102 cm) SID.

Proximal Forearm:
• CR **perpendicular to forearm**, (angle CR as needed) directed to a point approximately **2 in. (5 cm) proximal or superior to olecranon process.**
• Minimum 40 in. (102 cm) SID.

Collimation: Collimate on four sides to area of interest.

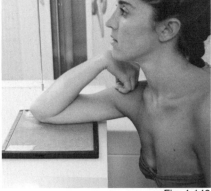

For Distal Humerus   Fig. 4-143

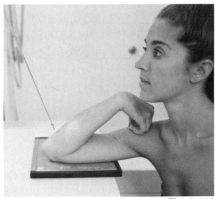

For Proximal Forearm   Fig. 4-144

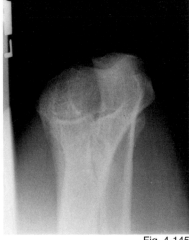

Distal Humerus   Fig. 4-145

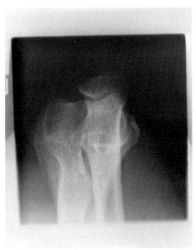

Proximal Forearm   Fig.4-146

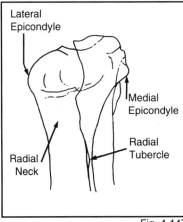

Distal Humerus   Fig. 4-147

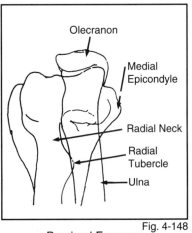

Proximal Forearm   Fig. 4-148

Evaluation Criteria:
• Four sided collimation borders should be visible.
• Patient ID information should be legible and R or L markers visible without superimposing anatomy.

Distal Humerus:
• Forearm and humerus should be directly superimposed.
• Medial and lateral epicondyles, distal margins of trochlea and capitulum and olecranon process all should be seen in profile.
• Joint space and articular surfaces of olecranon process and trochlea should be visualized.

• Optimum exposure will visualize (without overexposure) soft tissues and the olecranon process and other structures of distal humerus in profile. Other parts of humerus and proximal forearm will appear underexposed.

Proximal Forearm:
• Proximal ulna and radius will be superimposed by distal humerus.
• Outline of radial head and neck should be visible clearly and undistorted through distal humerus.
• Joint space of olecranon process will not appear open due to angle of CR.
• Optimum exposure will clearly visualize outlines of proximal ulna and radius superimposed over humerus. Soft tissues will not be readily visible and structures in profile will appear dark and overexposed.

• Coyle[1] Trauma Methods

Special projections taken for pathology or trauma to the area
of the radial head and/or the coronoid process of ulna.

Elbow
Optional
• Acute Flexion
(Jones Position)
• **Coyle Trauma Method**
• Radial head projections

Structures Best Shown:

1. Radial head, neck and tuberosity and articular margin of capitulum.
2. Coronoid process and articular margin of trochlea.

Technical Factors:

• Film Size - 8 x 10 in. (18 x 24 cm) crosswise.
• Detail screen, table top.
• 70 ± 6 kVp range. (See NOTE below.)

Patient Position:

• Supine or erect seated at end of table.

Shielding: Place lead shield over gonadal area.

1. Part Position - Radial Head

• Flex elbow 90° if possible, pronate hand.
• CR - angle **45° toward shoulder,** centered to radial head.
• Minimum 40 in. (102 cm) SID.

2. Part Position - Coronoid Process

• Elbow flexed **only 80°** from extended position (more than 80° will obscure coronoid process), pronate hand.
• CR - angle **45° away from shoulder**, into elbow joint.
• Minimum 40 in. (102 cm) SID.

Collimation: Collimate on four sides to area of interest.

NOTE: • Increase exposure factors by 4-6 kVp from lateral elbow because of angled CR.
• These projections are effective with or without splint.

Evaluation Criteria for Specific Anatomy:

1. Radial Head

• The joint space between radial head and capitulum should be open and clear.
• The radial head, neck and tuberosity should be in profile free of superimposition except for a small part of the coronoid process.
• The distal humerus and epicondyles will appear distorted due to the 45° angle.

2. Coronoid Process

• The distal portion of the coronoid will appear elongated but in profile.
• The joint space between coronoid process and trochlea should be open and clear.
• The radial head and neck will be superimposed by ulna.
• Optimum exposure factors should clearly visualize the coronoid process in profile. Bony margins of superimposed radial head and neck will be faintly visualized through the proximal ulna.

[1] Coyle, George F.: "Radiographing Immobile Trauma Patients, Unit 7, Special Angled Views of Joints—Elbow, Knee, Ankle" Multi-Media Publishing, Inc., Denver, Co., 1980.

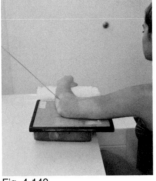
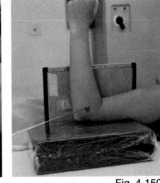

Fig. 4-149   Erect   Supine   Fig. 4-150
1. Angled for Radial Head

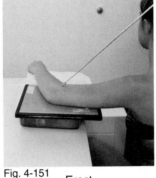

Fig. 4-151   Erect   Supine   Fig. 4-152
2. Angled for Coronoid Process

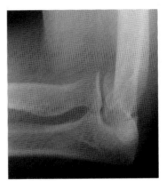
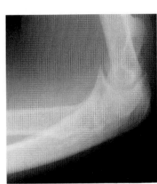

Fig. 4-153   Fig. 4-154
1. For Radial Head   2. For Coronoid Process

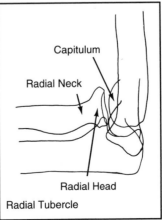
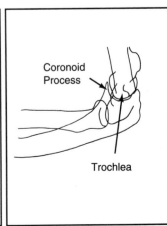

Fig. 4-155   Fig. 4-156
1. For Radial Head   2. For Coronoid Process

• Radial Head Projections

Structures Best Shown:

Radial head and neck projected in profile, with entire head and neck demonstrated without superimposition with varying degrees of rotation.

Technical Factors:

• Film Size - 8 x 10 in. (18 x 24 cm).
    Divide in half.
    or
  - 10 x 12 in. (24 x 30 cm).
    Divide in fourths.
• Detail screen, table top.
• 66 ± 6 kVp range.

Patient Position:

• Patient seated at end of table, arm **flexed 90°** resting on cassette with humerus, forearm and hand on same horizontal plane.

Shielding: Place lead shield over gonadal area.

Part Position:

• Center radial head area to center of the unmasked portion of film positioned so that distal humerus and proximal forearm are placed "square" with, or at right angles with the borders of cassette.
• Four projections are taken with the only difference being the rotation of the hand and wrist from maximum (1) external rotation to (4) maximum internal rotation, demonstrating different parts of the radial head projected clear of the coronoid process. (Near complete rotation of radial head occurs in these four projections.)
  1. Supinate hand (palm up), externally rotate as far as can be tolerated.
  2. Place hand in true lateral position (thumb up).
  3. Pronate hand (palm down).
  4. Internally rotate hand (thumb down) as far as can be tolerated.

Central Ray:

• CR **perpendicular** to film, directed to **radial head** (approximately 1 in. or 2 - 3 cm distal to lateral epicondyle).
• Minimum 40 in. (102 cm) SID.

Collimation: Collimate on four sides to area of interest (include at least 3 - 4 in. (10 cm) of proximal forearm as well as distal portion of humerus).

Evaluation Criteria:

• Elbow should be flexed 90° in true lateral position evidenced by direct superimposition of epicondyles.
• Radial head and neck will be partially superimposed by ulna but should be completely visualized in profile in the various projections.
• Optimum exposure with no motion should clearly visualize sharp bony margins and clear trabecular markings of the radial head and neck area.
• Patient ID should be clear and legible and R or L markers visible on lateral border without superimposing anatomy.

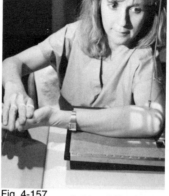
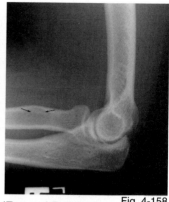

Fig. 4-157   1. Hand Supinated (External Rotation)   Fig. 4-158

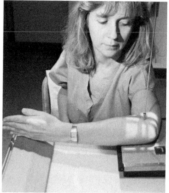
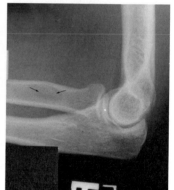

Fig. 4-159   2. Hand Lateral   Fig. 4-160

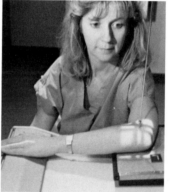
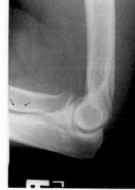

Fig. 4-161   3. Hand Pronated   Fig. 4-162

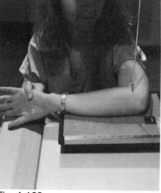
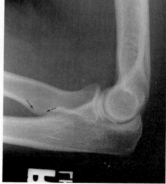

Fig. 4-163   4. Hand Internally Rotated   Fig. 4-164

• AP Projection

Warning: Do **NOT** attempt to rotate arm if fracture
or dislocation is suspected - see trauma routine.

Humerus
Basic
• **AP**
• Rotational Lateral

Structures Best Shown
Frontal view of entire humerus.

Technical Factors:
- Film Size - lengthwise, (large enough to include entire humerus)
  - 7 x 17 in. (18 x 43 cm), if available
  - or
  - 14 x 17 in. (35 x 43 cm), larger patient
  - or
  - 11 x 14 in. (28 x 35 cm), smaller patient.
- Moving or stationary grid (non-grid , detail screen may be used for smaller patient).
- 70 ± 6 kVp range.
- Minimize anode-heel effect if possible; shoulder at cathode end of x-ray beam.

Patient Position:
- May be taken erect or supine.
- Adjust height of cassette so that shoulder and elbow joints are the same distance from ends of film.
- Rotate body toward affected side as needed to bring the shoulder and proximal humerus in contact with cassette.

Shielding: Secure or place lead shield over pelvic area.

Part Position:
- Align humerus to long axis of film, unless diagonal placement is needed to include both shoulder and elbow joints.
- Extend hand and forearm as far as can be tolerated.
- Abduct arm slightly and gently supinate hand so that **epicondyles of elbow are parallel** to the film.

Central Ray:
- CR **perpendicular** to film, directed to **midpoint of humerus.**
- Minimum 40 in. (102 cm) SID.

Collimation: Collimate on four sides to soft tissue borders of humerus and shoulder. (Lower margin of collimation field to include elbow joint and up to 1 in. or 2.5 cm of proximal forearm.)

Respiration: Suspend respiration during exposure.

Alternate Routine: (To include one joint only)
If your department routine is to include only the joint nearest the site of injury, use a 10 x 12 in. (24 x 30 cm) or an 11 x 14 (28 x 35 cm) film and center the cassette so the joint in question is at least 1.5 or 2 in. (4-5 cm) from end of film.

Evaluation Criteria:
- Entire humerus including shoulder and elbow joints and about 1 in. or 3 cm of proximal forearm should be visualized, with collimation margins on all four sides.

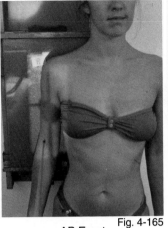

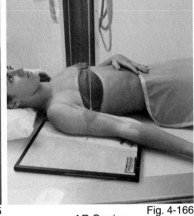

AP Erect Fig. 4-165   **AP Supine** Fig. 4-166

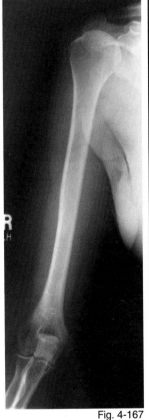

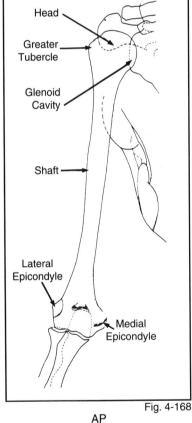

Fig. 4-167   Fig. 4-168
AP   AP

- True AP projection as evidenced by:
  - Greater tubercle is seen in profile laterally.
  - Humeral head is seen in profile medially with only minimal superimposition of glenoid cavity.
  - Outline of lesser tubercle is seen just medially to greater tubercle.
  - Lateral and medial epicondyles of distal humerus are seen in profile.
- Optimum exposure with no motion will visualize sharp borders and fine trabecular markings of the entire humerus. The proximal and distal portions of the humerus should appear near equal in exposure density. (Correct utilization of anode-heel effect will facilitate this.)
- Patient ID information should be legible; R or L marker placed on the lateral border of collimation field should be visible without superimposing the humerus.

• Rotational Lateral Projection

Warning: Do **NOT** attempt to rotate arm if fracture or dislocation is suspected - see trauma routine.

<table>
<tr><td>
Humerus
Basic
• AP
• **Rotational Lateral**
</td></tr>
</table>

Structures Best Shown
Lateral view of entire humerus.

Technical Factors:
- Film Size - lengthwise, (large enough to include entire humerus)
  - 7 x 17 in. (18 x 43 cm), if available
  - or
  - 14 x 17 in. (35 x 43 cm), larger patient
  - or
  - 11 x 14 in. (28 x 35 cm), smaller patient.
- Moving or stationary grid (non-grid, detail screen may be used for smaller patient).
- 70 ± 6 kVp range.
- Minimize anode-heel effect if possible; shoulder at cathode end of x-ray beam.

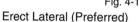

Patient and Part Position:
- May be taken erect or supine. (Erect may be easier for patient.)
- Preferred erect position is with patient facing film *(Fig. 4-169)* which allows close contact of humerus to cassette; flex elbow 90° as shown.
- May also be taken erect with back to film and elbow partially flexed, with body rotated toward affected side as needed to bring humerus and shoulder in contact with cassette. Internally, rotate arm as needed for lateral position *(Fig. 4-170)*.
- If taken supine, extend elbow, internally rotate arm into true lateral. *(Fig. 4-171)*.
- Adjust cassette so shoulders and elbow joints are the same distance from the ends of cassette.
- Epicondyles should be directly superimposed as viewed from the x-ray tube for a true lateral.

Central Ray:
- CR **perpendicular** to film, centered to **mid point of humerus**.
- Minimum 40 in. (102 cm) SID.

Collimation: Collimate on four sides to soft tissue border of humerus, insuring that all of shoulder and elbow joints are included.

Respiration: Suspend respiration during exposure.

Alternate Routine: (To include one joint only.)
- Positioning is same as above with centering similar to AP projection on preceding page.

Evaluation Criteria:
- Entire humerus including elbow and shoulder joints should be included with collimation margins on all four sides.
- True lateral projection as evidenced by:
  - Epicondyles are directly superimposed.
  - Lesser tubercle is shown in profile medially, partially superimposed by the lower portion of the glenoid cavity.
- Optimum exposure with no motion will visualize sharp borders and fine trabecular markings of the entire humerus. The proximal and distal parts of the humerus should appear near equal in exposure density. (Correct utilization of anode-heel effect will facilitate this.)

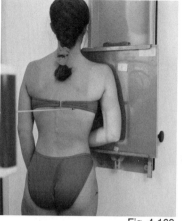

Fig. 4-169
Erect Lateral (Preferred)

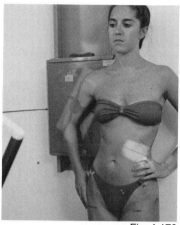

Fig. 4-170
Erect Lateral (Elective)

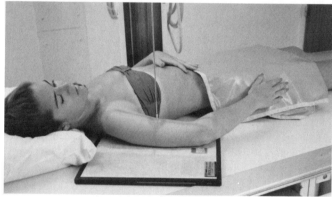

Supine Lateral — Fig. 4-171

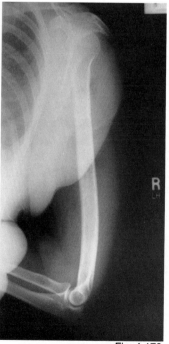

Fig. 4-172
Lateral

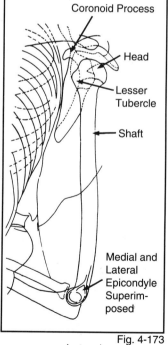

Fig. 4-173
Lateral

Coronoid Process
Head
Lesser Tubercle
Shaft
Medial and Lateral Epicondyle Superimposed

- Patient ID information should be legible; R or L marker placed on the lateral border of collimation field should be visible without superimposing the humerus.

• AP Projection

Warning: Do **NOT** attempt to rotate arm if fracture or dislocation is suspected. (This AP and the trama lateral should be taken at 90°to each other without arm rotation.

> **Humerus**
> (Trauma Routine)
> Basic
> • **AP (Neutral Rotation)**
> • Lateral (mid or distal)
> (Proximal Humerus - Ch. 5)

Structures Best Shown:
Frontal view of entire humerus.

Technical Factors:
- Film Size - lengthwise, (large enough to include entire humerus)
  - 7 x 17 in. (18 x 43 cm), if available
  - or
  - 14 x 17 in. (35 x 43 cm), larger patient
  - or
  - 11 x 14 in. (28 x 35 cm), smaller patient.
- Moving or stationary grid (non-grid , detail screen may be used for smaller patient).
- 70 ± 6 kVp range.
- Minimize anode-heel effect if possible - shoulder at cathode end of x-ray beam.

Patient Position:
- May be taken erect or supine. (Erect may be less painful for patient if already in an erect position.)
- Adjust cassette so that shoulder and elbow joints are the same distance from ends of film.
- Rotate body toward affected side as needed to bring proximal humerus in contact with cassette.

Shielding: Secure or place lead shield over pelvic area.

Part Position:
- Align humerus to long axis of film - unless diagonal placement is needed to include both shoulder and elbow joints.
- Gently extend elbow as far as can be tolerated.
- Abduct arm slightly away from body - **do not** attempt to rotate arm with possible fracture or dislocation. However, a lateral should then also be taken at a right angle or 90° from this AP. (If patient can rotate arm without discomfort, use non-trauma routine and gently rotate arm externally so that epicondyles of elbow are parallel to the film.)

Central Ray:
- CR **perpendicular** to film, directed to **mid point of humerus**.
- Minimum 40 in. (102 cm) SID.

Collimation: Collimate on four sides to area of humerus. (Include shoulder joint and elbow joint with up to 1 in. or 3 cm of proximal forearm.)

Respiration: Suspend respiration during exposure.

Alternate Routine: (To include one joint only.)
- Positioning is same as above with centering similar to non-trauma AP projection as described on page 141.

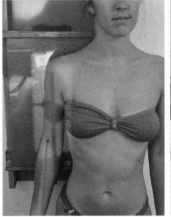
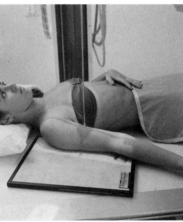

AP Erect   Fig.4-174   AP Supine   Fig. 4-175

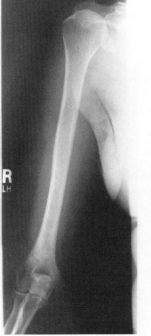

AP   Fig. 4-176

Evaluation Criteria:
- Entire humerus including shoulder and elbow joints and about 1 in. or 3 cm of proximal forearm should be visualized, with collimation margins on all four sides.
- Trauma routine may be taken with humerus as is rather than attempting to rotate into a true AP projection, but a lateral should then also be taken at a right angle or 90° from this AP projection.
- Optimum exposure with no motion will visualize sharp borders and fine trabecular markings of the entire humerus. The proximal and distal portions of the humerus should appear near equal in exposure density. (Correct utilization of anode-heel effect will facilitate this.)
- Patient ID information should be legible; R or L marker placed on the lateral border of collimation field should be visible without superimposing the humerus.

Humerus (Trauma Routine)

• Lateral Position - Mid and Distal Humerus

Warning: Do **NOT** attempt to rotate arm
if fracture or dislocation is suspected.

Proximal Humerus: see transthoracic lateral, p 160.

Humerus
(Trauma Routine)
Basic
• AP (Neutral Rotation)
• **Lateral (mid or distal)**
(Proximal Humerus - Ch. 5)

Structures Best Shown:
Lateral view of mid and distal humerus including elbow joint.

Technical Factors:
• Film Size - 11 x 14 in. (28 X 35 cm)
      or
     - 10 x 12 in. (24 x 30 cm),
            smaller patient.
• Detail screen, non-grid.
• 66 ± 6 kVp range.

Patient and Part Position:
• With patient recumbent, may be taken as a crosstable lateral *(Fig. 4-177)* or if necessary in a lateral decubitus body position *(Fig. 4-178* without attempting to rotate arm. (Should be 90° from AP projection.)
• Gently place cassette between arm and thorax (top of film to the axilla) with arm aligned to midline of cassette.

Shielding:
Place lead shield **over thorax and pelvis,** between the cassette and patient.

Central Ray:
• CR **perpendicular** to the **mid point of film.**
• Minimum 40 in. (102 cm) SID.

Collimation:
Collimate to soft tissue margins.

Respiration:
Suspend respiration during exposure. (This is important to prevent movement of cassette during the exposure.)

Evaluation Criteria:
• Distal two-thirds of humerus and elbow joint should be well visualized with collimation visible on lateral borders.
• This lateral view should be 90° or at right angle to the AP trauma projection.
• Optimum exposure with no motion should visualize sharp bony borders and fine trabecular markings of humerus and proximal forearm.
• Patient ID information should be legible; R or L marker placed on lateral border should be visualized without superimposing the humerus.

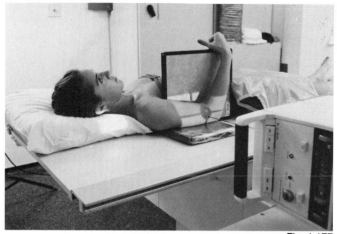

Lateral, Crosstable   Fig. 4-177

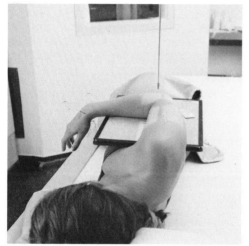

Lateral, Decubitus   Fig. 4-178

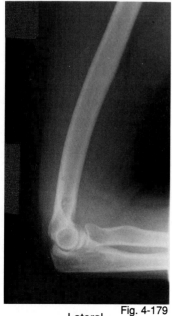

Lateral   Fig. 4-179

Chapter 5
Radiographic Anatomy and Positioning of the
Proximal Humerus and Shoulder Girdle

Contents

Proximal Humerus

Part I Radiographic Anatomy

Upper Limb (Extremity)

The first and second groups of bones of the upper limb are the hand and wrist, and the forearm respectively, as described in Chapter 4.

The third and fourth groups of bones of the upper limb are the arm or **humerus,** and the **shoulder girdle,** which includes the **clavicle** and **scapula**.

Humerus

The **humerus** is the largest and the longest bone of the upper limb. Its length on an adult equals approximately one-fifth of the body height. The humerus articulates with the **scapula** (shoulder blade) at the shoulder joint.

The anatomy of the mid and distal humerus was included in Chapter 4 with the elbow joint.

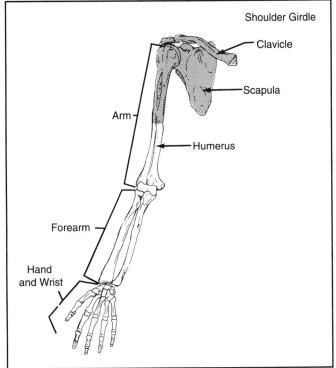

Upper Limb   Fig. 5-1

Proximal Humerus:

The proximal humerus is that part of the upper arm which articulates with the scapula, making up the shoulder joint. The most proximal part is the rounded **head** of the humerus. The slightly constricted area directly below the head is the **anatomical neck.** The process directly below the anatomical neck on the anterior surface is the **lesser tubercle,** *(tu'ber-k'l)* (tuberosity in earlier literature) and the larger lateral process is the **greater tubercle.** The deep groove between these two tubercles is the **intertubercular** *(in"ter-tu-ber'ku-lar)* **groove** (bicipital groove). The tapered area below the head and tubercles is the **surgical neck,** and distal to the surgical neck is the long **shaft** or **body** of the humerus.

The surgical neck is so named because it is the site of frequent fractures requiring surgery of the proximal humerus. Fractures at the anatomical neck are rare.

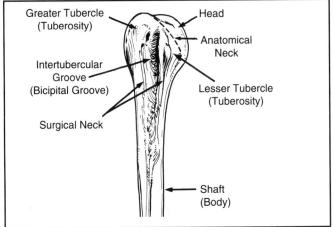

Frontal View of Proximal Humerus   Fig. 5-2
(Neutral Rotation, Oblique Position)

Anatomy of Proximal Humerus on Radiograph:

Figure 5-3 is an AP radiograph of the shoulder taken with **external rotation,** which places the humerus in a **true AP** or frontal position. Note that the drawing in *Fig. 5-2* represents a neutral rotation (natural position of arm without internal or external rotation). This places the humerus in an oblique position midway between an AP (external rotation) and a lateral (internal rotation).

Some of the parts are more difficult to clearly visualize on radiographs than on drawings, but a good understanding of locations and relationships between various anatomical parts aids in this identification.

  A. Head of humerus
  B. Greater tubercle
  C. Intertubercular groove
  D. Lesser tubercle
  E. Anatomical neck
  F. Surgical neck
  G. Shaft

The relative location of the greater and lesser tubercles is significant as a way of determining a true frontal view or a true AP projection of the proximal humerus. **The lesser tubercle is located anteriorly, and the greater tubercle is located laterally** in a true AP projection.

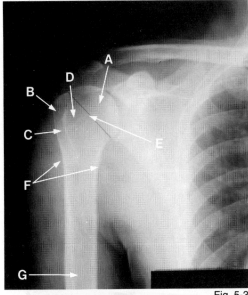

AP Shoulder – External Rotation   Fig. 5-3

Shoulder Girdle

The shoulder girdle consists of two bones, the **clavicle** and the **scapula**. The function of the clavicle and scapula is to connect each upper limb to the trunk or axial skeleton. Anteriorly the shoulder girdle connects to the trunk at the upper sternum, but posteriorly the connection to the trunk is incomplete in that the scapula is connected to the trunk by muscles only. Each shoulder girdle and upper limb connect at the shoulder joint between the scapula and the humerus. Each clavicle is located over the upper, anterior rib cage. Each scapula is situated over the upper, posterior rib cage.

The upper margin of the scapula is at the level of the **second posterior rib** and the lower margin is at the level of the **posterior seventh rib.**

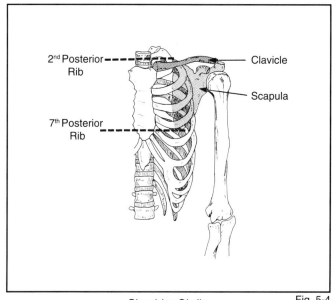

Shoulder Girdle   Fig. 5-4

Clavicle (collarbone)

The clavicle is a long bone with a double curvature having three main parts, the two ends and the long central portion. The lateral or **acromial** *(ah-kro'me-al)* **end** (extremity) of the clavicle articulates with the acromion of the scapula. This joint or articulation is termed the **acromioclavicular** *(ah-kro"me-o-klah-vik'u-lar)* **joint** and can be readily palpated or it may even be visible. The medial or **sternal end** (extremity) articulates with the manubrium, which is the upper part of the sternum. This articulation is termed the **sternoclavicular** *(ster"no-klah-vik'u-lar)* **joint.** This joint is also easily palpated and the combination of the sternoclavicular joints on either side of the manubrium help form an important positioning landmark called the **jugular** *(jug'u-lar)* **notch**, also called the suprasternal or manubrial notch in earlier literature.

The **body** or **shaft** of the clavicle is the elongated portion between the two ends.

The acromial end of the clavicle is flattened and has a downward curvature at its attachment with the acromion. The sternal end is more triangular in shape and is also directed downward to articulate with the sternum.

In general, there is a difference in size and shape of the clavicle between male and female. The female clavicle is usually shorter and less curved than is the male clavicle. The clavicle in the male tends to be thicker and more curved in shape, usually being most curved in heavily muscled males.

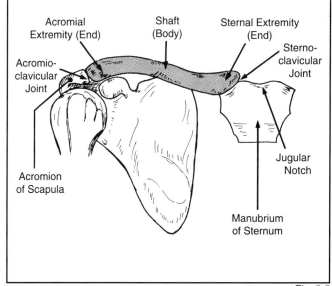

Clavicle   Fig. 5-5

Radiograph of the Clavicle

The AP radiograph of the clavicle in *Fig. 5-6* identifies the two joints and the three parts of the clavicle.

    A. Sternoclavicular joint

    B. Sternal end

    C. Body (shaft)

    D. Acromial end

    E. Acromioclavicular joint

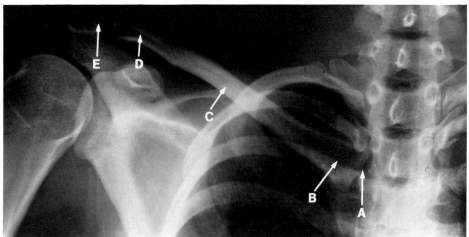

AP Radiograph of Clavicle   Fig. 5-6

Scapula (Shoulder Blade)

The scapula, which forms the posterior part of the shoulder girdle is a flat triangular bone with three borders, three angles and two surfaces. The three borders include the **medial** (vertebral) **border**, which is the long edge or border near the vertebrae; the **superior border**, the uppermost margin of the scapula; and the **lateral** (axillary) **border**, the border nearest the axilla (ak-sil'ah). Axilla is the medical term for the armpit.

Anterior View: The three corners of the triangular shaped scapula are called angles. The **lateral angle**, sometimes called the head of the scapula, is the thickest part of the scapula and ends laterally in a shallow depression called the **glenoid cavity** (fossa). The humerus articulates with the glenoid cavity of the scapula to form the glenohumeral or shoulder joint. The constricted area between the head and the body of the scapula is the **neck.**

The **superior** and **inferior angles** refer to the upper and lower ends of the medial or vertebral border. The **body** (blade) of the scapula is arched for greater strength. The thin, flat, lower part of the body is sometimes referred to as the "wing" or ala of the scapula, although these are not preferred anatomical terms.

The anterior surface of the scapula is termed the **costal** (kos'tal) **surface** because of the proximity to the ribs (costa, literally meaning rib). The mid area of the costal surface presents a large concavity or depression, the **subscapular fossa.**

The **acromion** is a long, curved process extending laterally over the head of the humerus. The **coracoid process** is a thick, beak-like process projecting anteriorly beneath the clavicle. The **scapular notch** is a notch on the superior border partially formed by the base of the coracoid process.

Posterior View: Figure 5-9 shows a prominent structure on the dorsal or posterior surface of the scapula, called the **spine.** The elevated spine of the scapula starts at the vertebral border as a smooth triangular area and continues laterally to end at the **acromion.** The acromion overhangs the shoulder joint posteriorly.

The posterior border or ridge of the spine is somewhat thickened and is termed the **crest** of the spine. The spine separates the posterior surface into an **infraspinous** (in"frah-spi'nus) **fossa** and **a supraspinous fossa.** Both of these fossae serve as surfaces of attachment for shoulder muscles. The names of these muscles are associated with the respective fossae, namely the infraspinous and supraspinous muscles.

Lateral View: The lateral view of the scapula, shown in *Fig. 5-10*, demonstrates relative positions of the various parts of the scapula. The thin scapula looks like the letter Y in this position. The upper parts of the Y are the acromion and coracoid process. The **acromion** is the expanded distal end of the spine extending superiorly and posteriorly to the **glenoid cavity** (fossa). The **coracoid process** is located more anteriorly in relationship to the glenoid cavity or shoulder joint.

The bottom leg of the Y is the body of the scapula. The posterior surface or back portion of the thin body portion of the scapula is called the **dorsal surface.** The spine extends from the dorsal surface at its upper margin. The anterior surface of the body is called the **costal surface.** The lower part of the thin body ends at the **inferior angle.**

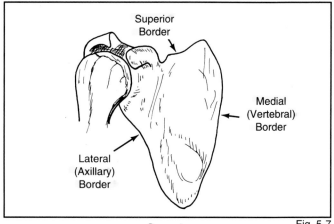

Scapula   Fig. 5-7

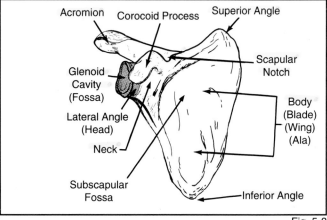

Scapula - Anterior or Costal Surface   Fig. 5-8

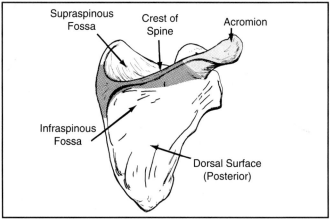

Scapula - Posterior or Dorsal Surface   Fig. 5-9

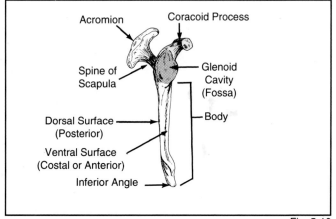

Scapula - Lateral View   Fig. 5-10

Review Exercise with Radiographs of Scapula

AP Projection: Figure 5-11 is an AP projection of the scapula taken with the arm abducted so as not to superimpose the scapula. Knowing shapes and relationships of anatomical parts should help in identifying each of these parts.

A. Acromion
B. Tip of arrow is about an inch below the coracoid process
C. Scapular notch
D. Superior angle
E. Medial (vertebral) border
F. Inferior angle
G. Lateral (axillary) border
H. Glenoid cavity (fossa)

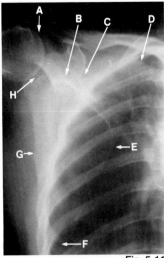

AP Projection Fig. 5-11

Lateral Position: This lateral position of the scapula is taken with the patient in an anterior oblique position with the upper body rotated until the scapula is separated from the rib cage in a true end-on or lateral position.

A. Acromion
B. Coracoid process
C. Inferior angle
D. Spine of scapula
E. Body of scapula

Note again that this lateral view of the scapula results in a Y shape wherein the acromion and the coracoid process make up the upper legs of the Y, and the body makes up the bottom leg.

The scapular Y position is named for this Y shape resulting from a true lateral view of the scapula.

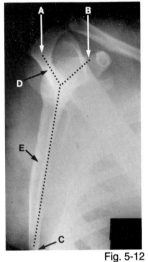

Fig. 5-12
Lateral Position

Proximal Humerus and Scapula

Inferosuperior Axial Projection: This projection (as illustrated in *Fig. 5-14*), results in a lateral view of the head and neck of the humerus. It also demonstrates the relationship of the humerus to the glenoid cavity, which makes up the shoulder joint.

The anatomy of the scapula may appear confusing in this position but knowing and understanding relationships of various parts of the scapula well will enable one to identify those labelled parts on this projection. This will also enable one to place this radiograph correctly on the illuminator (viewbox) for viewing with the correct side up.

Part **A** of *Fig. 5-13* is the tip of the **coracoid process**, which is located anterior to the shoulder joint and would therefore be uppermost on the radiograph if the film is placed on the viewbox as the x-ray tube sees it, with the anterior shoulder to the top.

Part **B** is the **glenoid cavity** which is the articulating surface of the **lateral angle** or **head** of the scapula.

Part **C** is the **spine** of the scapula which would be located posteriorly with the patient lying on her back as shown in *Fig. 5-14*.

Part **D** is the **acromion** which is the extended portion of the spine superimposed over the humerus in this position.

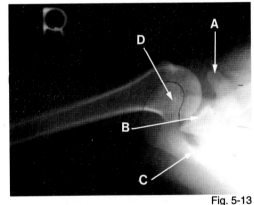

Fig. 5-13
Inferosuperior Axial Projection

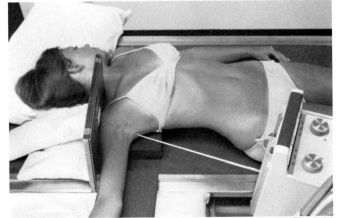

Inferosuperior Axial Projection Fig. 5-14

Classification of Joints

There are only three joints or articulations of the shoulder girdle. The **classification, mobility type** and **movement type** are as follows:

Classification
All three joints of the shoulder girdle are classified as **synovial joints**, characterized by a fibrous capsule containing synovial fluid.

Mobility Type
The mobility type of all three of these joints is **freely moveable** or **diarthrodial.** All symovial joints are by nature of their structure freely moveable. Therefore, the only difference between these three joints is the movement type.

Movement Type
The **glenohumeral** or **shoulder joint** involves articulation between the head of the humerus and the glenoid cavity of the scapula. The movement type is a **ball and socket** joint which allows great freedom of movement. These movements are **flexion, extension, abduction, adduction, circumduction, medial** (internal) and **lateral** (external) **rotation.**

The glenoid cavity is very shallow allowing the greatest freedom in mobility of any joint in the human body, but at some expense to its strength and stability. Even though the strong ligaments, tendons and muscles surrounding the joint provide stability, some stretching of the muscles and tendons can occur causing separation or dislocation of the humeral head from the glenoid cavity. Dislocations at the shoulder joint occur more frequently than at any other joint in the body requiring the need for frequent radiographic shoulder exams to evaluate for structural damage.

The shoulder girdle also includes two joints involving both ends of the clavicle. These are the sternoclavicular and acromioclavicular joints.

The **sternoclavicular joint** is a **double gliding or plane joint** in that the sternal end of the clavicle articulates with both the manubrium or upper portion of the sternum, as well as with the cartilage of the first rib. This allows a limited amount of gliding motion in nearly every direction.

The **acromioclavicular joint** is also a small synovial joint of the **gliding** or **plane movement type**, between the acromial end of the clavicle and the medial aspect of the acromion of the scapula. There are actually two types of movement at this joint. The primary movement is a gliding action between the end of the clavicle and the acromion. There is also some secondary rotary movement as the scapula moves forward and backward with the clavicle. This allows the scapula to adjust its position as it remains in close contact with the posterior chest wall. The rotary type movement however is limited and this joint is generally termed a gliding type joint.

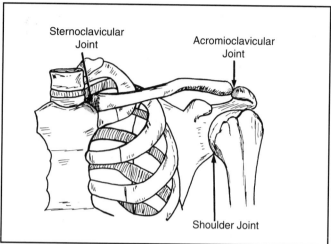

Joints of Shoulder Girdle   Fig. 5-15

Summary of Shoulder Girdle Joints

Classification: *Synovial*
(articular capsule containing synovial fluid)

Mobility Type: *Diarthrodial*
(freely movable)

Movement Types:
1. Shoulder joint (glenohumeral joint)
   - **Ball and socket**
2. Sternoclavicular Joint
   - **Gliding** (plane)
3. Acromioclavicular Joint
   - **Gliding** (plane)

Part II Radiographic Positioning

Radiographs of Shoulder Girdle for Proximal Humerus and Related Anatomy

Rotational views of the proximal humerus or shoulder girdle are commonly taken on non-trauma patients when fractures or dislocations of the humerus have been ruled out. These AP rotational projections demonstrate the glenohumeral joint well for possible calcium deposits or other pathology. Note specifically the location and shapes of (A) the **greater tubercle** and (B) the **lesser tubercle** on these external, internal and neutral rotation radiographs.

By studying the position and relationships of the greater and lesser tubercles on a radiograph of the shoulder, one can determine the rotational position of the arm. This understanding will enable one to know which rotational view is necessary to visualize specific parts of the proximal humerus.

External Rotation: The external rotation position represents a true **AP projection** or frontal view of the humerus in the anatomical position as determined by the epicondyles of the distal humerus. The arm and elbow are rotated externally until the palm of the hand is forward. This places an imaginary line between the medial and lateral epicondyles **parallel** to the film. (You can check this on yourself by dropping your arm at your side and externally rotating your hand and arm while palpating the epicondyles of your distal humerus.)

With this external rotation view (A) the **greater tubercle**, which is located anteriorly in a neutral position, **is now positioned in profile laterally.** The lesser tubercle (B) is now located anteriorly just medial to the greater tubercle.

Internal Rotation: The internal rotation results when the hand and arm are rotated internally until the epicondyles of the distal humerus are **perpendicular** to the film, thus placing the humerus in a **true lateral position**. The palm of the hand is back, or outward as needed to place the epicondyles perpendicular to the film.

The AP projection of the shoulder taken in the internal rotation position is therefore a lateral position of the humerus in which the **greater tubercle** is now rotated around to the anterior and medial aspect of the proximal humerus. The lesser tubercle is seen in profile medially.

Neutral Rotation: The neutral rotation AP projection of the shoulder as taken on a trauma patient when rotation views cannot be taken generally places the epicondyles of the distal humerus at an **approximate 45° angle** to the film. This results in a 45° oblique position of the humerus when the **palm of the hand is facing inward** against the thigh. The neutral position therefore is about midway between the external and internal positions. This places the greater tubercle anteriorly but still lateral to the lesser tubercle, as seen on the radiograph in *Fig. 5-21*.

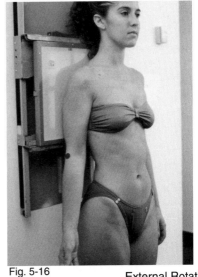
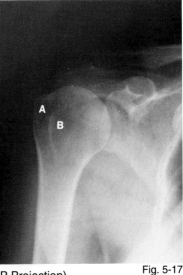

Fig. 5-16   External Rotation (AP Projection)   Fig. 5-17

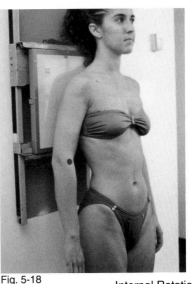
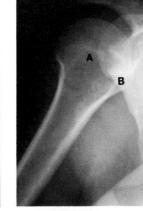

Fig. 5-18   Internal Rotation (Lateral Position)   Fig. 5-19

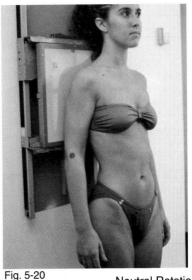
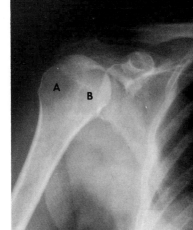

Fig. 5-20   Neutral Rotation (Oblique Position)   Fig. 5-21

National Survey:

Departmental standard and optional operating procedures (departmental routines) for the proximal humerus and shoulder girdle were with a few exceptions similar throughout all regions of the United States as shown. The regional differences are summarized below. (The number in parentheses in each regional box indicates the number of institutions which responded to this survey.)

Shoulder Routine:

Shoulder (Non-Trauma Routine)	U.S. Average (517)		East (197)		Midwest (243)		West (77)	
	Basic	Optional	Basic	Optional	Basic	Optional	Basic	Optional
• AP (Int. & Ext. Rotation)	92%		94%		89%		96%	
• Inferosuperior, Axial	20%	(15%)	19%	(16%)	19%	(15%)	21%	(10%)
• Post. Oblique for Glenoid Cavity	20%	(9%)	15%	(11%)	25%	(6%)	20%	(8%)
• Tangential for Intertubercular Groove[1]	1%							
Shoulder: (Trauma Routine-possible fracture or dislocation)								
• AP (Neutral Rotation)	93%		90%		94%		95%	
• Transthoracic Lateral	54%	(19%)	54%	(22%)	58%	(19%)	41%	(16%)
• Scapular Y	41%	(19%)	39%	(18%)	41%	(20%)	41%	(9%)
• Apical Oblique 45° Post. Obl. 45° Caudad	7%	(10%)	**6%**	(9%)	**6%**	(10%)	**12%**	(9%)

[1] Write-in's by survey respondents

Shoulder Routine: The shoulder **non-trauma routines** were very consistent throughout all regions of the United States.

The **trauma routines** for the shoulder however did show some regional differences. The selection of the **apical oblique** position as basic for the trauma shoulder routine was twice as high in the West (12%) as compared to the East or Midwest (6%). However those selecting it as optional were very consistent throughout the U.S. This is a relatively new position not previously described by the more common technology positioning references but it will be included in this chapter because of the high number indicating it as either basic or optional for the trauma shoulder routine.

Clavicle Routine

Clavicle:	U.S. Average (537)	
	Basic	Optional
• AP, CR perpendicular	88%	
or		
CR 15° cephalad	86%	
• PA, CR perpendicular	5%	(12%)
or		
CR 15° caudal	5.5%	(9%)
• AP, CR 25-30° cephalad[1]		8%

[1] Write-in's by survey respondents

AC Joints Routine

AC Joints:	U.S. Average (535)	
	Basic	Optional
• AP, Bilateral with weights	96%	
• AP, Bilateral without weights	92%	

Scapula Routine

Scapula:	U.S. Average (537)	
	Basic	Optional
• AP	99%	
• Lateral (Ant. Obl.)	93%	
• Lateral (Post. Obl.)		6%
• Scapular Y[1]		4%

[1] Write-in's by survey respondents

Summary

Clavicle Routine: The survey indicates that for the clavicle the **AP projection** is much more common than the PA projection. This was consistent throughout all regions of the U.S.

The choice of a **15° cephalic** angle or a **perpendicular CR** was very evenly divided. The recommended projection in this text however, is the angled CR to project the mid and distal clavicle above the ribs and scapula. The amount of CR angle varies depending on the shoulder thickness with a greater angle needed for a thinner shoulder.

AC Joints and Scapula Routines: The routines for both the AC joints and the scapula were very consistent throughout all regions of the United States.

The survey did not ask a specific question concerning the use of weights for the bilateral AC joints. The author has found however that it is a common practice in most regions of the United States to have the patient hold on to the weights rather than tying the weights to the wrists to allow for complete relaxation of the arms and shoulders. Some authorities believe this may result in false negative radiographs. (See page 164.)

Standard and Optional Operating Procedures

Certain basic and optional projections or positions for the humerus and shoulder girdle are demonstrated and described on the following pages as suggested standard and optional departmental procedures.

Basic Projections

Standard or basic projections, also sometimes referred to as routine projections or departmental routines are **those projections or positions commonly taken on average patients who are helpful and can cooperate in performing the procedure.**

Optional Projections

Optional projections are **those more common projections or positions taken as extra or additional projections to better demonstrate certain pathologic conditions or specific body parts.** (This does not mean they are optional as to whether or not they are important, or whether or not they need to be learned and mastered.)

Basic and Optional Projections

Shoulder
Basic
• AP Int. Rotation
• AP Ext. Rotation
Optional
• Inferosuperior Axial
• Glenoid Cavity (Post. Oblique)

Shoulder
(Trauma Routine - poss.
  fracture or dislocation)
Basic
• AP (Neutral Rotation)
• Transthoracic Lateral
  or
• Scapular Y
Optional
• Apical Oblique

Clavicle
Basic
• AP
  or
Optional
• PA

AC Joints
Basic
• AP, Bilateral with weights
• AP, Bilateral without weights

Sternoclavicular Joints: See sternum in Chapter 10.

Scapula
Basic
• AP
• Lateral

• AP Projection – Internal Rotation

Warning: Do **NOT** attempt to rotate arm if fracture or dislocation is suspected (see trauma routine).

> Shoulder
> Basic
> • **AP Int. Rotation**
> • AP Ext. Rotation

Structures Best Shown:
Lateral view of proximal humerus and lateral 2/3 of clavicle and upper scapula, including relationship of humeral head to glenoid cavity. Also demonstrates possible calcium deposits in muscles, tendons or bursal structures of shoulder.

Technical Factors:
• Film Size - 10 x 12 in. (24 x 30 cm), crosswise (or lengthwise to show more of humerus if injury includes proximal 1/2 of humerus).
• Moving or stationary grid.
• 75 ± 5 kVp range.

Patient Position:
• May be taken erect or supine. (Erect is usually less painful for patient if condition allows.)
• Rotate body slightly toward affected side if necessary to place shoulder in contact with cassette or table top.

Shielding: Secure lead shield at waist to shield pelvic area.

Part Position:
• Position patient so that coracoid process is at mid point of cassette. (Top of film 2 in. or 5 cm above top of shoulder.)
• Abduct extended arm slightly, then **internally rotate arm** (pronate hand) until epicondyles of distal humerus are **perpendicular** to film.

Central Ray:
• CR **perpendicular** to film, directed to **coracoid process.**
• Minimum 40 in. (102 cm) SID.

Collimation: Collimate on four sides, with lateral and upper borders adjusted to soft tissue margins.

Respiration: Suspend respiration during exposure.

Evaluation Criteria:
• Proximal 1/3 of humerus, upper scapula and lateral 2/3 of clavicle should be included with collimation visible on four sides.
• Center of collimation field should be to coracoid process indicating correct CR placement.
• Lateral view of proximal humerus evidenced by the **lesser tubercle** being visualized in profile **medially** partially superimposed by the lower portion of the glenoid cavity. A profile of the greater tubercle should be seen superimposed over the humeral head.
• Optimum exposure with no motion as evidenced by sharp borders and fine trabecular markings. Correct exposure will visualize the outline of the medial aspect of humeral head through the glenoid cavity, and visualize soft tissue detail to show possible calcium deposits.
• Patient ID information should be legible; R or L marker placed on the lateral border should be visible without superimposing the humerus.

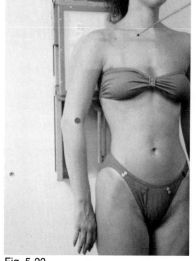
Fig. 5-22

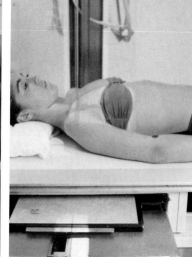
Patient and Part Position: Internal Rotation   Fig. 5-23

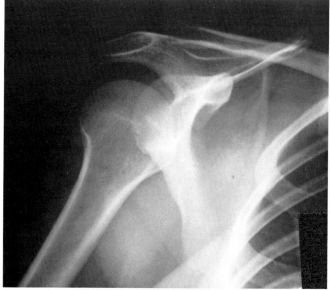
Internal Rotation   Fig. 5-24

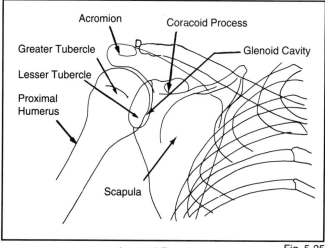

Acromion   Coracoid Process
Greater Tubercle   Glenoid Cavity
Lesser Tubercle
Proximal Humerus
Scapula

Internal Rotation   Fig. 5-25

• AP Projection – External Rotation

Warning: Do **NOT** attempt to rotate arm if fracture or dislocation is suspected (see trauma routine).

Shoulder
Basic
• AP Int. Rotation
• **AP Ext. Rotation**

Structures Best Shown:

Frontal view of proximal humerus and lateral 2/3 of clavicle and upper scapula, including relationship of humeral head to glenoid cavity. Also demonstrates possible calcium deposits in muscles, tendons or bursal structures of shoulder.

Technical Factors:

• Film Size - 10 x 12 in. (24 x 30 cm), crosswise (or lengthwise to show more of humerus if injury includes proximal 1/2 of humerus).
• Moving or stationary grid.
• 75 ± 5 kVp range.

Patient Position:

• May be taken erect or supine. (Erect is usually less painful for patient if condition allows.)
• Rotate body slightly toward affected side if necessary to place shoulder in contact with cassette or table top.

Shielding: Secure lead shield at waist to shield pelvic area.

Part Position:

• Position patient so that coracoid process is at mid point of cassette. (Top of film is about 2 in. or 5 cm above top of shoulder.)
• Abduct extended arm slightly, then **externally rotate arm** (supinate hand) until epicondyles of distal humerus are **parallel** to film.

Central Ray:

• CR **perpendicular** to center of film, directed to **coracoid process.** (With injury site at proximal humerus and film vertical, CR will be about 2 in. below coracoid process.)
• Minimum 40 in. (102 cm) SID.

Collimation: Collimate on four sides, with lateral and upper borders adjusted to soft tissue margins.

Respiration: Suspend respiration during exposure.

Evaluation Criteria:

• Proximal 1/3 of humerus, upper scapula and lateral 2/3 of clavicle should be included with collimation visible on four sides.
• Center of collimation field should be to coracoid process indicating correct CR placement.
• Frontal view of proximal humerus evidenced by the **greater tubercle** being visualized in profile **laterally.** A slight profile of the lesser tubercle should be seen superimposed over the proximal humerus about midway between the greater tubercle laterally. The humeral head which is shown in profile medially, should be partially superimposed by the glenoid cavity.
• Optimum exposure with no motion as evidenced by sharp borders and fine trabecular markings. Correct exposure will visualize the outline of the medial aspect of humeral head through the glenoid cavity, and

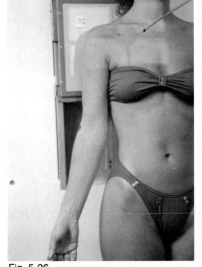
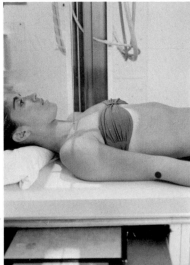

Fig. 5-26   Patient and Part Position: External Rotation   Fig. 5-27

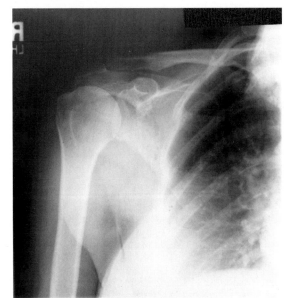

External Rotation   Fig. 5-28

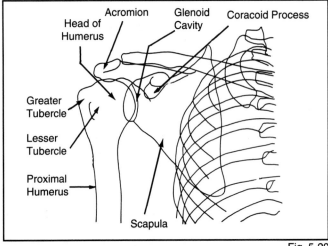

External Rotation   Fig. 5-29

visualize soft tissue detail to show possible calcium deposits.
• Patient ID information should be legible; R or L marker placed on the lateral border should be visible without superimposing the humerus.

• Inferosuperior, Axial Projection

(Lawrence Method)

Warning: Do **NOT** attempt this position if fracture or dislocation of proximal humerus is suspected.

Shoulder
Optional:
• **Inferosuperior Axial**
• Glenoid Cavity

Structures Best Shown:

Lateral view of proximal humerus and relationship to glenoid cavity. With exaggerated rotation the Hill-Sachs defect is demonstrated.

Technical Factors:

- Film Size - 8 x 10 in. (18 x 24 cm) crosswise.
- Stationary grid. (Must be crosswise to prevent grid cut-off due to CR angle.)
- 70 ± 6 kVp range.

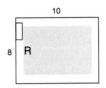

Patient Position:

- Patient supine with shoulder raised about 2 in. (5 cm) from table top by nonopaque support, with pillow under head.
- Move patient toward the front edge of table top.

Shielding: Place lead shield over pelvis.

Part Position:

- Abduct arm 90° from body; keep in **external rotation**, palm up with support under arm and hand extended over the edge of table.
- Rotate head toward opposite side.
- Place vertical cassette on table as close to neck as possible, adjust cassette perpendicular to CR and support with sand bags or other support.

Central Ray:

- With x-ray tube as close to patient's body as possible, direct CR **horizontally to axilla and humeral head.**
- Minimum 40 in. (102 cm) SID.

Collimation: Collimate closely on four sides.

Respiration: Suspend respiration during exposure.

Alternate Position: Exaggerated **external** rotation.[1] An anterior dislocation of the humeral head may result in a compression fracture of the articular surface of the humeral head, termed the Hills-Sachs defect. This is best demonstrated with this exaggrated external rotation wherein the thumb is pointed down and posteriorly about 45°.

Evaluation Criteria:

- The neck and head of humerus should be well visualized in a lateral position, evidenced by the lesser tubercle in profile superiorly.
- The relationship of the humeral head and glenoid cavity should be clearly visualized. The spine of the scapula should be seen on edge below the glenohumeral joint.
- The acromion and distal clavicle and AC joint outline should be seen faintly superimposed by the humeral head.
- Optimum exposure without motion should visualize sharp borders and fine trabecular markings of the proximal humerus and lateral aspects of scapula. The bony margins of the acromion and distal clavicle should be visible as well as the AC joint through the humeral head. Soft tissue will not be well visualized.
- Collimation borders should be visible on all four sides with wider upper and lower margins.

[1] Rafert, JA, et al,:Axillary Shoulder with Exaggerated Rotation: The Hill-Sachs Defect, Radiol Technol, **62**:18-21, Sept/Oct,1990

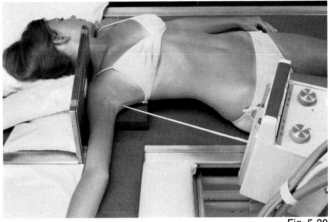

Inferosuperior Axial   Fig. 5-30

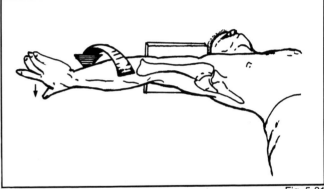

Alternate Position – Exaggerated Rotation   Fig. 5-31

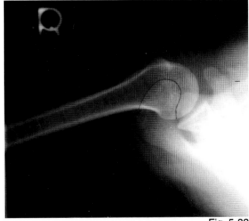

Inferosuperior Axial   Fig. 5-32

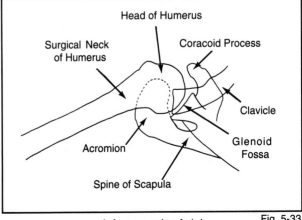

Inferosuperior Axial   Fig. 5-33

• Glenoid Cavity (Fossa) Position
(Grashey Method)

Structures Best Shown:
Glenoid cavity in profile and open glenohumeral joint space.

Technical Factors:
• Film Size - 8 x 10 in. (18 x 24 cm), crosswise.
• Moving or stationary grid.
• 75 ± 5 kVp range.

Patient Position:
• Erect or supine. (Erect is usually less painful for patient if condition allows.)
• Rotate body 35-45° toward affected side. (See NOTE.) If done supine, place supports under elevated shoulder and hip to maintain this position.

Shielding: Place gonadal shielding over pelvic area.

Part Position:
• Adjust cassette so top of film is about 2 in. (5 cm) above shoulder, and side of film is about 2 in. (5 cm) from lateral border of humerus.
• Abduct arm slightly with arm in neutral rotation.

Central Ray:
• CR **perpendicular** to film, **centered to glenohumeral joint**. (Approximately 2 in. or 5 cm distal and 2 in. or 5 cm medial to superior and lateral borders of shoulder.
• Minimum 40 in. (102 cm) SID.

Collimation: Collimate so upper and lateral borders of the light field are to the soft tissue margins.

Respiration: Suspend respiration during exposure.

NOTE: The degree of rotation will vary depending on how flat or round shouldered the patient is. Rounded or curved shoulder and back requires more rotation to place body of scapula parallel to film.

Evaluation Criteria:
• Glenoid cavity should be seen in profile without superimposition of humeral head (joint space should appear open).
• Optimum exposure without motion should visualize sharp bony borders and fine trabecular markings of humeral head and the lateral angle or head of scapula. Soft tissue detail in the area of joint space and axilla should be visualized.
• Collimation borders should be visible on four sides to area of soft tissue outer margins. The center of the collimation field should be to the area of the glenohumeral joint.
• Patient ID information should be legible and R or L marker visible on lateral margin without superimposing humerus.

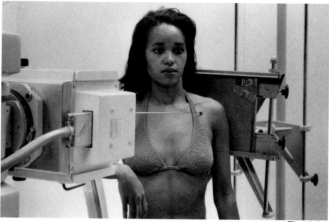

Glenoid Cavity Position   Fig. 5-34

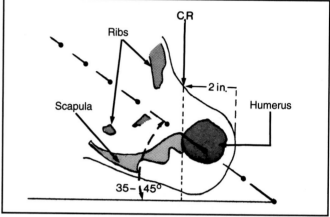

Glenoid Cavity Position   Fig. 5-35

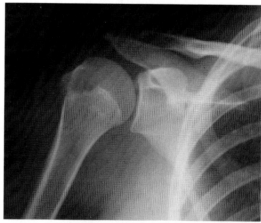

Glenoid Cavity Position   Fig. 5-36

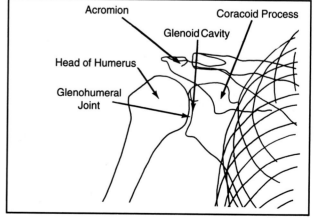

Glenoid Cavity Position   Fig. 5-37

• AP Projection – Neutral Rotation

Warning: Do **NOT** attempt to rotate arm if fracture or dislocation is suspected.

Shoulder
(Trauma Routine)
Basic
• **AP** (Neutral Rotation)
• Transthoracic Lateral
or
• Scapular Y
Optional
• Apical Oblique

Structures Best Shown:
Frontal view of proximal humerus; lateral 2/3 of clavicle and upper scapula, including relationship of humeral head to glenoid cavity. Also demonstrates possible calcium deposits in muscles, tendons or bursal structures of shoulder.

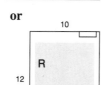

Technical Factors:
• Film Size - 10 x 12 in. (24 x 30), crosswise (or lengthwise to show more of humerus if injury includes proximal 1/2 of humerus).
• Moving or stationary grid.
• 75 ± 5 kVp range.

Patient Position:
• May be taken erect or supine. (Erect is usually less painful for patient if condition allows.)
• Rotate body slightly toward affected side if necessary to place shoulder in contact with film holder or table top.

Shielding: Secure lead shield at waist to shield pelvic area.

Part Position:
• Position patient so that coracoid process is at mid point of film holder. (Top of film 2 in. or 5 cm above top of shoulder.)
• Place patient's arm at side in neutral rotation. (Epicondyles are approximately 45° to plane of film.)

Central Ray:
• CR **perpendicular** to film holder, directed to **coracoid process.**
• Minimum 40 in. (102 cm) SID.

Collimation: Collimate on four sides, with lateral and upper borders adjusted to soft tissue margins.

Respiration: Suspend respiration during exposure.

Evaluation Criteria:
• Proximal 1/3 of the humerus, upper scapula and a minimum of lateral 2/3 of clavicle should be included with collimation visible on four sides.
• Center of collimation field should be to coracoid process indicating correct CR placement.
• With neutral rotation greater tubercle will be primarily superimposed over humeral head.
• Optimum exposure with no motion as evidenced by sharp borders and fine trabecular markings. Correct sxposure will visualize the outline of the medial aspect of humeral head through the glenoid cavity, and visualize soft tissue detail to show possible calcium deposits.
• Patient ID information should be legible; R or L marker placed on the lateral border should be visible without superimposing the humerus.

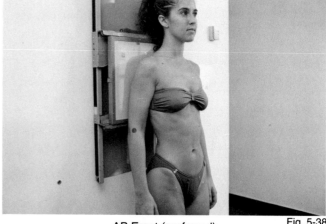

AP Erect (preferred)   Fig. 5-38

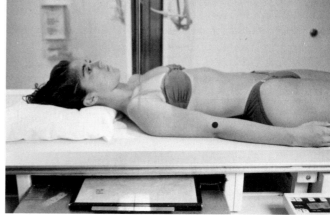

AP Supine   Fig. 5-39

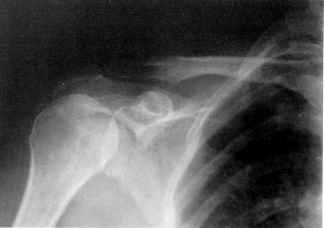

AP Projection   Fig. 5-40

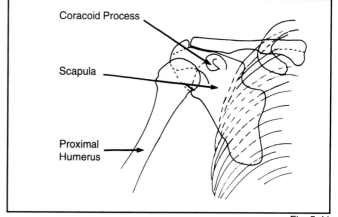

Coracoid Process

Scapula

Proximal Humerus

AP Projection   Fig. 5-41

• Transthoracic Lateral Position

Shoulder
(Trauma Routine)
Basic
• AP (Neutral Rotation)
• **Transthoracic Lateral**
  or
• Scapular Y
Optional
• Apical Oblique

Structures Best Shown:
Lateral view of proximal humerus and relationship of glenohumeral joint.

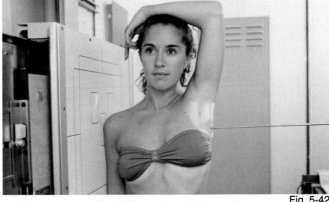

Erect Transthoracic Lateral   Fig. 5-42

Technical Factors:
• Film size - 10 x 12 in. (24 x 30 cm), lengthwise.
• Moving or stationary grid.
• 75 ± 5 kVp range.
• Minimum of 3 sec. exposure time with breathing technique (4 or 5 sec. is desirable).

Patient Position:
• May be taken erect or supine. (Erect preferred, which also may be more comfortable for patient.)
• Place patient in lateral position with side of interest against cassette with humerus aligned to midline of cassette.
• Insure that thorax is in a true lateral position so humerus is not superimposed by thoracic vertebrae or by sternum.

Shielding: Secure gonadal shield at waist to cover pelvic area.

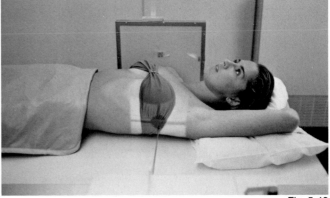

Supine Transthoracic Lateral   Fig. 5-43

Part Position:
• Affected arm at patient's side in neutral rotation, drop shoulder if possible.
• Raise opposite arm and place hand over top of head, elevate shoulder as much as possible to prevent superimposing affected shoulder.
• Position top of cassette about 2.5 - 3 in. (7 cm) above top of shoulder.

Central Ray:
• CR perpendicular to film directed through thorax to **surgical neck.**
• Minimum 40 in. (102 cm) SID.

Alternate CR Projection: If patient is in too much pain to drop injured shoulder sufficiently and elevate uninjured arm and shoulder high enough to prevent superimposition of shoulders, then angle CR 10 to 15° cephalad.

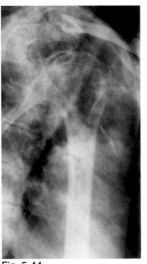

Fig. 5-44

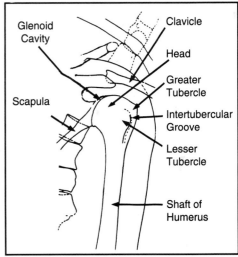

Transthoracic Lateral   Fig. 5-45

Collimation: Collimate on four sides to area of interest, remembering the divergence of x-ray beam.

Respiration: Breathing technique is preferred if patient can cooperate. Patient should be asked to gently breathe short shallow breaths without moving affected arm or shoulder. (This will best visualize proximal humerus by blurring out ribs and lung structures.)

NOTE: With possible fracture or dislocation, arm should not be rotated but taken as is which will result in a 90° or right angle view of proximal humerus, compared to the AP projection also taken without arm rotation. (Forced rotation of arm with a fracture may result in displacement of fractured humeral head or neck.)

Evaluation Criteria:
• Proximal half of humerus and glenohumeral joint should be visualized without superimposition by opposite shoulder.
• The outline of proximal humerus should be clearly visualized midway between thoracic vertebrae posteriorly and sternum anteriorly. Ribs and lung structures should appear blurred if breathing technique was used correctly.
• The relationship of the humeral head and glenoid cavity of scapula should be well demonstrated.
• Optimum exposure should visualize the entire border outlines of the humeral head and the proximal half of the humerus.
• This may not be a true lateral view of humerus because with possible humeral fracture or dislocation this is taken with arm in "as is" position, but it should present a view which is 90° or right angle to the AP projection also taken without forced rotation.

• Scapular Y Position
(Anterior Oblique Position)

Warning: Do **NOT** attempt to rotate arm if fracture or dislocation is suspected.

Shoulder
(Trauma Routine)
Basic
• AP (Neutral Rotation)
• Transthoracic Lateral
  or
• **Scapular Y**
Optional
• Apical Oblique

Structures Best Shown:
An oblique lateral view of the shoulder and proximal humerus superimposed over a lateral view of the scapula. Demonstrates relationship of humeral head to glenoid cavity.

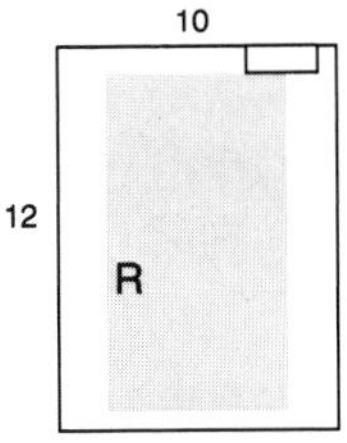

Technical Factors:
• Film size - 10 x 12 in. (24 x 30 cm), lengthwise.
• Moving or stationary grid.
• 75 ± 5 kVp range.

Patient Position:
• May be taken erect or recumbent but erect is usually more comfortable for patient.
• With patient facing the cassette, rotate into an anterior oblique position as for a lateral scapula. The average patient will be in a 60° anterior oblique position. (30° from a lateral.)

Shielding: Shield pelvic area with lead shield.

Part Position:
• Place top of cassette about 2 in. (5 cm) above top of shoulder.
• Center proximal humerus to midline of cassette.
• Abduct arm slightly so as not to superimpose proximal humerus over ribs.
• Do not rotate arm, take in neutral rotational position.

Central Ray:
• CR **perpendicular** to film, directed to the **glenohumeral joint.** (Approximately 2 or 2.5 in. (5-6 cm) below the top of the shoulder.)
• Minimum 40 in. (102 cm) SID.

Collimation: Collimate on four sides, to upper and lateral soft tissue margins of proximal humerus and shoulder.

Respiration: Suspend respiration during exposure.

NOTE: With severe injury when patient cannot be placed in erect or an anterior oblique position table top, this may be taken in the opposite posterior oblique position with injured shoulder elevated. This however, results in magnification and loss of definition.

Evaluation Criteria:
• The thin body of the scapula should be seen on end, **not** superimposed by ribs.
• The acromion and coracoid processes should appear as nearly symmetrical upper limbs of the **"Y".**
• The thin end-on view of the body of the scapula should appear superimposed over the mid portion of the proximal humerus, **if** the humerus is not dislocated. The proximal humerus will appear medial to the body of the scapula on an anterior dislocation (*Fig. 5-48*).
• Optimum exposure without motion should visualize well the "Y" appearance of the lateral scapula including the outline of the body of

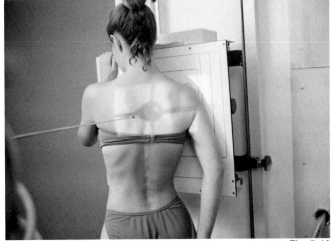

Scapular Y Projection

Fig. 5-46

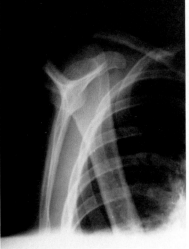

Fig. 5-47
Without Dislocation

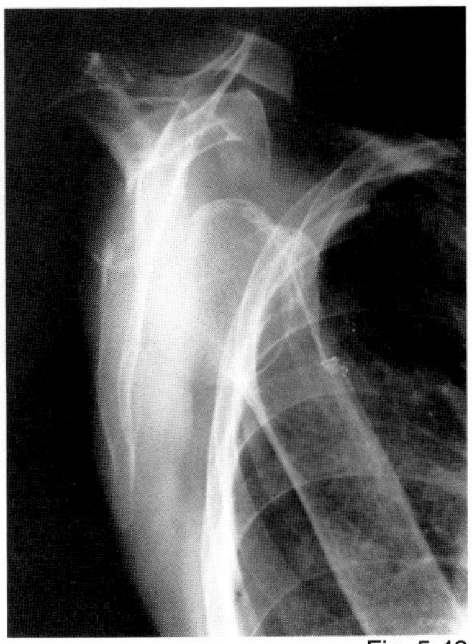

Fig. 5-48
With Anterior Dislocation

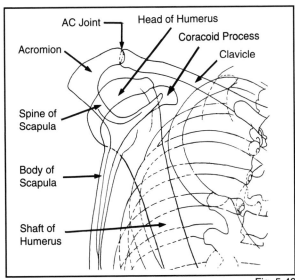

Scapular Y Projection
(Without Dislocation)

Fig. 5-49

the scapula through the humerus. Bony borders of ribs, scapula and humerus should appear clear and sharp.
• Patient ID information should be legible; R or L marker placed on lateral border should be visualized without superimposing the humerus.

• Apical Oblique Projection
(Posterior Oblique Position)

Shoulder
(Trauma Routine)
Basic
• AP (Neutral Rotation)
• Transthoracic Lateral
or
• Scapular Y
Optional
•**Apical Oblique**

Structures Best Shown:
The humeral head, glenoid cavity and scapular head and neck are well demonstrated. A good projection for possible glenohumeral dislocations (especially posterior dislocations) glenoid fractures, Hill-Sachs lesions and soft tissue calcifications. This is a recommended projection for acute shoulder trauma radiography.[1]

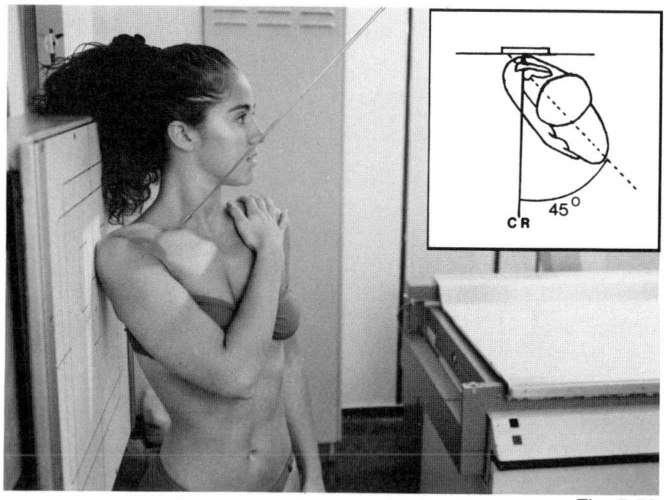

This view was first described by *Garth* et. al. in 1984 to demonstrate glenohumeral instability.[2]

Technical Factors:
• Film Size - 8 x 10 in. (18 x 24 cm), lengthwise.
• Moving or stationary grid.
• 75 ± 5 kVp range.

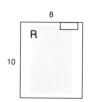

Patient Position:
• Erect or supine. (Erect is usually less painful if patient's condition allows.)
• Rotate body 45° toward affected side. (Posterior surface of affected shoulder against cassette.)

Shielding: Place gonadal shielding over pelvic area.

Part Position:
• Adjust cassette so the 45° angled CR will direct the glenohumeral joint to the center of the film.
• Flex elbow and place arm across chest, palm down.

Central Ray:
• CR **45° caudal,** centered to a point about **1 in. (2.5 cm) medial to the glenohumeral joint.**
• Minimum 40 in. (102 cm) SID.

Collimation: Collimate on four sides with lateral and upper borders adjusted to soft tissue margins.

Respiration: Suspend respiration during exposure.

Evaluation Criteria:
• The humeral head, glenoid cavity and neck and head of the scapula are well demonstrated free of superimposition except for the coracoid process, which should be visible as projected over the mid-glenohumeral joint region. The clavicle will appear curved and distorted and the acromion and AC joint should be projected superior to the humeral head.
• **Dislocations:** A posterior dislocation of the humerus will project the humeral head superior or cephalic to the glenoid cavity; an anterior dislocation will project the humeral head inferiorly or caudally.
• The center of the collimation field should be to the lateral angle (head) of the scapula.

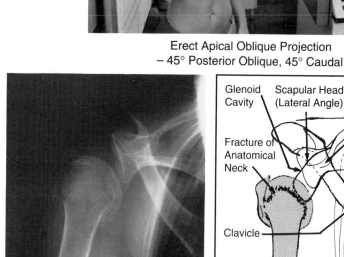

Erect Apical Oblique Projection
– 45° Posterior Oblique, 45° Caudal

Fig. 5-50

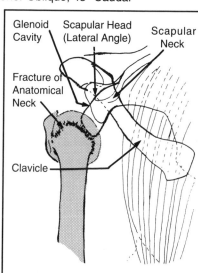

Fig. 5-51
Apical Oblique Projection (Note fracture of humeral head)

Glenoid Cavity / Scapular Head (Lateral Angle) / Scapular Neck / Fracture of Anatomical Neck / Clavicle

Fig. 5-52

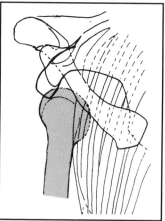

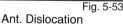

Fig. 5-53
Ant. Dislocation

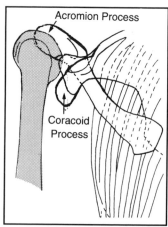

Acromion Process / Coracoid Process

Fig. 5-54
Post. Dislocation

• Optimum exposure with no motion will be evidenced by sharp borders and fine trabecular markings. Correct exposure will visualize the outline of the scapular spine and coracoid process and soft tissue detail to show possible calcifications.
• Patient ID information should be legible; R or L marker placed on the lateral border should be visible without superimposing the humerus.

[1] Sloth, C., and Lundgren, Just, S.: The Apical Oblique Radiograph in Examination of Acute Shoulder Trauma. Europ. J. Radiol. **9**:147-151, 1989
[2] Garth Jr., W.P., Slappey, C.E., and Ochs, C.W.: Roentgenographic Demonstration of Instability of the Shoulder: The Apical Oblique Projection. Bone Joint Surg. **66-A**:1450-1453, 1984

Clavicle

• AP Projection

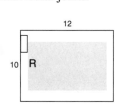

Clavicle
Basic
• **AP**
Optional
• **AP or PA Axial**

Structures Best Shown:
Clavicle, including acromioclavicular and sternoclavicular joints.

Technical Factors:
• Film Size - 10 x 12 in. (24 x 30 cm) crosswise.
• Moving or stationary grid.
• 75 ± 5 kVp range.

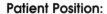

Patient Position:
• Erect or supine with arms at sides, chin raised looking straight ahead.

Shielding: Place gonadal shielding over pelvic area.

Part Position:
AP (Erect or supine)
• Posterior shoulder should be in contact with cassette or table top, without rotation of body.
• Center clavicle to center of cassette considering cephalic CR angle. (Clavicle can readily be palpated with medial aspect at jugular notch and lateral portion at AC joint above shoulder.)

Alternate PA (Erect)
Warning: Do **NOT** attempt prone position in cases of obvious trauma or pain to clavicle region to prevent possible fragment displacement and/or additional injury.
• Position patient facing film with anterior shoulder against cassette without rotation of body.
• Extend chin and turn head away from side of interest.
• Center clavicle to center of cassette considering caudal CR angle.

Central Ray:
• CR to **mid-clavicle**, AP - **10 to 20° cephalic**; PA - **5-15° caudal.** (See NOTE.)
• Minimum 40 in. (102 cm) SID.

Collimation: Collimate to area of clavicle. (Insure that both acromioclavicular and sternoclavicular joints are included.)

Respiration: Suspend respiration at end of exhalation.

NOTE: • CR Angle: Thin patients, angle CR 15°, average patient 10°, and heavy, thick shouldered patients angle only 5°.
• The AP erect or supine position is generally easier for patients and thus preferred over the PA projection. The PA projection however, is recommended for patients with rounded shoulders or kyphosis if their condition allows to decrease the OID resulting in less magnification and increased definition.

Alternate AP or PA Axial Projections: The CR may be increased to **25-30° cephalic (AP)** or **caudal (PA)** which will result in more shape distortion of the clavicle but may be used as an additional projection resulting in less superimposition of the clavicle over the scapula and thorax.

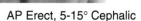
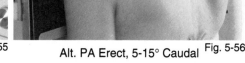

AP Erect, 5-15° Cephalic Fig. 5-55   Alt. PA Erect, 5-15° Caudal Fig. 5-56

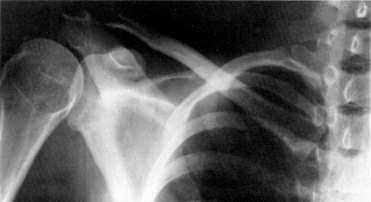

AP Clavicle, 5-15° Cephalic   Fig. 5-57

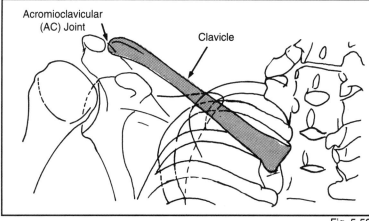

AP Clavicle   Fig. 5-58

Evaluation Criteria:
• Collimation borders should be visible with entire clavicle visualized including both AC and sternoclavicular joints.
• Correct angulation of CR will project distal clavicle just above the acromion of the scapula with minimum shape distortion. Only a small portion of the superior angle of the scapula will superimpose the clavicle. The medial portion of clavicle will be superimposed by the first and second ribs.
• Optimum exposure will visualize the distal clavicle and AC joint without excessive density. The bony margins of the medial clavicle and sternoclavicular joint should also be visualized through the thorax.
• Patient ID information should be legible and R or L marker visible without superimposing essential anatomy.

Acromioclavicular (AC) Joints

• AP Projection
(Bilateral – with and without weights)

AC Joints
Basic
• **AP, Bilateral with weights**
• **AP, Bilateral without weights**

Structures Best Shown:
Both AC joint spaces for comparison with and without stress. Demonstrates possible separation of joint spaces.

Technical Factors:
• Film Size - One 7 x 17 in. (18 x 43 cm) crosswise (or 14 x 17 in. if 7 x 17 in. is not available).
• Use "with weight" and "without weight" markers.
• Detail screen, non-grid.
• 50-60 kVp with screen; 70-75 with grid on larger patients.
• For broad shouldered patients, use two 8 x 10 in. (18 x 24 cm) cassettes crosswise placed side by side and exposed simultaneously to include both AC joints on one exposure.

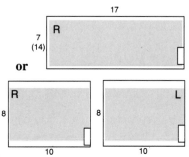

Patient Position:
• Erect, posterior shoulders against cassette with equal weight on both feet, arms at side, no rotation of shoulders or pelvis, looking straight ahead. (May be taken seated if patient's condition requires.)
• **Two sets** of bilateral AC joints are taken in the same position, one **without weights** and one **stress view with weights.**

Shielding: Secure gonadal shield around waist.

Part Position:
• With both shoulders against cassette, adjust height to place center of cassette to level of AC joints.

Central Ray:
• Direct CR to a **mid point between AC joints** (1.5 in. or 4 cm above jugular notch) **perpendicular** to film.
• 72 in. (180 cm) SID.

Collimation: Collimate with a long narrow light field to area of interest; upper light border should be to upper shoulder soft tissue margins.

Respiration: Suspend respiration during exposure.

Weights: After the first exposure is made without weights and cassette(s) have been changed, tie a minimum of 10 to 15 lb. weights to each wrist and with shoulders relaxed, **gently** allow weights to hang from wrists pulling down on each arm and shoulder. The same amount of weight must be used on each wrist. (Large muscular patients require more weight.)

NOTE: Patients should **NOT** be asked to hold on to the weights with their hands, rather the **weights must be tied to the wrists so the hands, arms and shoulders are relaxed**, to determine possible AC joint separation. (Holding on to weights may result in false negative radiographs.)[1]

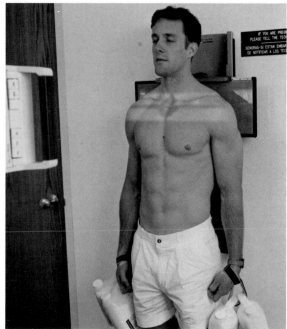

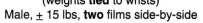

Stress View with Weights   Fig. 5-59
(weights **tied** to wrists)
Male, ± 15 lbs, **two** films side-by-side

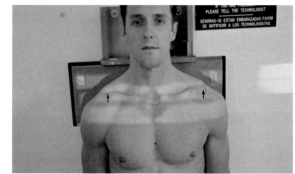

AC Joints Marked by Arrows   Fig. 5-60

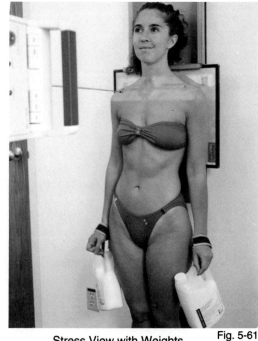

Stress View with Weights   Fig. 5-61
(weights **tied** to wrists)
Female, ± 10 lbs, **one** film crosswise

---

[1] James A. Rand, M.D. Mayo Clinic, Rochester, MN, 1990

• **AP Projection** – continued
(Bilateral – with and without weights)

Alternate Supine Position: If patient's condition requires, may be taken supine by tying both ends of a long strip of gauze to patient's wrists and placing around patient's feet with knees partially flexed, then slowly and gently straighten legs pulling down on shoulders. May also be done by an assistant **gently** pulling down on arms and shoulders. (Should only be done by qualified personnel to prevent additional injury.)

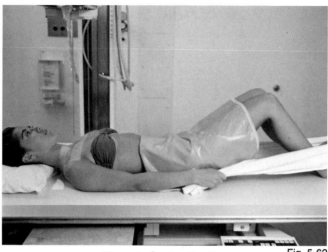

Alternate Supine Position   Fig. 5-62

Evaluation Criteria:

- Long narrow collimation field should visualize both AC joints as well as the entire clavicles and sternoclavicular joints on one or two separate radiographs exposed simultaneously.
- No rotation, as evidenced by symmetrical appearance of sternoclavicular joints on each side of vertebral column.
- Both AC joints should be on the same horizontal plane.
- Optimum exposure without motion should clearly visualize AC joints and soft tissue without excessive density.
- R and L markers as well as markers indicating stress (with weights) and non stress (without weights) should be visible without superimposing essential anatomy. Patient ID information should be clear and legible.

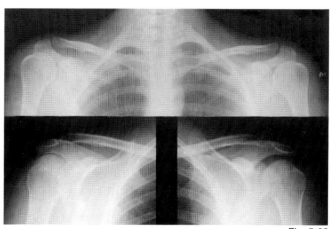

AP Acromioclavicular Joints   Fig. 5-63
(single film and two films exposed simultaneously)

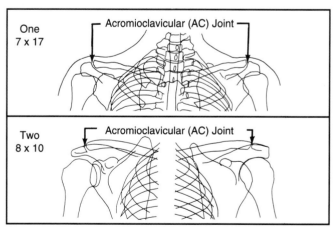

AC Joints   Fig. 5-64

Scapula

• AP Projection

Scapula
Basic
• **AP**
• Lateral

Structures Best Shown:

Frontal view of scapula with lateral border free from rib superimposition.

Technical Factors:

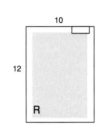

- Film Size - 10 x 12 in. (24 x 30 cm) lengthwise.
- Moving or stationary grid.
- 75 ± 5 kVp range.
- Minimum of 3 sec. exposure time with breathing technique. (4 or 5 sec. is desirable).

Patient Position:

- May be taken erect or supine. (Erect may be more comfortable for patient.)
- Posterior surface of shoulder in direct contact with table top or cassette **without rotation** of thorax. (Rotation toward affected side will place scapula into a truer frontal position but it will also result in greater superimposition of rib cage.)

Shielding: Place gonadal shield over pelvic area.

Part Position:

- Position patient and/or film holder so that the center point of the film is to **mid-scapula area, which is 2 in. (5 cm) inferior to coracoid process**. (Top of film about 2 in. or 5 cm above shoulder and lateral border of film about 2 in. or 5 cm from lateral margin of rib cage.)
- Gently **abduct arm 90°** and supinate hand. (Abduction will move scapula laterally to clear more of thoracic structures.)

Central Ray:

- Direct CR **to mid-scapula**, 2 in. (5 cm) inferior to coracoid process, **perpendicular** to film.
- Minimum 40 in. (102 cm) SID.

Collimation: Collimate on four sides to area of scapula.

Respiration: Breathing technique is preferred if patient can cooperate. Ask patient to gently breathe short shallow breaths without moving affected shoulder or arm.

Evaluation Criteria:

- The entire scapula should be visualized. (Approximately half of scapula will be seen through blurred thoracic structures with breathing technique.)
- Collimation borders should be visible on four sides with center of collimation field to about 2 in. or 5 cm inferior to coracoid process.
- Entire lateral portion of scapula should be visible without superimposition of ribs and lung. (Indicates correct abduction of arm and no rotation or obliquity of thorax.)
- Optimum exposure will visualize bony margins and trabecular markings of lateral portion of scapula. The medial aspect of the scapula should be visualized without excessive density wherein

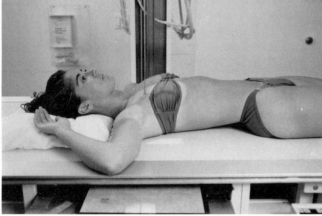

AP Supine   Fig. 5-65

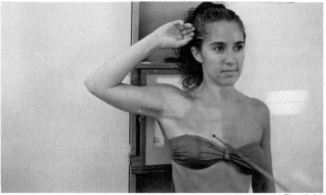

AP Erect   Fig. 5-66

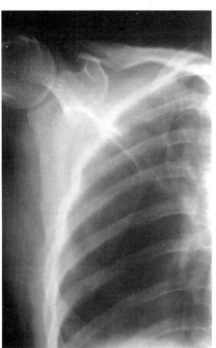

AP Scapula   Fig. 5-67

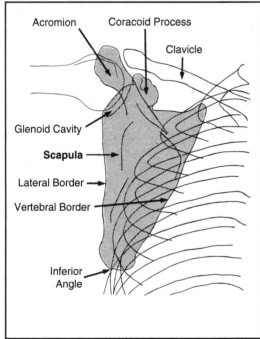

AP Scapula   Fig. 5-68

the bony margins of the vertebral border should be visible through the lung field along its entirety. Ribs and lung structures will appear blurred with proper breathing technique.

- Patient ID information should be legible and R or L marker visible without superimposing any portion of scapula.

•Lateral Position

Scapula
Basic
• AP
• **Lateral**

Structures Best Shown:
Lateral scapula projected clear of the rib cage. A fracture of the body of the scapula is best demonstrated in this position.

Technical Factors:
- Film Size - 10 x 12 in. (24 x 30 cm) lengthwise.
- Moving or stationary grid.
- 75 ± 5 kVp range.

Patient Position:
- Erect or recumbent position. (Erect position preferred if patient's condition allows. Can also be done recumbent with similar positioning but this is more painful and uncomfortable for patient.)
- Patient facing cassette in an anterior oblique position.

Shielding: Secure gonadal shield around waist.

Part Position:
- Have patient reach across front of chest and grasp opposite shoulder. (Figure 5-69 best demonstrates **body** of scapula.)
  or
  Have patient drop affected arm, flex elbow and place arm behind lower back with arm partially abducted. (Figure 5-71 best demonstrates **acromion and coracoid processes.**)
- Palpate borders of scapula and rotate patient until the scapula is in a true lateral position. (The flat posterior surface of scapula should be perpendicular to film.)
- The average patient will be rotated **30 to 40° from the lateral position.** (Results in a **50 to 60° anterior oblique** position.)
- Align scapula to midline of cassette.
- Place top of cassette about 2 in. (5 cm) above top of shoulder.

Central Ray:
- Direct CR to **mid vertebral border of scapula, perpendicular** to film.
- Minimum 40 in. (102 cm) SID.

Collimation: Collimate to area of scapula.

Respiration: Suspend respiration during exposure.

NOTE: May also be taken in the opposite posterior oblique if patient's condition requires. The affected shoulder would then be at an increased distance from the film resulting in some magnification and loss of definition.

Evaluation Criteria:
- Entire scapula should be visualized within collimation field in a lateral position, as evidenced by direct superimposition of vertebral and lateral borders.
- Body of scapula should be seen in profile, free of superimposition by ribs.
- As much as possible the humerus should not superimpose area of interest of the scapula.
- Optimum exposure should visualize the entire scapula without excessive density in area of inferior angle. Bony borders of both the acromion and coracoid processes should be seen through the head of the humerus.
- Patient ID information should be legible and R or L marker visible without superimposing any portion of scapula.

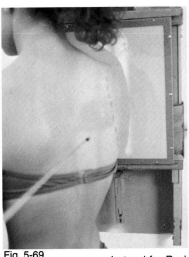
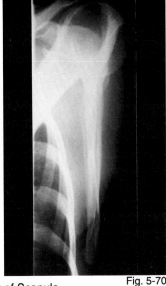

Fig. 5-69   Lateral for Body of Scapula   Fig. 5-70

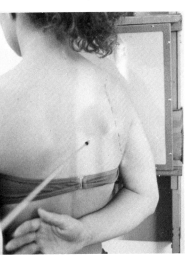
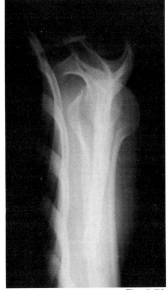

Fig. 5-71   Lateral for Acromion or Coracoid Process   Fig. 5-72

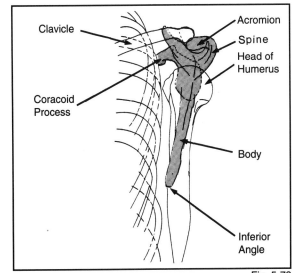

Clavicle — Coracoid Process — Acromion — Spine — Head of Humerus — Body — Inferior Angle

Lateral Scapula   Fig. 5-72

Chapter 6
Radiographic Anatomy and Positioning of the Lower Limb

Contributions by: Eugene D. Frank, MA, RT(R), FASRT
J. Fred Price, MS, RT(R), FASRT

Contents

Lower Limb (Foot)

Part I Radiographic Anatomy

Lower Limb (Extremity)

The bones of the lower limb are divided into four main groups: foot, leg, femur and hip. This chapter includes a thorough study of the anatomy and positioning for the first two groups, the **foot** and the **leg**. The **ankle joint** is also included in this chapter as well as the **knee joint** along with the distal femur.

Foot

The bones of the foot are fundamentally very similar to the bones of the hand and wrist as studied in Chapter 4.

The 26 bones of one foot are divided into three groups:

Phalanges (Toes)	14
Metatarsals (Instep)	5
Tarsals	7
Total	26

Phalanges - Toes (digits)

The most distal bones of the foot are the **phalanges**, which make up the digits or toes. The five digits of each foot are numbered one through five starting on the medial or big toe side of the foot. Note that the large toe or first digit has only two phalanges, similar to that of the thumb. These are the **proximal phalanx** and the **distal phalanx**. Each of the second, third, fourth and fifth digits has a **middle phalanx** in addition to a proximal and a distal phalanx. Since the first toe has two phalanges, and digits two through five have three apiece, there are **14** phalanges in each foot.

The similarities to the hand are obvious in that there are also 14 phalanges in each hand. However, there are two noticeable differences in that the phalanges of the foot are smaller and their movements are more limited than those of the hand.

When describing any of the bones or joints of the foot, the specific digit and foot should also be identified. For example, the distal phalanx of the first digit of the right foot would leave no doubt as to which bone is in question.

It should be noted that the distal phalanges of the second through fifth toes are very small and may be difficult to identify as separate bones on a radiograph.

Metatarsals

The five bones of the instep are the **metatarsal** bones. These are numbered as the digits with number one on the medial side and number five on the lateral side.

Each of the metatarsals is composed of three parts. The small, rounded, distal part of each metatarsal is the **head**. The centrally located, long, slender portion is termed the **shaft** or **diaphysis**. The expanded, proximal end of each metatarsal is the **base**.

The base of the fifth metatarsal is expanded laterally into a prominent rough **tuberosity**, which provides for the attachment of a tendon. This tuberosity is readily visible on radiographs and is a common trauma site for the foot.

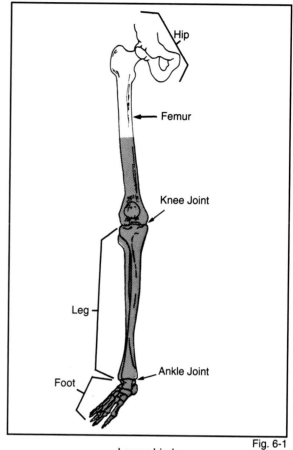

Lower Limb

Fig. 6-1

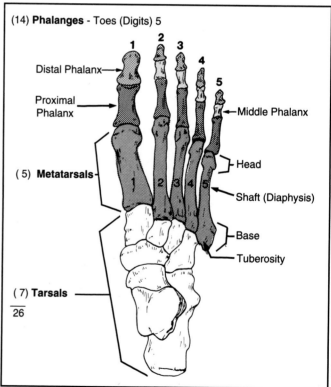

Bones of Foot

Fig. 6-2

Viewing Radiographs: Radiographs of the hands and feet are generally placed on an illuminator with the toes or fingers pointing up, viewing it as the x-ray tube sees it. Knowing the parts of the metatarsals will help in remembering this in that the **head** of each metatarsal or metacarpal will always be up and the **base** will be toward the bottom of the radiograph.

Radiogaphs of other parts of the body including the ankle and limbs are routinely placed on the illuminator (view box) in the anatomical position, with the limbs hanging down (*Fig. 6-3*).

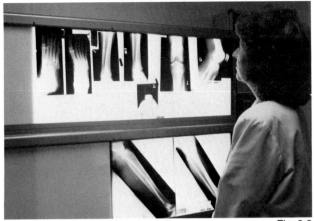

Viewing Radiographs of Limbs   Fig. 6-3

Joints (Articulations)

Joints of Digits: The joints or articulations of the digits of the foot are important to identify since fractures may involve the joint surfaces. Each joint of the foot has a name derived from the two bones on either side of that joint. Between the proximal and distal phalanges of the first digit is the **interphalangeal** or **IP joint**.

Since digits two through five each have one more bone, these digits have three joints each. Between the middle and distal phalanges is the **distal interphalangeal joint** or **DIP** joint. Between the proximal and middle phalanges is the **proximal interphalangeal joint** or **PIP joint.** The joint between each metatarsal and its respective proximal phalanx is the same for all five digits.

Joints of Metatarsals: Each of the joints at the head of the metatarsal is a **metatarsophalangeal** or **MP joint,** while each of the joints at the base of the metatarsal is a **tarsometatarsal joint** or **TM joint.** The base of the third metatarsal or the third tarsometatarsal joint is important because this is the centering point or central ray (CR) location for an AP and oblique foot.

When describing joints of the foot, it is important to state the name of the joint first, then include which digit or metatarsal as well as which foot. For example, an injury or fracture may be described as near the distal interphalangeal joint of the fifth digit of the left foot.

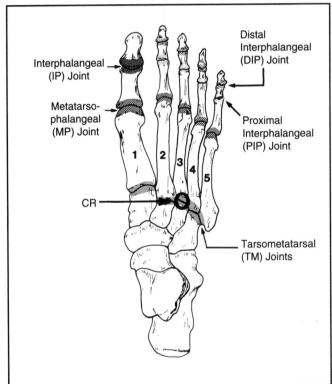

Joints of Right Foot   Fig. 6-4

Sesamoid Bones

Several small detached bones, called **sesamoid** bones, are often found in the feet and hands. These extra bones , which are embedded in certain tendons, are often present near various joints. In the upper limbs sesamoid bones are quite small and most often found on the palmar surface near the metacarpophalangeal joints, or occasionally at the interphalangeal joint of the thumb.

In the lower limbs, sesamoid bones tend to be larger and more significant radiographically. The largest sesamoid bone in the body is the patella or knee cap as described later in this chapter. Also the two sesamoid bones illustrated in *Fig. 6-5* are almost always present on the posterior or plantar surface of the first metatarsophalangeal joint. Sesamoid bones may also be found near other joints of the foot. Sesamoid bones are important radiographically, because it is possible to fracture these small bones. Due to their plantar location, they can be quite painful and cause discomfort. Special positioning may be necessary to demonstrate a fracture of a sesamoid bone.

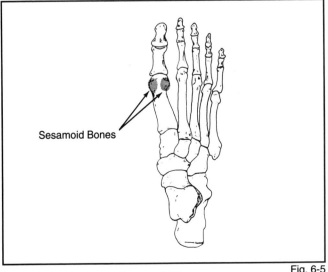

Sesamoid Bones   Fig. 6-5

Tarsals

The seven large bones of the proximal foot are termed tarsal bones. The names of the tarsals can be remembered with the aid of a mnemonic: **Come To Colorado (the) Next 3 Christmases.**

(1) **Come**	- **Calcaneus** (Os Calcis)
(2) **To**	- **Talus** (Astragalus)
(3) **Colorado**	- **Cuboid**
(4) **Next**	- **Navicular** (Scaphoid)
(5-6-7) **3 Christmases**	- **1st, 2nd, 3rd Cuneiforms**

Note above that the calcaneus, talus, and navicular bones are also known by the alternative names: os calcis, astragalus, and scaphoid. Correct usage however, dictates that the tarsal bone of the foot should be called the navicular, while the carpal bone of the wrist, which has a similar shape, should be called the scaphoid. (The carpal bone, unfortunately has more often been called the navicular rather than the preferred scaphoid.)

The similarities to the upper limb are less obvious with the tarsals in that there are only **seven tarsal bones** compared to the **eight carpal bones** of the wrist. Also, the tarsals are larger and less mobile because they provide a basis of support for the body in an erect position, compared to the eight smaller and more mobile carpals of the hand and wrist.

The seven tarsal bones are sometimes referred to as the ankle bones although only one of the tarsals, the talus, is directly involved in the ankle joint.

Calcaneus

The largest and strongest bone of the foot is the calcaneus. The posterior portion is often called the heel bone. The most posterior-inferior part of the calcaneus contains a process called the **tuberosity.** Certain large tendons are attached to this rough and striated process which at its widest points has two small rounded processes. The largest of these is labelled as the **lateral process**. The **medial process** is smaller and less pronounced.

Another ridge of bone which varies in size and shape is visualized laterally on the axial projection as the **peroneal trochlea** *(per"o-ne'al trok'le-ah)*. Sometimes in general this is also called the **trochlear process.** On the medial proximal aspect is a larger more prominent bony process called the **sustentaculum tali** *(sus"ten-tak'u-lum)*, literally meaning a support for the talus.

Knowing which bones each tarsal articulates with aids in understanding the relative position and the relationships of these tarsal bones.

Articulations: The calcaneus articulates with **two** bones; anteriorly with the **cuboid** and superiorly with the **talus.** The superior articulation with the talus forms the important **talocalcaneal** (subtalar) joint. There are three specific articular facets at this joint with the talus through which the weight of the body is transmitted to the ground in an erect position. These are the larger **posterior articular facet** and the smaller **anterior** and **middle articular facets.** Note that the middle articular facet is the upper portion of the prominent sustentaculum tali, which provides the medial support for this important weight-bearing joint.

The deep depression between posterior and middle articular facets is called the **calcaneal sulcus** *(Fig. 6-7).* This combined with a similar groove or depression of the talus forms an opening for certain ligaments to pass through. This opening or space is called the **tarsal sinus** or **sinus tarsi** *(Fig. 6-8).*

Talus

The talus is second largest tarsal bone and is located between the lower leg and the calcaneus. Therefore, the weight of the body is transmitted by this bone through the important ankle and talocalcaneal joints.

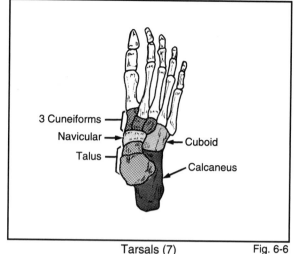

Tarsals (7)   Fig. 6-6

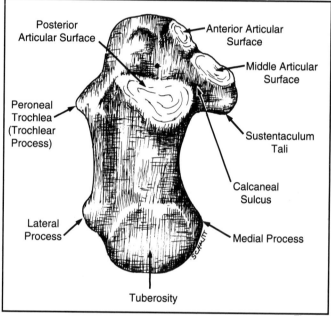

Left Calcaneus   Fig. 6-7
(Superior or Proximal Surface)

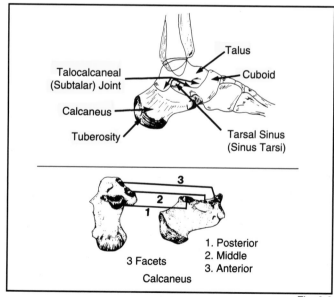

Calcaneus and Talus   Fig. 6-8
(With Ankle and Talocalcaneal Joints)

Articulations: The talus articulates with **four** bones; superiorly with the **tibia** and **fibula**, inferiorly with the **calcaneus** and anteriorly with the **navicular.**

Navicular

The navicular is a flattened, oval shaped bone located on the medial side of the foot between the talus and the three cuneiforms.

Articulations: The navicular articulates with **four** bones, posteriorly with the **talus** and anteriorly with the **three cuneiforms.**

Cuneiforms (3)

The three cuneiforms (meaning wedge shaped) are located on the medial and mid aspects of the foot between the first three metatarsals distally and the navicular proximally. The **first** and largest cuneiform, articulating with the first metatarsal, is the **medial** (internal) cuneiform. The **second** or **intermediate** (middle) cuneiform which articulates with the second metatarsal is the smallest of the cuneiforms. The **third** or **lateral** (external) cuneiform articulates with the third metatarsal distally and with the cuboid laterally. All three cuneiforms articulate with the navicular proximally.

Articulations: The **1st** or **medial (internal) cuneiform** articulates with **four** bones, the **navicular** proximally, the **first** and **second metatarsal** distally and the **intermediate** laterally.

The **2nd** or **intermediate (middle) cuneiform** also articulates with **four** bones, the **navicular** proximally, the **second metatarsal** distally and the **medial** and **lateral cuneiforms** on each side.

The **3rd** or **lateral (external) cuneiform** articulates with **six** bones, the **navicular** proximally, the **second, third,** and **fourth metatarsals** distally, the **intermediate cuneiform** medially and the **cuboid** laterally.

Cuboid

The cuboid is located on the lateral aspect of the foot, distal to the calcaneus and proximal to the fourth and fifth metatarsals.

Articulations: The **cuboid** articulates with **four** bones, the **calcaneus** proximally, the **3rd** or **lateral cuneiform** medially, and the **fourth** and **fifth metatarsals** distally. (Occasionally it will also articulate with a fifth bone, the navicular.)

Arches

The bones of the foot are arranged in **longitudinal** and **transverse arches** providing a strong shock absorbing type support for the weight of the body. The springy, longitudinal arch is composed of a medial and a lateral component with most of the arch on the medial and mid aspects of the foot.

The transverse arch is located primarily along the plantar surface of the distal tarsals and the tarsometatarsal joints. The transverse arch is primarily made up by the wedge shaped cuneiforms, especially the smaller second and third cuneiforms *(Fig. 6-10)* in combination with the larger first cuneiform and the cuboid.

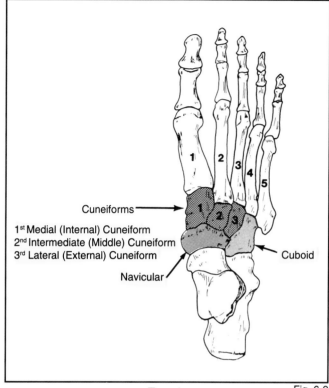

Cuneiforms
1st Medial (Internal) Cuneiform
2nd Intermediate (Middle) Cuneiform
3rd Lateral (External) Cuneiform
Cuboid
Navicular

Tarsals   Fig. 6-9

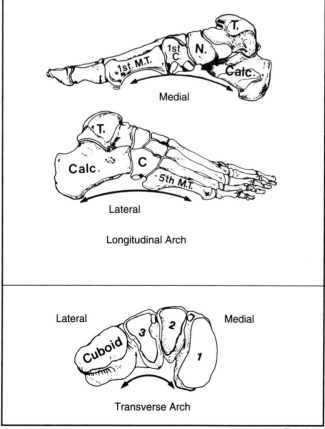

Medial

Lateral

Longitudinal Arch

Lateral   Medial

Transverse Arch

Arches   Fig. 6-10

Ankle Joint[1]

Frontal View

The **ankle joint** is formed by three bones, the two long bones of the lower leg, the **tibia** and **fibula**, and one tarsal bone, the **talus**. The expanded distal end of the slender fibula, which extends well down alongside the talus is termed the **lateral malleolus**.

The distal end of the larger and stronger tibia has a broad articular surface for articulation with the similarly shaped broad upper surface of the talus. The medial elongated process of the tibia which extends down alongside the medial talus, is termed the **medial malleolus**.

The inferior portions of the tibia and fibula form a deep socket or **mortise** into which the upper **talus** fits. The entire joint space of the ankle mortise however, is not seen on a true frontal view (AP projection) due to overlapping of portions of the distal fibula and tibia by the talus. This is caused by the more posterior position of the distal fibula, as shown on these drawings.

The anterior tubercle is an expanded process at the distal anterior and medial tibia, shown to articulate with the talus anteriorly *(Fig. 6-12)*.

Lateral View

The ankle joint is shown in a true lateral position in *Fig. 6-12*. This demonstrates that the **distal fibula is located slightly posterior in relationship to the distal tibia**. This relationship becomes important in evaluation for a **true lateral** radiograph of the leg, ankle or foot., A common misconception is to position and rotate the ankle so the medial and lateral malleoli are directly superimposed. This however will result in a slightly oblique ankle as these drawings illustrate. Therefore a true lateral requires the lateral malleolus to be about 15-20° **posterior** to the medial malleolus.

Note also that the more slender lateral malleolus generally extends **lower** or **more distal** than its counterpart, the medial malleolus.

Posterior malleolus is a radiologic term describing the distal posterior margin of the tibia. Serious fractures of the ankle may involve all three malleoli and would be termed a trimalleolar fracture.

Axial View

An axial view of the inferior margin of the distal tibia and fibula is shown in *Fig. 6-13*. This axial view visualizes an "end on" view of the ankle joint looking from the bottom up, demonstrating the concave inferior surface of the tibia. Also demonstrated are the relative positions of the **lateral** and **medial malleoli** of the fibula and tibia respectively. The smaller **fibula** is again shown to be **more posterior.** A line drawn through the mid portions of the two malleoli will be approximately 15° - 20° from the coronal plane (the true side-to-side plane of the body). Therefore, the lower leg and ankle must be rotated 15°-20° to bring the intermalleolar line parallel to the coronal plane. This relationship of the distal tibia and fibula becomes important in positioning for various views of the ankle joint or ankle mortise as described in the positioning pages of this chapter.

Ankle Joint

The ankle joint is a **synovial joint** of the **hinge type** with flexion and extension (dorsiflexion and plantar flexion) movements only. This requires strong collateral ligaments extending from the medial and lateral malleoli to the calcaneus and talus. Lateral stress can result in a "sprained" ankle with stretched or torn collateral ligaments as well as torn muscle tendons.

An articular capsule lined with synovial membrane encloses the entire ankle joint.

[1] Frank, E.D., et. al: Radiography of the Ankle Mortise, Radiologic Technology 62-5: 354-359, 1991.

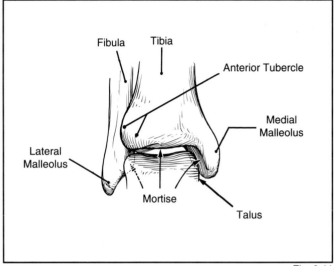

Right Ankle Joint – Frontal View   Fig. 6-11

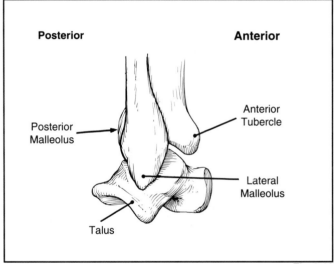

Right Ankle Joint – True Lateral View   Fig. 6-12

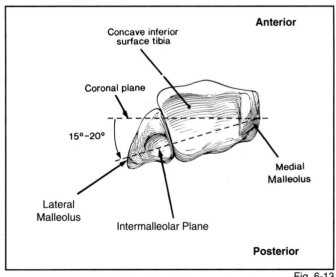

Ankle Joint – Axial View   Fig. 6-13
(Figs. 6-11, 12, 13 Courtesy of Mayo Foundation)

Foot and Ankle

Review Exercise with Radiographs

Three common projections of the foot and ankle are shown with labels for an anatomy review of the bones and joints. A good review exercise is to cover up the answers below and identify or write out all the parts as labelled before checking the answers as listed below.

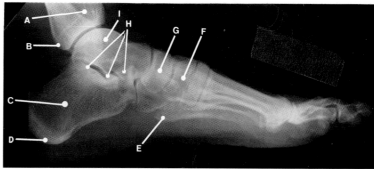

Lateral Left Foot   Fig. 6-14

Lateral Left Foot

A. Tibia
B. Posterior malleolus of tibia
C. Calcaneus
D. Tuberosity of calcaneus
E. Tuberosity at the base of
   5th metatarsal

F. 1st or medial cuneiform
G. Navicular
H. Talocalcaneal joint
I. Talus

Oblique Right Foot

A. Interphalangeal joint of 1st digit of right foot
B. Proximal phalanx of 1st digit of right foot
C. Metatarsophalangeal (MP joint of 1st digit of right foot)
D. Head of first metatarsal
E. Shaft of first metatarsal
F. Base of first metatarsal
G. 2nd or intermediate cuneiform (partially superimposed over 1st or medial cuneiform)
H. Navicular
I. Talus
J. Tuberosity of Calcaneus
K. Cuboid
L. Tuberosity of the base of the 5th metatarsal
M. Fifth metatarsophalangeal (MP) joint of right foot
N. Proximal phalanx of 4th digit of right foot
   (Note fracture in area of proximal 5th metatarsal.)

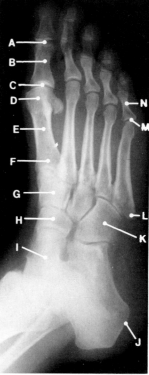

Fig. 6-15
Oblique Right Foot

AP Right Ankle

A. Fibula
B. Lateral malleolus
C. Mortise joint of ankle

D. Talus
E. Medial malleolus
F. Tibia

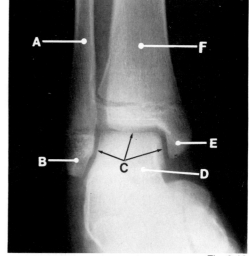

AP Right Ankle   Fig. 6-16
(Mortise View – 15° Medial Oblique)

Leg (Tibia and Fibula)

Starting distally, the first group of bones of the lower limb studied in this chapter were those of the foot. The second group are the two bones of the lower leg, the **tibia** and **fibula.** The third grouping is the single large bone of the thigh, namely the **femur.** The distal femur will be included in this chapter which includes the knee joint. The **patella** is a large sesamoid bone protecting the anterior part of the knee joint.

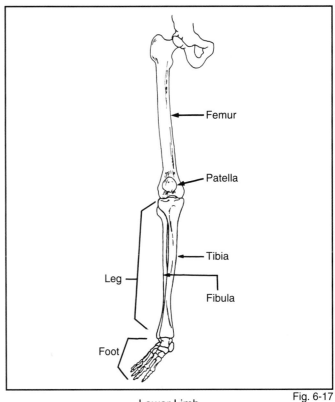

Lower Limb   Fig. 6-17

Tibia

The tibia, as one of the larger bones of the body, is the weight-bearing bone of the lower leg. The tibia can easily be felt through the skin in the anteromedial part of the leg. It is made up of three parts, the central **body** or **shaft** and **two extremities.**

The **medial** and **lateral condyles** are the two large processes making up the medial and lateral aspects of the proximal tibia.

The **intercondyloid eminence**, sometimes called the tibial spine, includes two small pointed prominences, called **intercondyloid tubercles**, located on the superior surface of the tibial head between the two condyles. The upper articular surface of the condyles includes two smooth concave **articular facets** (tibial plateau) which articulate with the femur.

The **tibial tuberosity** is a rough-textured prominence located on the mid-anterior surface of the tibia just distal to the condyles. This tuberosity is the distal attachment of the patellar tendon which connects to the large muscle of the anterior thigh. Sometimes in young persons, the tibial tuberosity separates from the shaft of the tibia, a condition known as Osgood-Schlatter disease.

The **body** or **shaft** is the long portion of the tibia between the two extremities. Along the anterior surface of the body, extending from the tibial tuberosity to the medial malleolus, is a sharp ridge called the **anterior crest** or **border.** This sharp anterior crest is just under the skin surface and is often referred to as the shin or shin bone.

The **distal extremity** of the tibia is smaller than the proximal and ends in a short pyramid-shaped process called the **medial malleolus.** The medial malleolus, located just under the skin, is easily palpated on the medial aspect of the ankle.

The lateral aspect of the distal extremity of the tibia forms a flattened, triangular shaped **fibular notch** for articulation with the distal fibula. The inferior smooth, concave-shaped articular surface is continuous with the articular surface of the medial malleolus for articulation with talus. This articulation makes up the ankle joint or ankle mortise.

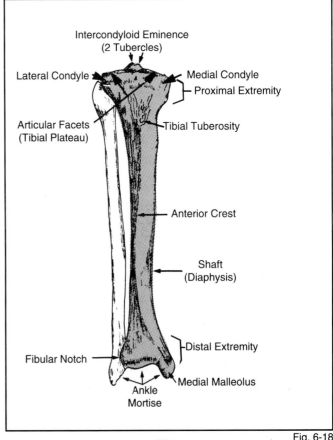

Tibia   Fig. 6-18

Fibula

The **fibula** or calf bone is a long slender bone located on the lateral aspect of the lower leg. It articulates with the tibia proximally and the tibia and talus distally. The proximal extremity of the fibula is expanded into a **head,** which articulates with the lateral aspect of the posteroinferior surface of the lateral condyle of the tibia. The extreme proximal aspect of the head is pointed and is known as the **apex** or **styloid process** of the head of the fibula. The tapered area just below the head is the **neck** of the fibula.

The **body** or **shaft** is the long, slender portion of the fibula between the two extremities. The enlarged distal end of the fibula can be felt as a distinct bump on the lateral aspect of the ankle joint and is known as the **lateral malleolus.** It's tip is about 1/2 in. (1.25 cm) lower or more distal than the medial malleolus. The medial surface of the lateral malleolus is smooth and oval shaped and articulates with the talus as part of the ankle joint or mortise as described on a previous page.

Distal Femur

The **femur** or thigh bone is the longest and strongest bone in the entire body. The femur is the only long bone between the **hip joint** and the **knee joint.** Similar to all long bones, the **body** or **shaft** of the femur is the slender, elongated portion of the bone.

Distal Femur (Anterior View)

The distal femur viewed anteriorly demonstrates the position of the patella or knee cap. The **patella,** which is the largest sesamoid bone in the body, is located anteriorly to the distal femur. Note that the most distal part of the patella is **above** or **proximal** to the actual knee joint by approximately 1/2 in. (1.25 cm) in this position with the lower leg fully extended. This relationship becomes important in positioning for the knee joint.

The **patellar surface** is the smooth and shallow, triangular shaped depression at the distal portion of the anterior femur. This depression is also sometimes termed the **intercondylar sulcus.** (Sulcus means a groove or depression.) Some literature also refers to this depression as the **trochlear groove.** (Trochlea means pulley or pulley-shaped structure in reference to the medial and lateral condyles.) All three of these terms should be recognized as referring to this smooth, shallow depression.

Note that the patella itself is mostly superior to the patellar surface with the leg fully extended. However, as the leg is flexed, the patella which is attached to large muscle tendons, moves distally or downward over the patellar surface. This is best shown on the lateral knee drawing *(Fig. 6-22)* on the following page.

Distal Femur (Posterior View)

The posterior view of the distal femur clearly demonstrates the two large rounded **condyles** which are joined anteriorly but are separated distally and posteriorly by the deep **intercondylar fossa** or **notch.** This posterior view demonstrates that the intercondylar fossa is primarily on the distal and posterior aspects of the femur.

The rounded distal portions of the **medial** and **lateral condyles,** contain smooth articular surfaces for articulation with the two articular surfaces of the tibia. Note that the medial condyle extends lower or more distally than the lateral when the femoral shaft is vertical as on this drawing *(Fig. 6-21)*. This explains why the CR must be angled 5 to 7° cephalic for a lateral knee to cause the two condyles to be directly superimposed when the femur is parallel to the film. The explanation for this is also seen in *Fig. 6-20* which demonstrates that in an erect anatomical position, wherein the distal femoral condyles are parallel to the floor at the knee joint, the femoral shaft is at an angle of approximately 10° from vertical for an average adult. The range is 5-15°.[1] This angle would be greater on a short person with a wider pelvis and less on a tall person with a narrow pelvis. Therefore, in general this angle is greater on a female than on a male. This is demonstrated further on page 218 *(Fig. 7-3)* of Chapter 7 on the proximal femur.

The **medial** and **lateral epicondyles,** which can readily be palpated, are rough prominences for muscle attachments and are located on the upper, outer portions of the condyles.

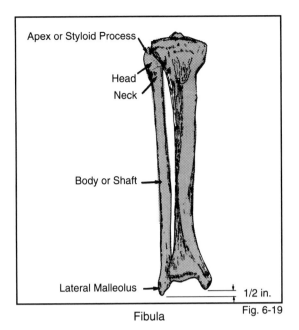

Fibula

Fig. 6-19

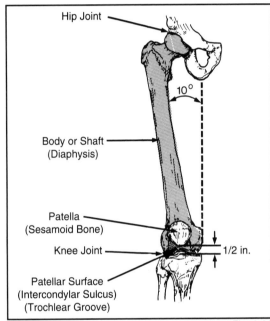

Femur (Anterior)

Fig. 6-20

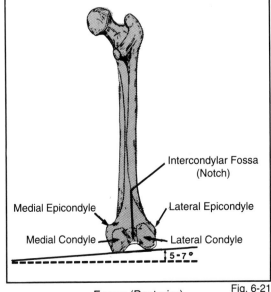

Femur (Posterior)

Fig. 6-21

---

[1] Keats, T.E., et al: Radiology 87:904, 1966

Distal Femur and Patella (Lateral View)

The lateral view in *Fig. 6-22* demonstrates the relationship of the patella to the patellar surface of the distal femur. The patella is a large sesamoid bone embedded in the tendon of the large quadriceps femoris muscle, and as the lower leg is flexed the patella moves downward and is drawn inward into the intercondylar groove or sulcus. A partial flexion of near 45°, as shown in this drawing, shows the patella being pulled only partially downward, but with 90° flexion the patella would move down further over the distal portion of the femur. This movement and the relationship of the patella to the femur becomes important in positioning for the knee joint and for the tangential projection of the **patellofemoral joint**. (Articulation between patella and distal femur.)

The posterior surface of the knee joint is termed the **popliteal region**.

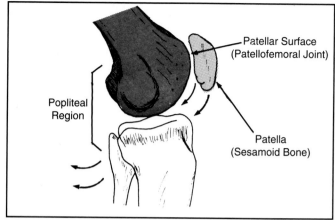

Distal Femur and Patella (Mediolateral)   Fig. 6-22

Distal Femur and Patella (Axial View)

The axial or end on view of the distal femur again demonstrates the relationship of the patella to the **patellar surface** (**intercondylar sulcus** or **trochlear groove**) of the distal femur. The **patellofemoral joint space** is visualized in this axial view (*Fig. 6-23*). Other parts of the distal femur are also well visualized.

The **intercondylar fossa** (notch) is shown to be very deep on the posterior aspect of the femur. The **epicondyles** are seen as rough prominences on the outermost tips of the large **medial** and **lateral condyles.**

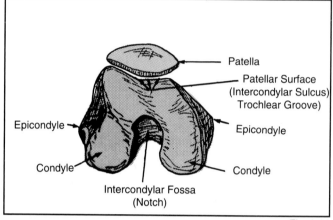

Distal Femur and Patella (Axial View)   Fig. 6-23

Patella

The **patella** (knee cap) is a flat triangular bone about 2 in. or 5 cm in diameter. The patella appears to be up-side down in that its pointed **apex** is located along the **inferior border** and its **base** is the **superior** or **upper border**. The outer or **anterior surface** is convex and roughened, while the inner **posterior surface** is smooth and oval shaped for articulation with the femur. The patella serves to protect the anterior aspect of the knee joint and acts as a pivot to increase the leverage of the large quadriceps femoris muscle, the tendon of which attaches to the tibial tuberosity of the lower leg. The patella is somewhat loose and movable in its more superior position when the leg is extended and the quadriceps muscles relaxed. However, as the leg is flexed and the muscles tighten, it moves distally and becomes locked into position. It should be noted that the patella articulates only with the femur, not with the tibia.

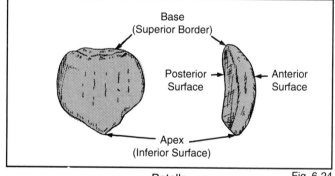

Patella   Fig. 6-24

Knee Joint

The knee joint proper is a large complex joint primarily involving articulation between the **femur** and the **tibia**, the **tibiofemoral joint.** The **patellofemoral joint** is also part of the knee joint wherein the patella articulates with the anterior surface of the distal femur.

Four major ligaments are identified on the posterior view drawing of *Fig. 6-25*. These are described and demonstrated further on the following page.

Proximal Tibiofibular Joint

The proximal tibia is not part of the knee joint in that it does not articulate with any aspect of the femur, even though a portion of one of the lateral ligaments does extend from the femur to the lateral proximal fibula. The head of the fibula however, does articulate with the lateral condyle of the tibia to which it is attached by certain posterior ligaments.

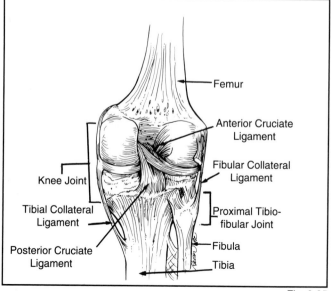

Fig. 6-25
Knee Joint and Proximal Tibiofibular Joint (Posterior View)

Knee Joint continued

Synovial Membrane and Cavity

The articular cavity of the knee joint is the largest joint space of the human body. The total knee joint is a synovial type enclosed in an **articular capsule** or **bursa** (a complex multifaceted saclike structure lined with synovial membrane closely integrated with certain fibrocartilage and ligaments, *Fig. 6-27*). This is also demonstrated in the arthrogram radiograph below *(Fig. 6-29)* wherein a combination negative and positive contrast media has been injected into the articular capsule or bursa.

The articular cavity or bursa of the knee joint extends upwards under and superior to the patella, identified as the **suprapatellar bursa** *(Fig. 6-27)*. Distal to the patella, the **infrapatellar bursa** is separated by a large **infrapatellar fat pad**, which can be identified on radiographs. Posteriorly the bursae continue as various subdivisions or recesses interspaced between certain ligaments and muscle tendons. These spaces posterior and distal to the femur can also be seen filled with negative contrast media on the lateral arthrogram radiograph.

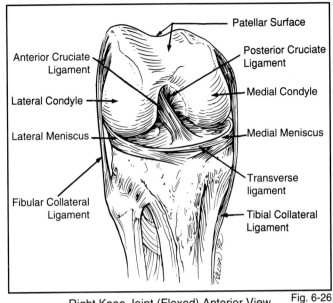

Right Knee Joint (Flexed) Anterior View   Fig. 6-26

Ligaments: The knee joint is highly dependent on ligaments for stability. There are two pair of major ligaments as well as various minor ligaments which maintain the knee joint. The two important pair of major ligaments are the two **collateral ligaments** (tibial and fibular), and the **two cruciate** *(kroo'she-at)* **ligaments** (anterior and posterior) *(Figs. 6-25 & 26)*.

The **patellar ligament** is shown as part of the tendon of insertion of the large quadriceps femoris muscle extending over the patella to the tibial tuberosity *(Fig. 6-27)*. The infrapatellar fat pad is posterior to this ligament which aids in protecting the anterior aspect of the knee joint.

The two collateral ligaments are strong bands at the sides of the knee which prevent adduction and abduction movements at the knee *(Figs. 6-25* and *6-26)*. The cruciate ligaments lie within the capsule of the knee joint. They are strong rounded cords which cross each other as they attach to the respective anterior and posterior aspects of the intercondylar eminence of the tibia. They stabilize the knee joint by preventing anterior or posterior movement of the tibia in relationship to the femoral condyles.

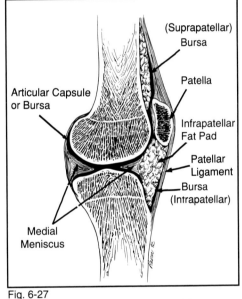

Fig. 6-27
Sagittal Section of Knee Joint
(Shows bursa, meniscus and fat pads)

Fig. 6-28
Superior View of Articular Surface of Tibia
(Shows menisci and cruciate ligament attachments)

Menisci (Articular Discs): The **medial and lateral menisci** *(me-nis'ci)* are fibrocartilage discs between the articular facets of the tibia (tibial plateau) and the femoral condyles *(Fig. 6-28)*. They are crescent-shaped and are thicker at their external margins and taper to a very thin center portion. They act as shock absorbers to reduce some of the direct impact and stress occurring at the knee joint. Along with the synovial membrane they are also believed to function in producing synovial fluid which acts as a lubricant for the articulating ends of the femur and tibia which are also covered with a tough, slick hyaline membrane.

Knee Trauma: The knee has the greatest potential for trauma injury of any joint in the human body, especially in contact sports such as football or basketball. For example, the most common type of knee injury in football from a blow to the lateral side of the knee is a rupture of the tibial collateral ligament. This injury is also often associated with a tearing of the anterior cruciate ligament and the medial meniscus (torn cartilage). These injuries typically come to the radiology department for either an MRI exam to visualize these soft tissue structures of the knee or for a knee arthrogram.

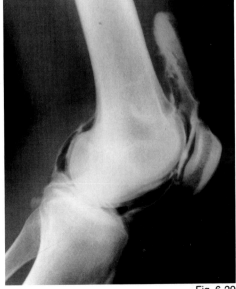

Fig. 6-29
Lateral Knee Arthrogram Radiograph
(Demonstrates articular capsule or bursa as outlined by a combination negative and positive contrast media)

Review Exercise with Radiographs

Common projections of the leg, knee and patella are shown with labels for an anatomy review.

AP – Right Leg
A. Medial condyle of the tibia
B. Body or shaft of tibia
C. Medial malleolus
D. Lateral malleolus
E. Body or shaft of the fibula
F. Neck
G. Head
H. Apex (styloid process) of head of fibula
I. Lateral condyle of tibia
J. Intercondylar eminence (tibial spine)

Lateral – Right Leg
A. Intercondylar eminence (tibial spine)
B. Tibial tuberosity
C. Body or shaft of tibia
D. Body or shaft of fibula
E. Medial malleolus
F. Lateral malleolus
G. Posterior malleolus (Posterior tip of distal tibia)

AP – Left Knee
A. Intercondyloid tubercles; together they make up the intercondyloid eminence (tibial spine)
B. Lateral epicondyle of femur
C. Lateral condyle of femur
D. Lateral condyle of tibia
E. Articular facets of tibia
F. Medial condyle of tibia
G. Medial condyle of femur
H. Medial epicondyle of femur
I. Patella (seen through femur)

Lateral – Left Knee
A. Base of patella
B. Apex of patella
C. Tibial tuberosity
D. Neck of fibula
E. Head of fibula
F. Apex (styloid process) of head of fibula
G. Intercondylar eminence (tibial spine)
H. Patellar surface (intercondylar sulcus or trochlear groove)

Tangential Projection (Patello-femoral Joint)
A. Patella
B. Patellofemoral joint
C. Lateral condyle
D. Patellar surface (Intercondylar sulcus, Trochlear groove, Femoral Trochlea)
E. Medial Condyle

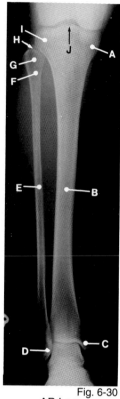

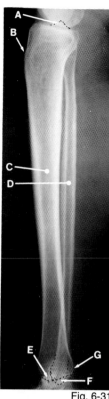

Fig. 6-30
AP Leg

Fig. 6-31
Lateral Leg

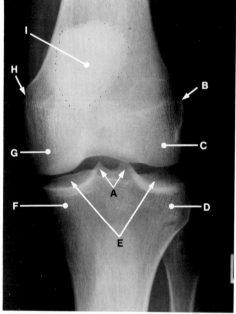
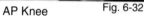

AP Knee   Fig. 6-32

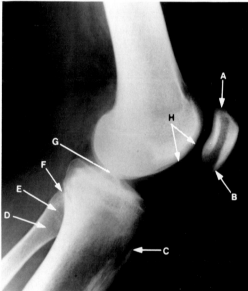

Lateral Knee   Fig. 6-33

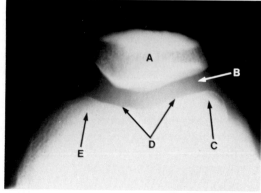

Fig. 6-34
Tangential Projection (Patellofemoral Joint)

Classification of Joints

The joints or articulations of the lower limb are (with one exception) all classified as **synovial joints** characterized by a fibrous type capsule containing synovial fluid. Therefore, they also are (with the one exception) **diarthrodial** or freely movable.

The one exception to the synovial joint is the **distal tibiofibular joint**, which is classified as a **fibrous joint** with fibrous interconnections between the surfaces of the tibia and fibula. It is of the **syndesmosis type** and is only **slightly movable**, or **amphiarthrodial**. The most distal part of this joint however, is smooth and lined with a synovial membrane that is continuous with the ankle joint.

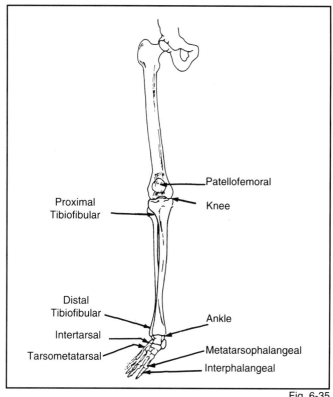

Joints of Lower Limb

Fig. 6-35

Summary of Foot, Ankle, Leg and Knee Joints

Classification: *Synovial* (Articular capsule containing synovial fluid)

Mobility Type: *Diarthrodial* (freely movable)

Movement Type:

1. Interphalangeal Joints — *Hinge*, flexion and extension movements

2. Metatarsophalangeal Joints — *Modified Condyloid*, flexion, extension, abduction and adduction. (Circumduction like that of the metacarpophalangeal joints of the hand are generally not possible.)

3. Tarsometatarsal Joints — *Gliding*, limited gliding movement

4. Intertarsal Joints — *Gliding*, subtalar in combination with some other intertarsal joints provides for gliding and rotation, results in **inversion** and **eversion** of the foot.

5. Ankle Joint — *Hinge*, dorsiflexion and plantar flexion only (side-to-side movements only occur with stretched or torn ligaments).

6. Knee Joint
   Tibiofemoral — *Special type Hinge*, flexion and extension and some gliding and rotational movements when knee is partially flexed.

   Patellofemoral — *Saddle*, considered a saddle type because of its shape and relationship of the patella to the distal femur.

7. Tibiofibular Joints:
   Proximal Tibiofibular — *Gliding*, limited gliding movement between lateral condyle and head of fibula.

   Distal Tibiofibular:
   Classification: — *Fibrous*
   Mobility Type: — *Amphiarthrodial* (slightly movable) of the **syndesmosis** type.

Motions of Foot and Ankle

Other confusing terminology involving the ankle and intertarsal joints are: **dorsiflexion, plantar flexion, inversion,** and **eversion.** To decrease the angle (flex) between the dorsum pedis and the anterior part of the lower leg is to dorsiflex at the ankle joint. Extending the ankle joint or pointing the foot and toe downward with respect to the normal position is termed plantar flexion.

Inversion is an inward turning of the ankle and talocalcaneal (subtalar) joints, while eversion is an outward turning. The lower leg does not rotate during inversion or eversion. Most sprained ankles result from an accidental and forced inversion or eversion.

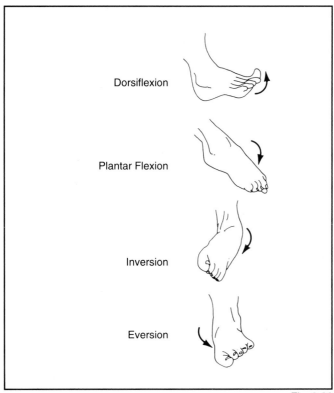

Dorsiflexion

Plantar Flexion

Inversion

Eversion

Motions of Foot and Ankle   Fig. 6-36

Surfaces and Projections of the Foot

Surfaces: The surfaces of the foot are sometimes confusing in that the top or **anterior surface** of the foot is called **dorsum.** Dorsal is usually the posterior part of the body. Dorsum, in this case, comes from the term **dorsum pedis** which refers to the upper surface, or the surface opposite the sole of the foot.

The sole of the foot is the **posterior** surface or **plantar surface.** Using these terms one can describe the common projections of the foot.

Projections: The **anteroposterior** or **AP projection** of the foot is the same as a **dorsoplantar projection.** The less common **postero-anterior** or **PA projection** can also be called a **plantodorsal projection.**

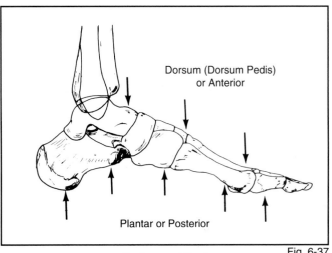

Dorsum (Dorsum Pedis) or Anterior

Plantar or Posterior

Surfaces of Foot   Fig. 6-37

Part II Radiographic Positioning

Positioning Considerations
Radiographic examinations involving the lower limb below the knee are generally done table top as shown in *Fig. 6-38*. Severe trauma cases or patients who are difficult to move can also be radiographed directly on the cart.

Distance
A common minimum SID (source-image receptor distance) is 40 in. or 102 cm. When radiographing with cassettes directly on the table top, to maintain a consant SID the tube height must be increased as compared to radiographs taken with the cassette in the Bucky tray. This difference is generally 3-4 in. (8-10 cm) for floating type table tops. The same minimum 40 in. (102 cm) SID should also be used when radiographing directly on the cart, unless exposure factors are adjusted to compensate for a change in SID.

NOTE: See page 35 for a discussion on the minimal 40 in. (102 cm) SID.

Gonadal Shielding
Gonadal shielding is important for exams of the lower limb because of the proximity of the gonads to the divergent x-ray beam as well as scatter radiation. Therefore, a lead vinyl covered shield should be draped over the patient's gonadal area as shown. Even though the gonadal rule states this should be done on patients of reproductive age when the gonads lie within or close to the primary field, it is a good practice to provide gonadal shielding for all patients.

Collimation
The collimation rule should again be followed, namely that **collimation borders should be visible on all four sides if the film is large enough to allow this without cutting off essential anatomy**. A general rule however, concerning film size is to **use the smallest film size possible for the specific part being radiographed.** Four-sided collimation is generally possible however, even with a minimal size film for most if not all radiographic exams of the lower limb.

Two or more projections may be taken on one film for some exams such as for the toes, foot, ankle or lower leg. This requires close collimation of the part being radiographed.

Four sided collimation allows for checking radiographs for accuracy of centering and positioning by placing a large imaginary "X" from the four corners of the collimation field. The center point of the "X" indicates the CR location.

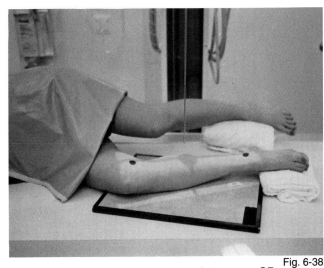

Fig. 6-38
Table top of lower limb, demonstrating correct CR location, good collimation and gonadal shielding

General Positioning
A general positioning rule especially applicable to both the upper and lower limbs is to **always place the long axis of the part being radiographed parallel to the long axis of the film.** If more than one projection is taken on the same film, the part should be parallel to the long axis of the part of the film being used. Also **all body parts should be oriented in the same direction,** when two or more projections are taken on the same film.

An exception to this rule is the lower leg of an adult. This limb generally has to be placed diagonally to include both the knee and the ankle joints as shown in *Fig. 6-38*.

Correct Centering
Accurate centering and alignment of the body part to the film and correct central ray location is especially important for exams of the upper and lower limbs where shape and size distortion must be avoided and the narrow joint spaces clearly demonstrated. Therefore, in general the part being radiographed should **be parallel to the plane of the film holder, the central ray should be 90° or perpendicular** and should be **directed to the correct centering point** as indicated on each positioning page. (Exceptions to the 90° or perpendicular CR do occur as indicated in the following pages.)

Exposure Factors

The principal exposure factors for radiographs of the lower limbs are:
1. Lower to medium kVp (50-70)
2. Short exposure time
3. Small focal spot
4. Adequate mAs for sufficient density

Correctly exposed radiographs of the lower limbs should generally visualize both soft tissue margins and fine bony trabecular markings of bones being radiographed.

Optional Technique for Foot: An increase to 70 or 80 kVp with accompanying decrease in mAs will increase exposure latitude to result in a more uniform exposure density between the phalanges and the tarsals.

Film Holders

For exams distal to the knee, detail extremity screens are used without grids. Single screen and single emulsion film are commonly used for adult extremities for better detail. A general rule states that grids should be used with body parts measuring over 10 cm. (Some references suggest a grid over 13 cm.) This places the average knee (measuring 9-13 cm) at a size where either a screen or grid may be used depending on patient size and departmental preferences. This text recommends a screen on smaller patients measuring 10 cm or less and a grid for larger patients measuring over 10 cm, especially on the AP knee. Anything proximal to the knee such as the mid or distal femur requires the use of a grid. When grids are used, either the moving Bucky grid under the table top may be used, or fine-lined portable grids.

Placement of Film Markers

At the top of each of the following positioning pages is a box drawing demonstrating the correct film holder size and placement (lengthwise or crosswise). A suggested corner placement for the patient ID information is shown for each film. The size and location of multiple projections on one film are also shown.

When evaluating final radiographs as part of the evaluation criteria, the patient ID information should always be checked to see if it is legible. R or L markers should be visible on the lateral margin of the collimation field on at least one projection on each film without superimposing any anatomy of interest.

Increase Exposure with Cast

A lower limb with a cast will require an increase in exposure. The thickness of the cast and the body part, as well as the type of cast will affect the increase in exposure required. A recommended conversion guide for casts is as follows:

• Small to medium dry plaster cast :	- increase 5-7 kVp

• Large or wet
  plaster cast:
	- double mAs **or**
	  increase 8-10 kVp.

• Fiberglass cast:	- increase 3-4 kVp

National Survey:

Departmental standard (basic) and optional routines for exams of the lower limbs were very consistent throughout the United States except for the patella routines which showed some regional differences. The results of this survey determined national norms for routines presented in the positioning pages of this text which follow. Approximately 530 responses were recieved to this survey.

Toe Routine

Toe	U.S. Average	
	Basic	Optional
• AP - CR Perpendicular	66%	
or		
- CR 10-15° toward heel	30%	
• Oblique	94%	
• Lateral	85%	

Foot Routine

Foot	U.S. Average	
	Basic	Optional
• AP, 10-15° toward heel	91%	
• Oblique - 30° oblique	75%	
or		
- 45° oblique	27%	
• Lateral - Mediolateral	80%	
or		
- Lateromedial	16%	5%

Calcaneus Routine

Calcaneus	U.S. Average	
	Basic	Optional
• Lateral	98%	
• Plantodorsal (axial)	90%	
or		
• Dorsoplantar (axial)	12%	11%
• Oblique		2%

Summary

Toes: The survey revealed some surprising results concerning routines for toes. For the AP projection, 66% indicated a perpendicular CR and only 30% a 10-15° CR angle toward the heel. Because of part-film alignment, the **10-15° CR angle is recommended** and demonstrated in this text.

The survey also revealed that 60% of departments take the AP of toe(s) only and 40% include the entire foot on the AP for possible secondary trauma or pathology to other aspects of the foot. Therefore, including the entire foot on the AP toe is listed as an alternate routine.

Foot: The results for the oblique foot also showed some discrepancies with 75% indicating a 30° oblique and 27% a 45° of the plantar surface to the film. (See page 192 on oblique foot where this is discussed under NOTE.) The **mediolateral** is shown to be the preferred lateral projection as also recommended in this text.

Ankle Routine

Ankle	U.S. Average	
	Basic	Optional
• AP (True AP, no rotation)	79%	3%
• AP Mortise (15 - 20° int. rotation)	51%	14%
• Oblique (45° internal)	72%	5%
• Lateral - Mediolateral	85%	2%
or		
- Lateromedial	16%	5%

Lower Leg Routine

Leg	U.S. Average	
	Basic	Optional
• AP	99%	
• Lateral	99%	

Knee Routine

Knee	U.S. Average	
	Basic	Optional
• AP : 5-7° Ceph.	72%	
or		
- No angle	13%	
or		
- PA	15%	
• AP Oblique		
- 45° medial Obli	45%	
or		
- 45° lateral Obli	5%	
or		
- PA 45° Obli	9%	
• Lateral		
- 10-15° flexion	14%	
or		
- 20-30° flexion	47%	
or		
- 35-40° flexion	30%	
Intercondyloid Fossa		
• PA Axial		
- Camp- Coventry	61%	
or		
- Kneeing, Holmblad	38%	10%
• AP Axial		10%

Ankle: The survey results suggest that there is some confusion in the ankle routine with the true **AP projection** and the **AP mortise 15-20° medial oblique** positions. Which of these should be included along with the 45° oblique and lateral positions for ankle routines? This text suggests that **both** be included for the ankle routines involving possible trauma or sprains to the ankle joint. (See page 198.)

Patella Routine:

Patella	U.S. Average		East (191)		Midwest (239)		West (77)	
	Basic	Optional	Basic	Optional	Basic	Optional	Basic	Optional
• Lateral	81%		81%		78%		91%	
• PA, CR perpendicular	65%		65%		62%		74%	
• Tangential								
- Pt prone, Settegast or Sunrise	68%		**75%**		67%		**53%**	
or								
- Pt supine, Merchant's method	13%	11%	11%	11%	13%	13%	**21%**	16%
• PA Oblique - CR perpendicular	9%	9%	8%	8%	10%	10%	9%	13%
or								
CR - 25-30° caudal	3%	3%	3%	3%	3%	3%	3%	3%

Knee: The survey results support a basic knee routine of an **AP**, a **45° medial oblique** and a **lateral**. The recommended flexion for the lateral knee by this text is only **15 to 20°** rather than 35 to 40°. The additional flexion will tighten the large anterior leg muscle drawing the patella into the intracondylar sulcus which will tend to obscure certain soft tissue information involving the joint space. (See page 206.)

This text also recommends a **90° CR** for the **AP knee** if the knee is fully extended, rather than a routine 5-7° cephalic angle. Studies by the authors supported by anatomists indicate that the tibial plateau is perpendicular to the tibial shaft on the average patient, therefore the knee joint space is best demonstrated by a CR that is **perpendicular to the long axis of the tibia**. (See page 204.)

Femur Routine:

Mid & Distal Femur	U.S. Average	
	Basic	Optional
• AP	99%	
• Lateral	99%	

Patella: The survey results for the patella routine indicated some regional differences in the U.S. The **tangential projection** is taken with the patient prone by 75% of departments in the East, but only by 53% in the western U.S. The percent taking this projection supine (such as the Merchant's method) is nearly twice as high in the West (21%) compared to the East (11%) and Midwest (13%). Both methods will be described in this text.

Standard and Optional Operating Procedures

Certain basic and optional projections or positions for the toes, foot, ankle, leg, knee and mid and distal femur are demonstrated and described on the following pages as suggested standard and optional departmental procedures.

Basic Projections
Standard or basic projections, at times referred to as routine projections or departmental routines are those projections or positions commonly taken on average patients who are helpful and can cooperate in performing the procedure.

Optional Projections
Optional projections are those more common projections or positions taken as extra or additional projections to better demonstrate certain pathologic conditions or specific body parts. (They are **not** optional as to whether or not they must be learned and mastered.)

Basic and Optional Projections

Toes
Basic
• AP
• Oblique
• Lateral
Optional
• Sesamoids
(Tangential)

Foot
Basic
• AP
• Oblique
• Lateral
Optional
• Lateral weight-
bearing

Calcaneus
Basic
• Plantodorsal
(Dorsoplantar)
• Lateral

Ankle
Basic
• AP
• AP Mortise
• Oblique (45°)
• Lateral
Optional
• AP Stress

Leg
Basic
• AP
• Lateral

Knee
Basic
• AP
• Oblique
• Lateral

Patella
Basic
• PA
• Lateral
• Tangential
Optional
• Oblique

Knee - Intercondyloid Fossa
Basic
• PA Axial
Optional
• AP Axial

Mid & Distal Femur
Basic
• AP
• Lateral

• AP Projection

Toes
Basic
• **AP**
• Oblique
• Lateral

Structures Best Shown:
Phalanges of digit(s) in question to include distal metatarsal(s) and associated joints.

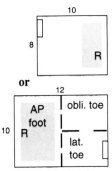

or

Alternate Routine

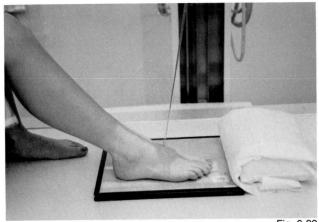

Fig. 6-39
AP – To Include All Digits (CR 10-15°)

Technical Factors:
• Film Size - 8 x 10 in. (18 x 24 cm) crosswise. (Divide in thirds or in half depending on the number of digits being included, see NOTE.)
• Detail screen, table top.
• 50-60 kVp range.

Alternate Routine (AP of entire foot)
• 10 x 12 in. (24 x 30 cm) crosswise.
• Divide in half.
(Some departments require the entire foot to be included for this AP projection for possible secondary trauma to other parts of the foot. (CR and collimation would be changed accordingly as for an AP foot.)

Patient Position:
• Patient supine with knee flexed, pillow under head.

Shielding: Place lead shield over pelvic area to shield gonads.

Part Position:
• Plantar surface of foot resting on cassette, with knee flexed as needed to rest foot firmly and easily on cassette. (If immobilization support is needed, flex opposite knee also to rest against and support the affected leg and knee.)
• Center and align long axis of digit(s) to long axis of unmasked cassette.

Central Ray:
• Angle CR **10-15° toward calcaneus** to align long axis of phalanges parallel to film.
• If a **15° wedge** is placed under foot for parallel part-film alignment, then the CR is **perpendicular** to film, *Fig. 6-41.*
• CR to **metatarsophalangeal (MP) joint(s)** in question.
• Minimum 40 in. (102 cm) SID.

Collimation: Collimate on four sides to area of interest. On side margins include a **minimum** of one digit on each side of digit(s) in question, or include all five digits if this is the department routine. (See NOTE.)

NOTE: Some departmental routines always include all the digits on the AP and obliques toes for possible trauma to other digits even if a specific toe is ordered. A recommended routine is to center to specific toe(s) of interest but open the collimation field wide enough to include a minimum of 1 or 2 digits on each side.

Evaluation Criteria:
• Digit(s) in question and distal half of metatarsals should be included.

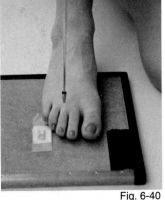

Fig. 6-40
AP 3rd Digit (CR 10-15°)

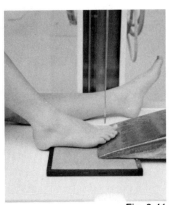

Fig. 6-41
AP 1st Digit With Wedge
(CR Perpendicular)

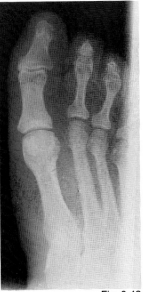

Fig. 6-42
AP 1st Digit

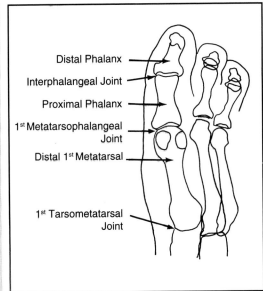

Distal Phalanx
Interphalangeal Joint
Proximal Phalanx
1st Metatarsophalangeal Joint
Distal 1st Metatarsal
1st Tarsometatarsal Joint

Fig. 6-43
AP 1st Digit

• Individual digits should be separated with no overlapping of soft tissues.
• Collimation borders should be visible on all four sides with the center at the MP joint(s) in question.
• No rotation as evidenced by symmetrical appearance of concavities on each side of shafts of phalanges and distal metatarsals.
• Interphalangeal and MP joints in question should appear open indicating correct CR centering and angle.
• Optimum exposure and contrast with no motion will visualize sharp borders and fine trabecular markings. Soft tissue margins and detail should be visible.
• Alternate routine - see AP foot.

• Oblique Position

Structures Best Shown:
Phalanges of digit(s) in question to include distal metartarsal(s) and associated joints.

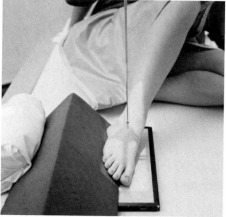

Fig. 6-44
Medial Oblique – To Include All Digits
(optional routine)

Technical Factors:
• Film Size - 8 x 10 in. (18 x 24 cm) crosswise.
  (Divide in thirds or in half depending on the number of digits being included, see NOTE.)
• Detail screen, table top.
• 50-60 kVp range.

Patient Position
• Patient supine with knee flexed, pillow under head.

Shielding: Place lead shield over pelvic area to shield gonads.

Part Position
• Place plantar surface of foot on cassette with knee flexed.
• Center and align long axis of digit(s) in question to long axis of unmasked portion of cassette.
• Rotate the leg and foot 30 to 45° medially for the 1st, 2nd and 3rd digits, and laterally for the 4th and 5th digits. (A medial oblique should be used if all digits are included, *Fig. 6-44*)
• Use 45° radiolucent support under elevated portion of foot to prevent motion.

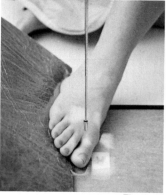

Fig. 6-45
Medial Oblique –
1st Digit

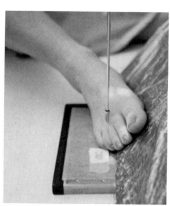

Fig. 6-46
Lateral Oblique –
4th Digit

Central Ray
• CR **perpendicular** to film, directed to MP joint(s) in question.
• Minimum 40 in. (102 cm) SID.

Collimation: Collimate on four sides to include phalanges and a minimum of distal 2/3 of metatarsals. On side margins include a **minimum** of one digit on each side of digit(s) in question, or include all five digits if this is the department routine. (See NOTE.)

NOTE: Some departmental routines always include all the digits on the AP and oblique toes for possible trauma to other digits even if a specific toe is ordered. A recommended routine however, is to center to specific toe(s) of interest but open the collimation field wide enough to include a minimum of 1 or 2 digits on each side.

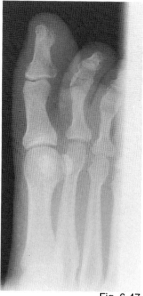

Fig. 6-47
Oblique –
1st Digit

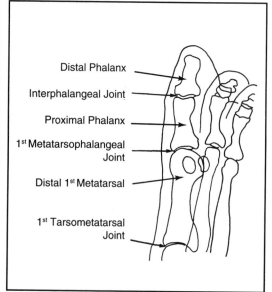

Distal Phalanx

Interphalangeal Joint

Proximal Phalanx

1st Metatarsophalangeal Joint

Distal 1st Metatarsal

1st Tarsometatarsal Joint

Fig. 6-48
Oblique –
1st Digit

Evaluation Criteria
• Digit(s) in question and distal half of metatarsals should be included without overlap (superimposition).
• Collimation borders should be visible on all four sides with the center at the MP joint(s) in question.
• Interphalangeal and MP joint spaces in question should appear open.
• Correct obliquity should be evident by increased concavity on one side of shafts and by overlapping of

soft tissues of digits. Heads of metatarsals should appear directly side by side with no (or only minimal) overlapping.
• Optimum exposure and contrast with no motion will visualize sharp borders and fine trabecular markings. Soft tissue margins and detail should be visible.

• Lateral Position

Toes
Basic
• AP
• Oblique
• **Lateral**

Structures Best Shown:
Phalanges of digit in question free of superimposition.

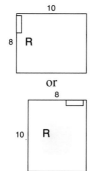

Technical Factors:
• Film Size - 8 x 10 in. (18 x 24 cm) crosswise. (Divide in thirds for individual digit routine, or separate film lengthwise if all digits were included in AP and obliques.)
• Detail screen, table top.
• 50-60 kVp range.

Patient and Part Position:
• Rotate affected leg and foot medially for 1st, 2nd and 3rd digits (patient turned up on unaffected side) and laterally for 4th and 5th digits (patient turned up on affected side).
• Adjust cassette to center and align long axis of toe in question to long axis of unmasked portion of film.
• Use tape, gauze or tongue blade to flex and separate unaffected toes to prevent superimposition.

Shielding: Place lead shield over pelvic area to shield gonads.

Central Ray:
• CR **perpendicular** to film.
• CR directed to **interphalangeal joint for 1st digit**, and to **PIP joint for 2nd-5th digits**.
• Minimum 40 in. (102 cm) SID.

Collimation: Collimate closely on four sides to affected digit.

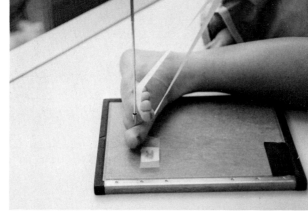

Lateral – 1st Digit

Fig. 6-49

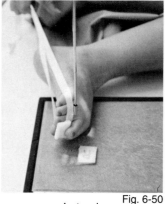

Lateral
2nd Digit

Fig. 6-50

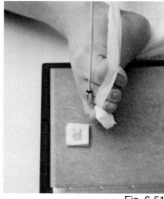

Lateral
4th Digit

Fig. 6-51

Evaluation Criteria:
• Phalanges of digit in question should be seen in lateral position free of superimposition by other digits. Toenail should be seen on edge in profile. (When total separation of toes is not possible, especially 3rd-5th digits, the proximal phalanx should be included and visualized through superimposed structures.)
• Interphalangeal joints should appear open and unobstructed. The MP joint should be visualized even if superimposed.
• Optimum exposure and contrast with no motion will visualize sharp borders and fine trabecular markings. Soft tissue margins and detail should be visible.

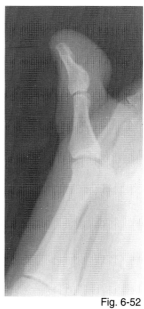

Fig. 6-52
Lateral – 1st Digit

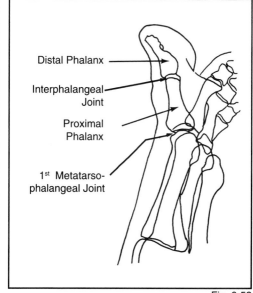

Distal Phalanx

Interphalangeal Joint

Proximal Phalanx

1st Metatarso-phalangeal Joint

Fig. 6-53
Lateral – 1st Digit

• Tangential Projection

Toes
Optional
• **Sesamoids**
(Tangential)

Structures Best Shown:
Sesamoids and head of 1st metatarsal in profile.
Note: A lateral of 1st digit in dorsiflexion may also be taken to visualize these sesamoids.

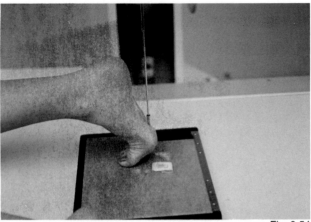

Tangential Projection - Patient Prone   Fig. 6-54

Technical Factors:
• Film Size - 8 x 10 in. (18 x 24 cm) crosswise.
   (Divide in half if combined with another projection.)
• Detail screen, table top.
• 50-60 kVp range.

Patient Position:
• Patient prone, provide pillow for head and small sponge or folded towel under lower leg for patient comfort.

Shielding: Place lead shield over pelvic area to shield gonads.

Part Position:
• Dorsiflex the foot so that the plantar surface of the foot forms about a **15-20° angle** from vertical.
• Dorsiflex the 1st digit (great toe), and rest on cassette to maintain position.
• Insure that long axis of foot is not rotated, place sandbags or other support on both sides of foot to prevent movement.

NOTE: This is an uncomfortable and often painful position, do not keep patient in this position longer than necessary.

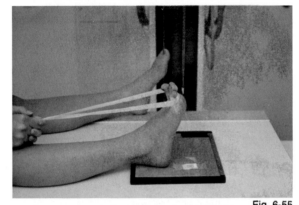

Alternate Projection - Patient Supine   Fig. 6-55

Central Ray:
• CR **perpendicular** to film, directed tangentially to posterior aspect of **head of 1st metatarsal**. (Depending on the amount of dorsiflexion of foot, may need to angle CR slightly for a true tangential projection.)
• Minimum 40 in. (102 cm) SID.

Collimation: Collimate closely to area of interest. Include at least the 1st, 2nd and 3rd distal metatarsals for possible sesamoids but with CR at 1st MP joint.

Alternate Projection: If patient cannot tolerate the above prone position, this may be taken in a reverse projection with patient supine by using a long strip of gauze for patient to hold the toes as shown. CR would again be directed tangential to head of 1st metatarsal. Use support to prevent motion. This however, is not a desirable projection because of the increased OID with accompanying magnification and loss of definition and should only be done if patient cannot tolerate prone position.

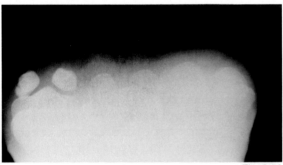

Tangential Projectiion   Fig. 6-56

Evaluation Criteria:
• Sesamoids should be seen in profile free of superimposition.
• A minimum of the first three distal metatarsals should be included in collimation field for possible sesamoids, with the center of the four sided collimation field at the distal portion of the head of 1st metatarsal.
• Optimum exposure without motion should visualize sharp borders and trabecular markings of sesamoid bones and distal portions of the heads of the metatarsals, without the sesamoids appearing overexposed.

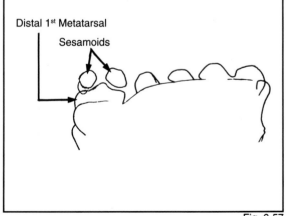

Distal 1st Metatarsal

Sesamoids

Tangential Projection   Fig. 6-57

Foot

• AP (Dorsoplantar) Projection

Structures Best Shown:
Phalanges, metatarsals, cuneiforms, cuboid and navicular.

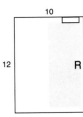

Technical Factors:
• Film Size - 10 x 12 in. (24 x 30 cm), lengthwise. (Divide in half for AP and oblique.)
• Detail screen, table top.
• 60 ± 5 kVp range; or 70-80 kVp for increased exposure latitude for more uniform density between phalanges and tarsals.

Patient Position:
• Patient supine, pillow for head.
• Flex knee and place plantar surface (sole) of affected foot flat on table.

Shielding: Place lead shield over pelvic area to shield gonads.

Part Position:
• Extend foot but maintain plantar surface resting flat and firmly on cassette.
• Align and center long axis of foot to long axis of unmasked portion of film. (Use sand bags if necessary to prevent cassette from slipping on table top.)
• If immobilization is needed, flex opposite knee also and rest against affected knee for support.

Central Ray:
• CR angled **10° toward heel** (so that CR is perpendicular to metatarsals).
• Direct CR to **base of 3rd metatarsal.**
• Minimum 40 in. (102 cm) SID.

Collimation: Collimate to outer margins of skin on four sides.

Evaluation Criteria:
• Entire foot should be visualized including all phalanges and metatarsals, as well as the navicular, cuneiforms and cuboids.
• Center of four-sided collimation field should be at the base of 3rd metatarsal.
• No rotation as evidenced by near equal distance between 2nd through 5th metatarsals. Bases of 1st and 2nd metatarsals are generally separated but bases of 2nd-5th metatarsals will appear to be overlapped.
• Sesamoid bones (if present) should be seen through head of 1st metatarsal.
• MP joints should generally appear open. IP joints however, may appear partially closed due to divergent rays.
• Optimum density and contrast with no motion should visualize sharp borders and trabecular markings of distal phalanges as well as tarsals distal to talus. (See optional technique for more uniform densities between phalanges and tarsals.)

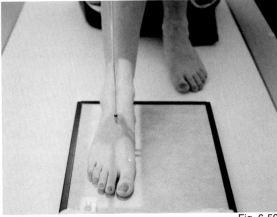

AP Foot — Fig. 6-58

AP Foot — Fig. 6-59

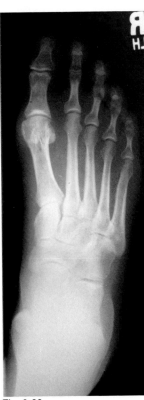

Fig. 6-60

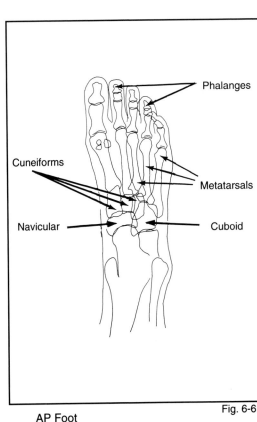

AP Foot — Fig. 6-61

Phalanges, Cuneiforms, Metatarsals, Navicular, Cuboid

• Oblique Position

<table>
<tr><td>

Foot
Basic
• AP
• **Oblique**
• Lateral

</td></tr>
</table>

Structures Best Shown:

Phalanges, metatarsals, cuboid, 3rd cuneiform, navicular and distal calcaneus with associated intertarsal spaces.

Technical Factors:
• Film Size - 10 x 12 in. (24 x 30 cm), lengthwise. (Divide in half for AP and oblique.)
• Detail screen, table top.
• 60 ± 5 kVp range; or 70-80 kVp for increased exposure latitude for more uniform density between phalanges and tarsals.

Patient Position:
• Patient supine, pillow for head. Flex knee, with plantar surface of foot on table.
• Body turned slightly away from side in question.

Shielding: Place lead shield over pelvic area to shield gonads.

Part Position: (Medial Oblique)
• Extend foot but maintain plantar surface resting flat and firmly on cassette.
• Align and center long axis of foot to long axis of unmasked portion of film. (Use sandbags if necessary to prevent cassette from slipping on table top.)
• Rotate foot **medially** to place **plantar surface 45° to plane of film.** (See NOTE.)
• Use 45° radiolucent support block to prevent motion.
• If additional immobilization is needed, place pillow or other support under and between knees and legs.

Central Ray:
• CR **perpendicular** to film, directed to **base of 3rd metatarsal.**
• Minimun 40 in. (102 cm) SID.

Collimation: Collimate to outer margins of skin on four sides.

NOTE: Some department routines call for a 45° medial oblique and others prefer only 30°. This text recommends 45° for the medial oblique which results in better separation at the bases of 2nd-5th metatarsals and between individual tarsals due to the natural transverse arch of the foot.

Alternate Lateral Oblique:
• Rotate the foot laterally 30° (less oblique required because of natural transverse arch).
• CR the same as for medial oblique.
• A lateral oblique will best demonstrate the space between 1st and 2nd metatarsals and between 1st and 2nd cuneiforms. The navicular will also be best visualized on the lateral oblique.

Evaluation Criteria:

Medial Oblique: (45°)
• Entire foot should be visualized from distal phalanges to posterior calcaneus and proximal talus.
• Center of four-sided collimation should be to base of 3rd metatarsal.
• Third through fifth metatarsals should be completely free of superimposition.

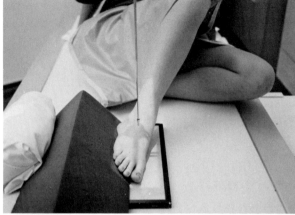

Patient Position: 45° Medial Oblique   Fig. 6-62

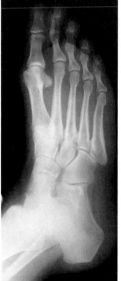

Fig. 6-63
45° Medial Oblique

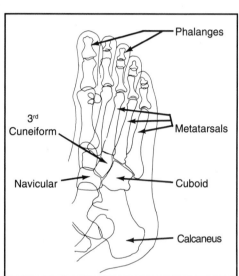

Fig. 6-64
45° Medial Oblique

(labels: Phalanges, 3rd Cuneiform, Navicular, Metatarsals, Cuboid, Calcaneus)

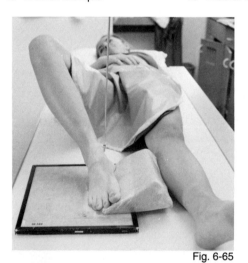

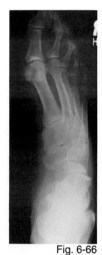

Fig. 6-65
Alternate 30° Lateral Oblique

Fig. 6-66
Lateral Oblique

• Tuberosity at base of 5th metatarsal should be well visualized.
• Optimum density and contrast with no motion should visualize sharp borders and trabecular markings of phalanges, metatarsals and tarsals.

Lateral Oblique: (30°)
• Bases of 1st and 2nd metatarsals should not overlap, and space between 1st and 2nd cuneiform should be open. Outline of the navicular should be seen in its entirety.

Foot

• Lateral Position

Foot
Basic
• AP
• Oblique
• **Lateral**

Structures Best Shown:
Tarsals are partially superimposed. Ankle joint and subtalar joint are seen partially superimposed, metatarsals and phalanges are superimposed.

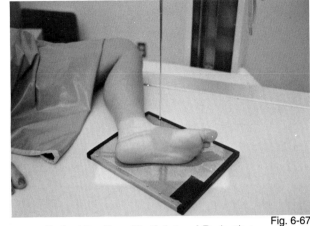

Patient Position: **Mediolateral** Projection
Fig. 6-67

Technical Factors:
• Film Size - 8 x 10 in. (18 x 24 cm) - smaller foot.
  or
  -10 x 12 in. (24 x 30 cm) - larger foot.
• Detail screen, table top.
• 60 ± 5 kVp range.

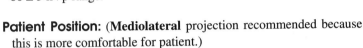

Patient Position: (**Mediolateral** projection recommended because this is more comfortable for patient.)
• Patient in lateral recumbent position, affected side down.
• Provide pillow for head.
• Flex knee of affected limb about 45°; place opposite leg **behind** the injured limb .

Shielding: Place lead shield over pelvic area to shield gonads.

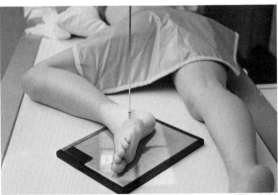

Alternate **Lateromedial**
Fig. 6-68

Part Position:
• Carefully dorsiflex the foot if possible to assist in positioning for a true lateral foot and ankle.
• Place support under leg and knee as needed so that **plantar surface is perpendicular to film.**
• Center cassette to foot and align long axis of foot to long axis of film.

Central Ray:
• CR **perpendicular** to film, directed to **first (medial) cuneiform.**
• Minimum 40 in. (102 cm) SID.

Collimation: Collimate to the outer skin margins of the foot, to include about 1 in. or 2-3 cm proximal to ankle joint.

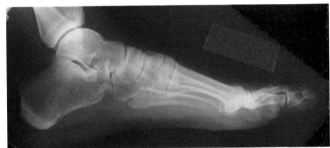

Mediolateral Foot
Fig. 6-69

Alternate Lateromedial Projection: May be taken as an alternate lateral. Is usually more uncomfortable or painful for patient and therefore, not recommended as a routine position even though it may be easier to achieve a true lateral in this position.

Evaluation Criteria:
• Entire foot should be visualized and a minimum of 1 in. or 2 cm of distal tibia-fibula.
• Center of four-sided collimation field should be at 1st (medial) cuneiform.
• Distal fibula should be seen superimposed over posterior portion of tibia.
• Tibiotalar joint space should be clearly visualized.
• Metatarsals should generally be superimposed with only a portion of the tuberosity at base of 5th metatarsal seen in profile distally.
• Optimum density and contrast should visualize borders of superimposed tarsals and metatarsals. Borders and trabecular markings of calcaneus and unsuperimposed parts of other tarsals should appear sharp and visible.

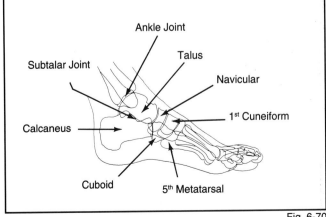

Lateral Foot
Fig. 6-70

• Lateral Weight-bearing Position

Foot
Basic
• AP
• Oblique
• Lateral
Optional
• **Weight-bearing**
Lateral

Structures Best Shown:

Lateral view of bones of the foot to show the condition of longitudinal arches with full weight of body. (Laterals of both feet are usually taken for comparison.)

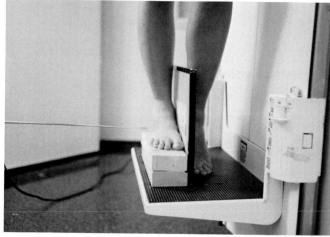

Patient Position: Weight-bearing Lateral   Fig. 6-71

Technical Factors:

- Film Size - 8 x 10 in. (18 x 24 cm), crosswise,
        or
        - 10 x 12 in. (24 x 30 cm) for larger feet.
- Detail screen.
- 60 ± 5kVp range.

Patient Position:

- Erect, standing on wood blocks on a step stool, or on a special wood box with a film slot for cassette. (Needs to be high enough to get x-ray tube down into a horizontal beam position.)
- Provide some support for patient to hold to for security.

Shielding: Secure lead shield around waist to shield gonadal area.

Part Position:

- Support vertical cassette between feet, with long axis of foot to long axis of film.
- Insure that cassette is low enough (or blocks are high enough) to include the entire plantar surface on the film.

Central Ray:

- CR directed **horizontally**, to **base of 5th metatarsal, perpendicular** to film.
- Minimum 40 in. (102 cm) SID.

Collimation: Collimate as for lateral foot (to outer skin margins of foot and to include distal tibia-fibula).

Comparison Lateral: After first lateral is taken, change cassettes for lateral of other foot for comparison.

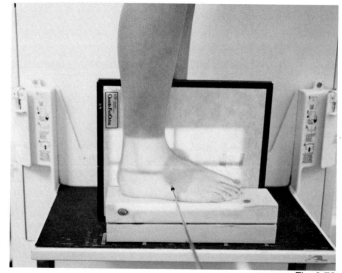

Part Position: Weight-bearing Lateral   Fig. 6-72

Evaluation Criteria:

- Entire foot should be visualized and a minimum of 1 in. or 2 cm of distal tibia-fibula.
- Center of collimation field should be to base of 5th metatarsal.
- Distal fibula should seem superimposed over posterior portion of tibia.
- Plantar surfaces of heads of metatarsals should appear directly superimposed.
- Optimum density and contrast should visualize borders of superimposed tarsals and metatarsals.

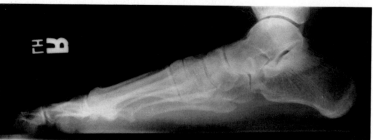

Weight-bearing Lateral   Fig. 6-73

•Plantodorsal (Axial) Projection

Calcaneus
Basic
• **Plantodorsal**
  (Dorsoplantar)
• Lateral

Structures Best Shown:
Calcaneus (os calcis).

Technical Factors:
- Film Size - 8 x 10 in. (18 x 24 cm)
- Divide in half, crosswise.
- Detail screen, table top.
- 65 ± 5 kVp range.
  (Increase 4-6 kVp from other foot projections to best visualize proximal calcaneus and/or calcaneo-talus relationship.)

Patient Position:
- Patient supine or seated on table.
- Leg fully extended.

Shielding: Place shielding over pelvic area to shield gonads.

Part Position:
- Center ankle joint to unmasked portion of cassette, with long axis of leg to long axis of unmasked film.
- Dorsiflex foot so that plantar surface is near perpendicular to film.
- Loop gauze around foot and ask patient to pull gently but firmly and hold the plantar surface of foot as near perpendicular to film as possible. (Do **not** keep in this position any longer than necessary as this may be very uncomfortable for patient.)

Central Ray:
- Direct CR to the **base of 3rd metatarsal.**
- Angle CR **40° cephalic from long axis of foot** (which would also be 40° from vertical **if** long axis of foot is perpendicular to film).
- Minimum 40 in. (102 cm) SID.

Collimation: Collimate closely to area of calcaneus.

Evaluation Criteria:
- Entire calcaneus should be visualized, from the tuberosity posteriorly, to the talocalcaneal joint anteriorly.
- No rotation. The bases of the 1st and 5th metatarsals should **not** be visible on either side. A portion of the sustentaculum tali should appear in profile medially.
- Optimum density and contrast will at least faintly visualize the talocalcaneal joint without overexposing the distal tuberosity area.

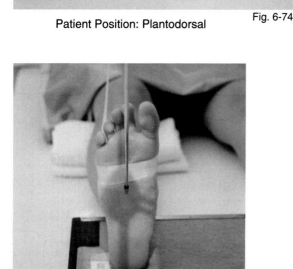

Patient Position: Plantodorsal   Fig. 6-74

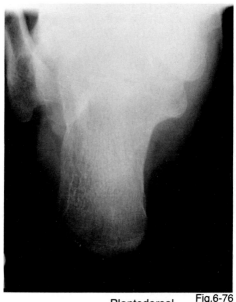

Plantodorsal   Fig. 6-76

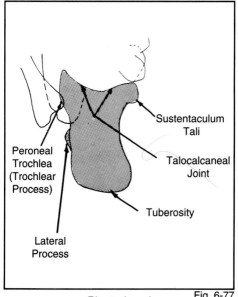

Part Position: Plantodorsal   Fig. 6-75

Sustentaculum Tali

Peroneal Trochlea (Trochlear Process)

Talocalcaneal Joint

Lateral Process

Tuberosity

Plantodorsal   Fig. 6-77

• Lateral Position

Calcaneus
Basic
• Plantodorsal
  (Dorsoplantar)
• **Lateral**

Structures Best Shown:
Calcaneus, talus and talocalcaneal joint.

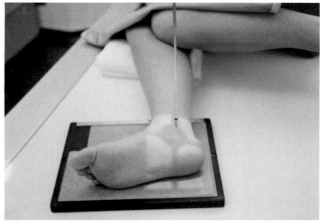

Patient and Part Position: Lateral Calcaneus   Fig. 6-78

Technical Factors:
• Film Size - 8 x 10 in. (18 x 24 cm)
• Divide in half, crosswise.
• Detail screen, table top.
• 60 ± 5 kVp range.

Patient Position:
• Lateral recumbent position, affected side down, pillow for head.
• Flex knee of affected limb about 45°; place opposite leg behind the injured limb.

Shielding: Place shielding over pelvic area to shield gonads.

Part Position:
• Adjust cassette to center calcaneus to unmasked portion of cassette, with long axis of foot parallel to long axis of film.
• Place support under knee and leg as needed to place plantar surface perpendicular to film.
• Position ankle and foot for a **true lateral** which places the lateral malleolus about 15-20° **posterior** to the medial malleolus.
• Dorsiflex foot so plantar surface is at right angle to leg and place support against ball of foot if needed to immobilize or to maintain this position.

Central Ray:
• CR **perpendicular** to film, directed to a point **3/4 in. or 2 cm inferior to medial malleolus.**
• Minimum 40 in. (102 cm) SID.

Collimation: Collimate to outer skin margins to include about 1 in. or 2 cm proximal to ankle joint.

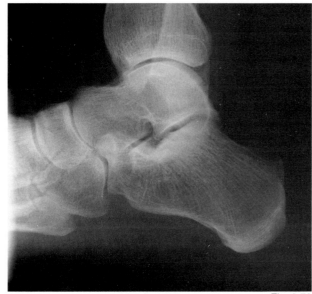

Lateral Calcaneus   Fig. 6-79

Evaluation Criteria:
• Calcaneus and talus should be visualized without rotation as evidenced by lateral malleolus superimposed over the posterior half of the tibia and talus. Tarsal sinus and calcaneocuboid joint space should appear open.
• Four sided collimation should include ankle joint proximally and talonavicular joint anteriorly.
• Optimum exposure will visualize soft tissue as well as more dense portions of calcaneus and talus. Trabecular markings will appear clear and sharp.

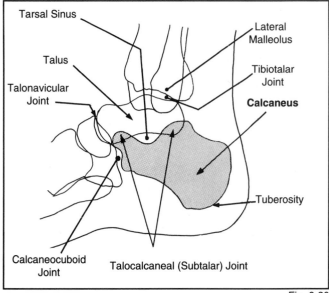

Lateral Calcaneus   Fig. 6-80

• AP Projection

<table>
<tr><td>

Ankle
Basic
• AP
• AP Mortise
• Oblique (45°)
• Lateral

</td></tr>
</table>

Structures Best Shown:

Frontal view of ankle joint, distal tibia and fibula and proximal talus. (The lateral portion of the ankle joint space will not appear open on this projection - see mortise projection on following page.)

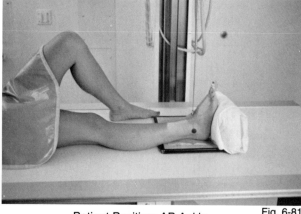

Patient Position: AP Ankle   Fig. 6-81

Technical Factors:
- Film Size - 10 x 12 in. (24 x 30 cm).
- Divide in half, crosswise.
- Detail screen, table top.
- 60 ± 5 kVp range.

Patient Position:
- Patient supine, pillow under head.
- Legs fully extended (small sand bag or other support under knee increases comfort of patient).

Shielding: Place shielding over pelvic area to shield gonads.

Part Position:
- Center ankle joint to unmasked portion of cassette, with long axis of leg to long axis of unmasked film.
- Dorsiflex foot so plantar surface is near perpendicular to film, place support under ball of foot.
- Adjust the **foot and ankle** for a **true AP projection**. (Insure that the entire lower leg is not rotated and that the long axis of the foot is in a vertical position.) The intermalleolar line will **not** be parallel to film. (See NOTE.)

Central Ray:
- CR **perpendicular** to film, directed to **a point midway between malleoli.**
- Minimum 40 in. (102 cm) SID.

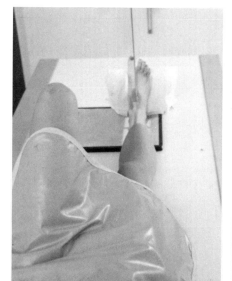

Part Position: AP Ankle   Fig. 6-82

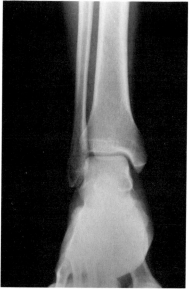

AP Ankle   Fig. 6-83
(Courtesy of E. Frank R.T.)

Collimation: Collimate to lateral skin margins, include proximal metatarsals and distal tibia-fibula.

NOTE: The malleoli will **not** be the same distance from the film in the anatomical position with a true AP projection. (The lateral malleolus will be about 15° more posterior.) The lateral portion of the mortise joint therefore should **not** appear open. If this portion of the ankle joint did appear open on a true AP, it may suggest a spread of the ankle mortise from ruptured ligaments.[1]

Evaluation Criteria:
- The center of four-sided collimation should be to mid-ankle joint. The area from the distal tibia-fibula to the proximal metatarsals should be included.
- The medial and upper portion of the ankle joint mortise should appear open, but the lateral portion will appear closed due to overlap of the distal fibula and a corner of the talus.
- Up to 1/2 the thickness of the distal fibula will overlap that of the medial tibia.
- Optimum exposure should visualize soft tissue, the lateral and medial malleoli, the talus and the distal tibia-fibula.
- With no motion and good exposure technique, trabecular markings and bony margins should appear sharp and clear.

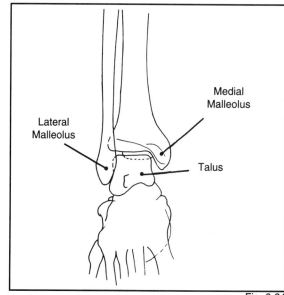

Fig. 6-84

AP Ankle

[1] Frank, E.D. et al, Mayo Clinic: Radiography of the Ankle Mortise, Radiologic Technology, 62-5: 354-359, 1991.

• Mortise Position (AP, Medial Oblique)

Ankle
Basic
• AP
• **AP Mortise**
• Oblique (45°)
• Lateral

Structures Best Shown:
Frontal view of entire ankle mortise.

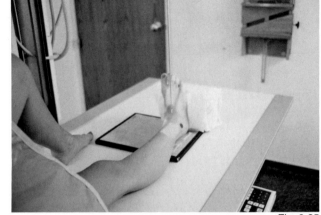
Patient Position: Mortise Position Fig. 6-85

Technical Factors:
• Film Size - 10 x 12 in. (24 x 30 cm).
• Divide in half, crosswise.
• Detail screen, table top.
• 60 ± 5 kVp range.

Patient Position:
• Patient supine, pillow under head.
• Legs fully extended (small sand bag or other support under knee increases comfort of patient).

Shielding: Place shielding over pelvic area to shield gonads.

Part Position:
• Center ankle joint to unmasked portion of cassette, with long axis of leg to long axis of unmasked film.
• Dorsiflex foot so plantar surface is near perpendicular to film, place support against ball of foot if needed to prevent motion.
• Internally rotate **entire leg and foot** about **15 to 20°** until the **intermalleolar line is parallel to film.**

Central Ray:
• CR **perpendicular** to film, directed to **a point midway between malleoli.**
• Minimum 40 in. (102 cm) SID.

Collimation: Collimate to lateral skin margins, include proximal metatarsals and distal tibia-fibula.

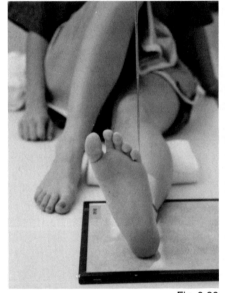
Part Position: Mortise Position Fig. 6-86

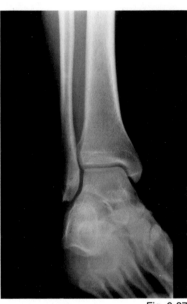
Mortise Position Fig. 6-87
(Courtesy of E. Frank R.T.)

NOTE: • This position should not be a substitute for either the AP projection or the oblique ankle position, but rather should be a separate position of the ankle taken routinely when potential trauma or sprains of the ankle joint are involved.[1]
• This is also a common projection taken during open reduction surgery of the ankle.

Evaluation Criteria:
• The center of four-sided collimation should be to mid ankle joint. The area from the distal tibia-fibula to the proximal metatarsals should be included.
• The entire ankle mortise should appear open with no overlap between distal fibula and talus, or between tibia and talus.
• There should only be minimal overlap at the distal tibiofibular joint space.
• Optimum exposure should visualize some soft tissue with sufficient density for the talus and distal tibia and fibula.
• With no motion and good exposure technique, trabecular markings and bony margins should appear sharp and clear.

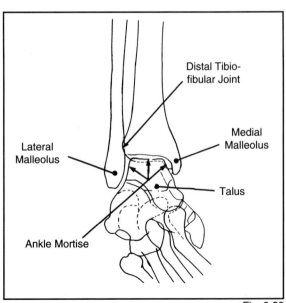
Mortise Position Fig. 6-88

Distal Tibio-fibular Joint
Medial Malleolus
Lateral Malleolus
Talus
Ankle Mortise

---

[1] Frank, E.D. et al, Mayo Clinic: Radiography of the Ankle Mortise, Radiologic Technology, 62-5: 354-359, 1991.

•Oblique Position

Structures Best Shown:
Distal tibiofibular joint and a more complete view of the distal fibula and lateral malleolus.

Technical Factors:
• Film Size - 10 x 12 in. (24 x 30 cm).
• Divide in half, crosswise.
• Detail screen, table top.
• 60 ± 5 kVp range.

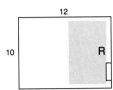

Patient Position:
• Patient supine, pillow under head.
• Legs fully extended (small sand bag or other support under knee increases comfort of patient).

Shielding: Place shielding over pelvic area to shield gonads.

Part Position:
• Center ankle joint to unmasked portion of cassette, with long axis of leg to long axis of unmasked film.
• Dorsiflex foot so plantar surface is near perpendicular to film, place support under ball of foot.
• Similar to mortise position except **rotate leg & foot** internally **45°** (45° between long axis of foot and surface of cassette. The interepicondylar line at the knee should also be 45° to the film).

Central Ray:
• CR **perpendicular** to film, directed to **a point midway between malleoli.**
• Minimum 40 in. (102 cm) SID.

Collimation: Collimate to lateral skin margins, include proximal metatarsals and distal tibia-fibula.

Alternate Lateral Oblique: Sometimes a lateral or external oblique is requested to rule out subtle fractures and/or to visualize parts of the talocalcaneal joint. The entire leg and long axis of the foot would be rotated **externally 45°.**

Evaluation Criteria:
• The center of four-sided collimation should be to mid-ankle joint. The area from the distal tibia-fibula to the proximal metatarsals should be included.
• The distal tibiofibular joint space should be primarily open with only minimal "touching" on an average ankle.
• Both the distal fibula and tibia may have some overlap with the talus.
• Optimum exposure should visualize soft tissue, the lateral and medial malleoli, the talus and the distal tibia and fibula.
• With no motion and good exposure technique, trabecular markings and bony margins should appear sharp and clear.

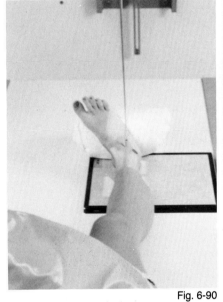

Patient Position: 45° Oblique Position   Fig. 6-89

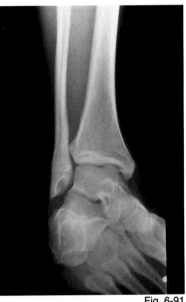

Fig. 6-90
Part Position: 45° Oblique Position

Fig. 6-91
45° Internal Oblique Position
(Courtesy of E. Frank R.T.)

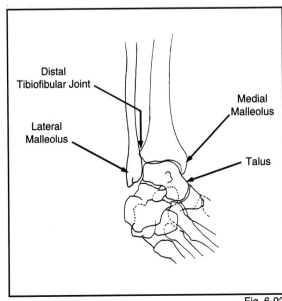

Distal Tibiofibular Joint

Lateral Malleolus

Medial Malleolus

Talus

Fig. 6-92
45° Internal Oblique Position

•Lateral Position

Structures Best Shown:
Lateral view of distal tibia and fibula, ankle joint, talus and calcaneus.

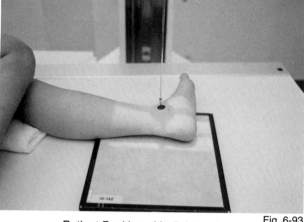

Patient Position: Mediolateral   Fig. 6-93

Technical Factors:
• Film Size - 10 x 12 in. (24 x 30 cm)
• Divide in half, crosswise.
• Detail screen, table top.
• 60 ± 5 kVp range.

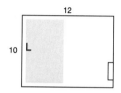

Patient Position:
• Lateral recumbent position, affected side down, pillow for head.
• Flex knee of affected limb about 45°; place opposite leg behind the injured limb.

Shielding: Place shielding over pelvic area to shield gonads.

Part Position: (Mediolateral Projection)
• Center ankle joint to unmasked portion of cassette, with long axis of leg aligned to long axis of unmasked film.
• Place support under knee as needed to place leg and foot in a **true lateral position.** The distal fibula and lateral malleolus will be about 15-20° **posterior** to distal tibia and medial malleolus. (See p. 178.)
• Dorsiflex foot so plantar surface is at a right angle to leg or as far as patient can tolerate. (This will help maintain a true lateral position.)

Central Ray:
• CR **perpendicular** to film, directed to **medial malleolus.**
• Minimum 40 in. (102 cm) SID.

Collimation:
Collimate to skin margins to include distal tibia and fibula and to mid-metatarsal area of foot.

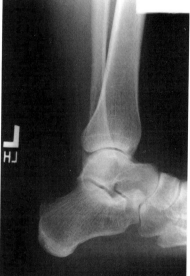

Fig. 6-94   Fig. 6-95
Part Position: Mediolateral   Lateral Position

Alternate Lateromedial Projection:
This lateral may also be taken even though generally it is not recommended because this position is more uncomfortable for patient. It would be positioned similarly to the above except patient is turned on opposite side (affected side up).

Evaluation Criteria:
• Center of four-sided collimation should be to mid-ankle joint.
• The upper arch of the tibiotalar joint should appear open with a uniform joint space.
• The lateral malleolus and distal fibula will appear superimposed over the posterior half of the talus, and the posterior 1/2 or 2/3's of the tibia.
• The talus and calcaneus should be seen in their entirety, as well as portions of the adjoining tarsal bones.
• Optimum exposure should visualize the outline of the distal fibula as well as some soft tissue detail. Trabecular markings and borders of all bones visualized should appear clear and sharp.

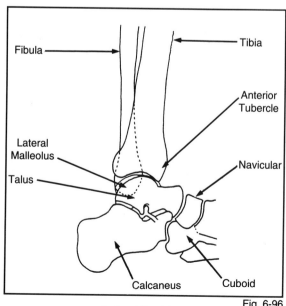

Fig. 6-96
Lateral Position

• AP Stress Projections

(Inversion and Eversion Positions)

Warning: Proceed with utmost care with injured patient.

Structures Best Shown:

Ankle joint for evaluation of joint separation and ligament tear or rupture.

Technical Factors:

• Film Size - 10 x 12 in. (24 x 30 cm).
• Divide in half, crosswise.
• Detail screen, table top.
• 60 ± 5 kVp range.

Patient Position:

• Patient supine, pillow under head.
• Leg fully extended, support under knee.

Shielding: Place shielding over gonadal area of patient. Supply lead gloves and a lead apron for physician if stress positions are hand held during exposures.

Part Position:

• Center ankle joint to unmasked portion of cassette with long axis of leg aligned to long axis of unmasked film.
• Dorsiflex the foot to as near right angle to the leg as possible.
• With leg and ankle in position for a **true AP** with no rotation, stress is applied wherein the entire plantar surface is turned medially for inversion, and laterally for eversion. (See NOTE.)

Central Ray:

• CR **perpendicular** to film, directed to a point **midway between malleoli**.
• Minimum 40 in. (102 cm) SID.

Collimate: Collimate to lateral skin margins, include proximal metatarsals and distal tibia-fibula.

NOTE: A physician or another health professional must be present to either hold the foot and ankle in these stress views, or to strap into position with weights, or to have patient hold this position with long gauze looped around ball of foot. If this is too painful for patient, local anesthesia may be injected by the physician.

Evaluation Criteria:

• The center of four-sided collimation should be to mid-ankle joint. The area from the distal tibia-fibula to the proximal metatarsals should be included.
• The appearance of the joint space may vary greatly depending on the severity of ligament damage.
• Optimum exposure should visualize soft tissue, the lateral and medial malleoli, the talus and the distal tibia and fibula.
• With no motion and good exposure technique, trabecular markings and bony margins should appear sharp and clear.

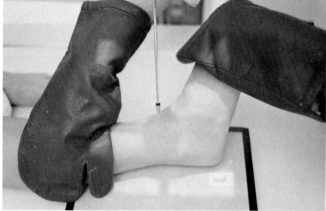

Inversion Stress Fig. 6-97

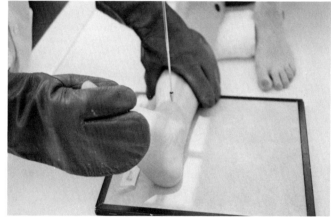

Eversion Stress Fig. 6-98

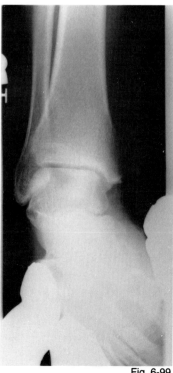

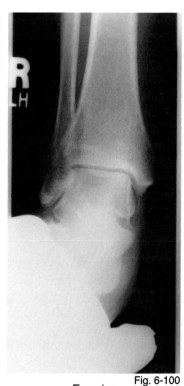

Fig. 6-99 Fig. 6-100
Inversion Eversion

Leg (Tibia and Fibula)

• AP Projection

Leg
• **AP**
• Lateral

Structures Best Shown:
Tibia and fibula and knee and/or ankle joints.

Technical Factors:
• Film Size - 14 x 17 in. (35 x 43 cm) divide in half lengthwise or diagonal.
• Detail screen, table top.
• 65 ± 5 kVp range.
• To make best use of the anode-heel effect, place the knee at cathode end of x-ray beam.

Patient Position:
• Patient supine, pillow for head.
• Leg fully extended.

Shielding: Place lead shielding over gonadal area.

Part Position:
• Adjust pelvis, knee and leg into a true AP with no rotation, (true anatomical position).
• Place sand bag against ball of foot for stabilization.
• Center and align mid line of unmasked portion of cassette to long axis of leg.
• Insure that both ankle and knee joints are 1-2 in. (3-5 cm) from ends of film (so that divergent rays will not project either joint off film).
• If necessary, place leg diagonally (corner to corner) on one 14 x 17 film to insure that both joints are included. (Also if needed a second smaller film may be taken of the joint nearest the injury site.)

Central Ray:
• CR **perpendicular** to film, directed to **mid point of film.**
• Minimum 40 in. (102 cm) SID.

Collimation: Collimate on both sides to skin margins, with full collimation at ends of film borders to include maximum knee and ankle joints.

Alternate Follow-up Exam Routine: The routine for follow up exams of long bones in some departments is to include only the one joint nearest the site of injury and to place this joint a minimum of 2 in. (5 cm) from the end of the film for better demonstration of this joint. However, for initial exams it is **especially important when the injury site is at the distal leg to also include the proximal tibiofibular joint area** because it is common to have a second fracture at this site. In this situation, for a large patient a second AP projection of the knee and proximal leg may be needed on a smaller film.

Evaluation Criteria:
• The entire tibia and fibula should be included with both the ankle and knee joints included on one (or two if needed) film(s). (Exception is alternate routine on follow up exams.)
• Close side collimation borders should be visible but only minimal if any border should be visible at the ends to maximize visualization of both joints.
• Overlap of the fibula and tibia will be visible at both the proximal and distal ends.
• Optimum exposure with correct use of the anode-heel effect will result in near equal density at both ends of the film.

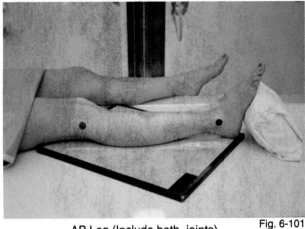

AP Leg (Include both joints)   Fig. 6-101

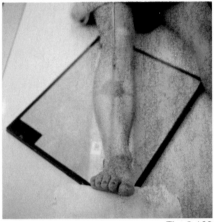

Fig. 6-102
AP Leg (Include both joints)

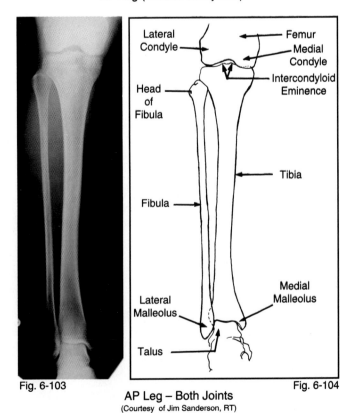

Fig. 6-103   Fig. 6-104
AP Leg – Both Joints
(Courtesy of Jim Sanderson, RT)

• Good exposure density without motion will result in visualization of sharp trabecular markings and sharp borders of entire tibia and fibula.

• Lateral Position

Leg
• AP
• Lateral

Structures Best Shown:
Tibia, fibula, knee and/or ankle joints.

Technical Factors:
- Film Size - 14 x 17 in. (35 x 43 cm) divide in half lengthwise or diagonal.
- Detail screen, table top.
- 65 ± 5 kVp range.
- To make best use of the anode-heel effect, place the knee (or head end of patient) at cathode end of x-ray beam.

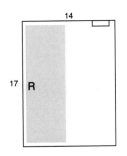

Patient Position:
- Patient in lateral recumbent position, injured side down, pillow for head.
- Generally the opposite leg may be placed behind the affected leg and supported with a pillow or sand bags.

Shielding: Place shield over pelvic and gonadal area.

Part Position:
- Flex knee about 45° and insure that leg is in a true lateral position. (Plane of patella should be perpendicular to film.)
- Center and align unmasked portion of cassette to long axis of leg. (Unless film is placed diagonally.)
- Insure that both ankle and knee joints are 1-2 in. (3-5 cm) from ends of film so that divergent rays will not project either joint off film.
- If necessary, place leg diagonally on 14 x 17 film to insure that both joints are included. (Also if needed, a second smaller film may be taken of the joint nearest the injury site.)

Central Ray:
- CR **perpendicular** to film, directed to **mid point of film.**
- Minimum 40 in. (102 cm) SID.

Collimation: Collimate on both sides to skin margins, with full collimation at ends of film borders to include maximum knee and ankle joints.

Alternate Follow-up Exam Routine: The routine for follow up exams of long bones in some departments is to include only the one joint nearest the site of injury and to place this joint a minimum of 2 in. (5 cm) from the end of the film for better demonstration of this joint. However, for initial exams it is especially important when the injury site is at the distal leg to also include the proximal tibiofibular joint area because it is common to have a second fracture at this site. In this situation for a large patient a second AP projection of the knee and proximal leg may be needed on a smaller film.

Crosstable Lateral: If patient cannot be turned, this can be taken crosstable with cassette placed on edge between legs. Place a support under injured leg to center leg to film, and direct horizontal beam from lateral side of patient.

Evaluation Criteria:
- The entire tibia and fibula should be included with both the ankle and knee joints included on one (or two if needed) film(s). (Exception is alternate routine on follow up exams.)
- Close side collimation borders should be visible but only minimal if any border should be visible at the ends to maximize visualization of both joints.
- A portion of the proximal head of the fibula will be superimposed by the fibula, and outlines of the distal fibula will be seen through the posterior 1/2 or 2/3's of the tibia. The majority of the shaft or body areas of the tibia and fibula will

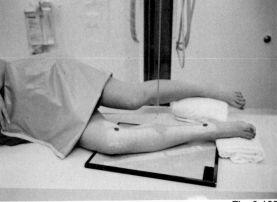

Patient Position – Lateral   Fig. 6-105

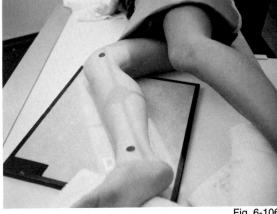

Part Position – Lateral   Fig. 6-106

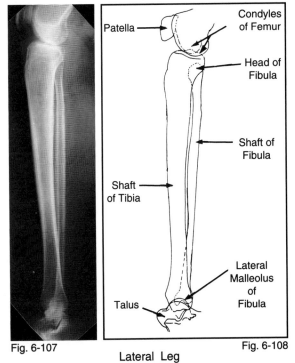

Fig. 6-107

Lateral Leg
(Courtesy of Jim Sanderson, RT.)

Fig. 6-108

Patella — Condyles of Femur — Head of Fibula — Shaft of Fibula — Shaft of Tibia — Lateral Malleolus of Fibula — Talus

lie parallel to each other not superimposed.
- Optimum exposure with correct use of the anode-heel effect will result in near equal density at both ends of the film.
- Good exposure density without motion will result in visualization of sharp trabecular markings and sharp borders of entire tibia and fibula.

• AP Projection

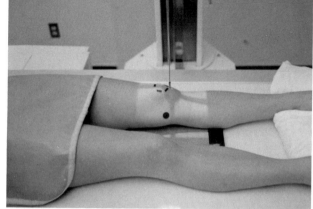
AP Knee   Fig. 6-109

Knee
Basic
• **AP**
• Lateral
• Oblique

Structures Best Shown:
Distal femur, proximal tibia and fibula, patella and knee joint.

Technical Factors:

• Film Size - 8 x 10 in. (18 x 24 cm), lengthwise.
• Moving or stationary grid, 70 ± 6 kVp range or for smaller patient, <10 cm, screen table top, 65 ± 5 kVp range.

Patient Position:
• Patient supine with no rotation of pelvis, pillow for head.
• Leg fully extended.

Shielding: Place shield over gonadal area.

Part Position:
• Align and center long axis of leg and knee to midline of table or cassette.
• Rotate leg internally about 5° for a true AP (or until **interepicondylar line is parallel** to plane of film). (Patella generally will be slightly medial to the center of distal femur.)
• Place sandbags by foot and ankle to stabilize and maintain this position.

Central Ray:
• Angle CR **perpendicular** to tibia shaft. (See NOTE.)
• Direct CR to a point **3/4 in. or 1 cm** distal to apex of patella.
• Minimum 40 in. (102 cm) SID.

Collimation: Collimate on both sides to skin margins, with full collimation at ends to film borders to include maximum femur and tibia/fibula.

NOTE:
• The CR should be 90° or **perpendicular to the long axis of the tibia** to best open up the knee joint space. A slight cephalic angle (3-5°) may be needed if the patient cannot fully extend the knee, or if the patient has a thick thigh and knee area wherein the tibial shaft is not parallel to the film. (The effect of too much angle wherein the CR is **not perpendicular** to tibial shaft is demonstrated in *Fig. 6-112*.)
• A common positioning error is centering too high. The CR must enter at the joint space which is distal to the patella.

Evaluation Criteria:
• The center of the collimation field should be to the mid-knee joint space.
• The femorotibial joint space should be open with the articular facets of the tibia seen on end with only minimal surface area visualized.
• No rotation will be evidenced by the symmetrical appearance of the femoral and tibial condyles and the joint space. The approximate medial half of the fibular

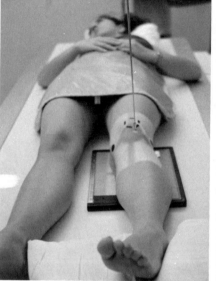
Part Position – AP Knee   Fig. 6-110

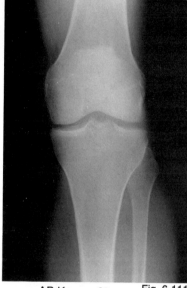
AP Knee – 0°   Fig. 6-111
(Courtesy of F. Price, RT)

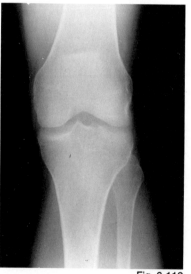
Fig. 6-112
AP Knee – 7° Cephalad
(Same patient as Fig. 6-111, CR now is not perpendicular to tibial shaft - see tibial plateau)
(Courtesy of F. Price, RT)

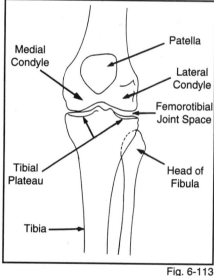
Fig. 6-113
AP Knee – 0°

head should be superimposed by the tibia.
• Optimum exposure will visualize the outline of the patella through the distal femur and the fibular head and neck will not appear overexposed.
• Trabecular markings of all bones should be visible and appear sharp. Soft tissue detail should be visible.

• Medial Oblique Position (AP)

Knee
Basic
• AP
• **Oblique**
• Lateral

Structures Best Shown: (Medial Oblique)
Distal femur, proximal tibia, fibular head and neck and lateral condyles of femur and tibia without superimposition. **Proximal tibiofibular joint** and femorotibial (knee) joint.

Technical Factors:
• Film Size - 8 x 10 in. (18 x 24 cm), lengthwise.
• Moving or stationary grid, 70 ± 6 kVp range or smaller patient, <10 cm, screen table top, 65 ± 5 kVp range.

Patient Position:
• Patient semi-supine with entire body and leg rotated partially away from side of interest.
• Place support under elevated hip, pillow for head.

Shielding: Place shield over gonadal area.

Part Position:
• Align and center long axis of leg and knee to midline of table or cassette.
• Rotate entire leg **internally 45°**. (Inter-epicondylar line should be 45° to plane of film.)
• If needed, stabilize foot and ankle in this position with sandbags.

Central Ray:
• Angle CR **5° cephalad**.
• Direct CR to **mid-point of the knee** at a level **3/4 in. (1 cm) distal to apex of patella.**.
• Minimum 40 in. (102 cm) SID.

Collimation: Collimate on both sides to skin margins, with full collimation at ends to film borders to include maximum femur and tibia/fibula.

Optional Lateral Oblique: A 45° lateral (external) rotation oblique may be taken as an optional position if a second oblique view of the knee area is desired. Positioning would be similar but with the entire leg **rotated laterally 45°**.

NOTE: The terms medial (internal) oblique or lateral (external) oblique positions refer to the direction of rotation of the anterior or patella surface of the knee. This is true for descriptions of both AP and PA oblique positions.

Evaluation Criteria:
AP Medial (internal) **Oblique**
• The proximal tibiofibular articulation should appear open, and the lateral condyles of femur and tibia are seen in profile with head and neck of fibula visualized without superimposition.
• Approximately 1/2 of the patella should be seen free of superimposition by the femur.
• Optimum exposure should visualize soft tissue in knee joint area and trabecular markings of all bones should appear clear and sharp. Head and neck area of fibula should not appear overexposed.

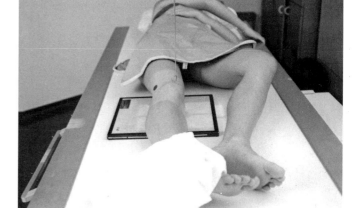

Medial Oblique (AP)   Fig. 6-114

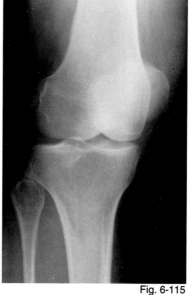

Fig. 6-115
Medial Oblique (AP)

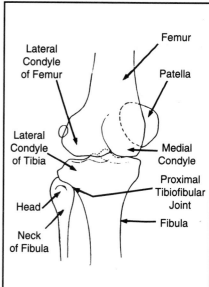

Fig. 6-116
Medial Oblique (AP)

Femur
Lateral Condyle of Femur
Patella
Lateral Condyle of Tibia
Medial Condyle
Head
Proximal Tibiofibular Joint
Neck of Fibula
Fibula

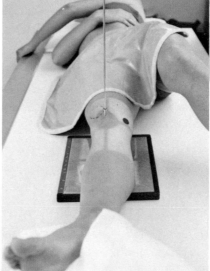

Fig. 6-117

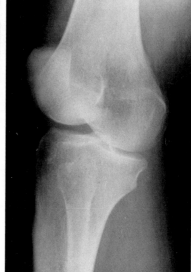

Optional Lateral Oblique (AP)   Fig. 6-118

AP Lateral (external) **Oblique**
• Medial condyles of femur and tibia are visualized in profile, and proximal fibula is seen superimposed over mid portion of proximal tibia.

• Lateral Position

Knee
Basic
• AP
• Oblique
• **Lateral**

Structures Best Shown:
Distal femur, proximal tibia, fibula, patella and tibiofemoral joint and patellofemoral joints.

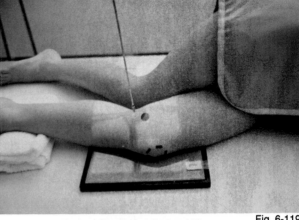
Patient Position – Lateral Knee   Fig. 6-119

Technical Factors:
• Film Size - 8 x 10 in. (18 x 24 cm), lengthwise.
• Moving or stationary grid, 70 ± 6 kVp range or smaller patient, <10 cm, screen table top, 65 ± 5 kVp range.

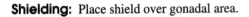

Patient Position:
• Patient in lateral recumbent position, affected side down, pillow for head.
• Provide support for knee of opposite limb placed behind knee being examined.

Shielding: Place shield over gonadal area.

Part Position:
• Adjust rotation of body and leg until knee is in a **true lateral** position (femoral epicondyles directly superimposed and plane of patella perpendicular to plane of film).
• Flex knee **15-20°**. (See NOTE.)
• Align and center long axis of leg and knee to midline of table or cassette.

Central Ray:
• Angle CR **5 to 10° cephalad**. (See NOTE.)
• Direct CR to a point **3/4 in. (1 cm) distal to** medial epicondyle.
• Minimum 40 in. (102 cm) SID.

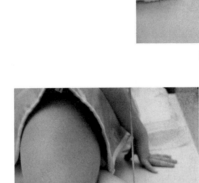
Fig. 6-120
Part Position – Lateral Knee

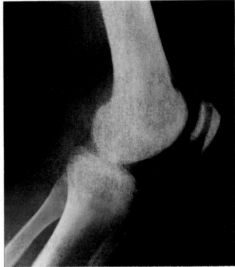
Fig. 6-121
Lateral Knee

Collimation: Collimate on both sides to skin margins, with full collimation at ends to film borders to include maximum femur and tibia/fibula.

Crosstable Lateral: If patient cannot be turned, this can also be taken crosstable with cassette placed on edge between legs. Place support under knee to center knee to film and direct horizontal beam from lateral side of patient.

NOTE: • Additional flexion will tighten muscles and tendons which may obscure important diagnostic information in the joint space. The patella will be drawn into the intercondylar sulcus also obscuring soft tissue information from effusion and/or fat pad displacement.   Additional flexion may also result in fragment separation of patellar fractures if present.
• Angle CR nearer 10° on short patient with wide pelvis, and only about 5° on tall, male patient with narrow pelvis. (See p. 177 for anatomy discussion.)

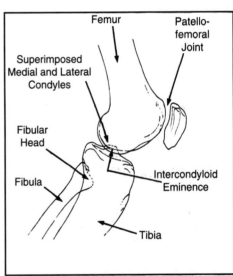
Fig. 6-122
Lateral Projection

Evaluation Criteria:
• **True Lateral:** Femoral condyles should be directly superimposed. The 5-10° cephalad angle of CR should result in direct superimposition of the **distal borders** of the condyles, and a true lateral without rotation will directly superimpose the **posterior borders.**
• The tibiofemoral joint space should be open with only the pointed intercondyloid eminence (tibial spines) superimposed by the femoral condyles.
• The patella should be seen in profile with the patellofemoral joint space open.

• For the average patient about one-half of the fibular head will be superimposed by the tibia.
• Optimum exposure will visualize important soft tissue detail and sharp trabecular markings.

• PA Axial Projection
(Tunnel View)

Knee - Intercondyloid
  Fossa
Basic
• PA Axial

Structures Best Shown:
Intercondyloid fossa shown in profile, femoral and tibial condyles, intercondyloid eminence and articular facets of tibia.

NOTE: Two methods are described for demonstrating these structures. This text recommends the prone position *(Fig. 6-123)* because this is an easier position for the patient. However, the Holmblad kneeling method provides another option with a slightly different projection of these structures with an increase in the amount of knee flexion.

Technical Factors:

- Film Size - 8 x 10 in. (18 x 24 cm), lengthwise.
- Moving or stationary grid (or screen, <10 cm).
- 75 ± 5 kVp range. (Increase 4-6 kVp from PA knee for increased penetration.)

Patient Position:
(1) Patient prone, pillow for head.
(2) Patient kneeling on x-ray table.

Shielding: Place lead shield over gonadal area. Secure around waist in kneeling position and extend shield down to at least the mid-femur level.

Part Position:
(1) Prone
- Flex knee **40-50°**, place support under ankle.
- Center cassette to knee joint considering projection of CR angle.

(2) Kneeling
- With patient kneeling on "all fours", place cassette under affected knee; film centered to popliteal crease.
- Ask patient to support body weight primarily on opposite knee.
- Place padded support under ankle and leg of affected limb to reduce pressure on injured knee.
- Ask patient to slowly **lean forward 20-30°**, and hold that position. (Results in 60-70° knee flexion.)

Central Ray:
(1) Prone - CR **perpendicular to lower leg** (40-50° caudal to match degree of flexion).
(2) Kneeling - CR **perpendicular to film and lower leg.**
- Direct CR to **mid-popliteal crease.**
- Minimum 40 in. (102 cm) SID.

Collimation: Collimate on four sides to knee joint area.

Evaluation Criteria:
- Center of four-sided collimation field should be to mid-knee joint area.
- For this projection it is most important that the intercondyloid fossa appear in profile, open without superimpositon by patella.
- No rotation will be evidenced by symmetrical appearance of the distal posterior femoral condyles and superimposition of approximately half of fibular head by tibia.

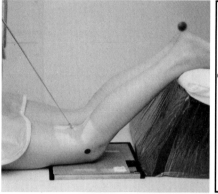
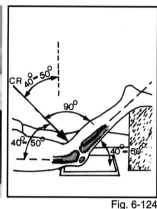

Fig. 6-123   Fig. 6-124
(1) Camp Coventry Method, Prone Position (40-50° Flexion)

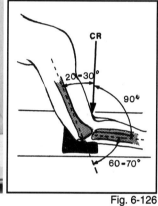

Fig. 6-125   Fig. 6-126
(2) Holmblad Method, Kneeling Position (60-70° Flexion)

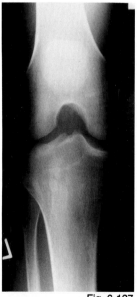
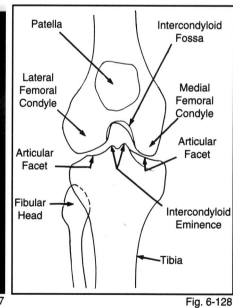

Fig. 6-127   Fig. 6-128
PA Axial Projection   PA Axial Projection

- Articular facets and intercondyloid eminence of tibia should be well visualized without superimposition.
- Optimum exposure should visualize soft tissue in the knee joint space and an outline of patella through the femur.
- Trabecular markings of femoral condyles and proximal tibia should appear clear and sharp.

• AP Axial Projection

Knee - Intercondyloid Fossa
Basic
• PA Axial
Optional
• **AP Axial**

Structures Best Shown:
Intercondyloid fossa shown in profile, femoral and tibial condyles, intercondyloid eminence (tibial spines) and articular facets of tibial (tibia plateau).

Fig. 6-129

AP Axial – 8 x 10 in. (18 x 24 cm) Cassette Crosswise
(40° Flexion, 40° CR Ankle)

NOTE: This is a reversal of the PA axial projection for those who cannot assume the prone position. This however, is **not** a preferred projection because of the distortion from the CR angle and increased part-film distance unless a curved cassette is available.

Technical Factors:
• Film Size - 8 x 10 in. (18 x 24 cm), crosswise.
• Curved cassette preferred if available to reduce part-film distance.
• Detail screen, small focal spot (65±5 kVp range), or
  Stationary grid (75 ± 5 kVp range) for larger patient.

Patient Position:
• Patient supine with support under partially flexed knee with entire leg in the anatomical position with **no rotation.**

Shielding: Place lead shield over pelvic area extending to mid-femur.

Part Position:
• Flex knee **40-45°** and place support under cassette as needed to place cassette firmly against posterior thigh and leg as shown in *Figs. 6-129* and *130.*
• If curved cassette is available, place under knee as shown in *Fig. 6-131.*
• Adjust cassette as needed to center film to mid-knee joint area.

Central Ray:
• CR **perpendicular** to lower leg (40-45° cephalad).
• Direct CR to a point **3/4 in. (2 cm) distal to apex of patella.**
• Minimum 40 in. (102 cm) SID.

Collimation: Collimate on four sides to knee joint area.

Evaluation Criteria:
• Center of four-sided collimation field should be to mid-knee joint area.
• The intercondyloid fossa should appear in profile, open without superimposition by patella. The intercondyloid eminence and tibial plateau and distal condyles of femur should be clearly visualized.
• **No rotation:** will be evidenced by symmetrical appearance of the distal posterior femoral condyles and superimposition of approximately half of fibular head by the tibia.

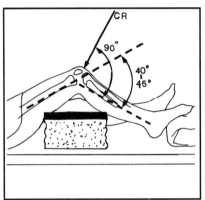

Fig. 6-130
With 8 x 10 Flat Cassette

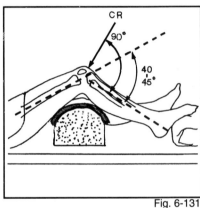

Fig. 6-131
With Curved Cassette
(Be'clere Method)

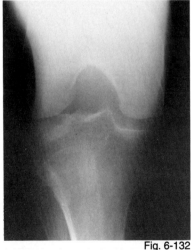

Fig. 6-132
AP Axial – 40° Flexion and CR Angle

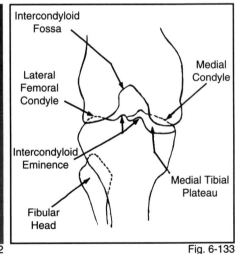

Fig. 6-133
AP Axial

• Optimum exposure should visualize soft tissue in the knee joint space and an outline of patella through the femur.
• Trabecular markings of femoral condyles and proximal tibia should appear clear and sharp.

Patella

• PA Projection

Patella
• **PA**
• Lateral
• Tangential

Structures Best Shown:
Knee joint and patella. (PA projection visualizes patella better than AP because of closer part-film distance.)

Technical Factors:
• Film Size - 8 x 10 in. (18 x 24 cm), lengthwise.
• Moving or stationary grid (or screen, <10 cm).
• 75 ± 5 kVp range.
  (**Increase 4-6 kVp** from PA knee technique for better patella visualization.)

Patient Position:
• Patient prone, legs extended, pillow for head.
• Place support under ankle and leg with smaller support under femur above knee to prevent direct pressure on patella.

Shielding: Place shield over gonadal area.

Part Position:
• Align and center long axis of leg and knee to mid- line of table or grid cassette.
• **True PA**: Inter-epicondylar line should be parallel to plane of film. (This usually requires about 5° internal rotation of anterior knee.)

Central Ray:
• CR **perpendicular** to film. Direct CR to **mid- patella area** (which is usually at approximately the mid-popliteal crease).
• Minimum 40 in. (102 cm) SID.

Collimation: Collimate closely on four sides to include just the area of the patella and knee joint.

NOTE:
• With a potential fracture of patella, extra care should be taken to **not flex knee** and **provide support under** thigh (femur) so as not to put direct pressure on patella area.
• May also be taken as an AP projection positioned like an AP knee if patient cannot assume a prone position.

Evaluation Criteria:
• Four-sided collimation field should include patella and knee joint area with the center at the mid-patella area.
• Sufficient exposure will visualize soft tissue in joint area and also clearly visualize the outline of patella as seen through the distal femur.
• No rotation as evidenced by symmetrical appearance of the condyles. The patella normally will be slightly off center toward the medial aspect of the femur.

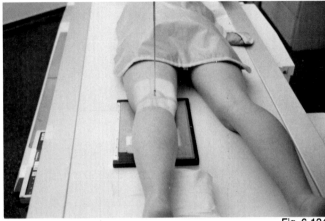

Fig. 6-134

Patient Position – PA Patella

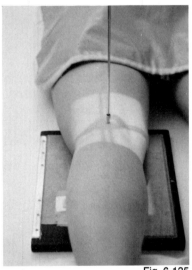

Fig. 6-135

Part Position – PA Patella

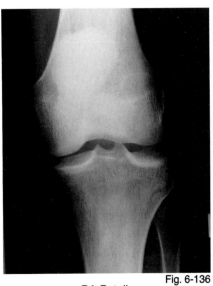

Fig. 6-136

PA Patella

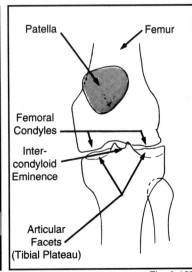

Fig. 6-137

PA Patella

Patella

• Lateral Position

Patella
• PA
• **Lateral**
• Tangential

Structures Best Shown:
Patella (in profile), patellofemoral joint and tibiofemoral joint.

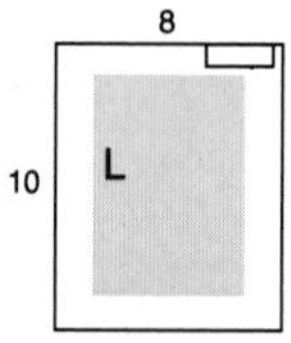

Technical Factors:
- Film Size - 8 x 10 in. (18 x 24 cm), lengthwise.
- Moving or stationary grid, 70 ± 6 kVp range or (smaller patient, <10 cm), screen table top, 60 ± 5 kVp range.
  (**Decrease 4-6 kVp** from lateral knee technique to avoid overexposing the patella.)

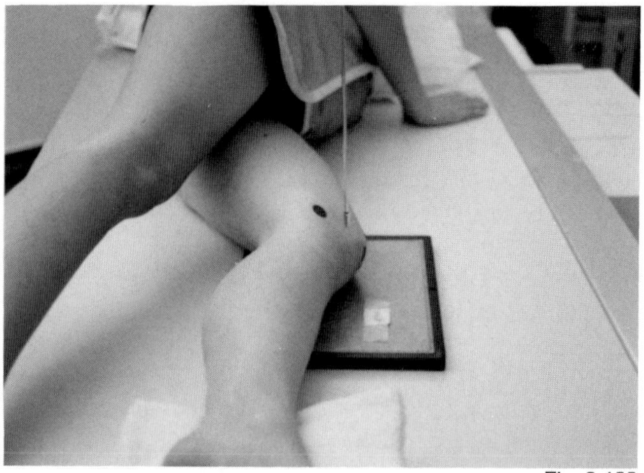

Patient Position:
- Patient in lateral recumbent position, affected side down, pillow for head.
- Provide support for knee of opposite limb placed either behind or in front of affected knee.

Shielding: Place shield over gonadal area.

Part Position:
- Adjust rotation of body and leg until knee is in a **true lateral** position (femoral epicondyles directly superimposed and plane of patella perpendicular to plane of film).
- Flex knee only 5 or 10°. (Additional flexion may separate fracture fragments if present.)
- Align and center long axis of patella to center line of table or cassette.

Central Ray:
- CR **perpendicular** to film. Direct CR to the **distal aspect of the patellofemoral joint.**
- Minimum 40 in. (102 cm) SID.

Collimation: Collimate closely on four sides to include just the area of the patella and knee joint.

NOTE: This can also be taken as a crosstable lateral with no knee flexion on a severe trauma patient.

Evaluation Criteria:
- Four-sided collimation should include patella and knee joint with the center to the distal aspect of the patellofemoral joint space.
- **True Lateral:** The anterior and posterior borders of the femoral condyles should be directly superimposed. The patellofemoral joint space should appear open.
- Optimum exposure will visualize the patella well without overexposure. Soft tissue detail of the knee joint should also be visible. The trabecular markings of the patella and other bones should appear clear and sharp.

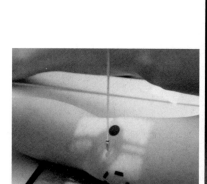
Fig. 6-138
Patient Position – Lateral Patella

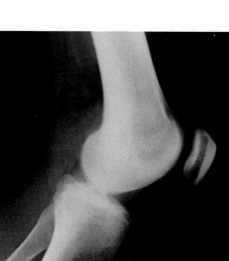

Fig. 6-139
Part Position – Lateral Patella

Fig. 6-140
Lateral Patella

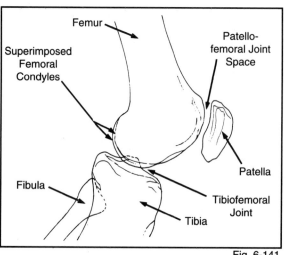
Fig. 6-141
Lateral Patella

• Tangential (Axial) Projection
Merchant Bilateral Method[1] (Patient supine - 45° knee flexion)

Patella
• PA
• Lateral
• **Tangential**

Structures Best Shown:
An axial view of patella, intercondylar sulcus, and patellofemoral joint with quadriceps femoris muscle in relaxed state.

Technical Factors:
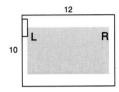

- Film Size - 10 x 12 in. (24 x 30 cm), crosswise.
- Detail screen, small focal spot.
  (Grid is not needed because of air gap due to increased OID.)
- 60 ± 5 kVp range.
- Some type of leg support and cassette holder should be used.

Patient Position:
- Patient supine with knees **flexed 45°** over the end of the table resting on a leg support. Place pillow under head. (Patient in general needs to be comfortable and relaxed for quadriceps muscles to be totally relaxed. (See NOTE.)

Shielding: Place lead shield over entire pelvic area.

Part Position:
- Place support under knees to raise distal femora so they are parallel to table top.
- Place knees and feet together and secure legs together below the knees to prevent rotation and to allow patient to be totally relaxed.
- Place cassette on edge against legs about 12 in. (30 cm) below the knees, **perpendicular** to x-ray beam.

Central Ray:
- Angle CR caudal, **30° from horizontal** (CR 30° to femora). Adjust CR angle if needed for true tangential projection of patellofemoral joint spaces.
- Direct CR to a point **midway between patellae.**
- 48 in.(120 cm) to 72 in.(180 cm) SID. (Increased SID reduces magnification.)

Collimation: Collimate **tightly** on all sides to area of patellae.

NOTE: Patient comfort and total relaxation is essential. The quadriceps femoris muscles must be relaxed for accurate diagnosis to prevent subluxation of patellae wherein they are pulled into the intercondylar sulcus or groove, which may result in false readings.[1]

Evaluation Criteria:
- Four-sided rectangular collimation field should be limited to area of patellae and anterior femoral condyles.
- The intercondyloid sulcus (trochlear groove) and patella of each distal femur should be visualized in profile.
- Patellofemoral joint space should be open with bony margins of condyles and patellae clearly defined.
- Optimum exposure should clearly visualize soft tissue and joint space margins and trabecular markings of patellae. Femoral condyles will appear underexposed with only the anterior margins clearly defined.

[1] Merchant, A C, et al: Reontgenographic Analysis of Patellofemoral Congruence, J Bone and Joint Surg., 56-A:1391-96, Oct. 1974.

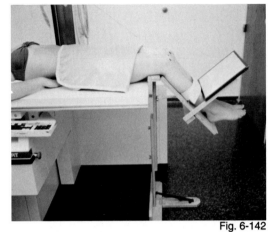

Fig. 6-142

Patient Position - Bilateral Tangential

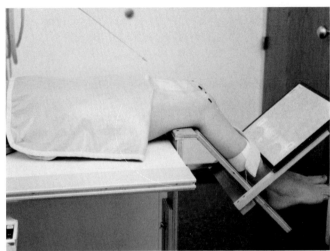

Part Position - Bilateral Tangential   **Fig. 6-143**

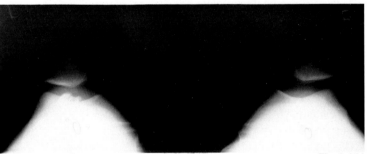

Tangential Bilateral   **Fig. 6-144**

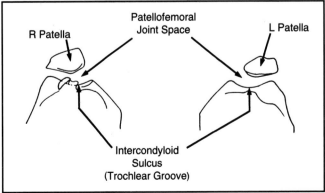

Tangential Bilateral   **Fig. 6-145**

• Tangential (Axial) Projection

1. Erect Position Method[1] (Patient erect, 40° knee flexion)
2. Hughston Method[2] (Patient prone, 55° knee flexion)
3. Settegast Method (Patient prone, 90° knee flexion)

Summary: Three additional methods for the tangential projection of the patella and patellofemoral joint are described and illustrated. Advantages and disadvantages of each are noted. This text recommends the Merchant method as described on the preceding page as a preferred method with the least disadvantages.

Technical Factors:
- Film Size - 8 x 10 in. (18 x 24 cm), crosswise.
- Detail screen, small focal spot.
- 65 ± 5 kVp range. (Increase to 70-75 kVp for erect position method due to increased OID.)

1. Erect Position Method: (Limited to those patients who are able to stand.)
- Patient standing with feet slightly spread. Feet are pointed directly ahead with foot of affected limb placed about 12 in. (30 cm) forward. Ask patient to lean back out of the way of the x-ray tube and support themselves by holding on to the x-ray table and/or hand rail on the stool. Film (cassette) is placed on stool horizontal to the floor with spacing blocks as needed to bring the film height midway to the knee. Ask patient to flex knee of affected limb about 40° and maintain that position. (Both knees may be taken individually on separate films for comparison.)

Central Ray:
- CR **perpendicular** to plane of film, directed to **mid-patellofemoral joint.**
- 48 in. (120 cm) to 72 in. (180 cm) SID. (Increased SID reduces magnification.)

NOTE: Patient stabilization may be a problem and relaxation of the quadriceps muscle is difficult to achieve with this method. However, no special equipment is needed and there is minimal distortion.

2. Hughston Method: (May be done bilaterally on one film for comparison.)
- Patient prone with cassette placed under knee. Slowly flex knee 55° and rest foot against collimator or other support. (Insure that collimator is not too hot for patient comfort.)

Central Ray:
- CR **45° cephalad.**
- Direct CR to **mid-patellofemoral joint**
- Minimum 40 in. (102 cm) SID.

NOTE: This is a relatively comfortable position for patient and relaxation of the quadriceps can be achieved. The major disadvantage is the image distortion caused by the film-body part-beam alignment.

3. Settegast Method: Warning: This acute flexion of knee should **not** be attempted until fracture of patella has been ruled out by other projections.

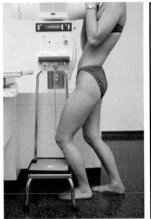 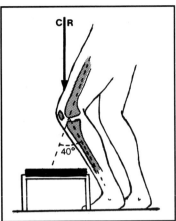

Fig. 6-146   Fig. 6-147
1. Erect Position - 40° Flexion of Knee

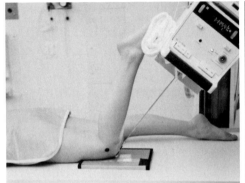 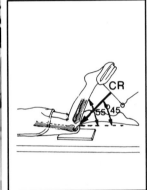

Fig. 6-148   Fig. 6-149
2. Hughston Method - 55° Flexion of Knee

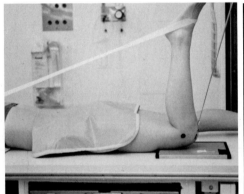 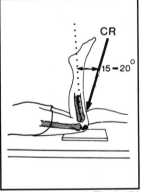

Fig. 6-150   Fig. 6-151
3. Settegast Method - 90° Flexion of Knee

- Patient prone with cassette under knee. Slowly flex knee to a **minimum of 90°.** Use gauze or tape to maintain position.

Central Ray:
- CR **perpendicular to patellofemoral joint space.** (The degree of angle is dependent on the amount of knee flexion but should be 15-20° from the long axis of the lower leg.)
- Minimum 40 in. (102 cm) SID.

NOTE: The major disadvantage to this method is that the acute knee flexion makes this impossible to use with knee trauma. Also the tightened quadriceps tend to center the patella and draw it into the intercondylar sulcus, thus reducing the diagnostic value of this projection.[1]

[1] Turner, GW, Burns, CB: Erect Position/Tangential Projection of the Patellofemoral Joint, Radiol Technol, 54-1:11-14, 1982.
[2] Hughston, AC: Subluxation of the Patella, J Bone and Joint Surg, 50-A:1003-26, 1958.

Patella

• Oblique Position (PA)

Patella
• PA
• Lateral
• Tangential
Optional
• Oblique

Structures Best Shown:

Oblique views of patella free of superimposition. (Each half of patella is shown free of superimposition in these two obliques.)

NOTE: These may be taken as optional projections to rule out small fissure fractures or other pathology not clearly demonstrated through the femur on the PA projection.

Technical Factors:

• Film Size - 10 x 12 in. (24 x 30 cm), crosswise.
• Divide in half for each oblique.
• Moving or stationary grid, 70 ± 5 kVp range or smaller patient, <10 cm, screen table top, 60 ± 5 kVp range.

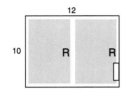

Patient Position:

External Oblique - Patient prone, turned up slightly oblique away from affected side with hand and arm of affected side up by head and opposite arm down by side. Provide pillow for head.

Internal Oblique - Same as above but patient turned into opposite oblique.

Shielding: Place shield over gonadal area.

Part Position:

External Oblique - Rotate the anterior or patella area of the leg externally. Generally a 45-55° rotation from a PA is required.

Internal Oblique - Same as above but rotate leg internally to displace the patella medially.

• Flex knee slightly to relax quadriceps muscles, place support under ankle.
• Center patella area to center of unmasked half of film.

Central Ray:

• CR **perpendicular** to film, directed to **mid-patella**.
• Minimum 40 in. (102 cm) SID.

Collimation: Collimate closely to area of patella and knee joint.

NOTE: Some references suggest a 25-30° caudal angle to result in an oblique axial projection.

Evaluation Criteria:

• Four-sided collimation field should include only the patella and knee joint area.
• Half or more of the patella should be seen in profile on each oblique not superimposed by femur.
• Optimum exposure should visualize the border outline of the patella through the femur and also clearly visualize the portion of the patella in profile without overexposure. Trabecular markings of that portion of the patella free of superimposition should be visible and appear clear and sharp.

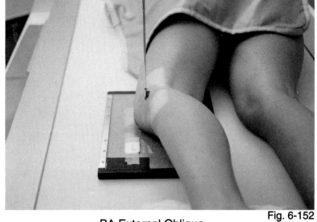

PA External Oblique
(Lateral half of patella free of superimpositions)
Fig. 6-152

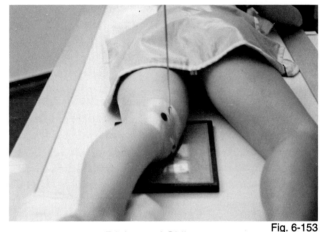

PA Internal Oblique
(Medial half of patella free of superimpositions)
Fig. 6-153

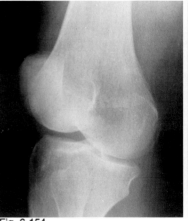

Fig. 6-154 External Oblique

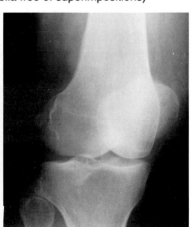

Internal Oblique Fig. 6-155

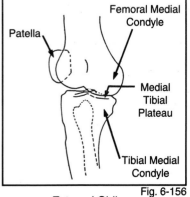

External Oblique Fig. 6-156

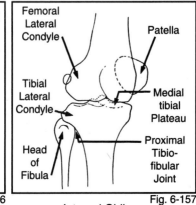

Internal Oblique Fig. 6-157

• AP Projection (Mid and Distal Femur)

NOTE: If site of interest is in area of proximal femur, a unilateral hip routine or a pelvis is recommended as described in Chapter 7.

Femur (Mid and Distal)
Basic
• **AP**
• Lateral

Structures Best Shown:

Mid and distal femur including knee joint.

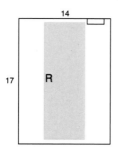

Technical Factors:

• Film Size - 14 x 17 in. (35 x 43 cm), lengthwise.
• Moving or stationary grid.
• 75 ± 5 kVp range.
• To make best use of the anode-heel effect, place the hip or head end of patient at cathode end of x-ray beam.

Patient Position:

• Patient supine, femur centered to midline of table, pillow for head. (May also be done on stretcher with portable grid placed under femur.)

Shielding: Place lead shield over pelvic area to insure correct gonadal shielding because of proximity to primary beam.

Part Position: (Mid and Distal Femur)

• Align femur to midline of table or film. (Mid and proximal femur tends to be in lateral part of thigh.)
• Rotate leg internally about 5° for a true AP as for an AP knee.
• Insure that knee joint is included on film considering the divergence of the x-ray beam. (Lower cassette margin should be about 2 in. or 5 cm below knee joint.)

Central Ray:

• CR **perpendicular** to femur and film, directed to **mid point of film.**
• Minimum 40 in. (102 cm) SID.

Collimation: Collimate closely on both sides to femur with end collimation to film borders.

Alternate Routine to Include Both Joints: Some departmental routines include both joints on at least one projection on all initial femur exams. For a large adult a second smaller film (10 x 12 in.) should then be used for an AP of either the knee or the hip insuring that both hip and knee joints are included. If the hip is included, the leg should be rotated 10-15° internally to place the femoral neck in profile.

Evaluation Criteria: (Mid and Distal Femur)

• Femur should be centered to collimation field with knee joint space a minimum of 1 in. (2.5 cm) from distal film margin. There should only be minimal collimation borders visible on proximal and distal margins of film.
• Knee joint space will not appear fully open due to divergent x-ray beam.
• **No rotation:** Femoral and tibial condyles should appear symmetrical in size and shape with the outline of patella near the center of distal femur (patella usually is slightly toward medial side of femur). The approximate medial half of fibular head should be superimposed by tibia.
• Optimum exposure with correct use of anode-heel effect will result in near uniform density of entire femur. Fine trabecular markings should be clear and sharp throughout length of femur.

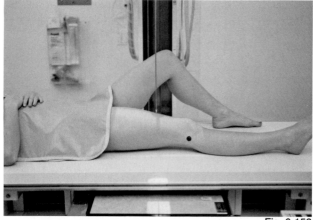

Patient Position – Mid and Distal Femur
Fig. 6-158

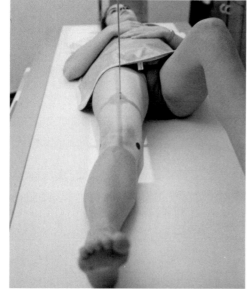

Part Position
Mid and Distal Femur
Fig. 6-159

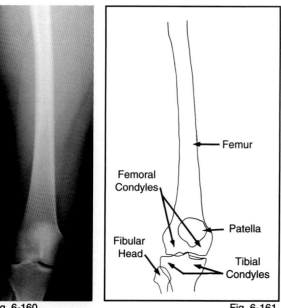

Fig. 6-160

Femur

Femoral Condyles

Patella

Fibular Head

Tibial Condyles

Fig. 6-161

AP – Mid and Distal Femur

• Lateral Position (Mid and Distal Femur)

NOTE: For possible trauma if site of interest is in area of proximal femur, a unilateral trauma hip routine is recommended as described in Chapter 7. For non-trauma lateral of mid and proximal femur, see following page.

Femur (Mid and Distal)
Basic
• AP
• **Lateral**

Technical Factors:
• Film Size - 14 x 17 in.
  (35 x 43 cm), lengthwise.
• Moving or stationary grid.
• 75±5 kVp range.
• To make best use of the anode-heel effect, place the hip of patient at cathode end of x-ray beam.

Patient Position:
• Lateral recumbent, or supine for trauma patient.

Shielding: Place lead shield over pelvic area to shield gonads.

Part Position:
Lateral Recumbent:
• **Warning -** Do not attempt this position with severe trauma.
• With patient on affected side, flex knee approximately 45° and align femur to midline of table or film (remember the femur tends to be in anterior part of thigh).
• Place unaffected leg behind affected leg (or in front of affected leg if this assists in a true lateral position).
• Adjust cassette to include knee joint on film (lower cassette margin should be about 2 in. or 5 cm below knee joint).

Supine: (Horizontal beam - Trauma)
• Place support under affected leg and support foot and ankle in true AP position.
• Place cassette on edge against lateral aspect of thigh to include knee with horizontal x-ray beam directed from medial side *(Fig. 6-163).*
• Elevate unaffected leg and place a high support under foot and ankle.

Alternate trauma projection for distal half of femur: Place vertical film against inside thigh with horizontal x-ray beam directed from lateral side *(Fig. 6-164).*

Central Ray:
• CR **perpendicular** to femur and film, directed to **mid point of film.**
• Minimum 40 in. (102 cm) SID.

Collimation: Collimate closely on both sides to femur with end collimation to film borders.

Evaluation Criteria: (Mid and Distal Femur)
• Femur should be centered to collimation field with knee joint space a minimum of 1 in. (2.5 cm) from distal film margin. There should only be minimal collimation borders visible on proximal and distal margins of film.
• Knee joint will not appear open and distal margins of the femoral condyles will not be superimposed due to divergent x-ray beam.
• **True lateral:** Anterior and posterior margins of femoral condyles should be superimposed and aligned. Patellofemoral joint space should be open.
• Optimum exposure with correct use of anode-heel effect will result in near uniform density of entire femur. Fine trabecular markings should be clear and sharp throughout length of femur.

Structures Best Shown:
Mid and distal femur including knee joint.

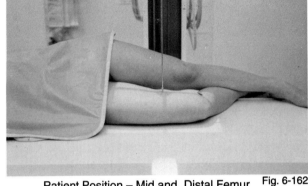

Patient Position – Mid and Distal Femur   Fig. 6-162

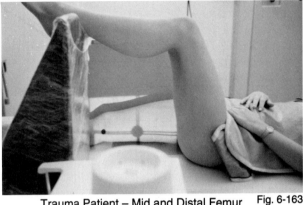

Trauma Patient – Mid and Distal Femur   Fig. 6-163

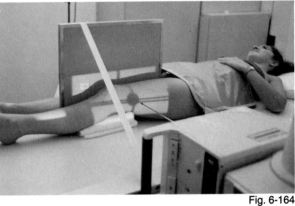

Fig. 6-164
Alternate Trauma Projection – **Distal Half** of Femur

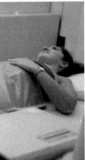

Fig. 6-165

Fig. 6-166
Part Position – Mid and Distal Femur

— Femur

— Patello-femoral Joint

Femoral Condyles

— Patella

• Lateral Position (Mid and Proximal Femur)

Warning: Do not attempt this position for patient with possible fracture of hip or proximal femur. Refer to trauma lateral hip routine in Chapter 7.

Femur (Mid and Distal)
Basic
• AP
• **Lateral**

Structures Best Shown:
Mid and proximal femur including lateral hip.

Technical Factors:
• Film Size - 14 x 17 in. (35 x 43 cm), lengthwise.
• Moving or stationary grid.
• 75 ± 5 kVp range.
• To make best use of the anode-heel effect, place the hip at cathode end of x-ray beam.

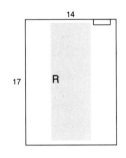

Patient Position:
• Patient in lateral recumbent position with affected side down, provide pillow for head.
• Ask patient to grasp the edge of table to maintain this position. (Do not pinch fingers when moving Bucky Tray.)

Shielding: Generally gonadal shielding is not possible on this projection without obscuring essential anatomy.

Part Position:
• Flex affected knee about 45° and align femur to midline of table.
• Place folded towel or other support under the affected leg for true lateral.
• With unaffected knee flexed, place leg behind affected leg for support, and have patient roll back (posteriorly) about 15° to prevent superimpositon of proximal femur and hip joint.
• Adjust cassette to include hip joint on film considering the divergence of the x-ray beam. (Palpate anterior superior iliac spine and place upper film margin at the level of this landmark.)

Central Ray:
• CR **perpendicular** to femur and film, directed to **mid point of film.**
• Minimum 40 in. (102 cm) SID.

Collimation: Collimate closely on both sides to femur with end collimation to film borders.

Alternate Routine to Include Both Joints: Some departmental routines include both joints on all initial femur exams. On a large adult this requires a second smaller film (10 x 12 in. or 24 x 30 cm) of the joint away from the site of injury insuring overlap of the two films.

Evaluation Criteria:
• Femur should be centered to collimation field with hip joint a minimum of 1 in. (2.5 cm) from proximal film margin.
• There should only be minimum collimation borders on proximal and distal margins of film.
• Proximal femur and hip joint should not be superimposed by opposite limb.
• **True lateral:** Evidenced by the superimposition of the greater and lesser trochanters by the femur with only a small part of the lesser trochanter visible on medial side. The greater trochanter should be nearly symmetrically superimposed by the neck of the femur.
• Optimum exposure should result in near uniform density of entire femur. Fine trabecular markings should appear clear and sharp throughout entire femur.

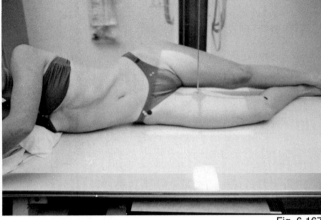

Patient Position – Mid and Proximal Femur   Fig. 6-167

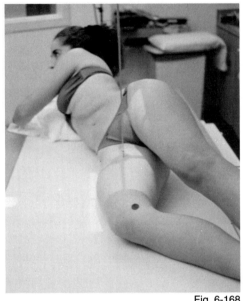

Part Position   Fig. 6-168
Mid and Proximal Femur

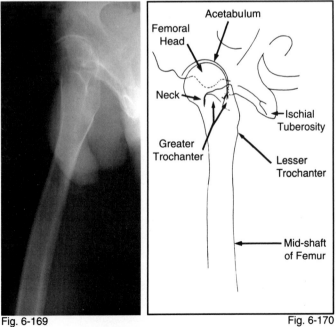

Fig. 6-169   Fig. 6-170
Mid and Proximal Femur

Chapter 7
Radiographic Anatomy and Positioning of the Proximal Femur and Pelvis

---

Contents

Proximal Femur and Pelvis

Part I Radiographic Anatomy

Lower Limb

The first two groups of bones of the lower limb, the foot and leg, were described in Chapter 6 along with the distal femur and the associated knee and ankle joints.

The third and fourth groups of lower limb bones to be discussed in this chapter are the **proximal femur** and the **bones of the hip**. The joints involving these two groups of bones which will also be included in this chapter are the important **hip joint** and the **sacroiliac** and **symphysis pubis** joints of the pelvic girdle.

Femur

The femur is the longest and strongest bone in the entire body   entire weight of the body is transferred through this bone and the ... ociated joints at each end. Therefore these joints are a frequent source of pathology when trauma occurs.

Proximal Femur

The proximal femur consists of four essential parts, the (1) head, (2) neck, and (3) greater and (4) lesser trochanters *(tro-kan´ters)*. The **head** of the femur is rounded and smooth for articulation with the hip bones. It contains a depression or pit near its center called the **fovea capitis** *(fo´ve-ah cap´itis)* wherein a ligament is attached to the head of the femur.

The **neck** of the femur is a strong pyramidal shaped process of bone connecting the head to the body or shaft in the region of the trochanters.

The **greater trochanter** is a large prominence located **superiorly** and **laterally** to the femoral shaft and is palpable as a bony landmark. The **lesser trochanter** is a smaller blunt conical shaped eminence which projects **medially** and **posteriorly** from the junction of the neck and shaft of the femur. The trochanters are joined posteriorly by a thick ridge called the **intertrochanteric** *(in˝ter-tro˝kan-ter´ik)* **crest**. The **body** or **shaft** of the femur is long and almost cylindrical in shape.

Angles of Proximal Femur: The angle of the neck to the shaft on an average adult is about **125°**, but this varies from 110-135° depending on the width of the pelvis and the length of the lower limbs. For a long-legged male with a narrow pelvis, the femur would be nearer vertical which would then change the angle of the neck also. On an average adult in the anatomical position, the longitudinal plane of the femur is about **10° from vertical.** This vertical angle would be nearer 15° on a female with a wide pelvis and shorter limbs, and near 5° on a long-legged male. (This angle also affects positioning and CR angles for a lateral knee as described in Chapter 6, *Figs. 6-20 and 21.*)

Another angle of the neck and head of the femur which is important radiographically is the **15-20° anterior** angle of the head and neck in relationship to the body of the femur. The head projects somewhat anteriorly or forward as a result of this angle. (This becomes important in radiographic positioning wherein the femur and leg must be rotated **15-20° internally** for a true AP projection of the proximal femur.)

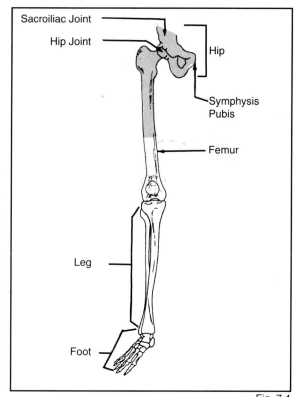

Lower Limb   Fig. 7-1

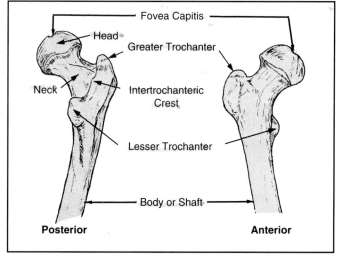

Proximal Femur   Fig. 7-2

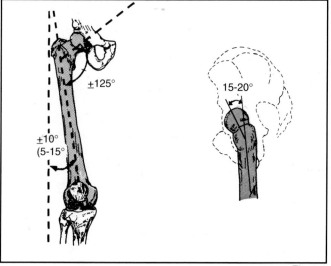

Angles of Proximal Femur   Fig. 7-3

Pelvis

The total **pelvis** serves as the base of the trunk and forms the connection between the vertebral column and the lower limbs. The pelvis consists of four bones: two **hip bones** or **ossa coxae** (also called innominatum), one **sacrum** *(sa'krum)* and one **coccyx** *(kok'siks)*.

It should be noted that sometimes the term **pelvic girdle** is used in reference to the total pelvis. This however is incorrect in that the **pelvic girdle consists only of the two ossa coxae or hip bones, and the term pelvis includes the sacrum and coccyx.**

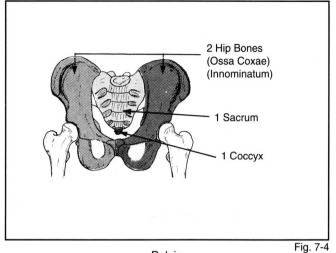

Pelvis

Fig. 7-4

Hip Bone

Each hip bone is composed of three divisions: (1) **ilium** *(il'e-um)*, (2) **ischium** *(is'ke-um)* and (3) **pubis** *(pu'bis)*. In a child, these three divisions are separate bones, but they fuse into one bone during the middle teens. The fusion occurs in the area of the **acetabulum** *(as"e-tab'u-lum)*. The acetabulum is a deep, cup-shaped cavity that accepts the head of the femur to form the hip joint. The ilium is the largest of the three divisions and is located superior to the acetabulum. The ischium is inferior and posterior to the acetabulum, while the pubis is inferior and anterior.

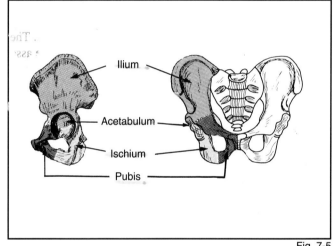

Hip Bone (Os Coxa)

Fig. 7-5

Ilium

Each **ilium** is composed of a **body** and an **ala** or wing. The body of the ilium is the more inferior portion near the acetabulum and includes the upper two-fifths of the acetabulum. The ala or wing portion is the thin, flared, upper part of the ilium.

The **crest** of the ilium is the upper margin of the ala and extends from the **anterior superior iliac spine** (ASIS) to the **posterior superior iliac spine** (PSIS). In radiographic positioning, the uppermost peak of the crest is often referred to as the **iliac crest** but it actually extends between the ASIS and PSIS.

Below the anterior superior iliac spine (ASIS) is a less prominent projection referred to as the **anterior inferior iliac spine**. Similarly, inferior to the posterior superior iliac spine is the **posterior inferior iliac spine**.

Positioning Landmarks: The two most important positioning landmarks of these borders and projections are the **crest of the ilium** (the iliac crest) and the **anterior superior iliac spine** (ASIS).

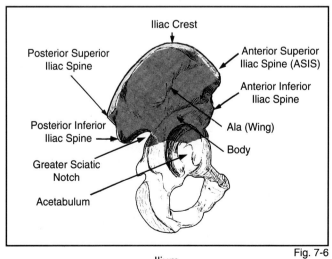

Ilium

Fig. 7-6

Ischium

The **ischium** is that part of the hip bone inferior and posterior to the acetabulum. Each ischium is divided into a **body** and a **ramus.** The upper portion of the body of the ischium makes up the posteroinferior two-fifths of the acetabulum. The lower portion of the body of the ischium (formerly called the superior ramus) projects caudally and medially from the acetabulum ending at the **ischial tuberosity.** Projecting anteriorly from the ischial tuberosity is the **ramus of the ischium.**

The rounded, roughened area near the junction of the superior and inferior rami is a landmark termed the **tuberosity** of the ischium or **ischial** *(is´ke-al)* **tuberosity.**

Directly posterior to the acetabulum is a bony projection termed the **ischial spine.** Directly above the ischial spine is a deep notch termed the **greater sciatic notch.** Below the ischial spine is a smaller notch termed the **lesser sciatic notch.**

Positioning Landmark: The ischial tuberosities bear most of the weight of the body when one sits and can be palpated through the soft tissues of each buttock when one is prone. However because of discomfort and possible embarrassment to the patient, this landmark is not as commonly used as the already described ASIS and crest of the ilium.

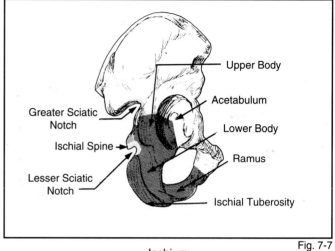

Ischium   Fig. 7-7

Pubis

The last of the three divisions of one hip bone is the **pubis** or **pubic bone.** The **body** of the pubis is anterior and inferior to the acetabulum and includes the anteroinferior one-fifth of the acetabulum.

Extending anteriorly and medially from the body of each pubis is a **superior ramus.** The two superior rami meet in the midline to form a slightly movable joint, the **symphysis pubis** *(sim´fi-sis pu´bis)*. Each **inferior ramus** passes down and posterior from the symphysis pubis to join the inferior ramus of the respective ischium.

The **obturator foramen** *(ob´tu-ra"tor fo-ra´men)* is a large opening formed by the rami of each ischium and pubis. The obturator foramen is the largest foramen in the human skeletal system.

Positioning Landmark: The superior margin of the symphysis pubis is a positioning landmark used in pelvis and hip positioning as well as positioning for the abdomen since this defines the lowermost margin of the abdomen.

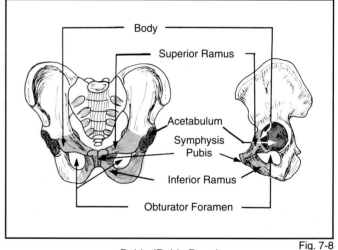

Pubis (Pubic Bone)   Fig. 7-8

Topographical Landmarks

Important positioning landmarks of the pelvis are reviewed in *Fig. 7-9*. The most superior aspect of the **iliac crest** and the **ASIS** are easily palpated. The ASIS is one of the most frequently used positioning landmarks of the pelvis. It is also most commonly used to check for rotation of the pelvis and/or lower abdomen by determining if the distance between the ASIS and table top is the same on both sides. The **greater trochanter** of the femur can be located in the soft tissues of the upper thigh. Note that the upper margin of the greater trochanter is about 1.5 in. (3.75 cm) above the upper border of the **symphysis pubis** while the **ischial tuberosity** is about the same distance below the symphysis pubis.

As previously stated, in chapter 3 on the abdomen, even though the ischial tuberosity is a palpable landmark, it is not commonly used in respect for the patient's comfort and modesty.

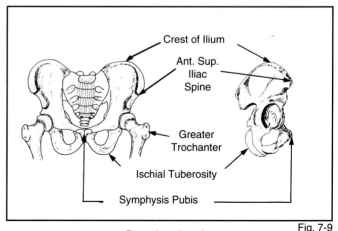

Bony Landmarks   Fig. 7-9

True and False Pelvis

A plane through the **brim** of the pelvis divides the pelvic area into two cavities. The pelvic brim is defined by the upper part of the symphysis pubis anteriorly and the upper, prominent part of the sacrum posteriorly. The general area above the oblique plane through the pelvic brim is termed the **greater** or **false pelvis**. The flared portion of the pelvis formed primarily by the alae or wings of the ilia form the lateral and posterior limits of the greater or false pelvis, while the abdominal muscles of the anterior wall define the anterior limits. The lower abdominal organs and a fetus within the pregnant uterus rest on the floor of the greater pelvis.

The area inferior to a plane through the pelvic brim is termed the **lesser** or **true pelvis**. The lesser or true pelvis is a cavity completely surrounded by bony structures. The size and shape of the true pelvis is of greatest importance during the birth process since the true pelvis forms the actual birth canal.

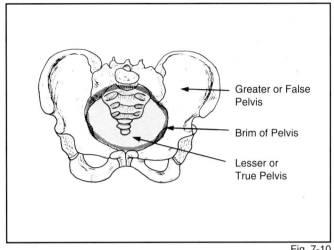

Pelvic Cavities

Fig. 7-10

True Pelvis

The oblique plane defined by the brim of the pelvis is termed the **inlet** of the true pelvis. The **outlet** of the true pelvis is defined by the two ischial tuberosities and the tip of the coccyx. The three sides of the triangularly shaped outlet are formed by a line between the ischial tuberosities and two lines between each ischial tuberosity and the coccyx. The area between the inlet and outlet of the lesser or true pelvis is termed the **cavity** of the true pelvis. During the birth process, the baby must travel through the inlet, cavity and outlet of the true pelvis.

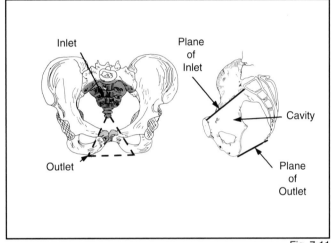

Lesser or True Pelvis

Fig. 7-11

Birth Canal

During a routine delivery, the baby's head first travels through the pelvic inlet, then to the midpelvis, and finally through the outlet to exit in a forward direction.

Because of the sensitivity to radiation by the fetus, radiographs of the pelvis generally are not taken during pregnancy. If the size or dimensions of the birth canal of the pelvis is in question, certain ultrasound procedures can be done to evaluate for potential problems during the birthing process.

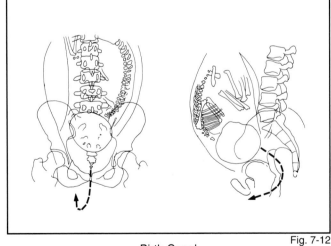

Birth Canal

Fig. 7-12

Male vs. Female Pelvis

The general shape of the female pelvis varies enough from the male pelvis to enable one to discriminate one from the other on pelvic radiographs. In general, the **female pelvis** is wider, deeper and more flared, while the **male pelvis** is narrower and less flared. In overall appearance, the female pelvis is deeper. Therefore the first difference between the male and female pelvis is the difference in the **overall general shape** of the pelvis.

A second major difference is the **angle of the pubic arch,** formed by the inferior rami of the pubes just below the symphysis pubis. In the female, this angle is usually obtuse or greater than 90 degrees, while in the male the pubic arch usually forms an acute angle, less than 90 degrees.

A third difference is the **shape of the inlet**. The inlet of the female pelvis is usually round, while in the male it is usually more oval or heart-shaped. The general shape of the pelvis does vary considerably from one individual to another, so that the pelvis of a slender female may resemble a male pelvis. In general, however, the differences are usually obvious enough that one can determine the sex of the patient from a radiograph of the pelvis.

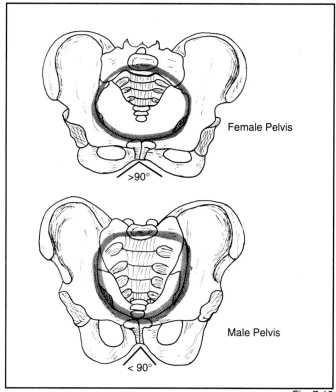

Pelvis - Male vs. Female   Fig. 7-13

Summary of Male, Female Pelvic Characteristics

	Male	Female
1. General shape	narrower, less flared	wider, deeper more flared
2. Angle of Pubic Arch	acute angle	obtuse angle
3. Shape of Inlet	oval	round

Male vs. Female Pelvis Radiographs

Figures 7-14 and 15 are pelvic radiographs of a male and a female subject. Note the three differences between this typical male and female pelvis.

First, in overall shape, the male pelvis appears narrower with a less flared appearance of the ilia.

Second, the acute angle of less than 90° of the pubic arch on the male is obvious, as compared to the greater than 90° angle on the female pelvis below. This is commonly one of the more noticeable differences.

Third, the shape of the inlet on the male pelvis is not as broad or rounded as compared to the female pelvis, even though the inlet on this male pelvis is more rounded and not as oval or heart shaped as on some males.

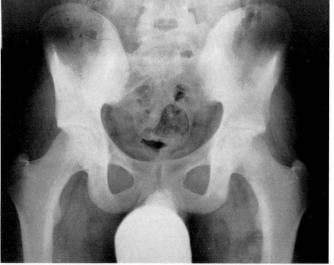

Male Pelvis   Fig. 7-14

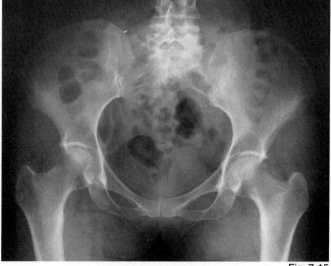

Female Pelvis   Fig. 7-15

Review Exercise with Radiographs

Key pelvic anatomy is labelled on the AP pelvis radiograph of *Fig. 7-16*. A good review exercise is to first cover up the answers while identifying these parts.

A. Iliac crest
B. ASIS (anterior end of crest)
C. Body of the left ischium
D. Ischial tuberosity
E. Symphysis pubis
F. Inferior ramus of the right pubis
G. Superior ramus of the right pubis
H. Right ischial spine
I. Acetabulum of right hip
J. Neck of right femur
K. Greater trochanter of right femur
L. Head of right femur
M. Ala or wing of right ilium

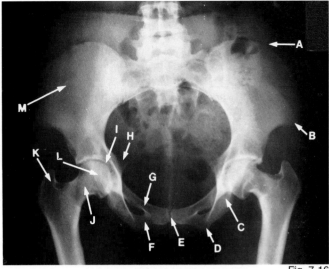

Pelvis - AP   Fig. 7-16

Lateral Hip

This demonstrates a good lateral radiograph of the proximal femur and hip taken with an inferosuperior projection (crosstable lateral) as demonstrated by the positioning drawing of *Fig. 7-18*.

A. Acetabulum
B. Femoral head
C. Femoral neck
D. Ischial tuberosity
E. Greater trochanter
F. Lesser trochanter
G. Shaft or body

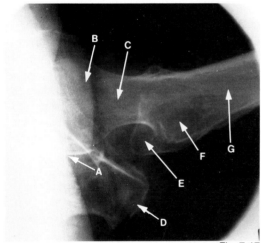

Inferosuperior Projection   Fig. 7-17

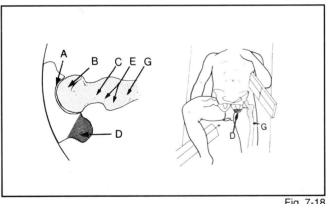

Proximal Femur and Hip - Lateral
(Inferosuperior Projection)   Fig. 7-18

Classification of Joints

The number of joints or articulations of the proximal femora and the pelvic girdle are limited with the hip joint being the most obvious. These joints of the pelvic girdle as listed below will again be described according to their **classification, mobility type and movement type.**

Sacroiliac Joints - Between sacrum and each ilium.
Symphysis Pubis - Between right and left pubic bones.
Union of Acetabulum - A temporary growth joint of the acetabulum which solidifies in mid teen years.
Hip Joints - Between head of femur and acetabulum of pelvis.

Sacroiliac Joints

The sacroiliac joints are wide, flat joints located obliquely between the sacrum and each ilium. These joints are situated at an unusual oblique angle requiring special positioning to visualize the joint spaces radiographically.

The sacroiliac joint is classified as a **synovial joint** in that it is enclosed in a **fibrous articular capsule** containing synovial fluid. The bones are joined by firm sacroiliac ligaments. Generally synovial joints by their nature are considered freely movable or diarthrodial joints. However the sacroiliac joint is a special type of synovial joint which permits little movement and is thus **amphiarthrodial**. The reason for this is the joint surfaces are very irregularly shaped and the interconnecting bones are snugly fitted since they serve a weight-bearing function. This restricts movement and the cavity of the joint or the joint space may be reduced in size or even be nonexistent in older persons, especially in males.

Symphysis Pubis

The pubic symphysis is the articulation of the right and left pubic bones in the midline of the anterior pelvis. The most superior, anterior aspect of this joint is palpable and is an important positioning landmark as already described.

The symphysis pubis is classified as a **cartilaginous joint** of the **symphyses sub-type** in that only limited movement is possible (**amphiarthrodial**). The two articular surfaces are separated by a **fibrocartilaginous disc** and held together by certain ligaments. This **interpubic disc** of fibrocartilage is a relatively thick pad (thicker in females than males) which is capable of being compressed or partially displaced thereby allowing some limited movement of these bones such as in pelvic trauma or during the birthing process in females.

Union of Acetabulum

The three divisions of each hip bone are separate bones in a child but come together in the acetabulum by fusing during the middle teens to become completely indistinguishable in an adult. Therefore this is classified as a **cartilaginous type** joint of the **synchondroses subtype** which are **immovable** or **synarthrodial** in an adult. This is considered a temporary type of growth joint similar to the joints between the epiphyses and diaphyses of long bones in growing children.

Hip Joint

The hip joint is classified as a **synovial type**, as truly characterized by a large fibrous capsule containing synovial fluid. It is a **freely movable** or **diarthrodial** joint and is the truest example of a **ball and socket** or **spheroidal** movement type.

The head of the femur forms more than half of a sphere as it fits into the relatively deep cup shaped acetabulum. This makes the hip joint inherently strong as it supports the weight of the body while still permitting a high degree of mobility. The articular capsule surrounding

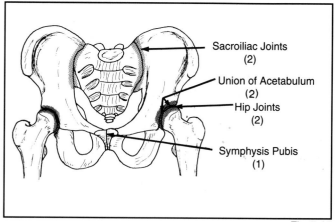
Joints of Pelvic Girdle   Fig. 7-19

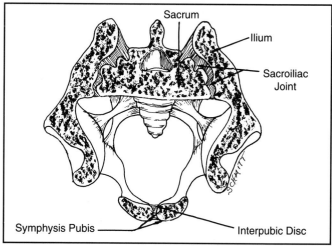
Coronal Section Showing Sacroiliac   Fig. 7-20
and Symphysis Pubis Joints

this joint is strong and dense with the thickest part being above, as would be expected since this is in line with the weight bearing function of the hip joints. A series of strong bands of ligaments surround the articular capsule and joint in general making this a very strong and stable joint.

Movements of the hip joint include **flexion** and **extension, abduction** and **adduction, medial** (internal) and **lateral** (external) **rotation** and **circumduction.**

Summary of Pelvic Girdle Joints

Classification:
- Sacroiliac Joint
- Symphysis Pubis } - *Synovial*
- Hip Joint

- Union of Acetabulum   - *Cartilaginous*

Mobility Type:
- Sacroiliac Joint
- Symphysis Pubis } - *Amphiarthrodial* (limited movement)

- Hip Joint   - *Diarthrodial* (freely movable)

Movement Type:
- Hip Joint   - *Ball and Socket* (spheroidal)

Part II Radiographic Positioning

Positioning Considerations

Location of Head and Neck

Radiographic positioning of the hip joint is a definite challenge for radiographers. Interrelationships of the pelvic girdle and the hip joint must be thoroughly understood. One must be able to find the exact location of the femoral head and femoral neck by two prominent positioning landmarks. These are the **ASIS** and the **upper border of the symphysis pubis.** To locate the head and neck of the femur, first locate the mid point of an imaginary line drawn between the ASIS and the symphysis pubis. The **neck** of the femur will lie along a line perpendicular to the mid point of the first line and approximately **2.5 in.** (6-7 cm) inferolateral the mid point. The **head** of the femur is approximately **1.5 in. (4 cm)** below the mid point of this imaginary line between the ASIS and the symphysis pubis.

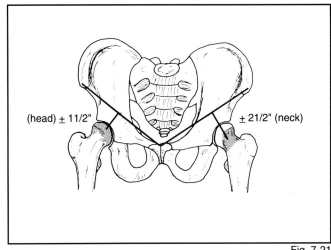
(head) ± 1 1/2"   ± 2 1/2" (neck)

Head or Neck Localization

Fig. 7-21

Appearance of Proximal Femur in Anatomical Position

As described earlier in this chapter under anatomy of the proximal femur, the head and neck of the femur project approximately 15-20° anteriorly or forward with respect to the rest of the femur and lower leg. Therefore when the leg is in the true anatomical position as for a true AP, the proximal femur is actually rotated posteriorly by 15 to 20 degrees. Therefore the femoral neck appears shortened and the lesser trochanter is visible when the leg and ankle are truly AP as in a true anatomical position.

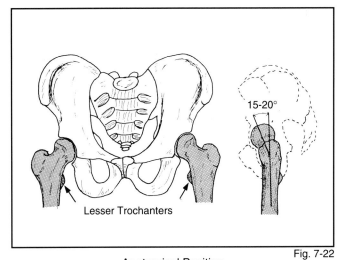
15-20°

Lesser Trochanters

Anatomical Position
(True AP of knee, leg and ankle)

Fig. 7-22

Internal Rotation of Leg

By **internally rotating** the **entire** leg, the proximal femur and hip joint will be projected in a true AP projection. The neck of the femur is now parallel to the imaging surface and will not appear foreshortened.

The key to proper placement of the leg is the **lesser trochanter.** If the entire leg is internally rotated a full 15 to 20 degrees, the outline of the lesser trochanter will generally not be visible at all as it is obscured by the shaft of the femur. If the leg is straight AP or externally rotated, then the lesser trochanter **is** visible. (See illustration on following page.)

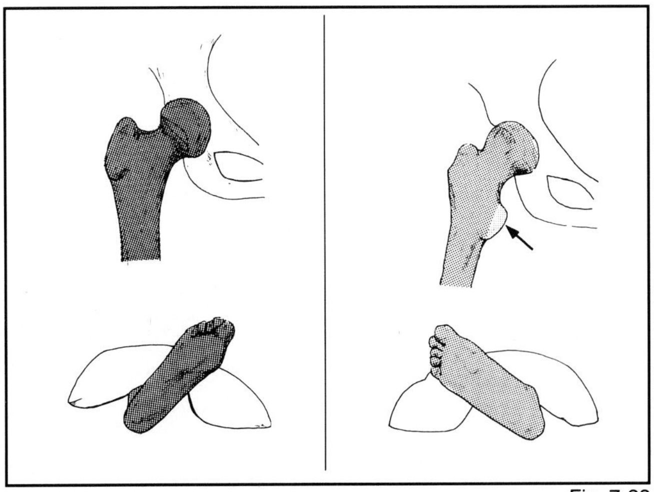

Evidence of Hip Fracture

The femoral neck is a common fracture site for an older patient who has fallen. The typical position of the foot for such a fracture is the **external rotation** of that lower limb as shown on your right and on the lower illustrations of the following page.

Positioning Warning: If such evidence of a hip fracture is present (external foot rotation), a pelvis radiograph should be taken "as is" **without** attempting to internally rotate the leg as would be necessary for a true AP hip projection. This radiograph should then be viewed by a radiologist to rule out a fracture. If this radiograph is negative, then standard hip or pelvis radiographs can be taken with internal leg rotation. Forcing an internal rotation of the leg with a fracture would be very painful, and even more important may displace the femoral head and/or neck at the fracture site.

Fig. 7-23

Internal Rotation
(True AP of hip)

External Rotation
(Typical hip
fracture position)

Summary: Effect of Lower Limb Rotation

These photos and associated pelvis radiographs demonstrate the effect of lower limb rotation on the appearance of the proximal femora.

1. Anatomical Position
- Long axes of feet vertical.
- Femoral necks partially foreshortened.
- Lesser trochanters **partially visible.**

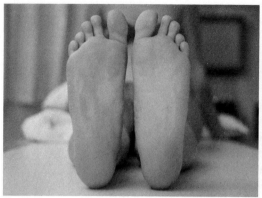
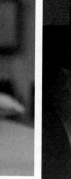

Fig. 7-24

1. Anatomical Position   Fig. 7-25

2. 15-20° Medial Rotation
(The desired position for visualizing pelvis and hips.)
- Long axes of feet and lower limbs rotated 15-20° internally.
- Femoral heads and necks in profile.
- True AP projection of proximal femurs.
- Lesser trochanters **not visible** or only slightly visible on some patients.

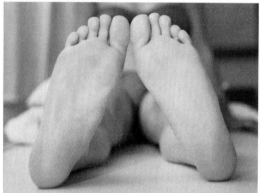

Fig. 7-26

2. 15-20° Medial Rotation   Fig. 7-27

3. External Rotation
- Long axes of feet and lower limbs equally rotated laterally in a normal relaxed position.
- Femoral necks greatly foreshortened.
- Lesser trochanters **visible in profile.**

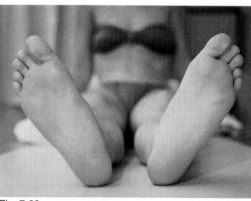
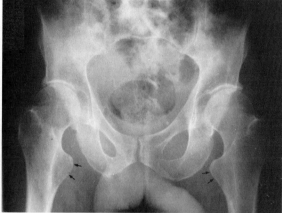

Fig. 7-28

3. External Rotation   Fig. 7-29

4. Typical Rotation with Hip Fracture
- Long axis of foot is externally rotated on side of hip fracture.
- Unaffected foot and limb in neutral position.
- Lesser trochanter on externally rotated limb is more visible.

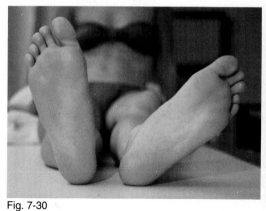
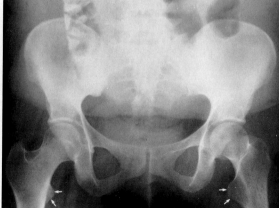

Fig. 7-30

4. Typical Rotation with Hip Fracture   Fig. 7-31

Gonadal Shielding Guidelines

Accurate gonadal shielding for pelvis and hip exams is especially critical because of the proximity of the radiation sensitive gonads to the primary rays. The gonadal shielding rule as described in Chapter One states for **all patients of reproductive age, gonadal shielding is needed if the gonads lie within or close to (2 in. or 5 cm) the primary x-ray field unless such shielding covers an area of primary interest on the image receptor.**

This is easier to apply for males in that small contact shields, such as the shaped contact shields shown in *Fig. 7-32* , should be used on **all males of reproductive age or younger**. The shields are placed over the area of the testes without covering up essential anatomy of the pelvis or hips. However care must be taken for pelvis radiographs that the shields cover the testes adequately without obscuring the pubic and ischial areas of the pelvis.

Ovarian contact shields for females of childbearing age or younger however require more critical placement to shield the area of the ovaries without covering up essential pelvic or hip anatomy. Vinyl covered lead material cut into various shapes and sizes can be used for this purpose for AP pelvis or bilateral hip radiographs. For a unilateral hip or proximal femur, larger contact shields can be used to cover the general pelvic area without covering the specific hip being radiographed as shown in *Fig. 7-33*. Accurate location of the femoral head and neck makes this type of gonadal shielding possible.

Gonadal shielding may be difficult for certain lateral pelvic or hip projections such as the lateral inferosuperior projection wherein shielding may obscure essential anatomy. However these are the exceptions and **close collimation must always be used** to reduce gonadal doses along with gonadal lead shielding whenever possible.

Exposure Factors and Patient Dosage
In the interest of reducing total radiation dose to the patient, a higher kVp range of 90 ± 5 is recommended for hip and pelvis exams. (This higher kVp technique with lower mAs results in a significantly lower radiation dose to the patient which is especially important for the pelvis and hip body areas because of their proximity to the gonads.)

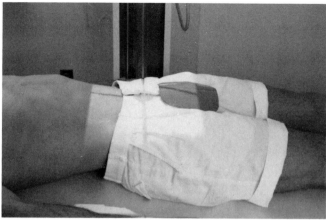

Fig. 7-32

Male Gonadal Shielding for
Hips and Pelvis

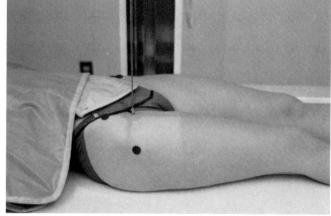

Fig. 7-33

Female Gonadal (Ovarian) Shielding
Unilateral Hip and Proximal Femur

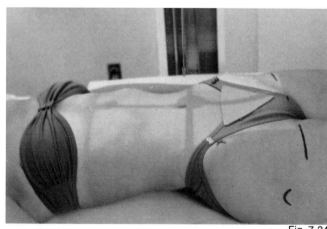

Fig. 7-34

Female Gonadal (Ovarian) Shielding
Pelvis or Bilateral Hips

National Survey

Departmental standard (basic) and optional routines for exams of the proximal femur and pelvis and the sacroiliac joints were very consistent throughout the United States.

Hip and Proximal Femur Routine

Hip	U.S. Average	
	Basic	Optional
• AP Pelvis	82%	
or		
AP Hip only	43%	
Non - Trauma		
• Lat. Frog-leg	82%	
Trauma		
• Axiolateral	36%	17%
Optional		
• Modified Inferosuperior		
(Clements - Nakayama Method)		11%

Pelvis Routine

Pelvis	U.S. Average	
	Basic	Optional
• AP	98%	
• Bilateral Frog-leg (non-trauma)	28%	17%

Sacroiliac Joints Routine

Sacroiliac Joints	U.S. Average	
	Basic	Optional
• Obli's - Post. 25°- 30°	69%	
or		
Ant. Obli's 25°- 30°	25%	
• AP 25° - 30° ceph.	62%	
or		
PA 25° - 30° caudal	5%	
• AP Pelvis	41%	

Summary:

Hip and Proximal Femur: The survey supported the routine of taking the **AP pelvis** to include both hips for comparison even when a single hip exam is requested.

For the lateral hip, the results support this text's recommended routine of a **lateral frog-leg for non-trauma**, and an **axiolateral for trauma patients.**

A question in the survey (results not included above) asked how positioning was done on a unilateral frog-leg (non-trauma) hip. **56%** indicated the knee is flexed and the thigh is abducted **without** rotation of the pelvis. Only **39%** indicated this is done **with** rotation of the pelvis as needed toward the affected side so the thigh is in contact with the table (Lowenstein and Hickey methods). This text recommends the latter method with the pelvis rotated as needed to place the femur parallel to the film.

Pelvis: The survey supported the **AP pelvis** as the common projection for the pelvis, with 28% indicating they also take the **bilateral frog-leg** routinely on non-trauma patients.

Sacroiliac Joints: The most common routine for the sacroiliac joints per this survey were the **posterior obliques** and an **AP with a 25-30° cephalic angle.** The anterior oblique and the AP pelvis are less frequently included as part of this routine. These will be described as optional projections in this chapter.

Certain basic and optional projections or positions for the pelvis, hips and proximal femora, and sacroiliac joints are demonstrated and described on the following pages as suggested routine and optional departmental procedures.

Basic and Optional Projections

Unilateral Hip
Basic
• AP Bilateral Hips
   or
  AP Unilateral Hip
• Lateral (unilateral hip)
  - Frog-leg (non-trauma)
   or
  - Axiolateral (trauma)
Optional
• Modified Axiolateral
  (Clements-Nakayama Method)

Pelvis
Basic
• AP
Optional
• Bilateral frog-leg
  (non-trauma)
• Ant. Oblique - Acetabulum
• AP Axial
  - Ant. Pelvic Bones
• Post. Oblique - Ilium

Sacroiliac Joints
Basic
• AP Axial
• Post. Obliques
Optional
• Ant. Obliques

• AP Projection

A recommended initial exam for unilateral hip trauma for comparison purposes.

| Unilateral Hip |
| • **AP Bilateral hips** |
| or |
| AP Unilateral hip |
| • Lateral (unilateral hip) |
| - Frog-leg (non-trauma) |
| - Axiolateral (trauma) |

Structures Best Shown:

Acetabulum, femoral heads, necks and greater trochanters and associated parts of the ilium, ischium and pubis.

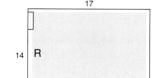

Technical Factors:

- Film Size - 14 x 17 in. (35 x 43 cm), crosswise.
- Moving or stationary grid.
- 90±5 kVp range. (See NOTE.)

Patient Position:

- Patient supine, arms at sides or across upper chest, provide pillow for head and support for under knees.

Shielding: Carefully shield gonads as much as possible without obscuring essential anatomy.

Part Position:

- Align midsagittal plane of patient to center line of table and/or cassette.
- Insure that pelvis is **not rotated**; the distance from table-top to each ASIS should be equal.
- Separate legs and feet, then **internally rotate** long axes of feet and lower limbs **15-20°**. (May need to place sandbag between heels and tape top of feet together or use additional sandbags against feet to retain this position.) **Warning:** Do **not** attempt to internally rotate legs if a hip fracture or dislocation is suspected. Take with affected leg "as is".
- Align center of cassette to level of the femoral heads which is at the upper margin of the greater trochanters. (See NOTE.)

Central Ray:

- CR **perpendicular**, directed to the **center of film** (level of superior margins of greater trochanters).
- Minimum 40 in. (102 cm) SID.

Collimation: Collimate on four sides to area of interest or to film margins on larger patients.

Respiration: Suspend respiration during exposure

NOTE: • The above centering is recommended for bilateral hips when taken as an initial exam for possible hip trauma for comparison purposes. Some departmental routines however suggest the entire pelvic girdle be centered to the film which as shown on page 234 centers the film to a level midway between the ASIS and the symphysis pubis.
- The higher kVp range of 90±5 is recommended to reduce patient dosage.

Evaluation Criteria:

- Proximal femora should be included in their entirety as well as bilateral pubis, ischium and at least the distal half of ilium.
- **No rotation:** The two obturator foramina and the bilateral ischial spines (if visible) should appear equal in size and shape.
- With bilateral full internal rotation, the femoral necks and greater

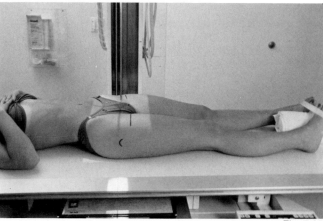

AP Bilateral Hips   Fig. 7-35

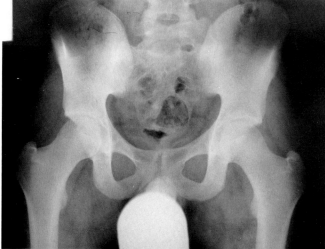

AP Bilateral Hips   Fig. 7-36

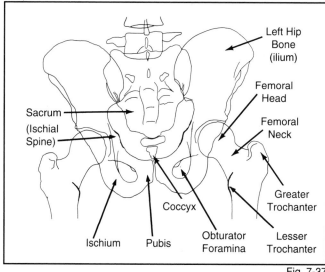

AP Bilateral Hips   Fig. 7-37

trochanters will appear in profile equal in size and shape. The lesser trochanters will not be seen at all or only small tips will be seen on medial femoral margins.
- Optimum exposure will visualize the margins of the femoral heads and acetabula through overlying pelvic structures without overexposing other parts of the proximal femora, pubis or ischium. Trabecular markings will appear clear and sharp if no motion is present.

• AP Projection

> **Unilateral Hip**
> Basic
> • AP Bilateral (Pelvis)
> or
> **AP Unilateral (Hip)**
> • Lateral (Unilateral Hip)
> - Frog-leg (non-trauma)
> - Axiolateral (trauma)

Structures Best Shown:
Acetabulum, femoral head, neck and greater trochanter.

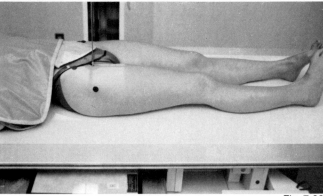
Patient Position - AP Hip   Fig. 7-38

Technical Factors:
• Film Size - 10 x 12 in. (24 x 30 cm), lengthwise.
• Moving or stationary grid.
• 90±5 kVp range.

Patient Position:
• Patient supine, arms at sides or across upper chest.
• Provide pillow for head and support under knees.

Shielding: Place shield over gonads and pelvic area insuring affected hip is not obscured.

Part Position:
• Locate **femoral neck** and align to **midline of table and/or film**. (Femoral neck is 2.5 in. or 6-7 cm inferior and perpendicular to midpoint of line between ASIS and symphysis pubis. Femoral neck can also be located on a longitudinal line about **2 in. or 5 cm medial to ASIS at level of greater trochanter.**)
• Insure **no rotation** of pelvis (equal distance from ASIS to table).
• Rotate affected leg **internally 15-20°** (only on non-trauma patient).

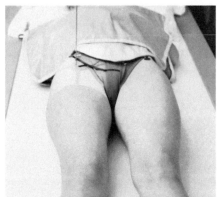
Part Position - AP Hip   Fig. 7-39

Central Ray:
• CR **perpendicular** to film, directed to **mid femoral neck** (center of film, see above).
• Minimum 40 in. (102 cm) SID.

Collimation: Collimate on four sides to area of interest or to film borders.

Respiration: Suspend respiration during exposure.

NOTE: The AP unilateral hip is generally done as a follow-up procedure. For hip trauma or pathology the **AP pelvis** (bilateral hips) should initially be taken for comparison as described on the preceding page.

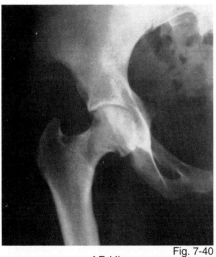
AP Hip   Fig. 7-40

Evaluation Criteria:
• The proximal 1/3 of the femur should be visualized along with the acetabulum and adjacent parts of the pubis, ischium and ilium.
• The hip joint space including the perimeter borders of the femoral head should be clearly visualized.
• The lesser trochanter should not project beyond the medial border of the femur at all or only its very tip is seen with sufficient internal rotation of leg, indicating the greater trochanter, femoral head and neck are seen in full profile without foreshortening.
• Optimum exposure will visualize the margins of the femoral head and the acetabulum through overlying pelvic structures without overexposing other parts of the proximal femur or pelvic structures. Trabecular markings of greater trochanter and neck areas will appear clear and sharp.

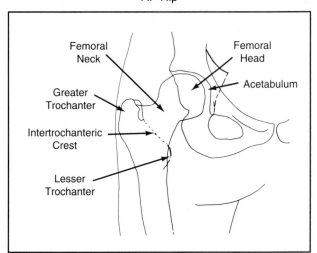
AP Hip   Fig. 7-41

• Lateral "Frog-leg" Position
(Modified Lauenstein and Hickey Method)

Warning: Do **not** attempt this position on patient with destructive hip disease or with potential hip fracture or dislocation. (This could result in significant displacement of fracture fragments. See lateral trauma projections on following pages.)

Unilateral Hip
Basic
• AP Bilateral (Pelvis)
   or
   AP Unilateral (Hip)
• **Lateral (Unilateral Hip)**
   - Frog-leg (non-trauma)
   - Axiolateral (trauma)

Structures Best Shown:
Lateral view of acetabulum and femoral head, neck and trochanteric area.

Technical Factors:
• Film Size - 10 x 12 in. (24 x 30 cm), crosswise.
• Moving or stationary grid.
• 90±5 kVp range.

Patient Position:
• Patient partially obliqued with pillow for head and a large support under unaffected knee.

Shielding: Place shield over gonads and pelvic area insuring affected hip is not obscured.

Part Position:
• Flex knee on affected side as thigh is drawn up to at least a 45° angle position.
• Abduct thigh and rotate toward affected side as needed to bring thigh in contact with table. (This is a very uncomfortable position, do not ask patient to remain in this position longer than necessary.)
• Center affected femoral neck to midline of table and/or mid point of film. (Femoral neck is 2.5 in. or 6-7 cm inferior and perpendicular to mid point of line between ASIS and symphysis pubis.)

Central Ray:
• CR **perpendicular** to film, directed to **mid-femoral neck.** (Center of film.)
• Minimum 40 in. (102 cm) SID.

Collimation: Collimate closely on four sides to area of interest.

Respiration: Suspend respiration during exposure.

Alternate Projection: A 20-25° cephalic CR angle is sometimes preferred wherein the greater trochanter will not superimpose as much of the proximal neck area.

Evaluation Criteria:
• Proximal 1/3 of femur should be visualized along with hip joint and acetabulum.
• The greater trochanter will superimpose most of femoral neck area.
• Lesser trochanter will be partially seen more distally than the greater trochanter projecting beyond the lower or medial margin of femur.
• Optimum exposure will visualize the margins of the femoral head and the acetabulum through overlying pelvic structures without overexposing other parts of the proximal femur. Trabecular markings of proximal femur should appear clear and sharp.

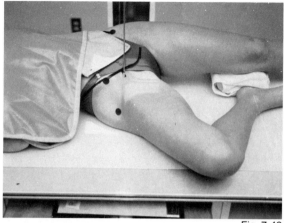

Unilateral Frog-leg position – No Angle   Fig. 7-42

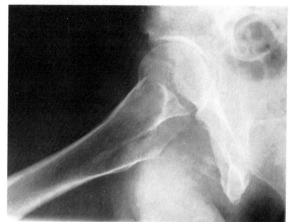

Unilateral Frog-leg – No Angle   Fig. 7-43

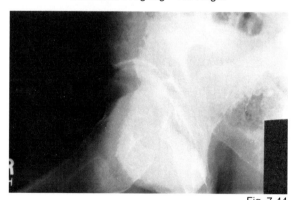

Unilateral Frog-leg 20-25° Cephalic Angle   Fig. 7-44

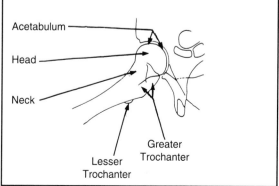

Acetabulum
Head
Neck
Greater Trochanter
Lesser Trochanter

Unilateral Frog-leg – No Angle   Fig. 7-45

• Axiolateral Position (Possible Trauma Projection)
(Inferosuperior Projection)
(Danelius-Miller Method)

Unilateral Hip
Basic
• AP Bilateral (Pelvis)
   or
   AP Unilateral (Hip)
• **Lateral (Unilateral Hip)**
   - Frog-leg (non-trauma)
   - **Axiolateral (trauma)**

Structures Best Shown:
Lateral view of acetabulum and femoral head, neck and trochanteric area.

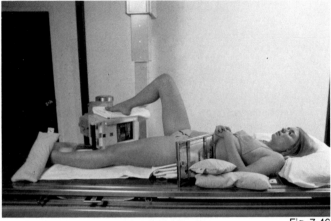
Axiolateral Hip   Fig. 7-46

Technical Factors:
• Film Size - 8 x 10 in. (18 x 24 cm), crosswise.
• Stationary grid cassette (lead strips must be in horizontal direction).
• 90±5 kVp range.

Patient Position: (May be done on stretcher if patient cannot be moved.)
• Patient supine, pillow for head.
• Elevate pelvis 2 in. or 5 cm if possible by placing supports under pelvis (more important for thin patient).

Shielding: Shield gonads as much as possible without obscuring essential anatomy.

Part Position:
• Flex and elevate unaffected leg so thigh is in near vertical position. Support in this position. If foot is rested on collimator as shown, provide folded sheets or padding to prevent burning of foot or coming in contact with electrical wires.
• Check to insure **no rotation** of pelvis (equal ASIS-table distance).
• Place cassette in crease above iliac crest and adjust so it is **parallel to femoral neck** and **perpendicular to CR.** Use cassette holder if available.
• Internally rotate affected leg 15-20° **unless contraindicated** by possible fracture or other pathology wherein any rotation should be performed **only** by a physician.

Central Ray:
• CR **perpendicular** to femoral neck and to film.
• Minimum 40 in. (102 cm) SID.

Collimation: Tight collimation on four sides to area of interest.

Respiration: Suspend respiration during exposure.

NOTE: This is a common projection for trauma, surgery, post surgery or other patients who cannot move or rotate legs.

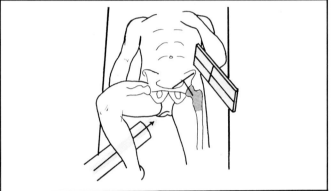
Axiolateral Hip   Fig. 7-47

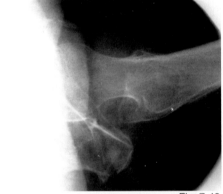
Axiolateral Hip   Fig. 7-48

Evaluation Criteria:
• Entire femoral head, neck and trochanter should be seen centered to mid film area.
• Only the most distal part of femoral neck should be superimposed by greater trochanter.
• Only a small part if any of lesser trochanter is visualized with inversion of affected leg.
• Optimum exposure will visualize femoral head and neck without overexposing proximal femoral shaft.

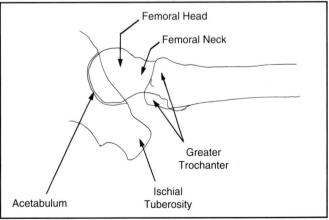
Femoral Head
Femoral Neck
Greater Trochanter
Ischial Tuberosity
Acetabulum
Axiolateral Hip   Fig. 7-49

• Modified Axiolateral (Possible Trauma Projection)
(Clements-Nakayama Method)[1]

Unilateral Hip
Optional
• **Modified Axiolateral**
 (Clements-Nakayama)

Structures Best Shown:
Lateral view of acetabulum and femoral head, neck and trochanteric area.

NOTE: This can be used with bilateral arthroplasty (surgery for plastic hip joints) with limited movement possible of both affected and unaffected legs and hips.

Technical Factors:
• Film Size - 8 x 10 in. (18 x 24 cm), lengthwise.
• Stationary grid cassette.
 (Cassette on edge with 15° tilt, grid lines parallel to table top.)
• 90±5 kVp range.

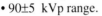

Patient Position:
• Supine, near edge of table (Bucky tray side) with both legs fully extended.
• Provide pillow for head, arms across upper chest.

Shielding: Shield gonads as much as possible without obscuring essential anatomy.

Part Position:
• Leg remains in neutral (anatomical) position. (15° posterior CR angle compensates for internal leg rotation.)
• Rest cassette on extended Bucky tray which places the bottom edge of cassette about 2 in. (5 cm) below the level of the table top.
• Tilt cassette about 15° from vertical and adjust alignment of cassette to insure that face of cassette is **perpendicular** to CR to prevent grid cutoff.

Central Ray:
• CR **perpendicular to** and **centered to femoral neck**, angled downward (posteriorly) **15°.**
• Cassette centered to CR.
• Minimum 40 in. (102 cm) SID.

Collimation: Collimate closely on four sides to area of interest.

Respiration: Suspend respiration during exposure.

Evaluation Criteria:
• Entire femoral head, neck and trochanters should be seen centered to mid film area.
• Femoral head and neck should be seen in profile with only minimal superimposition by greater trochanter.
• Lesser trochanter is seen projecting below femoral shaft. (With leg in neutral or anatomical position the amount of lesser trochanter seen will be minimal but with increased external rotation of leg this will increase.)
• Optimum exposure will visualize femoral head and neck without overexposing proximal femoral shaft.

[1] Clements, RS, Nakayama, HK; **Radiographic Methods in Total Hip Arthroplasty**; Radiologic Technology, 51: 589-600;1980.

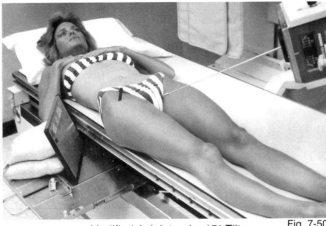
Modified Axiolateral – 15° Tilt   Fig. 7-50

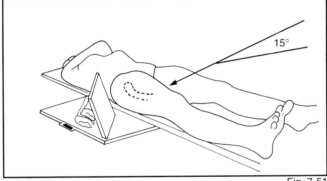
Modified Axiolateral   Fig. 7-51

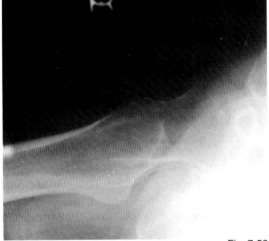
Modified Axiolateral   Fig. 7-52

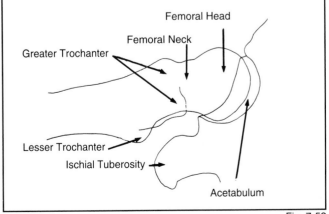
Modified Axiolateral   Fig. 7-53

• AP Projection

Pelvis
Basic
• AP

Structures Best Shown:
Pelvic girdle, L5, sacrum and coccyx, femoral heads, necks and greater trochanters.

Technical Factors:
- Film Size - 14 x 17 in. (35 x 43 cm), crosswise.
- Moving or stationary grid.
- 90±5 kVp range.

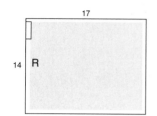

Patient Position:
- Patient supine, arms at sides or across upper chest, provide pillow for head and support for under knees.

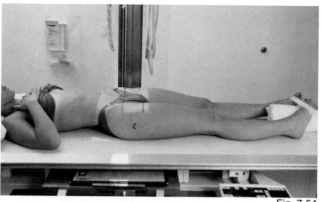

Patient and Part Position – AP Pelvis   Fig. 7-54

Shielding: Gonadal shielding should be done on all males of reproductive age. Ovarian shielding on females however is generally not possible without obscuring essential pelvic anatomy (unless interest is in areas of hips only).

Part Position:
- Align midsagittal plane of patient to center line of table and/or cassette.
- Insure that pelvis is **not rotated**; the distance from table-top to each ASIS should be equal.
- Separate legs and feet, then **internally rotate** long axes of feet and lower limbs **15-20°**. (May need to place sandbag between heels and tape top of feet together or use additional sandbags against feet to retain this position.) **Warning:** Do **not** attempt to internally rotate legs if a hip fracture or dislocation is suspected. Take with affected leg "as is".
- Center cassette to entire pelvis by aligning CR and the midline of cassette to a point midway between the level of the ASIS and the superior border of the symphysis pubis. (See NOTE.)

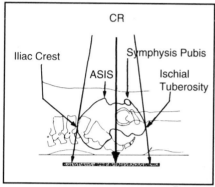

Fig. 7-55
CR and Pelvis Alignment

Central Ray:
- CR **perpendicular**, directed to the **center of film** (mid point of pelvis).
- Minimum 40 in. (102 cm) SID.

Collimation: Collimate to lateral skin margins and to upper and lower film borders.

Respiration: Suspend respiration during exposure.

NOTE: •If the area of interest is primarily in the hips and proximal femora, it is suggested that the center of the film be lowered to the level of the greater trochanters to center the hip joints and include more of the proximal femora.
  • The higher kVp range of 90±5 is recommended to reduce patient dosage.

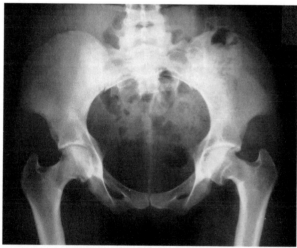

AP Pelvis   Fig. 7-56

Evaluation Criteria:
- Entire pelvis and proximal femora should be included and centered on film.
- Collimation borders will be minimal on larger patients. Smaller patients should show equal lateral collimation borders just lateral to greater trochanters.
- **No rotation:** The iliac ala or wings should appear symmetrical. The right and left ischial spines should appear equal in size as well as the two obturator foramina.
- Lesser trochanters should not be visible at all or only tips be visible, and greater trochanters should appear equal in size and shape.
- Optimum exposure will visualize L5 and sacrum area and margins of the femoral heads and acetabula as seen through overlying pelvic structures without overexposing the ischium and pubic bones. Trabecular markings of proximal femora and pelvic structures will appear clear and sharp.

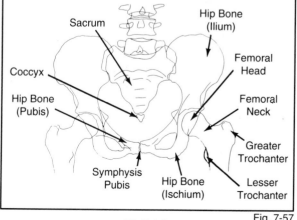

AP Pelvis   Fig. 7-57

• Bilateral "Frog-leg" Position
(Modified Cleaves Method)

Pelvis
Optional
• **Bilateral Frog-leg**
(non-trauma)
• Ant. Oblique
- Acetabulum
• AP Axial (Semi-axial)
- Ant. Pelvic Bones
• Post. Oblique - Ilium

Structures Best Shown:
Femoral heads, necks, and trochanteric areas on one radiograph for purpose of comparison. Entire pelvis is shown.

Technical Factors:
• Film Size - 14 x 17 in. (35 x 43 cm), crosswise.
• Moving or stationary grid.
• 75-80 kVp range.

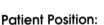

Patient Position:
• Patient supine, pillow for head, arms across upper chest.

Shielding: Shield gonads without obscuring essential anatomy (see NOTE).

Part Position:
• Align patient to midline of table and/or cassette.
• Pelvis must not be rotated (ASIS-table distance the same on both sides).
• Center midline of cassette to the level of femoral heads or 1 in. (2.5 cm) cephalad to symphysis pubis.
• Flex both hips and knees as far as is comfortable.
• Finalize all positioning, shield placement, tube placement, etc. and be ready to make exposure immediately after patient assumes this final uncomfortable position.
• Place the plantar surfaces of feet together and abduct both thighs as far as possible (40° from vertical if possible but more importantly insure that **both** thighs are **abducted** the **same amount**).

Central Ray:
• CR **perpendicular** to film, directed to a point **1 in. (2.5 cm) cephalad to symphysis pubis.**
• Minimum 40 in. (102 cm) SID.

Collimation: Collimate to film borders on four sides.

Respiration: Suspend respiration during exposure.

NOTE: • This position is frequently done on non-trauma pediatric patients for possible congenital hip deformities wherein carefully placed gonadal shields should be used for both male and females insuring that hip joints are not covered.

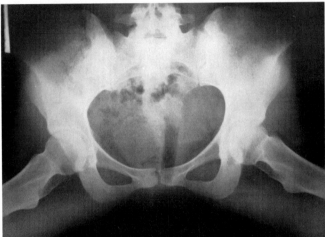

Bilateral "Frog-leg"   Fig. 7-58

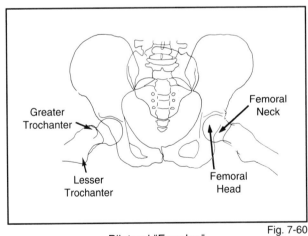

Bilateral "Frog-leg"   Fig. 7-59
(Courtesy of Kathy Martensen, R.T.)

Greater Trochanter

Lesser Trochanter

Femoral Neck

Femoral Head

Bilateral "Frog-leg"   Fig. 7-60

Evaluation Criteria:
• The pelvic girdle should be centered to the film or collimation field from right to left with the mid point being at about 1 in. (2.5 cm) superior to the symphysis pubis.
• **No rotation**, as evidenced by the symmetrical appearance of the pelvic bones, especially the ala of the ilium and the two obturator foramina.
• The lesser trochanters should appear equal in size as projected beyond the lower or medial margin of the femora.

• The femoral heads, necks and greater trochanters should appear symmetrical if both thighs were abducted equally.
• Optimum exposure will visualize the margins of the femoral head and the acetabulum through overlying pelvic structures without overexposing other parts of the proximal femur or pelvic structures. Trabecular markings of greater trochanter and neck areas will appear clear and sharp.

• Anterior Oblique – Acetabulum
(Teufel Method)

Pelvis
Optional
• Bilateral Frog-leg
  (non-trauma)
• **Ant. Oblique**
  - Acetabulum
• AP Axial (Semi-axial)
  - Ant. Pelvic Bones
• Post. Oblique - Ilium

Structures Best Shown:
Acetabulum and femoral head margin including the fovea capitis.

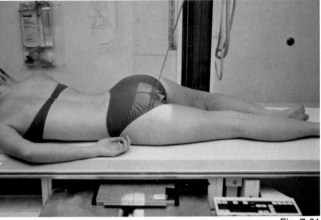

LAO Acetabulum   Fig. 7-61

Technical Factors:
• Film Size - 8x10in. (18x24cm), lengthwise.
• Moving or stationary grid.
• 75-80 kVp range.

Patient Position:
• Patient semiprone, pillow for head, **affected side down,** supported by partially flexed knee and arm of elevated side.

Shielding: Carefully shield gonads without obscuring area of acetabula and femoral heads.

Part Position:
• Adjust the patient into a 35- 40°anterior oblique (anterior pelvis surface and thorax 35- 40° from table top).
• Align femoral head area to midline of table and/or cassette. (Femoral head area is approximately 2 in. or 5 cm lateral of midsagittal plane, or 2 in. medial to ASIS of affected side.)
• Center cassette to about 1 in. (2.5 cm) superior to level of greater trochanter, or about 3 in. (8 cm) superior to the level of the ischial tuberosity. (Palpating this may be uncomfortable for patient.)

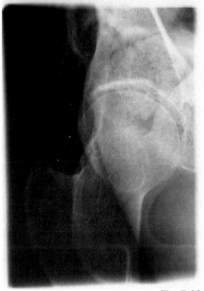

LAO Acetabulum   Fig. 7-62

Central Ray:
•CR **12° cephalic,** directed to **acetabulum** (center of film).
• 40 in. (102 cm) SID.

Collimation: Collimate closely on four sides to area of interest.

Respiration: Suspend respiration during exposure.

Evaluation Criteria:
• Acetabulum should be centered to film and/or collimation field.
• Femoral head and neck should appear in profile with superior articular margin of head including the area of the fovea capitis clearly defined, as well as the margins of the acetabulum and the joint space.
• Optimum exposure should clearly demonstrate the acetabulum and femoral head region. Trabecular markings of distal head and the neck area should appear clear and sharp.

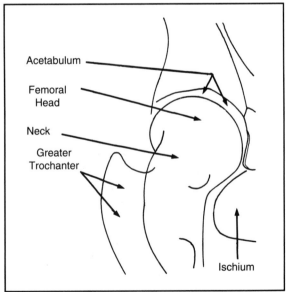

Acetabulum

Femoral
Head

Neck

Greater
Trochanter

Ischium

LAO Acetabulum   Fig. 7-63

• AP Axial Projection – (Anterior Pelvic Bones)

Pelvis
Optional
• Bilateral Frog-leg
  (non-trauma)
• Ant. Oblique
  - Acetabulum
• **AP Axial (Semi-axial)**
  - Ant. Pelvic Bones
• Post. Oblique - Ilium

Structures Best Shown:
Elongated and magnified view of pubic and ischial rami.

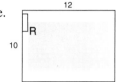

Technical Factors:
• Film Size - 10 x 12 in. (24 x 30 cm), crosswise.
• Moving or stationary grid.
• 90±5 kVp range.

Patient Position:
• Patient supine, pillow for head, legs extended with support under knees for comfort.

Shielding: Gonadal shielding may be done on males with care taken not to obscure essential anatomy. Ovarian shielding for females is more difficult without obscuring area of interest.

Part Position:
• Align midsagittal plane to midline of table and/or cassette.
• Insure **no rotation** of pelvis (ASIS-table distance the same on both sides).

Central Ray:
• Angle CR **cephalad, 20-30° for males** and **30-45° for females.** (These different angles are due to differences in shapes between male and female pelves.)
• Direct CR to a midline point **2 in. (5 cm) distal to** the superior border of the **symphysis pubis**.
• Align center of cassette to CR.
• Minimum 40 in. (102 cm) SID.

Collimation: Collimate closely on four sides to area of interest.

Respiration: Suspend respiration during exposure.

Evaluation Criteria:
• Elongated and magnified pubic and ischial bones superimposed over the sacrum and coccyx should be centered to film and/or collimation field.
• Lateral margins of collimation field should extend equally on both sides to just lateral to the femoral heads and acetabula.
• **No rotation**: Obturator foramina should appear equal in size and shape.
• Optimum exposure will visualize the femoral head margins and the acetabula through overlying pelvic structures without overexposing other parts of the pubis and ischial bones. With no part motion the trabecular markings of pubic and ischial bones will appear clear and sharp.

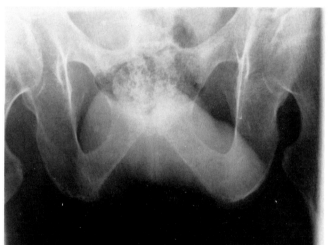

AP Axial (Semiaxial) of
Anterior Pelvic Bones

Fig. 7-64

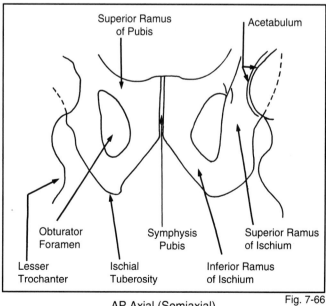

AP Axial (Semiaxial)

Fig. 7-65

Superior Ramus
of Pubis

Acetabulum

Obturator
Foramen

Symphysis
Pubis

Superior Ramus
of Ischium

Lesser
Trochanter

Ischial
Tuberosity

Inferior Ramus
of Ischium

AP Axial (Semiaxial)

Fig. 7-66

• Posterior Oblique – Ilium

Pelvis
Optional
• Bilateral Frog-leg
  (non-trauma)
• Ant. Oblique
  - Acetabulum
• AP Axial (Semi-axial)
  - Ant. Pelvic Bones
• **Post. Oblique - Ilium**

Structures Best Shown:
Broad surface of iliac wing and acetabulum in profile.

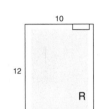

Technical Factors:
• Film Size -10 x 12 in. (24 x 30 cm), lengthwise.
• Moving or stationary grid.
• 75-80 kVp range.

Patient Position:
• Patient supine, pillow for head.

Shielding: Carefully place gonadal shielding for males. Ovarian shielding on females is not possible because such shielding would directly obscure area of interest.

Part Position:
• Turn into 40°posterior oblique position, **affected side down**.
• Place support under elevated pelvis and ask patient to reach across and hold onto edge of table to maintain this position.
• Center ilium being radiographed to center of table and/or cassette. (Note CR location as described below.)

Central Ray:
• CR perpendicular to film, directed to **mid ilium** or **center of film**.
  - Longitudinal midline of ilium is approximately 2 in. (5 cm) medial to ASIS.
  - Transverse midline of ilium is at the level of ASIS.
• Minimum 40 in. (102 cm) SID.

Collimation: Collimate on four sides to area of interest.

Respiration: Suspend respiration during exposure.

Evaluation Criteria:
• Entire ilium should be visualized and centered to film and/or collimation field. The full acetabulum should be included on lower margin and the sacrum on the medial margin.
• Broad surface view of wing of ilium should be seen without rotation.
• Optimum exposure should clearly visualize sacroiliac joint and acetabulum regions without overexposing lateral portion of iliac wing. Trabecular markings of ilium should be clear and sharp where not superimposed by bowel or other abdominal structures.

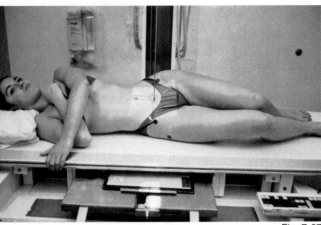

RPO Ilium   Fig. 7-67

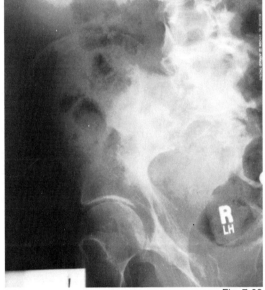

RPO Ilium   Fig. 7-68

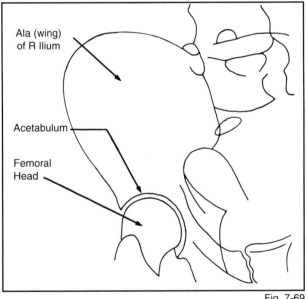

Ala (wing) of R Ilium

Acetabulum

Femoral Head

RPO Ilium   Fig. 7-69

• AP Axial Projection

Sacroiliac Joints
• **AP Axial**
• Post. Obliques
Optional
• Ant. Obliques

Structures Best Shown:
Sacroiliac joints, L5-S1 junction, sacrum and coccyx.

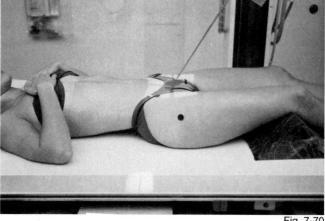

AP Axial

Fig. 7-70

NOTE: The urinary bladder should be emptied before beginning this procedure. It is also desirable to have the lower colon free of gas and fecal material which may require a cleaning enema as ordered by a physician.

Technical Factors:
• Film Size - 10 x 12 in. (24 x 30 cm), lengthwise.
• Moving or stationary grid.
• 90±5 kVp range.
  (Increase 6-10 kVp due to axial projection.)

Patient Position:
• Patient supine, pillow for head, legs extended with support under knees for comfort.

Shielding: Carefully place gonadal shielding for males. Ovarian shielding on females is not possible because such shielding would directly obscure area of interest.

Part Position:
• Align midsagittal plane to midline of table and/or cassette.
• Insure **no rotation** of pelvis (ASIS-table distance the same on both sides).

Central Ray:
• Angle **CR 30-35° cephalad** (generally males require about 30° and females or those with an increase in the lumbosacral curve require nearer 35°).
• Direct CR to a midline point **midway between the level of the ASIS and the symphysis pubis.** This is also about 1.5 to 2 in. (4-5 cm) below or distal to a bisecting line between the ASIS's.
• Align center of cassette to CR.
• Minimum 40 in. (102 cm) SID.

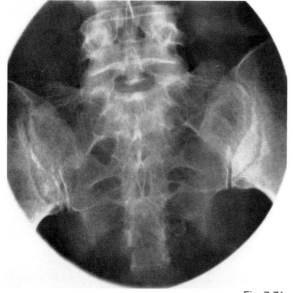

AP Axial

Fig. 7-71

Collimation: Collimate to area of interest but insure that side margins do not cut off sacroiliac joints.

Respiration: Suspend respiration during exposure.

Alternate AP Pelvis: Some departmental routines indicate a full AP pelvis with no CR angle as part of a SI joint routine in addition to or in place of this AP axial.

Alternate PA Projection: If patient cannot assume the supine position, this can also be taken as a PA with patient prone using a 30-35° **caudal** angle. The CR would be centered to the level of the iliac crest.

Evaluation Criteria:
• The sacroiliac joints and the first two segments of the sacrum should be centered to the collimation field and/or film.
• The sacroiliac joint spaces and the L5-S1 junction should appear open indicating correct CR angulation.
• Optimum exposure should visualize the margins of the sacroiliac joint spaces.

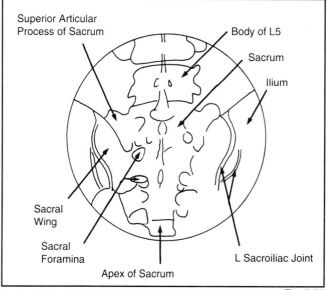

AP Axial

Fig. 7-72

239

• Posterior Oblique Positions (LPO and RPO)
(Bilateral)

Sacroiliac Joints
• AP Axial
• **Post. Obliques**
Optional
• Ant. Obliques

Structures Best Shown:
Sacroiliac joints **farthest from film**.
Both sides are done for comparison.

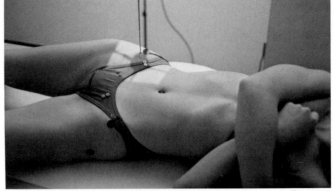
Posterior Oblique Position (LPO)   Fig. 7-73

Technical Factors:
• Film Size - 2 each 10 x 12 in. (24 x 30 cm),
  lengthwise.
• Moving or stationary grid.
• 90±5 kVp range.

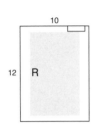

Patient Position:
• Patient supine, pillow for head.

Shielding: Carefully shield gonads without obscuring
  sacroiliac joint area. (Can readily be done on males but
  requires more care with females.)

Part Position:
• Turn into **25-30°** posterior oblique, **side of interest is el-
  evated**.
• **LPO** will visualize **right joint**.
• **RPO** will visualize **left joint**.
• Use some angle measuring device to insure correct and
  consistent angles on **both** obliques.
• Place support under elevated hip and flex elevated knee.
  Ask patient to reach across and grasp edge of table to help
  maintain this position.
• Align joint of interest to midline of table and/or cassette.
  (Note CR entrance point as described below.)
• Center film to level of ASIS.

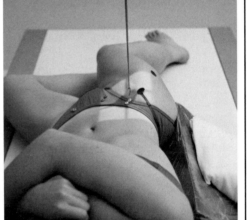
Fig. 7-74
Posterior Oblique Position (LPO)   Fig. 7-75

Central Ray:
• CR **perpendicular**, directed to a point **1 in. (2 .5
  cm) medial** to upside ASIS. (See NOTE for
  optional cephalic angle.)
• Minimum 40 in. (102 cm) SID.

Collimation: Collimate closely on four sides to
  area of interest.

Respiration: Suspend respiration during exposure.

NOTE: To demonstrate the inferior or distal part of
  the joint more clearly, the CR may be angled 15-
  20° cephalad.

Evaluation Criteria:
• Joint space on side of interest should appear open.
• The ala of the ilium and the sacrum should have no
  overlap indicating the correct obliquity. (Overlap
  indicates too much obliquity.)
• Optimum exposure will clearly visualize the
  margins of the joint space along its entirety.

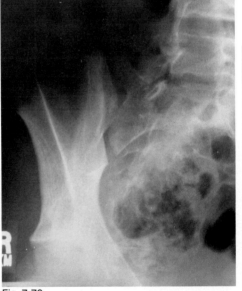
Fig. 7-76

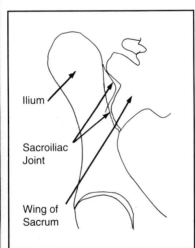
Ilium

Sacroiliac
Joint

Wing of
Sacrum

Posterior Oblique Position
(Courtesty of Kathy Martensen, R.T.)   Fig. 7-77

• Anterior Oblique Positions (LAO and RAO)

Sacroiliac Joints
• AP Axial (Semi-axial)
• Post. Obliques
Optional
• **Ant. Obliques**

Structures Best Shown:
Profile view of sacroiliac joint **closest to film. Both sides** are done for comparison.

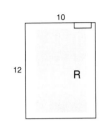

Technical Factors:
- Film Size - 2 each 10 x 12 in. (24 x 30 cm), lengthwise.
- Moving or stationary grid.
- 90±5 kVp range.

Patient Position:
- Patient in semiprone position, **affected side down**, pillow for head.
- Flex elevated knee, place elevated arm in front of head with opposite arm down behind back.

Shielding: Carefully place gonadal shielding for males. Ovarian shielding on females is more difficult without obscuring area of interest.

Part Position:
- Adjust body into 25-30° anterior oblique, **side of interest down.**
- **LAO** will visualize **left** joint.
- **RAO** will visualize **right** joint.
- Plane between ASIS should form a 25-30° angle with table top.
- Align joint of interest to midline of table and/or cassette. (Note CR entrance point as described below.)
- Center film to level of ASIS.

Central Ray:
- CR **perpendicular**, directed to a point **1 in. (2.5 cm) lateral** (below) the **vertebral spinous processes at level of the ASIS.** This will exit at a point 1 in. (2.5 cm) medial to downside ASIS. (See NOTE for optional caudal angle.)
- Miniumum 40 in. (102 cm) SID.

Collimation: Collimate closely on four sides to area of interest.

Respiration: Suspend respiration during exposure.

NOTE: To best demonstrate the inferior or distal aspect of the joint, the CR may be angled 15-20° caudad.

Evaluation Criteria:
- Joint space closest to the film should appear open.
- The ala of the ilium and the sacrum should have no overlap indicating the correct obliquity. (Overlap indicates too much obliquity.)
- Optimum exposure will clearly visualize the margins of the joint space along its entirety.

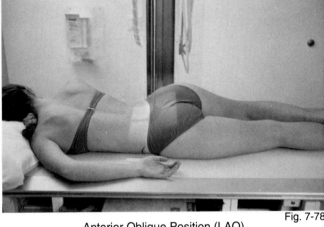

Anterior Oblique Position (LAO)

Fig. 7-78

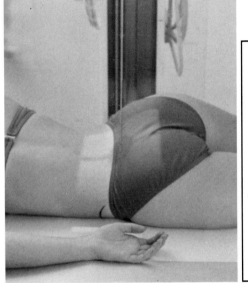

Fig. 7-79

Anterior Oblique Position
(LAO)

Fig. 7-80

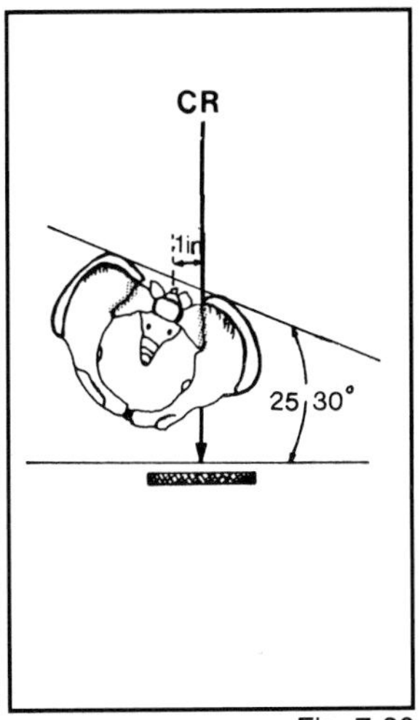

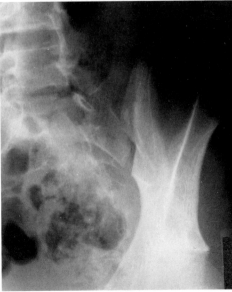

Fig. 7-81

Anterior Oblique Position

Fig. 7-82

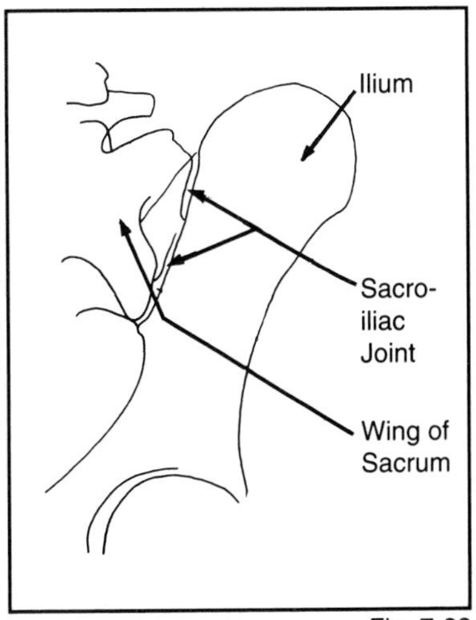

Ilium

Sacro-
iliac
Joint

Wing of
Sacrum

Chapter 8
Radiographic Anatomy and Positioning of the
Coccyx, Sacrum and Lumbar Spine

Contributions by: Alex Backus, MS, RT(R)

Contents

Part I Radiographic Anatomy

Vertebral Column

The vertebral *(ver´te-bral)* column is a complex succession of many bones called **vertebrae** *(ver´te-bre)*, singular is **vertebra** *(ver´te-brah)*. It provides a flexible supporting column for the trunk and head; and also transmits the weight of the trunk and upper body to the lower limbs. This column is located in the midsagittal plane, forming the posterior or dorsal aspect of the bony trunk of the body.

Spinal cord: The vertebral column encloses and protects the spinal cord which begins with the medulla oblogata of the brain. It passes through the foramen magnum of the skull and continues to the **first lumbar vertebra** where it tapers off. The spinal canal containing certain sacral nerves, (and also filled with cerebrospinal fluid) continues on into the sacrum.

Intervertebral Discs: The typical adult vertebrae are separated by tough but elastic **intervertebral discs**. These cushion-like discs are tightly bound to the vertebrae for spinal stability but also allow for flexibility and movement of the vertebral column.

Divisions

The entire vertebral column is divided by regions into five groups or divisions. Within each of these five regions there are a certain number of vertebrae that have distinctive characteristics of that particular region.

(1) Cervical Vertebrae: The first seven have similarities that group them as **cervical vertebrae**. While there may be a slight variation in the height of each vertebra from one individual to another, the average human has seven cervical vertebrae.

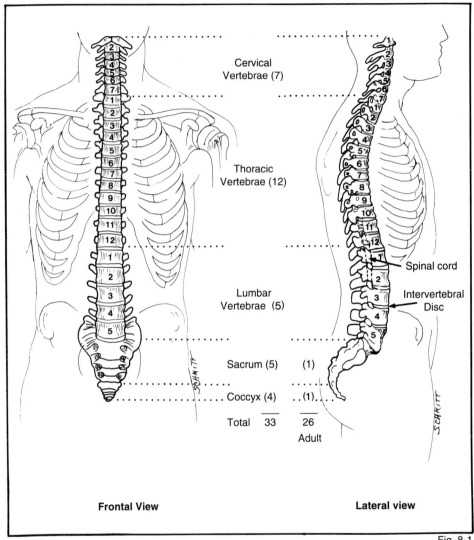

Cervical Vertebrae (7)

Thoracic Vertebrae (12)

Spinal cord

Lumbar Vertebrae (5)

Intervertebral Disc

Sacrum (5) (1)

Coccyx (4) (1)

Total 33 26
Adult

Frontal View

Lateral view

Vertebral Column

Fig. 8-1

(2) Thoracic Vertebrae: The next twelve vertebrae each connect to a pair of ribs. Since there are twelve pairs of ribs, there are **twelve thoracic vertebrae**. An older and incorrect term for the thoracic vertebrae is dorsal vertebrae. However, all of the vertebrae, being located on the posterior or dorsal aspect of the body, could correctly be called dorsal vertebrae; therefore, the twelve vertebrae of the upper back should correctly be called thoracic vertebrae. The specific anatomy of the cervical and thoracic vertebrae will be covered in chapter 9 which follows.

(3) Lumbar Vertebrae: The largest and most massive individual vertebrae are the **five lumbar vertebrae**. These vertebrae are the largest and strongest in the vertebral column because the entire body weight as supported by the vertebrae increases toward the lower end of the column. For this reason the discs between the lower lumbar vertebrae are common sites for stress and pathology creating pain and back problems, especially for mammals such as humans who walk in an upright position.

(4 and 5) Sacrum and Coccyx: Each of the vertebrae in the cervical, thoracic and lumbar regions forms as a separate vertebra in the child, and is retained as a separate bone in the adult. The sacrum *(sa´krum)* and coccyx *(kok´siks)*, however are different. In children there are **five sacral** (sa´kral) **segments** and from **three to five coccygeal** *(kok-sij´e-al)* **segments**. Some references suggest **four** coccygeal segments as normal, for an average total of **33 separate bones** in the vertebral column of a child.

In the adult however the sacrum and coccyx tend to fuse into two single bones. Counting the sacrum and coccyx as single bones, the adult vertebral column therefore is composed of **26 separate bones**.

Spinal Curvatures

The vertebral column forms a series of anteroposterior curves. These curves, as viewed from the side or on a lateral radiograph, are illustrated in *Fig. 8-2*. Soon after birth the **thoracic** and **sacral** (pelvic) **curves** begin to develop. These two posterior **convex** curves are called **primary curves.** As a child begins to raise his head and later begins to sit up, a **compensatory** or **secondary curve** forms in the opposite direction in the cervical region. This **cervical curve** is the least pronounced of the four curves, and is described as a posterior **concave** curve. (The terms concave and convex, meaning hollow and arched respectivly, are in relationship to the posterior surface.)

The fourth and final curve to form is the **lumbar curvature**, also a **concave** curve. This lumbar curvature develops when the child learns to walk. Both of the lower curves, the lumbar and sacral (pelvic) curvatures are usually more pronounced in the female than they are in the male.

These primary and secondary or compensatory curvatures are normal and serve an important function by increasing the strength of the vertebral column and by helping maintain balance along a center line of gravity in the upright position.

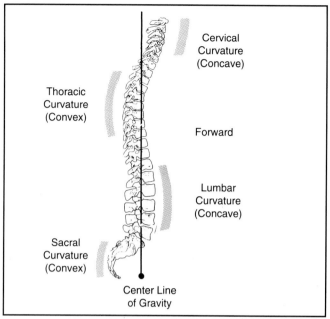

Normal Adult Curvature (Side View)   Fig. 8-2

Lordosis

The term lordosis *(lor-dō'sis)*, meaning swayback, is a condition wherein the **lumbar curvature is exaggerated**. This **abnormal increased concavity** of the lumbar spine, may result from pregnancy or extreme obesity by the increased weight of the abdominal contents. It may also be caused by poor posture, rickets or tuberculosis of the spine.

Kyphosis

Kyphosis *(ki-fō'sis)* is an **abnormal** or **exaggerated thoracic "humpback" curvature** with **increased convexity**, in reference to the posterior. This greater than normal curvature of the thoracic spine may also be caused by poor posture, rickets or tuberculosis of the spine.

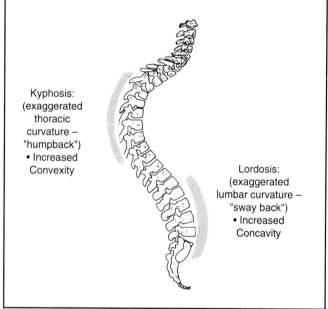

Lordosis – Kyphosis   Fig. 8-3

Scoliosis

An abnormal or exaggerated sideways or **lateral curvature** is called **scoliosis** *(sko˝le-ō'sis)*. If the spine is viewed from the back (illustrated in *Fig. 8-4*), the vertebral column is usually near straight with little lateral curvature. Occasionally, there is a slight lateral curvature in the upper thoracic region of a healthy adult. This curvature is usually associated with the dominant extremity, so the curvature is convex to the right in a right-handed person and convex to the left in a left-handed person.

A more serious type of problem occurs when there is a pronounced S-shaped lateral curvature. This deformity, is termed scoliosis and may cause severe deformity of the entire thorax. The effect of scoliosis is more obvious if it occurs in the lower vertebral column where it may create a tilting of the pelvis with a resulting effect on the lower limbs, creating a "limp" or uneven walk.

Summary: Lordosis refers to an abnormal or exaggerated lumbar or "swayback" type curvature with increased convexity. **Kyphosis** describes an abnormal or exaggerated thoracic or "humpback" type curvature with increased concavity, and **scoliosis** refers to an abnormal pronounced sideways or lateral curvature.

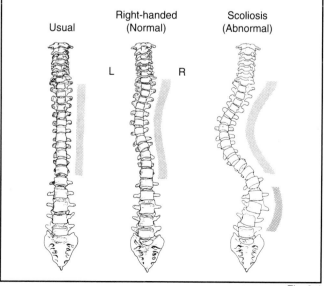

Scoliosis – Lateral Curvatures   Fig. 8-4
(Posterior View)

Typical Vertebra

Although the vertebrae in the different regions vary in size and shape, all are similar in basic structure. A typical vertebra consists of two main parts as follows:

(1) Body
The body is the thick, weight-bearing anterior part of the vertebra. Its superior and inferior surface are flat and rough for attachment of the intervertebral discs.

(2) Vertebral Arch
The second part of a typical vertebra consists of a ring or arch of bone extending posteriorly. With the body anteriorly, the vertebral arch forms a circular opening containing the spinal cord. This opening is called the **vertebral foramen.**

When a number of vertebrae are stacked, as they are in the normal articulated vertebral column, the succession of vertebral foramina forms a tubelike opening along the complete length of the spine. This opening, called the **vertebral** (spinal) **canal**, encloses and protects the spinal cord.

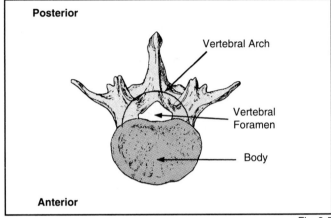

Typical Vertebra – Superior View   Fig. 8-5

Superior View: Part of the vertebral arch is formed by two projections, termed **pedicles**, *(ped´i-kuls)* that extend posteriorly from either side of the body. Pedicle is a Latin term meaning "little foot. "The pedicles form most of the sides of the vertebral arch. The posterior part of the vertebral arch is formed by two flat layers of bone termed laminae. Each **lamina** *(lam´i-na)* extends posteriorly from each pedicle to unite in the midline.

Extending laterally from approximately the junction of each pedicle and lamina is a projection termed the **transverse process**. At the midline junction of the two laminae, extending posteriorly, is another process called the **spinous process**. The spinous processes are the most posterior extensions of the vertebrae and can often be palpated along the dorsal surface of the neck and back.

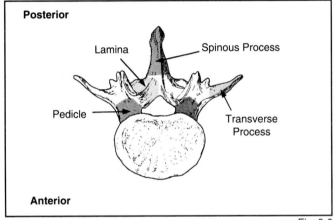

Typical Vertebra – Superior View   Fig. 8-6

Lateral View: A typical vertebra as seen from the side is illustrated in *Fig. 8-7*. The large **body** is most anterior and the **spinous process** is most posterior. Extending posteriorly from the body is one **pedicle**, which terminates in the area of the **transverse process**. Continuing posteriorly from the origin of the transverse process is one **lamina.**

Along the upper surface of each pedicle is a notch termed the **superior vertebral notch**, and along the lower surface of each pedicle is another deeper notch termed the **inferior vertebral notch.**

Summary: The typical vertebra has **two pedicles** and **two laminae** that form the vertebral arch and enclose the vertebral foramen containing the spinal cord, **two transverse processes** extending laterally, and **one spinous process** extending posteriorly.

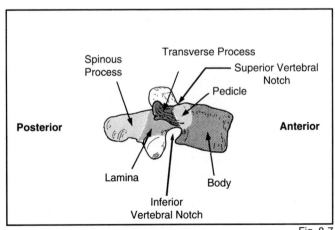

Typical Vertebra – Lateral View   Fig. 8-7

Typical Vertebra continued

Articular Processes

Each typical vertebra has **four articular processes** projecting from approximately the area of the junction of the pedicles and laminae. As seen from the side in *Fig. 8-8*, the process projecting upward is called the **superior articular process** and the process projecting downward is the **inferior articular process.** Two similar processes are also found on the opposite side of the typical vertebra. The importance of these processes becomes apparent when vertebrae are stacked together to form the vertebral column. The two superior articular processes of one vertebra articulate with the two inferior articular processes of the vertebra above, forming joints called **zygapophyseal** *(zi″gah-po-fiz′e-al)* **joints**. In earlier literature these were called apophyseal *(ah″po-fiz′e-al)* joints.

Zygapophyseal (apophyseal) Joints

Since there are two superior and two inferior articular processes on each vertebra, there are also two zygapophyseal joints between any two vertebrae, one on each side. It is often necessary to demonstrate these joints on certain radiographs of the vertebral column.

The term **facet** *(fas′et)* is sometimes used interchangeably with the term zygapophyseal joint; however, this is incorrect because the facet is actually only the **articulating surface** of the superior and inferior articular processes. The superior facets or articulating surfaces are only seen on either a posterior or oblique view. The inferior facets are seen on anterior, oblique and lateral views.

The intervertebral foramina and zygapophyseal joints must be demonstrated radiographically by the appropriate position in each of the three major portions of the vertebral column.

Intervertebral Foramina

In the articulated vertebral column, the inferior vertebral notches of the vertebra above and the superior vertebral notches of the vertebra below form the important openings, the **intervertebral foramina.** Between every two vertebrae there are two intervertebral foramina, one on each side. It is through these intervertebral foramina that spinal nerves and blood vessels are transmitted.

Intervertebral Disc

Intervertebral discs are found between the bodies of any two vertebrae. These fibrocartilage discs provide a resilient cushion between the vertebrae, helping to absorb shock such as received from jumping or other types of vigorous exercises. The vertebral column would be rigidly immovable without the intervertebral discs and zygapophyseal joints.

Each disc consists of an outer fibrous portion termed the **annulus fibrosus** *(an′u-lus fi-bro′sis)* and a soft, semigelatinous inner part called the **nucleus pulposus.** *(nu′kle-us pul′po-sus)*. Each intervertebral disc is similar to a donut, with the outer part being the annulus fibrosus and the hole of the donut, when filled, being similar to the nucleus pulposus. If, due to injury, the soft inner part protrudes to press on the spinal cord or spinal nerves, the condition is termed a "slipped disc" or, more properly, herniated nucleus pulposus (HNP).

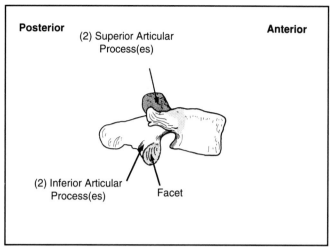

Typical Vertebra – Articular Process   Fig. 8-8

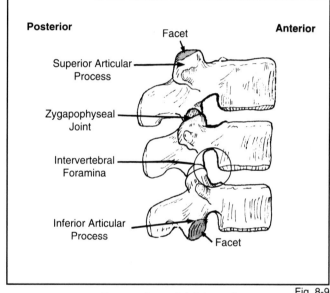

Zygapophyseal Joints and
Intervertebral Foramina   Fig. 8-9

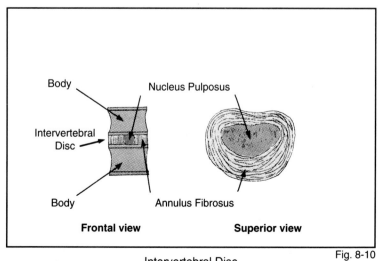

Intervertebral Disc   Fig. 8-10

Coccyx

Anterior Coccyx

Each division of the vertebral column will be studied in detail beginning distally. The most distal portion of the vertebral column is the **coccyx.** The anterior surface of the "tailbone" or coccyx is illustrated in *Fig. 8-11.* This portion of the vertebral column has greatly regressed in the human so there remains little resemblance to vertebrae. Three to five coccygeal segments (an average of four) have fused in the adult to form the single coccyx.

The most superior segment is the largest and broadest of the four sections and even has two lateral projections that are small **transverse processes.** The distal pointed tip of the coccyx is termed the **apex,** while the broader, superior portion is termed the **base.** Occasionally the second segment does not fuse solidly with the larger first segment; however, the coccyx usually is one, small, fairly insignificant end of the vertebral column.

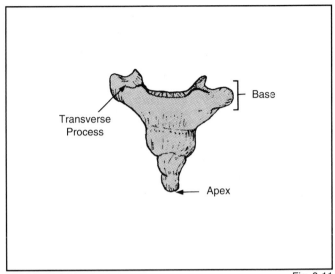

Coccyx – Anterior View   Fig. 8-11

Posterior Coccyx

The posterior aspect of an actual coccyx is pictured in *Fig. 8-12* along with a common U.S. postage stamp to allow a size comparison of the two. (Note that there is a small piece of bone missing on the right upper surface of the transverse process on this specimen.)

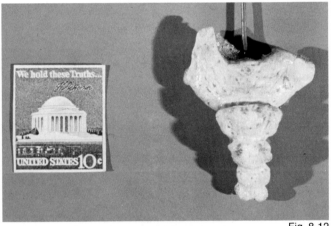

Coccyx – Posterior View (actual size)   Fig. 8-12

Lateral Coccyx

Ordinarily the coccyx curves forward as seen and identified on this lateral radiograph, so the apex points toward the symphysis pubis of the anterior pelvis. This forward curvature is more pronounced in males and less pronounced, or straighter, in females. The coccyx projects into the birth canal in the female and, if angled excessively forward, it can impede the birth process.

The most common injury associated with the coccyx results from a direct blow to the lower vertebral column when a person is in a sitting position. A wild ride on a toboggan might provide the type of force required to angulate the coccyx more forward than normal and make sitting down an action to be avoided for a period of time.

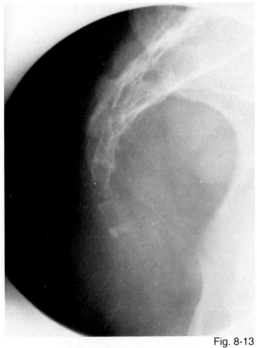

Fig. 8-13

Lateral Sacrum and Coccyx

Sacrum

Anterior Sacrum

Immediately superior to the coccyx is the **sacrum.** The anterior surface of a sacrum is illustrated in *Fig. 8-14*. The bodies of the original five segments can be seen, but they have fused into a single bone in the adult. The sacrum is shaped somewhat like a shovel, with the **apex** the most inferior portion. The anterior or pelvic surface is concave thereby adding to the capacity of the pelvic cavity.

Four sets of foramina or holes are shown on the anterior surface. These foramina serve to transmit nerves and blood vessels and are termed the **pelvic** (anterior) **sacral foramina.**

The large masses of bone lateral to the **body** of the first sacral segment are called the **alae** or wings of the sacrum. The upper surface of the sacrum closely resembles the last lumbar vertebra with which it articulates. Each **superior articular process** of the sacrum forms a zygapophyseal (apophyseal) joint with the inferior articular process of the fifth lumbar vertebra.

The anterior ridge of the body of the first sacral segment helps to form the inlet of the true pelvis and is termed the **promontory** of the sacrum, best demonstrated on a lateral view.

Lateral Sacrum and Coccyx

A lateral drawing of both the sacrum and the coccyx in *Fig. 8-15* clearly illustrates the dominant curve of the sacrum and the forward projection of the coccyx. These curves determine how the central ray must be angled for a true AP projection of the sacrum or the coccyx.

The **sacral promontory** is the anterior projecting ridge portion of the sacrum. The sacral promontory is seen anterior to the body of the first sacral segment. Directly posterior to the body of the first segment is the opening to the **sacral canal**, which is a continuation of the vertebral canal and contains certain sacral nerves. The **median sacral crest** is formed by the fused spinous processes of the sacral vertebrae.

As seen in *Figs. 8-15* and *8-16*, the posterior surface of the sacrum is much rougher and more irregular than the smooth anterior or pelvic surface.

The sacrum articulates with the ilium of the pelvis at the **auricular surface** (called this because of it's resemblance in shape to the auricle of the ear). This large auricular surface which projects posteriorly is best demonstrated on the posterior view of the sacrum (*Fig. 8-16*).

The **sacral horns** (cornua) are the small tubercles representing the inferior articular processes projecting down on each side of the fifth sacral segment. This is best seen on the lateral view of the sacrum where they are seen to project inferiorly and posteriorly to join the corresponding **horns** (cornua) of the **coccyx.**

Posterior Sacrum

Figure 8-16 is a photograph of an actual sacrum as seen from the posterior aspect. Clearly seen is the large, wedge-shaped (A) **auricular surface** which articulates with a similar surface on the ilium to form the **sacroiliac joint.** Each sacroiliac joint opens **obliquely posteriorly at an angle of 30 degrees.**

The **articulating facets of the superior articular processes** (B), also open to the rear and are shown on this photograph. There are eight, four on each side, **posterior sacral foramina** (C), corresponding to the same number of anterior sacral foramina.

The **sacral horns** (cornua) (D) are seen as small bony projections at the very inferoposterior aspect of the sacrum. Remnants of the enclosed sacral canal (E) can also be seen. (Deteriorating bone structure leaves this canal partially open on this bone specimen.)

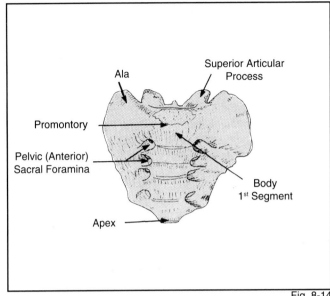

Sacrum – Anterior View   Fig. 8-14

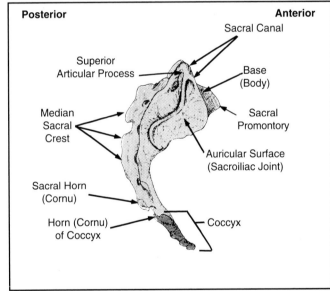

Sacrum and Coccyx – Lateral View   Fig. 8-15

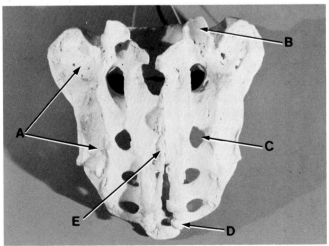

Sacrum – Posterior View   Fig. 8-16

Lumbar Vertebrae

Lateral and Superior Views

Joining the sacrum superiorly are the five large **lumbar vertebrae**. A typical lumbar vertebra as seen from the side is illustrated in *Fig. 8-17*. The **bodies** of the lumbar vertebrae are large in comparison to the vertebral bodies in the thoracic and cervical regions, with the last body, L5, being largest of all. The **transverse processes** are fairly small, while the posteriorly projecting **spinous process** is quite large and blunt. The palpable lower tip of each lumbar spinous process lies at the level of the intervertebral disc space inferior to each vertebral body.

Intervertebral Foramina: The **intervertebral foramina** are well seen from the side and are best visualized on a **true lateral** of the lumbar spine. This is demonstrated on the superior view of *Fig. 8-18* which shows the 90° orientation of the intervertebral foramen in relationship to the midsagittal plane. The intervertebral foramen would be the spaces or openings on each side of the central vertebral foramen formed when two vertebra are stacked on each other. These intervertebral foramina are shown in the circles on the lateral view drawing *(Fig. 8-17)* to demonstrate the area where they are located.

Zygapophyseal Joints: The **superior** and the **inferior articular processes** are best shown on a lateral view. These processes form the **zygapophyseal** (apophyseal) **joints** when several vertebrae are stacked on top of each other. The articular facets making up this joint form an angle of from **30° to 50°** to the midsagittal plane as shown in *Fig. 8-18*. The upper lumbar are nearer the 50° angle and the lower or distal lumbar are nearer the 30°. The average angle for the lumbar spine is 45°.

The **laminae** are large sturdy structures in a lumbar vertebra as demonstrated on a superior view. The portion of each lamina lying between the two articular processes has a special name, the **pars interarticularis** and is best shown on the posterior view of *Fig. 8-19*. Occasionally the pars interarticularis fails to unite the front and back of an individual vertebra. This condition allows the front part of one vertebra to slip forward on the vertebral body below it, a condition known as **spondylolisthesis** *(spon´di-lo-lis´the-sis)*.

Posterior View

The posterior view in *Fig. 8-19* is the general appearance of a lumbar vertebra as seen on an AP radiograph of the lumbar spine. Since the **spinous process** is being seen on end, just the outline of this process shows through the **body** on an AP radiograph. The **transverse processes** extending to each side are clearly shown on this view. The **superior and inferior articular processes** are also visualized; however, the actual zygapophyseal joint is best seen on an oblique radiograph of the lumbar vertebral column because of the angle of the articular facets as described above.

A common defect, most often seen in the fifth lumbar vertebra, is the failure of two lamina to unite, leaving a space or opening where the spinous process is usually found. This condition, termed **spina bifida,** *(spi´nah bif´i-da)* generally causes no problems as long as the structures within the vertebral canal remain in place. However, sometimes the soft tissues of the spinal cord coverings herniate posteriorly through this opening.

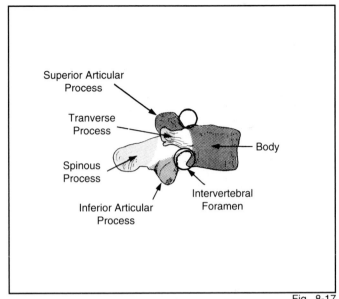

Lumbar Vertebra – Lateral View   Fig.. 8-17

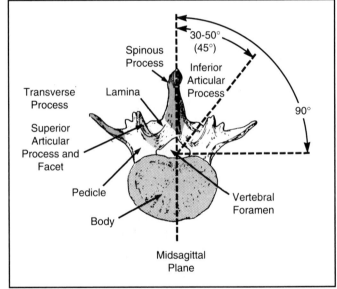

Lumbar Vertebra – Superior View   Fig. 8-18

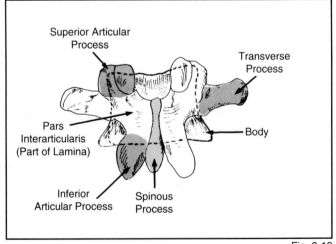

Lumbar Vertebra – Posterior View   Fig. 8-19

Anatomy Review

Superoinferior Projection

Certain parts on the superoinferior projection of a lumbar vertebra are labeled in *Fig. 8-20* on this radiograph of an individual lumbar vertebra taken from a disarticulated skeleton. These labeled parts are:

  A. Spinous process
  B. Lamina
  C. Pedicle
  D. Vertebral foramen
  E. Body
  F. Transverse process

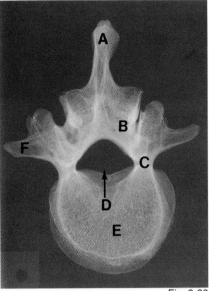

Lumbar Vertebra   Fig. 8-20
(Superoinferior Projection)

Lateral Position

Parts labeled A through F on the lateral view of a disarticulated lumbar vertebra are as follows:

  A. Body
  B. Inferior vertebral notch
  C. Area of the articulating facet of the inferior articular process, (actual articular facet not shown on this lateral view)
  D. Spinous process
  E. Superior articular process
  F. Pedicle

Note that this lateral view would "open up" and demonstrate the intervertebral foramina well, (the larger round opening directly under B, the inferior vertebral notch). However, it would not demonstrate the zygapophyseal joints. This would require a 45° oblique view.

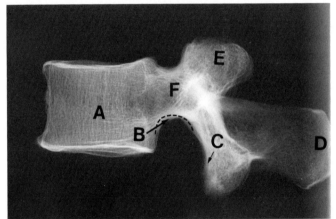

Lumbar Vertebra   Fig. 8-21
(Lateral Position)

AP Projection

Individual structures are more difficult to identify when the vertebrae are superimposed by the soft tissues of the abdomen as demonstrated on this AP lumbar spine radiograph. Those structures labeled A through E are:

  A. Transverse process of L5,
  B. Lower lateral portion of the body of L4,
  C. Lower part of the spinous process of L4 as visualized on end.
  D. One inferior articular process of L3, and
  E. Superior articular process of L4.

The facets of the inferior and superior articular processes (D and E) make up one zygapophyseal joint not visualized on this AP projection.

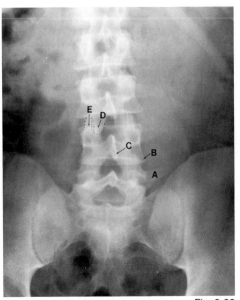

Lumbar Spine   Fig. 8-22
(AP Projection)

Anatomy Review continued

Lateral Lumbosacral Spine (Fig. 8-23)
Radiograph of entire lumbosacral spine in lateral position:
  A. Body of first lumbar vertebra
  B. Body of third lumbar vertebra
  C. Area of intervertebral disc between 4th and 5th lumbar vertebral bodies
  D. Body of fifth lumbar vertebra
  E. Spinous process of L4
  F. Superimposed intervertebral foramina between L2 and L3.

AP Lumbosacral Spine (Fig. 8-24)
AP projection of entire lumbosacral spine labeled as follows:
  A. Last thoracic vertebra (T12)
  B. First lumbar vertebra
  C. Third lumbar vertebra
  D. Fifth lumbar vertebra
  E. Sacrum
  F. Coccyx

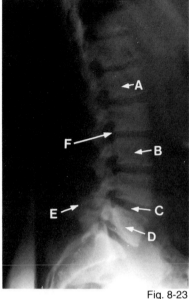

Fig. 8-23
Lumbosacral Spine, Lateral

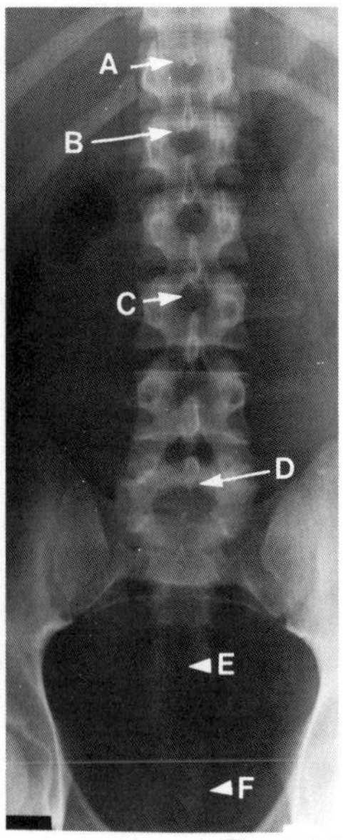

Fig. 8-24
Lumbosacral Spine, AP

Oblique Lumber Vertebrae

Appearance of "Scotty Dog"
Any bone and its parts, when seen in an oblique position, are more difficult to recognize than the same bone seen in the conventional frontal or lateral view. A vertebra is no exception; however, imagination can help us in the case of the lumbar vertebrae. A good 45° oblique will project the various structures in such a way that a "Scotty dog" seems to appear. The drawing in *Fig. 8-25* shows the various components of the "Scotty dog." The head and neck of the dog are probably the easiest features to recognize. The neck is one **pars interarticularis.** The **ear** of the dog is one **superior articular process,** while the **eye** is formed by one **pedicle.** One **transverse process** forms the **nose. The front legs** are formed by one **inferior articular process.**

Oblique Lumbar - Radiograph
The radiograph in *Fig. 8-26* shows the "Scotty dog" appearance that should be visible on a good oblique radiograph of the lumbar spine.
  A. Nose of the "Scotty dog," formed by one transverse process.
  B. Eye is one pedicle seen on end.
  C. Collar around the neck of the dog, which is the area of the pars interarticularis.
  D. Front leg of the animal, formed by one inferior articular process.
  E. Pointed ear, which is actually one of the superior articular processes.

Each of the five lumbar vertebrae should assume a similar "Scotty dog" appearance on a good oblique radiograph.

Classification of Joints

There are two types or classifications of joints or articulations involving the vertebral column.

(1) Zygapophyseal (Apophyseal) Joints
The zygapophyseal joints between the superior and inferior articular processes are classified as **synovial joints,** which are **diarthrodial** or freely movable, with a **gliding type** movement.

(2) Intervertebral Joints
The intervertebral joints between the bodies of any two vertebrae containing intervertebral discs which are made up of fibrocartilage are only slightly movable. These joints which are tightly bound by cartilage are thus classified as **cartilaginous joints**. They are **amphiarthrodial**

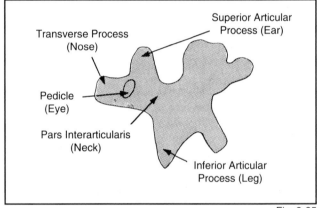

The "Scotty Dog"

Fig. 8-25

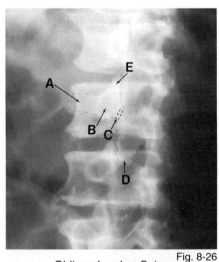

Fig. 8-26
Oblique Lumbar Spine
(The "Scotty Dog")

(slightly movable) of the **symphyses** subclass, similar to the symphysis pubis of the pelvis.

There is not a great deal of motion between any two vertebrae, however the combined effect of all the vertebrae in the column does allow a considerable range of motion. The possible movements are flexion, extension, lateral flexion (bending) and rotation. Certain radiographic exams of the spinal column involving hyperflexion and hyperextension and/or right and left bending routines can measure this range of motion.

Part II Radiographic Positioning

Topographical Landmarks

Correct positioning for the small coccyx and the larger sacrum and lumbar spine require a thorough understanding of certain topographical landmarks which can be easily and accurately palpated.

The most reliable topographical landmarks for the spine are the various palpable bony prominences that are fairly constant from one person to another. However, it should be emphasized that the landmarks as presented refer to an average healthy, erect, normally developed adult male or female. These landmarks will vary in subjects with anatomical and, especially, skeletal anomalies. The very young and the very old will also have slightly different features than the average adult.

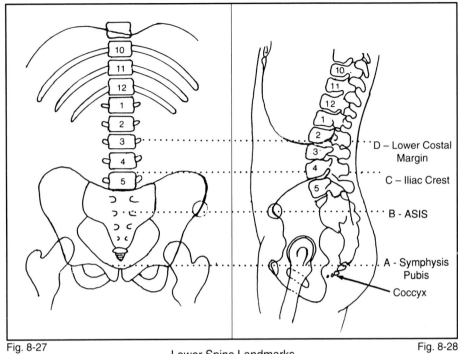

Fig. 8-27

Lower Spine Landmarks

Fig. 8-28

Lower Spine Landmarks

The drawings on the right and the photographs below illustrate various landmarks relative to the lower vertebral column.

Level A corresponds to the easily palpable superior margin of the **symphysis pubis**. The size and shape of the **coccyx** varies greatly but the mid-coccyx is approximately at the level of the **greater trochanter**, which is also near the level of the symphysis pubis. Although the coccyx may be palpated directly, this may not be advisable since this can be embarrassing to the patient.

Note on the photographs below that the greater trochanters are approximately 1 or 1.5 in. (3-4 cm) above the upper border of the symphysis pubis.

The **anterior superior iliac spine** (ASIS) is at about the same **level (B)** as the **second sacral segment**.

Level C is the most superior portion of the **iliac crest** and is at approximately the same level as the junction of the **fourth and fifth lumbar vertebrae**.

The lowest margin of the ribs or **lower costal margin** (D) is at the approximate level of L2 or 3.

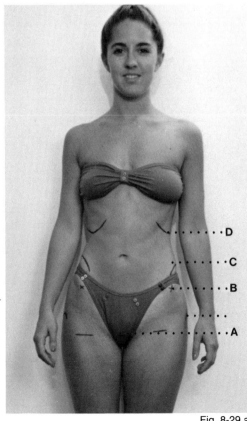

Fig. 8-29 a

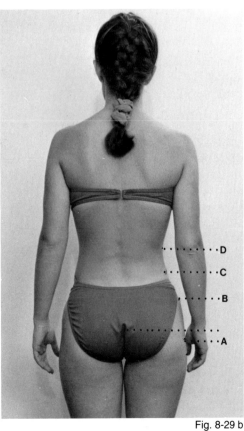

Fig. 8-29 b

Lower Spine Landmarks

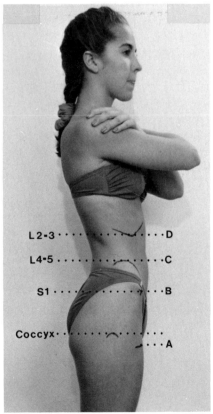

Fig. 8-29 c

Positioning Considerations

Oblique Lumbar Spine

Oblique positions which are routinely taken with the lumbar spine require a good understanding of the anatomy of the vertebra and the zygapophyseal joints to know how much to oblique and to know which side is being demonstrated since they can be taken in either anterior or posterior oblique positions.

Posterior Oblique: As the drawing and photographs of the skeleton demonstrate, the **downside** joints are visualized on **posterior** obliques. The downside zygapophyseal joints are not visible on the skeleton since they are "under" the bodies of the vertebra, *(Fig. 8-30)* but as seen on the inferosuperior sectional drawing, the downside or right joints would be demonstrated on a right posterior oblique (RPO). This is seen on the RPO radiograph in *Fig. 8-31* which clearly shows the "scotty dogs ", or the right zygapophyseal joints.

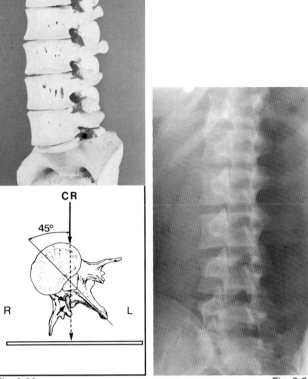

Fig. 8-30

Fig. 8-31

Posterior Oblique Lumbar Spine
RPO – downside or **right** joints

Anterior Oblique: Anterior obliques of the lumbar spine may be more comfortable for the patient and allows the natural lumbar curvature of the spine to coincide with the divergence angle of the x-ray beam.

As demonstrated, an **anterior** oblique visualizes the **upside** joints. Therefore, a right anterior oblique (RAO) visualizes the upside or left zygapophyseal joints *(Figs. 8-32 and 33)*.

The degree of obliquity depends on which area of the lumbar spine is of specific interest. A 45° oblique is for the general lumbar region but if interest is specifically in L1 or L2, the degree of obliquity should be **increased** to 55 or 60°. If interest is in the L5 - S1 area, the obliquity would be only 35° to 40° from an AP or PA.

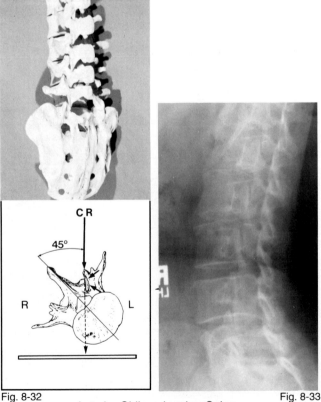

Fig. 8-32

Fig. 8-33

Anterior Oblique Lumbar Spine
RAO – upside or **left** joints

Positioning Considerations continued

Gonadal Shielding

Gonadal shielding and other protection practices such as close collimation are especially important because of the proximity of the lumbar spine, sacrum and coccyx to the gonads. Gonadal shielding can and should **always** be used on males of reproductive age on coccyx, sacrum or lumbar spine radiographs. If the area of interest is the sacrum and/or coccyx, gonadal shielding for females may not be possible without obscuring essential anatomy. However if the area of interest is the lumbar spine and proximal sacrum, gonadal shields should always be used on all children and males and females of reproductive age.

AP Projection - Lumbar spine

Frontal lumbar spine radiographs are commonly taken as AP projections with the **knees and hips flexed** to straighten the spine. Flexing the knees and hips *(Fig. 8-36)* reduces the lumbar curvature and brings the back in contact with the table, and the lumbar vertebral column nearer parallel to the film. The incorrect position is shown in *Fig. 8-35* wherein the pelvis is tipped forward slightly when the lower limbs are extended, which exaggerates the lumbar curvature. The flexing of the knees and hips is a simple positioning step but important because it straightens the spine and opens up the intervertebral spaces on an AP lumbar projection.

PA vs. AP Projections

Even though the AP projection with knees and hips flexed is a common routine for the lumbar spine, there are two reasons or advantages of taking these as PA projections in a prone position.

First, it reduces gonadal exposure significantly (20-30%) on females wherein the ovaries are located more anteriorly in the pelvic area. This is also true for frontal views of the coccyx and sacrum which can be taken PA rather than AP.[1]

The second reason is that the prone position places the lumbar spine with its natural lumbar curvature in such a way that the intervertebral disc spaces are nearer parallel to the divergent x-ray beam. This opens up and provides better visualization of the margins of the intervertebral disc spaces.

The one negative factor against the PA, especially for patients with large abdomens, is the increased OID with accompanying magnification and loss of detail. This however can be minimized with the use of a small focal spot and with increased SID. Each radiographer should determine departmental policy regarding the question of PA vs. AP lumbar spine, sacrum and coccyx.

The prone position also may be more comfortable for the patient, especially with back pain. However, the erect position is often the most comfortable for the patient already in an erect position and the lumbar spine can be taken erect with either AP or PA projections.

SID

A common minimum SID is 40 in. (102 cm), but an increased SID of 42, 44, or even 46 in. (107, 112 or 117 cm) not only reduces magnification and increases detail but also results in less skin dose to the patient.

Other advantages of increased SID for radiography of the spine are a decrease in the anode-heel effect and less angle of divergence of the x-ray beam, which facilitates in the "opening up" of intervertebral spaces when the vertebral column is parallel to the film.

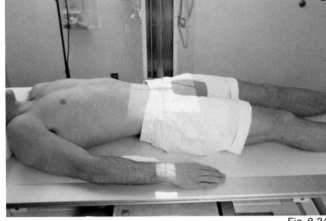
Gonadal shielding – Lumbar Spine   Fig. 8-34

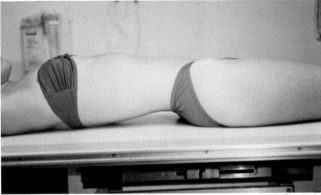
Incorrect – Lower Limbs Extended   Fig. 8-35

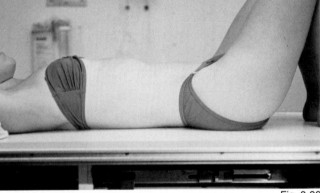
Correct – Knees and Hips Flexed   Fig. 8-36

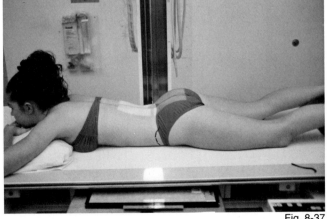
PA – Lumbar Spine with 44 in. (112 cm) SID   Fig. 8-37

---

[1] Handbook of selected tissue doses for projections common in diagnostic radiology. HEW Publication (FDA 89-8031) December, 1988.

National Survey
Departmental standard (basic) and optional routines of the coccyx, sacrum and lumbar spine were very consistent throughout the United States.

Sacrum and Coccyx Routine

Sacrum and Coccyx	U.S. Average	
	Basic	Optional
• AP sacrum (15-25°ceph.)	98%	
• AP coccyx (10°-20° caudal)	96%	
• Lateral sacrum	95%	
• Lateral coccyx	90%	

Lumbosacral Spine Routine

L.S. spine	U.S. Average	
	Basic	Optional
•AP	98%	
• Lateral	99%	
• L5 - S1 lateral spot	90%	
• Obliques (45°)	69%	
• AP L5 - S1 (30-35° ceph.)	16%	8%
• Lateral flexion and extension[1]		2%

[1] Write in's by respondents

Summary
The results did not reveal anything unexpected or unusual.

Standard and Optional Operating Procedures

Certain basic and optional projections or positions for the coccyx, sacrum and lumbar spine are demonstrated and described on the following pages as suggested standard and optional departmental procedures.

Basic Projections
Standard or basic projections, also sometimes referred to as routine projections or departmental routines are **those projections or positions commonly taken on average patients who are helpful and can cooperate in performing the procedure.**

Optional Projections
Optional projections are **those more common projections or positions taken as extra or additional projections to better demonstrate certain pathologic conditions or specific body parts.**

Basic and Optional Projections

Coccyx
Basic
• AP
• Lateral

Sacrum
Basic
• AP
• Lateral

Lumbar Spine
Basic
• AP
• Obliques (R and L)
• Lateral
• Lateral, L5-S1
Optional
• AP, L5-S1

Scoliosis Series
Basic
• PA Erect and/or Supine
• Erect Lateral
Optional
• PA Ferguson Method
• AP, R and L Bending

Spinal Fusion Series
Basic
• Lateral, Hyperextension
  and Hyperflexion
• AP, R and L Bending
  (same as for scoliosis
  series)

• AP Projection

Structures Best Shown:
Coccyx free of self-superimposition and superimposition of symphysis pubis.

NOTE: The urinary bladder should be emptied before beginning this procedure. It is also desirable to have the lower colon free of gas and fecal material which may require a cleaning enema as ordered by a physician.

Technical Factors:
• 8 x 10 in. (18 x 24 cm), lengthwise.
• Use moving or stationary grid.
• 70-75 kVp range (or 80-85 kVp and reduce mAs and dose in half).

Patient Position:
• Supine, pillow for head, legs extended with support under knees for comfort.

Shielding:
Use gonadal shielding for males. Ovarian shielding on females is not possible without obscuring area of interest.

Part Position:
• Align **midsagittal plane to midline of table** and/or cassette.
• Assure there is **no rotation** of pelvis.

Central Ray:
• CR angled **10° caudad**, to enter **2 in.** (5 cm) **superior to symphysis pubis**.
• Center cassette to CR.
• Minimum 40 in. (102 cm) SID.

Collimation:
Close four-sided collimation to area of interest. (Close collimation is important for adequate contrast and detail to clearly visualize all segments of the coccyx, and for radiation protection purposes.)

Respiration:
Suspend breathing on expiration.

NOTE: • May need to increase CR angle to 15° caudad with a greater anterior curvature of the coccyx if this is apparent by palpation or as evidenced on the lateral.
• May be done prone (angle **10° cephalad**) if necessary with CR centered to the coccyx which is easily palpable. This will result in increased OID but will **decrease** ovarian exposure on females.

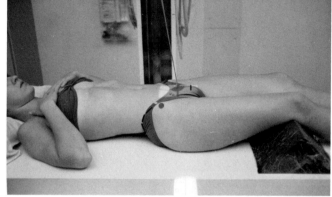

AP – 10° Caudad

Fig. 8-38

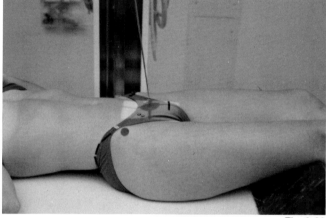

AP – 10° Caudad

Fig. 8-39

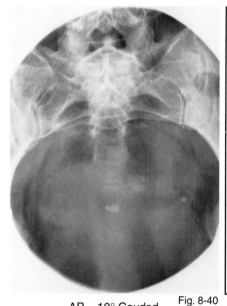

AP – 10° Caudad

Fig. 8-40

(Courtesy of Jim Sanderson, RT)

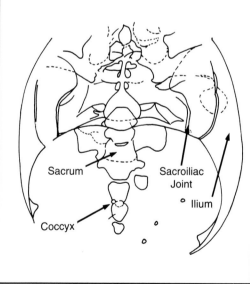

Sacrum   Sacroiliac Joint

Ilium

Coccyx

AP – 10° Caudad

Fig. 8-41

Evaluation Criteria:
• Coccyx should be seen free of superimposition and projected superior to pubis. (Repeat exam and increase angle of CR if superimposition is present.)
• Coccygeal segments should be open. If not, they may be fused or CR angle may need to be increased. (The greater the curvature of the coccyx, the greater the degree of angulation needed.)

• Coccyx should be equidistant from the lateral walls of the pelvic opening indicating no rotation.
• Coccyx should be in center of collimation field and film.
• Optimum exposure with relatively high (short scale) contrast should clearly visualize all segments of the coccyx without overexposing the most distal segment.
• Patient ID information and R or L marker should be visible without superimposing essential anatomy.

• Lateral Position

Coccyx
Basic
• AP
• **Lateral**

Structures Best Shown:
Coccyx (anterior angulation is best demonstrated in this position).

Technical Factors:
• Film Size - 8 x 10 in. (18 x 24 cm), lengthwise.
• Use moving or stationary grid.
• 75-80 kVp range.
• Place lead shield on table behind patient to reduce scatter to the film.

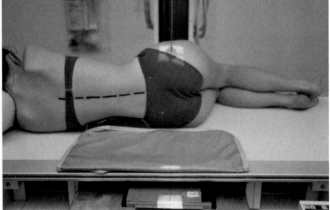

Lateral Coccyx   Fig. 8-42

Patient Position:
• Lateral recumbent, pillow for head.

Shielding: Shield gonads without obscuring area of interest. Ovarian shielding on females may not be possible without obscuring area of interest.

Part Position:
• Flex hips and knees.
• Place support under small of waist, and between knees and ankles.
• Align **long axis of coccyx with midline of table** and/or cassette. (Remember the superficial location of coccyx.)
• Place pelvis and body in **true lateral** position.
• The distal coccyx is at level of greater trochanter, which can generally be palpated.

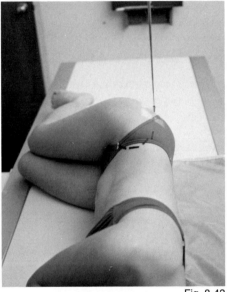

Lateral Coccyx   Fig. 8-43

Central Ray:
• CR **perpendicular** to table.
• Center CR to **level of about 1 or 1.5 in.** (3-4 cm) **superior to the greater trochanter.**
• Center cassette to CR.
• Minimum 40 in. (102 cm) SID.

Collimation: Close four-sided collimation to area of interest.

Respiration: Suspend breathing on expiration.

NOTE: • Do not overexpose. Requires less exposure (5-7 kVp) than lateral sacrum.
• Manual exposure time control is recommended because phototiming may result in improper density levels.

Evaluation Criteria:
• Coccyx should be seen in lateral profile in center of collimation field and film. (Close four-sided collimation should be evident.)
• If visible, the femoral heads should be superimposed indicating no rotation of pelvis.
• Segment interspaces should be open if not fused.

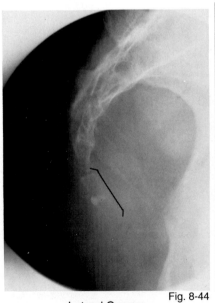

Lateral Coccyx   Fig. 8-44
(Courtesy of Jim Sanderson , RT)

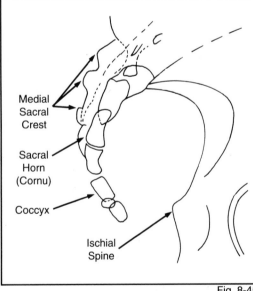

Lateral Coccyx   Fig. 8-45

• Optimum exposure with relatively high (short scale) contrast should clearly visualize all segments of the coccyx.
• Patient ID information and R or L marker should be visible without superimposing essential anatomy.

• AP Projection

Sacrum
Basic
• **AP**
• Lateral

Structures Best Shown:
Frontal view of sacrum not foreshortened, SI joints and the L5-S1 junction.

NOTE: The urinary bladder should be emptied before beginning this procedure. It is also desirable to have the lower colon free of gas and fecal material which may require a cleaning enema as ordered by a physician.

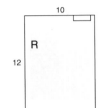

Technical Factors:
• Film Size - 10 x 12 in. (24 x 30 cm), lengthwise.
• Use moving or stationary grid.
• 75-80 kVp range (or 85-92 kVp and reduce mAs and dose in half).

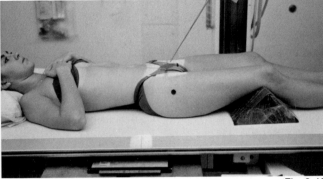
AP – 15° Cephalad

Fig. 8-46

Patient Position:
• Supine, pillow for head, legs extended with support under knees for comfort.

Shielding: Use gonadal shielding for males. Ovarian shielding on females is not possible without obscuring area of interest.

Part Position:
• Align **midsagittal plane to midline of table** and/or cassette.
• Assure there is **no rotation** of pelvis.

Central Ray:
• CR angled **15° cephalad**, to enter at **midsagittal plane midway between symphysis pubis and ASIS level.**
• Center cassette to CR.
• Minimum 40 in. (102 cm) SID.

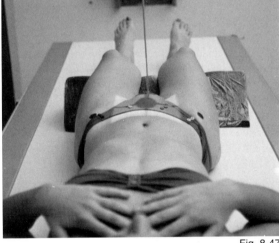
AP – 15° Cephalad

Fig. 8-47

Collimation: Close four-sided collimation to area of interest.

Respiration: Suspend breathing on expiration.

NOTE: • May need to increase CR angle to 20° cephalad for females or patients with an apparent greater posterior curvature or tilt of the sacrum and pelvis.
• Female sacrum is generally shorter and wider than male sacrum (a consideration in close four-sided collimation).
• May be done prone (angle **15° caudad**) if necessary. Will increase OID but will **decrease** ovarian exposure on females.

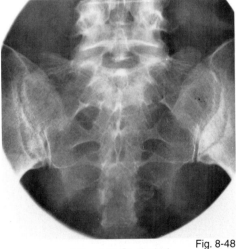
AP – 15° Cephalad

Fig. 8-48

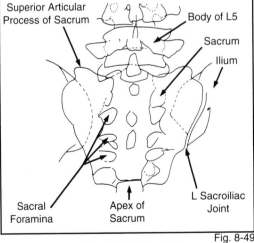

Superior Articular Process of Sacrum

Body of L5

Sacrum

Ilium

Sacral Foramina

Apex of Sacrum

L Sacroiliac Joint

AP – 15° Cephalad

Fig. 8-49

Evaluation Criteria:
• Sacrum should be centered to film and collimation field.
• Sacrum should be free of foreshortening and superimposition by pubis.

• Inferior portion of sacrum should be centered in the pelvic opening indicating no rotation of pelvis.
• Optimum exposure should demonstrate sufficient contrast and density to clearly visualize the area of the sacrum.
• Patient ID and R or L marker should be visible without superimposing essential anatomy.

• Lateral Position

Sacrum
Basic
• AP
• **Lateral**

Structures Best Shown:
Sacrum and L5-S1 joint.

Technical Factors:
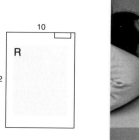

• Film Size - 10 x 12 in. (24 x 30 cm), lenthwise.
• Use moving or stationary grid.
• 80-85 kVp range.
• Place lead shield on table behind patient to reduce scatter to film.

Patient Position:
• Lateral recumbent, pillow for head.

Shielding:
Shield gonads without obscuring area of interest. (Complete ovarian shielding on females may obscure a portion of sacrum.)

Part Position:
• Flex hips and knees.
• Place support under small of waist and between knees and ankles.
• Align **long axis of sacrum with midline of table** and/or cassette.
• Place pelvis and body in **true lateral position**.

Central Ray:
• CR **perpendicular** to table and film.
• Center CR **2 in.** (5 cm) **anterior to posterior sacral surface at level of ASIS (S2).**
• Center cassette to CR.
• Minimum 40 in. (102 cm) SID.

Collimation:
Close four-sided collimation to area of interest.

Respiration:
Suspend breathing on expiration.

NOTE: • High amounts of secondary and scatter radiation is generated. Use higher ratio grids if possible.

Evaluation Criteria:
• Sacrum should be seen in lateral profile in center of film and center of four-sided collimation field.
• Posterior margins of pelvis should be superimposed and femoral heads aligned indicating no rotation of pelvis.
• Optimum exposure should clearly visualize the entire sacrum. (The distal coccyx segments will generally appear slightly overexposed.)
• Patient ID information and R or L marker should be visible without superimposing essential anatomy.

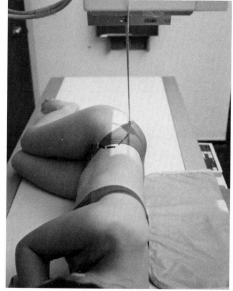

Lateral Sacrum   Fig. 8-50

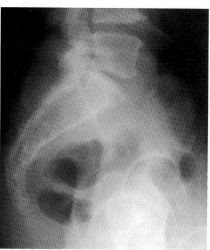

Lateral Sacrum   Fig. 8-51

Lateral Sacrum   Fig. 8-52

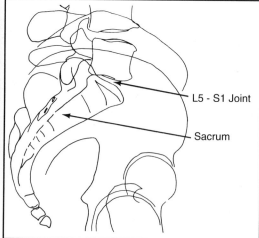

L5 - S1 Joint

Sacrum

Lateral Sacrum   Fig. 8-53

• AP (or PA) Projection

Lumbar Spine
Basic
• **AP**
• Obliques (R & L)
• Lateral
• Lateral L5-S1
Optional
• AP L5-S1

Structures Best Shown:

Lumbar vertebral bodies, intervertebral joints, spinous and transverse processes, laminae, SI joints and sacrum.

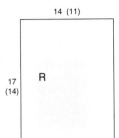

14 (11)

17 (14)   R

Technical Factors:

• Film Size - 14 x 17 in. (35 x 43 cm), lengthwise,
   or
   - 11 x 14 in. (30 x 35 cm)
• Use moving or stationary grid.
• 75-80 kVp range (or 85-92 kVp and reduce mAs and dose in half).

Patient Position:

• Supine with **knees and hips flexed** and head on pillow. (May also be done prone or erect, see NOTE below.)

Shielding:

Place contact shield over gonads without obscuring area of interest. Female ovarian shielding will obscure portions of sacrum and coccyx.

Part Position:

• Align **midsagittal plane to midline of table.**
• Place arms at side or up on chest.
• Assure **no rotation** of torso or pelvis.

Central Ray:

• CR **perpendicular** to film centered to:

Larger film (14 x 17): Center to **level of iliac crest** (L 4-5 interspace). This will include lumbar vertebrae, sacrum and possibly coccyx. Center cassette to CR.

Smaller film (11 x 14): Center to **level of 1-1.5 in.** (3-4 cm) **above iliac crest** (L3).
This will include primarily the five lumbar vertebrae. Center cassette to CR.
• Minimum 40 in. (102 cm) SID.

Collimation:

Four-sided collimation with superior and inferior borders to film margins to include maximum vertebral column.

Respiration:

Suspend breathing on **expiration**.

NOTE: • Presence of scoliosis may result in unavoidable rotation of spine.
• Flexion of knees and hips straightens the spine which helps open up intervertebral spaces.
• May be done prone since PA projection will open up interspaces better. This increases OID, therefore, use small focal spot. It may be more comfortable for patient, and it also significantly reduces ovarian dose for females. (See page 255.)
• Can also be done erect if necessary as an AP or PA projection.

Evaluation Criteria:

• The spinal column from approximately T11 to the distal sacrum should be seen if 14 x 17 film is used centered

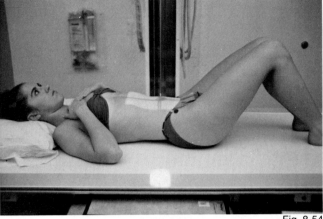

AP Projection   Fig. 8-54

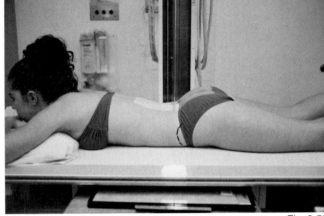

Alternate PA Projection   Fig. 8-55

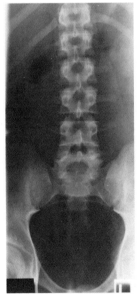

Fig. 8-56
AP Projection

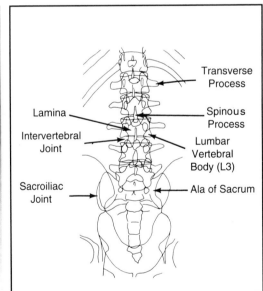

Transverse Process

Lamina

Intervertebral Joint

Sacroiliac Joint

Spinous Process

Lumbar Vertebral Body (L3)

Ala of Sacrum

Fig. 8-57
AP Projection

to midline of film and collimation field. (With 11 x 14 film, T12 to S1 should be visible.)
• SI joints should be equidistant from spine indicating no pelvic rotation. Spinous processes should appear in midline of vertebral column and R and L transverse processes should appear equal in length.
• Lateral margins of collimation field should include psoas muscle outlines.
• Optimum exposure should clearly visualize the lumbar vertebral body margins and intervertebral joint spaces without overexposing psoas muscle outlines and/or transverse processes.

• Oblique Position

Structures Best Shown:
Zygapophyseal (apophyseal) joints. (RPO and LPO show downside. RAO and LAO show upside.) "Scotty dogs" should be visualized on good oblique.

Both right and left obliques are taken.

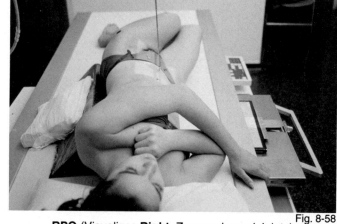
RPO (Visualizes **Right** Zygapophyseal Joints)
Fig. 8-58

Technical Factors:
• Film Size - 2 ea. 11 x 14 in. (30 x 35 cm), lengthwise.
    or
    - 10 x 12 in. (24 x 30 cm)
• Use moving or stationary grid.
• 75-80 kVp range (or 85-92 kVp and reduce mAs and dose in half).
• Use small focal spot if equipment allows.

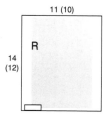

Patient Position:
• Semisupine (RPO and LPO) or semiprone (RAO and LAO).

Shielding: Place contact shield over gonads without obscuring area of interest.

Part Position:
• Position patient and **rotate body 45°** so as to put spinal column directly over midline of table.
• Flex knee for stability as shown.
• Arm should grasp edge of table. (Don't pinch fingers.)
• Support lower back and pelvis with radiolucent sponges to maintain position.

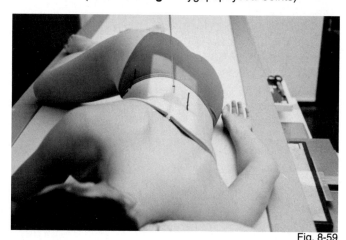
LAO (Visualizes **Right** Zygapophyseal Joints)
Fig. 8-59

Central Ray:
• CR **perpendicular** to film.
• Center **midway between the iliac crest and inferior rib margin** (L3).
• Center 2 in. (5 cm) laterally from midline of patient (2 in. lateral to spinous process).
• Center cassette to CR.
• Minimum 40 in. (102 cm) SID.

Collimation: Four-sided collimation to near borders of film. Slight additional collimation on lateral borders, especially on larger film.

Respiration: Suspend breathing on expiration.

NOTE: A 35-40° oblique best visualises the zygapophyseal joints at L1 - L2, and 55-60° for L5 - S1.

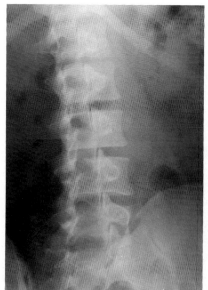
Oblique
Fig. 8-60

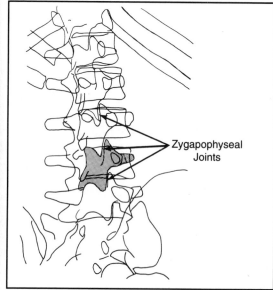
Zygapophyseal Joints

Oblique
Fig. 8-61

Evaluation Criteria:
• The spinal column from T11 to S1 should be seen.
• "Scotty dogs" (zygapophyseal joints closest to the film on posterior obliques) should be visualized on all five vertebral vertebrae.
• Spinal column should be in midline of collimation field and film.
• A properly 45° obliqued patient puts the pedicle (eye and nose of Scotty dog) in the center of the vertebral body, equidistant from the vertebral body borders. (Posterior placement of the pedicle indicates too much obliquity and anterior placement indicates not enough obliquity.)
• Optimum exposure should clearly visualize the zygapophyseal joints from L1 to L5 without overexposing other vertebral margins.

• Lateral Position

Lumbar Spine
Basic
• AP
• Obliques (R and L)
• **Lateral**
• Lateral L5-S1
Optional
• AP L5-S1

Structures Best Shown:
Lumbar vertebrae, intervertebral joints, spinous processes, L5-S1 junction, sacrum and first four intervertebral foramina.

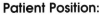

Technical Factors:
• Film Size - 14 x 17 in. (35 x 43 cm), lengthwise.
or
- 11 x 14 in. (30 x 35 cm).
• Use moving or stationary grid.
• 90-100 kVp range.
• To make best use of the anode-heel effect, place pelvis at the cathode end; or use wedge filter.
• Place lead shield on table behind patient to reduce scatter to the film.
• Use small focal spot if equipment allows.

Patient Position:
• Lateral recumbent, pillow for head, knees and hips flexed with support between knees and ankles and under knee resting on table to better maintain a true lateral position.

Shielding: Place contact shield over gonads without obscuring area of interest. Complete ovarian shielding for females will obscure a portion of sacrum.

Part Position:
• Align **coronal plane to midline** of table.
• Place radiolucent support under small of waist, as needed to place the long axis of the spine near parallel to the table (palpate spinous processes to determine this). See NOTE.
• Place pelvis and torso in **true lateral position.**

Central Ray:
• CR **perpendicular** to long axis of spine centered to:

Larger film (14 x 17): Center to **level of iliac crest** (L4). This will include lumbar vertebrae, sacrum and possibly coccyx. Center cassette to CR.

Smaller film (11 x 14): Center 1.5 in. (4 cm) **above iliac crest** (L3). This will include primarily the five lumbar vertebrae. Center cassette to CR.
• Minimum 40 in. (102 cm) SID.

Collimation: Closely collimate on lateral borders. (Light field will appear small due to divergent rays and the distance from the upside skin surface to the film.)

Respiration: Suspend breathing on expiration.

NOTE: • A slight sag of the spine will help open up the intervertebral joints considering the divergence of the x-ray beam if both ends of the lumbar spine are the same distance from table. The average male and some females require no CR angle. A female with a wider pelvis and narrow thorax may require a 3°- 5° caudal angle even with support, as shown in *Fig. 8-63.*
• If patient has a natural side curvature (scoliosis) of the lower spine, as determined by viewing the spine from the back with hospital gown open and patient standing evenly on both feet, the patient should be placed in whichever lateral position that places the sag or convexity of the spine down to better open the intervertebral spaces.

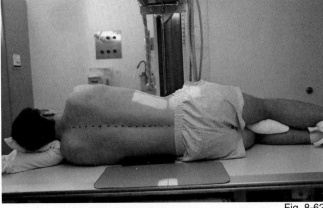

Male Lateral (CR Perpendicular to Film)   Fig. 8-62

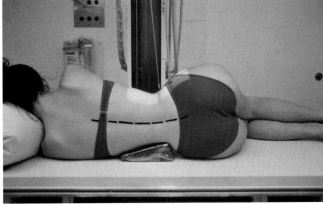

Female Lateral (CR 5° Caudal)   Fig. 8-63

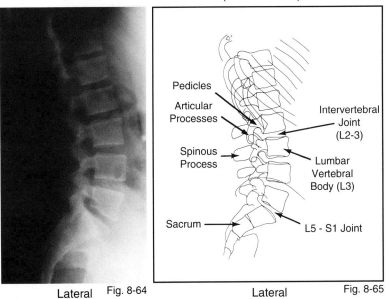

Lateral   Fig. 8-64   Lateral   Fig. 8-65

Pedicles

Articular Processes

Spinous Process

Sacrum

Intervertebral Joint (L2-3)

Lumbar Vertebral Body (L3)

L5 - S1 Joint

Evaluation Criteria:
• Using larger 14 x 17 in. film, vertebra from T12 to the distal sacrum should be seen in lateral profile centered to the film and the collimation field.
• Using smaller 11 x 14 in. film, T12 through S1 should be visualized.
• First four intervertebral foramina should be open. The fifth foramina will be open on the oblique views.
• Intervertebral joint spaces should appear open from T12 to S1.
• Optimum exposure should clearly visualize the vertebral bodies and joint spaces without overexposure of other vertebral structures.

• Lateral L5-S1 Position

<table>
<tr><td>
Lumbar Spine
Basic
• AP
• Obliques (R and L)
• Lateral
• **Lateral L5-S1**
Optional
• AP, L5 -S1
</td></tr>
</table>

Structures Best Shown:
L5-S1 joint space in lateral position.

Technical Factors:
• Film Size - 8 x 10 in. (18 x 24 cm), lengthwise.
• Use moving or stationary grid.
• 90-100 kVp range.
• Place lead shield on table behind patient to reduce scatter to film.

Patient Position:
• Lateral recumbent, pillow for head, knees and hips flexed with support between knees and ankles and under knee resting on table to better maintain a true lateral position.

Shielding:
Place contact shield over gonads without obscuring area of interest. Complete ovarian shielding for females will obscure a portion of sacrum.

Part Position:
• Align **coronal plane to midline of table.**
• Flex knees and hips.
• Place radiolucent support under small of waist. (See NOTE.)
• Place pelvis and torso in **true lateral** position.

Central Ray:
• CR **perpendicular** to film with sufficient waist support; or **angle 5-8° caudad** without sufficient support. (See NOTE below.)
• Center CR **1.5 in.** (4 cm) **inferior to iliac crest** and **1.5 in.** (4 cm) **anterior to posterior surface** of body. Center cassette to CR.
• Minimum 40 in. (102 cm) SID.

Collimation:
Close four-sided collimation to area of interest. Use extension cylinder cone if available; if not available, collimate closely.

Respiration:
Suspend breathing on expiration.

NOTE:
• If waist is not supported resulting in a sagging of the spinal column, the the CR is angled caudad an average of 5° for males and 8° for females.
• High amounts of secondary/scatter radiation is generated. Use close collimation, higher ratio grids and lead masking.

Evaluation Criteria:
• L5-S1 joint space should be open and in center of exposure field and film.
• There should be no rotation of torso and pelvis.
• At least L5-S1 should be seen in their entirety.
• Optimum exposure should clearly visualize the L5-S1 joint space through the superimposed ilia of the pelvis without excess burnout of other vertebral structures.

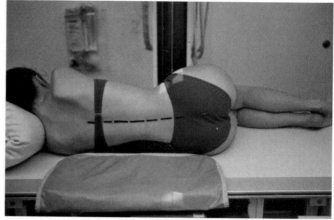

Lateral L5-S1 With Sufficient Support (0° Angle)   Fig. 8-66

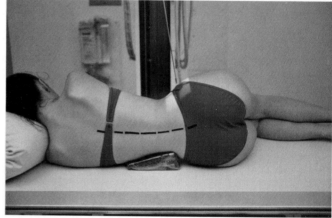

Lateral L5-S1 Without Sufficient Support (8° Caudad)   Fig. 8-67

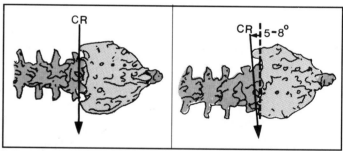

0° Angle   5-8° Angle   Fig. 8-68

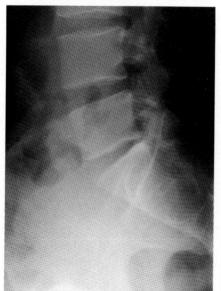

Lateral L5-S1   Fig. 8-69

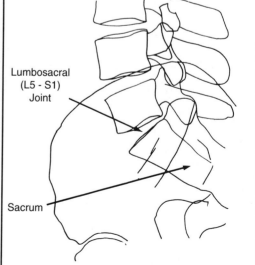

Lumbosacral (L5 - S1) Joint

Sacrum

Lateral L5-S1   Fig. 8-70

• AP L5-S1 Projection

Structures Best Shown:
L5-S1 joint space and sacroiliac joints in AP projection.

Technical Factors:
• 8 x 10 in. (18 x 24 cm), lengthwise.
• Use moving or stationary grid.
• 80-85 kVp range.
  (Increase 6-8 kVp from AP due to axial projection)

Patient Position:
• Supine, pillow for head, legs extended with support under knees for comfort.

Shielding: Place contact shield over gonads without obscuring area of interest. Female ovarian shielding will obscure portion of sacroiliac joints.

Part Position:
• Place arms at side or up on chest.
• Align **midsagittal plane to midline of table** and/or cassette.
• Assure **no rotation** of torso or pelvis.

Central Ray:
• Angle CR **cephalad, 30° (males)** to **35° (females).**
• CR should enter at the **level of the ASIS** centered to the **midline of the body.**
• Center cassette to CR.
• Minimum 40 in. (102 cm) SID.

Collimation: Close four-sided collimation to area of interest.

Respiration: Suspend breathing during exposure.

NOTE: • Angled AP projection opens up L5-S1 joint.
• Lateral projection is generally more informative than AP projection.
• May be done **prone** with similar **caudal** angle of CR. (Increases OID but **decreases ovarian dose** on females.)

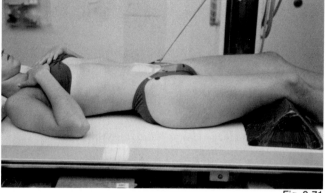

AP L5-S1   Fig. 8-71

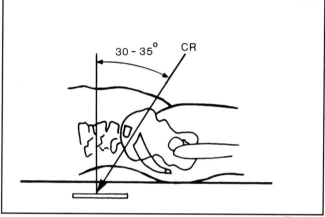

30 - 35°   CR

AP L5-S1   Fig. 8-72

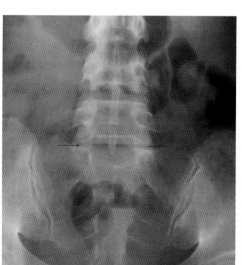

AP L5-S1 (30° Cephalad)   Fig. 8-73

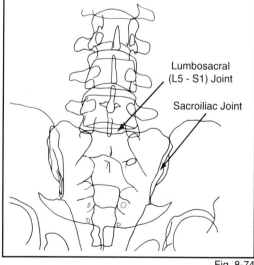

Lumbosacral (L5 - S1) Joint

Sacroiliac Joint

AP L5-S1   Fig. 8-74

Evaluation Criteria:
• L5-S1 joint should be demonstrated and in center of exposure field and film.
• Sacroiliac joints should be demonstrated and be equidistant from spine indicating no pelvic rotation.
• Optimum exposure should clearly visualize both the L5-S1 joint space and the sacroiliac joints.

• PA Projection

Structures Best Shown:

Thoracic and lumbar spine in the PA projection to evaluate for abnormal lateral curvature (scoliosis) of the spine.

Two films may be taken for comparison, one erect and one supine.

Technical Factors:

• Film Size - 14 x 17 in. (35 x 43 cm), lengthwise. Larger patients - use 14 x 36 in. if available. (A long cassette with two films placed end to end may also be used.)
• Use moving or stationary grid.
• Use erect marker for erect position.
• Relatively high kVp (80-100) range for long scale contrast. (See NOTE.)
• Use compensating filters for more uniform density.

Patient Position:

• Erect position (weight evenly distributed on both feet). May be taken AP (see NOTE).

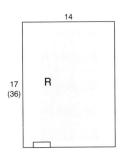

PA Erect   Fig. 8-75

Shielding:
Place contact shield over gonads without obscuring area of interest (upper edge of shield to level of ASIS). Use breast shields for young females. Shadow shields may be used as shown in *Fig. 8-76* and as evident in *Fig. 8-78.*)

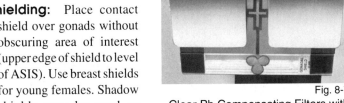

Fig. 8-76

Clear Pb Compensating Filters with Breast and Gonadal Shields
(Courtesy of Nuclear Associates, Carle, NY)

Part Position:

• Align **midsagittal plane to midline of film holder**. Arms at side.
• **No rotation** of torso or pelvis if possible. (Scoliosis may be accompanied with twisting and rotation of vertebrae making rotation unavoidable.)
• **Lower margin of cassette** is placed a minimum of **1 in.** (2.5 cm) **below iliac crest.**

Central Ray:

• CR **perpendicular,** directed to **mid point of film.**
• Minimum 40 in. (102 cm) SID.

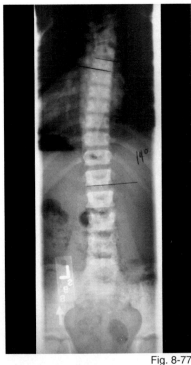
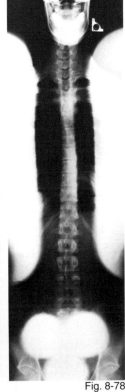

Fig. 8-77   Fig. 8-78
PA Erect   PA Erect
– 14 x 17 in. film   – 36 in. (90 cm) film

(Courtesy of Nuclear Associates.)

Collimation:
Collimate on four sides to area of interest. (Too narrow side collimation is not recommended on initial film since deformities of adjacent areas of ribs and pelvis also need to be evaluated.)

Respiration:
Suspend breathing on **expiration.**

NOTE: • A relative high kVp will result in a longer scale contrast and a more uniform density between thoracic and lumbar vertebrae. A second benefit of higher kVp is a reduction in total radiation dose to patient.
• A PA rather than AP projection is recommended because of the significantly reduced dosage to radiation sensitive areas such as ovaries, breasts and thyroid gland. Studies have shown this results in approximately 90% reduction in dosage to the breasts[1].
• Scoliosis generally requires repeat examinations over a period of time on young patients emphasizing the need for careful shielding.

Evaluation Criteria:

• Vertebral column should be in center of collimation field and film.
• Iliac crests should be a minimum of 1 in. or 2.5 cm above bottom edge of film.
• The distal lumbar vertebra should be included at the lower margin of the film and the total thoracic spine on upper film. (Younger and smaller patients will include the entire lumbar and thoracic vertebrae on one 14 x 17 in. [35 x 43 cm] film.)
• Optional 36 in. (90 cm) film will generally include entire thoracic and lumbar spine on older or larger patients.

[1] Frank Ed, Sterns JG, Gray JE, et al: Use of the Postero-anterior Projection; A method of reducing x-ray exposures to Radiosensitive Organs. Radiol. Technol; 54:343-347.

• Erect Lateral

Structures Best Shown:
Thoracic and lumbar spine in lateral projection to demonstrate possible spondylolisthesis (anterior displacement of one vertebra over another) or degrees of kyphosis or lordosis.

Technical Factors:
• Film Size - 14 x 17 in. (35 x 43 cm), lengthwise, or 14 x 36 in on larger patients if available. (A long cassette with 2 films placed end to end may also be used.)
• Use stationary or moving grid.
• Use erect marker.
• Use compensating filter for more uniform density.
• 90-100 kVp range. (See NOTE.)

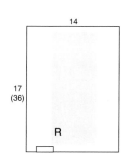

Patient Position:
• Patient in erect lateral position with arms folded above head, or if unsteady grasping a support in front of patient.
• The side of the convexity of primary curve should be against film.

Shielding: Place contact shield or shadow shield over gonads without obscuring area of interest. Use breast shields for young females.

Part Position:
• Place pelvis and torso in as **true a lateral position** as possible.
• **Align coronal plane of body to midline of film.**
• Lower margin of cassette a minimum of **1 in.** (2.5 cm) **below level of iliac crests.**

Central Ray:
• CR **perpendicular** directed to **mid point of film**.
• Minimum 40 in. (102 cm) SID.

Collimation: Four-sided collimation to area of interest. Use side collimation to area of vertebral column, however, use caution to **not** cut off a portion of vertebral column due to the increase in curvature.

Respiration: Suspend breathing on **expiration.**

NOTE: • A relative high kVp will produce a long scale contrast for a more uniform density of thoracic and lumbar vertebrae.

Evaluation Criteria:
• Thoracic and lumbar vertebra should be demonstrated in as true a lateral position as possible. (Some rotation of pelvis and/or thorax may be apparent since scoliosis generally is accompanied by a twisting or rotation of involved vertebrae.)
• One inch (2.5 cm) minimum of the iliac crests should be seen on lower margin of film.
• Vertebral column should be in center of collimation field and film.
• Optimum exposure and long scale contrast will visualize outline of distal lumbar vertebrae without overexposing thoracic vertebrae.
• Right or left and erect markers must be visible without superimposing essential anatomy.

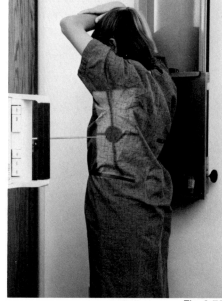

Erect Lateral   Fig. 8-79

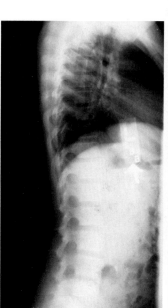

Fig. 8-80

Erect Lateral

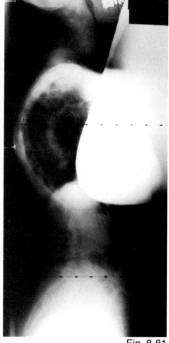

Fig. 8-81

Erect Lateral, full spine scoliosis exam. Clear Pb lateral thoracic compensating filter and breast shadow shield in place.
(Courtesy of Nuclear Associates, Carle, NY)

• AP Ferguson Method[1]

Scoliosis Series
Basic
• AP Erect and/or Supine
• Erect Lateral
Optional
• **AP Ferguson Method**
• AP, R and L Bending

Structures Best Shown:

Thoracic and lumbar spine in the AP projection to identify deforming (primary) curve from compensatory curve.

Two films are taken (one standard erect AP and one with the foot or hip on the convex side of the curve elevated).

Technical Factors:

- Film Size - 2 each 14 x 17 in. (35 x 43 cm), lengthwise.
- Use moving or stationary grid.
- Use erect marker.
- Relatively high kVp (80-100) range for long scale contrast and wider exposure latitude.
- Use compensating filters for more uniform density.

Patient Position:

- Patient in AP position, either seated or standing with arms at side.
- For second film, place a block under foot (or hip) if seated on convex side of curve enough so patient can barely maintain position **without assistance**. (A 3-4 in. or 8-10 cm block of some type may be used under buttock or foot as shown in *Fig. 8-83*.)

Shielding: Place contact shield or shadow shield over gonads without obscuring area of interest. Use breast shields for young females.

Part Position:

- Align **midsagittal plane to midline of table**. Arms at side.
- **No rotation** of torso or pelvis if possible.
- Bottom edge of cassette is placed a minimum 1 in. (2.5 cm) below level of iliac crest.

Central Ray:

- CR **perpendicular**, centered to **mid point of film**.
- Minimum 40 in. (102 cm) SID.

Collimation: Four-sided collimation to area of interest.

Respiration: Suspend breathing on **expiration**.

NOTE: • No form of support (i.e. compression band) is to be used in this exam. For second film patient should stand or sit with block under one side unassisted.
- May be done as PA projections which reduces dosage to radiation sensitive areas.

[1] Ferguson, AB: Roentgen Diagnosis of the Extremities and Spine, New York, 1939, Harper & Row Publishers

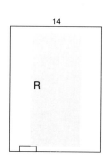
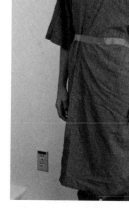

Fig. 8-82
AP Erect

Fig. 8-83
AP with Block Under Foot on Convex Side of Curve

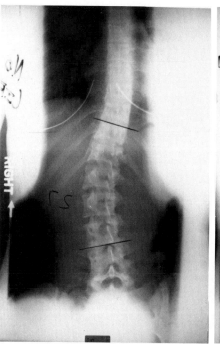
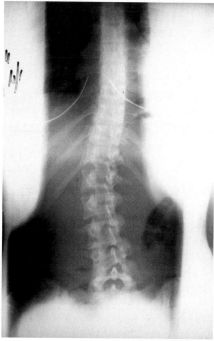

Fig. 8-84
AP Erect, with No Lift

Fig. 8-85
AP Erect, with Lift

Evaluation Criteria:

- All of thoracic and lumbar vertebra should be demonstrated in AP position.
- A minimum of one inch (2.5 cm) of iliac crest should be seen on lower film margin.
- Vertebral column should be in center of film and/or collimation field.
- Optimum exposure should clearly visualize the distal lumbar region without overexposure of the proximal thoracic region.
- Correct placement of gonad shields (and breast shields on females) should be evident.
- Right or left and erect markers must be visible but not superimposed by essential anatomy.

• AP (PA) Right and Left Bending

Scoliosis Series
Basic
• PA Erect and/or Supine
• Erect Lateral
Optional
• AP Ferguson Method
• **AP, R and L Bending**

Structures Best Shown:
Thoracic and lumbar spine in the AP (or PA) projection.

Two films are taken (one bending to right and one bending to left).

Technical Factors:
• Film Size - 2 each 14 x 17 in. (35 x 43 cm), lengthwise.
• Use moving or stationary grid.
• Use erect marker for erect position.
• Relatively high kVp (80-100) range for long scale contrast and wider exposure latitude.

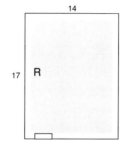

Patient Position:
• May be taken erect or supine.
• Patient in as true an anatomical position as possible.

Shielding: Place contact shield over gonads without obscuring area of interest. Use breast shields for young females.

Part Position:
• Start by aligning midsagittal plane to midline of table, arms at side.
• **No rotation** of torso or pelvis if possible.
• Bottom edge of cassette is placed **1 in.** (2.5 cm) **below iliac crest.**
• With the pelvis acting as a fulcrum, have patient bend (lateral flexion) **as far as possible** to either side.
• Both the upper torso and the legs may be moved to achieve maximum lateral flexion.
• Repeat above when doing opposite side.

Central Ray:
• CR **perpendicular**, directed to **mid point of film.**
• Minimum 40 in. (102 cm) SID.

Collimation: Four-sided collimation to near borders of film.

Respiration: Suspend breathing on **expiration.**

NOTE: • The pelvis must remain as stationary as possible during positioning.
• Pelvis acts as a fulcrum (pivot point) during changes of position.
• May be done as PA projections if taken erect which significantly reduces exposure to radiation sensitive areas.

Evaluation Criteria:
• Thoracic and lumbar vertebra should be demonstrated in extreme lateral flexion (both R and L) on two separate films.
• Iliac crests should be at least 1 inch or 2.5 cm above bottom of radiograph.
• Rotation of pelvis and/or thorax may be apparent since scoliosis generally is accompanied by rotation of involved vertebrae.

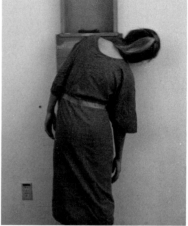

R Bending   Fig. 8-86

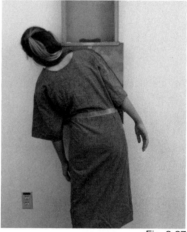

L Bending   Fig. 8-87

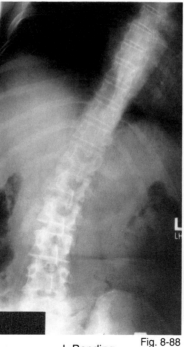

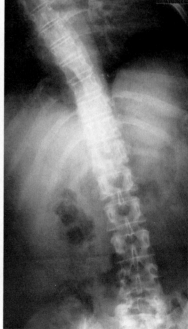

L Bending   Fig. 8-88   R Bending   Fig. 8-89

• Optimum exposure should clearly visualize the distal lumbar region without overexposure of the proximal thoracic region.
• Right or left markers must be visible not superimposed by essential anatomy.

• Lateral, Hyperextension and Hyperflexion

Structures Best Shown:
Two lateral projections of the lumbar spine at the site of the fusion.

Purpose: To demonstrate movement (if any) at fusion site.

Two films are taken (one with hyperflexion and one with hyperextension).

Right & Left bending positioning is similar to that for scoliosis series.

Technical Factors:
• Film Size - Two each 10 x 12 in. (24 x 30 cm), lengthwise.

or
  - 11 x 14 in. (30 x 35 cm)
or
  - 14 x 17 in. (35 x 43 cm)
• Use stationary or moving grid.
• 85-90 kVp range.
• Use hyperextension and hyperflexion markers.

10 (11) (14)

12
(14)
(17)   R

Patient Position:
• Patient in lateral recumbent position with pillow for head and support between knees. (See NOTE for possible erect position.)

Shielding: Place contact shield over gonads without obscuring area of interest.

Part Position:
• Start by aligning coronal plane to midline of table.
• Hyperflexion - using pelvis as fulcrum, have patient get into fetal position (bend forward) and draw legs up **as far as possible.**
• Hyperextension - using pelvis as fulcrum, have patient move torso and legs posteriorly **as far as possible** to hyperextend long axis of body.
• Assure there is no rotation of thorax or pelvis.

Central Ray:
• CR **perpendicular** to film.
• Center CR to **site of fusion** if known, or to level of **L3** (level of lower costal margin or about 1-1.5 in. or 3-4 cm above iliac crest).
• Center cassette to CR.
• Minimum 40 in. (102 cm) SID.

Collimation: Four-sided collimation to near borders of film (if 10 x 12). Larger films require more collimation, especially side collimation.

Respiration: Suspend respiration on expiration.

NOTE: • May also be done erect sitting on a stool, first leaning forward as far as possible gripping the stool legs; then leaning backwards as far as possible gripping the back of the stool to maintain this position.
• Pelvis must remain as stationary as possible during positioning.
• Pelvis acts as a fulcrum (pivot point) during changes of position.

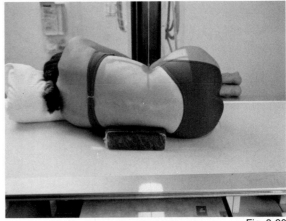

Lateral – Hyperflexion   Fig. 8-90

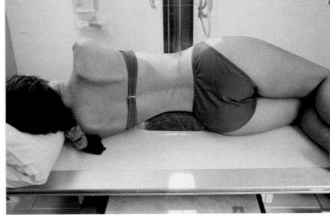

Lateral – Hyperextension   Fig. 8-91

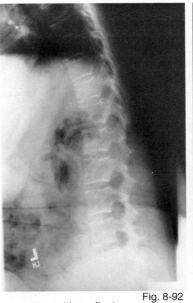

Fig. 8-92   Fig. 8-93
Hyperflexion   Hyperextension

Evaluation Criteria:
• Site of fusion should be in center of collimation field and film.
• Lower lumbar vertebra should be demonstrated in extreme hyperflexion and hyperextension on two separate films.
• L5 should be in midline of film.
• There should be no rotation of thorax or pelvis.
• Optimum exposure will clearly visualize outlines of lumbar vertebra and intervertebra joint spaces.
• R or L and hyperextension/hyperflexion markers should be visible without superimposing essential anatomy.

Chapter 9
Radiographic Anatomy and Positioning
of the
Thoracic and Cervical Spine

Contributions by: Alex Backus, MS, RT(R)

Contents

Part I Radiographic Anatomy

Upper Thoracic Column

The upper or cephalic portion of the vertebral column is divided into two portions, the **thoracic vertebrae** and the **cervical vertebrae.** Typically, there are 12 thoracic vertebrae and 7 cervical vertebrae.

Thoracic Vertebrae

The lumbar vertebrae, presented in the preceding chapter, most closely resemble typical vertebrae. As one progresses farther up the vertebral column, there are greater and greater differences compared to the lumbar vertebrae. The middle four thoracic vertebrae, numbers 5, 6, 7 and 8, are considered typical thoracic vertebrae. The lower four assume some of the characteristics of the lumbar vertebrae, while the upper four gradually assume features of the cervical region.

Rib Articulations

The one feature of all thoracic vertebrae that serves to distinguish them from all others is that **all thoracic vertebrae have facets for articulation with ribs.** Each thoracic vertebra is closely associated with one pair of ribs. Since there are 12 pairs of ribs, there are also 12 thoracic vertebrae.

Costovertebral Joints: All 12 vertebrae have either a full **facet** *(fas'et)* or two partial facets, termed **demifacets** *(dem"e-fas'et)*, on each side of the body. Each facet or combination of two demifacets accepts the head of a rib to form a **costovertebral joint**.

Costotransverse Joints: In addition, each of the first ten thoracic vertebrae have facets (one on each transverse process) that articulate with the tubercles of ribs 1 through 10. These articulations are termed **costotransverse joints**.

As the first ten pairs of ribs flare out away from the upper ten vertebrae, the tubercle of each rib articulates with one transverse process to form a costotransverse joint.

The costovertebral joint and costotransverse joint of one rib are shown in *Fig. 9-3.* Those vertebrae with two demifacets share the heads of two ribs, one on the right and one on the left. The demifacet on the bottom of one vertebra articulates with the superior portion of the head of a particular rib, while the demifacet near the top of the next vertebra articulates with the inferior part of the same head.

The first thoracic vertebra (T1) has on each side of its body a superior whole facet and an inferior demifacet. This indicates that the heads of the **first pair of ribs** articulate with the **upper part of T1** vertebra, (top of *Fig. 9-2*). This fact becomes important when identifing T1 vertebrae by association with the posterior first pair of ribs, which are readily seen on radiographs of the cervical and thoracic spine.

Thoracic vertebrae 10, 11 and 12 (T10-12) have a single costal facet on each side indicating the heads of the 10th, 11th & 12th ribs articulate with the respective vertebrae at these facets. This again provides a means of identifying these specific vertebrae. This will be demonstrated on the anatomy review of the thoracic and cervical spine on page 276.

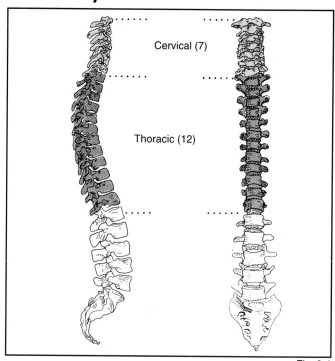

Cervical (7)

Thoracic (12)

Upper Vertebral Column　　　　　　　Fig. 9-1

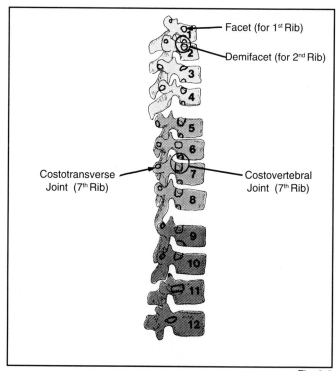

Facet (for 1st Rib)

Demifacet (for 2nd Rib)

Costotransverse Joint (7th Rib)

Costovertebral Joint (7th Rib)

Thoracic Vertebrae (Rib Articulations)　　Fig. 9-2

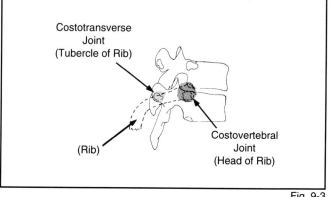

Costotransverse Joint (Tubercle of Rib)

(Rib)

Costovertebral Joint (Head of Rib)

Fig. 9-3

Costovertebral and Costotransverse Joints

Typical Thoracic Vertebrae

Lateral View

A side view of two typical thoracic vertebrae is shown in *Fig. 9-4*. As the thoracic vertebrae progress upward from twelve to one, they look less and less like typical lumbar vertebrae. The thoracic vertebrae are smallest near T1 and largest near T12.

Each thoracic vertebra possesses the seven processes of the typical lumbar vertebra. The large **spinous process** of each thoracic vertebra is longer and points more downward compared to the thick, blunt lumbar spinous process. The two **transverse processes** of thoracic vertebra T1 through T10 are unique in that each of these has a facet near its end.

The **superior articular processes** and the **inferior articular processes** serve to connect the successive thoracic vertebrae to form the **zygapophyseal** (apophyseal) joints.

On each side, between any two thoracic vertebrae, is an **intervertebral foramen**. The intervertebral foramina of the thoracic region are well seen on a direct lateral view such as *Fig. 9-4*. The main distinguishing characteristic of the thoracic vertebrae, however, is the fact that each thoracic vertebra possess facets for rib articulation.

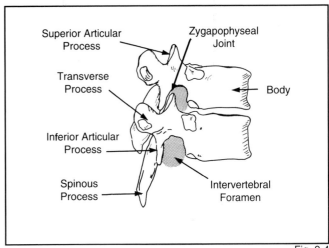

Fig. 9-4

Typical Thoracic Vertebrae
(Lateral View)

Superior View

A typical thoracic vertebra as seen from above is illustrated. The usual features of a typical vertebra plus the distinguishing characteristics of the **facets** are well shown. The **body** is the most anterior structure, while the **spinous process** is the most posterior structure. The spinous process seems fairly short when viewed in this direction, but remember that it is projected primarily downward.

The vertebral arch is composed of the two **pedicles** projecting from the body and the two **laminae**. Each **transverse process** projects from the junction of the pedicle and the lamina on each side. A single **rib** is shown in position to demonstrate the **costovertebral joint** and the **costotransverse joint** on one side.

An end on view of the articular **facet of the superior articular process** is shown which articulates with the inferior process of the adjoining vertebrae to form the zygapophyseal joint.

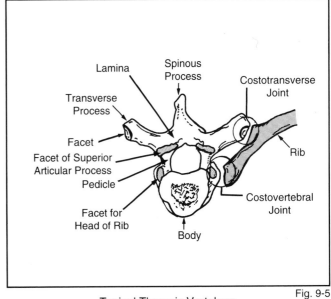

Fig. 9-5

Typical Thoracic Vertebrae
(Superior View)

Zygapophyseal Joints

The structure and angles of the facets of the inferior and superior articular processes making up the zygopophyseal joints differ markedly from that of the lumbar vertebrae. These joints on the lumbar vertebrae form an angle of approximately 45°, but on the thoracic vertebrae, this angle is from 15° to 20° from the coronal plane. Therefore, to demonstrate these joints radiographically on the thoracic spine requires a **70° to 75° oblique**, which is **15°-20° from the lateral position** *(Fig. 9-6)*.

Intervertebral Foramina

The location of the intervertebral foramina can be identified on these drawings by the pedicles which make up the roof of these foramina or openings. As demonstrated in *Fig. 9-6*, the intervertebral foramina on the thoracic vertebra are located at right angles or 90° to the midsagittal plane, similar to the lumbar vertebra. Therefore, to demonstrate them radiographically, **a true lateral position** is required, the same as for the lumbar spine.

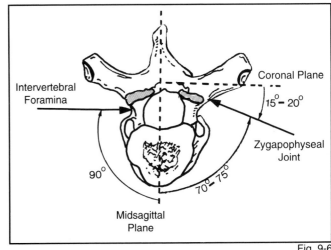

Fig. 9-6

Typical Thoracic Vertebrae
– Intervertebral Foramina
– Zygapophyseal Joints

Cervical Vertebrae

Typical Cervical Vertebrae

The cervical vertebrae show little resemblance to either the lumbar or thoracic vertebrae. In fact, the upper two cervical vertebrae, C1 and C2, are quite unusual. **C1** is often termed the **atlas**, a name derived from the Greek god who bore the world upon his shoulders. The **second cervical** is called the **axis**, since much of the rotation of the head occurs between C1 and C2.

The third through sixth cervical vertebrae are typical cervical vertebrae. The last or **seventh cervical vertebra** assumes many of the features of the thoracic vertebrae, including an extra long spinous process that gives C7 its special name, the **vertebra prominens**.

Superior View

Figure 9-8 shows a typical cervical vertebra as viewed from above. While the parts forming the vertebral arch are all present and the vertebra has the usual seven processes, they are somewhat different from those of either the typical lumbar or thoracic vertebra.

The **transverse processes** are quite small and arise from both the **pedicle** and the **body**, rather than from the pedicle-lamina junction. In addition, there is a hole in each transverse process called a **transverse foramen**. Important blood vessels and nerves pass through these successive transverse foramina. Thus one unique characteristic of all cervical vertebrae is that they each have **three** foramina; the two transverse foramina and the single large vertebral foramen.

The **spinous processes** of C2 through C6 are fairly short and usually end in two tips rather than only one. This double or forked tip is termed a **bifid tip**. The bodies are small and oblong in shape with some overlapping when they are stacked in the cervical vertebral column.

Lateral View

A typical cervical vertebra as viewed from the side illustrates that the **body** is the most anterior structure and the **spinous process** is the most posterior structure. Located behind the transverse process at the junction of the pedicle and the lamina is a short column of bone that is much more supportive than the similar area in the rest of the spinal column. This column of bone is termed the **articular pillar**, sometimes shortened to just pillar. Located on top of each pillar is the **superior articular process**. On the bottom is found the **inferior articular process** for formation of the zygapophyseal joint.

Each cervical vertebra and vertebral body continues to get smaller, progressing up from the seventh cervical to the third cervical vertebra.

Zygapophyseal Joints

The superior and inferior articular processes, as located over the articular pillars, are directly lateral to the large vertebral foramen. Therefore, the zygapophyseal joints of the second through seventh cervical vertebrae are located at right angles or **90°** to the midsagittal plane and would be visualized radiographically in a **true lateral position**. The exception to this is the zygopophyseal joints between C1 and C2 which are visualized only on a true frontal view.

Intervertebral Foramina

The intervertebral foramina can again be identified by the pedicles which make up the floor of these foramina as shown in *Figs. 9-8* and *9-10*. The intervertebral foramina are situated at a **45°** angle to the midsagittal plane, and open anteriorly as shown on this drawing. They are also directed at a **15°** inferior angle due to the shape and the overlapping of the cervical vertebrae. Therefore, to "open up" and visualize these foramina radiographically, a **45° oblique position** is required, and a **15° cephalic angle** of the x-ray beam.

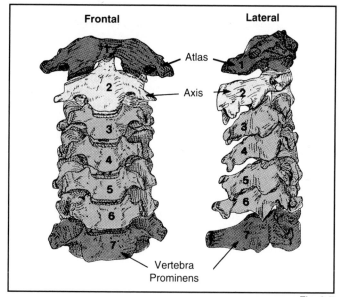

Cervical Spine — Fig. 9-7

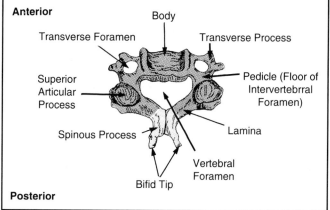

Typical Cervical Vertebra (Superior View) — Fig. 9-8

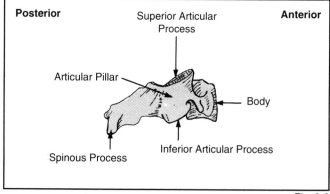

Typical Cervical Vertebra (Lateral View) — Fig. 9-9

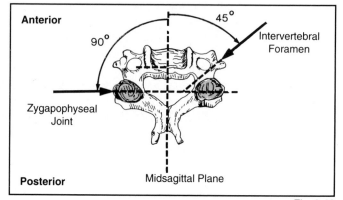

Typical Cervical Vertebra (Superior View) — Fig. 9-10
– Intervertebral Foramina
– Zygapophyseal Joints

Axis (C2)

The most distinctive feature of the second cervical vertebra, the **axis**, is the strong conical process projecting from the upper surface of the **body**. This radiographically important process is called the **dens (odontoid process)**.

Rotation of the head primarily occurs between C1 and C2, with the dens helping to make this type of motion possible. The **superior articular processes** are large flat surfaces assisting in rotation of the head. Severe stress as the possible result of a forced flexion-hyperextension "whip-lash" type of injury may cause a fracture of the dens. Any fracture of the vertebral column at this level could result in serious damage to the spinal cord as well.

The **inferior articular process** for articulation with C3 lies inferior to the **lamina.** Below the superior articular process is the transverse process with its **transverse foramen.** The blunt **spinous process** extends posteriorly.

Atlas (Cl)

The first cervical vertebra, the **atlas**, as seen from above, least resembles a typical vertebra. Anteriorly, there is no body, but simply an arch of bone termed the **anterior arch.** The dens is actually the body of C1, but embryologically the C1 body fuses to C2 and becomes the dens. Therefore, in an adult, the dens of C2 projects up through the large central opening of C1. This is demonstrated on the frontal open-mouth view of *Figs. 9-13* and *14.*

Posteriorly, another arch of bone, the **posterior arch,** may bear a small tubercle at the midline. This tubercle is all that remains of a spinous process. Each **superior articular process** presents a large depressed surface for articulation with the respective occipital condyle of the skull. The **transverse processes** are smaller, but still contain the **transverse foramina** distinctive of all cervical vertebrae. Lateral to the arches, on each side of C1, is a large area of bone termed the **lateral mass.**

Relationship of Cl and C2

The relationship of C2, with its dens, to C1, and the relationship of C1 to the base of the skull, are highly important. Figure 9-13 demonstrates the view as seen on an AP radiograph of the upper cervical spine taken with the mouth wide open *(Fig. 9-14)*. The anterior arch of C1, which lies in front of the dens, is not visible on this frontal view because it is a fairly thin piece of bone and is not well visualized on a frontal radiograph.

Normally, the various articulations between C2 and C1, and between C1 and the skull, are perfectly symmetrical. Accordingly, the relationship of the **dens** to C1 must also be perfectly symmetrical. Both injury and improper positioning can render these areas asymmetrical. For this reason, a perfectly positioned radiograph of this area can be of utmost importance.

The **lateral masses** of C1 are well demonstrated on this view, with their inferior articular processes on the lower borders. The joint between the **inferior** and the **superior articular processes**, the **zygapophyseal joint** is also well visualized on this frontal view. Extending laterally from each lateral mass of C1 are the **transverse processes** of C1.

The parts labelled A–D on the radiograph correspond to those parts labelled on the drawing, *(Fig. 9-13).*

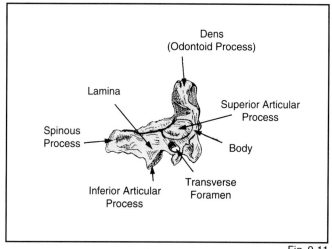

Axis (Lateral View)   Fig. 9-11

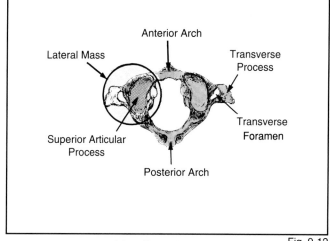

Atlas (Superior View)   Fig. 9-12

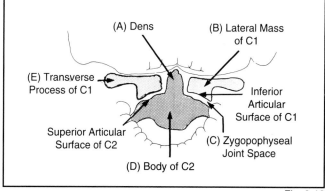

C1 and C2, Frontal Open-mouth View   Fig. 9-13

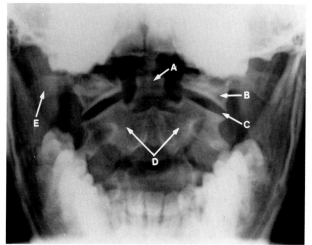

AP Open Mouth Radiograph   Fig. 9-14

Anatomy Review

AP and Lateral Thoracic Spine

Individual thoracic vertebrae can best be identified on the AP projection because of rib associations. The posterior ribs 1–12 can be readily seen and counted thus identifying specific thoracic vertebra. This is more difficult on the lateral thoracic spine unless the sternum can also be seen.

AP T Spine

A. 1st posterior rib
B. 10th posterior rib
C. Spinous process of T11
D. Body of T12
E. Intervertebral disc space between T8 and T9
F. Body of T7 (center of T spine and of average chest)
G. Body of T1 (remember head of 1st ribs articulate with upper portion of T1)

Lateral T spine

A. Body of T3
B. Body of T7 (center of T spine and of chest)
C. Intervertebral foramina between T11 and 12

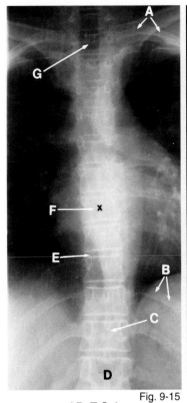

Fig. 9-15
AP T Spine

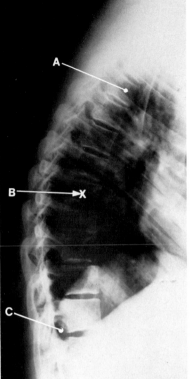

Fig. 9-16
Lateral T Spine

AP Cervical Spine

A conventional AP radiograph of the cervical spine is illustrated in *Fig. 9-17*. Usually, the first two or three thoracic vertebrae, as well as C7 up to C3, are seen well on this projection. Identifying specific vertebrae can be difficult, but T1 is probably the easiest to find. T1 should have the first pair of ribs attached to it. Therefore, to localize T1, locate the most superior ribs and find the vertebra to which they appear to connect. After locating T1, the visible cervical vertebrae can be identified by starting at C7 and counting upward.

Part **A** on this radiograph is the first thoracic vertebra, determined by discovering that part **B** is the first rib on the patient's right side.

Part **C** is the fourth cervical vertebra.

Part **D** is the articular pillar of C 3. The white area at the top of the radiograph is created by the combined shadows of the base of the skull and the mandible. These structures effectively cover up the first two cervical vertebrae on this type of radiograph.

Part **E** is the spinous process of C 3 seen on end.

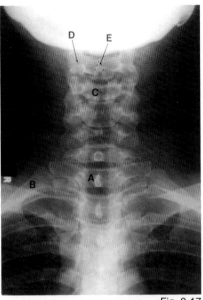

AP C Spine
Fig. 9-17

Anatomy Review continued

Lateral Cervical Spine

The single most important radiograph in any cervical spine series is a good lateral. A lateral cervical spine radiograph is demonstrated in *Fig. 9-18.* Radiographers should always try to show all seven cervical vertebrae on any lateral cervical spine radiograph if this is possible. At times this is difficult on those patients with thick shoulders and a short neck and a special "swimmers" lateral may need to be taken to include C7. In order to determine if all seven cervical vertebrae are being shown, locate the atlas, or C1, and count downward. The seventh cervical vertebra is marked with an X.

The lower anterior margins of the last four or five cervical vertebral bodies have a slight lipped appearance which, along with the general shape of the bodies, requires that the central ray be angled approximately **20 degrees cephalic** (toward the head) to "open up" these lower intervertebral spaces.

    A. Dens (odontoid process) enhanced with dotted lines
       on this visual
    B. Posterior arch of the atlas
    C. Body of C3
    D. Zygapophyseal joint between C4 and C5
    E. Spinous process of C6

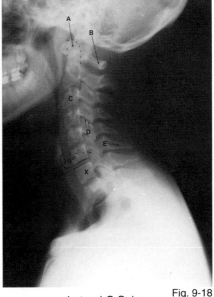

Lateral C Spine   Fig. 9-18

Oblique Cervical Spine

A good **oblique cervical spine** radiograph is shown in *Fig. 9-19.* An important purpose of the oblique position is to show the **intervertebral foramina.** Spinal nerves to and from the spinal cord are transmitted through these intervertebral foramina. Remember this is taken in a 45° oblique position with the central ray angled 15° cephalic, if taken as posterior obliques.

    A. Posterior arch of C1
    B. Intervertebral foramen between C4 and C5
    C. Pedicle of C6
    D. Body of C7

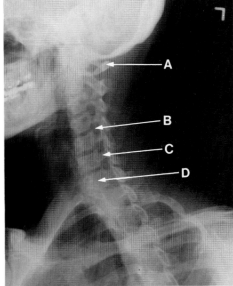

Oblique C Spine   Fig. 9-19

MRI Images of Lateral Cervical Spine

The MRI image of a lateral cervical spine clearly demonstrates not only bony structure but soft tissue as well *(Fig. 9-20).*

The vertebral canal containing the spinal cord is seen as the light, tube-like column directly posterior to the cervical vertebrae. The spinal cord (light gray) is seen to be a continuation of the medulla oblogata of the brain. A herniation of the disc between C5 and C6 is demonstrated with a slight posterior displacement causing mild spinal cord displacement (see arrows).

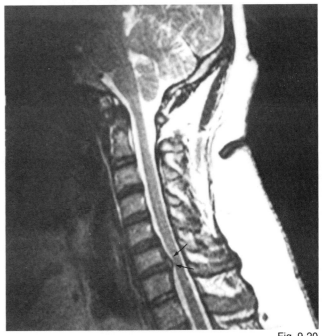

MRI Lateral C Spine Image   Fig. 9-20

Intervertebral Foramina vs. Zygapophyseal Joints

Two anatomical areas of the spine that must be demonstrated by the proper radiographs are the **intervertebral foramina** and the **zygapophyseal joints**. The physician gains important information concerning the relationship of consecutive vertebrae by studying these two areas on the appropriate radiograph. To complicate matters, however, depending on the part of the spine to be radiographed (cervical, thoracic, or lumbar), a different body position is required to best show each anatomical area.

Thoracic Spine

Thoracic Spine Skeleton: Two photographs of the thoracic vertebrae are shown in *Figs. 9-21* and *22*. The thoracic vertebrae on the left are in a lateral position, and on the right, an oblique position. A 70-degree oblique is necessary to open up the zygapophyseal joints on the thoracic spine. The lateral position of the thoracic spine best shows the intervertebral foramina. The **posterior** oblique position on the right shows the zygapophyseal joint on the **upside**. **Anterior** obliques would demonstrate the **downside** joints.

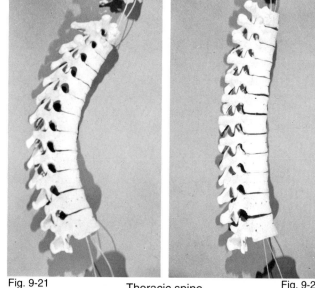

Fig. 9-21   Thoracic spine   Fig. 9-22
Left Lateral   Oblique (LPO)

Thoracic Spine Radiographs: Radiographs of the thoracic spine in the lateral position, and in the 70° oblique position correspond to the position of the thoracic skeleton directly above. Observe that the round openings of the superimposed **intervertebral foramina** are best visualized on the **lateral** radiograph on the left.

The **zygapophyseal joints** are best visualized on the **oblique** radiograph on the right. The oblique radiograph is in a 70° LPO position, which should best visualize the zygapophyseal joints on the **upside,** or those farthest away from the film. The LPO position best shows the **right zygapophyseal** joints.

Remember if the obliques were taken as **anterior** obliques, the opposite would be true, the **downside** joints would be demonstrated. An **LAO** would demonstrate the **left** zygapophyseal joints. Therefore, an LAO would demonstrate the same side joints as an RPO.

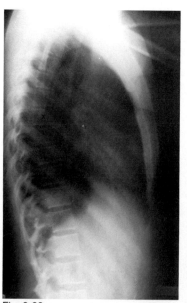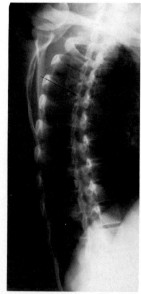

Fig. 9-23   Thoracic spine   Fig. 9-24
Left Lateral   Oblique (LPO)
– Intervertebral Foramina   – Zygapophyseal Joints

Intervertebral Foramina vs. Zygapophyseal Joints continued

Cervical Spine

Cervical Spine Skeleton *(Figs. 9-25 and 9-26)*

Two photographs of the cervical vertebrae are shown. On the left is a cervical section of the vertebral column in a left lateral position, while to the right is a 45° left posterior oblique position (LPO). The zygapophyseal joints visualize well on the lateral position.

On the right, the posterior oblique with a 45° rotation shows that the intervertebral foramina are clearly opened. It is important to know that the **left posterior oblique** position opens up the foramina on the **right side,** and a 15° CR **cephalic angle** is needed. Therefore, on a **posterior oblique** cervical spine radiograph, the **upside** is the side on which the intervertebral foramina are opened well.

If this were taken in an **anterior** oblique position, the foramina **closest** to the film, the downside would be open, and a 15° **caudal angle** would be required.

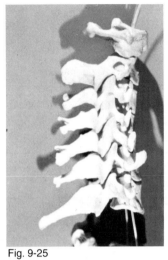 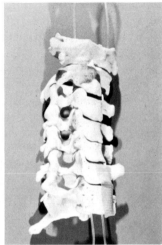

Fig. 9-25

Fig. 9-26

Left Lateral
– Zygapophyseal Joints

Oblique (LPO)
– Right Intervertebral
Foramina

Cervical Spine Radiographs *(Figs. 9-27 and 9-28)*

The two radiographs of the cervical spine illustrate the same anatomy in the same two positions as shown on the skeleton above. The lateral position on the left best shows the zygapophyseal joints. The joint on each side is superimposed upon the joint on the opposite side. One should remember that the zygapophyseal joints are located between the articular pillars of each vertebra.

The oblique cervical spine radiograph on the right shows the circular intervertebral foramina opened. In each oblique radiograph only one set of foramina are opened, while the ones on the opposite side are closed. Since this position is a left **posterior** oblique, the **right intervertebral foramina** or those on the **upside** are being shown.

It is important to remember that the LPO will show the same anatomy as the RAO. Therefore, if the patient were placed in an anterior oblique position, the downside foramina to the film will be shown. Thus in either case, LPO or RAO, the right intervertebral foramina will be visualized.

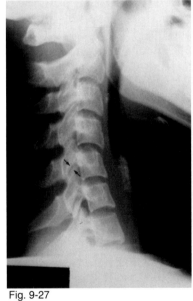 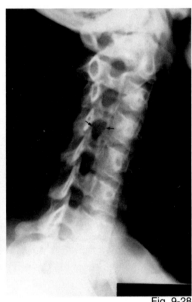

Fig. 9-27

Fig. 9-28

Lateral (Left)
– Zygapophyseal Joints

Oblique (LPO)
– Right Intervertebral Foramina

Summary of Intervertebral Foramina and Zygapophyseal Joints

The chart on the right summarizes which position of each region of the spine best visualizes either the intervertebral foramina or the zygapophyseal joints. The **intervertebral foramina** are best shown on the **oblique cervical**, and on the **lateral thoracic or lumbar**.

The zygapophyseal joints are best seen on the **lateral cervical**, the near **lateral thoracic (70°)** and the **45° oblique lumbar**.

The **upper body**, the cervical and thoracic regions, shows the **upside** best, while the **lower body** shows the **downside** best when radiographed anterior to posterior.

	Cervical	Thoracic	Lumbar
Intervertebral Foramina	• Oblique 45° • Upside (LPO or RPO)	• Lateral	• Lateral
Zygapophyseal Joints	• Lateral	• Oblique 70° • Upside (LPO or RPO)	• Oblique 45° • Downside (LPO or RPO)

Summary

Part II Radiographic Positioning

Topographical Landmarks

Sternum

The sternum provides some useful landmarks for locating various levels of the thoracic spine. The sternum is divided into three basic sections. The upper section is called the **manubrium.** The very top part of the manubrium, the **jugular** (suprasternal) **notch,** can be easily felt. The central portion of the sternum is called the **body.** The manubrium and body connect at a slight, easily located angle termed the **sternal angle.** The most inferior end of the sternum is called the **xiphoid process.** It takes some pressure to locate the xiphoid process on a patient.

With careful palpation or probing of these topographic landmarks, certain anatomical structures and relationships between structures can be determined. For example, the level of specific thoracic vertebrae can be determined from these three sternal landmarks—the jugular notch, the sternal angle and the xiphoid process. Both the sternal angle and the xiphoid process can be palpated, although they are not as easy to locate as the jugular notch.

Thoracic Spine

The bottom part of the xiphoid process, the **xiphoid tip,** is at the level of **T10** as indicated by line **A**. The **sternal angle** (line **C**) locates the **junction of T4 and T5.** The sternal angle is most easily located if one first locates the jugular notch and then follows the manubrium down about 2 in. or 5 cm until a slight bump is felt. The slight bump on the surface of the sternum should be the sternal angle. The second pair of ribs attach just lateral to the sternal angle.

One of the most important centering points for the thoracic spine is line **B** which locates **T7** at a level of **3 to 4 in.** (8-10 cm) **below the jugular notch.** The approximate center of the thoracic portion of the vertebral column is at the level of T7. The mid seventh thoracic vertebra is the center of the 12 thoracic vertebrae since the lower thoracic vertebrae are larger in size than the upper thoracic vertebrae.

The jugular notch, the easiest palpated anterior landmark, is identified by line **D** which is at the same level as the **disc space between T2 and T3.** Often, on a prepared skeleton, the jugular notch is closer to T 1, but this is not true on a person standing upright. On an average, standing adult, T1 is located 1.5 in. or (3.75 cm) above the jugular notch, marked as Line **E.**

The first thoracic vertebra can also be located by palpating posteriorly at the base of the neck for the prominent spinous process of C7, the **vertebra prominens.** Note that the long sloping vertebra prominens extends downward with its tip at the level of the body of T1.

Cervical Spine

The prominent topographical landmarks of the cervical region are illustrated. The prominent spinous process of the last cervical vertebra, **C7** (vertebra prominens), is at about the same level as the **body of T1.** On an average patient this is slightly above the level of the shoulders as shown on the model on the following page. The shoulders occasionally superimpose the last cervical vertebra on a lateral cervical spine radiograph. When this problem occurs, the shoulders must be depressed as much as possible.

The most prominent part of the **thyroid cartilage** or "Adam's apple" **(B)**, is at an approximate level of C5. This is not a reliable bony landmark, however, and varies between the level of C4 to C6. With the head in a neutral position, the angle of the jaw or **gonion (C)** is at the same level as **C3.** The **mastoid tip (D)** corresponds to the level of **C1.** The **EAM** (external acoustic meatus) **(E)** is easy to locate on any person and is about **1 inch or 2.5 cm above the level of C1.**

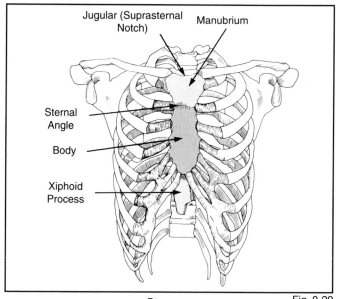

Sternum   Fig. 9-29

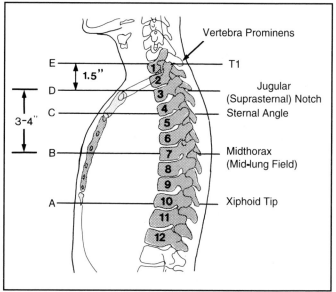

T Spine Landmarks   Fig. 9-30

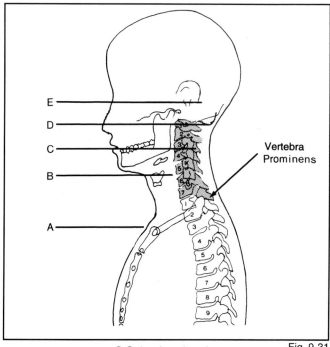

C Spine Landmarks   Fig. 9-31

Topographical Landmarks continued

Sternum and T spine Landmarks

The standard landmarks for the sternum and thoracic spine are illustrated on this model as follows: Line **A** is at the level of the **xiphoid tip**, which locates **T10**.

An important centering point is represented by line **B**, which anteriorly is 3 to 4 inches (8-10 cm) below the jugular notch at the level of **T7**. This is the center of the thoracic spine as well as the center of the lungs. Posteriorly this is about a handspread 7-8 inches (18-20 cm) below the vertebra prominens. On a well developed male such as this model, anteriorly this would be 4-5 in. (8-10 cm) below the jugular notch and posteriorly 8 in. (20 cm) below the vertebra prominens as described in Chapter 2 (page 63) on chest positioning. For a smaller male and for the average female these would be 3-4 in. (8-10 cm) anteriorly and about 7 in. (18 cm) posteriorly.

Line **C,** is at the **sternal angle** and corresponds to the disc space between **T4** and **T5**.

The **jugular notch** which corresponds to line **D** is at the level of the junction between **T2 and T3**. Line **E** corresponds to **T1**, the vertebra prominens, about 1-2 in. or (2.5-5 cm) above the jugular notch.

The sternum and the vertebra prominens can be used to locate individual thoracic vertebra. The use of these landmarks becomes necessary when well collimated radiographs are required of specific thoracic vertebrae.

C spine landmarks

These cervical spine landmarks are also identified on this model. The tops of the shoulders on an average adult are located slightly below the level of C7. This landmark does vary on different people, however, since on a very thin patient the shoulders may go down to T2 or T3. For a well developed male, such as this model, the shoulders slope and vary in such a way that they do **not** present a reliable positioning landmark. Since the spinous process of C7, the **vertebra prominens,** is very prominent (especially with head tipped forward), it should be used to help locate C7 rather than the top of the shoulders.

The **thyroid cartilage** of the larynx or "Adam's apple" localizes the **approximate** level of **C4** or **C5**. On most patients the upper margin of the thyroid cartilage corresponds nearer to the level of C4.

The **angle** or **gonion** of the mandible is at the level of **C3** when the head is in a neutral position.

The top of the cervical spine, or **C1**, is at the level of the **mastoid tip**. The mastoid tip can also be used to find the most inferior level of the base of the skull. The occipital condyles and foramen magnum are basal skull structures in line with the mastoid tip.

The **EAM** is about 1 inch (2.5 cm) above the level of C1.

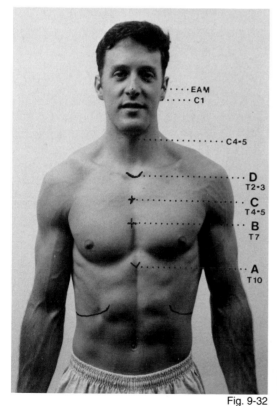
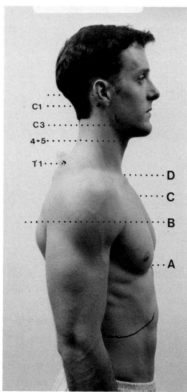
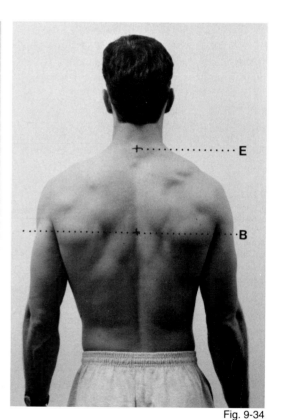

Fig. 9-32   Fig. 9-33   Fig. 9-34

Sternum, T Spine and C Spine Landmarks

National Survey

Departmental standard (basic) and optional routines of the thoracic spine did not show a significant difference in the different regions of the U.S. There were some regional differences for the cervical spine and especially the swimmers and AP "chewing" positions as shown below.

Thoracic Spine Routine

Thoracic Spine	U.S. Average	
	Basic	Optional
• AP	98%	
• Lateral	98%	
• Oblique	2%	13%

Cervical Spine Routine

Cervical Spine	U.S. Average		East		Midwest		West	
	Basic	Optional	Basic	Optional	Basic	Optional	Basic	Optional
• AP – 20° cephalic	95%		94%		91%		94%	
• Lateral	93%		93%		95%		91%	
• Obliques	90%		94%		86%		92%	
• AP- open mouth (C1 & C2)	93%		94%		91%		99%	
• Swimmers lateral (cervicothoracic)	59%	26%	46%	35%	66%	21%	67%	18%
• Lateral – flexion & extension	22%	31%	21%	30%	19%	34%	26%	31%
• AP "chewing" ("wagging jaw")	2%	10%	3%	13%	2%	7%	0	13%
• AP pillars (25-30° caudal)		2%						

Summary

The survey demonstrated a significant regional difference for the **AP "chewing"** or "wagging jaw" position. In the **midwest** only **7%** indicated it as an optional position compared to almost twice as many **(13%)** in both the **east** and the **west.**

There was also a significant regional difference for the **swimmers** position wherein the **total combined frequency for basic and optional** is similar in all regions. However, in the **midwest** and **west** a much higher percent indicated it as routine, **66 and 67%** respectively, as compared to only **46%** in the **east**. Overall the majority of respondents indicated it as part of the basic routine rather than optional which is the way it is presented in this text.

Standard and Optional Operating Procedures

Certain basic and optional projections or positions for the thoracic and cervical spine are demonstrated and described on the following pages as suggested standard and optional departmental procedures.

Basic Projections

Standard or basic projections, also sometimes referred to as routine projections or departmental routines are **those projections or posi-** tions commonly taken on average patients who are helpful and can cooperate in performing the procedure.

Optional Projections

Optional projections are **those more common projections or positions taken as extra or additional projections to better demonstrate certain pathologic conditions or specific body parts.** (These are not optional as to their importance.)

Basic and Optional Projections

Thoracic Spine
Basic
• AP
• Lateral
Optional
• Obliques

Cervical Spine
Basic
• AP
• AP Open Mouth
 (C1 and C2)
• Lateral
• Obliques
• Swimmers Lateral
 (Cervicothoracic)
Optional
• Lateral – hyperflexion and hyperextension
• AP "chewing," "wagging jaw"

Cervical Spine (Trauma series)
Basic
• Lateral (Horizontal Beam)
Optional
• AP
• Obliques
• Swimmers Lateral
 (Cervicothoracic)

• AP Projection

Thoracic Spine
Basic
• **AP**
• Lateral
Optional
• Obliques

Structures Best Shown:
Thoracic vertebral bodies, intervertebral joint spaces, distance between pedicles, spinous and transverse processes, posterior ribs and costovertebral articulations.

Technical Factors:
• Film Size - 14 x 17 in. (35 x 43 cm), lengthwise.
• Moving or stationary grid.
• 80-90 kVp range.
• Use wedge compensation filter with thicker part of filter at head end for more uniform density.

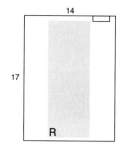

Patient Position:
• Supine with head at anode end of table. This orientation will utilize the anode-heel effect in addition to the wedge filter to result in a more uniform density on the film from T1 to T12. Arms at side. Head on table or on a thin pillow.

Shielding: Place lead shield over pelvic area to shield gonads. Breast shields may also be used for young females without obscuring the area of interest.

Part Position:
• Align **midsagittal plane to midline of table.**
• **Flex knees and hips** to reduce thoracic curvature.
• Assure there is **no rotation** of the pelvis or thorax.

Central Ray:
• CR **perpendicular** to film.
• Center to **T7**, which is 3 to 4 in. (8-10 cm) below jugular notch, or 2 in. (5 cm) below sternal angle.
• Center cassette to CR (top of cassette should be about 1 in. or 2.5 cm. above level of shoulder).
• Minimum 40 in. (102 cm) SID.

Collimation: Collimate on lateral margins to expose a field 4 or 5 in. (10-12 cm) wide on the film, with upper and lower borders to film margins. (Close collimation not only reduces patient exposure but improves contrast and visibility of anatomy.)

Respiration: Suspend respiration on **expiration** if breathing is labored; otherwise normal respiration can be allowed.

NOTE:
• T7 is center of thoracic spine since lower vertebrae are larger.

Evaluation Criteria:
• The spinal column from C7 to L1 should be seen centered to the midline of the film.
• Good collimation will include side collimation borders medial to female breast shadows.
• Sternoclavicular joints should be seen equidistant from the spine indicating no rotation.
• Vertebral bodies should be well penetrated from T1 to T12.
• Optimum exposure and the use of a wedge filter in addition to correct use of the anode-heel effect should clearly visualize the lower thoracic vertebral body margins and intervertebral joint spaces without overexposing the upper thoracic vertebrae.

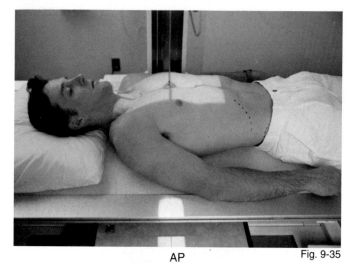

AP   Fig. 9-35

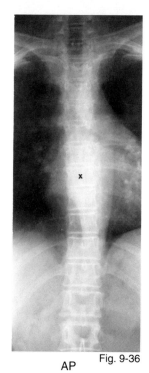

AP   Fig. 9-36

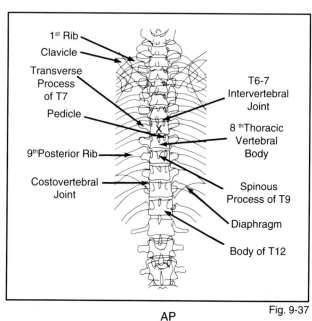

AP   Fig. 9-37

• Lateral Position

Structures Best Shown:

Thoracic vertebral bodies, intervertebral joint spaces and intervertebral foramina. Upper 2 or 3 vertebrae are not well visualized.

Take (swimmers) lateral (page 291) if upper thoracic vertebrae are of special interest.

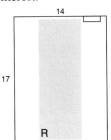

Technical Factors:

- Film Size - 14 x 17 in. (35 x 43 cm), lengthwise.
- Moving or stationary grid.
- 80-90 kVp range.
- With breathing technique use low mA and 3 to 4 sec exposure.
- Place lead shield on table behind patient to reduce scatter to film.

Patient Position:

- Left lateral recumbent, head on pillow (or erect if patient's condition requires this).

Shielding: Place lead shield over pelvic area to shield gonads. Breast shields may also be used for young females without obscuring area of interest.

Part Position:

- Align **mid-coronal plane to midline of table**.
- Raise arms to right angles to body with elbows flexed.
- Support waist so entire spine is parallel to table (palpate spinous processes to determine this).
- Flex hips and knees for stability with support between knees.

Central Ray:

- CR **perpendicular** to film.
- Center to **T7**, which is 3 to 4 in. (8-10 cm) below jugular notch or 7 - 8 in. (18 - 21 cm) below the vertebra prominens (see chest positioning).
- Center cassette to CR (top of cassette should be about 1 in. or 2.5 cm above level of shoulders).
- Minimum 40 in. (102 cm) SID.

Collimation: Collimate on lateral margins to expose a field 5 or 6 in. (13-15 cm) wide, with upper and lower borders to film margins. (Close collimation not only reduces patient exposure but improves contrast and visibility of anatomy.)

Respiration: Use breathing technique or suspend respiration after full expiration.

NOTE:

- If entire spine is not parallel to table, it may be necessary to angle 5 to 10° cephalad (broad shouldered patient).

Evaluation Criteria:

- The spinal column from C7 to L1 should be seen centered to the midline of the film. For most patients the upper vertebra will be underexposed due to superimposition of shoulders.
- Intervertebral disk spaces should be open.
- Vertebral bodies should be in lateral profile without rotation as indicated by superimposed posterior ribs.
- Optimum exposure should demonstrate the lower two-thirds of the thoracic spine with blurring of the ribs and lung markings if breathing technique is used.

Lateral   Fig. 9-38

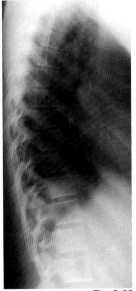

Lateral   Fig. 9-39

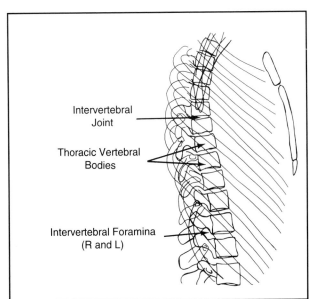

Intervertebral Joint

Thoracic Vertebral Bodies

Intervertebral Foramina (R and L)

Lateral   Fig. 9-40

• Oblique Position

Thoracic Spine
Basic
• AP
• Lateral
Optional
• **Obliques**

Structures Best Shown:
Zygapophyseal joints: RPO and LPO demonstrate upside joints (farther from film). RAO and LAO demonstrate downside joints (closest to film).

Technical Factors:
• Film Size - 14 x 17 in. (35 x 43 cm), lengthwise.
• Moving or stationary grid.
• 80-90 kVp range.

Patient Position:
• Lateral recumbent, head on pillow (or erect if patient's condition requires this).

Shielding: Place lead shield over pelvic area to shield gonads.

Part Position:
• Align **midaxillary plane to midline of table**.
• Rotate the body 20° from true lateral to create a **70° oblique** from plane of table.
• Flex hips, knees, and arms for stability as needed:
 - For posterior oblique (LPO or RPO), arm nearest table should be up and forward; arm nearest tube should be down and posterior.
 - For anterior oblique (LAO or RAO), arm nearest table should be down and posterior; arm nearest tube should be up and forward.

Central Ray:
• CR **perpendicular** to film.
• Center to **T7**, which is 3 to 4 in. (8-10 cm) below jugular notch or 2 in. (5 cm) below sternal angle.
• Center cassette to CR (top of cassette should be about 1 in. or 2.5 cm above level of shoulders).
• Minimum 40 in. (102 cm) SID.

Collimation: Close four-sided collimation to area of interest.

Respiration: Suspend breathing on full expiration.

NOTE:
• Patient's thorax is almost lateral for each oblique, some type of angle guide may be used to determine correct rotation (*Fig. 9-42*).
• May take as posterior or anterior oblique.

Evaluation Criteria:
• All twelve thoracic vertebra should be seen and centered to the midline of the film.
• The zygapophyseal joints should be open and well demonstrated, but the amount of kyphosis will determine how many apophyseal joints will be seen.
• Optimum exposure should demonstrate wide exposure latitude to visualize all parts of the 12 thoracic vertebrae.

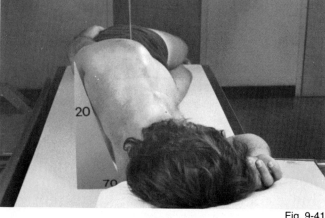

Oblique (RPO)   Fig. 9-41

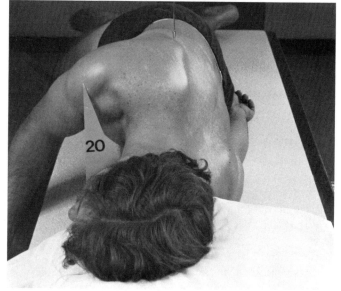

Oblique (LAO)   Fig. 9-42

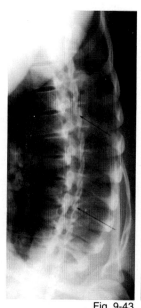

Fig. 9-43
Oblique

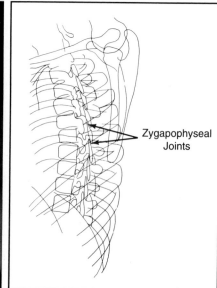

Zygapophyseal Joints

Fig. 9-44
Oblique

• AP Projection

Structures Best Shown:
Cervical vertebra 3 through 7 to include vertebral bodies, space between pedicles, intervertebral disc spaces and spinous processes.

8

10 R

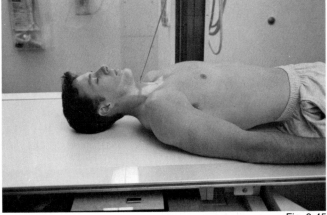

AP - 20° Cephalic Angle   Fig. 9-45

Technical Factors:
• Film Size - 8 x 10 in. (18 x 24 cm), lengthwise.
• Moving or stationary grid.
• 75-80 kVp range.

Patient Position:
• Supine or erect, with arms by sides.
• Head on table surface, provide immobilization if needed.

Shielding: Place lead shield over pelvic area to shield gonads. Use breast shielding on young females.

Part Position:
• Align **midsagittal plane to midline of table**.
• Adjust head so that a line from the occlusal plane to the base of the skull (mastoid tips) is perpendicular to table and/or (chewing surface of maxillary teeth) film.
• Immobilize head.
• Assure there is **no rotation** of the head or body.

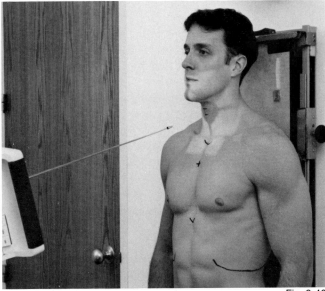

AP - 20° Cephalic Angle   Fig. 9-46

Central Ray:
• CR angled **15-20° cephalad** to enter at the level of the lower margin of the thyroid cartilage (**C5-6**).
• Center cassette to CR (top of cassette should be about 1 in. (2.5 cm) above level of EAM).
• Minimum 40 in. (102 cm) SID.

Collimation: Close four-sided collimation to area of interest.

Respiration: Suspend respiration during exposure.

NOTE:
• Patient should not swallow during exposure.
• Cephalad angulation will open up intervertebral disc spaces and project mandible superiorly.

Evaluation Criteria:
• C3 to T1 should be clearly seen.
• No rotation; spinous processes should be equidistant from the spinal borders.
• Intervertebral disc spaces should be open indicating correct CR angle.
• The mandible and base of the skull will be superimposed over the first two cervical vertebra.
• Optimum exposure should demonstrate both bone and soft tissue density.

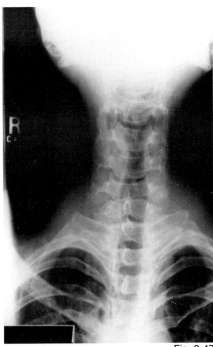

Fig. 9-47

AP - 20° Cephalic Angle

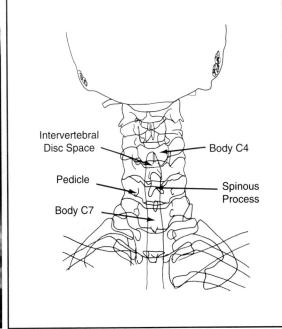

Intervertebral Disc Space

Pedicle

Body C7

Body C4

Spinous Process

Fig. 9-48

AP

• AP "open mouth" Projection (C1 and C2)

Cervical Spine
Basic
• AP
• **AP Open Mouth (C1 & 2)**
• Lateral
• Obliques
• Swimmers Lateral

Structures Best Shown:
Dens (odontoid process) and vertebral body of C2, lateral masses of C1 and zygapophyseal joints between C1 and C2.

Technical Factors:
• Film Size - 8 x 10 in. (18 x 24 cm), lengthwise.
• Moving or stationary grid.
• 75-80 kVp range.

Patient Position:
• Supine (or erect) with arms by sides.
• Head on table surface, provide immobilization if needed.

Shielding: Place lead shield over pelvic area to shield gonads. Use breast shielding on young females.

AP – "Open Mouth", C1-2   Fig. 9-49

Part Position:
• Align **midsagittal plane to midline of table**.
• Adjust head so that a line from **lower margin of upper incisors to the base of the skull** (mastoid tips) **is perpendicular** to table and/or film.
• Immobilize head to prevent rotation.
• Assure there is **no rotation** of the head or body.
• Assure that **mouth is wide open** during exposure. (Do this as the last step and work quickly as it is difficult to maintain this position.)

Central Ray:
• CR **perpendicular to film**, directed through **center of open mouth**.
• Center cassette to CR.
• Minimum 40 in. (102 cm) SID.

Collimation: Close four-sided collimation to area of interest.

Respiration: Suspend respiration during exposure.

NOTE:
 • Make sure that when patient is instructed to open mouth that only the lower jaw moves.
• Instruct the patient to keep the tongue in the lower jaw to prevent its shadow from being over the atlas and axis.

AP – "Open Mouth", C1-2   Fig. 9-50

Evaluation Criteria:
• The atlas and axis should be clearly demonstrated through the open mouth.
• Optimum head position if the lower margin of the **upper incisors** and the **base of the skull are superimposed**.
• Optimum exposure should demonstrate both bone and soft tissue density.
• The C1-2 zygapophyseal joint space and the dens (odontoid process) in its entirety should be clearly visible.

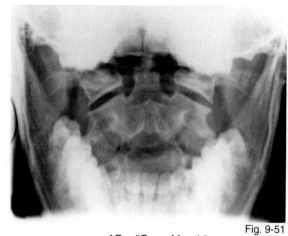

AP – "Open Mouth"   Fig. 9-51

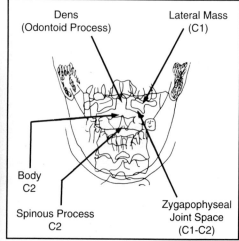

Dens (Odontoid Process)
Lateral Mass (C1)
Body C2
Spinous Process C2
Zygapophyseal Joint Space (C1-C2)

AP – "Open Mouth"   Fig. 9-52

• Lateral Position

Cervical Spine
Basic
• AP
• AP Open Mouth (C1 & 2)
• **Lateral**
• Obliques
• Swimmers Lateral

Structures Best Shown:
Cervical vertebral bodies, intervertebral joint spaces, articular pillars, spinous processes and zygapophyseal joints.

Trauma Patients: See trauma routine, page 294.

Technical Factors:
- Film Size - 10 x 12 in. (24 x 30 cm), lengthwise. or for smaller patient - 8 x 10 in. (18 x 24 cm) lengthwise.
- Moving or stationary grid (optional).
- 75-80 kVp range.

```
          10 (8)
        ┌─────────┐
12      │ R       │
(10)    │         │
        └─────────┘
```

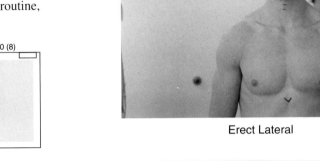

Erect Lateral   Fig. 9-53

Patient Position:
- Erect lateral, either sitting or standing with shoulder against vertical film holder.

Shielding: Secure lead shield around waist to shield gonads.

Part Position:
- Align **mid-coronal plane** to **midline** of table and/or cassette holder.
- Place top of cassette about 2 in. (5 cm) above EAM.
- Depress shoulders (hold equal weights in both hands, see NOTE).
- Ask patient to relax and **drop shoulders as far as possible**. (Do this as the last step before exposure as this is a difficult position to maintain.)
- Extend chin forward (to prevent superimposition of upper cervical by mandible).

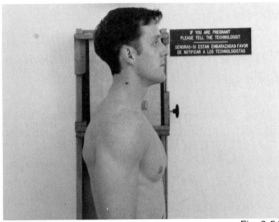

Erect Lateral   Fig. 9-54

Central Ray:
- CR **perpendicular** to film, directed horizontally to **C4-5** (level of upper margin of thyroid cartilage).
- Center cassette to CR.
- 72 in. (183 cm) SID.

Respiration: Suspend respiration on **full expiration** (for maximum shoulder depression).

Collimation: Four-sided collimation to area of interest. (With smaller film, collimate to near upper and lower film borders.)

NOTE:
- Adding 5-10 lb. weights to each arm may help in pulling down shoulders.
- Long (72 in.) SID compensates for loss of image sharpness and increased magnification caused by increased OID.

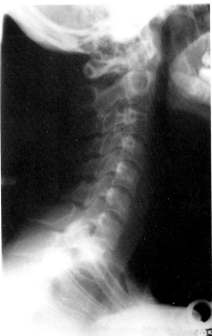

Fig. 9-55

Lateral

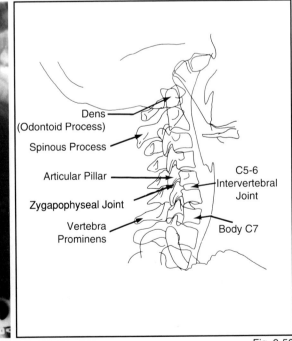

Dens (Odontoid Process)
Spinous Process
Articular Pillar
Zygapophyseal Joint
Vertebra Prominens
C5-6 Intervertebral Joint
Body C7

Fig. 9-56

Lateral

Evaluation Criteria:
- C1 through C7 should be clearly seen. If C7 is not seen, a special view (Swimmers) should be done of the cervicothoracic region.
- The rami of the mandible should not be superimposed over the upper cervical vertebra.
- No rotation is indicated by having both rami of the mandible superimposed.
- Optimum exposure should demonstrate soft tissue including margins of the air column, as well as proper bone density of the entire cervical vertebrae.

• Oblique Positions

Cervical Spine
Basic
• AP
• AP Open Mouth (C1 & 2)
• Lateral
• **Obliques**
• Swimmers Lateral

Structures Best Shown:

Anterior obliques - intervertebral foramina and pedicles closest to film.
Posterior obliques - intervertebral foramina and pedicles farthest from the film.

Trauma Routine: See page 295.

Both right and left obliques must be taken as either anterior or posterior obliques.

Technical Factors:

• Film Size - 8 x 10 in. (18 x 24 cm), lengthwise. or 10 x 12 in. (24 x 30 cm), lengthwise.
• Moving or stationary grid.
• 75-80 kVp range.

Patient Position:

• Erect position preferred (sitting or standing), or may be taken recumbent if patient's condition requires.

Shielding: Secure lead shield around waist to shield gonads.

Part Position:

• Center spine to **midline** of table and/or cassette.
• Place top of cassette about 2 in. (5 cm) above EAM.
• Arms at side; if recumbent, place arms as needed to help maintain position.
• Rotate body and head 45°. (Use protractor or other angle gauge to assure 45°.) See NOTE about head rotation.
• Extend chin to prevent mandible from superimposing vertebrae, but not too much to cause base of skull to superimpose C1.

Central Ray:

• Anterior obliques - **15°-20° caudad** to **C4** (level of upper margin of thyroid cartilage).
• Posterior obliques - **15°- 20° cephalad** to **C4**.
• Center cassette to central ray.
• Minimum 40 in. (102 cm) SID. (May also be taken at 72 in. as for lateral cervical.)

Collimation:

Four-sided collimation to area of interest. (With smaller film, collimate to near upper and lower film borders.)

Respiration: Suspend respiration.

NOTE: Departmental option: The head may be turned to true lateral position. (This results in some rotation of upper vertebrae but prevents superimposition of vertebra by mandible.)

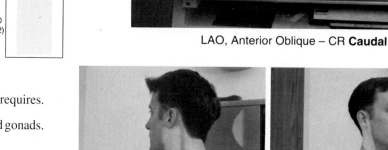

LAO, Anterior Oblique – CR **Caudal**   Fig. 9-57

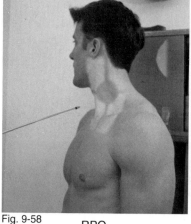

Fig. 9-58   RPO   Posterior Oblique   LPO   Fig. 9-59
– CR **Cephalad**

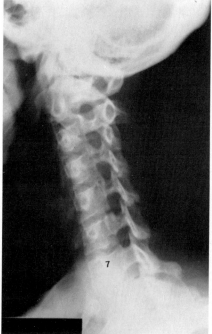

Oblique   Fig. 9-60

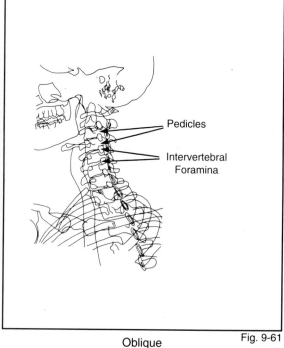

Pedicles

Intervertebral
Foramina

Oblique   Fig. 9-61

Evaluation Criteria:

• C1 through C7 should be clearly seen with open intervertebral foramina and open intervertebral disc spaces.
• The rami of the mandible should not superimpose the upper cervical vertebra.
• The base of the skull should not superimpose C1.
• Cervical pedicles should be demonstrated.
• Optimum exposure should demonstrate soft tissue including margins of the air column, as well as proper bone density of the entire cervical vertebrae.

• Swimmers Lateral Position

(Twining Method)

<table>
<tr><td>

Cervical Spine
Basic
• AP
• AP Open Mouth (C1 & 2)
• Lateral
• Obliques
• **Swimmers Lateral**

</td></tr>
</table>

Structures Best Shown:
Lower cervical and upper thoracic vertebral bodies, intervertebral disc spaces, and zygapophyseal joints.
Trauma Routine: See page 295.

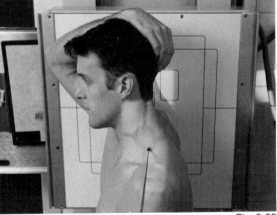

Swimmers Lateral   Fig. 9-62

Technical Factors:
• Film Size - 8 x 10 in. (18 x 24 cm), lengthwise.
• Use moving or stationary grid.
• 85-90 kVp range. (Increase 5-10 kVp from lateral cervical.)

Patient Position:
• Erect position preferred (sitting or standing), or may be done recumbent if patient's condition requires.

Shielding: Secure lead shield around waist to shield gonads.

Part Position:
• Align **mid-coronal plane to midline** of table or cassette holder.
• Place arm and shoulder nearest film **up** and slightly anterior, or posterior, whichever appears best for that specific patient. Rest this hand or arm on head for support.
• Position arm and shoulder away from film **down** and slightly posterior or anterior (opposite to shoulder nearest film). (This will separate humeral heads from vertebrae.)
• Maintain thorax and head in as true a lateral position as possible.

Central Ray:
• CR **perpendicular** to film. (See NOTE.)
• Center to **T1**, which is about 1.5 in. (4 cm) above level of jugular notch anteriorly, and at level of vertebra prominens posteriorly.
• Minimum 40 in. (102 cm) SID.

Swimmers Lateral   Fig. 9-63

Collimation: Close four-sided collimation to area of interest (about 5 x 6 in.). Close collimation improves contrast and the visibility of anatomy.

Respiration: Suspend breathing on full **expiration**.

NOTE: A caudal angulation of 5° may be necessary to help separate the two shoulders, especially on a heavily muscled patient or one who cannot sufficiently depress the shoulder away from the film.

Evaluation Criteria:
• Vertebral rotation should appear to be minimal.
• C4 to T3 should be clearly seen in outline when properly exposed.
• The humeral heads should be separated vertically.
• The magnified humeral head which was depressed and farthest from the film should appear distal to T4 or T5 area.

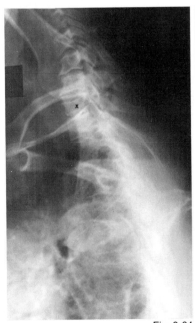

Swimmers Lateral   Fig. 9-64

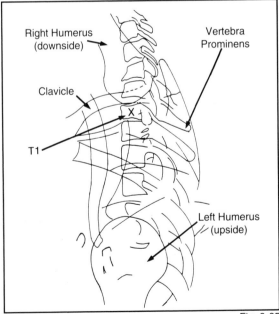

Right Humerus (downside)

Vertebra Prominens

Clavicle

T1

X

Left Humerus (upside)

Swimmers Lateral   Fig. 9-65

Cervical Spine

• Lateral, Hyperflexion / Hyperextension

> **Cervical Spine**
> Optional
> • **Lateral - hyperflexion &
> hyperextension**
> • AP Chewing ("Wagging
> Jaw")

Structures Best Shown:
Functional study to demonstrate motion or lack of motion of cervical vertebra.

Warning: **Never** attempt these positions on trauma patient before cervical fracture has been ruled out.

Technical Factors:
- Film Size - 10 x 12 in. (24 x 30 cm), lengthwise.
     or - 8 x 10 in. (18 x 24 cm), lengthwise.
- Moving or stationary grid (optional).
- 75-80 kVp range.

Patient Position:
- Erect lateral, either sitting or standing, arms at sides.

Shielding: Secure lead shield around waist to shield gonads.

Part Position:
- Align **midcoronal plane of vertebrae to midline** of film.
- Assure a **true lateral position**, no rotation of pelvis, shoulders or head.
- Adjust height of film so top of cassette is about 2 in. (5 cm) above EAM.
- Depress shoulders as far as possible (weights in each hand may be used).
- For **hyperflexion**: Chin should be depressed until it touches the chest or as much as patient can tolerate (do not allow shoulders to move forward and be sure that entire cervical is included on film).
- For **hyperextension**: Chin should be raised and head leaned back as much as possible (do not allow shoulder to move backward and be certain that entire cervical is included on film).

Central Ray:
- CR **perpendicular** to film, directed horizontally to area of **C4-5** (to center of film).
- 72 in. (183 cm) SID.

Collimation: Four-sided collimation to area of interest.

Respiration: Suspend respiration on full expiration.

NOTE: These are uncomfortable for patient, do not keep in these positions longer than necessary.

Evaluation Criteria:
- C1 through C7 should be included on film.
  (C7 however, may not be completely visualized on some patients.)
- No rotation is indicated by having both rami of the mandible superimposed.
- Optimum exposure should demonstrate soft tissue as well as proper bone density of entire cervical vertebrae.
- For hyperflexion: Spinous processes should be separated.
- For hyperextension: Spinous processes should be in close proximity.

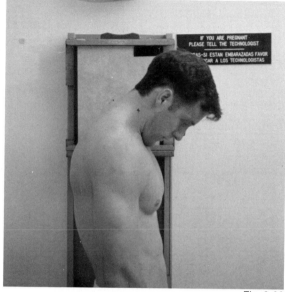

Hyperflexion   Fig. 9-66

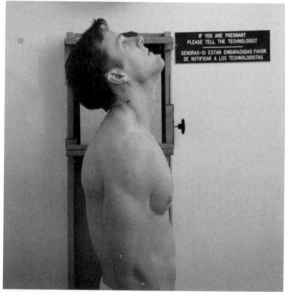

Hyperextension   Fig. 9-67

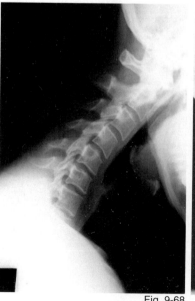

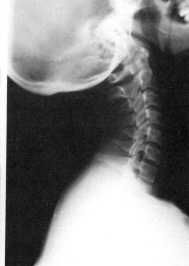

Hyperflexion   Fig. 9-68   Hyperextension   Fig. 9-69

• AP "Chewing" "Wagging Jaw" Projection
(Ottonello Method)

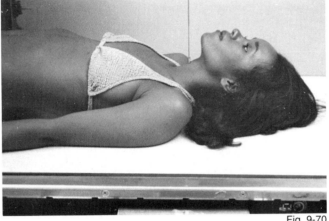

Position for AP "Chewing" Fig. 9-70

Cervical Spine
Optional
• Swimmers Lateral
• Lateral - hyperflexion & hyperextension
• **AP Chewing ("Wagging Jaw")**

Structures Best Shown:
Entire cervical spine with mandible blurred.

Technical Factors:
• Film Size - 8 x 10 in. (18 x 24 cm), lengthwise.
• Moving or stationary grid.
• Use low mA and long (> 3 sec) exposure time.
• 75-80 kVp.

Patient Position:
• Supine with arms at side.
• Head on table surface, provide immobilization.

Shielding: Secure lead shield around waist to shield gonads.

Part Position:
• Align **midsagittal plane to midline** of table.
• Adjust head so that a line drawn from **lower margin of upper incisors to the base of the skull is perpendicular** to table.
• Immobilize head.
• Assure there is **no rotation** of the head or body.
• Mandible must be in **continuous motion** during exposure.
• Assure that only the mandible moves. The upper jaw and head must not move.

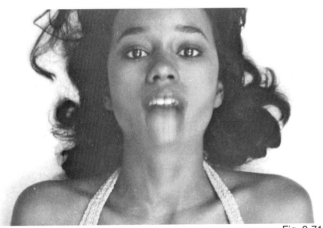

AP "Chewing" Fig. 9-71

Central Ray:
• CR **perpendicular** to film, centered to **C4-5** (upper margin of thyroid cartilage).
• Center film to CR.
• Minimum 40 in. (102 cm) SID.

Collimation: Four-sided collimation to area of interest.

Respiration: May be suspended, or fully exhaled while saying "AHHH".

NOTE:
• Practice with patient prior to exposure. Having the patient say "AHHHH" during exposure prevents the tongue from moving.
• Increase 2-4 kVp to compensate for mandibular and tongue shadow.

Evaluation Criteria:
• All seven vertebae should be clearly seen with mandibular blurring.
• The C1-2 area should be lighter but still well visualized.
• There should be no motion of the cranium or the cervical spine.
• Optimum exposure should demonstrate both the upper and lower cervical regions even though lower vertebrae will appear somewhat darker.

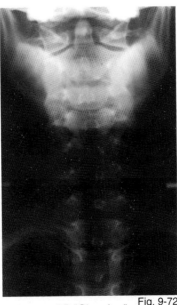

AP "Chewing" Fig. 9-72

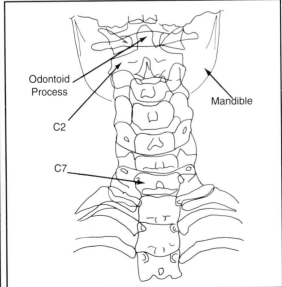

AP "Chewing" Fig. 9-73

Odontoid Process

C2

Mandible

C7

Cervical Spine - Trauma Series

• Lateral, Horizontal Beam

Warning: Severe trauma to head and/or neck area requires a horizontal beam cervical lateral taken first **without** moving patient's head and neck. Cervical collar, if present, should **NOT** be removed. This radiograph should be viewed by physician **before** attempting to move patient's head or neck for other cervical and/or skull trauma projections.

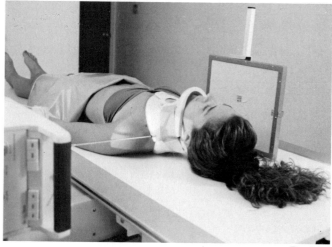
Lateral – Horizontal Beam   Fig. 9-74

Cervical Spine
(Trauma Series)
Basic
• **Lateral (horizontal beam)**

Structures Best Shown:
Cervical vertebral bodies, intervertebral joint spaces, articular pillars, spinous processes and zygapophyseal joints.

Technical Factors:
• Film Size - 10 x 12 in. (24 x 30 cm), lengthwise.
• Stationary or moving grid, or non grid cassette (see NOTE).
• 75-80 kVp range.

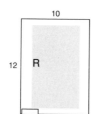

Patient Position:
• Supine on stretcher.

Shielding: Place lead shield over pelvic area to shield gonads.

Part Position:
• Do **not** manipulate or move head or neck.
• Support cassette vertically near shoulder, or place stretcher next to vertical grid device.
• Place top of cassette about 2 in. (5 cm) above EAM.
• Depress shoulders. (See NOTE.)
• Assure that inferior border of cassette is lower than posterior aspect of cervical spine (spinous processes).

Central Ray:
• CR **perpendicular** to film, directed horizontally to **C4** (level of upper margin of thyroid cartilage).
• 72 in. (183 cm) SID.

Collimation: Four-sided collimation to area of interest.

Respiration: Suspend respiration on full **expiration**.

NOTE:
• Traction on arms will help depress shoulders but should only be done with the consent or assistance of physician.
• Exposure is done on expiration to help depress shoulders.
• Long SID (72 in.) compensates for increased magnification caused by an increase in OID with resultant loss of image sharpness.
• Cervical collars should be left in place unless removed by physician.
• A **nongrid cassette** can be used due to the increased OID which provides an "air-gap" to prevent scatter radiation from reaching the film. This results in 75 to 80% reduction in exposure from the grid technique.

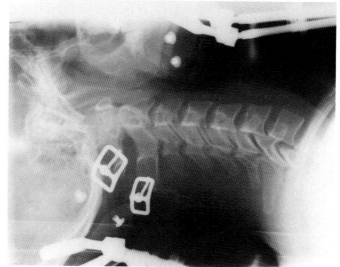
Lateral – Horizontal Beam   Fig. 9-75

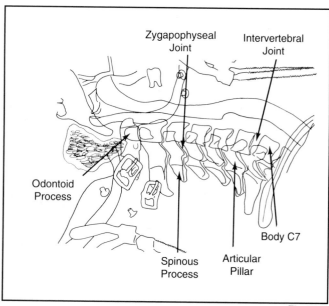
Lateral – Horizontal Beam   Fig. 9-76

Evaluation Criteria:
• C1 through C7 should be clearly seen. If C7 is not seen, the physician must review the film and grant permission before any additional (or special) views are obtained involving patient movement.
• Optimum exposure should demonstrate soft tissue as well as proper bone density of all aspects of the cervical vertebrae.

• AP   • Obliques   • Swimmers Lateral (Cervicothoracic)

Warning: Complete the basic lateral (horizontal beam) trauma cervical **before** removing cervical collar or moving patient's head and/or neck for these optional cervical trauma projections.

> **Cervical Spine**
> Trauma Series
> Optional
> • **AP**
> • **Obliques**
> • **Swimmers Lateral**

Structures Best Shown:
Frontal, oblique and lateral views of cervical vertebrae to rule out fractures and/or other trauma pathology.

Technical Factors:
- Film Size - 8 x 10 in. (18 x 24 cm) or
  10 x 12 in. (24 x 30 cm)
  lengthwise - AP and lateral
  crosswise - obliques
- Stationary or moving grid.
- 75-80 kVp range.

```
         10 (8)
        ┌────────┐
12      │        │
(10)    │  R     │
        │        │
        └────────┘
```

Patient Position:
- Supine, on stretcher or on x-ray table, arms at sides.

Shielding: Place lead shield over pelvic area to shield gonads.

Part Position:
- Stabilize patient's head when lifting enough to place cassette under patient.

AP Projection:
- Adjust midline of grid cassette to midsagittal plane.
- Place top of cassette about 1 in. (2.5 cm) above level of EAM.
- Adjust head so that a line from the occlusal plane to the base of skull is perpendicular to film.
- Assure no rotation of head or body.
- **CR** angled **15-20° cephalad**, directed to level of **C5** (lower margin of thyroid cartilage).
- Minimum 40 in. (102 cm) SID.

Oblique Positions:
- Both right and left posterior obliques are taken.
- Place grid cassette **crosswise** to prevent grid cutoff.
- Place top of cassette about 2 in. (5 cm) above level of EAM, centered so the 45° angled CR will be directed to center of cassette.
- Extend chin to prevent mandible from superimposing cervical.
- CR angled **45° medial** and **15-20° cephalad**, centered to level of **C4**, (upper margin of thyroid cartilage).
- Minimum 40 in. (102 cm) SID.

Swimmers Lateral:
- Cassette lengthwise, supported vertically near shoulder or place stretcher next to vertical grid device.
- Center cassette and CR to level of **C7/T1** (about 1.5 in. or 4 cm above level of jugular notch).
- Place support under shoulders if needed to assure that posterior aspect of vertebrae are included.
- Raise arm nearest film above head (if patient is able); depress opposite shoulder as much as possible to separate humeral heads.
- CR **horizontal**, and for most patients **perpendicular** to film (unless patient is unable to adequately separate shoulders by raising one and depressing the other wherein a 5° caudal angle may be necessary).
- 72 in. (183 cm) SID.

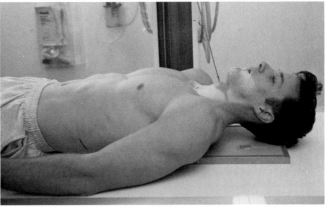

AP   Fig. 9-77

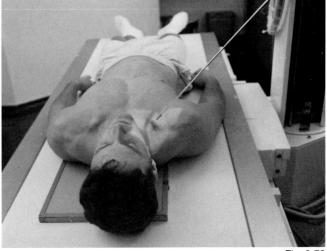

Oblique   Fig. 9-78

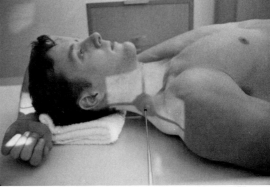

Swimmers Lateral   Fig. 9-79

Collimation: Four-sided collimation to area of interest.

Respiration: Suspend respiration during exposure, and for lateral take on full expiration to depress shoulders.

NOTE:
- These optional trauma cervical projections can be taken when specifically indicated or requested. The horizontal beam lateral (preceding page) is the most important position when the patient has spinal injury or trauma to the neck or head area.
- It is important to remember to angle the CR with the grid lines or along the long dimension of the grid to prevent grid cut off.

Evaluation Criteria:
- These would be the same as indicated on preceding pages for these specific projections.

Chapter 10
Radiographic Anatomy and Positioning of the Bony Thorax (Sternum and Ribs)

Contributions by: John Lampignano, M Ed, RT (R)

Contents

Part I Radiographic Anatomy

Bony Thorax

The bony thorax consists of the **sternum** anteriorly, the **thoracic vertebrae** posteriorly, and the **12 pairs of ribs** connecting the sternum to the vertebral column. The bony thorax serves to protect important organs of the respiratory system and vital structures within the mediastinum, such as the heart and great vessels.

The main function of the bony thorax however is to serve as an expandible bellows-like chamber wherein the interior capacity expands and contracts during inspiration and expiration respectively. This is caused by alternate action of muscles attached to the rib cage and atmospheric pressure causing the air to move in and out of the lungs during respiration.

Also the red marrow of the ribs and sternum are primary sites of red blood cell formation. Therefore, since these are areas of blood production, it is **very important** to protect **all** of the sternum when shielding with a lead apron.

The sternum is also a common site for marrow biopsy wherein under a local anesthetic, a needle is inserted into the marrow cavity of the sternum to withdraw a sample of red bone marrow. This is called a sternal puncture.

The drawing in *Fig. 10-1* shows the relationship of the sternum to the 12 pairs of ribs and 12 thoracic vertebrae. As demonstrated in this drawing, the thin sternum superimposes the thick and very dense thoracic spine in a direct frontal position. Therefore an AP or PA projection radiograph would show the thoracic spine well, but would show the sternum only faintly, if at all.

Sternum

The adult sternum is a thin, narrow, flat bone with three divisions. The upper portion is termed the **manubrium** *(mah-nu´bre-um)*, which is from the Latin meaning handle. The adult manubrium averages 2 inches or 5 centimeters in length.

The longest part of the sternum is the **body,** which is about 4 inches or 10 centimeters long. The Latin word for body is corpus. Another, but older, term for the body is gladiolus, which means sword. The union of the four segments of the body begins during puberty and is not completed until about the age of 25.

The most distal portion of the sternum is the **xiphoid process** *(zi´foid)*, which consists of cartilage during infancy and youth and usually doesn't become totally ossified until about age 40. The xiphoid process is generally rather small; although it can be quite variable in size, shape, and degree of ossification.

Palpable Landmarks

The uppermost border of the manubrium is an important external landmark that is very easy to palpate. This border is termed the **jugular notch.** Other secondary names for this area are **suprasternal or manubrial notch,** all of which describe the slightly notched area between the two clavicles along the upper border of the sternum. The jugular notch is at the same level as the disc space between **T2 and T3.**

Each **clavicle** joins the manubrium lateral to the jugular notch on each side at the **clavicular notch.** The joint formed is called the **sternoclavicular joint.** The only bony connection between each upper limb and the bony thorax is at the sternoclavicular joint.

The lower end of the manubrium joins the body of the sternum to form a palpable angle, the **sternal angle.** This is also an easily palpated landmark used for location of other structures of the bony thorax. The sternal angle is at the level of the disc space between **T4 and T5** in an average-shaped, upright adult.

The **xiphoid** can also be palpated and corresponds to approximately the level of **T10.**

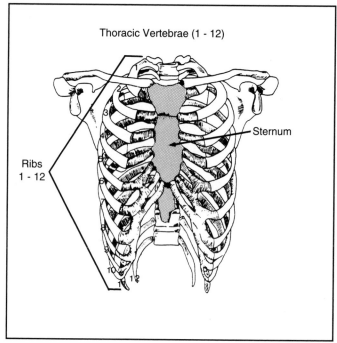

Bony Thorax — Fig. 10-1

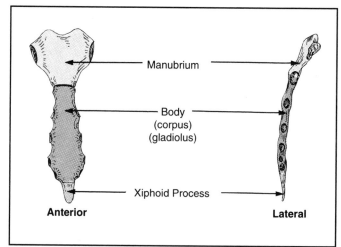

Sternum — Fig. 10-2

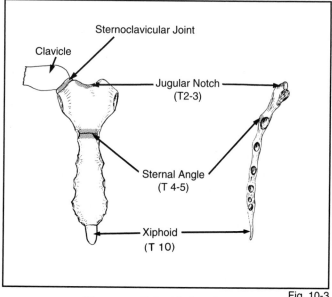

Sternum – Palpable Landmarks — Fig. 10-3

Sternal Rib Articulations

The **clavicles** and the **cartilages** of the **first seven pairs of ribs** connect directly to the sternum. Below each clavicular notch and sternoclavicular joint is a depression or **facet** for articulation with the cartilage of the first rib.

The drawing in *Fig. 10-4* illustrates that the ribs do not unite directly with the sternum, but do so with a short piece of cartilage termed **costocartilage.** The costocartilages and ribs have been added to one side of this drawing to show this relationship.

The second costocartilage connects to the sternum at the level of the sternal angle. An easy way to locate the anterior end of the second rib is to locate the sternal angle first, then feel laterally along the cartilage and the bone of the rib.

The third through the seventh costocartilages connect directly to the body of the sternum.

Ribs 8, 9 and 10 also possess costocartilage, but these connect to the number 7 costocartilages, which then connect to the sternum.

Ribs

Each rib is numbered according to the thoracic vertebra to which it attaches; therefore the ribs are numbered from the top down. The first seven pairs of ribs are considered **true ribs.** Each true rib attaches directly to the sternum by its own costocartilage. The term **false ribs** applies to the last five pairs of ribs, numbered 8, 9, 10, 11 and 12.

The drawing in *Fig. 10-5* again clearly shows that, although ribs 8 through 10 have costocartilages, they connect to the costocartilage of the seventh rib.

The last two pairs of false ribs are unique in that they do not possess costocartilage. The term **floating ribs** can be used to designate these last two pairs of ribs. Therefore, the last two pairs of ribs, in addition to being false ribs, can also be called floating ribs.

Summary: Ribs **1-7** are termed **true ribs** and connect directly to the sternum. The last five pair of ribs, number **8-12** are termed **false ribs**. The last two pair of ribs, number **11 and 12** which are also false ribs are termed **floating ribs** because they are not connected anteriorly.

Typical Rib

Inferior View: A typical rib viewed from its inferior surface is illustrated. A central rib is used to show the common characteristics of a typical rib. Each rib has two ends, a posterior or **vertebral end,** and an anterior or **sternal end.** Between the two ends is the **shaft** or body of the rib.

The vertebral end consists of a **head,** which articulates with one or two thoracic vertebral bodies, and a flattened **neck.** Lateral to the neck is an elevated **tubercle** that articulates with the transverse process of a vertebra and allows for attachment of a ligament. The shaft extends laterally from the tubercle, then angles forward and downward. The area of forward angulation is termed the **angle** of the rib.

Posterior View: Seen on this posterior view are the **head, neck** and **tubercle** at the vertebral end of the rib. Progressing laterally, the angle of the rib is where the shaft bends forward and downward toward the sternal end. As seen in *Fig. 10-5*, the posterior or vertebral end of a typical rib is 3 to 5 inches (7.5 to 12.5 cm) **higher** than the anterior or sternal end. Therefore, when viewing a radiograph of a chest or ribs, one must remember that the part of a rib most superior is the posterior end or the end nearest the vertebrae. The anterior end is more inferior.

The lower inside margin of each rib protects an **artery**, a **vein** and a **nerve**; therefore, rib injuries are very painful and may be associated with substantial hemorrhage. This inside margin, containing the blood vessels and nerves, is termed the **costal groove.**

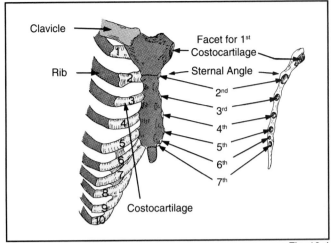

Sternal – Rib Articulations   Fig. 10-4

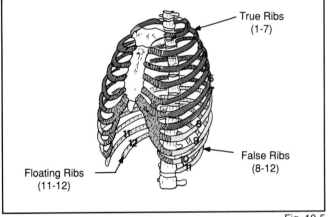

Ribs   Fig. 10-5

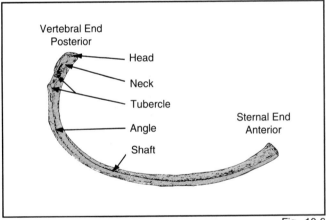

Typical Rib (Inferior View)   Fig. 10-6

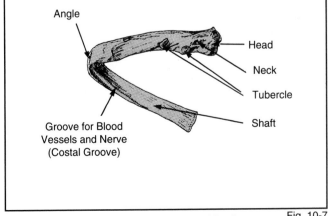

Typical Rib (Posterior View)   Fig. 10-7

Rib Cage

The drawing in *Fig. 10-8* illustrates the bony thorax with the sternum and costocartilages removed. The fifth ribs have been shaded to better illustrate the downward angulation of the ribs.

Not all ribs have the same appearance. The first ribs are short and broad, and are the most vertical of all the ribs. Counting downward from the short first pair, the ribs get longer and longer down to the seventh ribs. From the seventh ribs down they get shorter and shorter through the fairly short twelfth or last pair of ribs. The first ribs are the most sharply curved. The bony thorax is **widest** at the lateral margins of the **eighth or ninth ribs.**

Articulations of Thorax

Anterior Articulations

A frontal view of an articulated thorax is illustrated in *Fig. 10-9*. The joints or articulations of the anterior bony thorax are identified on this photograph. The joints along with the classification and the types of motion allowed are as follows:

Part **A** is the joint between costocartilage and the sternal end of the fourth rib, and is called a **costochondral** union or junction. These are a unique type of union wherein the cartilage and bone are bound together by the periosteum of the bone itself. This permits **no motion**, therefore, they are **synarthrodial.**

Part **B** is one **sternoclavicular joint.** The sternoclavicular joints are **synovial** joints containing articular capsules which permit **a gliding motion** and are therefore **diarthrodial** joints.

Part **C** is the **sternocostal joint** of the first rib. The cartilage of the first rib attaches directly to the manubrium with no synovial capsule and allows **no motion (synarthrodial).** Therefore this is a **cartilaginous** class joint of the **synchondrosis** type, similar to the epiphyseal joints of long bones.

Part **D** is the fourth sternocostal joint, typical of the second through the seventh joints between costocartilage and sternum. These are **synovial** joints which allow a slight **gliding motion**, making them **diarthrodial** joints.

Part **E** represents the continuous borders of the **interchondral joint** between the costal cartilage of the anterior sixth through tenth ribs. These are all interconnected by a **synovial** type joint with a long thin articular capsule lined by synovial membrane. These allow a slight **gliding type movement (diarthrodial)**, facilitating movement of the bony thorax during the breathing process.

Posterior Articulations

The remaining posterior types of joints in the bony thorax, parts F and G, are illustrated in *Fig. 10-10*. The joints between the ribs and the vertebral column, (F) the **costotransverse joints** and the **costovertebral joints** are **synovial** joints with articular capsules lined by synovial membrane which allow a **gliding motion,** and are therefore **diarthrodial.**

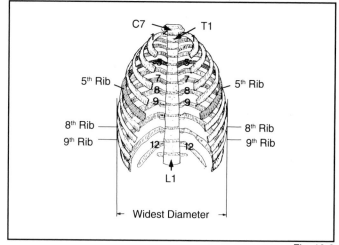

Rib Cage   Fig. 10-8

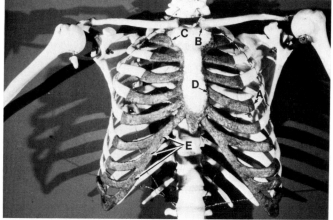

Articulated Thorax   Fig. 10-9

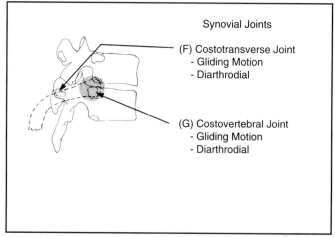

Synovial Joints

(F) Costotransverse Joint
  - Gliding Motion
  - Diarthrodial

(G) Costovertebral Joint
  - Gliding Motion
  - Diarthrodial

Posterior Articulations   Fig. 10-10

Summary of Thorax Articulations

Joints	Classification	Movement Type
1st Sternocostal Joint (between 1st rib and sternum)	Cartilaginous - synchondrosis	Immovable - synarthrodial
2nd - 7th Sternocostal Joints (between 2nd - 7th ribs and sternum)	Synovial	Gliding- diarthrodial
1st - 10th Costochrondral Unions (between costocartilage and ribs)	Unique type of union	Immovable - synarthrodial
6th - 10th Interchondral Joints (between anterior 6-10th costal cartilages)	Synovial	Gliding- diarthrodial
1st - 12th Costovertebral Joints (between heads of ribs and T vertebrae)	Synovial	Gliding- diarthrodial
1st - 12th Costotransverse Joints (between ribs and transverse process of T vertebrae)	Synovial	Gliding- diarthrodial

Anatomy Review

Sternum

The sternum is both difficult to radiograph sucessfully and difficult to study anatomically on the finished radiograph. The parts of the sternum listed A through G on the photograph of an actual sternum in *Fig. 10-11* are:

    A. Jugular (suprasternal) notch
    B. Clavicular notch
    C. Facet for the costocartilage of the first rib
    D. Manubrium
    E. Sternal angle
    F. Body or corpus

Part B is the area of articulation of the clavicle to the sternum. Remember that the clavicle articulates just lateral to the jugular notch and just above the articulation of the cartilage of the first rib.

Also, on this particular sternum the xiphoid process has not ossified, but the lower bracket indicates the area where it would normally be found if it were cartilaginous or osseous.

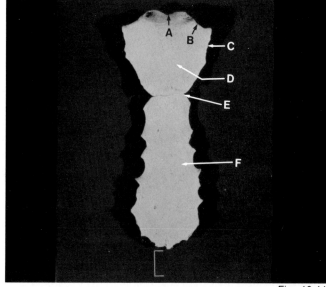

Sternum   Fig. 10-11

Sternum Radiographs

RAO: Radiographs of the sternum in the frontal position are illustrated in *Figs. 10-12* and *13*. These are conventional frontal radiographs of the sternum taken in a slight right anterior oblique position. The slight degree of obliquity tends to project the thoracic vertebrae to one side of the sternum.

The various parts of the sternum are difficult to visualize on radiographs of the sternum, so parts of the radiograph in *Fig. 10-12* have been enhanced. The labeled parts are:

    A. Sternal end of one clavicle
    B. Jugular notch
    C. Manubrium
    D. Sternal angle
    E. Body
    F. Area of the xiphoid process

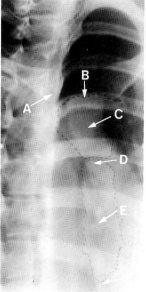
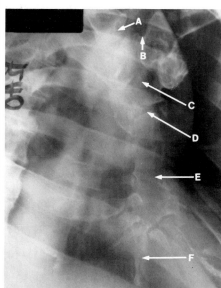

Fig. 10-12
RAO Sternum   RAO Sternum   Fig. 10-13

Typical Rib

A photograph of a typical rib as viewed from the undersurface is illustrated in *Fig. 10-14*. **A, B** and **C** are structures at the posterior or vertebral end of the rib.

    A. Head
    B. Neck
    C. Tubercle of this rib
    D. Angle of the rib
    E. Portion of the costal groove

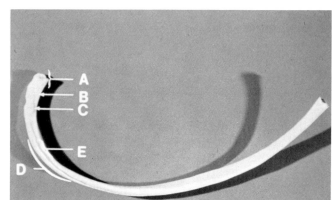

Fig. 10-14
Typical Rib

Positioning Considerations for the Sternum

The sternum is difficult to radiograph due to its bony composition and position within the thorax. The sternum is made up primarily of spongy bone with a thin layer of hard, compact bone surrounding it. Therefore, it is easy to overexpose. Also the sternum is an anterior midline structure that is in the same plane as the thoracic spine. Since the thoracic spine is much more dense, it is virtually impossible to see the sternum in a true AP or PA projection. Therefore a frontal view is obtained in a 15 to 20° RAO position to shift the sternum just to the left of the thoracic vertebrae and into the homogenous heart shadow. (See *Fig. 10-15.*)

The degree of obliquity is dependent upon the size of the thoracic cavity. A shallow or thin chest requires more obliquity than a deep one to cast the sternum away from the thoracic spine. For example a patient with a large, barrel-chested thorax with a greater anteroposterior measurement requires **less** rotation (~ 15°). A thin-chested patient requires **more** rotation (~20°). This principle is illustrated by the drawings in *Figs. 10-16 and 17.*

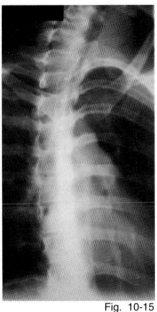

Fig. 10-15
RAO Sternum, Breathing Technique

Breathing Technique

A breathing technique involves the patient taking short, shallow breaths during the exposure. If performed properly, the lung markings overlying the sternum will become obscured, while the image of the sternum remains sharp and well defined. This requires a low kVp range, low mA, and a long exposure time of 3 or 4 seconds. The radiographer must be sure the thorax in general isn't moving during the exposure other than from the gentle breathing motion.

Because of the low bony density of the sternum, even if the breathing technique is not used, a relatively low kVp and adequate mAs technique is required.

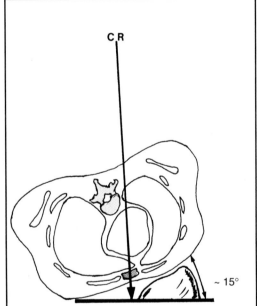

Fig. 10-16
Large, Barrel-Chested Thorax, ~ 15°

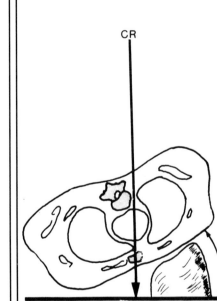

Fig. 10-17
Thin-Chested Thorax, ~ 20°

Use a safe SID

It has been a common practice to lower the source-image-receptor distance (SID) to a minimal range to create magnification with resultant blurring of overlying posterior ribs. While this produces visible images of the sternum, it also results in an increase in the radiation exposure to the patient. A safe and practical SID of **no less than 30 inches** should be used and a **minimum of 6 inches** (15 cm) between the collimator and the skin surface should always be maintained.

Tomography

Tomography, if such equipment is available, is a common method for radiographing the sternum in a frontal view without loss of detail from overlying structures.

Positioning Considerations for Ribs

Specific positions performed in a rib series are generally determined by the patient's clinical history and the department protocol.

The radiographer must obtain a complete clinical history that includes the nature of the trauma or pathology, the location of the rib pain or injury, if the patient has been coughing up blood or fluid, and whether the patient is able to stand.

The following positioning tips are provided to assist the radiographer in producing a diagnostic study of the ribs:

Above or below Diaphragm

The location of the trauma determines which region of the ribs are radiographed. Ribs above the diaphragm require a different technique, different breathing instructions, and generally different body positions than ribs located below the diaphragm.

The upper ten posterior ribs are generally the minimum ribs above the dome or central portion of the diaphragm on a full inspiration as described in chapter two on the chest. However with painful rib injuries the patient may not be able to take as full an inspiration and only nine, or even eight posterior ribs may be seen above the diaphragm on inspiration.

Above Diaphragm: To best demonstrate these above diaphragm ribs, the radiographer should:

(a) Take the radiographs **erect**, if patient is able to stand. This allows better inspiration of the lungs with the diaphragm dropping to its lowest position. Also most rib injuries are very painful and body movement creating pressure against the rib cage such as from movements on the x-ray table can cause severe pain and discomfort.

(b) Suspend respiration and expose upon **inspiration**. This should project the diaphragm below the eighth or ninth, or even tenth ribs on full inspiration.

(c) Select a relatively **low kVp** technique. Since the upper ribs are surrounded by lung tissue, a lower kVp will preserve radiographic contrast and visualize the ribs through the air-filled lungs. However if the site of injury is over the heart area, a higher kVp may be be used to obtain a longer scale contrast to visualize ribs both through the heart shadow and through the lung fields.

Below Diaphragm: To best demonstrate these ribs below the diaphragm, the radiographer should:

(a) Take the radiographs with patient **recumbent.** This will allow the diaphragm to rise to the highest position to provide a uniform background density for the lower ribs.

(b) Suspend respiration and expose upon **expiration.** This should allow the diaphragm to rise to the level of the sixth or seventh ribs, again providing a uniform background density.

(c) Select a **medium kVp** technique. Since the lower ribs are surrounded by the muscular diaphragm and must be demonstrated through dense abdominal structures, a medium kVp will insure proper penetration of these tissues.

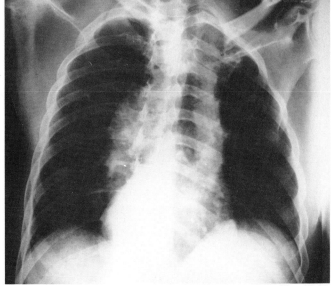

Fig. 10-18

Ribs Above Diagragm
- Erect if possible
- Inspiration
- Low kVp

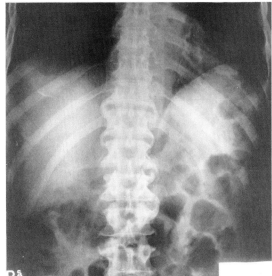

Fig. 10-19

Ribs Below Diagragm, Injury to Left Side
- Recumbent
- Expiration
- Medium kVp

Recomended Projections

Departmental routines for ribs may vary depending on the preference of radiologists. One recomended routine is as follows:

Select the projections that will place the **area of interest closest to the film,** and **rotate the spine away from the area of interest.**

For example, if a patient has a history of trauma to the **left posterior ribs** two preferred projections are a straight **AP** and a **left posterior oblique.** (Above or below diaphragm technique would be determined by the level of injured ribs.) The LPO position will move the spinous processes **away from** the left side. The left posterior ribs are closest to the film and also placed nearer parallel to the film to reduce foreshortening of these ribs.

A second example is a patient who has trauma to the **right anterior ribs.** Two preferred projections would be a straight **PA** and a **left anterior oblique.** The **PA** will place the site of injury closest to the film and the **LAO** position will rotate the spinous process **away from** the site of trauma.

Marking the site of injury

Some departments prefer that the radiographer tape a small, metallic "BB" or some other small type of marker over the site of injury. This will give the radiologist the general location of the trauma or pathology. This policy varies in different departments and each radiographer should know their departmental policy regarding this.

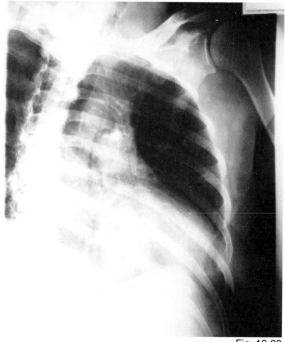

Fig. 10-20

LPO Ribs
– Injury to right posterior ribs
– Metallic marker to site of injury (Optional)

Chest Radiographs

Departmental policy and routines also vary concerning the inclusion of chest x-rays as part of a rib exam routine. However injury to the thorax often creates respiratory dysfunctions and patients with a history of rib injuries should have an erect PA (and lateral) projection of the chest taken with lung technique to rule out a possible pneumothorax and hemothorax. If the patient cannot assume an erect position for this, a decubitus position using a horizontal beam should be included if possible to determine air-fluid levels.

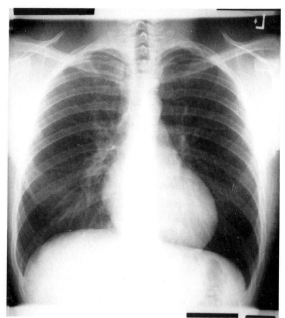

Fig. 10-21

PA chest

National Survey

A survey of the operating procedures (department routines) was conducted throughout the United States. The following information was compiled from the survey indicating the national norm for basic and optional projections of the sternum and ribs. In regard to ribs, specific projections / positions are often determined by the location of the trauma.

Sternum Routine

Sternum	U.S. Average	
	Basic	Optional
• Lateral	97%	
• RAO (15-20°)	95%	
• LAO*		5%
• Tomograms*		2%

* Write-ins by survey respondents

Ribs Routine

Ribs	U.S. Average	
	Basic	Optional
• AP or PA (Above or Below Diaphragm)	89%	
• Single Oblique (Ant or Post)	66%	
• PA Chest (to rule out pneumothorax or hemo-thorax)	66%	
• Two Obliques	27%	5%

Standard and Optional Operating Procedures

Certain basic and optional projections or positions for the sternum and ribs are demonstrated and described on the following pages as suggested standard and optional departmental procedures.

Basic Projections

Standard or basic projections, also sometimes referred to as routine projections or departmental routines are those projections or positions commonly taken on average patients who are helpful and can cooperate in performing the procedure.

Optional Projections

Optional projections are those more common projections or positions taken as extra or additional projections to better demonstrate certain pathologic conditions or specific body parts.

Basic and Optional Projections

Sternum
Basic
• RAO
• Lateral

Ribs
• Posterior Ribs (AP)
(Above or Below Dia.)
or
Anterior Ribs (PA)
(Above or Below Dia.)
• Axillary Ribs (Ant or Post Obli's)
(Above or Below Dia.)
• PA Chest (page 66)*

*The PA chest for lung field technique will not be demonstrated specifically in this chapter on the ribs as this projection is the same as described in chapter 2 on the chest and similar to the PA projection for ribs (page 309).

• RAO Position

Sternum
Basic
• **RAO**
• Lateral

Structures Best Shown:
Entire sternum superimposed over heart shadow.

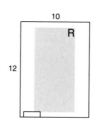

Technical Factors:
• Film Size - 10 x 12 in. (24 x 30 cm), lengthwise.
• Moving or stationary grid.
• Minimum 3 sec. exposure with breathing technique.
• 60-70 kVp range.

Patient Position:
• Erect (preferred), or semiprone position slightly obliqued, right arm down by side, left arm up.

Shielding: Place lead shield over gonadal region.

Part Position:
• Oblique patient **15 to 20°** to the right side, RAO (See NOTE).
• Align long axis of sternum to midline of x-ray table and/or film.
• Place top of cassette about 1.5 in. (4 cm) above the jugular notch.

Central Ray:
• CR **perpendicular** to film holder.
• CR directed to **center of film**, (midway between the jugular notch and xiphoid process).
• 30 to 40 in. (77-102 cm) SID. (See NOTE)

Collimation: Collimate to area of sternum (should result in about a 5 in. or 13 cm wide collimation field).

Respiration: Breathing technique preferred if patient can cooperate (for blurring of overlying lung markings).

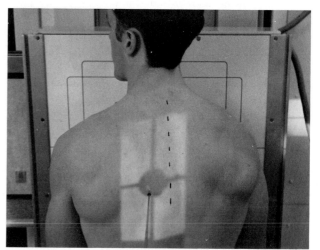

Erect – RAO   Fig. 10-22

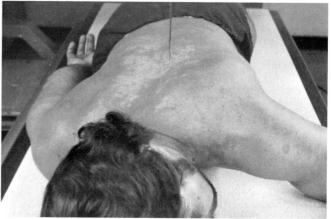

Recumbent – RAO   Fig. 10-23

NOTE: • A large deep-chested thorax requires less rotation than a thin-chested patient to shift the sternum just to the left of vertebral column superimposed over the homogenous heart shadow. The amount of required rotation can also be determined by placing one hand on the sternum and the other on the spinous processes and determining that these two points are not superimposed as viewed from the position of the x-ray tube.

• Shorter SID causes magnification and loss of recorded detail of overlying posterior thoracic structures resulting in better visibility of sternum. However, a shorter SID results in increased skin dosage and a **minimum of 6 in.** (15 cm) between collimation and skin surface must be maintained for radiation safety purposes.

Severe Trauma: Can be taken in LPO position if patient cannot turn in a semiprone position.

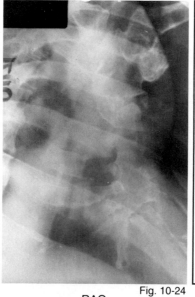

RAO   Fig. 10-24
(Courtesy of Bill Collins, RT)

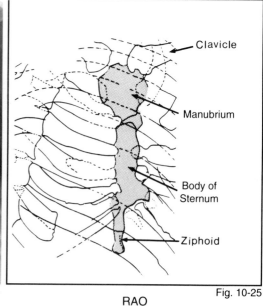

RAO   Fig. 10-25

Clavicle

Manubrium

Body of Sternum

Ziphoid

Evaluation Criteria:
• Entire sternum visualized, superimposed over the heart shadow.
• Correct rotation places entire sternum alongside vertebral column without superimposition of any part of sternum by vertebrae.

• Optimum exposure visualizes outline of sternum through overlying ribs. Lung markings should appear blurred with breathing technique.

• Lateral Position

<table>
<tr><td>**Sternum**
Basic
• RAO
• **Lateral**</td></tr>
</table>

Structures Best Shown:
Entire sternum with minimal overlap of soft tissues.

Technical Factors:
• Film Size - 10 x 12 in. (24 x 30 cm), lengthwise.
• Moving or stationary grid.
• 70 - 75 kVp range.

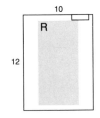

Patient Position:
• Erect (preferred), or lateral recumbent.

Shielding: Place lead shield over gonadal region.

Part Position:
Erect
• Standing or seated with shoulders and arms **drawn back** as far as possible.
Lateral Recumbent
• Lying on side with arms up above head, keep shoulders back.
• Place top of cassette 1.5 in. (4 cm) above the jugular notch.
• Align long axis of sternum to midline of table and/or film.
• Insure a true lateral, **no rotation.**

Central Ray:
• CR **perpendicular** to film holder.
• CR directed to **center of film**, (midway between the jugular notch and xiphoid process).
• Minimum 40 in. (102 cm) SID, or 72 in. (183 cm) to reduce magnification of sternum.

Collimation: Close four-sided collimation to area of sternum.

Respiration: Suspend and expose upon **inspiration**.

NOTE: Large pendulous breasts of female patients may be drawn to the sides and held in position with a wide bandage.

Severe trauma: Can be taken crosstable with patient supine on stretcher, as a lateral dorsal decubitus position *(Fig. 10-28).*

Evaluation Criteria:
• Entire sternum is visualized without superimposition by ribs or soft tissue of arms or shoulders.
• No rotation of the sternum.
• Optimum exposure and contrast to visualize sternum, from proximal manubrium to distal xiphoid.

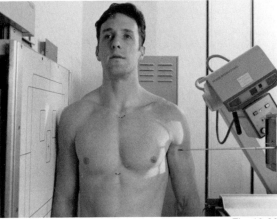

Lateral – Erect   Fig. 10-26

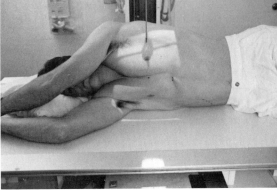

Lateral – Recumbent   Fig. 10-27

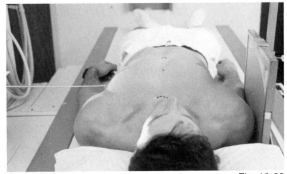

Dorsal Decubitus   Fig. 10-28

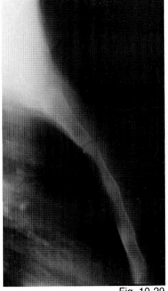

Lateral   Fig. 10-29

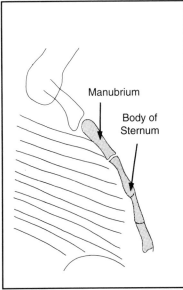

Manubrium

Body of Sternum

Lateral   Fig. 10-30

• AP Projection
(Above or Below Diaphragm)

Ribs
- **Posterior Ribs (AP)**
  (Above or Below Dia.)
  or
  Anterior Ribs (PA)
  (Above or Below Dia.)
- Axillary Ribs (Ant or Post Obli's)
  (Above or Below Dia.)
- PA Chest (page 66)

Structures Best Shown:
Posterior ribs, above or below the diaphragm.

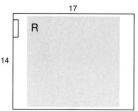

Technical Factors:
- Film Size - 14 x 17 in. (35 x 43 cm).
- Film crosswise (see NOTE).
- Moving or stationary grid.
- Above diaphragm: 65-75 kVp.
- Below diaphragm: 75-85 kVp.

Patient Position:
- Erect preferred for above diaphragm if patients condition allows; or supine for below diaphragm.

Shielding: Place lead shield over gonadal region.

Part Position:
- Align **midsagittal plane to midline** of table and/or film holder.
- Rotate shoulders anteriorly to remove scapulae from lung fields.
- **Raise chin** to prevent superimposing upper ribs, look straight ahead.
- **No rotation** of thorax or pelvis.

Central Ray:

Above Diaphragm:
- CR **perpendicular** to film holder, centered to **3 or 4 in.** (8-10 cm) **below jugular notch** (level of T 7).
- Center cassette to level of CR (top of cassette should be about 1.5 in. or 4 cm above shoulders).

Below Diaphragm:
- CR **perpendicular, centered to midway between xiphoid and lower rib cage.**
- Center cassette to level of CR (bottom of cassette should be about at the level of iliac crest).
- Minimum 40 in. (102 cm) SID.

Collimation: Collimate to outer margins of thorax.

Respiration: Suspend and expose upon **inspiration** for **above** diaphragm, and **expiration** for **below** diaphragm.

NOTE: Place film crosswise for both above and below diaphragm ribs except for small patients because average width of thorax is greater than height as discussed in chapter 2. (This is more important at shorter SID with greater magnification than at a 72 in. (183 cm) SID as for chests.)

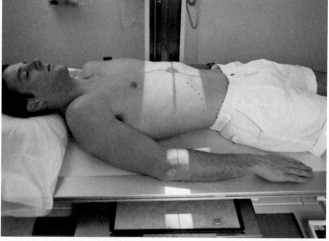

AP Erect – Above Diaphragm   Fig. 10-31

AP Supine – Below Diaphragm   Fig. 10-32

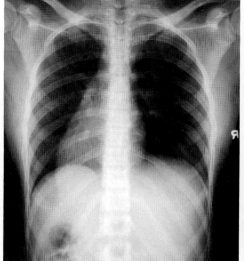

AP – Above Diaphragm   Fig. 10-33

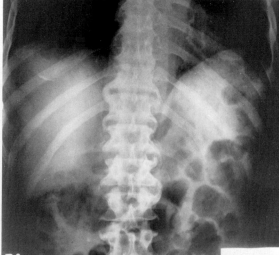

AP – Below Diaphragm   Fig. 10-34

Evaluation Criteria:
- The first through eighth or ninth posterior ribs should be visualized above the diaphragm.
- No motion is seen on the radiograph.
- No rotation of the thorax is evident.
- Optimum exposure and penetration should visualize ribs through the heart shadow without overexposing mid-posterior ribs through the lung fields.

• PA Projection
(Above Diaphragm)

Ribs
• Posterior Ribs (AP)
  (Above or Below Dia.)
    or
Anterior Ribs (PA)
  (Above or Below Dia.)
• Axillary Ribs (Ant or Post Obli's)
  (Above or Below Dia.)
• **PA Erect Chest** (page 66)

Structures Best Shown:
Anterior ribs, above the diaphragm. (Below diaphragm rib injuries are generally to posterior ribs and AP projections are taken.)

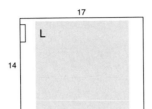

Technical Factors:
• Film Size - 14 x 17 in. (35 x 43 cm), crosswise.
• Moving or stationary grid.
• 65-75 kVp range (above diaphragm).

Patient Position:
• Erect preferred, or prone if necessary, with arms down to the side.

Shielding: Place lead shield over gonadal region.

Part Position:
• Align midsagittal plane to midline of film holder.
• **No rotation** of thorax or pelvis.

Central Ray:
• CR **perpendicular** to film holder, centered to **T7** (7-8 in. or 18-20 cm below vertebra prominens as for PA chest).
• Center cassette to level of CR. (Top of cassette should be about 1.5 in. or 4 cm above shoulders.)
• Minimum 40 in. (102 cm) SID (or 72 in, 180 cm, SID as per chest projections).

Collimation: Collimate along lateral margins of thorax, and to upper and lower margins of film.

Respiration: Suspend and expose upon **inspiration.**

PA Erect Chest: It is common departmental policy to include an erect PA chest projection with lung exposure techniques to rule out respiratory dysfunctions such as a pneumothorax or hemothorax which may accompany rib injuries *(Fig. 10-37).* Positioning is similar to that for PA ribs, above diaphragm, as shown in *Fig. 10-35* and described above.

Evaluation Criteria:
• The first through eighth or ninth posterior ribs should be visualized above the diaphragm.
• No motion of the ribs as seen on the radiograph.
• No rotation of the thorax.
• Optimum exposure and penetration should visualize outlines of all ribs above the diaphragm, including ribs through the heart shadow with-out excessive burnout of other ribs.

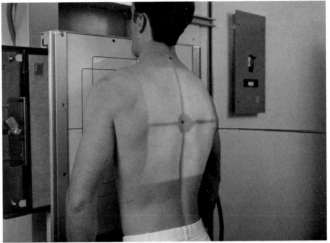

PA Ribs – Above Diaphragm   Fig. 10-35

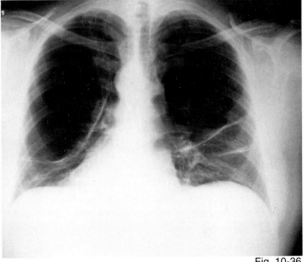

Fig. 10-36
PA Ribs

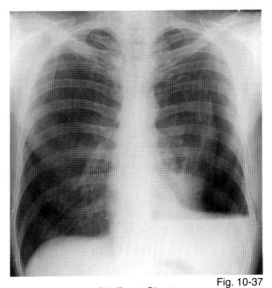

Fig. 10-37
PA Erect Chest
(Demonstrates a combination hemo and pneumo thorax on left side)

• Posterior or Anterior Oblique Position
(Above or Below Diaphragm)

Ribs
- Post Ribs (AP)
  (Above or Below Dia.)
  or
  Ant Ribs (PA)
  (Above or Below Dia.)
- **Axillary Ribs (Ant or Post Obli's)**
  (Above or Below Dia.)
- PA Chest (page 66)

Structures Best Shown:
Axillary margin of ribs on the side of interest projected without self-superimposition.

Posterior/lateral injury - posterior obliques, affected side toward film. Anterior/lateral injury - anterior obliques, affected side away from film.

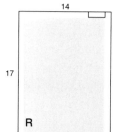

Technical Factors:
- Film Size - 14 x 17 (35 x 43 cm), lengthwise.
- Moving or stationary grid.
- 70-75 kVp range above diaphragm, or 80-85 kVp below diaphragm.
- Attach metallic marker to area of injury if this is part of departmental routine.

Patient Position:
- Erect preferred for above diaphragm if patients condition allows; or supine for below diaphragm.

Shielding: Place lead shield over gonadal region.

Part Position:
- Rotate patient into 45° posterior or anterior oblique, **affected side closest to film** on **posterior** oblique; and **affected side away from film** on **anterior** oblique. (Rotate spine **away** from site of injury.)
- Raise elevated side arm above head; extend opposite arm down and behind patient away from thorax.
- If recumbent, flex knee of elevated side to help maintain this position.
- Support body with positioning blocks if needed.
- Align a plane of the thorax midway between the spine and the lateral margin of thorax on side of interest to the midline of the table and/or film (insure that side of interest is **not** cut off).

Central Ray:
- CR **perpendicular** to film holder, centered midway between lateral margin of ribs and spine.

Above Diaphragm:
- CR to level 3 or 4 in. (8-10 cm) below jugular notch **(T 7)**. (Top of cassette about 1.5 in or 4 cm above shoulders.)

Below Diaphragm:
- CR to level midway between xiphoid and lower rib cage. (Bottom of cassette should be about at level of iliac crest.)
- 72 in. (183 cm), or minimum 40 in (102 cm) SID.

Collimation: Collimate to near film borders on all four sides to not cut off rib cage for possible primary and secondary sites of rib injuries.

Respiration: Suspend and expose on **inspiration** for above diaphragm ribs, and on **expiration** for below diaphragm ribs.

NOTE: • For this recommended routine, an injury to the **right** side would require an **RPO** or an **LAO**.
- Injury to the **left** side would require an **LPO** or an **RAO**.
- Some departmental routines include taping a small metallic "BB" directly on the patient at the injury site to assist in locating possible rib fractures.

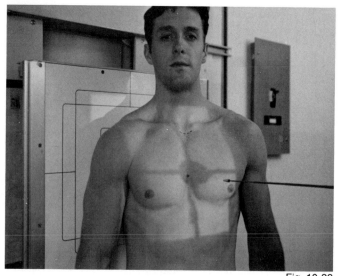

Fig. 10-38

RPO
(Injury to the **right posterior** ribs, above diaphragm)

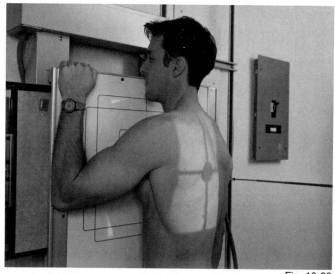

Fig. 10-39

RAO
(Injury to **left anterior** ribs, above diaphragm)

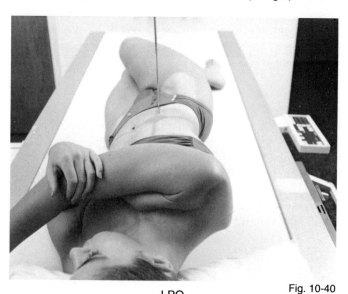

Fig. 10-40

LPO
(Injury to **left posterior** ribs, below diaphragm)

Posterior or Anterior Oblique Position (Above or Below Diaphragm) continued

Evaluation Criteria:
• A 45° oblique should be evident in that the distance between the vertebral column and the lateral rib margin on the affected side should be about twice the distance on the unaffected side.
• No motion of the rib margins should be evident on the radiograph.
• The axillary portion of the ribs, involving the site of injury (above or below diaphragm), should be elongated, clearly seen and included in the collimation field.

Above Diaphragm Ribs
• Upper nine or ten pairs of ribs should be included and seen above the diaphragm.
• Optimum exposure and contrast should visualize the ribs through the heart shadow and lateral rib margins without overexposing ribs through the mid-lung fields.

Below Diaphragm Ribs
• Lower ribs, the eighth through twelfth, should be included and seen below the diaphragm.
• Optimum exposure and contrast should clearly visualize the ribs below the diaphragm as seen through the dense abdominal structures. (Ribs above the diaphragm in the mid-lung field area will appear dark and overexposed.)

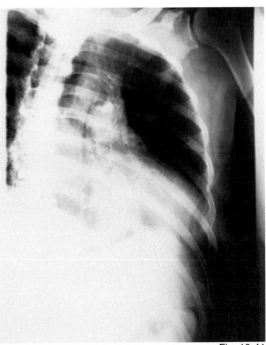

Fig. 10-41

RPO, Above Diaphragm

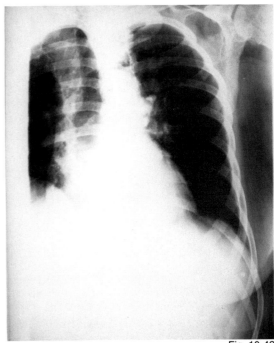

Fig. 10-42

RAO, Above Diaphragm

Chapter 11
Radiographic Anatomy and Positioning
of the
Cranium
(Skull Series and Sella Turcica)

Contributions by: Kathy M. Martensen, BS, RT (R)
Barry T. Anthony, RT (R)

Contents

Part 1 Radiographic Anatomy

Skull

The skull or bony skeleton of the head rests on the superior end of the vertebral column and is divided into two main sets of bones; the **cranium,** which consists of eight bones, and the fourteen **facial bones.**

The cranium is that part of the skull that surrounds and protects the brain, while that portion anterior and inferior to the brain case is termed the facial skeleton or the facial bones.

The **eight cranial bones** will be studied in this chapter and will be referred to as the cranium.

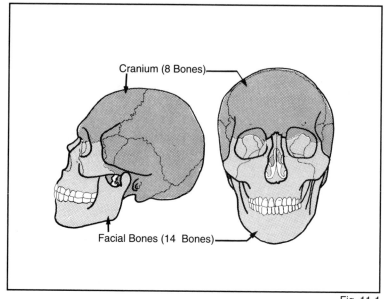

Skull – Bony Skeleton of Head   Fig. 11-1

Cranial Topography (surface landmarks)

Certain surface landmarks and localizing lines must be used for accurate positioning of the cranium. Each of the following topographical structures can either be seen or palpated:

The **glabella** *(glah-bel'ah)* is the smooth, slightly depressed triangular area between the eyebrows and above the bridge of the nose.

The **acanthion** *(ah-kan'the-on,* little thorn) is the midline point at the junction of the upper lip and the nasal septum. This is the point where the nose and upper lip meet.

A flat triangular area projects forward as the chin (mentum) in the human. The mid point of this triangular area of the chin as it appears from the front is termed the **mental point.**

Extending across the forehead directly above each eye is a ridge or arch of bone called the **superciliary ridge** (arch).

Slightly above this ridge is a slight groove or depression termed the **supraorbital groove** or SOG. The SOG is important because it corresponds to the highest level of the facial bone mass, which is also the **level of the floor of the anterior fossa** of the cranial vault.

Note: The superciliary arch and the SOG can be located on yourself by placing your finger firmly against the length of your eyebrow and feeling the slightly raised arch of bone; then allow your finger to slide upward and feel it drop slightly into the SOG, the slight groove above your eyebrow.

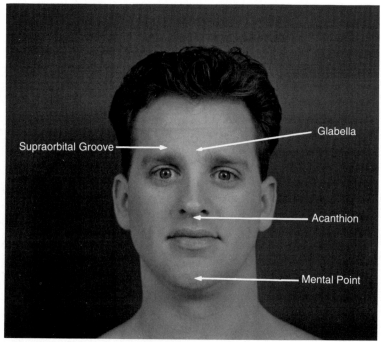

Surface Landmarks   Fig. 11-2

Surface Landmarks continued

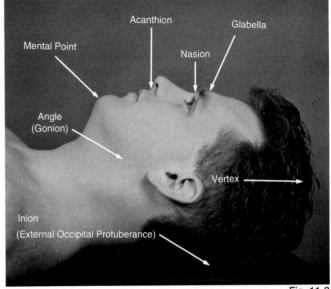

Surface Landmarks   Fig. 11-3

The **glabella, acanthion** and **mental point** are shown as seen on a side view of the head.

The **nasion** *(na′ze-on)* is the depression at the bridge of the nose. Anatomically, the nasion is the junction of the two nasal bones and the frontal bone.

The **angle**, sometimes called **gonion** *(go′ne-on)*, refers to the lower posterior angle on each side of the jaw or mandible.

The **vertex** is the most superior portion of the skull, or the very top of the cranium.

The **inion** *(in′e-on)*, the most prominent point of the **external occipital protuberance,** is the bump along the midline of the lower back of the head at the junction of the head and neck, the area where posterior neck muscles attach. The approximate locations of the vertex and inion are also shown in *Figs. 11-4* and *5.*

The **superciliary arch** and the **supraorbital groove** (SOG) are again identified on this side view.

Base of Orbit

Landmarks directly associated with the eye or base of the bony orbit are shown in this frontal and lateral drawing. The **base of the orbit** is the circle of bone forming the outermost ridge of the bony socket, termed the orbit. The orbit, as will be described and illustrated in chapter 12 on facial bones which follows, is conical in shape and extends posteriorly from the base.

The junctions of the upper and lower eyelids are termed **canthi** *(kan′thi).* Thus the **inner canthus** *(kan′thus)* is where the eyelids meet near the nose, while the more lateral junction of the eyelids is termed the **outer canthus.**

The superior rim of the orbital base is termed the **supraorbital margin** or **SOM**, and the inferior rim is termed the **infraorbital margin** or **IOM.** Another landmark is the **mid-lateral orbital margin,** that portion of the lateral rim near the outer canthus of the eye.

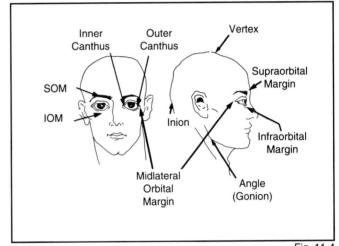

Surface Landmarks   Fig. 11-4

Ear

Various localizing lines utilize the **external acoustic (auditory) meatus** *(me-a′tus)* **(EAM)** as a reference point. The EAM is the opening of the external ear canal. The center point of the EAM is termed the **auricular point.** As a positioning landmark, however, this is generally referrred to as just the EAM.

The **auricle** or **pinna** is that portion of the external ear not contained within the head, that is, the larger flap of the ear made up of cartilage. The **tragus** is the small cartilaginous flap of the external ear covering the EAM.

The **top of ear attachment (TEA)** is the most superior attachment of the auricle to the scalp or that point where the side-frames of one's eyeglasses rest. The top of ear attachment is an important landmark because it corresponds to the **level of the petrous ridge** on each side.

The **inion** is shown to be slightly above an extension of a line connecting the infraorbital margin and the EAM.

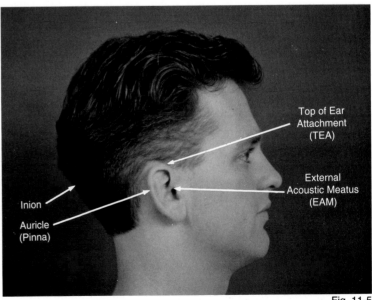

Surface Landmarks   Fig. 11-5

Lines and Planes

The **midsagittal** or **median plane** divides the body into left and right halves. This plane is important in accurate positioning of the cranium since, for every **frontal** or **lateral** position, **the midsagittal plane is either perpendicular to, or parallel to, the plane of the film.**

The **interpupillary** or **interorbital line** is a line connecting either the pupils or the outer canthi of the patient's eyes. When the head is placed in a **true lateral** position, the **interpupillary line must be exactly perpendicular to the plane of the film.**

Frontal Skull Positioning Lines

Certain positioning lines are important in skull radiography. These lines are formed by connecting certain anterior landmarks to the mid point of the external acoustic meatus (EAM). The most superior of these lines is the **glabellomeatal line,** which is not as precise as the other four since the glabella is an area and not a specific point.

The **orbitomeatal line (OML)** is a frequently used positioning line located between the outer canthus or mid-lateral orbital margin and the EAM.

The **infraorbitomeatal line (IOML)** is formed by connecting the middle of the infraorbital margin to the EAM. An older term identifying the same line is Reid's base line. Sometimes this is also refered to as just the base line of the cranium, although these terms are not used in this text.

There is an average **7-8 degree** angle difference between the orbitomeatal and the infraorbitomeatal lines. There is also an approximate **7-8 degree** average angle difference between the orbitomeatal and glabellomeatal lines. Knowing the angle differences between these three lines is helpful in making positioning adjustments for specific projections of the cranium and facial bones.

The **acanthiomeatal** and **mentomeatal lines** are important in radiography of the facial bones. These lines are formed by connecting the acanthion and the mental point, respectively, to the EAM.

The **glabelloalveolar line** connects the glabella to a point at the anterior aspect of the alveolar process of the maxilla. This line is used for positioning a tangential projection for the nasal bones.

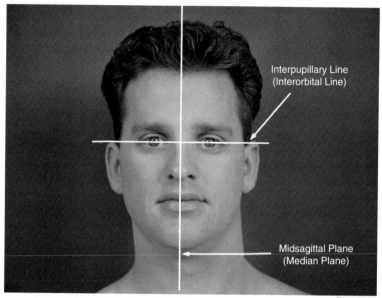

Lines and Planes

Fig. 11-6

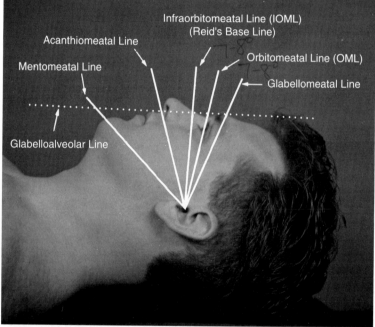

Positioning Lines

Fig. 11-7

Skull Positioning Aids

An angle indicator or protractor can be used, or a cardboard straight-edge cut at a specific angle, to accurately position the cranium. In this case, a 90° straight-edge is shown to determine that the orbitomeatal line has been placed perpendicular to the film plane by depressing the chin as needed, or by placing a support under the back of the head if the chin cannot be depressed far enough. The chin can be raised or lowered to change the perpendicular reference line to be used.

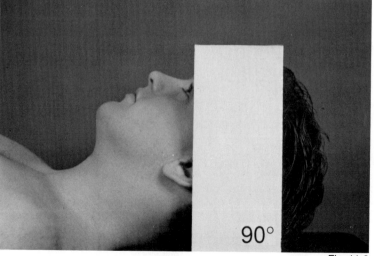

Frontal Positioning

Fig. 11-8

Cranium

The eight bones of the cranium are divided into calvarium or skull cap, and floor. Each of these areas more or less consists of four bones.

Calvarium (Skull Cap)
(1) Frontal Bone
(2) Left Parietal Bone *(pa-ri′-i-tal)*
(3) Right Parietal Bone
(4) Occipital Bone *(ok-sip′-i-tal)*

Floor
(5) Left Temporal Bone
(6) Right Temporal Bone
(7) Sphenoid Bone *(sfe′noid)*
(8) Ethmoid Bone *(eth ′moid)*

The eight bones making up the calvarium or skull cap and floor or base of the cranium are demonstrated on these frontal, lateral and superior cut-away view drawings. These eight cranial bones are fused in an adult to form a protective enclosure for the brain. Each of these cranial bones will be demonstrated and described individually in the pages which follow.

Joints of the Cranium (Sutures)

The articulations or joints of the cranium are called **sutures** and belong in the class of joints termed **fibrous joints.** Since in an adult they are **immovable,** they are called **synarthrodial.**

The **coronal** *(ko-ro′nal)* **suture** separates the frontal bone from the two parietals. Separating the two parietal bones in the midline is the **sagittal suture.**

Posteriorly, the **lambdoidal** *(lam′doy-dal)* **suture** separates the two parietals from the occipital bone.

The **squamosal** *(skwa-mo′sal)* **suture** is formed by the inferior junction of each parietal bone with the respective temporal bone. This suture is visible only on the lateral view.

Each end of the sagittal suture is identified as a point or area with a specific name as labeled. The anterior end of the sagittal suture is termed the **bregma** *(breg′mah,)* while the posterior end is the **lambda** *(lam′dah).* The **pterion** *(ter′re-on)* is a point at the junction of the parietal, temporal and the greater wing of the sphenoid. The **asterion** *(as-te′re-on)* is a point posterior to the ear where the squamosal and lambdoidal sutures meet. These four recognizable bony points are used in surgery or other cases where cranial measurements are necessary.

Fontanels: Early in life, the bregma and lambda are not bony, but are soft spots. These soft spots are termed the **anterior** and **posterior fontanels** *(fon″tah-nels′)* in the newborn.

Two smaller lateral fontanels are the **sphenoid** (pterion in an adult) and **mastoid** (asterion in an adult) **fontanels,** located respectively at the sphenoid and mastoid angles of the parietal bones on each side of the head. Thus there are a total of **six fontanels** or unossified membranous areas in a newborn.

The lateral and posterior fontanels close within several months after birth. The anterior fontanel, however, which is the largest fontanel measuring about 2.5 x 4 cm at birth, doesn't completely close until about 18 months of age.

Certain irregular bones called **sutural** or **Wormian bones** sometimes develop in the adult at these fontanels.

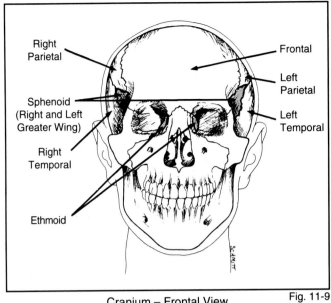

Cranium – Frontal View   Fig. 11-9

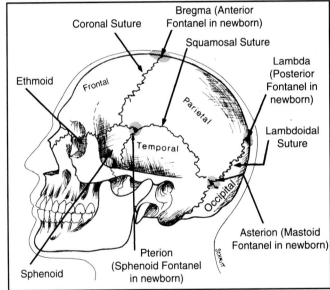

Cranium – Lateral View   Fig. 11-10

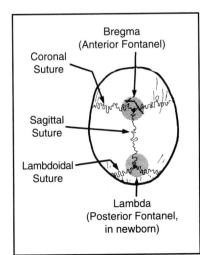

Sutures – Superior View   Fig. 11-12

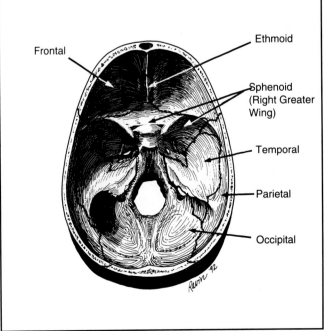

Cranium – (Superior Sectional View)   Fig. 11-11

Cranial Bones

Each of the cranial bones will be separated and studied individually. After the description of each of these eight bones will be a listing of those specific adjoining bones with which they articulate, or with which they are joined since in an adult they are all fused or immovable. Some of the bones with which the cranial bones articulate are facial bones which are described in the chapter which follows. Knowing all of these "articulations" helps in learning the specific locations and relationships of each of these bones beginning with the frontal bone.

(1) Frontal Bone

As viewed from the front, the only bone of the calvarium readily visible is the **frontal bone.** This bone, which forms the forehead and the superior part of each orbit, consists of two main parts. The **squamous** or **vertical portion** forms the forehead, while the **orbital** or **horizontal portion** forms the superior part of the orbit.

Squamous or vertical portion: The **glabella** is the smooth prominence between the eyebrows and above the bridge of the nose. The **supraorbital groove (SOG)** is the depression above each eyebrow.

The superior rim of each orbit is the **supraorbital margin** or **SOM.** The **supraorbital notch** (foramen) is a small hole or opening within the supraorbital margin slightly medial to its mid point. A nerve and an artery pass through this small opening.

That ridge of bone beneath each eyebrow is termed the **superciliary ridge** (arch). Between the superciliary arches is the **glabella.** On each side of the squama, above the supraorbital grooves, is a larger rounded prominence termed the **frontal tuberosity** (eminence).

Orbital or horizontal portion (inferior view): As seen from the inferior aspect, the frontal bone shows primarily the horizontal or orbital portion. The **supraorbital margins,** the **superciliary ridges,** the **glabella** and the **frontal tuberosities** can all be seen.

The **orbital plate** on each side forms the superior part of each orbit. Below the orbital plates lie facial bones, and above the orbital plates is the anterior part of the floor of the brain case. The **supraorbital groove (SOG),** not seen on this inferior view, is the external landmark at the level of the orbital plates.

Each orbital plate is separated from the other by the **ethmoidal notch.** The ethmoid bone, one of the bones of the floor of the cranium, fits into this notch. The **nasal (frontal) spine** is found at the anterior end of the ethmoidal notch.

Articulations: The frontal bone articulates with **4** cranial bones; right and left parietals, the sphenoid and the ethmoid. (The frontal bone also articulates with 8 facial bones.)

(2 & 3) Parietal Bones

The paired **right** and **left parietal bones** are well demonstrated on these side and top view drawings. The lateral walls of the cranium and part of the roof are formed by the two parietal bones. Each of the parietals is roughly square in shape and has a concave internal surface.

The widest portion of the entire skull is located between the **parietal tubercles (eminences)** of the two parietal bones. The frontal bone is primarily anterior to the parietals, the occipital is posterior, the temporals inferior and the greater wings of the sphenoid inferior and anterior.

Articulations: Each parietal articulates with **5** cranial bones; the frontal, the occipital, a temporal, the sphenoid and the opposite parietal.

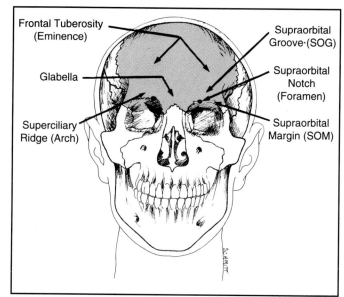

Squamous Portion of Frontal Bone

Fig. 11-13

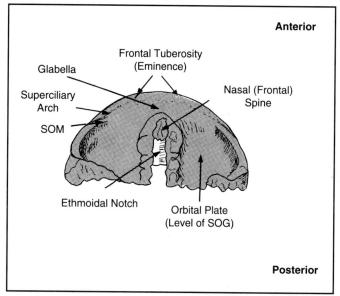

Orbital Portion of Frontal Bone (Inferior View)

Fig. 11-14

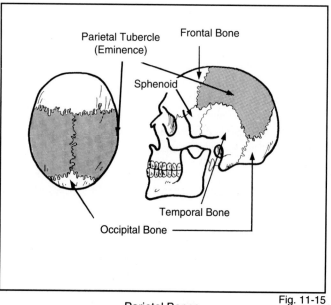

Parietal Bones

Fig. 11-15

(4) Occipital Bone

The inferoposterior portion of the calvarium or skull cap is formed by the single occipital bone. The external surface of the occipital bone presents a rounded part termed the **squamous portion.** The squamous portion forms most of the back of the head and is that part of the occipital bone superior to the **foramen magnum.** Foramen magnum literally means "great hole" and is the avenue by which the spinal cord leaves the brain.

The two **lateral condylar portions** (occipital condyles) are oval processes with convex surfaces, one on each side of the foramen magnum. These articulate with depressions on the first cervical vertebra, the atlas. This two-part articulation between the skull and the cervical spine is called the **occipito-atlantal joint(s).**

The prominent bump on the squamous portion of the occipital bone is the **external occipital protuberance** or **inion.**

Articulations: The occipital articulates with **6** bones; the two parietals, the two temporals, the sphenoid and the atlas (first cervical vertebra).

(5 & 6) Temporal Bones

Lateral view: The paired **right** and **left temporal bones** are complex structures housing the delicate organs of hearing and balance. As seen from the side in this lateral view drawing, the left temporal bone is situated between the greater wing of the sphenoid bone anteriorly, and the occipital bone posteriorly. The thin upper portion of each temporal forms part of the wall of the cranium, termed the **squamous** portion. This part of the skull is quite thin and is therefore the most vulnerable portion of the entire skull to fracture which may result in hemorrhage beneath the bony surface.

Extending anteriorly from the squamous portion of the temporal bone is an arch of bone termed the **zygomatic** *(zi'go-mat'ik)* **process.** This process meets the temporal process of the zygomatic bone (one of the facial bones) to form the easily palpated **zygomatic arch.**

Inferior to the zygomatic process and just anterior to the **EAM** (external acoustic meatus) is the **temporomandibular fossa,** into which the mandible fits to form the **TMJ** or **temporomandibular joint.**

Between the mandible and the EAM is a slender bony projection called the **styloid process.**

The second main portion of the temporal bone is that area posterior and inferior to the EAM, the **mastoid** portion. This is sometimes also called the **petromastoid portion** of the temporal bone since internally this includes the petrous portion. Extending downward from this portion is the easily palpated **mastoid process** or **tip.** Many air cells of the mastoid sinus are located within the mastoid process.

Superior View: The floor of the cranium is well visualized in this drawing. The single occipital bone resides between the paired temporal bones. The third main portion of each temporal bone is the **petrous** *(pet'rus)* **portion,** often termed the **petrous pyramid** or **pars petrosa.** This pyramid-shaped portion of the temporal bone is the thickest and densest bone in the cranium. The petrous pyramid projects forward and toward the midline from the area of the **external acoustic meatus.**

The delicate organs of hearing and balance are housed in and protected by the **petrous pyramids.** The upper edges of the pyramids are often called the **petrous ridges.** The petrous ridge corresponds to the level of the external landmark, the TEA or top of the ear attachment. Medially, each petrous pyramid ends with the **internal acoustic meatus,** which serves to transmit the nerves of hearing and equilibrium.

Articulations: Each temporal articulates with **3** cranial bones; a parietal, the occipital and the sphenoid. (Each temporal also articulates with 2 facial bones.)

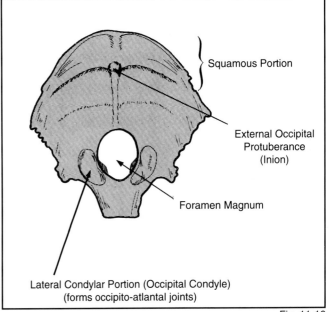

Occipital Bone (Inferior View)   Fig. 11-16

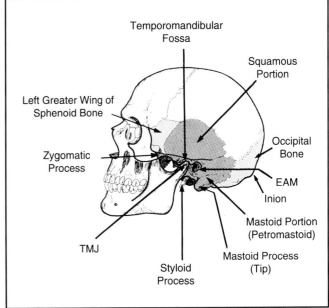

Temporal Bone (Lateral View)   Fig. 11-17

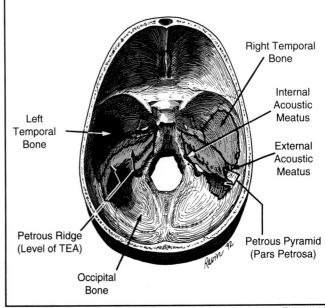

Temporal Bone (Superior View)   Fig. 11-18

(7) Sphenoid Bone

Superior View: The single centrally located **sphenoid bone** forms the anchor for all eight cranial bones. The central portion of the sphenoid is the body, which lies in the midline of the floor of the cranium and contains the sphenoid sinuses as best shown on the medial sectional drawing of *Fig. 11-23* on the following page. The central depression on the body is termed the **sella turcica** *(sel'a-tur'si-ka)*. This depression looks like a saddle from the side as shown in *Fig. 11-21* and derives its name from words meaning Turkish saddle. The sella turcica partially surrounds and protects a major gland of the body, the **hypophysis** or pituitary gland. Posterior to the sella turcica is the back of the saddle, the **dorsum sellae** *(dor'sum sel'e)*, also best seen on the lateral drawing of *Fig. 11-21*.

The **clivus** *(kli'vus)* is a shallow depression just posterior to the base of the dorsum sellae. This depression is continuous with a similar groove at the base of the occipital bone sloping upward from the foramen magnum to where it joins the sphenoid. This area forms a base of support for the pons portion of the brain. Thus a portion of the clivus is formed by the base of the occipital bone and a portion by the posterior surface of the body of the sphenoid.

Extending laterally from the body to either side are two pairs of wings. The smaller pair, termed the **lesser wings**, are triangular in shape and are nearly horizontal. They project laterally from the upper, anterior portion of the body and extend to about the middle of each orbit. The **greater wings** extend laterally from the sides of the body and form a portion of the floor of the cranium, as well as a portion of the sides of the cranium.

There are **three pairs** of small openings in the greater wings for passage of certain nerves and blood vessels. Lesions which can cause erosion of these foramina can be detected radiographically. The **foramen rotundum** *(ro-tun'dum)* is not well visualized on the superior view, but the **foramen ovale** *(ova'le)*, which is located just lateral and posterior to the foramen rotundum, is clearly demonstrated. The location of the small rounded **foramen spinosum** *(spino'sum)* is also seen on the superior view drawing *(Fig. 11-19)*.

Oblique View: An oblique drawing of the sphenoid bone demonstrates the complexity of this bone. Using one's imagination, the shape of the sphenoid has been compared to a bat with its wings and legs extended as in flight. The centrally located depression, the **sella turcica**, is better seen on this view.

Arising from the most posterior aspect of the **lesser wings** are two more bony projections termed **anterior clinoid processes**. The anterior clinoids are somewhat larger and are spread further apart than are the **posterior clinoid processes**, which extend superiorly from the **dorsum sellae**, best seen on the lateral drawing in *Fig. 11-21*.

Between the anterior body and the lesser wings on each side are groove-like canals through which the optic nerve and certain arteries pass into the orbital cavity. This begins in the center as the **chiasmatic** *ki-az-mat'ik)* or **optic groove**, which leads on each side to an **optic canal**, which ends at the **optic foramen** or opening into the orbit. The optic foramina can be demonstrated radiographically with frontal oblique projections of the orbits.

Slightly lateral and posterior to the optic foramina on each side are irregular shaped openings, seen best on this oblique

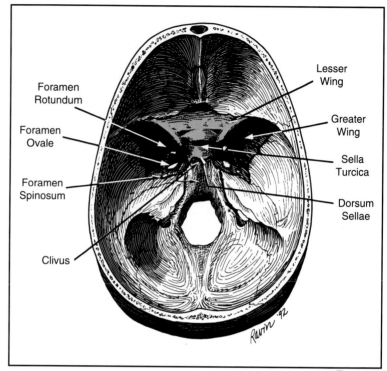

Sphenoid Bone (Superior View)   Fig. 11-19

Labels: Foramen Rotundum, Foramen Ovale, Foramen Spinosum, Clivus, Lesser Wing, Greater Wing, Sella Turcica, Dorsum Sellae

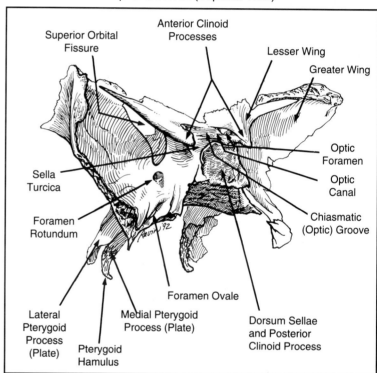

Sphenoid Bone (Oblique View)   Fig. 11-20

Labels: Superior Orbital Fissure, Anterior Clinoid Processes, Lesser Wing, Greater Wing, Optic Foramen, Optic Canal, Chiasmatic (Optic) Groove, Dorsum Sellae and Posterior Clinoid Process, Foramen Ovale, Medial Pterygoid Process (Plate), Pterygoid Hamulus, Lateral Pterygoid Process (Plate), Foramen Rotundum, Sella Turcica

view, called **superior orbital fissures**. These openings provide additional communication with the orbits for numerous nerves and blood vessels. The foramen rotundum is seen again on this oblique view.

Projecting downward from the inferior surface of the body are four processes that correspond to the legs of the imaginary bat. The more lateral, somewhat flat extensions are termed the lateral **pterygoid** *(ter 'i-goyd)* **processes**, sometimes called plates. Directly medial to these are the two **medial pterygoid processes** or plates. Inferior to these are small hook-like processes called **pterygoid hamuli**. The pterygoid processes or plates form part of the lateral walls of the nasal cavities.

Articulations: Because of its central location the sphenoid articulates with **all 7** of the other cranial bones. (The sphenoid also articulates with 5 facial bones.)

Sella Turcica - lateral view: In a true lateral position, the sella turcica would look similar to this drawing. Deformity of the sella turcica is often the only clue that a lesion exists intracranially; therefore, radiography of the sella turcica may be very important.

The depression of the **sella turcica** and the **dorsum sellae** are best seen from the side. The **anterior clinoid processes** are seen anterior to the sella turcica, while the **posterior clinoid processes** are demonstrated superior to the dorsum sellae.

(8) Ethmoid Bone

The eighth and last cranial bone to be studied is the **ethmoid bone.** The single ethmoid bone lies primarily below the floor of the cranium. The top of the ethmoid is shown on the left in *Fig. 11-22*, situated in the ethmoidal notch of the frontal bone.

Magnified posterior and lateral views of the entire ethmoid are shown on the right. The small upper horizontal portion of the bone is termed the **cribriform plate** and contains many small openings or foramina through which pass the olfactory nerves, the nerves of smell. Projecting superiorly from the cribriform plate, similar to a rooster's comb, is the **crista galli** *(kris'ta gal'le)*.

The major portion of the ethmoid lies beneath the floor of the cranium. Projecting downward in the midline is the **perpendicular plate** which helps to form the bony nasal septum. The two **lateral labyrinths** (masses) are suspended from the under surface of the cribriform plate on each side of the perpendicular plate. The lateral masses contain many air cells and help to form the medial walls of the orbits and the lateral walls of the nasal cavity. Extending medially and downward from the medial wall of each labyrinth are thin scroll-shaped projections of bone. These projections are termed the **superior** and **middle nasal conchae** *(kong'ha)* or **turbinates.**

Articulations: The ethmoid articulates with **2** cranial bones, the frontal and the sphenoid. (It also articulates with 11 facial bones.)

Cranium – Medial Sectional View

The drawing on the right represents the right half of the skull, sectioned near the midsagittal plane. The centrally located sphenoid and ethmoid bones are well demonstrated on this drawing showing their relationship to each other and to the other cranial bones.

The **ethmoid bone** is located anterior to the sphenoid bone. The **crista galli** and **cribriform plate** are shown with the **perpendicular plate** extending inferiorly. The perpendicular plate forms the upper portion of the bony nasal septum.

The **sphenoid bone**, containing the saddle shaped **sella turcica,** is located directly posterior to the ethmoid bone. Shown again is one of the two long slender shaped **pterygoid processes** or plates extending down and forward ending with the small pointed process called the **pterygoid hamulus.** The center body portion of the sphenoid bone in this sectional view demonstrates a hollow-like area containing the **sphenoid sinus.**

The larger **frontal bone** also demonstrates a cavity in this sectional view directly posterior to the glabella containing the **frontal sinus.**

An interior view of the large rounded **parietal bone** is shown making up most of the lateral and superior portion of the calvarium or skull cap.

The **squamous portion** of the **temporal bone** is demonstrated just inferior to the parietal bone where it also forms part of the lower wall of the cranium.

The large **occipital bone** is shown to make up the lower posterior/inferior wall and floor of the cranium.

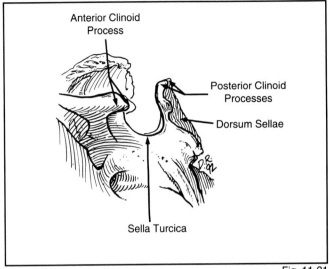

Sella Turcica (Lateral View)

Fig. 11-21

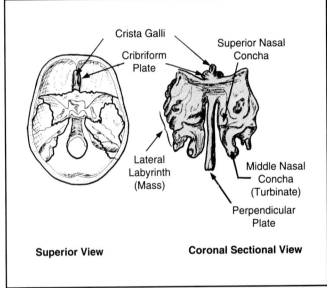

Superior View **Coronal Sectional View**

Ethmoid Bone

Fig. 11-22

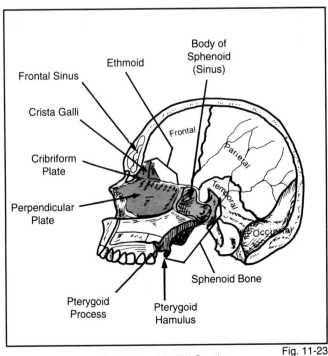

Cranium – Medial Section

Fig. 11-23

Anatomy Review

Following are review exercises for anatomy of the cranium as labelled on radiographs.

A recommended method of review and reinforcement is to cover up the answers below and first attempt to identify each of the labelled parts from memory. Specific anatomical parts may be more difficult to recognize on radiographs as compared to drawings but knowing locations as well as relationships to surrounding structures and bones should aid in identifying these parts.

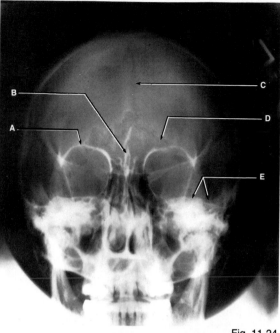

PA Caldwell Projection   Fig. 11-24

Cranial Bones – PA Caldwell Projection
A. Supraorbital margin of R orbit
B. Crista galli of ethmoid
C. Sagittal suture
D. Lambdoidal suture (Posterior skull)
E. Petrous ridge

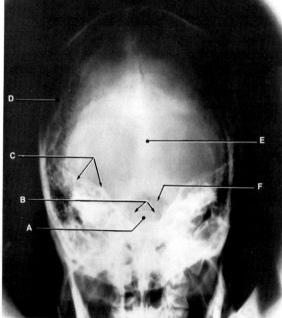

AP Axial Projection   Fig. 11-25

Cranial Bones – AP Axial Projection
A. Dorsum sella of sphenoid
B. Posterior clinoid processes
C. Petrous ridge or petrous pyramid
D. Parietal bone
E. Occipital bone
F. Foramen magnum

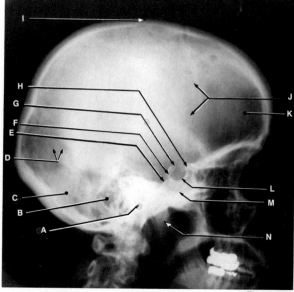

Lateral Position   Fig. 11-26

Cranial Bones – Lateral Position
A. External acoustic meatus (EAM)
B. Mastoid portion of temporal bone
C. Occipital bone
D. Lambdoidal suture
E. Clivus
F. Dorsum sellae
G. Posterior clinoid processes
H. Anterior clinoid processes
I. Vertex of cranium
J. Coronal suture
K. Frontal bone
L. Sella turcica
M. Body of sphenoid (sphenoid sinus)
N. Mandibular rami

Anatomy Review continued

Cranial Bones – Submentovertex (SMV) Projection

This projection is taken with the head tipped back until the top of the cranium (vertex) is against the film. The central ray enters below the chin or mentum, thus the term submentovertex projection. This results in an inferior view of the cranium with the facial bones superimposing the anterior portion of the cranium.

A. Petrous pyramid
B. Mastoid portion of temporal bone
C. Ramus of mandible
D. Vomer (Vomer is a facial bone which along with the perpendicular plate of the ethmoid makes up the midline structure of the nasal cavity - will be demonstrated in Chapter 12.)
E. Foramen ovale
F. Foramen spinosum
G. Dens (Odontoid process)
H. Foramen magnum

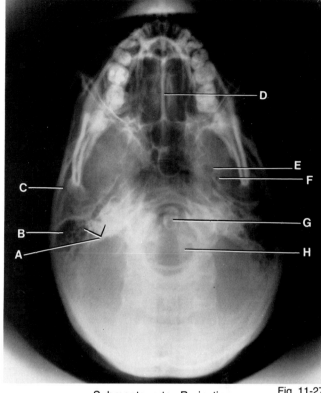

Submentovertex Projection   Fig. 11-27

Skull Morphology
(Skull Classifications by Shape and Size)

Mesocephalic Skull

The shape of the average head is termed **mesocephalic** *(mes'o-se-fal'ik)*. The average caliper measurements of the adult skull are 15 centimeters between the parietal eminences, 19 centimeters from frontal eminence to external occipital protuberance, and 23 centimeters from vertex to beneath the chin. While most adults have a skull of the average size and shape, there are exceptions to the rule.

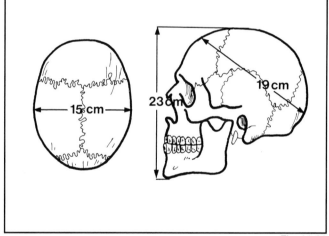

Average Skull (Mesocephalic)   Fig. 11-28

Brachycephalic - Dolichocephalic Skulls

Variations of the average-shaped or mesocephalic skull include the **brachycephalic** *(brak'e-o-se-fal'ik)* and the **dolichocephalic** *(dol'i-ko-se-fal'ik)* designations. The short, broad head is termed brachycephalic; while the long, narrow head is called dolichocephalic. The most common radiographic positions and projections are based on the mesocephalic standard, so persons with other skull shapes will require different angulations and rotations than those normally used.

The main variation to remember is the angle difference between the petrous pyramids and the midsagittal plane. In the average shaped, mesocephalic head, the petrous pyramids form an angle of 47 degrees. An angle greater than 47 degrees (approximately 54 degrees) is found in the brachycephalic skull; while an angle less than 47 degrees (approximately 40 degrees) is found in the dolichocephalic designation.

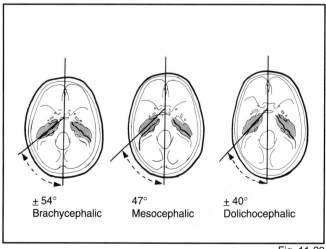

± 54°   47°   ± 40°
Brachycephalic   Mesocephalic   Dolichocephalic

Variable Shapes

Fig. 11-29

Cranium

Part II Radiographic Positioning

Positioning Considerations

Erect vs. Recumbent

Projections of the skull should be taken erect whenever the patient's condition allows. This can be accomplished by ultilizing an upright head unit, a standard x-ray table in the vertical position or an erect grid-film holder. The erect position allows the patient to be quickly and easily positioned and permits a horizontal beam to be utilized. A horizontal beam is necessary to visualize any existing air fluid levels within the inner cranial or sinus cavities.

Patient Comfort

Patient motion almost always results in an unsatisfactory radiograph. During skull radiography the head must be placed in precise positions and held there long enough to obtain a motionless exposure. Always remember that there is a patient attached to the other end of the skull being manipulated. If every effort is made to make the body comfortable and to utilize positioning aids such as sponges, sandbags and compression devices, radiographic positioning of the head will be much easier. Except for severe trauma patients, patients should be asked to suspend respiration (hold their breath) during the exposure to help in preventing motion of the head from breathing movements of the thorax, especially if the patient is in a prone position. This, however, generally is not necessary for erect skull radiographs.

Exposure Factors

The principal exposure factors for radiographs of the skull are:
- Medium kVp, 70-80. (Some departments use in the 80-90 range to better penetrate the petrous pyramid regions.)
- Short exposure time.
- Small focal spot should be used on all skull radiographs if equipment allows.
- Adequate mAs for anatomical area of interest.

SID

Certain types of head unit type equipment as demonstrated in this chapter have a fixed SID of 36 in. (91cm). A common table top SID is listed as 40 in. (102 cm) **minimum distance.** Some departments routinely increase this to 42 or 44 in. (107-112 cm) resulting in a reduction in skin dose exposure to the patient and improved definition on radiographs due to less magnification.

Radiation Protection

The best protection for minimizing radiation exposure to the patient in skull radiography is first, to use **good collimation practices**, and second to **minimize repeats**. The special head units generally utilize a circle or rectangular diaphragm to limit the exposure field to approximately the size of film. Adjustable collimators are used with conventional table units and collimation borders should be adjusted closely on four sides to the outer margins of the skull.

There is some question as to whether gonadal shielding should be used in skull radiography. According to publication HEW 76-8031, "Handbook of Selected Organ Doses for Projections Common in Diagnostic Radiology" with accurate collimation there is no detectable contribution to gonadal exposure when radiographing the skull. If gonadal shields are used for table-top skull procedures, some references suggest that such shields should be placed on the table top under the patient rather than on top of the patient to absorb possible scatter and secondary radiation.

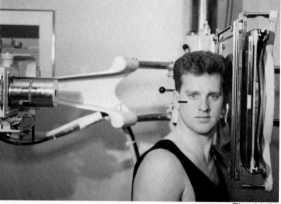
Erect, Head Unit   Fig. 11-30

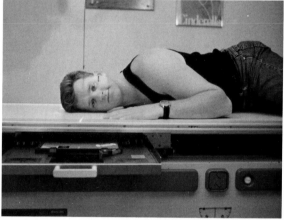
Recumbent, Table Top   Fig. 11-31

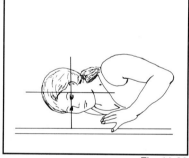
Rotation   Fig. 11-32

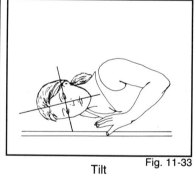
Tilt   Fig. 11-33

Causes of Positioning Errors

When positioning a patient's head, it is necessary to look at various facial features and palpate numerous anatomical landmarks in order to place certain planes precisely in relation to the plane of the film. Although the human body is supposed to be bilaterally symmetrical, (that is, the right half is supposed to be exactly like the left half), this supposition is not always true. The ears, nose and jaw are often asymmetrical. The nose frequently deviates to one side of the midsagittal plane, while the ears are not necessarily in the same place nor of the same size on each side. The lower jaw or mandible is also often asymmetrical. Bony parts, such as the mastoid tips and the orbital margins, are safer landmarks to use. While you often look at the patient's eyes during positioning, it is best not to look at the nose in between.

Common Positioning Errors

Rotation and **tilt** are two very common positioning errors. Rotation of the skull almost always results in a retake, therefore it is important that the head is not turned to one side. Tilt is a tipping or slanting to one side, even though rotation is not present. Both rotation and tilt must be avoided in skull positioning.

National Survey

Departmental standards (basic) and optional routines for exams of the cranium and sella turcica were somewhat consistent throughout the United States as shown below. The results of this survey determined national norms for routines as presented in the positioning pages which follow.

Skull Series Routine:

Cranium - Skull Series	U.S. Average		East		Midwest		West	
	Basic	Optional	Basic	Optional	Basic	Optional	Basic	Optional
• AP Axial (Towne)	95%		98%		94%		91%	
• Lateral	89%		90%		88%		88%	
• PA - 15° caudal (Caldwell)	57%		65%		53%		49%	
or PA - 0°	55%		50%		59%		51%	
• Basilar (SMV)	21%	8%	21%	9%	19%	8%	24%	7%
• PA Waters[1]		7%						
Trauma Skull Series								
• Lateral (crosstable)	51%	22%						
• AP	43%	20%						
• AP Axial	20%	13%						

[1] Write in's by respondents

Summary:

Skull Series: The survey indicated some regional differences in the basic PA projection for the skull series. The PA Caldwell with 15° caudal angle is more common in the eastern states with **65%** indicating it as basic and only **50%** indicated a 0° PA. This is reversed in both the midwestern and western states where the 0° PA is more frequently considered basic than the 15° Caldwell. These results however do not suggest a major difference in departmental routines but it does indicate that overall departmental routines are almost evenly divided as to which of these projections is considered to be part of their basic skull series. Therefore **both** are presented in this text as possible basic projections for the skull series.

The frequency of the basilar (SMV) projection as part of a skull series is a little more common in the west (24%) than in the midwest (19%) or the East (21%).

Sella Turcica Routine:

Sella Turcica	U.S. Average	
	Basic	Optional
• Lateral	96%	
• AP Axial - 37°	30%	
or AP Axial - 30°	20%	
• PA - 0° cephalic	24%	
• PA Axial (Haas)	13%	

Sella Turcica: The lateral as expected was the most common basic projection for the sella turcica with other less frequent AP or PA projections indicated. Each of these will be included as possible optional projections for the sella turcica in this chapter.

The **37° AP axial** is shown to be more frequently taken (30%) than the **30°** AP axial (20%).

Survey Questions on Possible Discontinued Procedures:
The national survey included questions on (I) the **expected trend** in the next three or four years, (II) the **quantity** of specific exams done in their departments during the past year, and (III) whether or not **the procedure should still be taught and included** in a basic student textbook. The results were as follows:

Responses for sella turcica exam:

Sella Turcica	U.S. Average (316)	East (114)	Midwest (147)	West (55)
I. Trend				
a. Increase	3%	3%	2%	2%
b. Decrease	29%	31%	24%	38%
c. No change	68%	66%	74%	60%
II. Annual Quantity				
a. 0-2	49%	51%	45%	59%
b. 3-9	31%	30%	36%	21%
c. 10-15	10%	11%	10%	9%
d. 16+	10%	8%	9%	11%
III. Be Included				
a. Yes	70%	76%	69%	60%
b. No	30%	24%	31%	40%

Summary (Sella Turcica):
These results indicate no change or a decrease in the number of these exams being done, especially in the western states. However the majority of survey respondents indicated this exam should still be taught and should therefore be included in a basic student positioning text such as this.

Results of these survey questions for other exams of the cranium and facial bones are included in chapters 12 and 13.

Standard and Optional Operating Procedures

Certain basic and optional projections or positions for the cranium (skull series) and the sella turcica are demonstrated and described on the following pages as suggested standard and optional departmental procedures.

Basic Projections

Standard or basic projections, also sometimes referred to as routine projections or departmental routines are those projections or posi-

tions commonly taken on average patients who are helpful and can cooperate in performing the procedure.

Optional Projections

Optional projections are those more common projections or positions taken as extra or additional projections to better demonstrate certain pathologic conditions or specific body parts. (These are not optional as to whether or not they are important or need to be learned and mastered by radiographers.)

Basic and Optional Projections

Skull Series
Basic
• AP Axial (Towne)
• Lateral
• PA - 0°
    or
 PA - 15° Caldwell
Optional
• Submentovertex (SMV)
  (basilar)

Skull Series
(Trauma)
• Lateral (Horizontal beam)
• AP 0°
    or
 AP "Reverse Caldwell"
• AP Axial (Towne)

Sella Turcica
Basic
• Lateral
Optional
• AP Axial (Towne)
• PA
• PA Axial (Haas)

•AP Axial Projection
(Occipital Position or Towne Method)

Skull Series
Basic
• **AP Axial (Towne)**
• Lateral
• PA - 0°
or
PA - 15° Caldwell

Structures Best Shown:
Occipital bone, petrous pyramids and foramen magnum with dorsum sellae and posterior clinoids in its shadow.

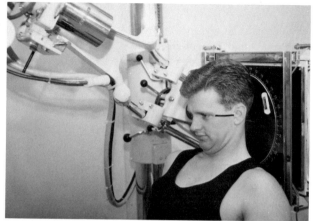

AP Axial – Erect   Fig. 11-34

Technical Factors:
• Film Size - 10 x 12 in. (24 x 30 cm), lengthwise
• Moving or stationary grid.
• 70-80 kVp range.
• Use small focal spot.

Patient Position:
• Remove all metal, plastic or other removable objects from head.
• Patient erect or supine.
• Erect may be done with dedicated head unit if available or with erect table or other erect grid-film holder device.
• Rest patient's posterior skull against head unit or table top.

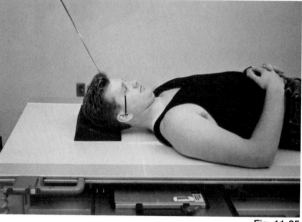

AP Axial – Supine   Fig. 11-35

Part Position:
• Depress chin, bringing **orbitomeatal line (OML) perpendicular** to film. (See NOTE).
• Align **midsagittal plane perpendicular** to midline of head unit or table top to prevent head rotation and/or tilt.

Central Ray:
• Angle CR **30° caudal to OML** (See NOTE).
• Center at midsagittal plane, **2.5 in.** (6 cm) **above the superciliary arch.**
• Center cassette to CR.
• SID: Head Unit, 36 in. (91 cm).
   Table Top, minimum 40 in. (102 cm).

Collimation: Use 10 x 12 in. circle diaphragm or collimate to outer margins of skull on all sides.

Respiration: Suspend respiration during exposure.

NOTE: If patient is unable to depress the chin sufficiently to bring the **OML** perpendicular to the film, the infraorbitomeatal line **(IOML)** can be placed perpendicular instead and the CR angle increased to **37° caudal.**
This maintains the **30° angle between OML and CR** and demonstrates the same anatomical relationships. (There is a 7° difference between the OML and IOML.)

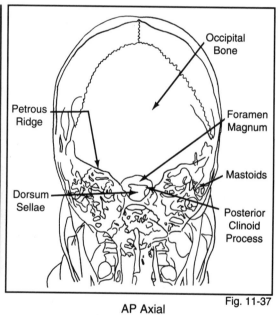

AP Axial   Fig. 11-36

AP Axial   Fig. 11-37

• Dorsum sella and posterior clinoids are projected into foramen magnum.
• Petrous ridges are symmetrical and visualized superior to the mastoids.
• Sufficient penetration and exposure, without motion, to visualize occipital bone.
• Patient ID information with R or L marker visible within collimated field without superimposing anatomy.

Evaluation Criteria:
• Entire skull visualized on radiograph.
• Equal distance from foramen magnum to lateral margin of skull on each side.

•Lateral Position

Skull Series
Basic
• AP Axial (Towne)
• **Lateral**
• PA - 0°
  or
PA - 15° Caldwell

Structures Best Shown:
Lateral cranium closest to film, sella turcica, anterior and posterior clinoids, dorsum sellae, and greater and lesser wings of sphenoid.

Technical Factors:
• Film Size - 10 x 12 in. (24 x 30 cm), crosswise.
• Moving or stationary grid.
• 70-80 kVp range.
• Use small focal spot.

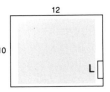

Patient Position:
• Remove all metal, plastic or other removable objects from head.
• Patient erect or prone.
• Erect may be done with dedicated head unit if available or with erect table or other erect grid-film holder device.

Part Position:
• Place head in a **true lateral position**, with side of interest closest to film, oblique body as needed for patient comfort. (A way to check for rotation is to palpate the external occipital protuberance posteriorly and the nasion or glabella anteriorly and insure that these two points are the same distance from the film.)
• Align **midsagittal plane parallel** to film, insuring no rotation or tilt.
• To prevent head tilting, bring **interpupillary line perpendicular** to film.
• Adjust chin to bring **infraorbitomeatal line perpendicular** to front edge of cassette.

Central Ray:
• Align CR **perpendicular** to film.
• Center to a point about **2 in**. (5 cm) **superior to EAM.**
• Center cassette to CR.
• SID: Head Unit, 36 in. (91 cm).
    Table Top, minimum 40 in. (102 cm).

Collimation: Use 10 x 12 in. circle diaphragm or collimate to outer margins of skull on all sides.

Respiration: Suspend respiration during exposure.

NOTE: For patients in the recumbent position, a radiolucent support placed under the chin will help in maintaining a true lateral position.

Evaluation Criteria:
• Entire skull visualized on radiograph.
• The cranium is seen without rotation or tilt when:
    - Mandibular rami, orbital roofs, greater and lesser wings of sphenoid and external auditory canals are superimposed.
    - Sella turcica and clivus are demonstrated in profile without rotation.
• Sufficient penetration and exposure, without motion, to visualize parietal region.
• Patient ID information with R or L marker visible within collimated field without superimposing anatomy.

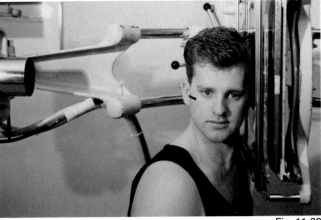

Lateral – Erect   Fig. 11-38

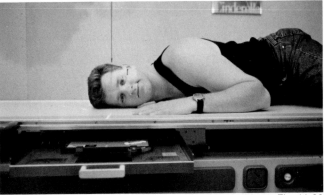

Lateral – Recumbent   Fig. 11-39

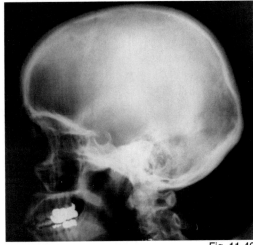

Lateral   Fig. 11-40

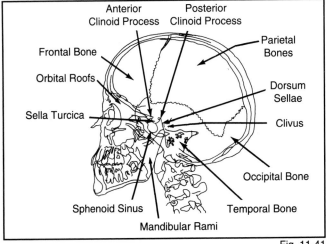

Lateral   Fig. 11-41

Anterior Clinoid Process
Posterior Clinoid Process
Parietal Bones
Frontal Bone
Orbital Roofs
Dorsum Sellae
Sella Turcica
Clivus
Sphenoid Sinus
Occipital Bone
Temporal Bone
Mandibular Rami

•PA Projection (0° CR)

Skull Series
Basic
• AP Axial (Towne)
• Lateral
• **PA - 0°**
or
PA - 15° Caldwell

Structures Best Shown:
Frontal bone, crista galli, internal auditory canals, frontal and ethmoid sinuses, petrous ridges, greater and lesser wings of sphenoid and dorsum sellae.

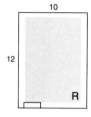

Technical Factors:
• Film Size - 10 x 12 in. (24 x 30 cm), lengthwise.
• Moving or stationary grid.
• 70-80 kVp range.
• Use small focal spot.

Patient Position:
• Remove all metal, plastic or other removable objects from head.
• Patient erect or prone.
• Erect may be done with dedicated head unit if available or with erect table or other erect grid-film holder device.

Part Position:
• Rest patient's nose and forehead against head unit or table top.
• Tuck chin bringing **orbitomeatal line (OML) perpendicular** to film.
• Align **midsagittal plane perpendicular** to midline of table preventing head rotation and/or tilting.
• Center cassette to **glabella**.

Central Ray:
• CR **perpendicular** to table and **centered to cassette.**
• SID: Head Unit, 36 in. (91 cm).
    Table Top, minimum 40 in. (102 cm).

Collimation: Use 10 x 12 in. circle diaphragm or collimate to outer margins of skull on all sides.

Respiration: Suspend respiration during exposure.

Evaluation Criteria:
• Entire skull visualized on radiograph.
• Petrous ridges superimpose superior orbital region.
• Petrous pyramids fill orbits.
• Distance from oblique orbital line to lateral margin of skull on each side is equal.
• Dorsum sellae and anterior clinoids are visualized superior to ethmoid sinuses.
• Sufficient penetration and exposure, without motion, to visualize frontal bone.
• Patient ID information with R or L marker visible within collimated field without superimposing anatomy.

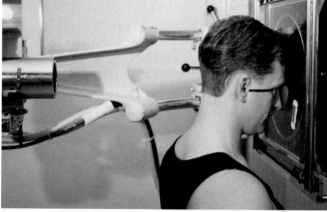

PA, 0° CR, OML Perpendicular   Fig. 11-42

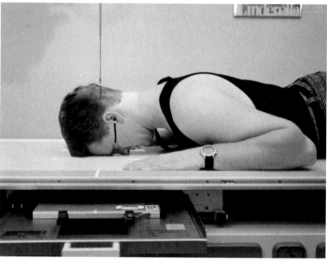

PA, 0° CR, OML Perpendicular   Fig. 11-43

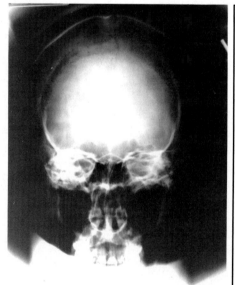

PA, 0° CR   Fig. 11-44

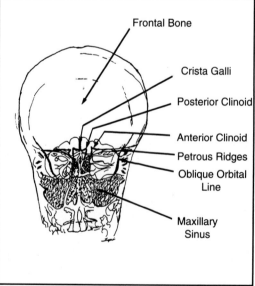

PA, 0° CR   Fig. 11-45

Frontal Bone
Crista Galli
Posterior Clinoid
Anterior Clinoid
Petrous Ridges
Oblique Orbital Line
Maxillary Sinus

•PA Projection (15° CR)
(Caldwell Method)

Skull Series
Basic
• AP Axial (Towne)
• Lateral
• PA - 0°
or
PA - 15° Caldwell

Structures Best Shown:
Greater and lesser sphenoid wings, frontal bone, superior orbital fissures, frontal and ethmoid sinuses, foramen rotundum, orbital margin, and cristi galli.

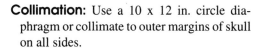

Technical Factors:
• Film Size - 10 x 12 in. (24 x 30 cm), lengthwise.
• Moving or stationary grid.
• 70-80 kVp range.
• Small focal spot.

Patient Position:
• Remove all metal, plastic or other removable objects from head.
• Patient erect or prone.
• Erect may be done with dedicated head unit if available or with erect table or other erect grid-film holder device.

Part Position:
• Rest patient's nose and forehead against head unit or table top.
• Tuck chin, bringing **orbitomeatal line (OML) perpendicular** to film.
• Align **midsagittal plane perpendicular** to midline of head unit or table top preventing head rotation and/or tilting.
• Center cassette to **nasion.**

Central Ray:
• CR angled **15° caudal** (see NOTE) and **centered to cassette.**
• SID: Head Unit, 36 in. (91 cm).
  Table Top, minimum 40 in. (102 cm).

Collimation: Use a 10 x 12 in. circle diaphragm or collimate to outer margins of skull on all sides.

Respiration: Suspend respiration during exposure.

NOTE: In some departments an alternate projection is a **30° caudal** tube angle to better visualize the inferior orbital rim area.

Evaluation Criteria:
• Entire skull visualized on radiograph.
• Distance from oblique orbital line to lateral margin of skull on each side is equal.
• Superior orbital fissures are symmetrically visualized within orbits.
• Sufficient penetration and exposure, without motion, to visualize frontal bone.
• Patient ID information with R or L marker visible within collimated field without superimposing anatomy.

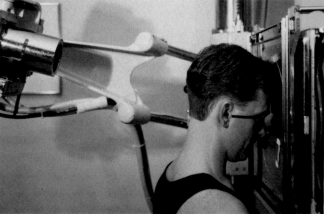

PA, CR 15° Caudal, OML Perpendicular   Fig. 11-46

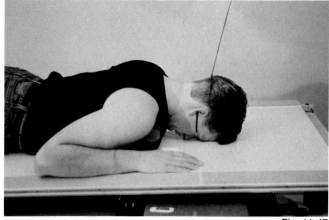

PA, CR 15° Caudal, OML Perpendicular   Fig. 11-47

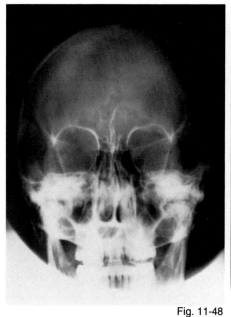

Fig. 11-48
PA, 15° Caudal (Caldwell)

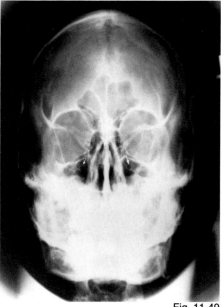

Fig. 11-49
Alternate PA, 30° Caudal

PA with 15° caudal angle:
• Petrous pyramids and internal auditory canals (if they can be visualized) are projected into the lower one-third of orbits.
• Superior orbital margin is visualized without superimposition.

PA with 30° caudal angle:
• Petrous pyramids are projected below the inferior orbital rim, allowing visualization of the entire orbital margin.
• Foramen rotundum adjacent to each inferior orbital rim is visualized (see arrows).

•Submentovertex (SMV) Projection
(Basilar Position)

Structures Best Shown:
Foramen ovale and spinosum, mandible, sphenoid and ethmoid sinuses, mastoid processes, petrous ridges, hard palate, foramen magnum, and occipital bone.

Technical Factors:
• Film Size - 10 x 12 in. (24 x 30 cm), lengthwise.
• Moving or stationary grid.
• 70-80 kVp range.
• Use small focal spot.

Patient Position:
• Remove all metal, plastic or other removable objects from head.

• Patient in an erect position (or supine if patient cannot maintain an erect position).

• Erect which is easier for patient may be done with dedicated head unit if available or with erect table or other erect grid-film holder device.

Part Position:
• Raise chin, hyperextending neck if possible until **infraorbitomeatal line (IOML) is parallel to film.** (See NOTE.)
• Head rests on vertex.
• Align **midsagittal plane perpendicular** to midline of head unit or table top, thus **avoiding tilt and/or rotation.**
• If taken supine, extend head over end of table and support cassette and head as shown keeping **IOML parallel to film** and **perpendicular to CR.**

Central Ray:
• CR directed **perpendicular to infraorbitomeatal line.**
• Center midway between angles of mandible at a level 2.5 - 3 in. (6-8 cm) inferior to mandibular symphysis.
• SID: Head Unit, 36 in. (91 cm).
  Table Top, min. 40 in. (102 cm).

Collimation: Use a 10 x 12 in. circle diaphragm or collimate to outer margins of skull on all sides.

Respiration: Suspend respiration during exposure.

NOTE: • If patient is unable to sufficiently extend neck, compensate by angling CR **perpendicular to IOML.** With head unit the film can also be angled as needed to maintain the film perpendicular to CR.
• Position is very uncomfortable for patient, move quickly.

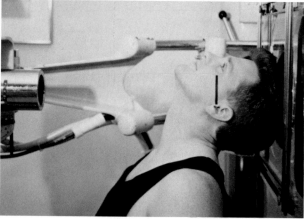
Submentovertex (SMV)　　Fig. 11-50

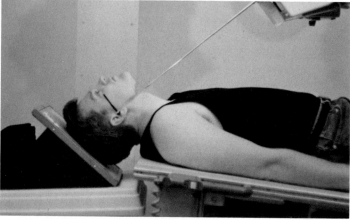
Submentovertex (SMV)　　Fig. 11-51

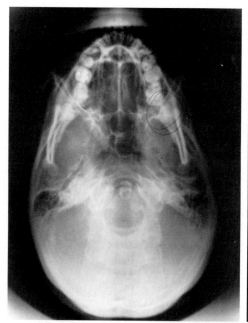
Submentovertex　　Fig. 11-52

Foramen Ovale and Spinosum — Sphenoid and Ethmoid Sinuses — Mandibular Condyles — Petrous Ridges — Mastoid Processes — Foramen Magnum — Occipital Bone

Submentovertex　　Fig. 11-53

Evaluation Criteria:
• Entire skull visualized on radiograph.
• Mandibular symphysis superimposes anterior frontal bone.
• Distance along coinciding mandibular surfaces to lateral border of skull are equal.

• Mandibular condyles are projected anterior to petrous pyramids.
• Foramen ovale and spinosum are visualized.
• Sufficient penetration and exposure, without motion, to visualize foramen magnum.
• Patient ID information and R or L marker visible within collimated field without superimposing anatomy.

• **Lateral Position** (Horizontal Beam)

Warning: It is essential that cervical spine fractures and dislocations are ruled out before attempting to move or manipulate the patient's head or neck.

Skull Series
Trauma
• **Lateral (Horizontal Beam)**
• AP 0° or AP "Reverse Caldwell"
• AP Axial (Towne)

Structures Best Shown:
Lateral cranium closest to film, sella turcica, anterior and posterior clinoids, dorsum sellae, and greater and lesser wings of sphenoid.

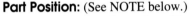

Technical Factors:
• Film Size - 10 x 12 in. (24 x 30 cm).
• Place grid cassette vertically against affected lateral cranium, crosswise to patient.
• 70-80 kVp range.
• Use small focal spot.

Patient Position:
• Remove all metal, plastic or other removable objects from head.
• Patient in a supine recumbent position.
• If patient's head can be manipulated, carefully elevate occiput on a radiolucent sponge. If one cannot manipulate head, position cassette 1 in. (2.5 cm) below occipital bone as shown in *Fig. 11-54*.

Part Position: (See NOTE below.)
• Place head in **true lateral position**, relative to cassette, with side of interest closest to cassette.
• Align **midsagittal plane parallel** with cassette.
• Place **interpupillary line perpendicular** to cassette.
• Adjust chin to bring **infraorbitomeatal line parallel** with long axis of cassette.
• Adjust cassette to assure that entire circumference of skull will be visualized on radiograph.

Central Ray:
• A **horizontal beam**, (which is essential for visualization of inner cranial air/fluid levels) is directed **perpendicular** to cassette.
• Center to a point **2 in.** (5 cm) **superior to EAM.**
• Minimum 40 in. (102 cm) SID.

Collimation: Collimate to outer margins of skull on all sides.

NOTE: On patient with cervical spine injury **do not** attempt to raise or adjust head, take "as is" *(Fig. 11-54).*

Evauation Criteria:
• Entire skull visualized on radiograph.
• The cranium is seen without rotation or tilt:
  - Mandibular rami, orbital roofs, greater and lesser wings of sphenoid and external auditory canals are superimposed.
  - Sella turcica and clivus are demonstrated in profile without rotation.

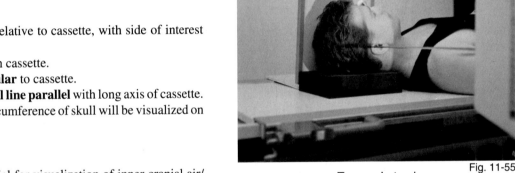

Fig. 11-54
Trauma Lateral
(without head manipulation)

Fig. 11-55
Trauma Lateral
(without cervical injury, head can be raised)

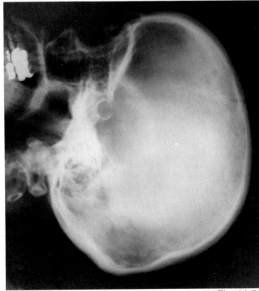

Trauma Lateral   Fig. 11-56

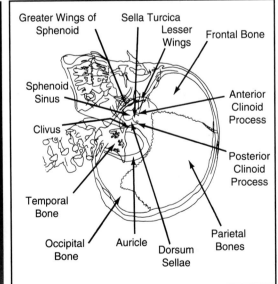

Trauma Lateral   Fig. 11-57

• Sufficient penetration and exposure, without motion, to visualize parietal region.
• Patient ID information with R or L marker visible within collimated field without superimposing anatomy.

• AP 0° Projection or AP "Reverse Caldwell" Projection
• AP Axial (Towne) Projection
(Positioning **with** possible cervical spine injury)

Warning: It is essential that cervical spine fractures and dislocations are ruled out before attempting to move or manipulate the patient's head or neck.

For all three of the projections demonstrated on this page the patient's head and neck are not moved. The degree of CR angulation is the only variation.

Exception: If a cervical spine injury has been ruled out, the chin can be depressed to bring the orbitomeatal line perpendicular to the film and the CR can then be adjusted accordingly.

> **Skull Series**
> Trauma
> • Lateral (Horizontal Beam)
> • **AP 0° or AP "Reverse Caldwell"**
> • **AP Axial (Towne)**

Structures Best Shown:
Same as nontrauma PA (which mirrors the AP), nontrauma Caldwell, and nontrauma AP axial projections.

Technical Factors:
- Film Size - 10 x 12 in. (24 x 30 cm), lengthwise.
- Moving or stationary grid.
- 70-80 kVp range.
- Use small focal spot.

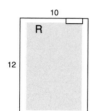

Patient Position:
- Patient in a supine recumbent position.
- If possible, slide patient onto x-ray table as one complete unit, do **NOT** move head or neck. It is not necessary to remove collar or backboard in order to obtain these projections.
- Remove all metal, plastic or other removable objects from head.

Part Position:
- On patient with suspected cervical injury **do not** attempt to adjust head, but compensate by adjusting CR angles.
- Slide patient's entire body to bring midsagittal plane to midline of table.

Central Ray:
- Minimum 40 in. (102 cm) SID.

AP 0° Projection
- Angle **CR parallel with OML.** On a patient in a cervical collar this is approximately 10 to 15° caudal.
- Center CR to **glabella**; then center cassette to CR.

AP "Reverse Caldwell" Projection
- Angle CR **15° more cephalic** than angle used for AP. (See NOTE.)
- Center CR to **nasion**; then center cassette to CR.

AP Axial (Towne) Projection
- Angle CR **30° more caudal** than angle used for AP. (See NOTE.)
- Center CR to **midsagittal plane 2.5 in. (6 cm) above superciliary arch**; then center cassette to CR.

Collimation: Collimate to outer margins of skull on all sides.

NOTE: If a 10° caudal angle is required for a trauma AP projection, the angle could be **5° cephalic** for the "Reverse Caldwell" position. This would be 15° more cephalic than the AP projection.

For the axial AP (Towne) projection one would therefore also need to angle 30° more caudal from the trauma AP projection, which would be **40° caudal.** The CR, for the AP axial, should not exceed 45° or excessive distortion will hinder the visualization of needed anatomy.

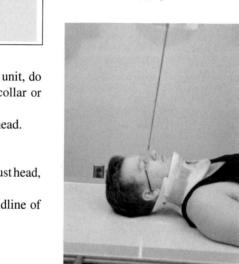

AP 0°   Fig. 11-58

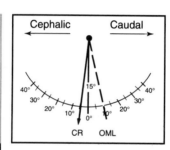

CR parallel to OML
(10° caudal)

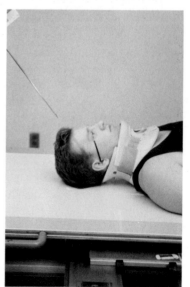

Fig. 11-59
AP "Reverse Caldwell"

CR 15° cephalic to OML
(total 5° cephalic)

AP Towne   Fig. 11-60

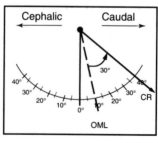

CR 30° caudal to OML
(total 40° caudal)

AP 0°, AP "Reverse Caldwell" and AP Axial (Towne) Projections continued

AP versus PA:

Trauma skull projections are performed AP while most of the nontrauma projections are taken PA. This variation will demonstrate reverse anatomical magnification. For example on a PA projection the orbits, being closest to the cassette, will be less magnified than the sagittal and lambdoidal sutures which are situated farther from the cassette. On the AP projection, the opposite is true, the orbits are more magnified than the sutures. The PA projection will also demonstrate more distance from the oblique orbital line to the lateral margin of the skull than the AP projection. This is illustrated in *Figs. 11-62* and *63* which compares an **AP reverse Caldwell** with a standard **PA Caldwell**.

Even though magnification differences exist between the PA and AP projections, causing them to look quite different from one another, the basic evaluation criteria remains the same.

Evaluation Criteria:

Trauma AP 0° Projection

- Entire skull visualized on radiograph.
- Petrous ridges superimpose superior orbital region.
- Petrous pyramids fill orbits with internal auditory canals seen horizontally through center of orbits.
- Distance from oblique orbital line to lateral margin of skull on each side is equal.
- Dorsum sellae and anterior clinoids are visualized superior to ethmoid sinuses.
- Sufficient penetration and exposure, without motion, to clearly visualize frontal bone.

Trauma AP "Reverse Caldwell" Position

- Entire skull visualized on radiograph.
- Distance from oblique orbital line to lateral margin of skull on each side is equal.
- Superior orbital fissures are symmetrically visualized within orbits.
- Petrous pyramids and internal auditory canals are projected into the lower one-third of orbits.
- Superior orbital margin is visualized without superimposition.
- Sufficient penetration and exposure, without motion, to clearly visualize frontal bone.

Trauma AP Axial (Towne) Projection

- Entire skull visualized on radiograph.
- Equal distance from foramen magnum to lateral margin of skull on each side.
- Dorsum sella and posterior clinoids are projected into foramen magnum. (See NOTE.)
- Petrous ridges are symmetrical and visualized superior to the mastoids.
- Sufficient penetration and exposure, without motion, to clearly visualize occipital bone.

NOTE: If one could not bring the CR 30° more caudal than the AP projection before the maximum angle of 45° was reached, the dorsum sella and posterior clinoids would be projected superior to the foramen magnum instead of within it as seen in *Fig. 11-64b*.

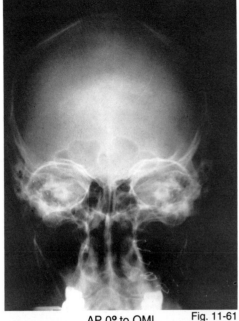

AP 0° to OML   Fig. 11-61

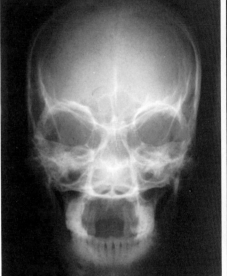

AP "Reverse Caldwell"   Fig. 11-62
(15° Cephalad to OML)

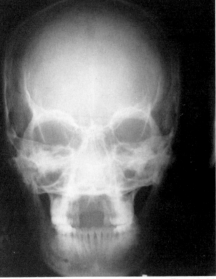

PA Caldwell (15° Caudal)   Fig. 11-63
Comparison Radiograph

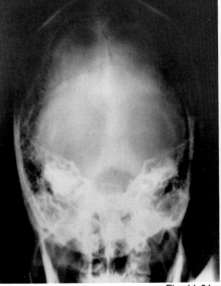

Fig. 11-64 a
Trauma AP Axial "Towne" (30° caudal to OML) (Maximum 45° angle)

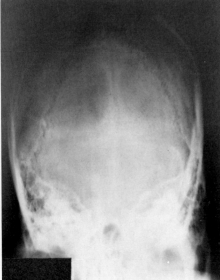

Fig. 11-64 b
Trauma AP Axial
(Less than 30° caudal to OML)

• Lateral Position

Sella Turcica
Basic
• **Lateral**

Structures Best Shown:
Sella turcica, anterior and posterior clinoid processes, dorsum sellae and clivus.

Technical Factors:
- Film Size - 8 x 10 in. (18 x 24 cm), crosswise.
- Moving or stationary grid.
- 70-80 kVp range.
- Use small focal spot.

Patient Position:
- Remove all metal, plastic or other removable objects from head.
- Patient in an erect or prone position (erect preferred).

Part Position:
- Place head in a **true lateral** position; oblique body as needed for patient's comfort.
- Align **interpupillary line perpendicular** to head unit or table top.
- Bring **midsagittal plane parallel** with head unit or table top.
- Place **infraorbitomeatal line perpendicular** to front edge of cassette.

Central Ray:
- Align CR **perpendicular** to film.
- Center to a **point 3/4 in.** (2 cm) **anterior** and **3/4 in. superior** to the external auditory meatus (EAM).
- Center cassette to CR.
- SID: Head Unit, 36 in. (91 cm).
    Table Top, minimum 40 in. (102 cm).

Collimation: Use a circle diaphragm or collimate on all sides to yield a field size of approximately 4 in. (10 cm).

Respiration: Suspend respiration during exposure.

NOTE: To obtain a sharply detailed image of the sella turcica, the utilization of a small focal spot and close collimation is essential.

Evaluation Criteria:
- The sella turcica is located in the center of the radiograph, with the body and lesser wings of the sphenoid and the clivus within the collimated field.
- Close four-sided collimation should be evident.
- The cranium is visualized without rotation or tilt:
  - The sella turcica and clivus are demonstrated in profile without rotation.
  - The anterior and posterior clinoids are superimposed.
  - The greater wings and lesser wings of sphenoid are superimposed.
- Sufficient penetration and exposure, without motion, to clearly visualize sella turcica and pituitary fossa.
- Patient ID information with R or L marker visible within collimated field without superimposing essential anatomy.

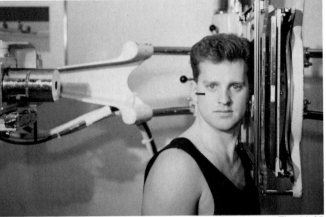

Lateral Sella Turcica   Fig. 11-65

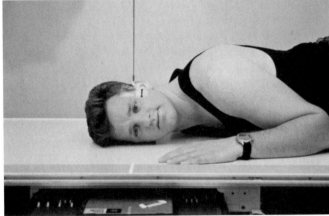

Lateral Sella Turcica   Fig. 11-66

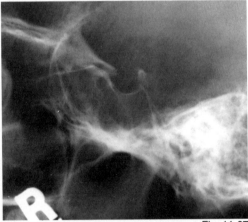

Lateral Sella Turcica   Fig. 11-67

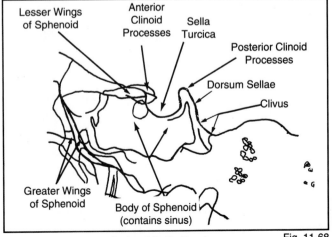

Lateral Sella Turcica   Fig. 11-68

• AP Axial Projection
(Towne Position)

> **Sella Turcica**
> Optional
> • **AP Axial (Towne)**
> • PA
> • PA Axial **(Haas)**

Structures Best Shown:
Dorsum sellae, anterior and posterior clinoids, foramen magnum, petrous ridges and occipital bone.

Technical Factors:
• Film Size - 8 x 10 in. (18 x 24 cm), lengthwise.
• Moving or stationary grid.
• 70-80 kVp range.
• Use small focal spot

Patient Position:
• Remove all metal, plastic or other removable objects from head.
• Patient in an erect or supine position.

Part Position:
• Rest patient's posterior skull against head unit or table top.
• Adjust chin to bring **infraorbitomeatal line perpendicular** to film.
• Align **midsagittal plane perpendicular** to midline of head unit or table.

Central Ray:
• Angle CR **37° caudal** if **dorsum sellae and posterior clinoids** are of interest.
• Angle CR **30° caudal** if the **anterior clinoids** are of interest.
• Center at midsagittal plane, **1.5 in**. (4 cm) **above superciliary arch**.
• Center cassette to CR.
• SID: Head Unit, 30 in. (91 cm); Table Top, minimum 40 in. (102 cm).

Collimation: Use a circle diaphragm or cylinder cone, collimate on all sides to size of approximately 4 in.(10 cm) square.

Respiration: Suspend respiration during exposure.

NOTE: To obtain a sharply detailed image of the dorsum sellae, a small focal spot and close collimation is essential.

Evaluation Criteria:
• The dorsum sellae is located in center of the radiograph, with petrous ridges and occipital bone within the collimated field.
• Sufficient penetration and exposure, without motion, to visualize dorsum sellae.
• Patient ID information with R or L marker visible within close four-sided collimation field without superimposing essential anatomy.

37° caudal angle:
• Cranium is seen without rotation or tilt:
 - Petrous ridges are symmetrical.
 - Equal distance from dorsum sellae to each side of foramen magnum.
• Dorsum sellae and posterior clinoids are projected into foramen magnum.

30° caudal angle:
• Cranium is seen without rotation or tilt:
 - Petrous ridges are symmetrical.
 - Equal distance from midsagittal plane, which can be identified by the perpendicular plate, to each anterior clinoid.
• Dorsum sellae is projected above the foramen magnum superimposing the occipital bone.
• Anterior clinoids are clearly visualized, adjacent to each petrous ridge, directly above the foramen magnum.

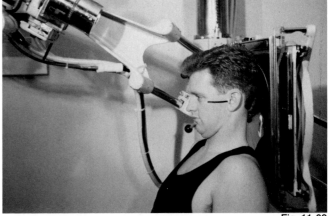
AP Axial, 30-37° Caudal, IOML Perpendicular   Fig. 11-69

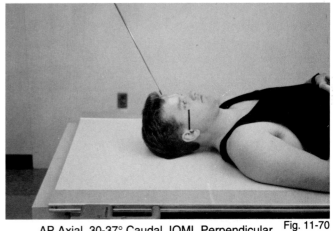
AP Axial, 30-37° Caudal, IOML Perpendicular   Fig. 11-70

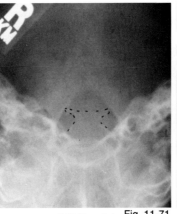
37° Caudal   Fig. 11-71

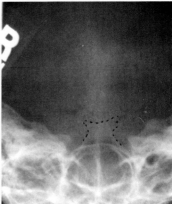
30° Caudal   Fig. 11-72

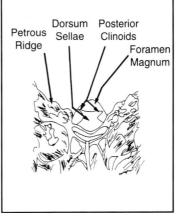
37° Caudal   Fig. 11-73

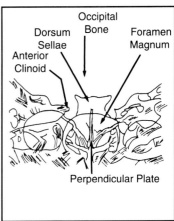
30° Caudal   Fig. 11-74

• PA Projection

Sella Turcica
Optional
• AP Axial (Towne)
• PA
• PA Axial (Haas)

Structures Best Shown:
Dorsum sellae, tuberculum sellae, anterior and posterior clinoids and petrous ridges.

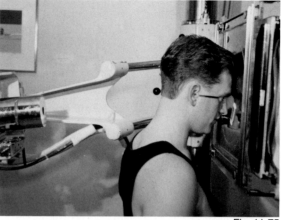
Fig. 11-75
PA, 10° Cephalic, OML Perpendicular

Technical Factors:
• Film Size - 8 x 10 in. (18 x 24 cm), lengthwise.
• Moving or stationary grid.
• 70-80 kVp range.
• Use small focal spot.

[diagram: 8 x 10 with R]

Patient Position:
• Remove all metal, plastic or other removable objects from head.
• Patient in an erect or prone position (erect preferred).

Part Position:
• Rest patient's nose and forehead against head unit or table.
• Tuck chin until **orbitomeatal line is perpendicular** to film.
• Align **midsagittal plane perpendicular** to midline of head unit or table.
• Center cassette to **glabella.**

Central Ray:
• Angle CR **10° cephalad**.
• Center CR to cassette.
• SID: Head Unit, 36 in. (91 cm).
      Table Top, minimum 40 in. (102 cm).

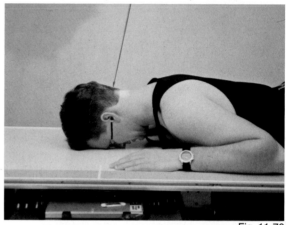
Fig. 11-76
PA, 10° Cephalic, OML Perpendicular

Collimation: Use a circle diaphragm, or cylinder cone, or collimate on all sides to yield a field size of approximately 4 in. (10 cm).

Respiration: Suspend respiration during exposure.

NOTE: To obtain a sharply detailed image of the dorsum sellae, the utilization of a small focal spot and close collimation is essential.

Evaluation Criteria:
• The dorsum sellae is located in the center of the radiograph, with the petrous ridges and frontal bone within the collimated field.
• Close four-sided collimation should be evident.
• Cranium is seen without rotation or tilt:
  - Petrous ridges are symmetrical.
  - Equal distance from midsagittal plane, which can be identified by the perpendicular plate, to each anterior clinoid.
• Dorsum sellae is projected above the foramen magnum superimposing the occipital bone.
• Anterior clinoids are clearly visualized adjacent to each petrous ridge, directly above the foramen magnum.
• Sufficient penetration and exposure, without motion, to visualize dorsum sellae.
• Patient ID information with R or L marker visible within collimated field without superimposing essential anatomy.

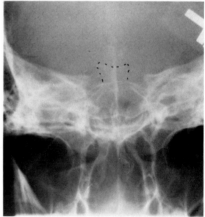
Fig. 11-77
PA, 10° Cephalic

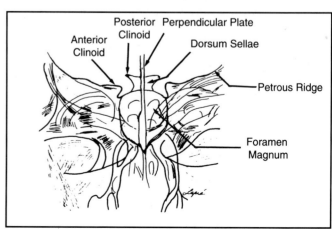

Anterior Clinoid — Posterior Clinoid — Perpendicular Plate — Dorsum Sellae — Petrous Ridge — Foramen Magnum

Fig. 11-78
PA, 10° Cephalic

• PA Axial Projection
(Haas Method)

Sella Turcica
Optional
• AP Axial (Towne)
• PA
• PA Axial (Haas)

Structures Best Shown:
Dorsum sellae, posterior clinoids, foramen magnum and petrous ridges.

Technical Factors:
• Film Size - 8 x 10 in. (18 x 24 cm), lengthwise.
• Moving or stationary grid.
• 70-80 kVp range.
• Use small focal spot

Patient Position:
• Remove all metal, plastic or other removable objects from head.
• Patient in an erect or prone position (erect preferred).

Part Position:
• Rest patient's nose and forehead against head unit or table.
• Depress chin until **orbitomeatal line is perpendicular** to film.
• Align **midsagittal plane perpendicular** to midline of head unit or table.

Central Ray:
• Angle CR **25° cephalic**.
• Center at midsagittal plane, **1 in.** (2.5 cm) **above superciliary arch.** (The CR will pass through a line connecting both EAM's.)
• Center CR to cassette.
• SID: Head Unit, 36 in. (91 cm).
       Table Top, minimum 40 in. (102 cm).

Collimation: Use a circle diaphragm or cylinder cone, or collimate on all sides to yield a field size of approximately 4 in. (10 cm).

Respiration: Suspend respiration during exposure.

NOTE: To obtain a sharp detailed image of the dorsum sellae, the utilization of a small focal spot and close collimation is essential.

Evaluation Criteria:
• The dorsum sellae is located in the center of the radiograph, with the petrous ridges and entire foramen magnum visualized within the collimated field.
• Close four sided collimation should be evident.
• Cranium is seen without rotation or tilt:
  - Petrous ridges are symmetrical.
  - Equal distance from dorsum sellae to each side of foramen magnum.
• Dorsum sella and posterior clinoids are projected into foramen magnum.
• Sufficient penetration and exposure, without motion, to visualize dorsum sellae.
• Patient ID information with R or L marker visible within collimated field without superimposing essential anatomy.

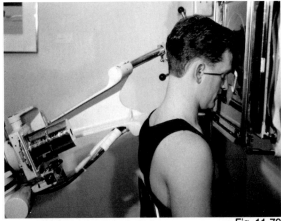

Fig. 11-79
PA Axial, CR 25° Cephalic, OML Perpendicular

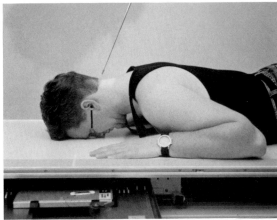

PA Axial, CR 25° Cephalic   Fig. 11-80

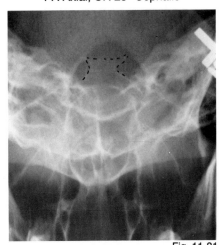

PA Axial, 25° Cephalic   Fig. 11-81

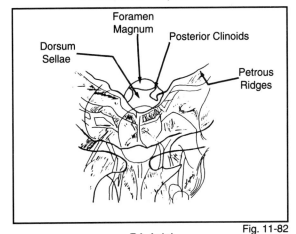

Foramen Magnum
Posterior Clinoids
Dorsum Sellae
Petrous Ridges

PA Axial   Fig. 11-82

Chapter 12
Radiographic Anatomy and Positioning of the Facial Bones

Contributions by: Kathy M. Martensen, BS, RT (R)
Barry T. Anthony, RT (R)

Contents

12 Facial Bones

Part I Radiographic Anatomy

Skull (Cranial and Facial Bones)

The skull or bony skeleton of the head consists of **14 facial bones** listed and described in this chapter, and **8 cranial bones** described in Chapter 11. The cranial bones are again identified on these drawing to demonstrate anatomical relationships of the total skull structure.

Each of the facial bones are identified on these frontal and lateral drawings *(Figs. 12-1 and 12-2),* except for the two palatine bones and the vomer which are internally located and not visible on a dry skeleton from the exterior. These are identified on sectional drawings later in this chapter.

The 14 facial bones to be studied in this chapter contribute to the shape and form of a person's face. In addition, the cavities of the orbits, nose and mouth are largely constructed from the bones of the face. Of the 14 bones making up the facial skeleton, only 2 are single bones. The remaining 12 consist of six pairs of bones with similar bones on each side of the face.

Facial Bones
    2 - **Maxillae** *(mak-sil 'e)* (Upper Jaw) or **Maxillary Bones**
    2 - **Zygomatic** or **Malar Bones** *(zi 'go-mat'ik, ma'lar)*
    2 - **Lacrimal Bones** *(lak'ri-mal)*
    2 - **Nasal Bones**
    2 - **Inferior Nasal Conchae** *(kong 'ke)*
    2 - **Palatine Bones** *(pal 'ah-tin)*
    1 - **Vomer** *(vo'mer)*
    1 - **Mandible** (Lower Jaw)
    ‾‾‾‾‾‾‾‾
    14 Total

Each of the facial bones will be separated and studied individually, or as pairs for those six paired bones. After the description of each of these facial bones will be a listing of those specific adjoining bones with which they articulate, or with which they are joined since in an adult they are all fused and immovable except for the mandible. Knowing these anatomical relationships helps in understanding the structure of the total skull or bony skeleton of the head.

Right and Left Maxillary Bones
The first pair of facial bones to be studied are the two **maxillae or maxillary bones** which are the largest immovable bones of the face. The only facial bone that is larger than the maxilla is the movable lower jaw or mandible. All of the other bones of the upper facial area are closely associated with the two maxillae, thus they are structurally the most important bones of the upper face. The right and left maxillary bones are solidly united at the midline below the nasal septum. Each maxilla assists in the formation of three cavities of the face : (1) the mouth, (2) the nasal cavity, and (3) one orbit.

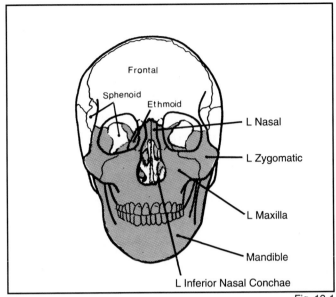

Facial Bones – Frontal View   Fig. 12-1

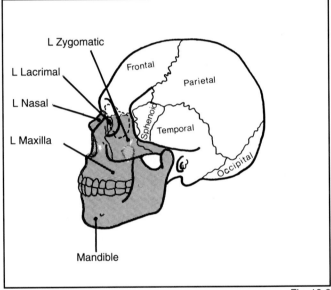

Facial Bones – Lateral View   Fig. 12-2

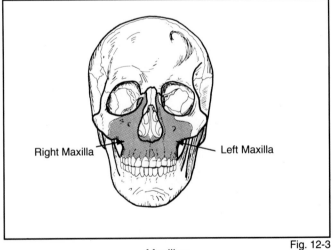

Maxillae   Fig. 12-3

Maxillary bones continued

Lateral View of Left Maxilla: Each maxilla consists of a centrally located **body** and **four processes** projecting from that body. Three of these processes are more obvious and are seen on these lateral and frontal drawings. The fourth process, the palatine process, is described below as part of the hard palate.

The **body** of each maxilla is the centrally located portion that lies lateral to the nose. One of the three processes is the **frontal process,** which projects upward along the lateral border of the nose toward the frontal bone. The **zygomatic process** projects laterally to unite with the zygomatic bone. The third process, the **alveolar process,** is the inferior or lower aspect of the body of each maxilla. The eight upper teeth on each side are embedded in cavities along the inferior margin of the alveolar process.

The two maxillae are solidly united in the midline anteriorly. At the upper part of this midline union is the **anterior nasal spine.** A blow to the nose sometimes results in this nasal spine being separated from the maxillae.

A point at the base of the anterior nasal spine is called the **acanthion,** described in chapter 11 as a surface landmark at the midline point where the nose and upper lip meet.

Frontal View: The relationship of the two maxillary bones to the remainder of the bones of the skull is well demonstrated in this frontal view (*Fig. 12-5*). Note again **three processes** as seen in the frontal view of the skull. Extending upward toward the frontal bone is the **frontal process.** Extending laterally toward the zygomatic bone is the **zygomatic process,** and supporting the upper teeth is the **alveolar process.**

The body of each maxillary bone contains a large air-filled cavity known as a **maxillary sinus.** There are several of these air-filled cavities found in certain bones of the skull. These sinuses communicate with the nasal cavity and are collectively termed paranasal sinuses and will be described further in the chapter which follows.

Hard Palate (inferior surface)

The **fourth process** of each maxillary bone is the **palatine process,** which can only be demonstrated on an inferior view of the two maxillae (*Fig. 12-6*). The two palatine processes form the anterior portion of the roof of the mouth, called the hard or bony palate. The two palatine processes are solidly united in the midline to form a synarthrodial or immovable joint. A common congenital defect called a cleft palate is an opening between the palatine processes, caused by an incomplete joining of the two bones.

The posterior part of the hard palate is formed by the horizontal portions of two other facial bones, the **palatine bones.** Note that the posterior part of the hard palate is formed by the two palatine bones, while the anterior part of the hard palate is formed by the palatine processes of the two maxillary bones.

Only the horizontal portions of the L-shaped palatine bones are visible on this view. The vertical portion is demonstrated later on a cut-away drawing in *Fig. 12-11.*

The two small inferior portions of the sphenoid bone of the cranium are also shown on this inferior view of the hard palate. These two processes, the **pterygoid hamuli,** are likened to the outstretched legs of a bat as described in chapter 11.

Articulations: Each maxilla articulates with **2 cranial bones,** the frontal and the ethmoid; and with **7 facial bones,** a zygomatic, a lacrimal, a nasal, a palatine, an inferior nasal concha, the vomer and the opposite maxilla.

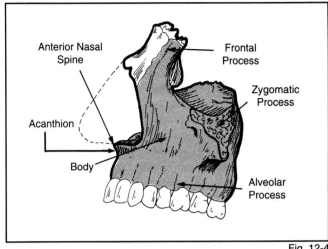

Left Maxilla (Lateral View)   Fig. 12-4

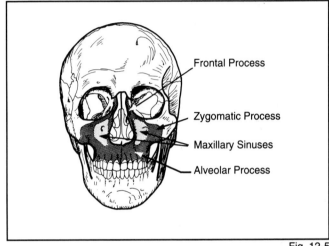

Maxillae (Frontal View)   Fig. 12-5

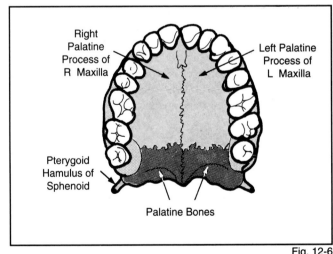

Maxillae and Palatine Bones (Inferior Surface)   Fig. 12-6

Right and Left Zygomatic (Malar) Bone

One **zygomatic bone** is located lateral to the zygomatic process of each maxilla. These bones form the prominence of the cheek and make up the lower outer portion of each orbit.

Projecting posteriorly from the zygomatic bone is a slender process connecting with the zygomatic process of the temporal bone to form the **zygomatic arch.** The zygomatic arch is a fairly delicate structure and is sometimes fractured or "caved in" by a blow to the cheek. Note that the anterior portion of the zygomatic arch is formed by the zygomatic bone and the posterior portion by the temporal bone. The **zygomatic prominence** is a positioning landmark and refers to this prominent portion of the zygomatic bone.

Articulations: Each zygomatic articulates with **3 cranial bones**, the frontal, the sphenoid, and a temporal; and with **one facial bone**, a maxilla.

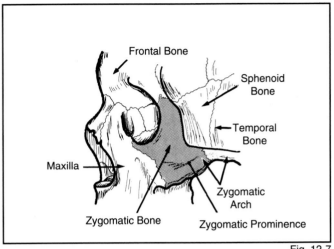

Fig. 12-7

Zygomatic (Malar) Bone – Lateral View

Right and Left Nasal and Lacrimal Bones

The lacrimal and nasal bones are the thinnest and most fragile bones in the entire body.

Lacrimal Bones: The two small and very delicate lacrimal bones (about the size and shape of a fingernail) lie anteriorly on the medial side of each orbit just posterior to the frontal process of the maxilla. Lacrimal, derived from a word meaning tear, is appropriate since the lacrimal bones are closely associated with the tear ducts.

Nasal Bones: The two fused nasal bones form the bridge of the nose and are somewhat variable in size. Some persons have very prominent nasal bones, while others are quite small. Much of the nose is made up of cartilage and only the upper portion at the bridge of the nose is formed by the two nasal bones. The nasal bones lie just anterior and superior to the frontal process of the maxillae and just inferior to the frontal bone. The point of junction of the two nasal bones with the frontal bone is a positioning landmark termed the **nasion.**

Articulations:

Lacrimal: Each lacrimal articulates with **2 cranial bones**, the frontal and the ethmoid; and with **2 facial bones**, a maxilla and an inferior nasal concha.

Nasal: Each nasal also articulates with **2 cranial bones**, the frontal and the ethmoid; and with **2 facial bones**, a maxilla and the opposite nasal bone.

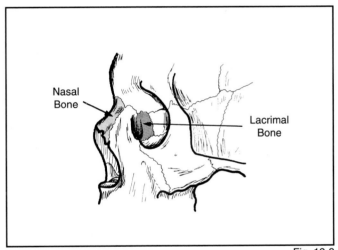

Fig. 12-8

Nasal and Lacrimal Bones – Lateral View

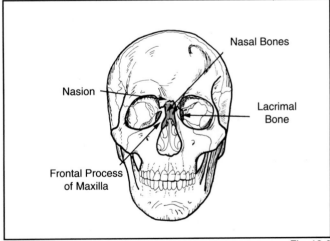

Fig. 12-9

Nasal and Lacrimal Bones – Frontal view

Right and Left Inferior Nasal Conchae

Within the nasal cavity are two thin, curved or scroll-shaped facial bones termed the **inferior nasal conchae** (turbinates). These two bones project from the lateral walls of the nasal cavity on each side and extend medially.

The **superior and middle nasal conchae** (turbinates) are similar scroll-like projections that extend from the ethmoid bone into the nasal cavities.

In summary, there are three pairs of nasal conchae or turbinates. **The superior and middle pairs are parts of the ethmoid bone**, while the **inferior pair are separate facial bones.**

The effect of the three pairs of turbinates is to divide the nasal cavities into various departments. These irregular compartments tend to break up or mix the flow of air coming into the nasal cavities before it reaches the lungs. In this way the incoming air is somewhat warmed and cleaned as it comes in contact with the mucous membrane covering the conchae, before it reaches the lungs.

Sectional Drawing

Inferior Nasal Conchae: The relationship between the various nasal conchae and the lateral wall of one nasal cavity is illustrated in this sectional drawing *(Fig. 12-11)*. The midline structures making up the nasal septum have been removed so that the lateral portion of the right nasal cavity can be seen. Note that the **superior and middle conchae** are part of the ethmoid bone, and the **inferior nasal conchae** are separate facial bones. The **cribriform plate** and the **crista galli** of the ethmoid bone help to separate the cranium from the facial bone mass.

Right and Left Palatine Bones

The two **palatine bones** are difficult to visualize when studying a dry skeleton because they are located internally and are not visible from the outside. Each palatine bone is roughly L-shaped. The vertical portion of the L extends upward between one maxilla and one pterygoid plate of the sphenoid bone. The horizontal portion of each L helps to make up the posterior portion of the hard palate as shown in *Fig. 12-6*.

Articulations:

Inferior Nasal Conchae: Each inferior nasal conche articulates with **one cranial bone**, the ethmoid; and with **3 facial bones,** a maxilla, a lacrimal and a palatine.

Palatine: Each palatine articulates with **2 cranial bones**, the sphenoid and the ethmoid; and **4 facial bones**, a maxilla, an inferior nasal conchae, the vomer and the opposite palatine.

Bony Nasal Septum

The midline structures of the nasal cavity, including the **bony nasal septum**, are shown on this sagittal view drawing. The bony nasal septum is formed by two bones, the **ethmoid** and the **vomer.** It is formed superiorly by the **perpendicular plate** of the ethmoid bone, and inferiorly by the single vomer bone. Anteriorly, the nasal septum is cartilaginous and is termed the **septal cartilage.**

The bony nasal septum, which can be demonstrated radiographically, is thus formed by the perpendicular plate of the ethmoid bone and the vomer bone. In severe trauma to the nasal bone area, the septum may get pushed to one side, away from the midline. This injury would be termed a deviated nasal septum.

Vomer

The single **vomer bone** (meaning plowshare) is a thin triangular shaped bone that forms the inferoposterior part of the nasal septum. The surfaces of the vomer are marked by small furrowlike depressions for

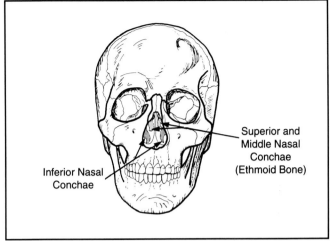

Inferior Nasal Conchae   Fig. 12-10

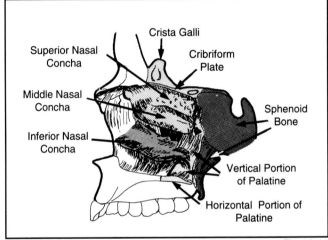

Inferior Nasal Conchae and Palatine Bones   Fig. 12-11

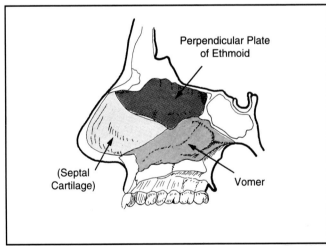

Bony Nasal Septum and Vomer   Fig. 12-12

blood vessels, a source of nose bleed with trauma to the nasal area. A deviated nasal septum describes the clinical condition wherein the nasal septum is deflected or displaced laterally from the midline of the nose. This deviation usually occurs at the site of junction between the septal cartilage and the vomer. A severe deviation can entirely block the nasal passageway making breathing through the nose impossible.

Articulations: The vomer articulates with **2 cranial bones**, the sphenoid and ethmoid; and with **4 facial bones**, the right and left palatine and the right and left maxilla. (The vomer also articulates with the septal cartilage.)

Mandible

The last and the largest of the facial bones is the lower jaw or
mandible. It is the only movable bone in the adult skull. This
large facial bone, which is a single bone in the adult, actually
originates as two separate bones. The two bones in the infant
join to become one bone at approximately one year of age.

The specific parts of the mandible will be described beginning
with a lateral view of a detached mandible.

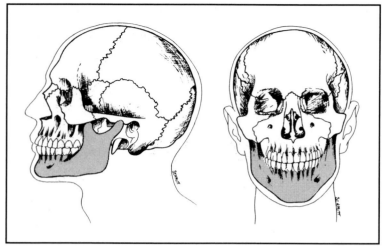

Mandible   Fig. 12-13

Lateral View: The **angle** (gonion) of the mandible divides each half of
the mandible into two main parts. That area anterior to the angle is
termed the **body** of the mandible, while that area superior to each angle
is termed the **ramus.** Since the mandible is a single bone, the body
actually extends from the left angle around to the right angle.

The lower teeth are rooted in the mandible; therefore, an **alveolar
process** or ridge extends along the entire superior portion of the body of
the mandible.

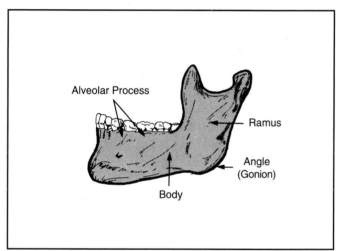

Mandible – Lateral View   Fig. 12-14

Frontal View: The anterior aspect of the adult mandible is shown on
this frontal view of a detached mandible. The single body forms from
each lateral half and unites at the anterior midline. The flat triangular
area projecting forward as the chin in the human is called the **mentum**
or **mental protuberance.** The center of the mental protuberance is
described as the **mental point.** Mentum and mental are Latin words
referring to the whole area known as the chin. The mental point is a
specific point of the chin whereas the mentum is the entire area.

Located on each half of the body of the mandible are the **mental foramina.** These foramina serve as passageways for nerves and blood
vessels.

The area of fusion of the two halves of the mandible is termed the
symphysis of the mandible or **symphysis menti.** This area of fusion is
just superior to the mental protuberance and extends upward to the
alveolar border.

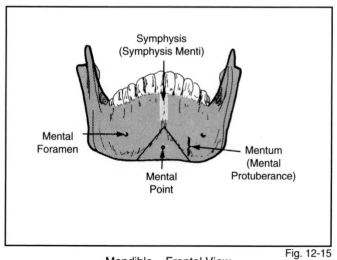

Mandible – Frontal View   Fig. 12-15

Mandible continued

Ramus: The upper portion of each **ramus** terminates in a U-shaped notch termed the **mandibular notch.** At each end of the mandibular notch is a process. The process at the anterior end of the mandibular notch is termed the **coronoid process.** The coronoid process does not articulate with another bone and cannot be easily palpated since it lies just inferior to the zygomatic arch. It serves as a site for muscle attachment.

Memory Aid: The **coronoid process** of the mandible must not be confused with the **coronoid process** of the proximal ulna of the forearm, or the **coracoid process** of the scapula. One way to remember these terms is to associate "n" in coronoid with the n's in ulna and in mandible.

The posterior process of the upper ramus is termed the **condyloid process** and consists of two parts. The rounded end of the condyloid process is called the **condyle** or **head,** while the constricted area directly below the condyle is the **neck.** The condyle of the condyloid process fits into the temporomandibular fossa of the temporal bone to form the **temporomandibular joint** or **TMJ.**

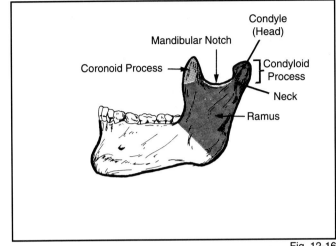

Mandible, Left Side Fig. 12-16

Axiolateral Position: The mandible, as illustrated, is rotated slightly and is tilted so that the left half of the mandible is projected above the right half. This is called an axiolateral or oblique position. Since both sides of the mandible would be superimposed on a true lateral, part of the routine mandible positioning series calls for tilting the mandible to show primarily one side, as seen in this illustration. The opposite axiolateral position shows the other side in the same way. These tilted lateral positions clearly demonstrate the **body** and entire **ramus,** including the **coronoid process, the condyle** and the **condyloid process.**

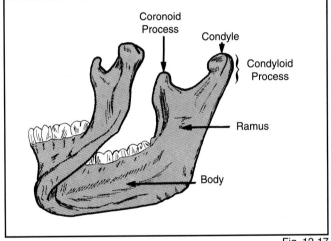

Mandible – Axiolateral (obli.) Position Fig. 12-17

Submentovertex Projection: The horseshoe shape of the mandible is well visualized on a **submentovertex** (SMV) projection. Note that the mandible is a fairly thin structure, which explains why it is susceptible to fractures. The area of the chin or **mentum** is well demonstrated as are the **body** and **rami** of the mandible. The relative positions of the upper ramus and its associated **coronoid process** and **condyle** are also demonstrated with this projection. Note that the condyles project inward on this view as is demonstrated on radiographs of this projection.

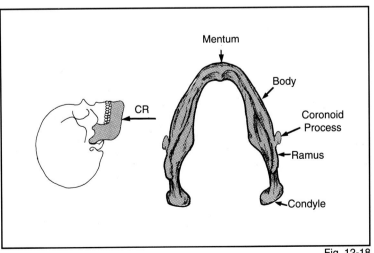

Submentovertex Projection of Mandible Fig. 12-18

Temporomandibular Joint (TMJ)

The temporomandibular joint (TMJ), the only movable joint in the skull, is shown on this lateral drawing and on the lateral view photograph of a dry skull *(Figs. 12-19 and 20)*. The relationship of the mandible to the temporal bone of the cranium is well demonstrated.

The TMJ is formed by the **condyle** or head of the condyloid process of the mandible fitting into the **temporomandibular fossa** of the temporal bone. The TMJ is located just anterior and slightly superior to the **external acoustic** (auditory) **meatus** or **EAM.**

Joint Classification (Skull and Mandible)

Synovial Joints (Diarthrodial)

The TMJ is classified as a **synovial type** joint which is **diarthrodial** or freely movable. This synovial joint is divided into upper and lower synovial cavities by a single articular fibrous disc. A series of strong ligaments join the condylar neck of the mandible to the lower borders of the zygomatic process of the temporal bone.

The two-part articular capsule is lined by synovial membrane and divided by the articular disc. This complete two-part synovial joint along with its fibrous articular disc allows for not only a **hinge type motion** but also a **gliding movement** wherein the mandibular condyle glides forward as the mouth is opened. This movement is further facilitated by a shallow temporomandibular fossa of the temporal bone with which the condyle or head of mandible articulates.

Fibrous Joints (Synarthrodial)

There are two types of **fibrous** joints involving the skull. These are both **synarthrodial** or immovable joints. First are the **sutures** between cranial bones as described in the preceding chapter. Second is a unique type of fibrous joint involving the teeth and the mandible and the maxillae. This is a **gomophysis** (*gom-fo'sis*) subclass type fibrous joint between the roots of the teeth and the alveolar processes of both the maxillae and the mandible.

TMJ Motion: These drawings illustrate the TMJ in both an **open and a closed mouth** position. When one opens the mouth widely, the condyle moves forward to the front edge of the fossa. If the condyle slips too far anteriorly, the joint may dislocate. If the TMJ dislocates, either by force or by jaw motion, it may be difficult or even impossible to close the mouth, which returns the condyle to its normal position.

Radiographs (open and closed mouth): Two axiolateral projections (Schuller method) of the TMJ are shown below in closed and open mouth positions. The range of anterior movement of the condyle in relationship to the temporomandibular fossa is clearly demonstrated.

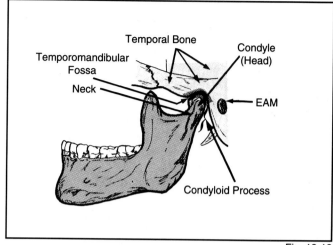

Temporomandibular Joint (TMJ)
Fig. 12-19

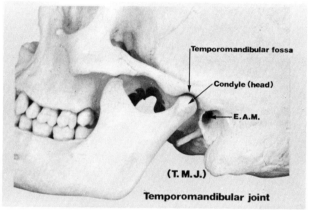

Joints of Mandible
Fig. 12-20

- **TMJ**: Classification - **Synovial** (diarthrodial)
  Movement type - Hinge
  - Gliding

- **Alveoli and Roots of Teeth**:
  Classification - **Fibrous** (synarthrodial)
  Subclass - **Gomophysis**

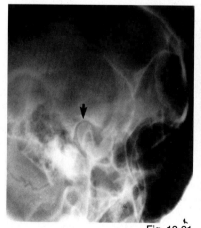

Closed Mouth
Fig. 12-21

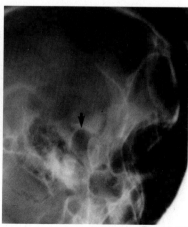

Open Mouth
Fig. 12-22

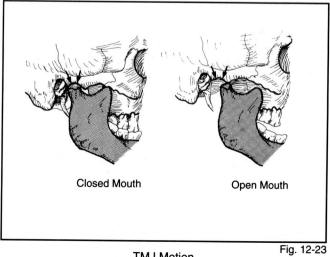

Closed Mouth   Open Mouth

TMJ Motion
Fig. 12-23

Orbits

The complex anatomy of the 14 facial bones helps to form several facial cavities. Those cavities formed in total or in part by the facial bones are the mouth or oral cavity, the nasal cavities and the bilateral orbits. The mouth and nasal cavities are primarily passageways and, as such, are not often examined specifically by radiographers. The orbits, however, containing the vital organs of sight and associated nerves and blood vessels, are frequently radiographed. The structure and shape of the orbits are illustrated in this simplified drawing. Each orbit is a **cone-shaped,** bony-walled structure composed of parts of **seven bones.**

The rim of the orbit, corresponding to the circular portion of the cone, is called the **base.** The base of the orbit is seldom a true circle, however, and may even look like a figure with four definite sides. The most posterior portion of the cone, the **apex,** corresponds to the **optic foramen** through which the optic nerve passes.

The long axis of the orbits project both upward and toward the midline. If one's head were placed in an upright AP or lateral position with the orbitomeatal line adjusted parallel to the floor, each orbit would project upward or superiorly at an angle of **30 degrees,** and toward the midsagittal plane at an angle of **37 degrees.** These two important angles are used during radiographic positioning of the optic foramina. Remember that each optic foramen is located at the apex of its respective orbit. In order to radiograph either optic foramen it is necessary to both extend the patient's chin by 30 degrees and rotate the head 37 degrees. The central ray is then projected through the base of the orbit along the long axis of the cone-shaped orbit.

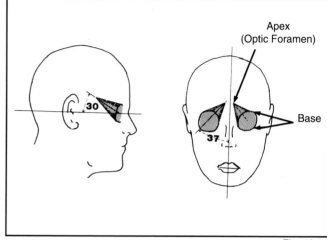

Orbits (Cone–shaped)   Fig. 12-24

Bony Composition of Orbits

Each orbit is composed of parts of seven bones. The circumference or circular base of each orbit is composed of parts of **three** bones, the **frontal bone (orbital plate)** from the cranium, and the **maxilla** and **zygomatic bone** from the facial mass. Inside each orbital cavity are a roof, a floor and two walls, parts of which are also formed by these three bones. The orbital plate of the frontal bone forms most of the roof of the orbit. The zygomatic bone forms much of the lateral wall and some of the floor of the orbit, while a portion of the maxilla helps to form the floor.

All seven bones that form each orbit are shown in *Fig. 12-26.* The **frontal bone, zygomatic bone** and **maxilla** make up the base of the orbit. Some of the medial wall of the orbit is formed by the thin **lacrimal bone.** The **sphenoid** and **ethmoid** bones make up most of the posterior orbit, while only a small bit of the **palatine** bone contributes to the very posterior portion of the floor of each orbit.

In summary, the **seven** bones making up each orbit include **three cranial bones**—the frontal, sphenoid and ethmoid; and **four facial bones**—the maxilla, zygomatic, lacrimal and palatine.

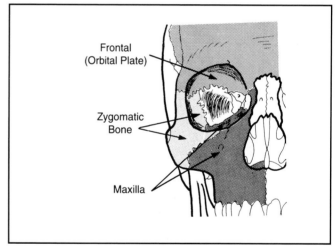

Base of Orbit – 3 bones   Fig. 12-25
(Direct Frontal View)

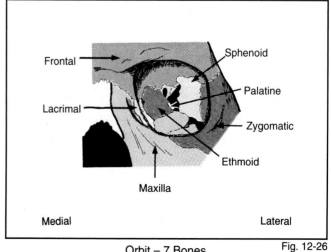

Orbit – 7 Bones   Fig. 12-26
(Slightly Obli. Frontal View)

Openings in Posterior Orbit

Each orbit also contains three holes or openings in the posterior portion of the orbit, as demonstrated. The **optic foramen** is a small hole in the sphenoid bone, located posteriorly at the apex of the cone-shaped orbit. The **superior orbital fissure** is a cleft or opening between the greater and lesser wings of the sphenoid bone, located lateral to the optic foramen. A third opening is the **inferior orbital fissure,** located between the maxilla, zygomatic bone and greater wing of the sphenoid.

The small root of bone separating the superior orbital fissure and the optic canal is known as the **sphenoid strut.** The optic canal is a small canal into which the optic foramen opens. Therefore, any abnormal enlargement of the optic nerve could cause erosion of the sphenoid strut, which is actually a portion of the lateral wall of the optic canal.

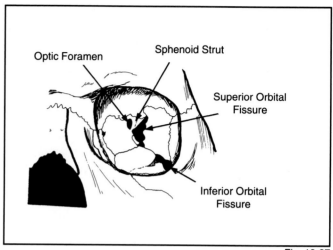

Orbits – Posterior Openings
(Slightly Obli. Frontal View)

Fig. 12-27

Orbital Fractures

"Blow-Out" Fracture: Due to the unique construction of the orbit (a closed cone) and to the fact that the orbit is filled with structures containing large amounts of water (water does not compress), certain fractures are common to the orbit. One type of fracture is called a **"blowout" fracture.** If the front of the orbit is struck solidly, such as with a ball or a fist, the contents of the cavity have no place to go. Since the bone along the floor of the orbit is quite thin, the orbital contents "blow-out" in that direction. Since the orbital contents involve vision, diagnosis of this type of fracture must be made early in treatment.

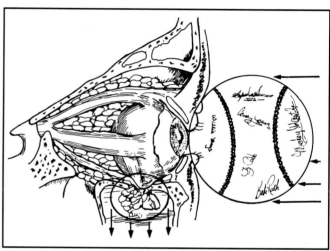

"Blow-out" Fracture

Fig. 12-28

"Tripod" Fracture: Another unique fracture of the facial bone area is called the **"tripod" fracture.** This fracture essentially involves the zygomatic bone and its three connections. If fractures were to occur at the three points of attachment with the maxilla, temporal and frontal bones, as might result from a direct blow to the cheek, then the result is a free-floating zygomatic bone or a "tripod" fracture. The bones in this area of the body are highly vascular. Healing is quite rapid, which can be both good and bad. If either a "blow-out'' or "tripod" fracture is not diagnosed early, the fracture may heal out of place and cause additional problems. The fracture might even have to be rebroken to be set properly.

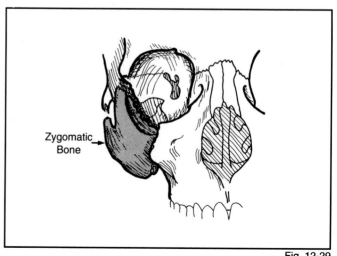

"Tripod" Fracture

Fig. 12-29

Anatomy Review

Review exercises for anatomy of the cranial and facial bones follow as demonstrated on both a dry skull and on radiographs. Not all specific anatomy shown on the dry skull can be identified on these radiographs but those parts that are identifiable are labeled as such. A good learning and/or review exercise is to carefully study both the dry skull illustrations and the radiographs, and identify each part before looking at the answers below.

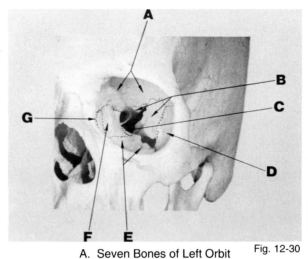

A. Seven Bones of Left Orbit   Fig. 12-30

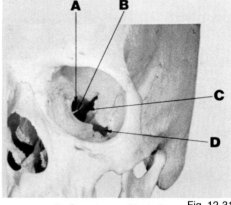

B. Openings of Left Orbit   Fig. 12-31

Orbital Structures and Openings:

A. Seven Bones of Left Orbit: *(Fig.12-30)*
A. Frontal bone (orbital plate)
B. Sphenoid bone
C. Small portion of palatine bone
D. Zygomatic bone
E. Maxillary bone
F. Ethmoid
G. Lacrimal

B. Openings of Left Orbit: *(Fig. 12-31)*
A. Optic foramen
B. Sphenoid strut
C. Superior orbital fissure
D. Inferior orbital fissure

C. Parieto-orbital Projection of Orbits: *(Fig. 12-32)*
A. Orbital plate of frontal bone
B. Sphenoid bone
C. Optic foramen and canal
D. Superior orbital fissure
E. Inferior orbital margin
F. Sphenoid strut (part of inferior and lateral wall of optic canal)
G. Lateral orbital margin
H. Superior orbital margin

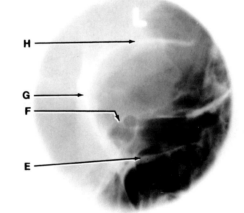
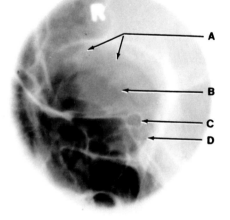

C. Parieto-orbital Projection of Orbits   Fig. 12-32

Facial Bones, Frontal View *(Fig. 12-33)*

A. Left nasal bone
B. Frontal process of left maxilla
C. Optic foramen
D. Superior orbital fissure
E. Inferior orbital fissure
F. Superior and middle nasal conchae of ethmoid bone
G. Vomer facial bone (lower portion of bony nasal septum)
H. Inferior nasal conchae facial bone
I. Anterior nasal spine of maxillary bones
J. Alveolar process of left maxilla

K. Alveolar process of left mandible
L. Mental foramen
M. Mentum or mental protuberance
N. Body of right mandible
O. Angle of right mandible
P. Ramus of right mandible
Q. Body of right maxilla (contain maxillary sinuses)
R. Zygomatic prominence of right zygomatic bone
S. Outer orbit portion of right zygomatic bone
T. Sphenoid bone (cranial bone)

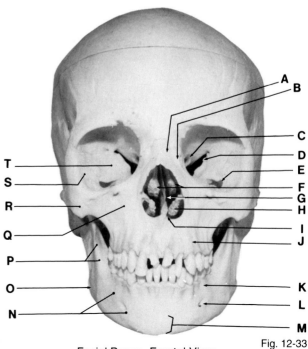

Facial Bones, Frontal View   Fig. 12-33

Anatomy Review continued

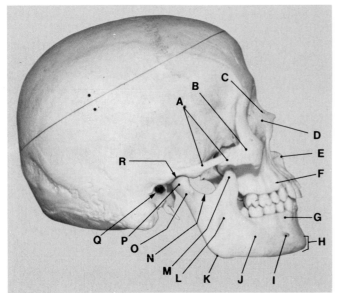

Fig. 12-34

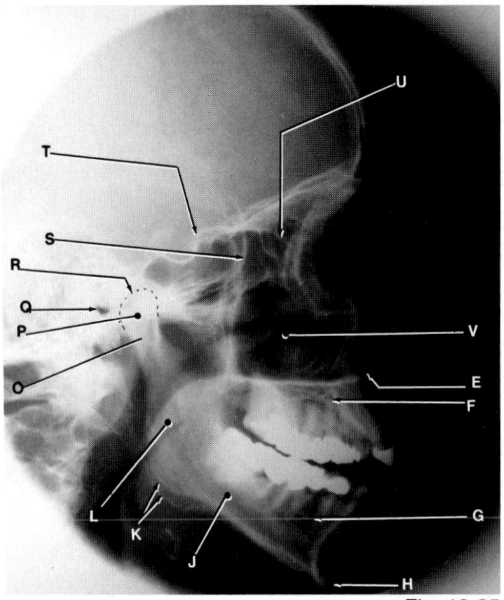

Facial Bones –Lateral

Fig. 12-35

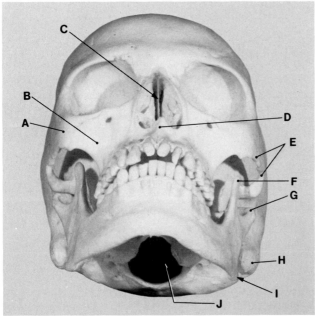

Fig. 12-36

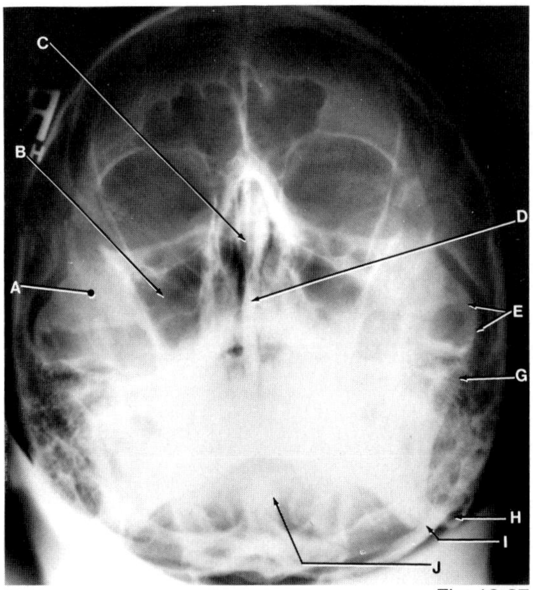

Facial Bones – Parietoacanthial projection (Waters)

Fig. 12-37

Facial Bones – Lateral
(Figs. 12-34 and 35)

A. Zygomatic arch
B. R Zygomatic
C. R Nasal bone
D. Frontal process of R maxilla
E. Anterior nasal spine
F. Alveolar process of maxilla
G. Alveolar process of mandible
H. Mentum or mental protuberance
I. Mental foramen
J. Body of mandible
K. Angle (gonion)

L. Ramus of mandible
M. Coronoid process
N. Mandibular notch
O. Neck of mandibular condyle
P. Condyle or head
Q. External acoustic meatus (EAM)
R. Temporomandibular fossa of temporal bone

Radiograph Only

S. Greater wings of sphenoid
T. Lesser wings of sphenoid with anterior clinoid processes
U. Ethmoid sinuses between orbits
V. Body of maxilla containing maxillary sinuses

Facial Bones – Parietoacanthial (Waters)
(Figs. 12-36 and 37)

The photograph *(Fig. 12-36)* represents the skull in a parietoacanthial projection, (Waters position) with the head tilted back. This results in a parietoacanthial projection which is one of the more common projections to visualize the facial bones.

A. Zygomatic prominence
B. Body of maxilla (contains maxillary sinuses)
C. Bony nasal septum (perpendicular plate of ethmoid and vomer bone)
D. Anterior nasal spine
E. Zygomatic arch
F. Coronoid process (not seen on radiograph)
G. Condyle (head)
H. Mastoid process of temporal bone
I. Angle of mandible
J. Foramen Magnum (radiograph demonstrates the dens or odontoid process within foramen magnum)

Anatomy Review continued

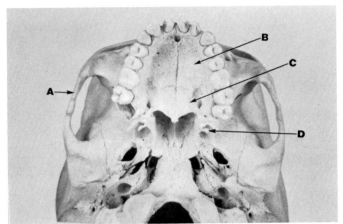

Facial Bones – Inferior View

Fig. 12-38

Facial Bones – SMV (Inferior View)

The photograph above illustrates an inferior view of the dry skull with the mandible removed. The submentovertex projection radiograph on the right is positioned with the top (vertex) of the head against the film with the central ray entering under the chin (mentum).

A. Zygomatic arch
B. Palatine process of maxilla
C. Horizontal process of palatine
D. Ptergoid hamulus of sphenoid

(Radiograph only:)
E. Foramen ovale of sphenoid
F. Foramen spinosum of sphenoid
G. Foramen magnum
H. Petrous pyramid of temporal bone
I. Mastoid portion of temporal bone
J. Sphenoid sinus in body of sphenoid
K. Head and condyle of mandible
L. Posterior border (vertical portion) of palatine bone
M. Vomer or bony nasal septum
N. Right maxillary sinuses
O. Ethmoid sinuses

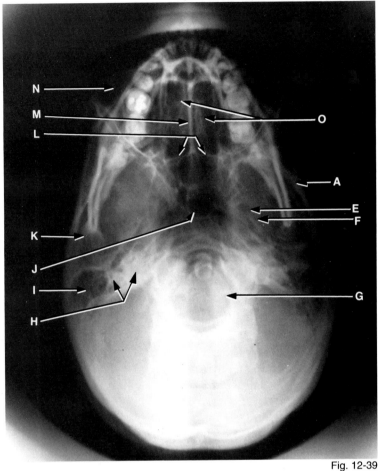

Fig. 12-39

Submentovertex (SMV) Projection

Part II Radiographic Positioning

Special Projections and Anatomical Relationships

PA Skull Projection: The PA skull on the right (*Fig. 12-41*) was taken with no tube angulation and with the OML (dotted line in *Fig. 12-40*) perpendicular to the plane of the film. The central ray is therefore parallel to the orbitomeatal line (OML). This results in the **petrous pyramids being projected directly into the orbits** so that the orbits appear totally filled by the petrous pyramids. Drawn on both radiographs (*Figs. 12-40 and 41*) is a line through the roof of the orbits and through the petrous ridges. With the orbits superimposed by the petrous pyramids, very little facial bone detail can be demonstrated radiographically. Therefore this PA projection has limited value for visualizing facial bones.

Parietoacanthial (Waters) Projection: In order to better visualize the facial bone mass, it is necessary to project the petrous pyramids inferiorly. The petrous pyramids are such dense, bony structures that they must be removed from the facial bone area of interest, either by tube angulation or by extending the neck. The radiographs to the right (*Figs. 12-42 and 43*) demonstrate how this can be accomplished. The neck is extended by raising the chin so that the **petrous pyramids will be projected just below the maxillary sinuses**. The central ray is now parallel to the mentomeatal line (dotted line). The radiograph on the right (Waters method), if done correctly as described later in this chapter, demonstrates the petrous ridges (see arrows) projected below the maxillae and maxillary sinuses. Thus except for the mandible, the facial bones are now projected superior to and **not** superimposed over the dense petrous pyramids.

Positioning Considerations

Erect vs. Recumbent: Positioning considerations for the facial bones are similar to that of the skull as described in the previous chapter.

Facial bone projections should also be taken erect if the condition of the patient allows. This can be done with an erect table or erect grid-film holder device such as the head unit in *Fig. 12-44*. It is generally easier to move the patient's entire body as needed in an erect position (especially obese or hypersthenic type patients) to accurately adjust the various planes and positioning lines of the head for accurate skull positioning.

Trauma patients generally need to be taken table top however, especially with possible neck injuries. Most of these facial bone projections can be

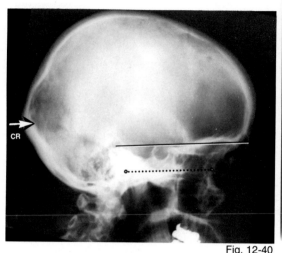

Fig. 12-40

(Lateral skull for comparison of bony relationships)

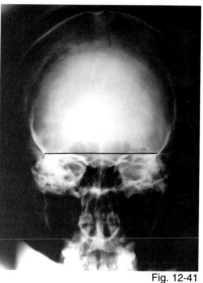

Fig. 12-41

Skull – PA projection

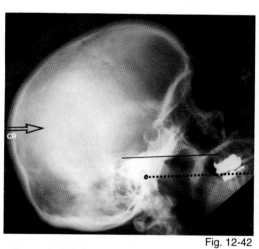

Fig. 12-42

(Lateral skull for comparison of bony relationships)

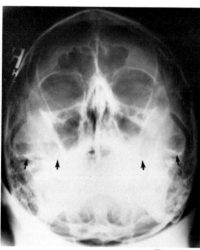

Fig. 12-43

Facial Bones – (Waters) Parietoacanthial projection

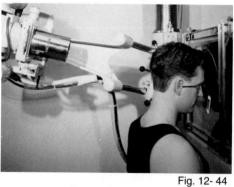

Fig. 12- 44

Erect – Head Unit

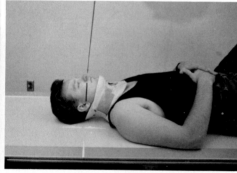

Fig. 12- 45

Supine – Trauma Patient

taken supine without moving the patient by compensating CR angles and/or CR-part-film alignments as will be demonstrated. However, AP skull or facial bones are only taken in emergencies when the patient cannot turn into the prone position since the lens of the eye receives about 95% more radiation with an AP projection than with an PA.

National Survey

Departmental standards (basic) and optional routines for exams of the facial bones were surprisingly consistent throughout the United States. The results of this survey determined national norms for departmental routines as presented in the positioning pages which follow:

Facial Bones Routine

Facial Bones	U.S. Average	
	Basic	Optional
• Lateral	94%	
• PA Waters (parietoacanthial)	87%	
• PA Caldwell	35%	
• PA Modified Waters	24%	
• SMV	13%	

Nasal Bones Routine

Nasal Bones	U.S. Average	
	Basic	Optional
• PA Waters	95%	
• Lateral - both sides or	81%	
• Lateral - one side	21%	
• PA Caldwell	20%	
• Superioroinferior (axial)	12%	

Optic Foramina Routine

Optic Foramina	U.S. Average	
	Basic	Optional
• Rhese Oblique (bilateral)	97%	
• PA Waters	14%	
• PA Caldwell	11%	
• Lateral	9%	

Mandible Routine

Mandible	U.S. Average	
	Basic	Optional
• Axiolateral - oblique	82%	
• PA - 0° angle	78%	
• AP Towne	46%	
• PA semiaxial (20-25°cephalic)	31%	
• Panorex	16%	
• PA modified Waters	13%	
• SMV (basilar)	12%	

Zygomatic Arch Routine Routine

Zygomatic Arch	U.S. Average	
	Basic	Optional
• SMV (basilar)	81%	
• PA Waters (parietoacanthial)	62%	
• AP Towne	42%	
• Oblique Axial (tangential)	33%	
• Lateral	30%	

Temporomandibular Joints Routine

TMJ	U.S. Average	
	Basic	Optional
• Lateral (Laws) or	57%	
• Lateral (Schuller)	48%	
• Tomograms	26%	
• AP Towne	13%	
• Panorex	7%	

Survey Questions on Possible Discontinued Procedures:

The national survey included questions on the **quantity** of specific exams being done in their departments during the past year, the **expected trend** in the next three or four years, and whether or not the procedure **should still be taught and included** in a basic student textbook. The results were as follows:

TMJ's	U.S. Average	East	Midwest	West
I. Trend				
a. Increase	8%	15%	4%	8%
b. Decrease	32%	27%	35%	33%
c. No change	60%	58%	61%	59%
II. Annual Quantity				
a. 0-5	22%	17%	21%	28%
b. 6-19	38%	36%	41%	33%
c. 20-30	20%	24%	20%	12%
d. 31+	20%	23%	18%	17%
III. Be Included				
a. Yes	92%	95%	90%	92%
b. No	8%	5%	10%	8%
Zygomatic Arches				
I. Trend				
a. Increase	14%	20%	11%	7%
b. Decrease	11%	11%	10%	11%
c. No change	75%	69%	79%	82%
II. Annual Quantity				
a. 0-4	15%	12%	17%	13%
b. 5-35	45%	48%	43%	50%
c. 36-140	19%	14%	22%	25%
d. 141+	21%	26%	18%	12%
III. Be Included				
a. Yes	96%	97%	94%	100%
b. No	4%	3%	6%	0%
Optic Foramina				
I. Trend				
a. Increase	11%	13%	10%	13%
b. Decrease	22%	19%	21%	27%
c. No change	67%	68%	69%	60%
II. Annual Quantity				
a. 0-4	46%	44%	47%	48%
b. 5-14	18%	19%	19%	17%
c. 15-87	21%	18%	23%	27%
d. 88+	15%	19%	11%	8%
III. Be Included				
a. Yes	81%	83%	76%	83%
b. No	19%	17%	24%	17%

Summary: These responses indicate a **decreasing trend or no change** expected in the number of these exams during the next three or four years. It also indicates that the current annual **quantity** of these exams is **very low** in a high percentage of U.S. hospitals and medical centers. This is very consistent throughout all regions of the United States. However, a strong majority in all regions indicated that these exams should still be taught and be included in a basic positioning text such as this. This suggests that all radiographers should still know how to take these exams when required.

Standard and Optional Operating Procedures

Certain basic and optional projections or positions for exams involving the facial bones are demonstrated and described on the following pages as suggested standard and optional departmental procedures.

Basic Projections
Standard or basic projections, also sometimes referred to as routine projections or departmental routines are those projections or positions commonly taken on average patients who are helpful and can cooperate in performing the procedure.

Optional Projections
Optional projections are those more common projections or positions taken as extra or additional projections to better demonstrate certain pathologic conditions or specific body parts. (These are **not** optional as to whether or not they are important or need to be learned and mastered by radiographers.)

Basic and Optional Projections

Facial Bones
Basic
• Lateral
• Parietoacanthial (Waters)
Optional
• Modified parietoacanthial
  (modified Waters)
• PA Caldwell

Facial Bones
Trauma
Basic
• Lateral (crosstable)
• Acanthioparietal (reverse Waters)

Nasal Bones
Basic
• Lateral
• Parietoacanthial (Waters)
Optional
• PA Caldwell
• Superioinferior (Axial)

Zygomatic Arches
Basic
• Submentovertex (SMV) (Basilar)
• Parietoacanthial (Waters)
Optional
• AP axial (Towne)
• Oblique axial
• Lateral

Optic Foramina
Basic
• Parieto-orbital (Rhese)

Orbits
Basic
• Modified acanthioparietal
  (modified Waters)

Mandible
Basic
• Axiolateral (oblique)
• PA
Optional
• AP axial (Towne)
• PA axial
• Panorex
• Submentovertex (basilar)

TMJ's
Basic
• Axiolateral 15° Oblique (Law)
  or
  Axiolateral (Schuller)
Optional
• AP axial (Towne)
• Tomography
• Panorex

•Lateral Position

Structures Best Shown:
Superimposed facial bones, greater wings of the sphenoid, orbital roofs, sella turcica, zygoma and mandible.

Technical Factors:
• Film Size - 8 x 10 in. (18 x 24 cm), lengthwise.
• Moving or stationary grid.
• 70-80 kVp range.
• Use small focal spot.

Patient Position:
• Remove all metal, plastic or other removable objects from head.
• Patient erect or prone. (Erect preferred if patient's condition allows.)

Part Position:
• Rest lateral side of head against head unit or table top, with side of interest closest to cassette.
• Adjust head into a **true lateral position**, oblique body as needed for patient's comfort. (A way to check for rotation is to palpate the external occipital protuberance posteriorly and the nasion or glabella anteriorly and insure that these two points are the same distance from the film.)
• Align **midsagittal plane parallel** to film.
• Align **interpupillary line perpendicular** to film.
• Adjust chin to bring the **infraorbitomeatal line perpendicular** to front edge of cassette.

Central Ray:
• Align CR **perpendicular** to head unit or table.
• Center CR to **zygoma**, at a level **half way between outer canthus and EAM.**
• Center cassette to CR.
• SID: Head unit, 36 in. (91 cm). Table Top, minimum 40 in. (102 cm).

Collimation: Use an 8 x 10 in. circle diaphragm or collimate on all sides to within 1 in. (2.5 cm) of nearest facial bone.

Respiration: Suspend respiration during exposure.

Evaluation Criteria:
• The superimposed zygomatic bones are located in the center of the radiograph, with the EAM's and orbital roofs visualized within the collimated field.
• The cranium is not rotated:
  - The mandibular rami, the orbital roofs and the greater wings of sphenoid are superimposed.
• Sufficient penetration and exposure, without motion, to visualize maxillary region.
• Patient ID information with R or L marker visible within collimated field without superimposing essential anatomy.

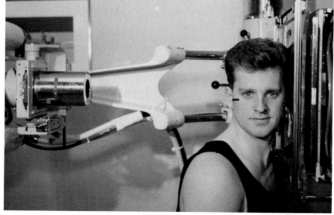
Lateral Erect — Fig. 12-46

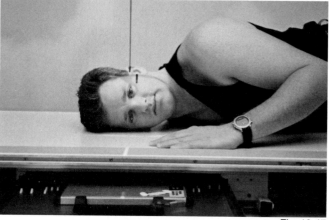
Lateral Recumbent — Fig. 12-47

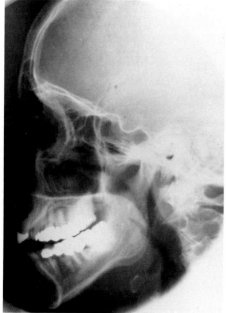
Lateral — Fig. 12-48

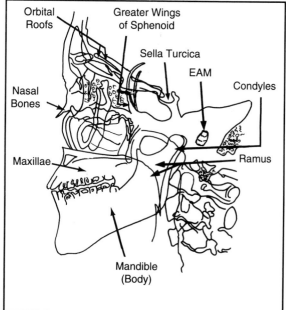
Lateral — Fig. 12-49

• Parietoacanthial Projection

(Waters Method)

Structures Best Shown:
Inferior orbital rim, maxillae, nasal septum, zygomatic bones, zygomatic arches and anterior nasal spine.

Technical Factors:
• Film Size - 10 x 12 in. (24 x 30 cm), lengthwise.
     or 8 x 10 in. (18 x 24 cm)
• Moving or stationary grid.
• 70-80 kVp range.
• Use small focal spot.

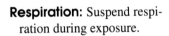

Patient Position:
• Remove all metal, plastic or other removable objects from head.
• Patient erect or prone. (Erect preferred if patient's condition allows.)

Part Position:
• Extend neck, resting chin against head unit or table top.
• Adjust head until **mentomeatal line is perpendicular.** OML will form a **37°** angle with the head unit or table top. (See NOTE).
• Position the **midsagittal plane perpendicular** to the midline of the head unit or table, preventing rotation and/or tilting of head. (A way to check for rotation is to palpate the mastoid processes on each side and the lateral orbital margins with the thumb and finger tips and insure that the lines between these points are perpendicular to the film.)
• Center cassette to **acanthion.**

Central Ray:
• Align CR **perpendicular** to head unit or table.
• Center CR to cassette.
• SID: Head Unit, 36 in. (91 cm); Table Top, minimum 40 in. (102 cm).

Collimation: Use a 10 x 12 in. circle diaphragm or collimate to outer margins of skull on all sides.

Respiration: Suspend respiration during exposure.

NOTE: In this position, the average patient's nose tip will be **approximately** 3/4 in. (2 cm) away from the head unit or table.

Evaluation Criteria:
• Entire skull visualized on radiograph.
• Cranium seen without rotation:
  - Equal distance from midsagittal plane, identified by the bony nasal septum, to the outer skull margin on each side.
  - Equal distance from lateral orbital margins to the lateral margins of the skull.
• Inferior maxillary sinuses are free from superimposing maxillary alveolar processes.
• **Petrous ridges are below the maxillary sinuses.**

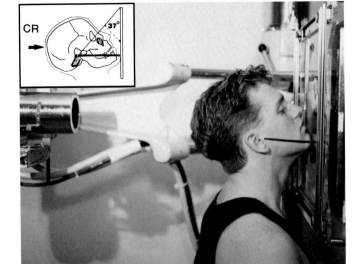

Parietoacanthial (Waters)   Fig. 12-50

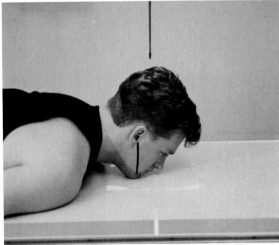

Parietoacanthial (Waters)   Fig. 12-51

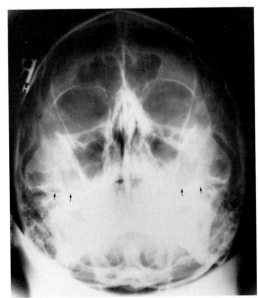

Parietoacanthial (Waters)   Fig. 12-52

Bony Nasal Septum

Inferior Orbital Rim

Zygomatic Bone

Zygomatic Arch

Petrous Ridge

Mastoid

Dens in Foramen Magnum

Maxillary Alveolar Process

Parietoacanthial (Waters)   Fig. 12-53

• Inferior orbital rim is clearly identified.
• Sufficient penetration and exposure, without motion, to visualize maxillary region.
• Patient ID information with R or L marker visible within collimated field without superimposing essential anatomy.

•Modified Parietoacanthial Projection
(Modified Waters Method)

Facial Bones
Optional
• **Modified Parietoacanthial**
  (Mod. Waters)
• PA Caldwell

Structure Best Shown:

Floor of orbits.

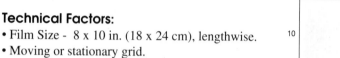

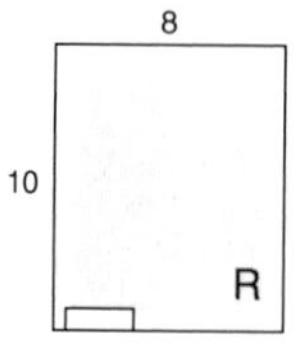

Technical Factors:
• Film Size - 8 x 10 in. (18 x 24 cm), lengthwise.
• Moving or stationary grid.
• 70-80 kVp range.
• Use small focal spot.

Patient Position:
• Remove all metal, plastic or other removable objects from head.
• Patient erect or prone. (Erect preferred if patient's condition allows.)

Part Position:
• Extend neck, resting chin and nose against head unit or table top.
• Adjust head until **OML forms a 55° angle** with the film. (A protractor should be used to determine precise angle.)
• Position **midsagittal plane perpendicular** to the midline of the head unit or table.
• Center cassette to **acanthion.**

Central Ray:
• Align CR **perpendicular** to head unit or table.
• Center CR to cassette.
• SID: Head Unit, 36 in. (91 cm).
        Table Top, minimum 40 in. (102 cm).

Collimation: Use an 8 x 10 in. circle diaphragm or collimate to within 1 in. (2.5 cm) of facial bones.

Respiration: Suspend respiration during exposure.

NOTE: This projection is excellent for evaluating the possibility of a "blow-out" fracture of the orbits.

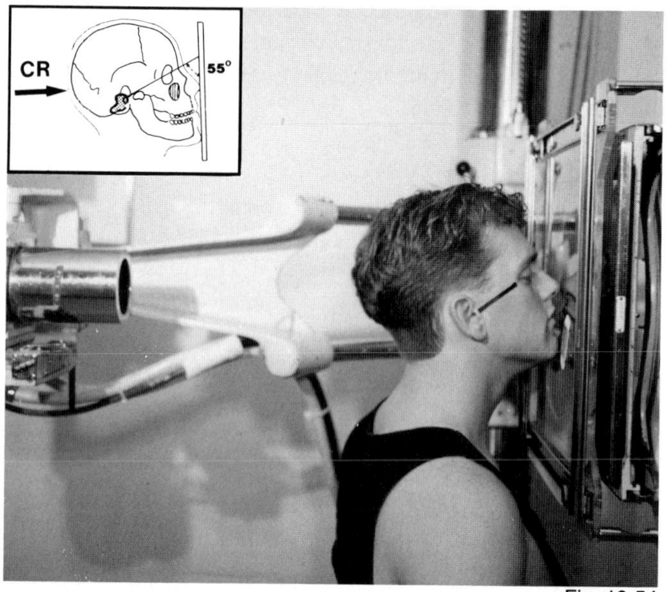

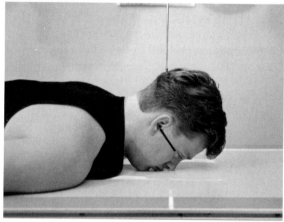

Modified Parietoacanthial (Waters)

Fig. 12-54

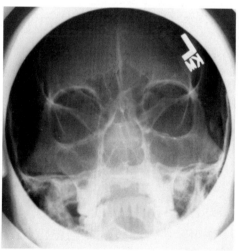

Fig. 12-55

Modified Parietoacanthial (Waters)

Evaluation Criteria:
• The inferior orbital rim is located in the center of the radiograph, with the entire orbital rim and maxillary bones within the collimated field.
• The cranium is not rotated:
  - Equal distance from the midsagittal plane, identified by the bony nasal septum, to the outer orbital margin on each side.
• **Petrous ridges** are projected into the **lower half of the maxillary sinuses, below the inferior orbital rim.**
• Sufficient penetration and exposure, without motion, to visualize the orbital floors.
• Patient ID information with R or L marker visible within collimated field without superimposing essential anatomy.

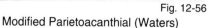

Fig. 12-56

Modified Parietoacanthial (Waters)

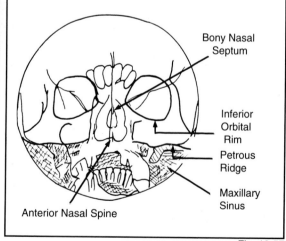

Bony Nasal Septum

Inferior Orbital Rim

Petrous Ridge

Maxillary Sinus

Anterior Nasal Spine

Fig. 12-57

Modified Parietoacanthial (Waters)

•PA Projection
(Caldwell Method)

Structures Best Shown:
Orbital rim, maxillae, nasal septum, zygomatic bones, and anterior nasal spine. (For floor of orbits, see NOTE below.)

Technical Factors:
• Film Size - 10 x 12 in. (24 x 30 cm), lengthwise.
  or
  8 x 10 in. (18 x 24 cm).
• Moving or stationary grid.
• 70-80 kVp range.
• Use small focal spot.

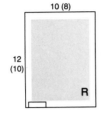

Patient Position:
• Remove all metal, plastic or other removable objects from head.
• Patient erect or prone. (Erect preferred if patient's condition allows.)

Part Position:
• Rest patient's nose and forehead against head unit or table top.
• Tuck chin, bringing **OML perpendicular** to head unit or table top.
• Align **midsagittal plane perpendicular** to midline of head unit or table top. (Insure no rotation or tilt of head.)
• Center cassette to **nasion.**

Central Ray:
• Angle **CR 15° caudal.** (See NOTE).
• Center CR to cassette.
• SID: Head Unit, 36 in. (91 cm).
  Table Top, minimum 40 in. (102 cm).

Collimation: Use an 8 x 10 in. circle diaphragm or collimate on all sides to within 1 in. (2.5 cm) of facial bones.

Respiration: Suspend respiration during exposure.

NOTE: Optional method if interest is in floor of orbits: Use a **30°** caudal angle to project the petrous ridges below the inferior orbital margin.

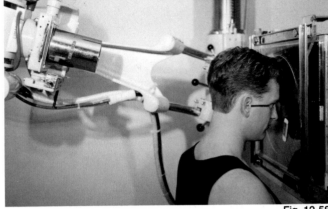
PA (Caldwell)   Fig. 12-58

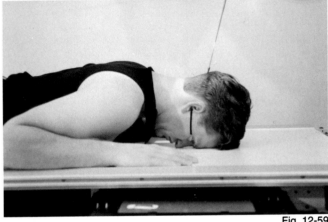
PA (Caldwell)   Fig. 12-59

Evaluation Criteria:
• The inferior orbital rim is located in the center of the radiograph, with the entire orbital rim and maxillary bones within the collimated field.
• Cranium is not rotated:
  - Equal distance from midsagittal plane, identified by the crista galli, to the outer orbital margin on each side.
  - Superior orbital fissures are symmetrically visualized within the orbits.

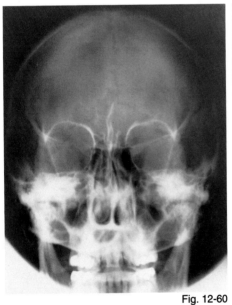
Fig. 12-60
PA (Caldwell)

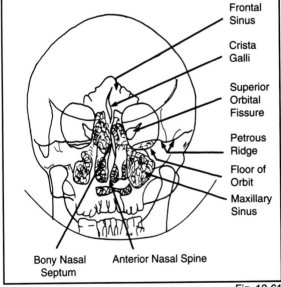
PA (Caldwell)   Fig. 12-61

Labels: Frontal Sinus, Crista Galli, Superior Orbital Fissure, Petrous Ridge, Floor of Orbit, Maxillary Sinus, Bony Nasal Septum, Anterior Nasal Spine

• **Petrous ridges** are projected into **lower one-third of orbits** with 15° caudal CR. (See NOTE.)
• Frontal sinus is projected above frontonasal suture.
• Sufficient penetration and exposure, without motion, to visualize maxillary region and orbital floor.
• Patient ID information with R or L marker visible within collimated field without superimposing essential anatomy.

•Trauma Lateral (Horizontal Beam)

Warning: It is essential that cervical spine fractures and dislocations are ruled out **before** attempting any manipulation of the patient's head or neck.

Facial Bones
Trauma
Basic
• **Lateral** (Horizontal Beam)
• Acanthioparietal
Optional
• Modified Acanthioparietal

Structures Best Shown:
Superimposed facial bones, greater wings of sphenoid, orbital roofs, sella turcica, and mandible.

Technical Factors:
- Film Size - 8 x 10 in. (18 x 24 cm).
- Place grid cassette on edge; lengthwise with patient.
- 70-76 kVp range.
- Use small focal spot.

Patient Position:
- Remove all metal, plastic or other removable objects from head.
- Patient in a supine recumbent position.
- Place grid cassette vertically against affected lateral cranium.

Part Position: (See NOTE below.)
- Adjust head into a **true lateral position**, relative to cassette.
- Align **midsagittal plane parallel** with grid cassette. (No rotation or tilt.)
- Position **interpupillary line perpendicular** to grid cassette.
- Adjust chin to align **infraorbitomeatal line perpendicular to front edge of cassette.**
- Adjust cassette, aligning cassette midline to **zygomatic prominence.**

Central Ray:
- A horizontal beam, which is essential for visualization of inner cranial air-fluid levels, is brought **perpendicular** to the cassette.
- Center CR to **cassette midline**, at a level **half way between outer canthus and EAM.**
- Minimum 40 in. (102 cm) SID.

Collimation: Use an 8 x 10 in. circle diaphragm or collimate on all sides to within 1 in. (2.5 cm) of nearest facial bone.

NOTE: Do not attempt to adjust or move head in any way with possible cervical spine injury.

Evaluation Criteria:
- The superimposed zygomatic bones are located in the center of the radiograph, with the EAM's and orbital roofs visualized within the collimated field.
- The cranium is not rotated:
  - The mandibular rami, the orbital roofs and the greater wings of the sphenoid are superimposed.
- Sufficient penetration and exposure, without motion, to visualize maxillary region.
- Patient ID information with R or L marker visible within collimated field without superimposing essential anatomy.

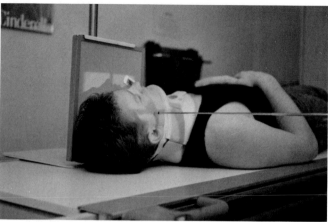

Trauma Lateral   Fig. 12-62

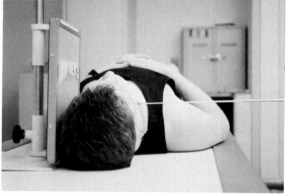

Trauma Lateral   Fig. 12-63

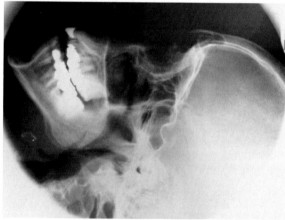

Trauma Lateral   Fig. 12-64

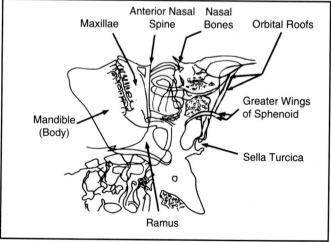

Trauma Lateral   Fig. 12-65

•Trauma Acanthioparietal
(Reverse Waters)

Facial Bones
Trauma
Basic
• Lateral (Horizontal Beam)
• **Acanthioparietal**

Warning: See following page for positioning with possible cervical spine injury wherein these same projections can be taken without any movement or adjustment of head or neck.

Structures Best Shown:
(Same as following page.)

Technical Factors:
- Film Size - 10 x 12 in. (24 x 30 cm), lengthwise.
  or 8 x 10 in. (18 x 24 cm).
- Moving or stationary grid.
- 70-80 kVp range.
- Use small focal spot.

Patient Position:
- Remove all metal, plastic or other removable objects from head.
- Patient in a supine recumbent position.
- If possible, slide patient onto x-ray table to utilize moving grid. If exam is performed on the cart, position a stationary grid under patient's head.

Part Position:
- Position the midsagittal plane **perpendicular** to the midline of the cassette.

Acanthioparietal: (Reverse Waters)
- Extend chin, bringing **mentomeatal line perpendicular** to cassette.
- OML will form a **37°** angle with the cassette.

Central Ray:
- Align CR **perpendicular** to cassette.
- Center CR to **acanthion.**
- Center cassette to CR.
- Minimum 40 in. (102 CM) SID.

Collimation: Use an 8 x 10 in. circle diaphragm or collimate to outer margins of skull on all sides.

Optional: A modified acanthioparietal (modified reverse Waters) may also be taken as shown in Fig. 12-67 by adjusting the head until the OML forms a **55° angle** with the cassette.

Evaluation Criteria:
- The inferior orbital rim is located in the center of the radiograph, with the entire orbital rim and maxillary bones within the collimated field.
- The cranium is visualized without rotation:
  - Equal distance from midsagittal plane, identified by the bony nasal septum, to the outer orbital margin on each side.
- Inferior orbital rim is clearly identified.
- Sufficient penetration and exposure, without motion, to visualize maxillary region.
- Patient ID information with R or L marker visible within collimated field without superimposing essential anatomy.

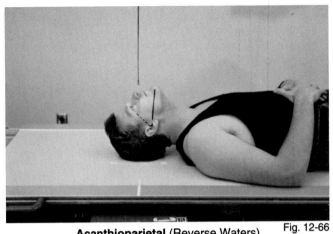

Acanthioparietal (Reverse Waters)   Fig. 12-66
– CR parallel to mentomeatal line and perpendicular to film.
– OML **37°** to film

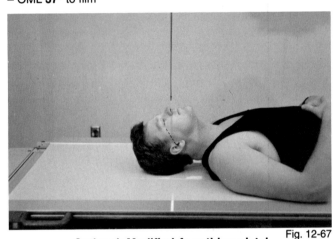

Fig. 12-67
Optional: Modified Acanthioparietal
(Modified Reverse Waters)
– CR perpendicular to film.
– OML **55°** to film

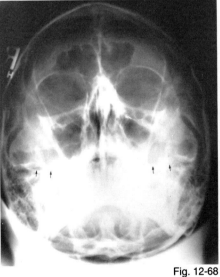

Fig. 12-68
Acanthioparietal

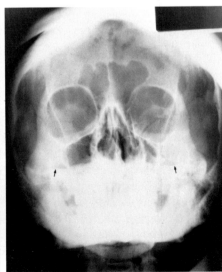

Fig. 12-69
Modified Acanthioparietal

Acanthioparietal:
- Petrous ridges (see arrows) are below the maxillary sinuses.

Modified Acanthioparietal:
- Petrous ridges are projected into the maxillary sinuses, below the inferior orbital rim.

•Trauma Acanthioparietal
(Reverse Waters)
Positioning **WITH** possible cervical spine injury

Warning: With possible cervical spine injury these two projections can be taken **without** any movement or adjustments of head or neck as described and demonstrated on this page.

Facial Bones
Trauma
Basic
• Lateral (Horizontal Beam)
• **Acanthioparietal**

Structures Best Shown:
Inferior orbital rim, maxillae, zygomatic bones, zygomatic arches, nasal septum, floor of orbits and anterior nasal spine.

Technical Factors:
* Film Size - 10 x 12 in. (24 x 30 cm), lengthwise.
  or 8 x 10 in. (18 x 24 cm).
* Moving or stationary grid.
* 70-80 kVp range.
* Use small focal spot.

Patient Position:
* Patient in a supine recumbent position.
* If possible, slide patient onto x-ray table as one complete unit. The head should never be raised to position a grid under patient. It is not necessary to remove cervical collar or backboard to obtain projections.
* Remove all metal, plastic or other removable objects from head.

Part Position:
* On patient with suspected cervical injury do **not** attempt to adjust head, mock position by angling the CR.
* Slide patient's entire body to bring midsagittal plane to midline of table.

Acanthioparietal Projection:
* Angle CR **cephalic** to align CR **parallel with mentomeatal line.** A **55°** angle will be formed between the CR and OML.

Central Ray:
* Center CR to **acanthion**, then center cassette to CR.
* Minimum 40 in. (102 cm) SID.

Collimation: Use an 8 x 10 in. circle diaphragm or collimate to within 1 in. (2.5 cm) of facial bones.

Optional: A modified trauma acanthioparietal (modified reverse Waters) may also be taken as shown in *Fig. 12-71* by first aligning the **CR parallel with the OML, then aligning 37° more cephalad.** If a 10° caudal angle is required to align the CR parallel with OML, then the final angle required for the modified acanthioparietal projection will be 27° cephalic. This results in 37° cephalic from OML.

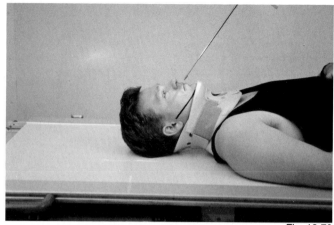

Acanthioparietal (Reverse Waters)
– CR parallel to mentomeatal line

Fig. 12-70

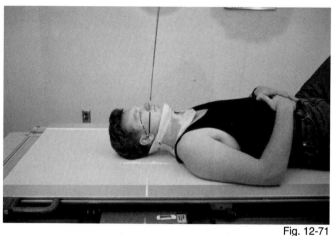

Fig. 12-71

Optional: Modified Acanthioparietal
(Modified Reverse Waters)
– CR 37° to OML

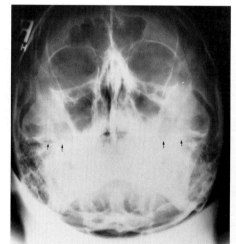

Fig. 12-72
Acanthioparietal

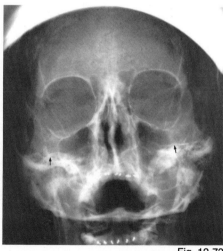

Fig. 12-73
Modified Acanthioparietal

Evaluation Criteria:
* The inferior orbital rim is located in the center of the radiograph, with the entire orbital rim and maxillary bones within the collimated field.
* The cranium is visualized without rotation:
  - Equal distance from midsagittal plane, identified by the bony nasal septum, to the outer orbital margin on each side.
* Inferior orbital rim is clearly identified.

* Sufficient penetration and exposure, without motion, to visualize maxillary region.
* Patient ID information with R or L marker visible within collimated field without superimposing essential anatomy.

Acanthioparietal:
* Petrous ridges are projected below the maxillary sinuses.

Modified Acanthioparietal:
* Petrous ridges are projected into the maxillary sinuses.

•Lateral Position

Structures Best Shown:

Nasal bone and soft tissue nose structures.

Both sides are generally taken for comparison, with the side closest to film demonstrated best.

Technical Factors:
- Film size - 8 x 10 in. (18 x 24 cm).
- Place film crosswise and divide in half.
- Detail screen, table top.
- 50-60 kVp range.
- Use small focal spot.

Patient Position:
- Remove all metal, plastic or other removable objects from head.
- Patient in an erect or prone position.

Part Position:
- Rest lateral side of head against head unit or table top, with side of interest closest to cassette.
- Position nasal bone to center of unmasked half of cassette.
- Adjust head into a **true lateral position,** oblique body as needed for patient's comfort.
- Align **midsagittal plane parallel** with head unit or table top.
- Align **interpupillary line perpendicular** to head unit or table top.
- Position **infraorbitomeatal line perpendicular** to front edge of cassette.

Central Ray:
- Align CR **perpendicular** to film.
- Center **1/2 in. (1.25 cm) inferior and posterior to nasion.**
- SID: Head Unit, 36 in. (91 cm).
    Table Top, minimum 40 in. (102 cm).

Collimation: Use a circle diaphragm or collimate on all sides to within 2 in. (5 cm) of nasal bone.

Respiration: Suspend respiration during exposure.

NOTE: To obtain a sharply detailed image of the nasal bone the utilization of a small focal spot, detail screen and close collimation is essential.

Evaluation Criteria:
- The nasal bone is located in the center of the unmasked half of film, with the nasal soft tissue, anterior nasal spine and frontonasal suture located within the collimated field.
- The nasal bone is demonstrated without rotation.
- Sufficient penetration and exposure, without motion, to visualize nasal bone and soft tissue structures.
- Patient ID information with R or L marker visible within collimated field without superimposing essential anatomy.

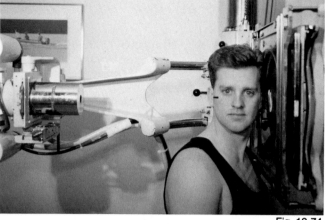

Lateral   Fig. 12-74

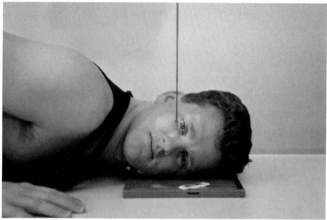

Lateral   Fig. 12-75

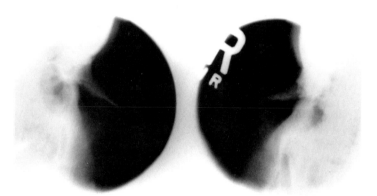

Lateral (R and L)   Fig. 12-76

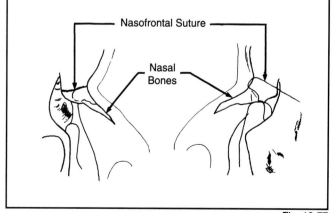

Lateral   Fig. 12-77

Nasal Bones

• Parietoacanthial Projection
(Waters Method)

Nasal Bones
Basic
• Lateral
• **Parietoacanthial (Waters)**

Structures Best Shown:
Bony nasal septum.

Technical Factors:
• Film Size - 8 x 10 in. (18 x 24 cm), lengthwise.
• Moving or stationary grid.
• 70-80 kVp range.
• Use small focal spot.

Patient Position:
• Remove all metal, plastic or other removable objects from head.
• Patient erect or prone. (Erect preferred if patient's condition allows.)

Part Position:
• Extend neck, resting chin against head unit or table top.
• Adjust head until **mentomeatal line is perpendicular** to film. OML will form a **37°** angle with head unit or table top. (See NOTE).
• Position the **midsagittal plane perpendicular** to the midline of the head unit or table (no rotation or tilt of head).
• Center cassette to **acanthion.**

Central Ray:
• Align CR **perpendicular** to film.
• Center CR to cassette.
• SID: Head Unit, 36 in. (91 cm).
    Table Top, minimum 40 in. (102 cm).

Collimation: Use an 8 x 10 in. circle diaphragm or collimate to outer margins of skull on all sides.

Respiration: Suspend respiration during exposure.

NOTE: In this position, the average patient's nose tip will be approximately 3/4 in. (2 cm) away from the head unit or table top. (However, do **NOT** use this nose-tip-film distance as a final positioning guage because of variations in nose size.)

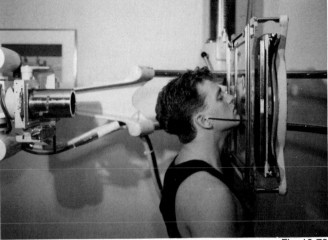

Parietoacanthial (Waters)   Fig. 12-78

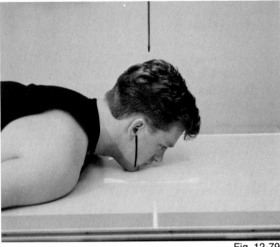

Parietoacanthial (Waters)   Fig. 12-79

Evaluation Criteria:
• The bony nasal septum is located in the center of the radiograph, with the maxillary and frontal sinuses visualized within the collimated field.
• Cranium is seen without rotation:
  - Equal distance from the midsagittal plane, identified by the bony nasal septum, to the outer orbital rim.
• Inferior maxillary sinuses are free from superimposing maxillary alveolar processes.
• Petrous ridges are below the maxillary sinuses.
• Inferior orbital rim is clearly identified.

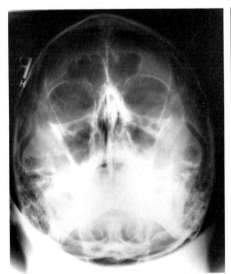

Parietoacanthial   Fig. 12-80

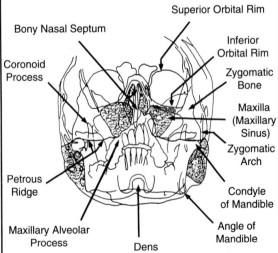

Parietoacanthial   Fig. 12-81

• Sufficient penetration and exposure, without motion, to visualize the bony nasal septum.
• Patient ID information with R or L marker visible within collimated field without superimposing essential anatomy.

•PA Projection
(Caldwell Method)

Nasal Bones
Optional
• **PA Caldwell**
• Superoinferior (Axial)

Structures Best Shown:
Bony nasal septum.

Technical Factors:
- Film Size - 8 x 10 in. (18 x 24 cm), lengthwise.
- Moving or stationary grid.
- 70-80 kVp range.
- Use small focal spot.

Patient Position:
- Remove all metal, plastic or other removable objects from head.
- Patient erect or prone. (Erect preferred if patient's condition allows.)

Part Position:
- Rest patient nose and forehead against head unit or table top.
- Tuck chin, bringing **OML perpendicular** to head unit or table top.
- Align **midsagittal plane perpendicular** to midline of head unit or table top. (Insure no rotation or tilt of head.)
- Center cassette to **nasion.**

Central Ray:
- Angle **CR 15° caudal.**
- Center CR to cassette.
- SID: Head Unit, 36 in. (91 cm).
       Table Top, minimum 40 in. (102 cm).

Collimation: Use an 8 x 10 in. circle diaphragm or collimate on all sides to within 1 in. (2.5 cm) of facial bones.

Respiration: Suspend respiration during exposure.

Evaluation Criteria:
- The bony nasal septum is located in the center of the radiograph, with the entire orbital rim and maxillary bones within the collimated field.
- Cranium is not rotated:
  - Equal distance from the midsagittal plane, identified by the crista galli, to the outer orbital margin on each side.
  - Superior orbital fissures are symmetrically visualized within the orbits.
- Petrous ridges are projected into lower one-third of orbits.
- Frontal sinus are projected above the frontonasal suture.
- Sufficient penetration and exposure, without motion, to visualize the bony nasal septum and vomer.
- Patient ID information with R or L marker visible within collimated field without superimposing essential anatomy.

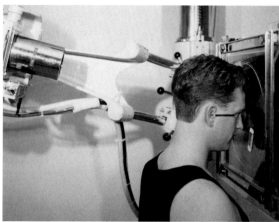

PA Caldwell — Fig. 12-82

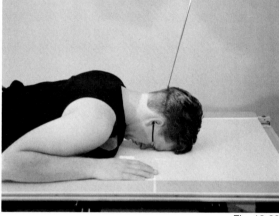

PA Caldwell — Fig. 12-83

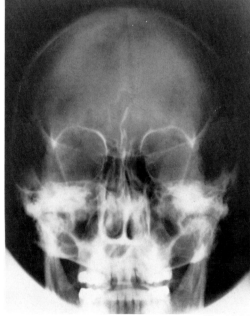

PA Caldwell — Fig. 12-84

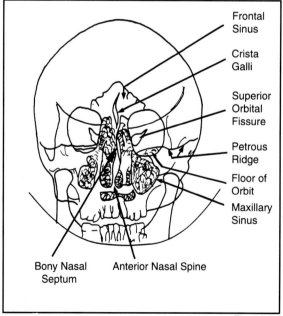

Frontal Sinus

Crista Galli

Superior Orbital Fissure

Petrous Ridge

Floor of Orbit

Maxillary Sinus

Bony Nasal Septum

Anterior Nasal Spine

PA Caldwell — Fig. 12-85

• Superoinferior (Axial) Projection

Nasal Bones
Optional
• PA Caldwell
• **Superoinferior (Axial)**

Structures Best Shown:
Nasal bones.

Technical Factors:
Film Size - Occlusal film packet.
        or 8 x 10 in. (18 x 24 cm), crosswise.
• Detail screen, table top.
• 50-60 kVp range.
• Use small focal spot.
• Accessories: Sponge or sand bag and occlusal film if available.

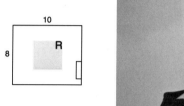

Patient Position:
• Remove all metal, plastic or other removable objects from head.
• Patient is seated in a chair at end of table or lying supine on table.

Part Position:
Upright Seated on Chair:
• Extend chin and rest on cassette. It may be necessary to incline cassette on sandbag as demonstrated to **place film perpendicular to glabelloaveolar line.** If occlusal film is used, have patient hold film between teeth extending it beyond nasal soft tissue.
• Align **midsagittal plane perpendicular** to cassette midline.
Supine:
• Elevate head on sponge.
• Position **midsagittal plane perpendicular** to table.
• If occlusal film is used, place between teeth, extend film beyond nasal soft tissue.
• Align film center to patient's midsagittal plane.
• **Glabelloalveolar line is perpendicular** to film.

Central Ray:
• Center CR to **glabelloalveolar line.** (CR must just skim glabella and anterior upper front teeth.)
• Minimum 40 in. (102 cm) SID.

Collimation: Collimate on all sides to within 1 in. (2.5 cm) of nasal bones.

Respiration: Suspend respiration during exposure.

NOTE: The occlusal film packet is the recommended method due to decreased OID.
• Any combination of prominent forehead, small nose or protruding front incisors may make visualization of the nasal bones impossible with this projection.

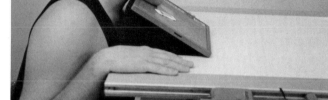
Superoinferior Projection   Fig. 12-86

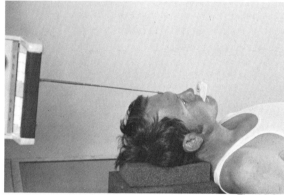
Fig. 12-87
Superoinferior Projection with Occlusal Film

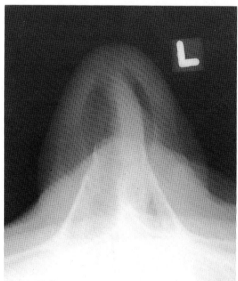
Superoinferior Projection   Fig. 12-88

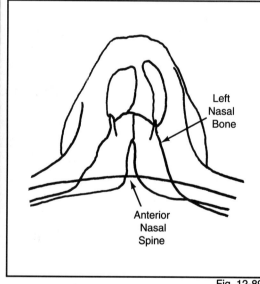

Left
Nasal
Bone

Anterior
Nasal
Spine

Superoinferior Projection   Fig. 12-89

Evaluation Criteria:
• Included on radiograph are nasal soft tissue and nasal bones.
• Nasal bones are visualized with little superimposition of the glabella or alveolar ridge.
• No rotation of nose: Equal distance from anterior nasal spine to outer soft tissue borders on each side.

• Sufficient penetration and exposure, without motion, to visualise nasal bones and nasal soft tissue.
• Patient ID information with R or L marker visible within collimated field without superimposing anatomy.

• Submentovertex (SMV) Projection
(Basilar Position)

> **Zygomatic Arch**
> Basic
> • **Submentovertex**
>   (Basilar)
> • Parietoacanthial
>   (Waters)

Structures Best Shown:
Bilateral zygomatic arches.

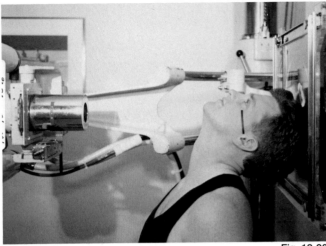

SMV Projection   Fig. 12-90

Technical Factors:
• Film Size - 8 x 10 in. (18 x 24 cm), lengthwise.
• Moving or stationary grid.
• 60-70 kVp range.
• Use small focal spot.

```
      8
   ┌──────┐
   │    R │
10 │      │
   │      │
   └──────┘
```

Patient Position:
• Remove all metal, plastic or other removable objects from head and neck.
• Patient in an erect position (or supine **only** if patient cannot maintain an erect position).
• Erect which is easier for patient may be done with dedicated head unit if available or with erect table or other erect grid-film holder device.

Part Position:
• Raise chin, hyperextending neck until **infraorbitomeatal line is parallel** to film. (See NOTE).
• Head rests on vertex of skull.
• Align **midsagittal plane perpendicular** to midline of head unit or vertical table, thus avoiding tilt and/or rotation.

Central Ray:
• Align CR **perpendicular** to film. (See NOTE).
• Center CR **midway between angles of mandible,** at a level **1.5 in.** (4 cm) **inferior to mandibular symphysis.**
• Center cassette to CR.
• SID: Head Unit, 36 in. (91 cm).
     Table Top, minimum 40 in. (102 cm).

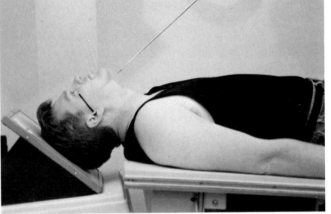

SMV Projection   Fig. 12-91

Collimation: Use an 8 x 10 in. circle diaphragm, or collimate to outer margins of skull on all sides.

Respiration: Suspend respiration during exposure.

NOTE: If patient is unable to sufficiently extend neck, angle CR **perpendicular to IOML.** With head unit the film can then also be angled as needed to maintain the film perpendicular to CR.
• Position is very uncomfortable for patient, move quickly.

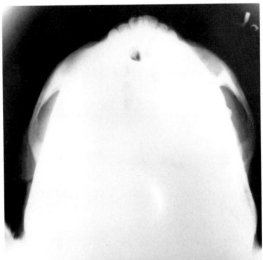

SMV Projection   Fig. 12-92

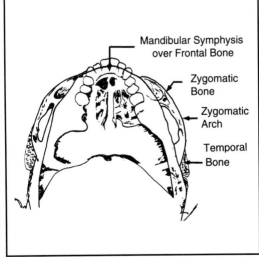

Mandibular Symphysis over Frontal Bone

Zygomatic Bone

Zygomatic Arch

Temporal Bone

SMV Projection   Fig. 12-93

Evaluation Criteria:
• Zygomatic arches are demonstrated, projecting laterally from each zygomatic and temporal bone, unless trauma prevents their visualization.
• Mandibular symphysis superimposes anterior frontal bone.
• Zygomatic arches are symmetrically visualized, without rotation.

• Sufficient penetration and exposure, without motion, to visualize zygomatic arches.
• Patient ID information and R or L marker visible within collimated field without superimposing essential anatomy.

• Parietoacanthial Projection
(Waters Method)

Zygomatic Arch
Basic
• Submentovertex
  (Basilar)
• **Parietoacanthial**
  (Waters)

Structures Best Shown:
Bilateral zygomatic bones and arches.

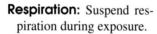

Technical Factors:
• Film Size - 8 x 10 in. (18 x 24 cm), lengthwise.
• Moving or stationary grid.
• 70-80 kVp range.
• Use small focal spot.

Patient Position:
• Remove all metal, plastic or other removable objects from head.
• Patient erect or prone. (Erect preferred if patient's condition allows.)

Part Position:
• Extend neck, resting chin against head unit or table top.
• Adjust head until **mentomeatal line is perpendicular** to head unit or table. OML will form a **37°** angle with head unit or table top. (See NOTE).
• Position the **midsagittal plane perpendicular** to the midline of the head unit or table (no rotation or tilt of head).
• Center cassette to **acanthion**.

Central Ray:
• Align CR **perpendicular** to film.
• Center CR to cassette.
• SID: Head Unit, 36 in. (91 cm).
        Table Top, minimum 40 in. (102 cm).

Collimation: Use an 8 x 10 in. circle diaphragm, or collimate to outer margins of skull on all sides.

Respiration: Suspend respiration during exposure.

NOTE: In this position, the average patient's nose tip will be **approximately** 3/4 in. (2 cm) away from the head unit or table.

Evaluation Criteria:
• Entire skull visualized on radiograph.
• Cranium seen without rotation:
  - Equal distance from midsagittal plane, identified by the bony nasal septum, to the outer skull margin on each side.
• Inferior maxillary sinuses are free from superimposing alveolar process.
• Petrous ridges are below the maxillary sinuses. Each ridge is seen projecting laterally, from the posterior alveolar process.
• Inferior orbital rim is clearly identified.

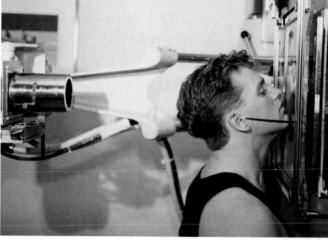

Parietoacanthial (Waters)   Fig. 12-94

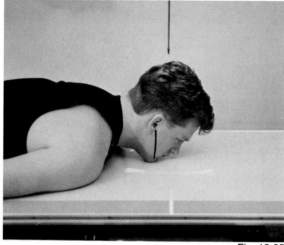

Parietoacanthial (Waters)   Fig. 12-95

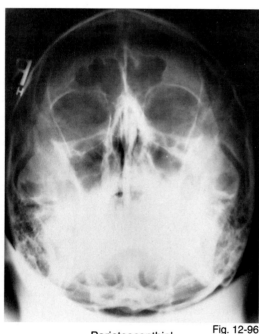

Parietoacanthial   Fig. 12-96

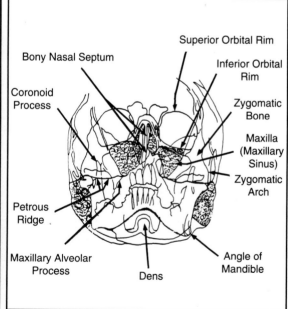

Parietoacanthial   Fig. 12-97

• Sufficient penetration and exposure, without motion, to visualize zygomatic bone and arches.
• Patient ID information with R or L marker visible within collimated field without superimposing essential anatomy.

• AP Axial Projection
(Modified Towne Method)

<table>
<tr><td>

Zygomatic Arch
Optional
• **AP Axial** (Towne)
• Oblique Axial
• Lateral

</td></tr>
</table>

Structure Best Shown:
Bilateral zygomatic arches.

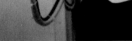

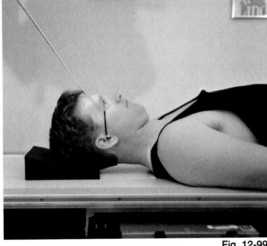

AP Axial   Fig. 12-98

Technical Factors:
• Film Size - 8 x 10 in. (18 x 24 cm), lengthwise.
• Moving or stationary grid.
• 60-70 kVp range.
• Use small focal spot.

Patient Position:
• Remove all metal, plastic or other removable objects from head.
• Patient in an erect or supine position.

Part Position:
• Rest patient's posterior skull against head unit or table top.
• Tuck chin, bringing **orbitomeatal line perpendicular** to film. (See NOTE below.)
• Align **midsagittal plane perpendicular** to midline of head unit or table top to prevent head rotation or tilting.

Central Ray:
• Angle CR **30° caudal**. (See NOTE).
• Center CR to 1 in. (2.5 cm) superior to **glabella.**
• Center cassette to CR.
• SID: Head Unit, 36 in. (91 cm).
  Table Top, minimum 40 in. (102 cm).

Collimation: Use an 8 x 10 in. circle diaphragm, or collimate to outer margins of skull on all sides.

Respiration: Suspend respiration during exposure.

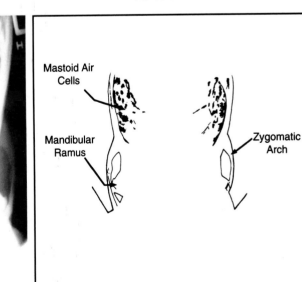

AP Axial   Fig. 12-99

NOTE: If patient is unable to depress the chin sufficiently to bring the OML perpendicular to the film, the infraobritomeatal line (**IOML**) can be placed perpendicular instead and the CR angle increased to 37° caudal. This maintains the 30° angle between OML and CR and demonstrates the same anatomical relationships. (There is a 7° difference between the OML and IOML.)

AP Axial   Fig. 12-100

Mastoid Air Cells

Mandibular Ramus

Zygomatic Arch

AP Axial   Fig. 12-101

Evaluation Criteria:
• Zygomatic arches are in center of radiograph, visualized lateral to each mandibular ramus.
• Zygomatic arches are seen without rotation:
  - Arches are not superimposing mandible.
  - Arches are symmetrical.

• Sufficient penetration and exposure, without motion, to visualize zygomatic arches.
• Patient ID information with R or L marker visible within collimated field without superimposing essential anatomy.

• Oblique Axial Position
(Tangential Projection)

Structures Best Shown:
Single zygomatic arch free of superimposition.

Both sides are generally taken for comparison.

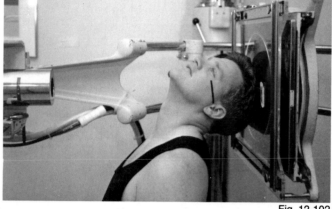

Oblique Axial   Fig. 12-102

Technical Factors:
• Film Size - 8 x 10 in. (18 x 24 cm), lengthwise. (May use one film crosswise divided in half or two single films lengthwise.)
• Moving or stationary grid.
• 60-70 kVp range.
• Use small focal spot.

Patient Position:
• Remove all metal, plastic or other removable objects from head.
• Patient in an erect position (or supine only if patient cannot maintain an erect position).
• Erect which is easier for patient may be done with dedicated head unit if available or with erect table or other erect grid-film holder device.

Part Position:
• Raise chin, hyperextending neck until **infraorbitomeatal line is parallel** to film. (See NOTE.)
• Rest head on vertex of skull.
• Turn head **15° toward side to be examined**; then tilt head to bring **midsagittal plane 15° toward side to be examined.**

Central Ray:
• Align **CR perpendicular** to film or IOML. (See NOTE):
• Center to **zygomatic arch of interest.** (CR will skim parietal eminence and body of mandible.)
• Center cassette to CR.
• SID: Head Unit, 36 in. (91 cm).
       Table Top, minimum 40 in. (102 cm).

Collimation: Use an 8 x 10 in. circle diaphragm or collimate on all sides to within 1 in. (2.5 cm) of zygomatic bone and arch.

Respiration: Suspend respiration during exposure.

NOTE: If patient is unable to sufficiently extend neck, angle CR **perpendicular to IOML.** With head unit the film can then also be angled as needed to maintain the film perpendicular to CR.
• Position is very uncomfortable for patient, move quickly.

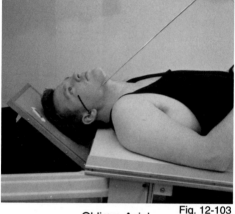

Oblique Axial   Fig. 12-103

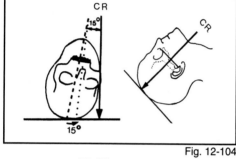

Fig. 12-104
− 15° Tilt
− 15° Rotation
− CR Perpendicular to IOML

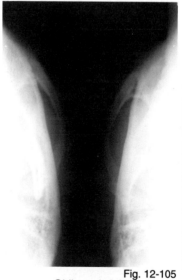

Fig. 12-105
Oblique Axial

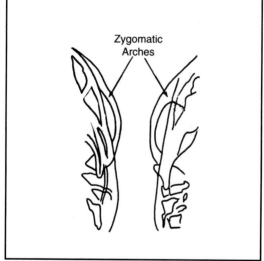

Zygomatic Arches

Fig. 12-106
Oblique Axial

Evaluation Criteria:
• Zygomatic arch visualized in the center of collimation field.
• Zygomatic arch is demonstrated **without superimposition of parietal or mandible.**
• Sufficient penetration and exposure, without motion, **to visualize zygomatic arch.**
• Patient ID information and R or L marker visible within collimated field without superimposing anatomy.

• Lateral Position

Zygomatic Arch
Optional
• AP Axial (Towne)
• Oblique Axial
• **Lateral**

Structures Best Shown:
Superimposed zygomatic arches.

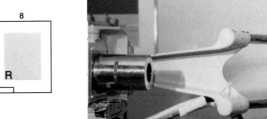

Technical Factors:
• Film Size - 8 x 10 in. (18 x 24 cm), lengthwise.
• Moving or stationary grid.
• 70-80 kVp range.
• Use small focal spot.

Patient Position:
• Remove all metal, plastic or other removable objects from head.
• Patient erect or prone. (Erect preferred if patient's condition allows.)

Part Position:
• Rest lateral side of head against head unit or table top, with side of interest closest to cassette.
• Adjust head into a **true lateral position,** oblique body as needed for patient's comfort.
• Align **midsagittal plane parallel** with head unit or table top.
• Align **interpupillary line perpendicular** to film.
• Adjust chin to bring **infraorbitomeatal line perpendicular** to front edge of cassette.

Central Ray:
• Align CR **perpendicular** to film.
• Center CR to the **zygomatic prominence.**
• Center cassette to CR.
• SID: Head Unit, 36 in. (91 cm).
          Table Top, minimum 40 in. (102 cm).

Collimation: Use an 8 x 10 in. circle diaphragm or collimate on all sides to within 1 in. (2.5 cm) of nearest facial bone.

Respiration: Suspend respiration during exposure.

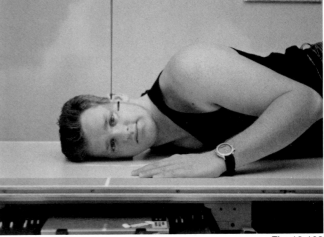

Lateral   Fig. 12-107

Lateral   Fig. 12-108

Evaluation Criteria:
• The superimposed zygomatic bones are located in the center of the radiograph, with the EAM's and orbital roofs visualized within the collimated field.
• The cranium is not rotated:
   - The mandibular rami, the orbital roofs and the greater wings of sphenoid are superimposed.
• Sufficient penetration and exposure, without motion, to visualize zygomatic bones.
• Patient ID information with R or L marker visible within collimated field without superimposing essential anatomy.

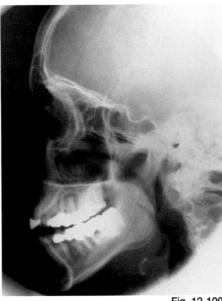

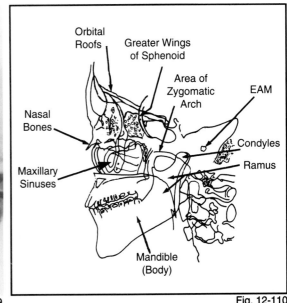

Orbital Roofs
Greater Wings of Sphenoid
Area of Zygomatic Arch
EAM
Nasal Bones
Condyles
Ramus
Maxillary Sinuses
Mandible (Body)

Fig. 12-109
Lateral

Fig. 12-110
Lateral

• Parieto-Orbital Projection
(Rhese Method)

Optic Foramina
Basic
• Parieto-orbital
(Rhese)

Structures Best Shown:
Cross section of each optic canal.

Both sides are generally taken for comparison.

Technical Factors:
- Film Size - 8 x 10 in. (18 x 24 cm).
- Crosswise, divided in half.
- Moving or stationary grid.
- 65-70 kVp range.
- Use small focal spot.

Patient Position:
- Remove all metal, plastic or other removable objects from head.
- Patient in an erect or supine position.
- Start by positioning patient as for a PA skull projection.

Part Position
- Oblique (rotate) head **37° toward side of interest.** Rest patient's **chin, cheek** and **nose** against head unit or table top. (See NOTE).
- Midsagittal plane will form a **53° angle** with film. (A protractor should be used to obtain an accurate angle.)
- Position **acanthiomeatal line perpendicular** to plane of film.
- Align entire interpupillary line on the same transverse plane.
- Center mid point of orbit, adjacent to head unit or table top, to center of unmasked half of cassette.

Central Ray:
- Align CR **perpendicular** to film.
- Center CR to unmasked half of cassette.
- SID: Head Unit, 36 in. (91 cm).
  Table Top, minimum 40 in. (102 cm).

Collimation: Use a circle diaphragm or collimate on all sides to yield a field size of approximately 4 in. (10 cm).

Respiration: Suspend respiration during exposure.

NOTE: • This is sometimes called a "three-point landing" position.
• A view of both orbits are taken for comparison on the same film. When positioning for the opposite orbit, oblique head in the opposite direction.
• To obtain a sharply detailed image of the optic foramen the utilization of a small focal spot and close collimation is essential.

Evaluation Criteria:
- The optic foramen is located in the center of unmasked half of film, with the orbital margins also included within the collimated field.
- **Optic foramen** is projected into the **lower outer quadrant of orbit.**
- Sufficient penetration and exposure, without motion, to visualize the optic foramen.
- Patient ID information with R or L marker visible within collimated field without superimposing essential anatomy.

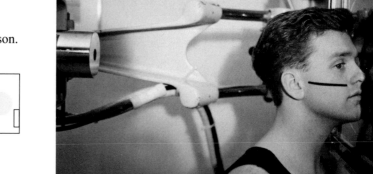

Parieto-orbital Projection — Fig. 12-111

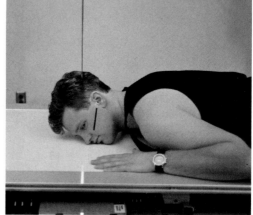

Parieto-orbital Projection — Fig. 12-112

- 37° Rotation
- Acanthiomeatal line 0°
- CR 0°

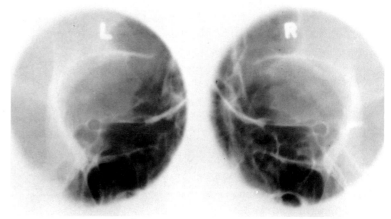

Bilateral Parieto-orbital — Fig. 12-113

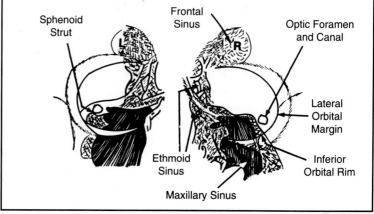

Sphenoid Strut · Frontal Sinus · Optic Foramen and Canal · Lateral Orbital Margin · Inferior Orbital Rim · Maxillary Sinus · Ethmoid Sinus

Bilateral Parieto-orbital — Fig. 12-114

• Modified Parietoacanthial Projection
(Modified Waters Method)

Structures Best Shown:
Floor of orbits and inferior orbital rim.

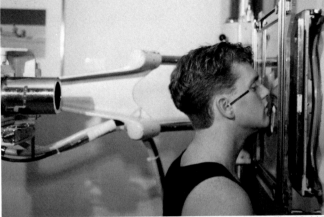

Modified Parietoacanthial   Fig. 12-115

Technical Factor:
• Film Size - 8 x 10 in. (18 x 24 cm), lengthwise.
• Moving or stationary grid.
• 70-80 kVp range.
• Use small focal spot.

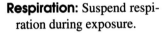

Patient Position:
• Remove all metal, plastic or other removable objects from head.
• Patient erect or prone. (Erect preferred if patient's condition allows.)

Part Position:
• Extend neck, resting chin and nose against head unit or table top.
• Adjust head until **OML forms a 55°** angle with the film. (A protractor should be used to determine precise angle.)
• Position **midsagittal plane perpendicular** to the midline of the head unit or table. (Insure no rotation or tilt of head.)
• Center cassette to **acanthion.**

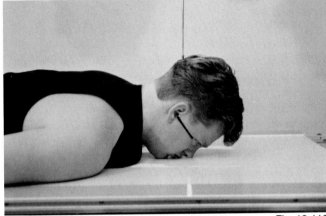

Modified Parietoacanthial   Fig. 12-116

Central Ray:
• Align CR **perpendicular** to film, then center CR to cassette.
• SID: Head Unit, 36 in. (91 cm).
       Table Top, minimum 40 in. (102 cm).

Collimation: Use an 8 x 10 in. circle diaphragm or collimate to within 1 in. (2.5 cm) of facial bones.

Respiration: Suspend respiration during exposure.

NOTE: This projection is excellent for evaluating the possibility of a "blow-out" fracture of the orbits.

Evaluation Criteria:
• The inferior orbital rim is located in the center of the radiograph, with the entire orbital rim and maxillary bones within the collimated field.
• The cranium is seen without rotation:
   - Equal distance from the midsagittal plane, identified by the anterior nasal spine and the bony nasal septum, to the outer orbital margin on each side.
   - Superior orbital fissures are symmetrically visualized within orbits.
• **Petrous ridges** are projected into **the lower maxillary sinuses, below the inferior orbital rim.**

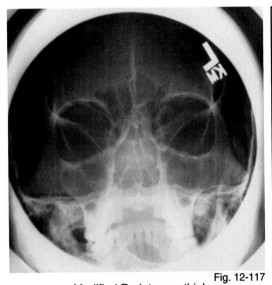

Modified Parietoacanthial   Fig. 12-117

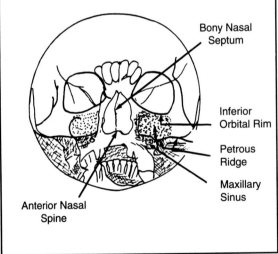

Modified Parietoacanthial   Fig. 12-118

(labels: Bony Nasal Septum, Inferior Orbital Rim, Petrous Ridge, Maxillary Sinus, Anterior Nasal Spine)

• Sufficient penetration and exposure, without motion, to visualize the orbital floors.
• Patient ID information with R or L marker visible within collimated field without superimposing essential anatomy.

• Axiolateral Projection
(Oblique Position)

Mandible
Basic
• **Axiolateral** (Oblique)
• PA

Structures Best Shown:
Mandibular rami, body and mentum of mandible positioned closest to film.

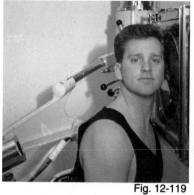

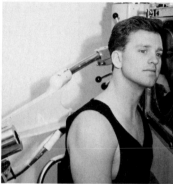

Fig. 12-119
Position for Ramus

Fig. 12-120
Position for Body

Technical Factors:
• Film Size - 8 x 10 in. (18 x 24 cm), crosswise.
• Moving or stationary grid.
• 70-80 kVp range.
• Use small focal spot

Patient Position:
• Remove all metal, plastic or other removable objects from head.
• Patient erect or supine. (Erect preferred if patient's condition allows.)

Part Position:
• Place head in a lateral position, with side of interest positioned closest to cassette.
• If possible, have patient close mouth and bring teeth together.
• Align **interpupillary line perpendicular** to head unit or table.
• Extend chin, to prevent cervical spine superimposition.
• Oblique (rotate) head. The degree of obliquity will depend on which section of the mandible is of interest. (Area of interest should be positioned parallel to film).
  - Head in **true lateral** position best demonstrates **ramus.**
  - Chin turned **30°** toward film best demonstrates **body.**
  - Chin turned **45°** toward film best demonstrates **mentum.**

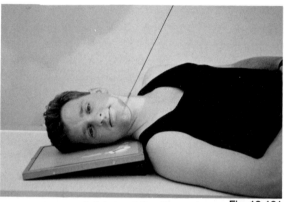

Axiolateral (for Ramus) Fig. 12-121

Central Ray:
• Angle CR **25° cephalic.**
• Direct CR to mandibular region of interest.
• Center cassette to CR.
• SID: Head Unit, 36 in. (91 cm).
    Table Top, minimum 40 in. (102 cm).

Collimation: Use a circle diaphragm or collimate on all sides to within 2 in. (5 cm) of mandible.

Respiration: Suspend respiration during exposure.

Evaluation Criteria:
• The mandible area of greatest interest is located in the center of the radiograph, with the entire mandible found within the collimated field.
• If radiograph taken in a true lateral position for the **ramus:**
  - Opposite mandible does not superimpose ramus of interest.
  - Ramus is visualized without superimposing the cervical spine.
  - Condylar and coronoid processes are well visualized.
  - Mandibular ramus is demonstrated without foreshortening.
• If radiograph is taken at 30° head rotation for the **body:**
  - Opposite mandible does not superimpose body of interest.

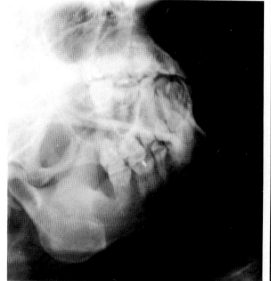

Axiolateral (for Ramus) Fig. 12-122

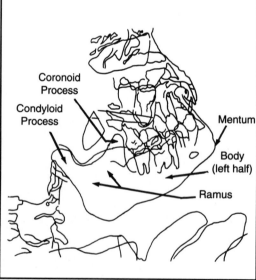

Coronoid Process
Condyloid Process
Mentum
Body (left half)
Ramus

Axiolateral (for Ramus) Fig. 12-123

  - Mandibular body is demonstrated without foreshortening.
• If radiograph is taken at 45° head rotation for the **mentum:**
  - Mentum area of interest is seen without superimposition.
  - Mandibular mentum is demonstrated without foreshortening.
• Sufficient penetration and exposure, without motion, to visualize the mandibular area of interest.
• Patient ID information with R or L marker visible within collimated field without superimposing essential anatomy.

Mandible

• PA Projection

Mandible
Basic
• Axiolateral (Oblique)
• **PA**

Structures Best Shown:
Mandibular rami and lateral portion of body.

Technical Factors:
- Film Size - 8 x 10 in. (18 x 24 cm), lengthwise.
- Moving or stationary grid.
- 70-80 kVp range.
- Use small focal spot.

Patient Position:
- Remove all metal, plastic or other removable objects from head.
- Patient erect or prone. (Erect preferred if patient's condition allows.)

Part Position:
- Rest patient's forehead and nose against head unit or table top.
- Tuck chin, bringing **OML perpendicular** to film.
- Align **midsagittal plane perpendicular** to midline of head unit or table top. (Insure no rotation or tilt of head.)
- Center cassette to **junction of lips**.

Central Ray:
- Align CR **perpendicular** to film.
- Center CR to cassette (to junction of lips).
- SID: Head Unit, 36 in. (91 cm).
      Table Top, minimum 40 in. (102 cm).

Collimation: Use an 8 x 10 in. circle diaphragm or collimate on all sides to within 1 in. (2.5 cm) of mandible.

Respiration: Suspend respiration during exposure.

Evaluation Criteria:
- Radiograph includes TMJ's, mandibular rami and mentum.
- Mandible is demonstrated without rotation:
  - Mandibular rami are symmetrically visualized on each side of the cervical spine.
- Midbody and mentum are faintly visualized, superimposing the cervical spine.
- Sufficient penetration and exposure, without motion, to visualize mandibular body and rami.
- Patient ID information with R or L marker visible within collimated field without superimposing essential anatomy.

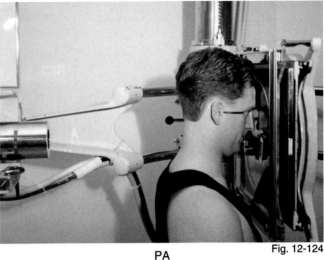

PA   Fig. 12-124

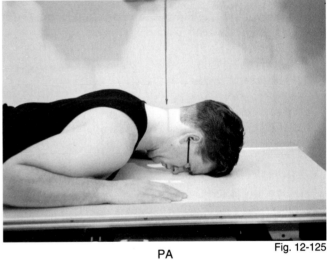

PA   Fig. 12-125

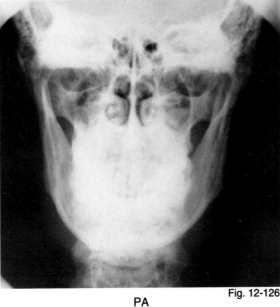

PA   Fig. 12-126

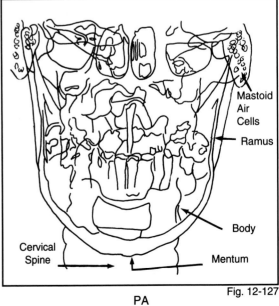

Mastoid Air Cells

Ramus

Body

Cervical Spine

Mentum

PA   Fig. 12-127

• AP Axial Projection
(Towne Method)

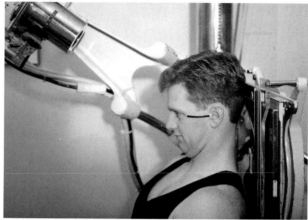

AP Axial   Fig. 12-128

Mandible
Optional
• **AP Axial (Towne)**
• PA Axial
• Panorex
•Submentovertex (basilar)

Structures Best Shown:
Condyloid processes of mandible and temporomandibular fossae.

Technical Factors:
• Film Size - 8 x 10 in. (18 x 24 cm), lengthwise.
• Moving or stationary grid.
• 70-80 kVp range.
• Use small focal spot.

Patient Position:
• Remove all metal, plastic or other removable objects from head.
• Patient in an erect or supine position.

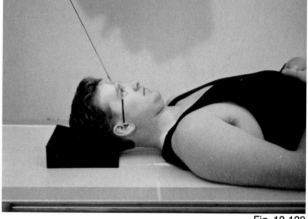

AP Axial   Fig. 12-129

Part Position:
• Rest patient's posterior skull against head unit or table top.
• Tuck chin, bringing **orbitomeatal line perpendicular** to film. (See NOTE).
• Align **midsagittal plane perpendicular** to midline of head unit or table top to prevent head rotation or tilting.

Central Ray:
• Angle CR **35-40° caudal**. (See NOTE).
• Center CR to **glabella**.
• Center cassette to CR.
• SID: Head Unit, 36 in. (91 cm).
        Table Top, minimum 40 in. (102 cm).

Collimation: Use an 8 x 10 in. circle diaphragm or collimate on all sides to within 1 in. (2.5 cm) of mandible.

Respiration: Suspend respiration during exposure.

NOTE: • If patient is unable to bring OML perpendicular to film, increase the CR angle as needed to result in 35-40° to the OML.
• If the area of interest is the TM fossae, angle 40° to the OML to reduce superimposing the TM fossae and mastoid portions of the temporal bone.

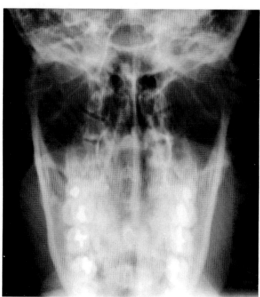

AP Axial   Fig. 12-130

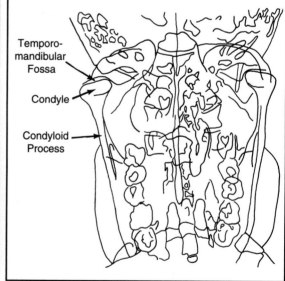

Temporo-mandibular Fossa

Condyle

Condyloid Process

AP Axial   Fig. 12-131

Evaluation Criteria:
• Included on the radiograph are the condyloid processes of the mandible and the temporomandibular fossae.
• Mandible is visualized without rotation:
  - Condyloid processes are symmetrically visualized on each side of cervical spine.
• Clear visualization of condyle and temporomandibular fossae relationship with minimal superimposition of the TM fossae and mastoid portions.
• Sufficient penetration and exposure, without motion, to visualize condyloid process and temporomandibular fossa.
• Patient ID information with R or L marker visible within collimated field without superimposing essential anatomy.

• PA Axial Projection
(Reverse Towne Method)

Structures Best Shown:
Mandibular condylar processes, rami and lateral portion of body.

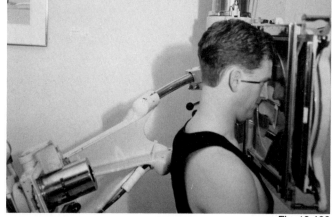

PA Axial — Fig. 12-132

Technical Factors:
• Film Size - 8 x 10 in. (18 x 24 cm), lengthwise.
• Stationary or moving grid.
• 70-80 kVp range.
• Use small focal spot.

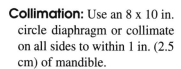

Patient Position:
• Remove all metal, plastic or other removable objects from head.
• Patient in an erect position or prone position.

Part Position:
• Rest forehead and nose against head unit or table top.
• Tuck chin, bringing **OML perpendicular** to film.
• Align **midsagittal plane perpendicular** to midline of head unit or table top to prevent rotation or tilt of the head.
• Center cassette to **acanthion.**

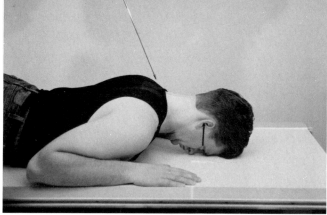

PA Axial — Fig. 12-133

Central Ray:
• Angle CR **20 to 25° cephalic** (see NOTE).
• Center CR to cassette.
• SID: Head Unit, 36 in. (91 cm).
          Table Top, minimum 40 in. (102 cm).

Collimation: Use an 8 x 10 in. circle diaphragm or collimate on all sides to within 1 in. (2.5 cm) of mandible.

Respiration: Suspend respiration during exposure.

NOTE: The 20-25° cephalic angle results in better visualization of the proximal rami and the condyles with less superimposition than with the basic PA projection and no angle.

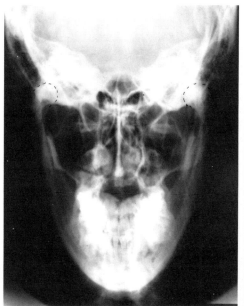

PA Axial — Fig. 12-134

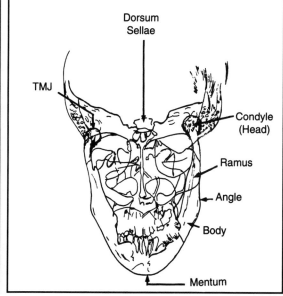

PA Axial — Fig. 12-135

Evaluation Criteria:
• Radiograph includes TMJ's, mandibular rami and mentum.
• Mandible is demonstrated without rotation. Mandibular rami are symmetrically visualized on each side of the cervical spine.
• Condylar processes are partially visualized. (Heads of condyles will be superimposed by mastoid processes.)
• Dorsum sellae is projected above the foramen magnum.
• Sufficient penetration and exposure, without motion, to visualize mandibular body and rami.
• Patient ID information with R or L marker visible within collimated field without superimposing essential anatomy.

• Panorex

Mandible
Optional
• AP Axial (Towne)
• PA Axial
• **Panorex**
• Submentovertex (basilar)

Structures Best Shown:
Teeth, mandible, nasal fossae, maxillary sinus, zygomatic arches and maxillae.

Technical Factors:
• Film Size - 9 x 12 in. (23 x 30 cm), crosswise.
• Curved nongrid cassette.
• 70-80 kVp range.

Unit Preparation:
• Attach cassette to panorex unit.
• Position tube and cassette at starting position.
• Raise chin rest to approximately same level as patient's chin.

Shielding: Wrap vest type lead apron around patient

Patient Position:
• Remove all metal, plastic or other removable objects from head and neck.
• Explain to patient how tube and film will rotate and the time span needed for exposure.
• Guide patient into unit resting patient's chin on bite block.
• Position patient's body, head and neck as demonstrated in *Figure 12-136*. Do not allow head and neck to stretch forward but have patient stand in close with spine straight and hips forward *(Fig. 12-139)*.

Part Position:
• Adjust height of chin rest until **IOML is aligned parallel with floor**. The occlusal plane (plane of biting surface of teeth) will decline 10° from posterior to anterior.
• Align **midsagittal plane** with the vertical center line of the chin rest.
• Position bite block between patient's front teeth. (See NOTE.)
• Instruct patient to place lips together and position tongue on roof of mouth.

Central Ray:
• X-ray beam direction is fixed and is directed slightly cephalic in order to project anatomical structures, positioned at the same height, on top of one another.
• Fixed SID as per panorex.

Collimation: A narrow vertical slit diaphragm is attached to tube, providing inherent collimation.

NOTE: When the temporomandibular joints are of interest, a second panorex is taken with the mouth open. This requires a larger bite block to be placed between the patient's teeth.

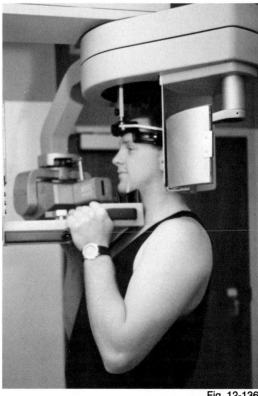

Fig. 12-136

Panorex – Head Correctly Positioned

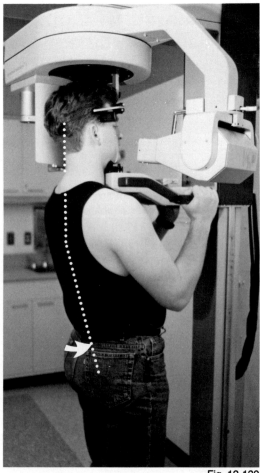

Fig. 12-139

Panorex – Correct Body Position

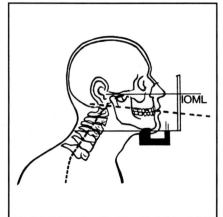

Incorrect Position   Fig. 12-137

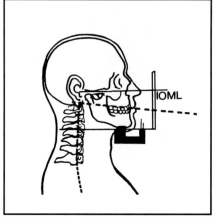

Correct Position   Fig. 12-138

(Courtesy of Siemens Co.)

Panorex continued

Evaluation Criteria:

- Included on radiograph is entire mandible, nasal fossae and maxillary sinuses.
- The mandible is oval in shape, with the mandibular symphysis projected slightly below the mandibular angles.
- The occlusal plane is aligned parallel with the long axis of radiograph.
- The upper and lower teeth are positioned slightly apart with no superimposition.
- A portion of the cervical spine is visualized on each side of the radiograph.
- The cervical spine is demonstrated erect without superimposing the temporomandibular joints.
- Mandible is visualized without rotation or tilting:
  - TMJ's are at the same level on the radiograph.
  - Rami and posterior teeth are equally magnified on each side.
  - Image is located in the center of film.
- The anterior and posterior teeth are sharply visualized with uniform magnification.
- Density of mandible and teeth are uniform across entire radiograph, no density loss is seen in center of radiograph.
- No artifacts are seen blurring over image.
- Patient ID information with R or L marker is visible within collimated field without superimposing essential anatomy.

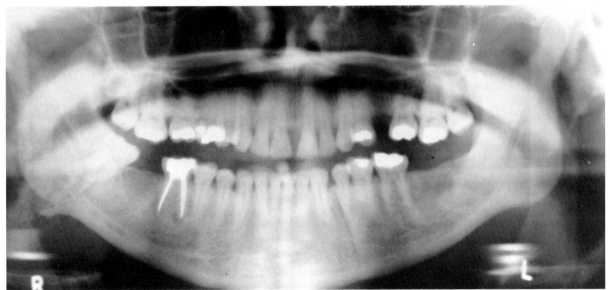

Panorex

Fig. 12-140

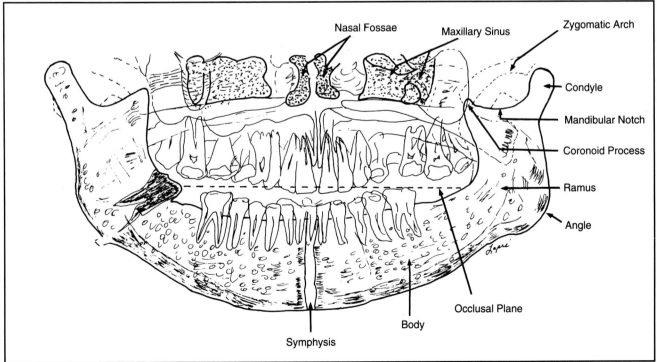

Nasal Fossae   Maxillary Sinus   Zygomatic Arch

Condyle

Mandibular Notch

Coronoid Process

Ramus

Angle

Occlusal Plane

Body

Symphysis

Panorex

Fig. 12-141

• Submentovertex (SMV) Projection
(Basilar Position)

Mandible
Optional
• AP Axial (Towne)
• PA Axial
• Panorex
• **Submentovertex** (basilar)

Structures Best Shown:
Mandible, coronoid and condyloid processes.

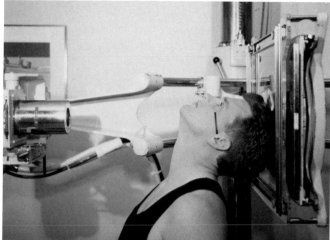
Submentovertex   Fig. 12-142

Technical Factors:
- Film Size - 8 x 10 in. (18 x 24 cm), lengthwise.
- Stationary or moving grid.
- 70-80 kVp range.
- Use small focal spot.

Patient Position:
- Remove all metal, plastic or other removable objects from head and neck.
- Patient in an erect position (or supine **only** if patient cannot maintain an erect position).
- Erect which is easier for patient may be done with dedicated head unit if available or with erect table or other erect grid-film holder device.

Part Position:
- Raise chin, hyperextending neck until **infraorbitomeatal line is parallel** to film.
- Rest head on vertex of skull.
- Align **midsagittal plane perpendicular** to midline of head unit or vertical table to prevent head rotation or tilt.

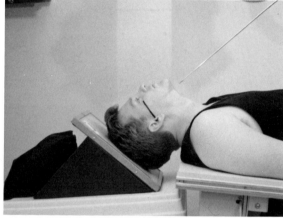
Submentovertex   Fig. 12-143

Central Ray:
- Align CR **perpendicular to film or IOML.** (See NOTE).
- Center CR to a point **midway between angles of mandible**, at a level **1.5 in.** (4 cm) **inferior to mandibular symphysis.**
- Center cassette to CR.
- SID: Head Unit, 36 in. (91 cm).
  Table Top, minimum 40 in. (102 cm).

Collimate: Use an 8 x 10 in. circle diaphragm or collimate to within 1 in. of mandible.

Respiration: Suspend respiration during exposure.

NOTE:
- If patient is unable to sufficiently extend neck, angle tube **perpendicular to IOML.** With head unit the film can then also be angled as needed to maintain the film perpendicular to CR.
- This position is very uncomfortable for patient, move quickly.

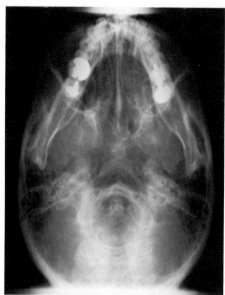
Fig. 12-144
Submentovertex

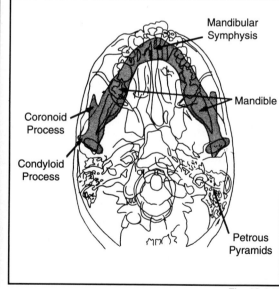
Submentovertex   Fig. 12-145

Mandibular Symphysis

Mandible

Coronoid Process

Condyloid Process

Petrous Pyramids

Evaluation Criteria:
- Entire mandible is visualized on radiograph.
- Mandibular symphysis superimposes anterior frontal bone.
- Cranium is not rotated: Distance along coinciding mandibular surfaces to lateral border of skull are equal.

- Mandibular condyles are projected anterior to petrous ridges.
- Mandibular coronoid processes are visualized, projecting lateral from the rami area, on each side of mandible
- Sufficient penetration and exposure, without motion, to visualize entire mandible.
- Patient ID information and R or L marker visible within collimated field without superimposing essential anatomy.

• Axiolateral Oblique Position
(Law Method)

TMJ's
Basic
• **Axiolateral Oblique**
(Law)
or
Axiolateral (Schuller)

Technical Factors:
• Film Size - 2 each 8 x 10 in. (18 x 24 cm), lengthwise.
      or 8 x 10 in. crosswise divided in half.
• Stationary or moving grid.
• 70-80 kVp range.
• Use small focal spot and detail screen.

Patient Position:
• Remove all metal, plastic or other removable objects from head.
• Patient erect or prone. (Erect preferred if patient's condition allows.)

Shielding: Secure lead shield around waist to protect gonads.

Part Position:
• Rest lateral side of head against head unit or table top, with side of interest closest to cassette.
• Adjust head into a **true lateral position,** oblique body as needed for patient's comfort.
• Align **midsagittal plane parallel** with head unit or table top.
• Align **interpupillary line perpendicular** to film.
• Position **infraorbitomeatal line perpendicular** to front edge of cassette.
• From lateral position, **rotate face toward head unit or table top 15°.**
• Do not allow chin to tilt inward toward cassette.
• Center cassette to TMJ positioned adjacent to cassette, located **1 in. anterior to EAM.**

Central Ray:
• Angle CR **15° caudal.**
• Center CR to cassette. Table Top, center CR 1.5 in. (4 cm) superior to upside EAM.
• SID: Head Unit, 36 in. (91 cm). Table Top, minimum 40 in. (102 cm).

Collimation: Use a circle diaphragm or collimate on all sides to yield a field size of approximately 4 in. (10 cm).

Respiration: Suspend respiration during exposure.

Structures Best Shown:
Temporomandibular joint closest to film. (Generally taken bilateral with open and closed mouth positions.)

or

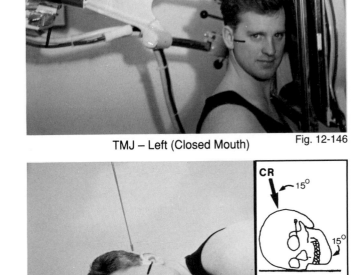

TMJ – Left (Closed Mouth)   Fig. 12-146

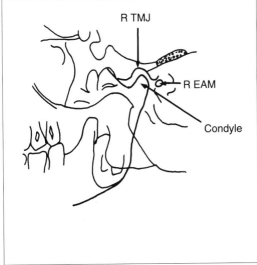

Fig. 12-147
TMJ – Right
– 15° Oblique (Head Rotation)
– 15° Caudal Angle

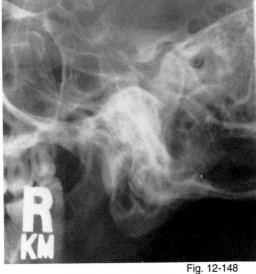

TMJ – Closed Mouth   Fig. 12-148

Fig. 12-149
TMJ – Closed Mouth

R TMJ

R EAM

Condyle

Evaluation Criteria:
• TMJ closest to film is located in the center of collimation field.
• TMJ closest to film is clearly demonstrated without superimposition of opposite TMJ.
• TMJ of interest does not superimpose cervical spine.
• On closed mouth radiograph, condyle will lie within mandibular fossa.

• On open mouth radiograph, condyle will move anterior within the mandibular fossa.
• Sufficient penetration and exposure, without motion, to visualize TMJ.
• Patient ID information with R or L marker visible within collimated field without superimposing essential anatomy.

• Axiolateral Position
(Schuller Method)

TMJ's
Basic
• Axiolateral Oblique
  (Law)
  or
Axiolateral (Schuller)

Structures Best Shown:
Temporomandibular joint closest to film. (Generally taken bilateral with open and closed mouth positions.)

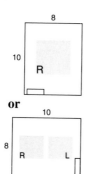

Technical Factors:
• Film Size - 2 each 8 x 10 in. (18 x 24 cm), lengthwise.
  or 8 x 10 in. crosswise divided in half.
• Moving or stationary grid.
• 70-80 kVp range.
• Use small focal spot and detail screen.

Patient Position:
• Remove all metal, plastic or other removable objects from head.
• Patient in an erect or prone position.

Part Position:
• Rest lateral side of head against head unit or table top, with side of interest closest to cassette.
• Adjust head into a **true lateral position**, oblique body as needed for patient's comfort.
• Align **interpupillary line perpendicular** to film.
• Align **midsagittal plane parallel** with head unit or table top.
• Position **infraorbitomeatal line perpendicular** to front edge of cassette.
• Center cassette to TMJ positioned adjacent to cassette, located **1 in. anterior to EAM.**

Central Ray:
• Angle CR **25° to 30° caudal.**
• Center CR to cassette. Table Top , center CR 1 in (2.5 cm) anterior and 2 in. (5 cm) superior to upside EAM.
• SID: Head Unit, 36 in. (91 cm).
  Table Top, minimum 40 in. (102 cm).

Collimation: Use a circle diaphragm or collimate on all sides to yield a field size of approximately 4 in. (10 cm).

Respiration: Suspend respiration during exposure.

Evaluation Criteria:
• TMJ closest to film is located in the center of the radiograph.
• TMJ closest to film is visualized anterior to EAM.
• On closed mouth radiograph, condyle will lie within mandibular fossa.
• On open mouth radiograph, condyle will move anterior within fossa.
• Sufficient penetration and exposure, without motion, to visualize TMJ.
• Patient ID information with R or L marker visible within collimated field without superimposing essential anatomy.

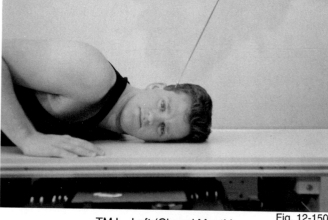

TMJ – Left (Closed Mouth)
– True Lateral
– 25-30° Caudal Angle   Fig. 12-150

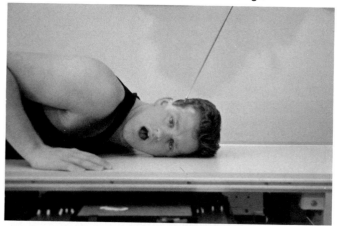

Open Mouth   Fig. 12-151

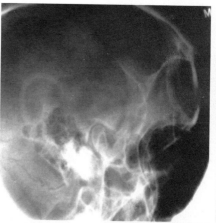

Closed Mouth   Fig. 12-152

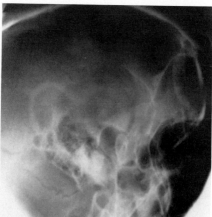

Open Mouth   Fig. 12-153

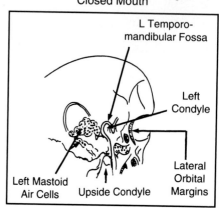

L Temporo-mandibular Fossa
Left Condyle
Lateral Orbital Margins
Left Mastoid Air Cells   Upside Condyle
Closed Mouth   Fig. 12-154

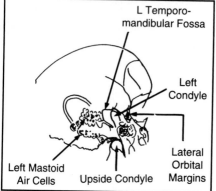

L Temporo-mandibular Fossa
Left Condyle
Lateral Orbital Margins
Left Mastoid Air Cells   Upside Condyle
Open Mouth   Fig. 12-155

• AP Axial Projection
(Towne Method)

> **TMJ's**
> Optional
> • **AP Axial** (Towne)
> • Tomography
> • Panorex

Structures Best Shown:
Condyloid processes of mandible and temporomandibular fossae.

Technical Factors:
• Film Size - 8 x 10 in. (18 x 24 cm), lengthwise.
• Moving or stationary grid.
• 70-80 kVp range.
• Use small focal spot.

Patient Position:
• Remove all metal, plastic or other removable objects from head.
• Patient in an erect or supine position.

Part Position:
• Rest patient's posterior skull against head unit or table top.
• Tuck chin, bringing **orbitomeatal line perpendicular** to head unit or table top. (See NOTE).
• Align **midsagittal plane perpendicular** to midline of head unit or table top to prevent head rotation or tilt.

Central Ray:
• Angle CR **35° caudal from the orbitomeatal line.** (See NOTE).
• Center CR to midsagittal plane at a level approximately 1.5 in. (3.75 cm) **above the superciliary arch.**
• Center cassette to CR.
• SID: Head Unit, 36 in. (91 cm).
   Table Top, minimum 40 in. (102 cm).

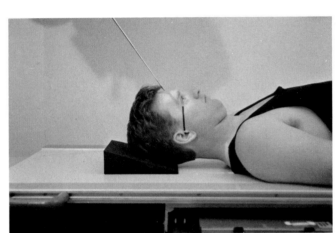

AP Axial – CR 35° to OML   Fig. 12-156

AP Axial – CR 35° to OML   Fig. 12-157

Collimation:
Use an 8 x 10 in. circle diaphragm or collimate on all sides to mandible.

Respiration:
Suspend respiration during exposure.

NOTE: • An increased CR angle to 40° may best demonstrate the TM fossae and joint area on some patients.

Evaluation Criteria:
• Included on the radiograph are the condyloid processes of the mandible and the temporomandibular fossae.
• Mandible is visualized without rotation:
 - Condyloid processes are symmetrically visualized on each side of cervical spine.
• Clear visualization of condyle and temporomandibular fossae relationship.

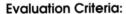

AP Axial   Fig. 12-158

Mastoid Air Cells
Temporomandibular Fossa
Condyle (Head)
Condyloid Process
Ramus

AP Axial   Fig. 12-159

• Sufficient penetration and exposure, without motion, to visualize condyloid process and temporomandibular fossa.
• Patient ID information with R or L marker visible within collimated field without superimposing essential anatomy.

•Tomography
•Panorex - see mandible pages

•Panorex - see mandible pages

TMJ's
Optional
• AP Axial (Towne)
• **Tomography**
• **Panorex**

Structures Best Shown:
Condyloid process of mandible and temporomandibular fossae. (Generally taken bilateral with open and closed mouth positions.)

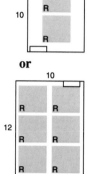

Technical Factors:
• Film Size - 8 x 10 in. (18 x 24 cm), or 10 x 12 in. (24 x 30 cm), lengthwise.
• Moving grid.
• Low kVp range to produce high contrast.
• Long exposure time to provide time for machine movement.
• Small focal spot.

Unit Preparation:
• With x-ray tube perpendicular to table, connect x-ray source to film holder.
• Set the most complex motion available in your facility.
• Use a wide tube angle in order to obtain thin cuts of the TMJ's.
• Place a pad on table for patient's comfort.

Shielding: Place a vest type lead shield over patient.

Patient Preparation:
• Remove all metal, plastic or other removable objects from head.
• Explain to patient how tube will move during the exposure and the importance of holding still while radiographs are being taken, as well as in between radiographs.
• Patient in a prone position.
• Rest lateral side of head against table top, with side of interest placed up, away from the cassette if this is the side to be in focus at the set fulcrum height.

Part Position:
• Adjust head into a **true lateral position**, oblique body as needed for patient's comfort.
• Align **interpupillary line perpendicular** to table top.
• Align **midsagittal plane parallel** with table top.
• Position **infraorbitomeatal line perpendicular** to front edge of cassette.
• Instruct patient to close mouth.
• Use radiolucent sponges, tape, etc. where needed to help patient maintain position.

Central Ray:
• Center to a point **1/2 in.** (1.3 cm) **anterior to the EAM.**
• Mark centering point on patient, with a water soluble marker, to assure centering between radiographs.
• Position tube and cassette to starting position.
• Take 3 scout tomograms, vary fulcrum height between exposures.
  - **1st radiograph**: take with the fulcrum set at the **level of the outer canthus** of affected TMJ.
  - **2nd radiograph**: take a cut **5 mm above** initial radiograph.
  - **3rd radiograph**: take a cut **5 mm below** initial radiograph.
• Mark radiograph with a R or L marker and fulcrum height used.

Collimation: Tightly collimate to TMJ.

Respiration: Suspend respiration during exposure.

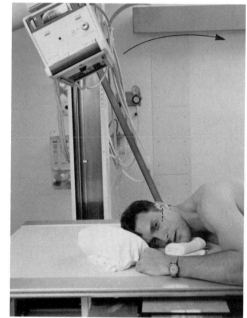

TMJ Tomogram   Fig. 12-160

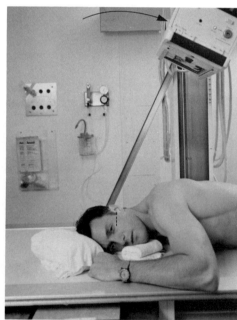

TMJ Tomogram   Fig. 12-161

Tomography continued

Evaluation Criteria:

- The TMJ is located in the center of the radiograph, with the condyloid process and EAM included within the collimated field.
- The cranium is visualized without rotation.
- The condyloid process and tempormandibular fossae are clearly visualized, in focus, on at least one radiographic cut.
- Sufficient penetration and exposure, without motion, to visualize temporomandibular joint.

- Patient ID information with R or L marker visible within collimated field without superimposing essential anatomy.

Closed Mouth:
- Condyle lies within the mandibular fossa.

Open Mouth:
- Condyle is visualized anterior to the mandibular fossa.

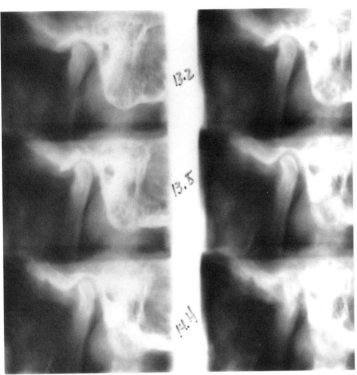

Fig. 12-162

Closed Mouth (Right TMJ)

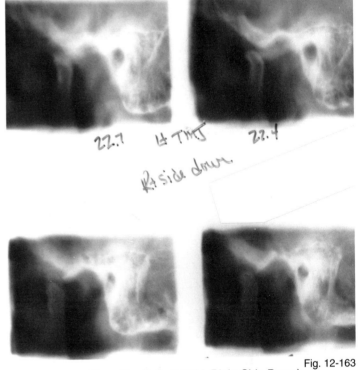

Fig. 12-163

Open Mouth (Left TMJ, Right Side Down)

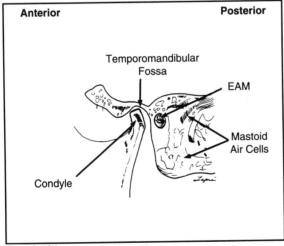

Fig. 12-164

Closed Mouth

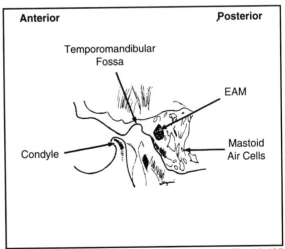

Fig. 12-165

Open Mouth

Chapter 13

Radiographic Anatomy and Positioning of the Paranasal Sinuses, Mastoids and Temporal Bone

Contributions by: Kathy M. Martensen, BS, RT (R)
Barry T. Anthony, RT (R)

Contents

Paranasal Sinuses

Part I Radiographic Anatomy

Skull

The skull is the bony skeleton of the head and includes the 8 cranial bones and the 14 facial bones, the anatomy of which were described in chapters 11 and 12. Two exceptions which were not described are the **paranasal sinuses** and portions of the temporal bone, namely the **mastoid** and **petrous portions**. The petrous portion contains the organs of hearing and equilibrium. This anatomy and related radiographic positioning for these parts will be described and illustrated in this chapter.

Paranasal Sinuses

The large, air-filled cavities of the paranasal sinuses are sometimes called the accessory nasal sinuses because they are lined with mucous membrane continuous with that of the nasal cavity. These sinuses are divided into four groups according to the bones wherein they are contained:

1. **Maxillary (2)**   - maxillary (facial) bones
2. **Frontal** (usually 2)   - frontal (cranial) bone
3. **Ethmoid** (many)   - ethmoid (cranial) bone
4. **Sphenoid** (1 or 2)   - sphenoid (cranial) bone

Only the maxillary sinuses are part of the facial bone structure. The frontal, ethmoid and sphenoid are contained within the respective cranial bones.

The paranasal sinuses begin developing in the fetus but only the maxillary sinuses exhibit a definite cavity at birth. The frontal and sphenoid sinuses begin to be visible on radiographs at age six or seven, and the ethmoid sinuses develop last. All the paranasal sinuses are generally fully developed by the late teenage years.

Each of these groups of sinuses will be studied beginning with the largest, the maxillary sinuses.

1. Maxillary Sinuses

The large **maxillary sinuses** are paired structures, one being located within the body of each maxillary bone. An older term for maxillary sinus is antrum, an abbreviation of "Antrum of Highmore". (Named after Nathaniel Highmore (1613-1685) an English physician.) Each maxillary sinus is shaped somewhat like a pyramid on a frontal view. Laterally they appear more cubical in shape. The average total vertical dimension is between 3 and 4 cm, and the other dimensions are between 2.5 and 3 cm.

The bony walls of the maxillary sinuses are thin. The floor of each maxillary sinus is slightly below the level of the floor of each nasal fossa, although the two sinuses are variable in size from one person to another and from one side to the other.

All of the paranasal sinus cavities communicate with each other and with the **nasal cavity,** which is divided into two equal chambers or **fossae.** In the case of the maxillary sinuses, this site of communication is located at the upper or superior aspect of the sinus cavity itself, as demonstrated in *Fig. 13-3*. Therefore, when a person is erect, any mucus or fluid trapped within the sinus will tend to stay there and layer out, forming an air-fluid level. Therefore radiographic positioning of the paranasal sinuses should be accomplished with the patient in the **erect position** to demonstrate any possible air-fluid levels.

Projecting into the floor of each maxillary sinus are several conical elevations relating to roots of the first and second upper molar teeth. Occasionally, the floor is perforated by one or more of these roots and infections originating in the teeth, particularly the molars and premolars, may travel upward into the maxillary sinus.

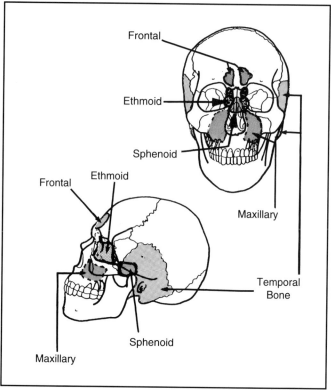

Skull – Paranasal Sinuses and Temporal Bone   Fig. 13-1

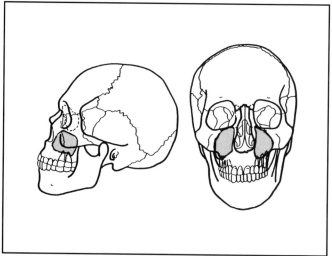

Maxillary Sinuses   Fig. 13-2

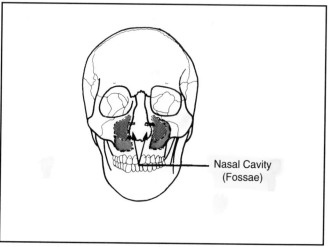

Maxillary Sinuses   Fig. 13-3

2. Frontal Sinuses

The **frontal sinuses** are located between the inner and outer tables of the skull, posterior to the glabella. Whereas the maxillary sinuses are always paired and are usually fairly symmetrical in size and shape, the frontal sinuses are rarely symmetrical. The frontal sinuses are usually separated by a septum which deviates from one side to the other or may even be absent entirely resulting in one single cavity. Generally however there are two cavities with a wide variation in their sizes and shapes. They are generally larger in men than in women.

The frontal sinuses which rarely become aerated before age six communicate with the nasal cavity by way of a duct which empties into the anterior part of the mid nasal cavity or meatus. The size or even the presence of of the frontal sinuses vary greatly among individuals. They may be only singular on either the right or left side only, or they may be paired as shown, or they may even be totally absent.

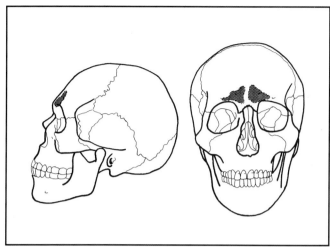

Frontal Sinuses

Fig. 13-4

3. Ethmoid Sinuses

The **ethmoid sinuses** are made up of many air cells contained within the lateral masses or labyrinths of the ethmoid bone. These air cells are grouped into anterior, middle and posterior collections, but they all intercommunicate. These cells also communicate with the nasal cavities via a single passageway from each side.

As seen from the side, it would appear that the anterior ethmoid sinuses fill the orbits. A portion of these sinuses are medial to the orbits, however, and are contained in the lateral masses of the ethmoid bone, which helps to form the medial wall of each orbit.

The ethmoid sinuses extend posteriorly within the labyrinths to communicate with the sphenoid sinuses contained in the sphenoid bone.

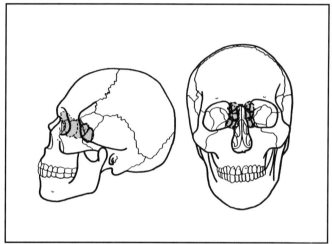

Ethmoid Sinuses

Fig. 13-5

4. Sphenoid Sinuses

The **sphenoid sinus** lies in the body of the sphenoid bone, directly below the sella turcica. The body of the sphenoid containing these sinuses is cubical in shape and is frequently divided by a thin septum to form two cavities. This septum may be incomplete or absent entirely, however resulting in only one cavity. If there are two cavities or sinuses, they are generally asymmetrical in shape. Anteriorly the sphenoid sinuses communicate through rounded openings with the spheno-ethmoidal recess of the nasal cavity.

Since the sphenoid sinuses are so close to the base or floor of the cranium, sometimes a pathologic process makes its presence known by its effect on these sinuses. An example of this occurrence is the demonstration of an air-fluid level within the sphenoid sinuses following skull trauma. This demonstration could be the only radiographic proof obtainable that the patient has a basal skull fracture, and that either blood or cerebrospinal fluid is leaking through the fracture into the sphenoid sinuses.

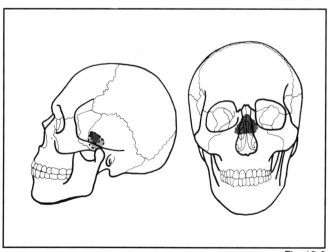

Sphenoid Sinuses

Fig. 13-6

Radiographs – Paranasal Sinuses

Drawings of the sinuses tend to show definite sizes and shapes of the sinuses with clear-cut borders. In actual radiographs these borders are not nearly as definite since the various sinuses overlap and superimpose each other as seen on these radiographs of four common sinus projections. Relative locations and relationships of each of these sinuses are clearly demonstrated on these labeled radiographs: (**F** - frontal sinuses, **E** - ethmoid sinuses, **M** - maxillary sinuses, **S** - sphenoid sinuses.)

Lateral Sinuses: *(Fig. 13-7)*

The frontal sinuses are clearly visualized between the inner and outer tables of the skull.

The sphenoid sinuses appear to be continuous with the ethmoid sinuses anteriorly.

The large maxillary sinuses are clearly visualized. Note that the roots of the upper teeth appear to extend up through the floor of the maxillary sinuses.

PA (Caldwell) Projection: *(Fig. 13-8)*

The frontal, ethmoid and maxillary sinuses are clearly illustrated in this frontal view radiograph. The sphenoid sinuses are not demonstrated specifically because they are located directly behind the ethmoid sinuses. This relationship is demonstrated on the lateral view.

PA Axial Transoral Projection: *(Fig. 13-9)*

All four groups of sinuses are clearly demonstrated on this projection taken with the head tipped back to separate and project the sphenoid sinuses below the ethmoids. The open mouth also removes the upper teeth from direct superimposition of the sphenoids. The pyramid shaped maxillary sinuses are clearly seen.

The mastoid air-cells also appear on each side, postero-lateral to the mandible (see arrows). They appear as small air-filled clusters within the mastoid portions of the temporal bone as described on following pages, but they are not part of the paranasal sinuses.

Submentovertex (SMV) Projection: *(Fig. 13-10)*

This projection is taken with head tipped back so the top (vertex) of the head is touching the table top and the CR is directed from below the chin (mentum).

The centrally located sphenoid sinuses are seen anterior to the large opening, the foramen magnum. The multiple clusters of ethmoid air cells are also clearly seen extending to each side of the nasal septum. Parts of the maxillary sinuses are seen on each side as superimposed by the mandible and teeth.

The mastoid portions containing air cells (labeled **A**), and the dense petrous portions of the temporal bones (labeled **B**), as described on the following page are also well demonstrated.

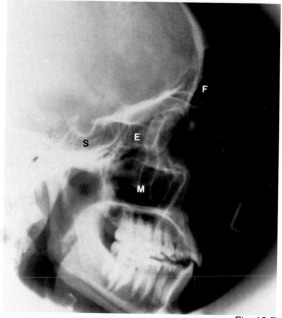

Fig. 13-7
Lateral Sinuses

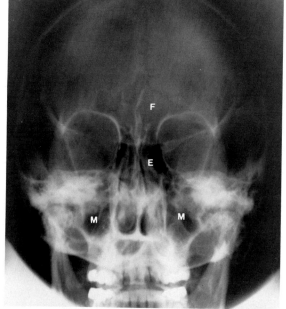

PA Caldwell
Fig. 13-8

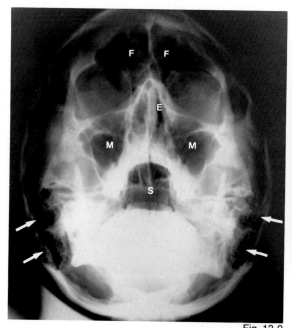

Fig. 13-9
PA Axial Transoral Projection (Open Mouth Waters)

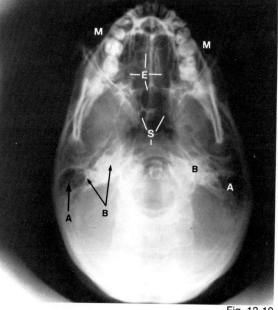

SMV Projection
Fig. 13-10

Temporal Bones

Each **temporal bone is** divided into three main portions. The thin upper portion forming part of the wall of the skull is the **squamous portion**. The area posterior to the external auditory meatus is the **mastoid portion**, with its prominent mastoid process or tip. The third main portion is the dense **petrous portion,** also called the **petrous pyramid** or **pars petrosa**. The upper border or ridge of the petrous pyramids are commonly called the **petrous ridges**.

Without resorting to body-section radiography or computed tomography, the temporal bone is probably the most difficult part of the entire body to radiograph with consistently high quality. Certain projections however can be taken to demonstrate the mastoid sinuses within the mastoid portion of each temporal bone. The very dense petrous pyramids are also demonstrated as seen on the following radiographs.

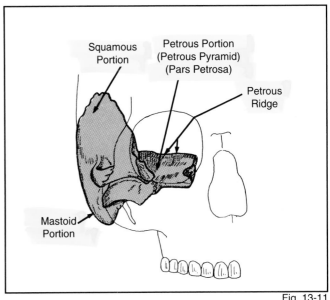

Fig. 13-11

Temporal Bone

Radiographs - Mastoids & Petrous Pyramids

Various structures of the temporal bone are labeled on these radiographs of two projections commonly taken to demonstrate the mastoids and petrous pyramids.

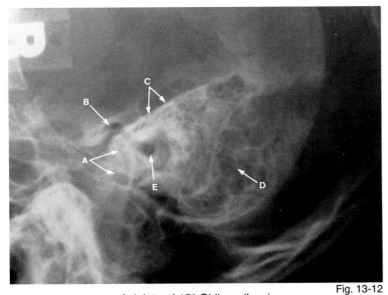

Fig. 13-12

Axiolateral 15° Oblique (Law)

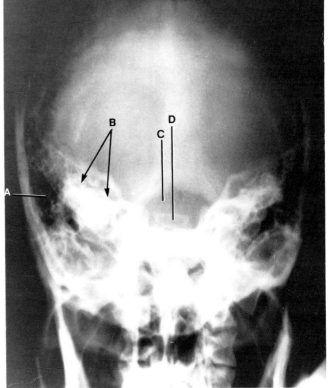

Fig. 13-13

AP Axial (Towne)

Axiolateral 15° Oblique Position (Law Method)
A. Condyle of mandible
B. Temporomandibular fossa
C. Petrous portion (petrous ridge), end-on view
D. Mastoid air cells
E. External acoustic meatus (EAM)

AP Axial (Towne Method)
A. Mastoid air cells
B. Petrous portions
C. Foramen magnum
D. Dorsum sellae

Anatomy of Organs of Hearing and Equilibrium
(contained within petrous portion of temporal bones)

Ear

The organs of hearing and equilibrium are the main structures found within the petrous portion of the temporal bones. These small, delicate structures are difficult to visualize radiographically, due not only to their small size, but also to the increased density of the temporal bones surrounding them. The internal structures of the temporal bone, including the three important divisions of the ear (the external, middle and internal portions) are illustrated in *Fig. 13-14.*

The **external ear** begins outside the head with the **auricle** or **pinna**, which channels sound waves into a tube-like opening, the **external acoustic (auditory) meatus (EAM).** This tube-like meatus ends at the eardrum, which is properly called the **tympanic membrane**.

The **middle ear**, located between the tympanic membrane and the inner ear, contains the **three** small bones called **auditory ossicles**. These small bones transmit sound vibrations from the tympanic membrane to the sensory apparatus of hearing in the **internal ear**. Certain nerves and blood vessels pass through the **internal acoustic meatus** to connect the inner ear with the brain.

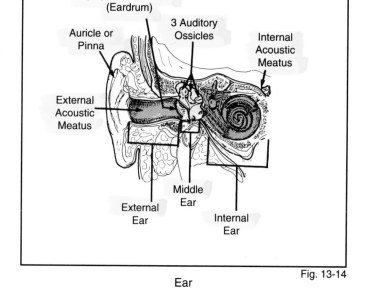

Ear   Fig. 13-14

External Ear

As previously described, the **external ear** begins with the **auricle** or **pinna** on each side of the head. The **tragus** is part of this external structure. It is the small liplike structure located anterior to the EAM, acting as a partial shield to the ear opening. The canal of the external ear is termed the **exterior acoustic (auditory) meatus.** Some references refer to the external opening as the external acoustic (auditory) meatus, and refer to the canal as the external acoustic (auditory) canal. In this text the entire canal is referred to as the external acoustic meatus. The meatus is about 2.5 centimeters long, half of which is bony in structure and half of which is cartilaginous.

The **mastoid tip** of the temporal bone is posterior and inferior to the external auditory meatus, while the **styloid process** is inferior and slightly anterior. The meatus narrows somewhat as it meets the tympanic membrane. The eardrum is situated at an oblique angle, forming a depression or well at the lower medial end of the meatus.

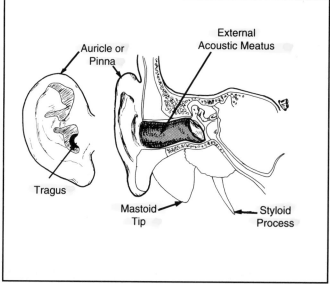

External Ear   Fig. 13-15

Middle Ear

The middle ear is an irregularly shaped, air-containing cavity located between the external and the internal ear portions. The three main components of the middle ear are the **tympanic membrane,** the **three** small bones called **auditory ossicles,** and the **tympanic cavity.** The tympanic membrane is considered part of the middle ear even though it serves as a partition between the external and middle ears.

The tympanic cavity, is further divided into two parts. The larger cavity opposite the eardrum is called the **tympanic cavity proper.** The area above the level of the external auditory meatus and the eardrum is called the **attic** or the **epitympanic recess.** A structure important radiographically is the **drum crest** or **spur.** The tympanic membrane is attached to this sharp, bony projection. The drum crest or spur separates the external acoustic meatus from the epitympanic recess. The tympanic cavity communicates anteriorly with the nasopharynx by way of the Eustachian tube or the auditory tube.

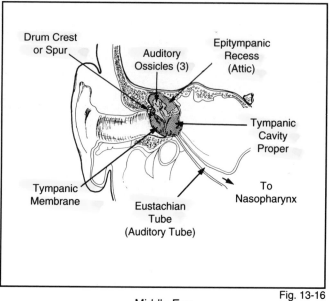

Middle Ear   Fig. 13-16

Temporal Bone

Middle Ear continued

The frontal drawing in *Fig. 13-17* illustrates the general relationships of the **external acoustic meatus** and **Eustachian tube** to the external features. The passageway between the middle ear and the **nasopharynx** is labeled as the **Eustachian** or **auditory tube**. This tube is about 4 centimeters long and serves to equalize the pressure within the middle ear to the outside atmospheric air pressure through the nasopharynx. The sensation of one's ears popping is caused by the pressure being adjusted internally in the middle ear to prevent damage to the eardrum.

A problem associated with this direct communication between the middle ear and the nasopharynx is that disease organisms have a direct passageway from the throat to the middle ear. Therefore, ear infections often accompany sore throats.

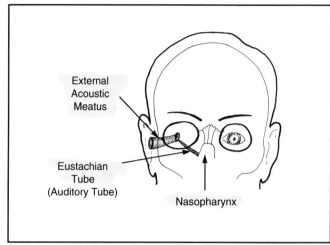

Middle Ear   Fig. 13-17

Internal Acoustic Meatus: The drawing in *Fig. 13-18* demonstrates the ear structures as they would appear in a modified PA (Caldwell) projection. A 10-degree caudal angle to the orbitomeatal line will project the petrous ridges to the mid orbital level. The result is a special transorbital view taken to demonstrate the **internal acoustic meatus**. The opening to the internal acoustic meatus is an oblique aperture, smaller in diameter than the opening to the external acoustic meatus. Certain auditory and facial nerves, as well as blood vessels, pass through the internal acoustic meatus.

Note that in this PA projection the internal acoustic meatus is projected into the orbital shadow slightly below the petrous ridge, allowing it to be visualized on radiographs taken in this position. Remember that the lateral portions of the petrous ridges are at approximately the level of the **TEA** (top of ear attachment). These external relationships to the internal structures are important to remember.

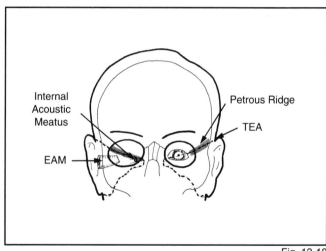

Modified PA Caldwell (10°)   Fig. 13-18

Mastoids: A second direct communication into the middle ear occurs posteriorly from the **mastoid air cells**. The schematic drawing in *Fig. 13-19* is a sagittal section showing the relationships of the mastoid air cells to the **attic** or **epitympanic recess** and the **tympanic cavity proper**. The **aditus** is the opening between the epitympanic recess and the mastoid portion of the temporal bone.

The aditus connects directly to a large chamber within the mastoid portion termed the **antrum**. The antrum then connects to the various mastoid air cells. This communication allows infection in the middle ear, which may have originated in the throat, to pass into the mastoid area. Once within the mastoid area, infection is separated from brain tissue by only thin bone. Before the common use of effective antibiotics, this was often a pathway for a serious infection of the brain, termed encephalitis. The thin plate of bone forming the roof of the antrum, aditus and attic area of the tympanic cavity is called the **tegmen tympani**.

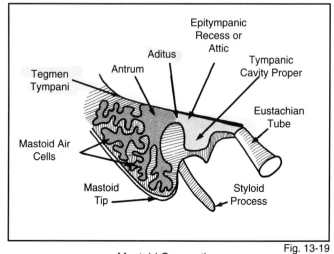

Mastoid Connection   Fig. 13-19

Auditory Ossicles: The **auditory ossicles** are three small bones that are prominent structures within the middle ear. The drawing in *Fig. 13-20* demonstrates that these three small bones are articulated to permit vibratory motion. The three auditory ossicles are located partly in the attic or epitympanic recess, and partly in the tympanic cavity proper. These delicate bones bridge the middle ear cavity to transmit sound vibrations from the **tympanic membrane** to the internal ear.

Vibrations are first picked up by the **malleus**, meaning hammer, which is attached directly to the inside surface of the tympanic membrane. The head of the malleus articulates with the central ossicle, the **incus**. The incus receives its name from a supposed resemblance to an anvil, but it actually looks more like a premolar tooth with a body and two roots. The incus then connects to the stirrup-shaped **stapes**, which is the smallest of the three auditory ossicles. The foot plate of the stapes is then attached to another membrane called the **oval window** leading into the inner ear.

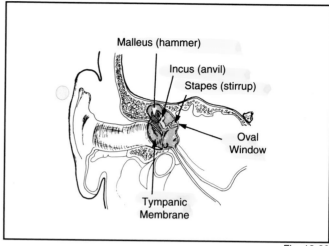

Auditory Ossicles   Fig. 13-20

The drawings in *Fig. 13-21* illustrate the relationship of the **auditory ossicles** to one another in both a frontal view and a lateral view. As seen from the front, the most lateral of the three bones is the **malleus**, while the most medial of the three bones is the **stapes**. The lateral-view drawing demonstrates how the ossicles would appear if one looked through the **external acoustic meatus** to see the bony ossicles of the middle ear. Note that the malleus, with its attachment to the eardrum, is located slightly anterior to the other two bones.

The resemblance of the **incus** to a premolar tooth with a body and two roots is well visualized in the lateral drawing. One root of the incus then connects to the stapes, which in turn connects to the oval window.

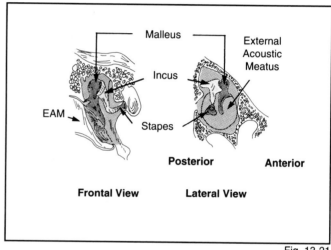

Auditory Ossicles   Fig. 13-21

Internal Ear

The very complex **internal ear** contains the essential sensory apparatus of both hearing and equilibrium. Lying within the densest portion of the petrous pyramid, it can be divided into two main parts, the **osseous** or **bony labyrinth**, important radiographically, and the **membranous labyrinth**. The osseous labyrinth is a bony chamber housing the membranous labyrinth, a series of intercommunicating ducts and sacs. One such duct is the **endolymphatic duct**, a blind pouch or closed duct contained in a small canal-like, bony structure. The canal of the endolymphatic duct arises from the medial wall of the vestibule and extends to the posterior wall of the petrous pyramid, located both posterior and lateral to the **internal acoustic meatus.**

Osseous (Bony) Labyrinth: The osseous or bony labyrinth is divided into **three** distinctly shaped parts, the **cochlea** (meaning snail shell), the **vestibule** and the **semicircular canals**. The osseous labyrinth completely surrounds and encloses the ducts and sacs of the membranous labyrinth. As illustrated in *Fig. 13-22,* the snail-shaped, bony cochlea houses a long coiled tube-like duct of the membranous labyrinth. The cochlea is the most anterior of the three parts of the osseous labyrinth. The vestibule is the central portion of the bony labyrinth and contains the **oval window**, sometimes called the vestibular window. The three semicircular canals are located posterior to the other inner ear structures.

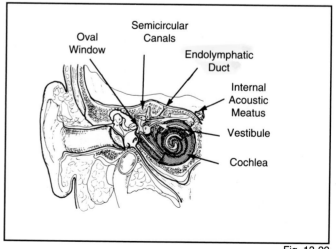

Internal Ear   Fig. 13-22

Osseous (Bony) Labyrinth - Lateral View: A lateral view of the **osseous labyrinth** is shown in *Fig. 13-23.* Included are the three main divisions of the osseous or bony labyrinth: the cochlea, vestibule and semicircular canals. The three semicircular canals are named according to their position, thus they are called the **superior, posterior** and **lateral semicircular canals.** Observe that each is located at right angles to the other two, allowing a sense of equilibrium as well as a sense of direction. It is important to remember that the semicircular canals relate to the sense of direction or equilibrium, and the cochlea relates to the sense of hearing.

"Windows" of Inner Ear: The two openings into the inner ear are covered by membranes. These are termed the **oval** or **vestibular window**, and the **round** or **cochlear window** (fenestra rotundum). The oval or vestibular window receives vibrations from the external ear through the foot plate of the stapes of the middle ear, and transmits these vibrations into the **vestibule** of the internal ear. The round or cochlear window is located at the base of the first coil of the cochlea. The round window is a membrane that allows movement of fluid within the closed duct system of the membranous labyrinth. As the oval window moves slightly inward with a vibration, the round window moves outward since this is a closed system and fluid does not compress.

Tomography - Anatomical Relationships

Tomography or body section radiography is usually required to adequately visualize the delicate structures of the middle and internal ear. Tomography requires a good understanding of not only the specific anatomy, but also of distances between various structures.

Superior View - AP Projection: Certain structures labeled **A** through **I** are identified in *Fig. 13-24.* Distances and relationships between these structures should be noted as positioned for this AP projection. Part **A** is the cochlea; **B** is the Eustachian or auditory tube; **C** is the bony ossicles in the tympanic cavity of the middle ear; **D** is the external acoustic meatus; **E** is the antrum; **F** is the semicircular canals; **G** is the endolymphatic duct; **H** is the vestibule; and **I** is the internal acoustic meatus.

It is important to note that almost all of the structures of the ear are located between the cochlea (toward the anterior) and the antrum (toward the posterior) in a distance of approximately 1 centimeter or 10 millimeters. The distance from the back of the head to the center of the external acoustic meatus is approximately 10 centimeters.

Average distances between structures are based on the average-shaped skull with the OML perpendicular to the tabletop, and they will vary with the shape and size of the skull. If the OML were not kept perpendicular to the tabletop, these distances would also vary.

Generally speaking, however, the most important structures of the middle and internal ear can be located in the **1 centimeter distance between 9.5 cm and 10.5 cm from the table top.**

Superior View - Lateral Position: *Figure 13-25* gives a top view of the head with the patient in a lateral position. The various ear structures are again shown with important distances identified. From the table top, the average distance to the midline is 7 centimeters, and to the internal acoustic meatus, 9 centimeters. The internal acoustic meatus extends 1 centimeter or 10 millimeters toward the inner ear. The inner ear extends another 1 centimeter and the middle ear extends approximately 5 millimeters farther. The distance from the tympanic membrane to the external acoustic opening is 2.5 centimeters or 25 millimeters.

These figures demonstrate that the **distance from the external opening of the external acoustic meatus to the internal acoustic meatus is approximately 5 centimeters** in the average-shaped skull.

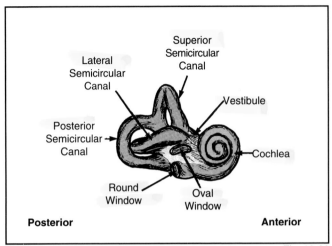

Osseous Labyrinth – Lateral View
Fig. 13-23

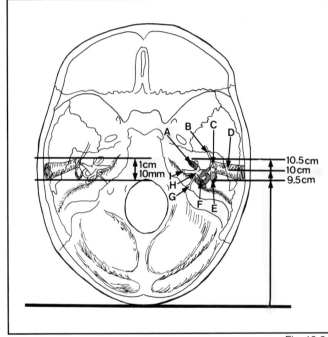

Ear Structures
Fig. 13-24

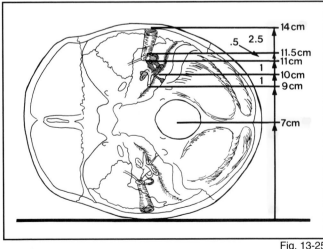

Ear Structures
Fig. 13-25

The interrelationships between the various structures of the middle and internal ear, as well as the various distances from the table top, are most important in tomography or body section radiography of these various structures.

Part II Radiographic Positioning

National Survey

Departmental routines for exams of the paranasal sinuses, mastoids and temporal bone were quite consistent throughout the United States as follows:

Paranasal Sinuses Routine

Paranasal Sinuses	U.S. Average	
	Basic	Optional
• Lateral	99%	
• PA Caldwell	97%	
• AP Waters	93%	
• Basilar (SMV)	57%	9%
• Open mouth Waters	30%	13%

Petrous Pyramids Routine

Petrous Pyramids	U.S. Average	
	Basic	Optional
• AP Axial (Towne)	83%	
• Basilar (SMV)	64%	7%
• Anterior Profile (Reverse Stenvers)	5%	9%

Mastoids Routine

Mastoids	U.S. Average	
	Basic	Optional
•Axiolateral 15° oblique (Laws)	81%	
• Posterior Profile (Stenvers)	84%	
• AP Axial* (Towne)	30%	
• Axiolateral 45° oblique* (Mayer)	12%	
• Schullers*	7%	
• Hickey *	5%	

* Write in's by survey respondents

Survey Questions on Possible Discontinued Procedures:

The national survey included questions on the **quantity** of specific exams being done in their departments during the past year, the **expected trend** in the next three or four years, and whether or not the procedure **should still be taught and included** in a basic student textbook. The results are shown on the chart at the right.

Mastoids	U.S. Average	East	Midwest	West
I. Trend				
a. Increase	7%	10%	4%	5%
b. Decrease	34%	32%	35%	39%
c. No change	59%	58%	61%	56%
II. Annual Quantity				
a. 0-3	21%	16%	17%	43%
b. 4-11	40%	41%	42%	32%
c. 12-22	19%	20%	21%	9%
d. 23+	20%	23%	20%	16%
III. Be Included				
a. Yes	88%	93%	90%	71%
b. No	12%	7%	10%	29%

Petrous Pyramids	U.S. Average	East	Midwest	West
I. Trend				
a. Increase	3%	2%	3%	5%
b. Decrease	24%	23%	23%	30%
c. No change	73%	75%	74%	65%
II. Annual Quantity				
a. 0-5	75%	72%	76%	79%
b. 6-20	17%	17%	18%	14%
c. 21+	8%	11%	6%	7%
III. Be Included				
a. Yes	57%	61%	56%	44%
b. No	43%	39%	44%	56%

Temporal Bone	U.S. Average	East	Midwest	West
I. Trend				
a. Increase	3%	4%	1%	7%
b. Decrease	16%	15%	18%	13%
c. No change	81%	81%	81%	80%
II. Annual Quantity				
a. 0-2	81%	81%	81%	85%
b. 3-20	10%	15%	9%	6%
c. 21+	9%	7%	10%	9%
III. Be Included				
a. Yes	37%	37%	36%	38%
b. No	63%	63%	64%	62%

Summary

The trend as indicated is strongly a **decrease** and **no change** for all three of these exams. The annual quantity for all of these exams is very low by a high percentage of institutions responding to this survey.

The positive response to the question as to whether or not the exams should still be included was the strongest for the mastoids in all areas of the country. This indicates there is a strong belief that radiographers should still know and be able to take mastoids when needed.

The petrous pyramids had a less positive response, and for the temporal bone survey the majority indicated it should no longer be taught and not included in this text. It therefore was dropped in this edition, but the mastoids and petrous pyramids are still included.

Standard and Optional Operating Procedures

Certain basic and optional projections or positions for the sinuses, mastoids and petrous pyramids are demonstrated and described on the following pages as suggested standard and optional departmental procedures.

Basic Projections
Standard or basic projections, also sometimes referred to as routine projections or departmental routines are those projections or posi-

tions commonly taken on average patients who are helpful and can cooperate in performing the procedure.

Optional Projections
Optional projections are those more common projections or positions taken as extra or additional projections to better demonstrate certain pathologic conditions or specific body parts. (They are not optional as to their importance.)

Basic and Optional Projections:

Paranasal Sinuses
Basic
• Lateral
• PA (Caldwell)
• Parietoacanthial (Waters)
• Submentovertex (basilar)
Optional
• Axial transoral
  (Open-mouth Waters)

Mastoids
Basic
• Axiolateral Oblique (Law)
• Posterior Profile (Anterior Oblique)
  (Stenvers)
Optional
• AP Axial (Towne)
• Axioposterior Oblique (Mayer)

Petrous Pyramids
Basic
• AP Axial (Towne)
• Submentovertex (basilar)

• Lateral Position

> **Sinuses**
> Basic
> • **Lateral**
> • PA (Caldwell)
> • Parietoacanthial (Waters)
> • Submentovertex (basilar)

Structures Best Shown:
Sphenoid sinuses, superimposed frontal, ethmoid and maxillary sinuses, sella turcica and orbital roofs.

Technical Factors:
• Film Size - 8 x 10 in. (18 x 24 cm), lengthwise.
• Moving or stationary grid.
• 70-80 kVp range.
• Use small focal spot.

Patient Position:
• Remove all metal, plastic or other removable objects from head.
• Patient in an **erect position**. (See NOTE).

Part Position:
• Rest lateral side of head against head unit or table top, with side of interest closest to cassette.
• Adjust head into a **true lateral** position, oblique body as needed for patient's comfort.
• Align **interpupillary line perpendicular** to film.
• Align **midsagittal plane parallel** with film.
• Adjust chin to bring IOML **perpendicular** to front edge of cassette.

Central Ray:
• Align a **horizontal CR perpendicular** to the film.
• Center to a point **midway between outer canthus and EAM.**
• Center cassette to CR.
• SID: Head Unit, 36 in. (91 cm).
      Table or upright grid unit, minimum 40 in. (102 cm).

Collimation: Use an 8 x 10 in. circle diaphragm, or collimate on all sides to area of sinus cavities.

Respiration: Suspend respiration during exposure.

NOTE: •To visualize air-fluid levels an erect position is required. Fluid within the paranasal sinus cavities is thick and gelatin like, causing it to cling to the cavity walls. In order to visualize this fluid a short time must be allowed for the fluid to settle after a patient's position has been changed. If an upright head or grid unit is not available, the table can be placed in a vertical position and used in the same manner as the erect grid unit.
• If patient cannot sit or stand, this can be taken with patient supine utilizing a cross-table horizontal x-ray beam.

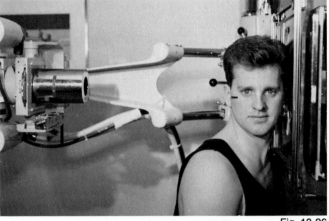
Erect Lateral (Head Unit)
Fig. 13-26

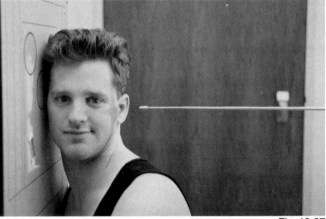
Erect Lateral (Upright Grid)
Fig. 13-27

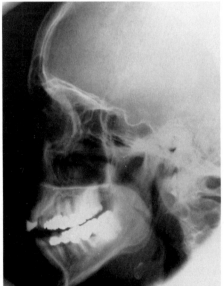
Lateral
Fig. 13-28

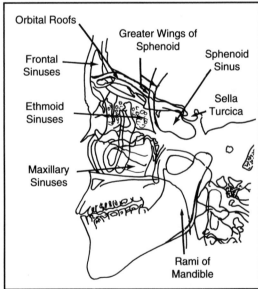
Lateral
Fig. 13-29

- The mandibular rami, the orbital roofs and the greater wings of the sphenoid are superimposed.
- The sella turcica is demonstrated without rotation.
• Sufficient penetration and exposure, without motion, to visualize the frontal and sphenoid sinuses.
• Patient ID information with R or L marker visible within the close four-sided collimation field without superimposing essential anatomy.

Evaluation Criteria:
• Included and centered to the collimation field and film are the frontal, sphenoid, ethmoid and maxillary sinuses. (Sphenoid sinuses are of primary interest in the lateral position.)
• The cranium is not rotated or tilted:

• PA Projection
(Caldwell Method)

<table>
<tr><td>
Sinuses
Basic
• Lateral
• PA (Caldwell)
• Parietoacanthial (Waters)
• Submentovertex (basilar)
</td></tr>
</table>

Structures Best Shown:
Frontal sinuses and anterior ethmoid sinuses.

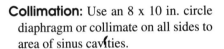

Technical Factors:
• Film Size - 8 x 10 in. (18 x 24 cm), lengthwise.
• Moving or stationary grid.
• 70-80 kVp range.
• Use small focal spot.
• Upright Head Unit is angled 15°, CR is horizontal. (See NOTE).

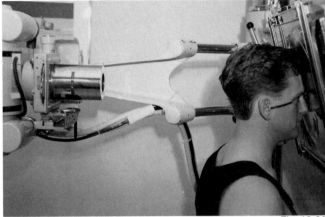
Fig. 13-30
PA – Horizontal CR, Film Tilted 15°

Patient Position:
• Remove all metal, plastic or other removable objects from head.
• Patient in an **erect position**. (See NOTE).

Part Position:
• Rest patient's nose and forehead against head unit.
• Adjust chin, bringing **OML perpendicular** to film.
• Align **midsagittal plane perpendicular to midline** of film.
• Center cassette to **nasion.**

Central Ray:
• Align **CR horizontal**, parallel with the floor. (See NOTE).
• Center CR to cassette.
• SID: Head Unit, 36 in. (91 cm).
    Table top or upright grid unit, minimum 40 in. (102 cm).

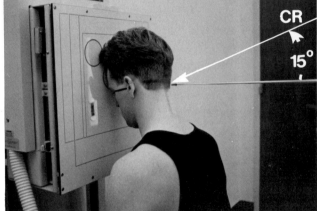
Fig. 13-31
Alternate PA – CR 15° Caudal

Collimation: Use an 8 x 10 in. circle diaphragm or collimate on all sides to area of sinus cavities.

Respiration: Suspend respiration during exposure.

NOTE: • To measure air-fluid levels, the **CR must be horizontal** and the **patient must be erect.**

Alternate PA: If the vertical grid unit angulation cannot be adjusted and remains vertical, angle the CR 15° caudal. However since the beam is not completely horizontal, air-fluid levels will not be demonstrated as clearly defined straight lines but will be seen as gradual density changes.

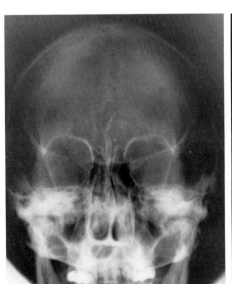
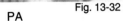
Fig. 13-32
PA

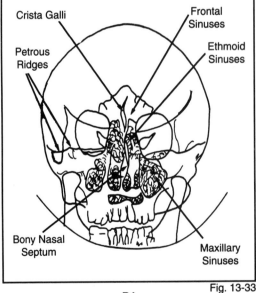
Fig. 13-33
PA

Evaluation Criteria:
•Included and centered to the collimation field and film are the frontal and anterior ethmoid sinuses.
•The cranium is not rotated or tilted:
- Equal distance from the midsagittal plane, identified by the crista galli, to the outer orbital margin.
- Superior orbital fissures are symmetrically visualized within the orbits.
• Petrous ridges are projected into lower one-third of orbits.

• Frontal sinuses are projected above the frontonasal suture.
• Anterior ethmoid air cells are visualized laterally adjacent to each nasal bone, directly below the frontal sinuses.
• Sufficient penetration and exposure, without motion, to visualize the frontal and ethmoid sinuses.
• Patient ID information with R or L marker visible within the closely collimated field without superimposing essential anatomy.

• Parietoacanthial Projection
(Waters Method)

Sinuses
Basic
• Lateral
• PA (Caldwell)
• **Parietoacanthial (Waters)**
• Submentovertex (basilar)

Structures Best Shown:
Maxillary sinuses and nasal fossae.

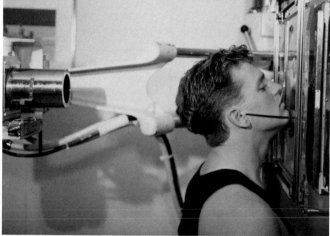

Parietoacanthial Projection   Fig. 13-34

Technical Factors:
• Film Size - 8 x 10 in. (18 x 24 cm), lengthwise.
• Moving or stationary grid.
• 70-80 kVp range.
• Use small focal spot.

Patient Position:
• Remove all metal, plastic or other removable objects from head.
• Patient in an **erect position**. (See NOTE).

Part Position:
• Extend neck, resting chin and nose against head unit.
• Adjust head until **mentomeatal line (MML) is perpendicular** to film, OML will form a 37° angle with head unit or table top.
• Position the **midsagittal plane perpendicular** to the midline of film.
• Center cassette to **acanthion.**

Central Ray:
• Align a **horizontal CR perpendicular** to the film.
• Center CR to cassette.
• SID: Head Unit, 36 in. (91 cm).
        Table top or upright grid unit, minimum 40 in. (102 cm).

Collimation: Use an 8 x 10 in. circle diaphragm, or collimate on all sides to area of sinus cavities.

Respiration: Suspend respiration during exposure.

NOTE: • CR must be horizontal and patient must be erect to demonstrate air-fluid levels within the paranasal sinus cavities.
• In this position the average patient's nose tip will be approximately 3/4 in. (2 cm) away from the head unit or table top.

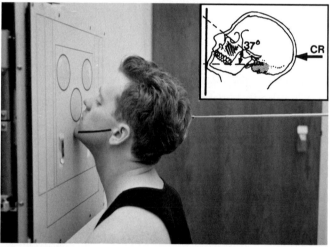

Parietoacanthial Projection   Fig. 13-35
- CR and MML perpendicular

Evaluation Criteria:
• Included on radiograph are the frontal and maxillary sinus.
• Cranium seen without rotation:
  - Equal distance from midsagittal plane, identified by the bony nasal septum, to the outer orbital margin.
• Inferior maxillary sinuses are free from superimposing alveolar processes.
• Inferior orbital rim is clearly identified.
• Petrous ridges are below the maxillary sinuses. Each ridge is seen projecting laterally, from the posterior maxillary alveolar process.

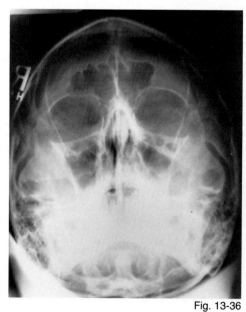

Fig. 13-36
Parietoacanthial Projection

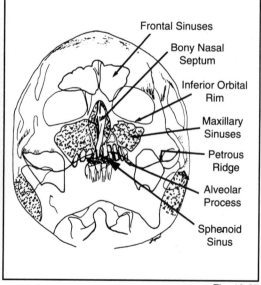

Frontal Sinuses

Bony Nasal Septum

Inferior Orbital Rim

Maxillary Sinuses

Petrous Ridge

Alveolar Process

Sphenoid Sinus

Fig. 13-37
Parietoacanthial Projection

• Sufficient penetration and exposure, without motion, to visualize maxillary sinuses.
• Patient ID information with R or L marker visible within collimated field without superimposing essential anatomy.

• Submentovertex (SMV) Projection
(Basilar Position)

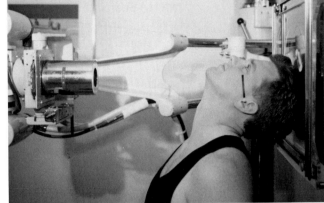

SMV Projection   Fig. 13-38

Sinuses
Basic
• Lateral
• PA (Caldwell)
• Parietoacanthial (Waters)
• **Submentovertex (basilar)**

Technical Factors:
• Film Size - 8 x 10 in. (18 x 24 cm), lengthwise.
• Moving or stationary grid.
• 70-80 kVp range.
• Use small focal spot.

Structures Best Shown:
Sphenoid sinuses, ethmoid sinuses and nasal fossae.

Patient Position:
• Remove all metal, plastic or other removable objects from head and neck.
• Patient in an **erect position** if possible to show air-fluid levels..

Part Position:
• Raise chin, hyperextending neck if possible until **IOML is parallel** to head unit or vertical table. (See NOTE).
• Head rests on vertex of skull.
• Align **midsagittal plane perpendicular** to midline of head unit or vertical table.

Central Ray:
• CR directed **perpendicular to IOML**. (See NOTE.)
• Center CR midway between angles of mandible, at a level 1.5 in. (4 cm) inferior to mandibular symphysis.
• Center CR to cassette.
• SID: Head Unit, 36 in. (91 cm). Table or upright grid unit, minimum 40 in. (102 cm).

Collimation: Use an 8 x 10 in. circle diaphragm, or collimate on all sides to area of sinus cavities.

Respiration: Suspend respiration during exposure.

NOTE: • If patient is unable to sufficiently extend neck, angle tube **perpendicular to IOML**. With head unit the film can then also be angled as needed to maintain the film perpendicular to CR.
• Position is very uncomfortable for patient, move quickly.

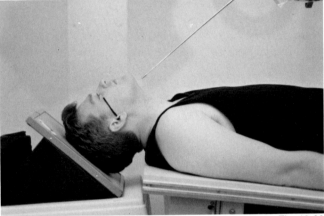

SMV Projection   Fig. 13-39

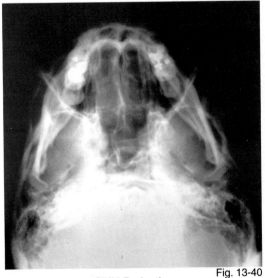

SMV Projection   Fig. 13-40

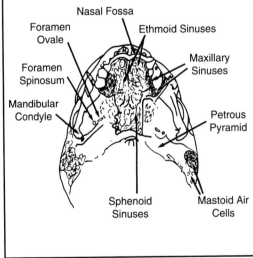

Nasal Fossa
Foramen Ovale
Ethmoid Sinuses
Foramen Spinosum
Maxillary Sinuses
Mandibular Condyle
Petrous Pyramid
Sphenoid Sinuses
Mastoid Air Cells

SMV Projection   Fig. 13-41

Evaluation Criteria:
• Anatomy anterior to foramen magnum visualized and centered to collimation field and film.
• Mandibular symphysis superimposes anterior frontal bone.
• The cranium is not rotated or tilted:
  - Distance along coinciding mandibular surfaces to lateral border of skull are equal.
  - Petrous pyramids are visualized symmetrically.

• Mandibular condyles are projected anterior to petrous ridges.
• Sufficient penetration and exposure, without motion, to visualize sphenoid and ethmoid sinuses and foramen ovale and spinosum.
• Patient ID information and R or L marker visible within collimated field without superimposing essential anatomy.

• Axial Transoral Projection
(Open-mouth Waters)

Sinuses
Optional
• **Axial Transoral**
(Open-mouth Waters)

Structures Best Shown:
Sphenoid and maxillary sinuses and nasal fossae.

Technical Factors:
• Film Size - 8 x 10 in. (18 x 24 cm), lengthwise.
• Moving or stationary grid.
• 70-80 kVp range.
• Use small focal spot.

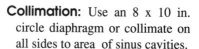

Patient Position:
• Remove all metal, plastic or other removable objects from head.
• Patient in an **erect position**. (See NOTE.)

Part Position:
• Extend neck, resting chin and nose against head unit.
• Adjust head until **mentomeatal line is perpendicular** to film. OML will form a 37° angle with head unit or table top (see NOTE).
• Position the **midsagittal plane perpendicular** to the midline of the head unit.
• Instruct patient to open mouth by telling him/her to "drop jaw without moving head". (Mentomeatal line is no longer perpendicular.)
• Center cassette to **acanthion.**

Central Ray:
• Align a **horizontal CR perpendicular** to the film.
• Center CR to cassette.
• SID: Head Unit, 36 in. (91 cm).
     Table or upright grid unit,
     minimum 40 in. (102 cm).

Collimation: Use an 8 x 10 in. circle diaphragm or collimate on all sides to area of sinus cavities.

Respiration: Suspend respiration during exposure.

NOTE: • CR must be horizontal and patient erect to demonstrate air-fluid levels within the paranasal sinus cavities.
• In this position the average patient's nose tip will be approximately 3/4 in. (2 cm) away from the head unit or table top.

Evaluation Criteria:
• Included on radiograph are the frontal, maxillary and sphenoid sinuses.
• Cranium seen without rotation or tilt:
  - Equal distance from the midsagittal plane (identified by the bony nasal septum) to the outer orbital margin.
• Inferior maxillary sinuses are free from superimposing alveolar processes.
• Inferior orbital rim is clearly identified.
• Petrous ridges are below the maxillary sinuses. Each ridge is seen projecting laterally, from the posterior maxillary alveolar process.

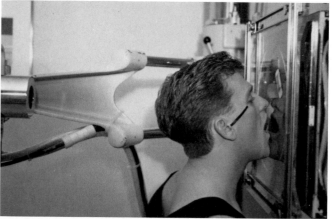
Axial Transoral Projection   Fig. 13-42

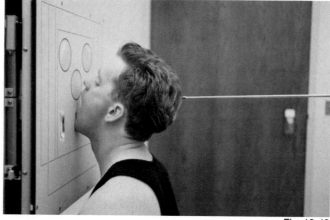
Axial Transoral Projection   Fig. 13-43

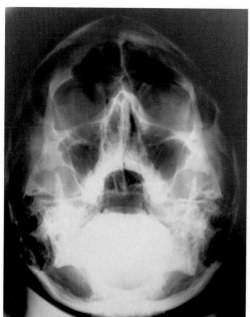
Fig. 13-44
Axial Transoral Projection

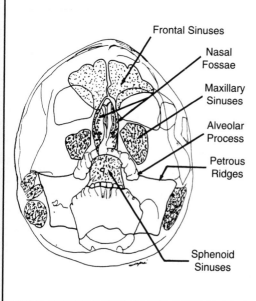
Frontal Sinuses
Nasal Fossae
Maxillary Sinuses
Alveolar Process
Petrous Ridges
Sphenoid Sinuses
Fig. 13-45
Axial Transoral Projection

• Sphenoid sinus is visualized within shadow of open mouth.
• Sufficient penetration and exposure, without motion, to visualize the maxillary and sphenoid sinuses.
• Patient ID information with R or L marker visible within collimated field without superimposing essential anatomy.

• Axiolateral Oblique Position
(Law Method)

Structures Best Shown:
Mastoid air cells closest to film.

Both sides are generally taken for comparison.

Technical Factors:
• Film Size - 2 each 8 x 10 in. (18 x 24 cm), lengthwise.
• Moving or stationary grid.
• 70-80 kVp range.
• Use small focal spot.

Patient Position:
• Remove all metal, plastic or other removable objects from head.
• Patient in an erect or prone position.
• Tape each auricle forward to prevent superimposing mastoid.

Part Position:
• Rest lateral side of head against head unit or table top, with side of interest closest to cassette; oblique body as needed for patient comfort.
• Align midsagittal plane parallel with head unit or table top in a true lateral position, then **rotate face 15° toward film.** (Do not allow chin to tilt inward, toward cassette.)
• Align **interpupillary line perpendicular** to head unit or table.
• Adjust chin to bring **IOML perpendicular** to front edge of cassette.
• Center cassette to **mastoid tip adjacent to cassette**, located **1 in.** (2.5 cm) **posterior to EAM.**

Central Ray:
• Angle CR **15° caudal.**
• Center CR to cassette. Table Top, center CR 1 in. (2.5 cm) posterior and superior to upside EAM.
• SID: Head Unit, 36 in. (91 cm).
       Table Top, minimum 40 in. (102 cm).

Collimation: Use a circle diaphragm or collimate on all sides to yield a field size of approximately 4 in. (10 cm).

Respiration: Suspend respiration during exposure.

NOTE: To obtain a sharply detailed image of the mastoid cells the utilization of a small focal spot and close collimation is essential.

Evaluation Criteria:
• The mastoid air cells of interest are located in the center of collimation field and film, posterior to the EAM.
• Opposite mastoid does not superimpose mastoid of interest but is seen inferior to it.
• Ear auricle does not superimpose mastoid.
• Temporomandibular joint is visualized anterior to mastoid cell of interest.

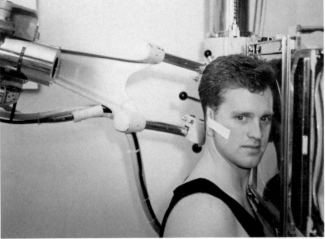

Axiolateral Oblique   Fig. 13-46

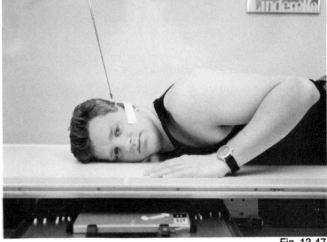

Axiolateral Oblique
- 15° Oblique (head rotation)
- 15° Caudal angle   Fig. 13-47

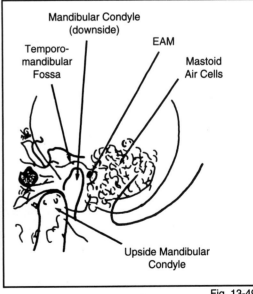

Axiolateral Oblique   Fig. 13-48

Mandibular Condyle
(downside)

Temporo-
mandibular
Fossa

EAM

Mastoid
Air Cells

Upside Mandibular
Condyle

Axiolateral Oblique   Fig. 13-49

• Sufficient penetration and exposure, without motion, to visualize mastoid air cells.
• Patient ID information with R or L marker visible within collimated field without superimposing essential anatomy.

• Posterior Profile (Anterior Oblique) Position
(Stenvers Method)

Structures Best Shown:
Petrous ridge in profile (positioned parallel to film) the bony labyrinth, the tympanic cavity, the internal auditory canal and the mastoid air cells.

Both sides are generally taken for comparison.

Technical Factors:
• Film Size - 2 each 8 x 10 in. (18 x 24 cm), lengthwise.
• Moving or stationary grid.
• 70-80 kVp range.
• Use small focal spot.

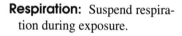

Patient Position:
• Remove all metal, plastic or other removable objects from head.
• Patient in an erect or prone position, facing the film as for a PA projection.

Part Position:
• Adjust chin to bring **IOML perpendicular** to plane of film.
• Rotate head **45° toward side of interest.** Rest patient's forehead, nose and zygoma against head unit or table top. (Side of interest is closest to film.)
• Looking through the head unit glass, center cassette to a point midway between the outer canthus and the EAM. (Table top - see NOTE.)

Central Ray:
• Angle CR 12° **cephalic.**
• Center CR to cassette. (Table Top - see NOTE.)
• SID: Head Unit, 36 in. (91 cm); Table Top, minimum 40 in. (102 cm).

Collimation: Use a circle diaphragm or collimate on all sides to yield a field size of approximately 4 in. (10 cm).

Respiration: Suspend respiration during exposure.

NOTE: • For table top, center CR about 2 in. (5 cm) posterior and slightly superior to elevated EAM.
• To obtain a sharply detailed image of the mastoid air cells the utilization of a small focal spot and close collimation is essential.

Evaluation Criteria:
• Included and centered to collimation field and film are the petrous ridge and mastoid process of side of interest.
• Petrous pyramid is clearly visualized in profile.
• Mastoid process is seen in profile below the cranial margin.
• Posterior margin of mandibular ramus borders the posterior margin of the cervical spine.
• Mandibular condyle superimposes cervical spine.

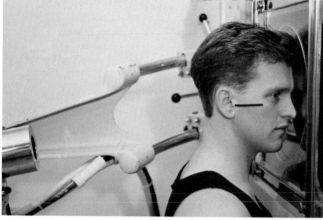

Posterior Profile Position   Fig. 13-50

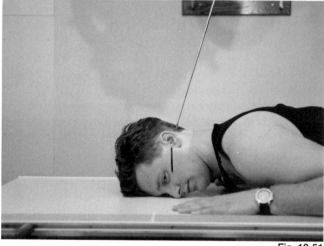

Posterior Profile Position   Fig. 13-51
- 45° Anterior oblique
- 12° Cephalic angle

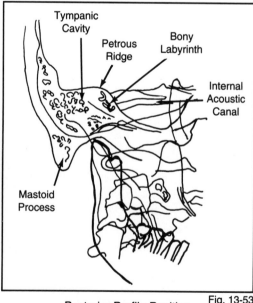

Posterior Profile Position   Fig. 13-52

Posterior Profile Position   Fig. 13-53

Tympanic Cavity
Petrous Ridge
Bony Labyrinth
Internal Acoustic Canal
Mastoid Process

• The internal acoustic canal, cochlea and semicircular canals (bony labyrinths) are visualized below petrous ridge.
• Sufficient penetration and exposure, without motion, to visualize the mastoid process and petrous ridge.
• Patient ID information with R or L marker visible within collimated field without superimposing essential anatomy.

• AP Axial Projection
(Towne Method)

Mastoids
Optional
• **AP Axial**
• Axioposterior Oblique
(Mayer)

Structures Best Shown:
Petrous pyramids, mastoid air cells, and bony labyrinth.

Technical Factors:
- Film Size - 8 x 10 in. (18 x 24 cm), lengthwise.
- Moving or stationary grid.
- 70-80 kVp range.
- Use small focal spot.

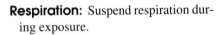

Patient Position:
- Remove all metal, plastic or other removable objects from head.
- Patient in an erect or supine position with posterior skull against head unit or table top.

Part Position:
- Depress chin, bringing **OML perpendicular** to film. (See NOTE.)
- Align **midsagittal plane perpendicular** to midline of head unit or table to prevent head rotation and/or tilt.

Central Ray:
- Angle **CR 30° caudal to OML**. (See NOTE.)
- Center CR to the **midsagittal plane,** at a level **2.5 in.** (6 cm) **above nasion**. (The CR will pass through a line connecting both EAM's.)
- Center cassette to CR.
- SID: Head Unit, 36 in. (91 cm); Table Top, minimum 40 in. (102 cm).

Collimation: Use an 8 x 10 in. circle diaphragm or collimate to outer margins of skull.

Respiration: Suspend respiration during exposure.

NOTE: • If patient is unable to depress the chin sufficiently to bring the **OML** perpendicular to the film, the **IOML** can be placed perpendicular instead and the CR angle increased to 37° caudal. This maintains the **30° angle between OML and CR** and demonstrates the same anatomical relationships. (There is a 7° difference between the OML and the IOML.)

• **Head Unit Option:** If patient cannot depress chin sufficiently, the top of the grid device can also be tilted back 7° from vertical to maintain the same CR-film relationship.

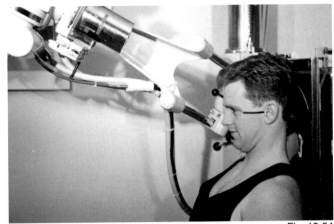

AP Axial

Fig. 13-54

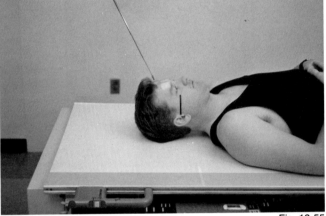

AP Axial
- OML perpendicular
- CR 30° caudal

Fig. 13-55

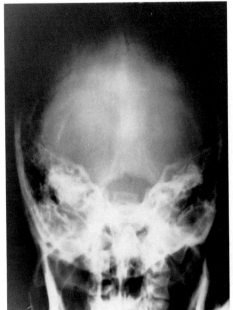

AP Axial

Fig. 13-56

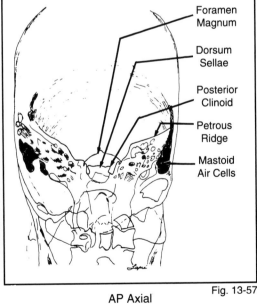

AP Axial

Fig. 13-57

Foramen Magnum
Dorsum Sellae
Posterior Clinoid
Petrous Ridge
Mastoid Air Cells

Evaluation Criteria:
- Included on the radiograph are both petrous ridges and both mastoid air cells.
- The cranium is seen without rotation or tilt:
  - Petrous ridges are symmetrical.
  - Equal distance from foramen magnum to lateral margin of skull on each side.

- Dorsum sellae and posterior clinoids are projected into foramen magnum.
- Sufficient penetration and exposure, without motion, to visualize bony labyrinth without overexposing mastoid air cells.
- Patient ID information with R or L marker visible within collimated field without superimposing essential anatomy.

• Axioposterior Oblique Position
(Mayer Method)

Mastoids
Optional
• AP Axial
• **Axioposterior Oblique**
(Mayer)

Structures Best Shown:
Provides an end-on view of petrous portion, visualizes the external acoustic meatus (canal), mastoid air cells, mastoid antrum and bony labyrinth.

(Both sides are generally taken for comparison.)

Technical Factors:
• Film Size - 2 each 8 x 10 in. (18 x 24 cm), lengthwise.
• Moving or stationary grid.
• 70-80 kVp range.
• Use small focal spot.

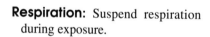

Patient Position:
• Remove all metal, plastic or other removable objects from head.
• Patient in an erect or supine position, back of head against table as for an AP projection.

Part Position:
• Adjust chin, bringing **IOML perpendicular** to front edge of cassette.
• Rotate head **45° toward side of interest.** (Side of interest is closest to film.)

Central Ray:
• Angle **CR 45° caudal.**
• Center the CR approximately **3 in.** (7.5 cm) **above the superciliary arch.** The CR should pass through the EAM of interest.
• Center cassette to CR.
• SID: Head Unit, 36 in. (91 cm).
       Table Top, minimum 40 in. (102 cm).

Collimation: Use a circle diaphragm or collimate on all sides to yield a field size of approximately 4 in. (10 cm).

Respiration: Suspend respiration during exposure.

NOTE: • To obtain a sharply detailed image of the mastoid air cells the utilization of a small focal spot and close collimation is essential.
    • A variation of this position is a double 30° angle; head is rotated 30° from lateral and CR 30° caudal (Owen modification of Mayer method).

Evaluation Criteria:
• The mastoid air cell of interest is located in the center of collimation field and film.
• The petrous portion is located inferior to the mastoid portion (as seen with end-on view).
• Sufficient penetration and exposure, without motion, to visualize the bony labyrinth without overexposing the mastoid air cells.
• Patient ID information with R or L marker visible within collimated field without superimposing essential anatomy.

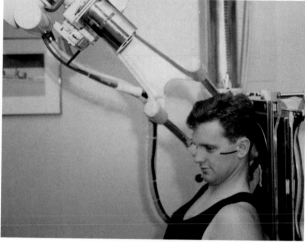

Axioposterior Oblique   Fig. 13-58

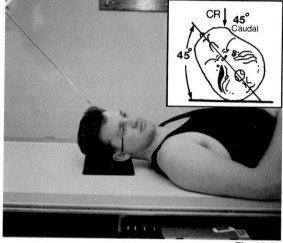

Axioposterior Oblique   Fig. 13-59
- 45° Posterior oblique
- 45° Caudal angle

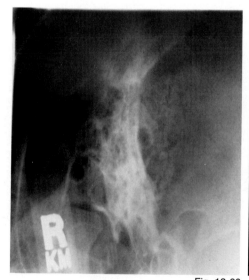

Axioposterior Oblique   Fig. 13-60

Fig. 13-61

Anterior   Posterior

Mastoid Air Cells

Bony Labyrinth

Mandibular Condyle

External Acoustic Canal

Axioposterior Oblique

Petrous Pyramids

- **AP Axial Projection** - (same positioning as for AP Axial Mastoids, page 407)
- **Submentovertex (SMV) Projection**

(Basilar Position)

> **Petrous Pyramids**
> Basic
> • **AP Axial** (Towne)
> • **Submentovertex** (basilar)

Structures Best Shown:
Bilateral petrous pyramids including internal acoustic canals, bony labyrinths and tympanic cavities.

Technical Factors:
- Film Size - 8 x 10 in. (18 x 24 cm), lengthwise.
- Moving or stationary grid.
- 70-80 kVp range.
- Use small focal spot.

Patient Position:
- Remove all metal, plastic or other removable objects from head and neck.
- Patient in erect position (or supine only if erect is not possible).

SMV Projection
Part Position:
- Raise chin, hyperextending neck if possible until IOML **is parallel** to head unit or vertical table. (See NOTE).
- Head rests on vertex of skull.
- Align **midsagittal plane perpendicular** to midline of head unit or vertical table.

Central Ray:
- CR directed **perpendicular to IOML**. (See NOTE.)
- Center CR midway between angles of mandible, at a level 2.5-3 in. (6-8 cm) inferior to mandibular symphysis.
- Center CR to cassette.
- SID: Head Unit, 36 in. (91 cm).
  Table or upright grid unit, minimum 40 in. (102 cm).

Collimation: Use an 8 x 10 in. circle diaphragm or collimate on all sides to area of interest.

Respiration: Suspend respiration during exposure.

NOTE: • If patient is unable to sufficiently extend neck, angle tube **perpendicular to IOML**. With head unit the film can then also be angled as needed to maintain the film perpendicular to CR.
• Position is very uncomfortable for patient, move quickly.

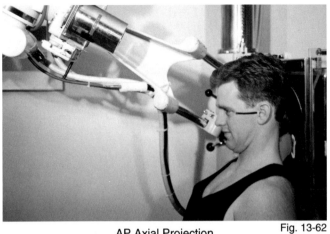

AP Axial Projection
- OML perpendicular
- CR 30° caudal

Fig. 13-62

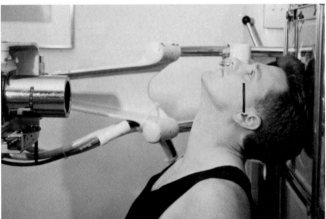

SMV Projection

Fig. 13-63

Evaluation Criteria:
SMV Projection
- Entire skull visualized and centered to collimation field and film.
- Mandibular symphysis superimposes anterior frontal bone.
- The cranium is not rotated or tilted:
  - Distance along coinciding mandibular surfaces to lateral border of skull are equal.
  - Petrous pyramids are visualized symmetrically.
- Mandibular condyles are projected anterior to petrous pyramids.

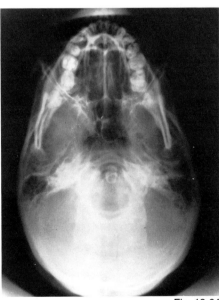

SMV Projection   Fig. 13-64

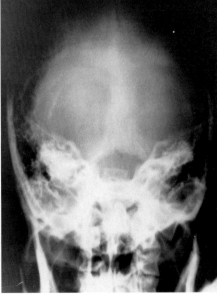

AP Axial Projection   Fig. 13-65

- Internal acoustic canal, foramen ovale and spinosum are visualized.
- Sufficient penetration and exposure, without motion, to visualize petrous pyramids.
- Patient ID information and R or L marker visible within collimated field without superimposing essential anatomy.
- **AP Axial Projection**: Similar to mastoids, p. 407.

Chapter 14
Radiographic Anatomy and Positioning of the
Upper Gastrointestinal System

Contributions by: John Lampignano, M Ed, RT (R)
Barry T. Anthony RT (R)

Contents

Part I Radiographic Anatomy

Digestive System

The digestive system includes the entire **alimentary canal** and several **accessory organs.** The alimentary canal begins at the (1) **mouth**, continues as the (2) **pharynx**, (3) **esophagus**, (4) **stomach**, (5) **duodenum** *(du´o-de´num)*, first part of the **small intestine** *(in-tes´tin)*, and ends as the (6) **large intestine**, which terminates as the (7) **anus** *(a´nus)*.

Accessory organs of digestion include the **teeth, salivary glands, pancreas, liver and gallbladder.**

Anatomy and positioning of parts (1) mouth, through (5) duodenum, will be covered in this chapter. The remainder of the small intestine, the large intestine and the anus will be covered in Chapter 15.

Functions: The digestive system performs three primary functions.
1. The first function is the intake of water, vitamins and minerals, plus the **intake and digestion** of food. Food is ingested in the form of carbohydrates, lipids and proteins. These complex food groups must be broken down or digested so that absorption can take place.
2. The second primary function of the digestive system is to **absorb** digested food particles, along with water, vitamins and essential elements from the alimentary canal into the blood or lymphatic capillaries.
3. The third function is to **eliminate** any unused material in the form of solid waste products.

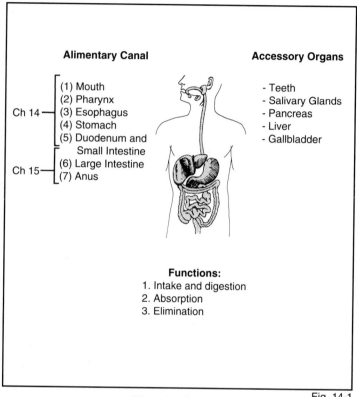

Alimentary Canal

Ch 14
- (1) Mouth
- (2) Pharynx
- (3) Esophagus
- (4) Stomach
- (5) Duodenum and Small Intestine

Ch 15
- (6) Large Intestine
- (7) Anus

Accessory Organs
- Teeth
- Salivary Glands
- Pancreas
- Liver
- Gallbladder

Functions:
1. Intake and digestion
2. Absorption
3. Elimination

Digestive System   Fig. 14-1

Common Radiographic Procedures

Two common radiographic procedures involving the upper gastrointestinal system are presented in this chapter. Common radiographic procedures are those examinations performed routinely in large and small radiology departments, as well as in certain clinics and physicians' offices. These common radiographic examinations involve the administration of a contrast medium.

1. **Esophagram** or Barium Swallow
   - Study of pharynx and esophagus.
     A radiographic examination specifically of the pharynx and esophagus is termed an **esophagram** or **barium swallow.** This procedure studies the form and function of the swallowing aspect of the pharynx and esophagus.

2. **Upper Gastrointestinal Series** (UGI) (Upper GI)
   - Study of distal esophagus, stomach and duodenum.
     The procedure designed to study the distal esophagus, stomach and duodenum in one examination is termed an **upper gastrointestinal series.** Alternative designations for upper gastrointestinal series include UGI, upper, GI or, most commonly, **upper GI.** A PA radiograph from an upper GI series is shown in *Fig. 14-2.* Barium sulfate mixed with water is the preferred contrast medium for the entire alimentary canal. The negative density area (white appearing) on the radiograph indicates the stomach and duodenum area filled with the barium sulfate contrast media.

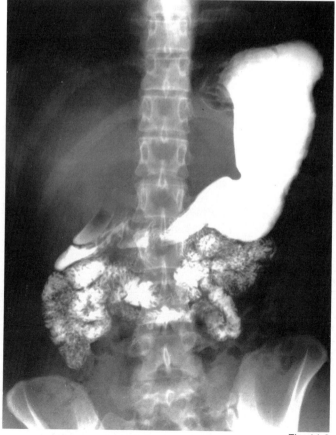

PA – Upper GI Series   Fig. 14-2

(1) Mouth
(Oral or Buccal Cavity)

The alimentary canal is a continuous hollow tube, beginning with the mouth. The **mouth** may also be referred to as the **oral cavity**, or **buccal** *(buk'al)* **cavity.** The mouth and surrounding structures are visualized in midsagittal section in *Fig. 14-3.*

The main cavity of the mouth is bounded in front and on the sides by the inner surfaces of the **upper and lower teeth.** The roof of the mouth is formed by the **hard and soft palates,** while the main part of the floor is formed by the **tongue.** The mouth or oral cavity connects posteriorly with the **pharynx.**

Accessory Organs in the Mouth

Accessory organs of digestion associated with the mouth are the **teeth** and the **salivary glands.** The teeth and tongue cooperate in chewing movements to reduce the size of food particles and to mix food with saliva. These chewing movements, termed **mastication** *(mas"ti-ka'shun),* initiate the mechanical part of digestion.

Three pairs of glands secrete most of the saliva in the mouth. These are: (1) **parotid** *(pah-rot'id,* meaning near the ear), (2) **submandibular** (sometimes called submaxillary, below mandible or maxilla) and (3) **sublingual** *(sub-ling'gwal,* below the tongue).

Saliva is 99.5% water and 0.5% solutes or salts and certain digestive enzymes. Between 1000 and 1500 milliliters are secreted daily by the salivary glands. Saliva dissolves foods so that digestion can begin. It also contains an enzyme to begin digestion of starch.

Specific salivary glands secrete a thickened fluid which contains mucus. This lubricates food being chewed so that the food can form into a ball or bolus for swallowing. The act of swallowing is termed **deglutition** *(deg"loo-tish'un).*

NOTE: The salivary glands may be the site of infection, especially the parotid glands. **Mumps** is an inflammation and enlargement of the parotid glands caused by the mumps virus, which on about 30% of males past puberty also results in inflammation of the testes.

(2) Pharynx

The alimentary canal continues as the pharynx posterior to the mouth. The **pharynx** *(far'inks)* is about 12.5 centimeters long, and is that part of the digestive tube found posterior to the nasal cavities, mouth and larynx. A midsagittal and a coronal section of the pharynx, as seen from the posterior, are shown in *Fig. 14-5.* The three parts of the pharynx are named according to their location.

The **nasopharynx** is posterior to the **bony nasal septum** and nasal cavities, and superior to the level of the soft palate.

The **oropharynx** is directly posterior to the oral cavity proper. The oropharynx extends from the **soft palate** to the **epiglottis** *(ep"i-glot'is).* The epiglottis is a membrane-covered cartilage that moves down to cover the opening of the larynx during swallowing.

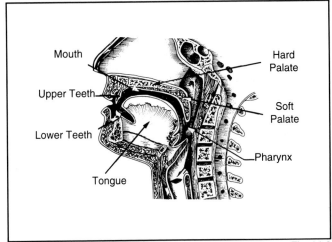

Midsagittal Section of Mouth (Oral or Buccal Cavity)   Fig. 14-3

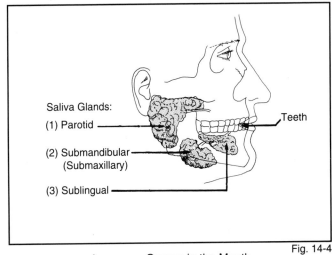

Accessory Organs in the Mouth   Fig. 14-4

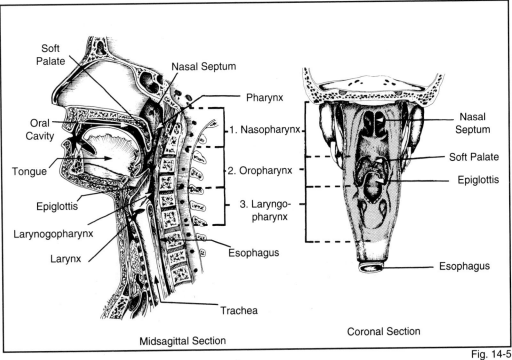

Midsagittal Section   Coronal Section

Pharynx   Fig. 14-5

The third portion of the pharynx is termed the **laryngopharynx** or hypopharynx. The laryngopharynx extends from the level of the epiglottis to the level of the lower border of the cricoid cartilage. From this point it continues as the **esophagus.** The **trachea** is seen anterior to the esophagus.

Pharynx continued

Cavities Communicating with the Pharynx

The surface drawing in *Fig. 14-6* illustrates that there are seven cavities or openings communicating with the three portions of the pharynx. The two **nasal cavities** and the two **tympanic cavities** connect to the **nasopharynx.** The tympanic cavities of the middle ears connect to the nasopharynx via the **auditory** or **Eustachian tubes**.

The mouth connects posteriorly to the oropharynx. Inferiorly, the **laryngopharynx** connects to the openings of both the **larynx** and the **esophagus.**

Deglutition (Swallowing)

It is most important that food and fluid travel from the oral cavity directly to the esophagus during the act of swallowing or deglutition. During swallowing, the soft palate closes off the nasopharynx to prevent swallowed substances from regurgitating into the nose. The tongue prevents the material from reentering the mouth.

During swallowing, the epiglottis is depressed to cover the laryngeal opening like a lid. The vocal folds or cords also come together to close off the epiglottis. These actions combine to prevent food and fluid from being aspirated (going down the "wrong pipe").

Also, respiration is inhibited during deglutition to help prevent swallowed substances from entering the trachea and lungs. Occasionally, bits of material pass into the larynx and trachea during deglutition. A forceful episode of reflex coughing is usually necessary to reject these offensive intruders.

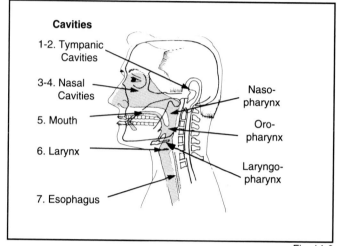

Pharynx

Fig. 14-6

(3) Esophagus

The third part of the alimentary canal is the **esophagus**, or gullet as it is sometimes called. The esophagus is a muscular canal, about 9.75 inches (25 cm) long, extending from the laryngopharynx to the stomach. The esophagus begins posterior to the level of the lower border of the **cricoid cartilage of the larynx,** which is at the level of **the sixth cervical vertebra** (C6). The esophagus terminates at its connection to the stomach, at the level of the **eleventh thoracic vertebra** (T 11).

In *Fig. 14-7*, one can see that the esophagus is located posterior to the larynx and trachea. The spatial relationship of the esophagus to both the trachea and the thoracic vertebrae is an important relationship to remember. The esophagus is both posterior to the trachea, and just anterior to the cervical and thoracic vertebral bodies.

The descending **thoracic aorta** is between the distal esophagus and the lower thoracic spine. The **heart, within its pericardial sac,** is immediately posterior to the **sternum,** anterior to the esophagus, and superior to the **diaphragm.**

The **esophagus** is essentially vertical as it descends to the stomach. This swallowing tube is the narrowest part of the entire alimentary canal. The esophagus is most constricted, first, at its proximal end where it enters the thorax, and, second, where it passes through the diaphragm at the esophageal hiatus or opening. The esophagus pierces the diaphragm at the level of **T10**. Just before passing through the diaphragm, the esophagus presents a distinct dilatation as shown in *Fig. 14-8.*

As the esophagus descends within the posterior aspect of the mediastinum, two indentations are present. One indentation occurs at the **aortic arch,** and the second is found where the esophagus crosses the **left bronchus.**

The lower portion of the esophagus lies close to the posterior aspects of the **heart.**

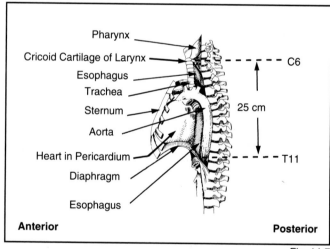

Esophagus

Fig. 14-7

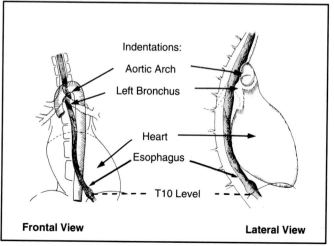

Esophagus in Mediastinum

Fig. 14-8

Esophagus continued

Diaphragm Openings

The **esophagus** passes through the **diaphragm** slightly to the left and somewhat posterior to the mid point of the diaphragm. The drawing on the left in *Fig. 14-9* represents the inferior surface of the diaphragm and indicates the relative positions of the **esophagus, inferior vena cava** and **aorta.**

The drawing on the right shows the short abdominal portion of the esophagus below the diaphragm. The **abdominal segment of the esophagus,** termed the **cardiac antrum,** measures between 1 and 2 centimeters. The cardiac antrum curves sharply to the left after passing through the diaphragm to attach to the stomach.

The opening between the esophagus and the stomach is termed the **esophagogastric junction** (cardiac orifice). This is best shown in the drawing on the following page, *Fig. 14-13.* Cardiac is an adjective denoting a relationship to the heart, therefore the cardiac antrum and the cardiac orifice are located near the heart.

The junction of the stomach and the esophagus is normally securely attached to the diaphragm, so the upper stomach tends to follow the respiratory movements of the diaphragm.

Swallowing and Peristalsis

The **esophagus** contains a well-developed muscular layer composed of skeletal muscle at its proximal or upper end, and smooth muscle consisting of both longitudinal and circular fibers in its mid and distal portions. Unlike the trachea, the esophagus is a collapsible tube that only opens when swallowing occurs. The process of deglutition continues in the esophagus after originating in the mouth and pharynx. Fluids tend to pass from the mouth and pharynx to the stomach primarily by gravity. A bolus of solid material tends to pass both by gravity and by peristalsis.

Peristalsis is a wave-like series of muscular contractions propelling solid and semi-solid materials through the tubular alimentary canal. The bolus of barium sulfate, seen in the esophagus in *Figs. 14-10 and 11,* is descending to the stomach both by gravity and by peristalsis. A peristaltic contraction is seen in the upper esophagus in *Fig. 14-10.* This patient also demonstrates some pathology involving the mid-esophagus area which is creating a constriction and partial blockage of the esophagus at this point.

The esophagus in *Fig. 14-11* is also seen filled with barium with a normal peristaltic constricture in the lower esophagus. This patient also has a pacemaker with attached wires evident in the upper mid-chest. Accumulation of barium in the stomach is seen on both of these radiographs.

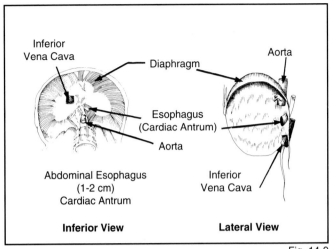

Fig. 14-9

Esophagus passing through diaphragm

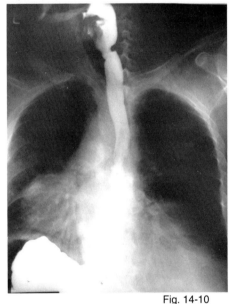

Fig. 14-10

PA Esophagram

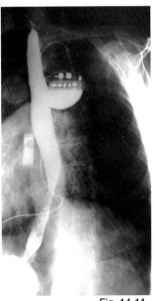

Fig. 14-11

RAO Esophagram

(4) Stomach

The **stomach,** located between the **esophagus** and the **small intestine,** is the most dilated portion of the alimentary canal. When empty, the stomach tends to collapse. When the stomach must serve as a reservoir for swallowed food and fluid, it is remarkably expandable. At times, the stomach may stretch almost to the point of rupture.

Synonyms for stomach are the Latin word *ventriculus,* meaning "little belly," and the Greek word *gaster,* meaning "stomach." *Gastro* is a common term denoting stomach.

Since the shape and position of the stomach are highly variable, the average shape and location will be utilized in the following illustrations, with variations to follow later in this chapter.

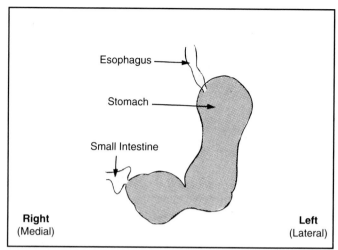

Right
(Medial)

Left
(Lateral)

Stomach (Frontal View)   Fig. 14-12

Stomach Openings and Lesser Curvature

The **esophagogastric junction** (cardiac orifice) is the aperture or opening between the esophagus and the stomach, which is guarded by circular muscles of the cardiac sphincter. In a similar fashion, the orifice leaving the distal stomach is termed the **pyloric orifice** or **pylorus.** The pyloric sphincter is a thickened muscular ring that relaxes periodically during digestion to allow stomach or gastric contents to move into the first part of the small intestine.

The **lesser curvature** forms a concave border as it extends between the cardiac and pyloric openings on the right or medial side of the stomach. An obvious notch, termed the **angular notch** (incisura angularis)**,** is located along the lesser curvature, closer to the pyloric orifice than to the cardiac orifice. This notch divides the stomach inferior to the cardiac orifice into a small right portion (pylorus region) and a large left portion (body). See *Fig. 14-14.*

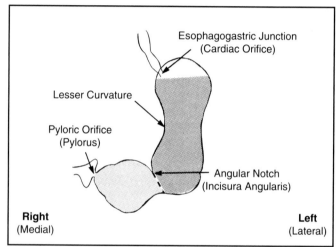

Right
(Medial)

Left
(Lateral)

Stomach (Frontal View)   Fig. 14-13

Stomach Subdivisions

The stomach is composed of three main subdivisions: (1) **the fundus,** (2) the **body** or **corpus,** and (3) the **pyloric portion.** The fundus is that ballooned portion lying lateral and superior to the cardiac orifice. The upper portion of the stomach, including the cardiac antrum of the esophagus, is relatively fixed to the diaphragm and tends to move with motion of the diaphragm. In the upright or erect position, the fundus is usually filled by a bubble of swallowed air.

Lateral to the angular notch (the patient's left) and inferior to the fundus is the large portion of the stomach called the body or corpus. The smaller terminal portion of the stomach to the right or medial of the angular notch is the pyloric portion of the stomach, which terminates at the pyloric valve or pylorus.

The pyloric portion is frequently divided into two parts, (1) the **pyloric antrum,** to the right of the angular notch, and (2) the narrowed **pyloric canal,** ending at the pyloric sphincter.

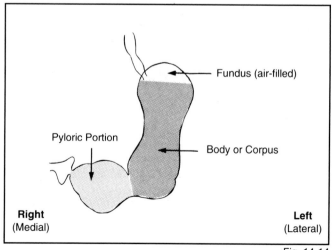

Right
(Medial)

Left
(Lateral)

Stomach (Frontal View)   Fig. 14-14

Stomach continued

Greater Curvature and Rugae

The **greater curvature** extends along the lateral border of the stomach from the **esophagogastric junction** (cardiac orifice) to the **pylorus.** This greater curvature is four to five times longer than the lesser curvature, and is convex rather than concave. The notch found at the junction of the esophagus and the greater curvature is termed the **cardiac notch** (incisura cardiaca).

When the stomach is empty, the internal lining is thrown into numerous longitudinal folds termed **gastric folds** or rugae, pronounced *roo'je,* (plural of ruga, *roo'gah*)**.** A gastric canal, formed by rugae along the lesser curvature, is believed to funnel fluids directly to the pylorus.

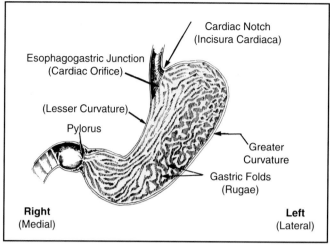

Stomach (Coronal Section)

Fig. 14-15

Stomach Position

The illustration in *Fig. 14-16* shows the typical orientation of an average, empty stomach in a frontal and lateral view. The **fundus**, in addition to being the most superior portion of the stomach, is located posterior to the **body** of the stomach. The body can be seen to curve inferior and anterior from the fundus.

The **plyoric portion** is directed posteriorly. The **pyloric valve** (sphincter) and the first part of the small bowel are very near the posterior abdominal wall. The relationship of these components of the stomach will be important in the distribution of air and barium in the stomach in specific body positions.

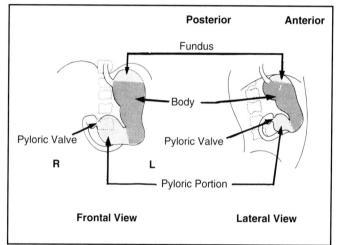

Average Empty Stomach Orientation

Fig. 14-16

Air-Barium Distribution in Stomach

If an individual were to swallow a barium sulfate and water mixture, along with some air, the position of the person's body would determine the distribution of the barium and air within the stomach. The illustration in *Fig. 14-17* shows air as black, and the barium sulfate mixture as white.

The drawing on the left depicts the stomach of a person who is in an **erect** position. In the erect position, air will rise to fill the fundus, while barium will descend by gravity to fill the pyloric portion of the stomach.

The middle drawing shows the stomach of a person in a **prone** position. Since the fundus is more posterior than the lower body of the stomach, air will be found primarily in the fundus, while barium will gravitate to the lower body and the pyloric portion of the stomach.

The drawing on the right depicts the stomach of a person in a **supine** position. In a supine position, barium will travel to the fundus, while air will locate toward the distal end of the stomach. When studying radiographs of a stomach containing both air and barium sulfate, one can determine the patient's position by the relative locations of air versus barium.

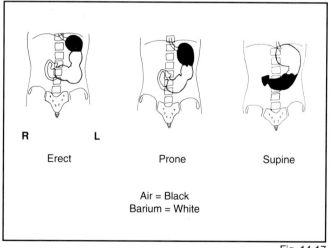

Air-Barium Distribution in the Stomach (Frontal Views)

Fig. 14-17

(5) Duodenum

The fifth and final part of the upper GI system to be studied in this chapter is the **duodenum,** which is the first portion of the small intestine. Since the duodenum is examined radiographically during the routine upper GI series, the duodenum will be studied in this chapter, while the remainder of the small bowel will be studied in Chapter 15.

The duodenum is about 10 inches (25 cm) long, and is the shortest, widest and most fixed portion of the small bowel.

The drawing in *Fig. 14-18* demonstrates that the C-shaped duodenum is closely related to the **head of the pancreas.** The head of the pancreas, nestled in the C-loop of the duodenum, has been affectionately labeled the "romance of the abdomen" by certain authors.

The duodenum and the pancreas are retroperitoneal structures , that is they are located posterior or behind the parietal peritoneum as described and illustrated in the following chapter on the lower GI system.

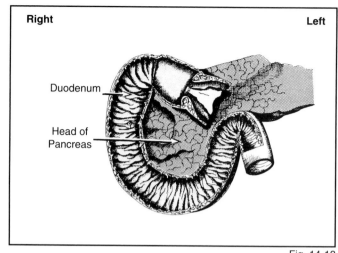

Right   Left

Duodenum

Head of Pancreas

Duodenum   Fig. 14-18

Four parts of the Duodenum

The duodenum is shaped like a letter C and consists of four parts. The **superior portion** begins at the **pylorus.** The first part of the superior portion is termed the **duodenal bulb** or **cap.** It is shaped somewhat like an arrowhead. The duodenal bulb is easily located during barium studies of the upper GI tract and must be carefully studied since this area is a common site of ulcer disease.

The second part of the duodenum is the **descending portion,** the longest segment. The descending portion of the duodenum receives both the common bile duct and the main pancreatic duct.

The third part of the duodenum is the **horizontal portion.** This horizontal portion curves back to the left to join the final segment, termed the **ascending portion.** The junction of the duodenum with the second portion of small bowel, the **jejunum,** is relatively fixed and held in place by a fibrous muscular band, the **ligament of Treitz**[1]. This is a significant reference point in certain radiographic small bowel studies.

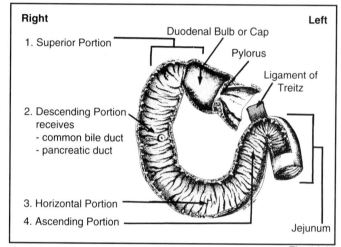

Right   Left

Duodenal Bulb or Cap

1. Superior Portion

Pylorus

Ligament of Treitz

2. Descending Portion receives
- common bile duct
- pancreatic duct

3. Horizontal Portion

4. Ascending Portion

Jejunum

Fig. 14-19

Duodenum (Cut away view to show internal surface)

Anatomy Review

Radiograph of Stomach and Duodenum

This PA radiograph of the stomach and duodenum provides a good review of important radiographic anatomy. Identify the structures labeled on the radiograph then compare your answers with those listed below:

A. Distal esophagus
B. Area of esophagogastric junction (cardiac orifice)
C. Lesser curvature
D. Angular notch (Incisura angularis)
E. Pyloric portion
F. Pyloric valve or sphincter
G. Duodenal bulb
H. Descending portion of duodenum
I. Gastric folds or rugae
J. Body of stomach
K. Greater curvature
L. Fundus

NOTE: A pathologic constricture termed a "Schatzke's ring" is evident at the distal esophagus (see arrow). This is a type of hiatal hernia wherein the esophagogastric junction has herniated through the diaphragmatic opening.

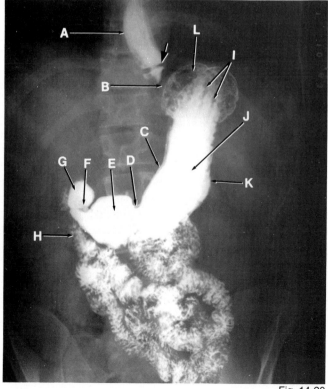

Fig. 14-20

PA Projection

---

1. Wendel Treitz (1819-1872), an Austrian physician and anatomist.

Digestion

Mechanical Digestion

Digestion can be divided into a mechanical process and a chemical component. Mechanical digestion includes all movements of the GI tract, beginning in the mouth with chewing or **mastication** (*mas"ti-ka'shun),* and continuing in the mouth, pharynx and esophagus with swallowing or **deglutition. Peristaltic activity** can be detected in the lower esophagus as well as in the remainder of the alimentary canal. The passage of solid or semisolid food from the mouth to the stomach takes from 4 to 8 seconds, while liquids pass in about 1 second.

The stomach, acting as a reservoir for food and fluid, also acts as a large mixing bowl. Peristalsis tends to move the gastric contents toward the pyloric valve, but this valve opens selectively. If it is closed, the stomach contents are churned or mixed with stomach fluids into a semifluid mass termed **chyme** *(kīm).* When the valve opens, small amounts of chyme are passed into the duodenum by stomach **peristalsis.** Gastric emptying is a fairly slow process, taking 2 to 6 hours to totally empty after an average meal. Food with high carbohydrate content leaves the stomach in several hours while food with high protein or fat content moves through much slower.

The small intestine continues mechanical digestion with a churning motion within segments of the small bowel. This churning or mixing activity is termed **rhythmic segmentation.** Rhythmic segmentation tends to thoroughly mix food and digestive juices, and to bring the digested food into contact with the intestinal lining or mucosa to facilitate absorption. **Peristalsis** is again present to propel intestinal contents along the alimentary canal. Peristaltic contractions in the small intestine, however, are much weaker and slower than in the esophagus and stomach and the chyme moves through the small intestine at about 1 cm/min. Therefore the chyme will normally take 3 to 5 hours to pass through the entire small intestine.

Chemical Digestion

Chemical digestion includes all of the chemical changes that food undergoes as it travels through the alimentary canal. Six different classes of substances are ingested: (1) **carbohydrates** or complex sugars, (2) **proteins,** (3) **lipids** *(lip'id)* or **fats,** (4) **vitamins,** (5) **minerals** and (6) **water.** Only the carbohydrates, proteins and lipids need to be chemically digested in order to be absorbed. Vitamins, minerals and water are used in the form in which the body ingests them.

Chemical digestion is speeded up by various **enzymes.** Enzymes are **biological catalysts** found in the various digestive juices which are produced by salivary glands in the mouth and by the stomach, small bowel and pancreas. The various enzymes are organic compounds which are proteins. They accelerate chemical changes in other substances without actually appearing in the final products of the reaction.

(1) **Carbohydrate** digestion of starches is begun in the mouth and stomach, and is completed in the small intestine. The end products of digestion of these complex sugars are **simple sugars**.

(2) **Protein** digestion is begun in the stomach and is completed in the small intestine. The end products of protein digestion are **amino acids.**

(3) **Lipid** or fat digestion essentially takes place only in the small bowel, although small amounts of the enzyme necessary for fat digestion are found in the stomach. **Bile,** manufactured by the liver and stored in the gallbladder, is discharged into the duodenum to assist in the breakdown of lipids. Bile contains no enzymes, but it does serve to emulsify fats. During emulsification, large fat droplets are broken down to small fat droplets which have greater surface area (to volume) and give enzymes greater access for the breakdown of lipids. The end products of fat or lipid digestion are **fatty acids** and **glycerol** *(glis'er-ol).*

Mechanical Digestion

Mouth (teeth and tongue)	- Mastication (chewing) - Deglutition (swallowing)
Pharynx	- Deglutition
Esophagus	- Deglutition - Peristalsis (waves of muscular contraction) (1-8 secs)
Stomach	- Mixing (chyme) - Peristalsis (2-6 hrs)
Small Intestine	- Rhythmic Segmentation (churning) - Peristalsis (3-5 hrs)

Summary

Chemical Digestion

Substances Ingested, Digested and Absorbed:

1) Carbohydrates (complex sugars) → Simple Sugars
2) Proteins → Amino Acids
3) Lipids (fats) → Fatty Acids and Glycerol (Small Bowel Only)

Substances Ingested but NOT Digested:

4) Vitamins
5) Minerals
6) Water

Enzymes (digestive juices)
- biological catalysts
Bile (from GB)
- emulsifies fats

Summary

Most absorption of digestive end products takes place in the small intestine. Simple sugars, amino acids, fatty acids, glycerol, H_2O and most salts and vitamins are absorbed into the bloodstream or the lymphatic system through the lining of the small intestine. Limited absorption takes place in the stomach and may include some water, alcohol and certain drugs but no nutrients. Any residues of digestion or any unabsorbed digestive products are eliminated from the large bowel as a component of feces.

Summary

In general, **three primary functions** of the digestive system are accomplished within the alimentary canal.

First, **ingestion** and/or **digestion** takes place in the mouth, pharynx, esophagus, stomach and small intestine.

Second, digestive end products along with water, vitamins and minerals are **absorbed** by the small intestine and, to a very small degree, by the stomach, and are transported into the circulatory system.

Third, unused or unnecessary solid material is **eliminated** by the large intestine. (Specific digestive functions of the individual small and large intestines are described in more detail in the following chapter on the lower GI system.)

Primary Functions Digestive System

1) **Ingestion** and/or **Digestion**
   (Mouth, Pharynx, Esophagus, Stomach and Small Intestine)

2) **Absorption**
   (Small Intestine)

3) **Elimination**
   (Large Intestine)

Summary

Body Habitus

A study of the radiographic anatomy of the GI system must include a discussion of the variations in body habitus.

The type of body habitus has a great effect on the location of the GI organs within the abdominal cavity. To be able to accurately and consistently position for these GI procedures, one must know and understand the characteristics of each of these classes of body habitus.

There are four general classes of bodily habitus: (1) **hypersthenic,** (2) **sthenic**, (3) **hyposthenic**, and (4) **asthenic.** The word sthenic *(sthen´ik)* actually means active or strong.

The hypersthenic type of body build is the massive type, representing about 5 percent of the total population. The average body type is the sthenic designation, describing about half or 50 percent of all individuals. Slightly more slender than the sthenic type is the hyposthenic habitus, representing about 35 percent of the total population. The very slender type is the asthenic category which comprises about 10 percent of all subjects.

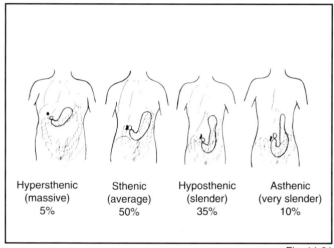

| Hypersthenic (massive) 5% | Sthenic (average) 50% | Hyposthenic (slender) 35% | Asthenic (very slender) 10% |

Bodily Habitus (Frontal View)　　Fig. 14-21

Hypersthenic vs. Asthenic

Hypersthenic: The two extremes of bodily habitus are the hypersthenic and the asthenic builds. The **hypersthenic** type designates the **massive body build,** with the chest and abdomen being very broad and deep from front to back. The lungs are short and wide, and the diaphragm is quite high. The heart is short and wide, and lies in a transverse axis. The transverse colon is quite high, and the entire large bowel extends to the periphery of the abdominal cavity.

The **gallbladder** (GB) is higher and more to the right compared to the average position. The gallbladder is almost transverse and lies well away from the midline. The **stomach** is also very high and assumes a transverse position.

Asthenic: The opposite extreme is the **extremely slender build or asthenic** type. In the asthenic habitus, the chest cavity is narrow, shallow and quite long, so that the diaphragm lies very low. The heart is long and slender.

The **large bowel** (LB) folds on itself, and is found very low and toward the midline. The **gallbladder** and **stomach** are both low, vertical and near the midline. The abdominal cavity is shallow, with its greatest capacity in the pelvic region.

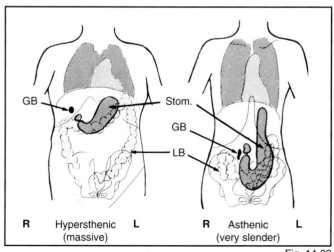

| R Hypersthenic L (massive) | R Asthenic L (very slender) |

Hypersthenic vs. Asthenic　　Fig. 14-22
(Frontal View)

Body Habitus continued

Sthenic vs. Hyposthenic

Sthenic: The **average body build** is the **sthenic** type, which is a more slender version of the hypersthenic classification. The **stomach** is more J-shaped and is located lower than in the massive body type. The **gallbladder** is less transverse and lies midway between the lateral abdominal wall and the midline. The **splenic flexure** of the **large bowel** is often quite high, resting under the left diaphragm.

Hyposthenic: The **hyposthenic** type is considered to be a modification of the more slender asthenic build. The **stomach** is elongated, J-shaped and extends to the iliac crest or below. The **gallbladder** is lower and more toward the midline compared to the sthenic type of build. The **large bowel** is located lower than in the average habitus, but the **splenic flexure** may still be found high in the upper left quadrant.

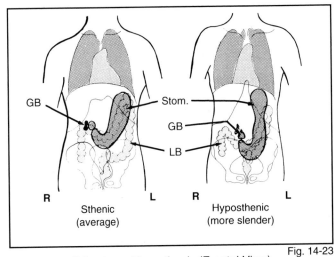

Fig. 14-23

Sthenic vs. Hyposthenic (Frontal View)

Summary of Factors Affecting Stomach and GB shape, size and /or location

Body Habitus:

Body habitus determines the relative size, shape, position, muscular tone and mobility of all organs. The two organs most dramatically affected by body habitus are the **stomach** and **gallbladder**. Many radiographic examinations are done daily on these two organs. It is necessary to assess the body habitus of each patient requiring radiographs of these two organs. The assessment requires a knowledge of body habitus and an ability to judge the relative position of the stomach and gallbladder from among the wide variations present in the general public such as the three examples shown on the following page. Most persons do not fall clearly into one of the distinct four possible body types but are combination types and one needs to be able to evaluate each patient for stomach and/or gallbladder locations.

Additional Factors:

In addition to body habitus, other factors affecting the position of the stomach include **posture, stomach contents** and **respiration**. Posture refers to the relative position of the body. Depending on whether one is upright, supine, prone, on one side, or in the Trendelenburg position, the position of various organs, especially the stomach, will change. Whether the stomach is empty, full or in some phase of digestion will affect stomach position.

Finally, since the upper stomach is attached to the diaphragm, whether one is in full inspiration or expiration, or somewhere in between will affect the cephalic extent of the stomach. As a radiographer, correct localization of all borders of the stomach and other organs will come with sufficient positioning practice.

Radiographs of Upper GI Demonstrating Body Types

The three body type examples below with radiographs demonstrate the position and location of the stomach on these three most common body types. The location of the stomach and duodenal bulb to specific vertebra should be noted in relationship to the level of the iliac crest and lower costal margin positioning landmarks.

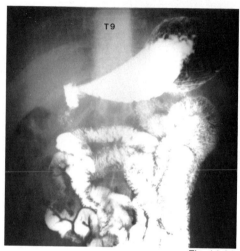

Fig. 14-24

Hypersthenic

General Stomach - high and transverse, Level T9 - 12

Pyloric Portion - Level of T11 - 12, at midline

Duodenal Bulb Location - Level of T 11-12, to right of midline.

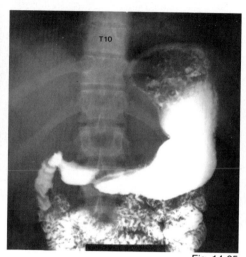

Fig. 14-25

Sthenic

General Stomach - Level T10 - L2

Pyloric Portion - Level of L2, near midline

Duodenal Bulb Location - Level of L2, at midline.

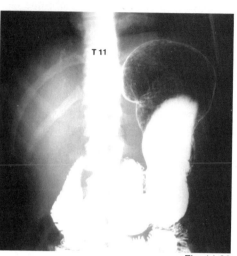

Fig. 14-26

Asthenic

General Stomach - low and vertical, Level T11 - L4

Pyloric Portion - Level of L3 - 4, to left of midline

Duodenal Bulb Location - Level of L3, at midline.

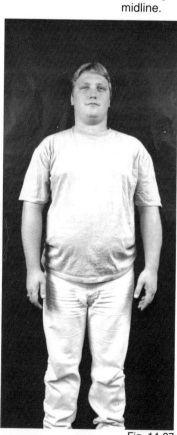

Fig. 14-27

Hypersthenic
- Generally shorter in height with broad shoulders and hips and short torso (less distance between lower rib cage and iliac crest)

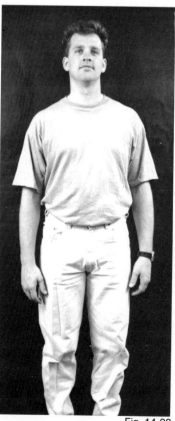

Fig. 14-28

Sthenic/Hyposthenic
- Near average in height, weight and length of torso (This example is taller and broader than average, therefore would be somewhere between sthenic and hyposthenic)

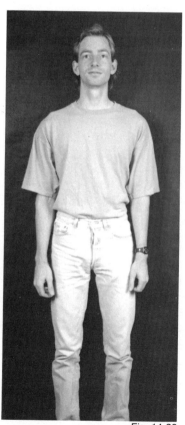

Fig. 14-29

Hyposthenic/ Asthenic
- Generally tall and thin with long torso (This example is some broader than a true asthenic, therefore would be somewhere between a hyposthenic and asthenic)

Part II Radiographic Procedures

Similarities

Radiographic procedures or examinations of the entire alimentary canal are similar in three general aspects.

First, since most parts of the GI tract are comparable in density to those tissues surrounding them, some type **of contrast medium** must be added to visualize these structures. Ordinarily, the only parts of the alimentary canal that can be seen on plain radiographs are the fundus of the stomach (in the upright position) due to the gastric air bubble, and parts of the large intestine due to pockets of gas and collections of fecal matter.

Most of the alimentary canal simply blends in with the surrounding structures and cannot be visualized without the use of contrast media. This fact is illustrated by comparing a plain abdominal radiograph *(Fig. 14-30)* to an upper GI series radiograph using barium sulfate as a contrast medium *(Fig. 14-31).*

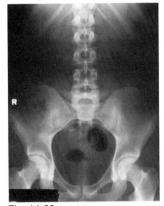
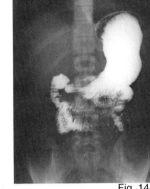

Fig. 14-30

Fig. 14-31

Use of Contrast Medium

A **second** similarity is that the initial stage of each radiographic examination of the alimentary canal is carried out utilizing **fluoroscopy.** Fluoroscopy allows the interested physician to (1) observe the GI tract in motion, (2) produce radiographs during the course of the examination, and (3) determine the most appropriate course of action to take for the complete radiographic examination. To be able to view organs in motion and to isolate anatomical structures is absolutely essential for radiographic examination of the upper GI tract. The structures in this area assume a wide variety of shapes and sizes depending on the body habitus of the individual involved.

In addition, the functional activity of the alimentary canal exhibits a wide range of differences that are considered within normal limits. In addition to these variations, a large number of abnormal conditions exist, making it important that these organs be viewed directly by fluoroscopy.

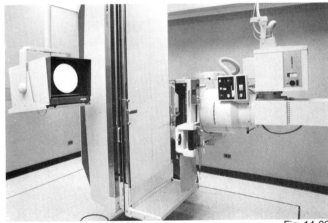

Fluoroscopy Room

Fig. 14-32

A **third** similarity is that **radiographs are produced during and after the fluoroscopic examination** of any specific parts of the alimentary canal to provide a permanent record of the normal or abnormal findings. A positive radiograph from an upper GI series is shown in *Fig. 14-33* demonstrating a duodenal ulcer, a type of mucosal erosion or "out pouching" (see arrow).

A spot radiograph of a barium enema of the lower GI tract is shown in *Fig. 14-34* demonstrating a carcinoma involving a segment of the large intestine.

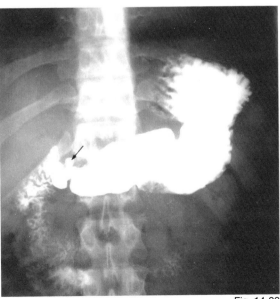
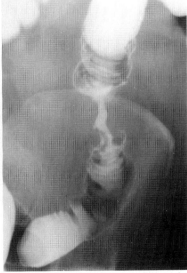

Fig. 14-33

Fig. 14-34

Duodenal Ulcer

Large Intestine Carcinoma

Contrast Media

Radiolucent and radiopaque contrast media are utilized to render the GI tract visible radiographically. **Radiolucent or negative contrast media** include **swallowed air**, **CO_2 gas crystals**, and the normally present **gas bubble** in the stomach. Calcium carbonate crystals are most commonly used in producing CO_2 gas.

Barium Sulfate (Barium)

The most common **positive or radiopaque contrast medium** used to visualize the gastrointestinal system is **barium sulfate**, ($BaSO_4$), commonly referred to as just **barium**. As illustrated in *Fig. 14-35* barium sulfate is a powdered, chalklike substance. The powdered barium sulfate is mixed with water prior to ingestion by the patient. This particular compound, which is a salt of barium, is relatively inert because of its extreme insolubility in water and other aqueous solutions, such as acids. All other salts of barium tend to be toxic or poisonous to the human system. Therefore, the barium sulfate used in radiology departments must be chemically pure.

A mixture of barium sulfate and water forms a colloidal **suspension,** not a solution. In order to be a solution, the molecules of the substance added to water must actually dissolve in the water. **Barium sulfate never dissolves in the water**. In a colloidal suspension, however, (such as barium sulfate and water) the particles suspended in the water may tend to settle out when allowed to sit for a period of time.

The radiograph shown in *Fig. 14-36* is of several cups of barium that were mixed with a ratio by volume of one part water to one part barium sulfate and then allowed to sit for 24 hours. Since different brands of barium sulfate were used, some cups exhibit more settling out than others. When the barium sulfate and water are mixed before they are actually needed, each cup must be well stirred before actual use.

Many special barium sulfate preparations are available commercially. Most of these preparations contain finely divided barium sulfate in a special suspending agent, so these preparations tend to resist settling out and, therefore, stay in suspension longer. Each of these suspensions must be well mixed before use, however. Various brands have different smells and different flavors, such as chocolate, chocolate malt, vanilla, lemon, lime or strawberry.

Thin Barium

Barium sulfate may be prepared or purchased in a relatively thin or thick mixture. The thin barium sulfate and water mixture, as illustrated in *Fig. 14-37,* contains one part $BaSO_4$ to one part of water. Thin barium is the consistency of cream and is used to study the entire GI tract.

The motility, or speed with which barium sulfate passes through the GI tract, depends on the suspending medium and additives, the temperature and the consistency of the preparation, as well as upon the general condition of the patient and the GI tract. It is most important to mix the preparation exactly according to radiologist preferences and departmental protocol. When the mixture is cold, the chalky taste is much less objectionable.

Thick Barium

Thick barium contains three or four parts of $BaSO_4$ to one part of water and should be the consistency of cooked cereal. Thick barium is well suited for use in the esophagus since it will descend slowly and will tend to coat the mucosal lining.

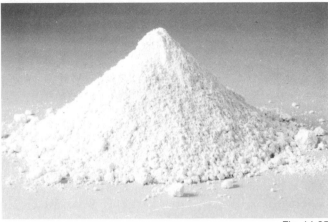

Barium Sulfate ($BaSO_4$)   Fig. 14-35

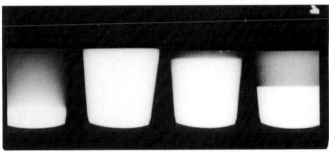

Cups of Barium (24 hrs.)   Fig. 14-36

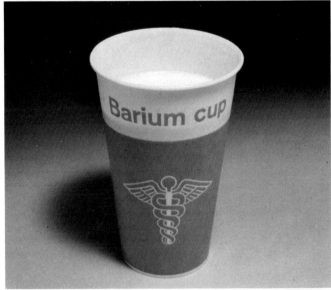

Thin Barium Sulfate and Water Mixture   Fig. 14-37

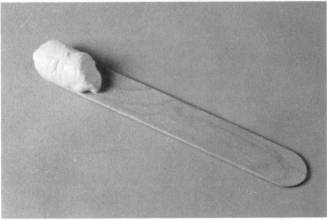

Thick Barium Sulfate Mixture   Fig. 14-38

Contrast Media continued

Contraindications to Barium Sulfate

Occasionally, barium sulfate mixtures are contraindicated. If there is any chance that the mixture might escape into the peritoneal cavity, such as through a perforated viscus, or if surgery is anticipated following the radiographic procedure, then **water-soluble, iodinated contrast media** are used. An example of this type is MD-Gastroview®, shown in *Fig. 14-39* in a 240 ml bottle. Other examples are Gastrografin® or Oral Hypaque®, all of which can be easily removed by aspiration before or during surgery. Should any of this water-soluble material escape into the peritoneal cavity, the body can readily absorb it. Barium sulfate, on the other hand, will not be absorbed and must be removed by the surgeon wherever it is found outside the alimentary canal. One drawback to the water-soluble materials is their bitter taste. Although these iodinated contrast media are sometimes mixed with carbonated soft drinks to mask the taste, they are often used "as is" or diluted with water. The patient should be forewarned that the taste may be slightly bitter.

The use of water-soluble iodinated contrast media however is contraindicated and should **not** be used if the patient is sensitive to iodine.

It has been reported that a small number of patients are hypersensitive to barium sulfate. Although this is a rare occurrence, the patient should be observed for any signs of allergic reaction.

Double Contrast

The use of double contrast techniques has been employed widely to enhance the diagnosis of certain diseases and conditions during upper GI's. Some departments are also performing double contrast esophagrams. The use of double contrast procedures employing both radiolucent and radiopaque contrast media was developed in Japan, where there is a high incidence of stomach carcinoma.

The **radiopaque** contrast medium is barium sulfate. A high density is used to provide good coating of the stomach mucosa. A pre-measured, commercially-produced cup of barium sulfate is often provided by the department, where the technologist needs only to add water and mix thoroughly.

The **radiolucent** contrast medium is either room air or carbon dioxide gas. To introduce room air, small pin prick holes are placed in the patient's straw. As the patient drinks the barium mixture, air is drawn in.

Carbon dioxide gas is created when the patient ingests gas-producing crystals. Two common forms of these crystals are calcium and magnesium citrate. Upon reaching the stomach these crystals form a large gas bubble. The gas forces the barium sulfate against the stomach mucosa providing better coating and visibility of the mucosa and its patterns *(Fig. 14-40)*. Potential polyps, diverticulae, and ulcers will be demonstrated better with a double contrast technique.

Post Exam Elimination (Defecation)

One of the normal functions of the large intestine is the absorption of water. Any barium sulfate mixture remaining in the large intestine after either an upper GI series or a barium enema may become hardened and somewhat solidified in the large bowel, and consequently be difficult to evacuate. Certain patients may require a laxative after these examinations to help remove the barium sulfate. If laxatives are contraindicated, the patient should force fluids or use mineral oil until stools are free from all traces of white.

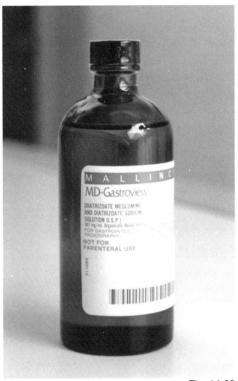

Fig. 14-39
Example of Water-Soluble
Iodinated Contrast Media

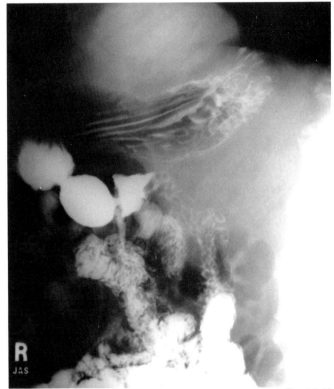

UGI-Double Contrast
(R Lateral Position)
Fig. 14-40

Radiography—Fluorography Equipment

General Fluoroscopy Unit

During fluoroscopy, the viewer is able to position a part so that the anatomy in question can be best seen by isolating it from objectionable overlying shadows. The fluoroscopic unit is equipped with a spot film device to permanently record optimum images. Cassettes of various sizes can be moved into position to permit a conventional, phototimed radiographic exposure. When fluoroscopy is being performed, these cassettes are in a leadprotected park position.

A conventional combination radiography-fluorography (R/F) unit is illustrated in *Fig. 14-41*. The modern general purpose fluoroscopy room is equipped with a variety of electronic devices. These include an **image intensifier and spot film device** which move as the table is tilted up or down. The electronically enhanced image can be viewed either with a **mirror optical system** or with a **television monitor.** This room utilizes the television monitor system. The television system is much more versatile and more widely accepted than the mirror system. Since these television systems are always closed-circuit systems, monitors can be placed outside the fluoro room for simultaneous viewing during the examination.

Many fluoroscopic systems utilize a **spot film camera** in addition to the direct filming methods related to the spot film device. This particular fluoroscopic unit is equipped with a 105 mm spot film camera in addition to a conventional spot film device. The spot film cameras are similar to movie cameras, but the framing frequency is slower and the film size is larger. Framing can be adjusted from a single exposure to 6 or 12 frames per second. The principal advantage of spot film cameras over direct filming methods is much less radiation exposure to the patient and better quality of the image.

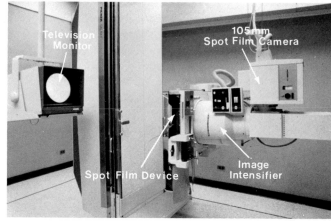

General Fluoroscopy Room   Fig. 14-41

Image Intensification

Conventional early fluoroscopy had two serious limitations: (1) the image was statistically inferior and (2) the amount of light given off prevented the use of daylight or photopic vision. In the early 1950's, the invention of the **image intensifier** revolutionized fluoroscopy.

The image intensifier utilizes the radiation that passes through the patient and enhances the resultant image by electronically making this image much brighter. The modern image intensifier produces an image at least 1,000 times brighter than the older fluoroscopy screen techniques, and, in some cases, as much as 6,000 times brighter. The image produced through image intensification is bright enough to be seen with photopic or day vision. The room lights are dimmed and the fluoroscopic examination is carried out in a comfortably illuminated room.

In *Fig. 14-42,* the image intensifier is located above the tabletop, while the x-ray tube is located beneath the tabletop.

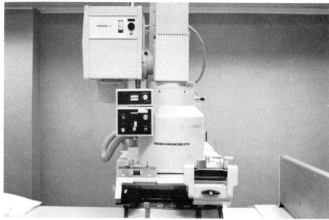

Image Intensifier Arrangement   Fig. 14-42

Esophagram

Two common radiographic procedures of the upper gastrointestinal system involving the administration of contrast media are the **esophagram**, or barium swallow as it is sometimes referred to, and the **upper GI series**. Each of these procedures will be described in detail beginning with the esophagram.

Definition

An esophagram or barium swallow is the common radiographic procedure or examination of the **pharynx** and **esophagus**, utilizing a radiopaque contrast medium. Occasionally a negative or radiolucent contrast medium may be used.

Purpose

The purpose of an esophagram is to study radiographically the form and function of the swallowing aspects of the pharnyx and esophagus.

Indications

Some clinical indications for an esophagram include:
- Anatomical anomalies
- Impaired swallowing mechanics
- Foreign body obstruction
- Esophageal reflux
- Esophageal varices

Anatomical anomalies may be congenital or acquired due to lifestyle or disease. Patients suffering from a stroke often develop **impaired swallowing mechanisms**. Patients may ingest a variety of **foreign bodies** that may include a bolus of food, metallic objects, and other materials. Their location and dimensions may be determined during the esophagram. Radiolucent foreign bodies such as fish bones may require the use of additional materials and techniques to detect them.

    Esophageal reflux is reported as heartburn by many patients. Gastric contents will return back through the gastric orifice and irritate the lining of the esophagus.

    Esophageal varices is the dilation of the veins in the distal esophagus. This condition is often seen with acute liver disease such as cirrhosis. In advanced cases the veins may begin to bleed.

Contraindications

No major contraindications exist for esophagrams except possible sensitivity to the contrast media used. The radiographer should determine if the patient has a history of sensitivity to barium sulfate, or water-soluble contrast media if it is utilized.

Patient Preparation

Radiographic examination of any part of the alimentary canal requires that the portion of the tract to be studied be empty. Since the esophagus is empty most of the time, there is no patient preparation for an esophagram unless an upper GI series is to follow. When combined with an upper GI, or if the primary interest is the lower esophagus, preparation for the UGI takes precedence.

    For an esophagram only, all clothing and anything metallic between the mouth and the waist should be removed and the patient should wear a hospital gown. Prior to the fluoroscopic procedure, a pertinent history should be taken and the examination should be carefully explained to the patient.

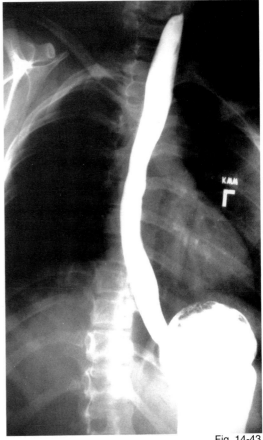

Fig. 14-43

RAO Esophagram

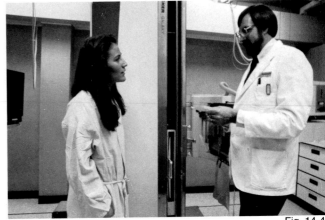

Fig. 14-44

Patient Preparation

Room Preparation

The first part of an esophagram involves fluoroscopy with a positive contrast medium. The examination room should be clean and tidy, and appropriately stocked before the patient is escorted to the room. The appropriate amount and type of contrast medium should be ready. Esophagrams utilize both thin and thick barium. Additional items useful in the detection of a radiolucent foreign body are: (1) cotton balls soaked in thin barium, (2) barium pills or gelatin capsules filled with $BaSO_4$ and (3) marshmallows followed by thin barium.

The control panel should be set for fluoroscopy with the appropriate technical factors selected. The fluoroscopy timer should be set for its maximum, usually five minutes. The spot film mechanism should be in proper working order and a supply of spot film cassettes should be handy. The appropriate number and size of conventional cassettes should be provided. The spot film camera should be loaded and in working condition.

Since the esophagram begins with the table in the vertical position, the footboard should be in place and tested for security. Lead aprons and lead gloves should be provided for the radiologist, as well as lead aprons for all other personnel to be in the room. Proper radiation protection methods must be observed at all times during fluoroscopy.

In most fluoroscopy units, the Bucky tray must be positioned at the foot end of the table. Appropriately place the radiation foot switch and provide the radiologist a stool, except where the examination is controlled from a remote area. Tissues, towels, emesis basins, spoons, drinking straws and a waste receptacle should be readily accessible.

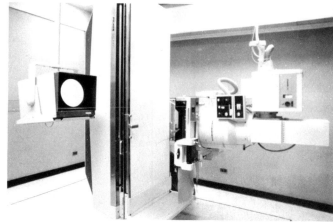

Room Preparation   Fig. 14-45

General Procedure

With the room prepared and the patient ready, the patient and radiologist are introduced, and the patient's history and the reason for the exam are discussed. The fluoroscopic examination usually begins with a general survey of the patient's chest, including heart, lungs and diaphragm, and the abdomen.

During fluoroscopy, the radiographer's duties, in general, are to follow the radiologist's instructions, to assist the patient as needed and to expedite the procedure in any manner possible. Since the examination is begun in the upright or erect position, a cup of thin barium is placed in the patient's left hand close to the left shoulder. The patient is then instructed to follow the radiologist's instructions concerning how much to drink and when. The radiologist will observe the flow of barium with the fluoroscope.

Swallowing (deglutition) of thin barium is observed with the patient in various frontal and oblique positions. Similar positions may be utilized while the patient swallows thick barium. The use of thick barium allows better visualization of mucosal patterns and any lesion within the esophagus. The type of barium mixture to be used, however, will be determined by the radiologist.

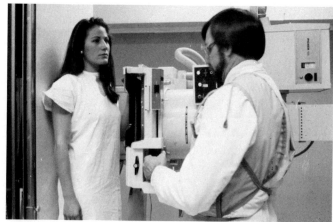

Fluoroscopy   Fig. 14-46

General Procedure continued

After the upright studies, horizontal and Trendelenburg positions with thick and thin barium may follow. A patient is shown in the **Trendelenburg position** (head lower than feet) with a cup of thin barium *(Fig. 14-47)*. The pharynx and cervical esophagus are usually studied fluoroscopically with spot films, while the main portion of the esophagus down to the stomach is studied both with fluoroscopy and with overhead radiographs. Radiographs using a spot film device or the spot film camera are exposed to document any abnormalities or suspicious areas.

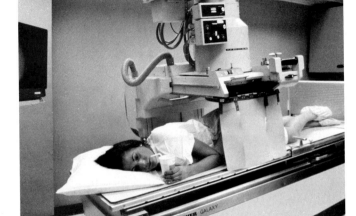

Trendelenburg Position

Fig. 14-47

Additional Fluoroscopy Procedures

The diagnosis of possible esophageal reflux or regurgitation of gastric contents may occur during fluoroscopy of an esophagram. The patient may be asked to perform one of the following procedures to detect esophageal reflux. They include:

(1) Breathing exercises
(2) The water test
(3) The toe-touch test

(1) Breathing Exercises

The various breathing exercises are all designed to increase both the intrathoracic and intra-abdominal pressures. The most common breathing exercise is the **Valsalva maneuver**. The patient is asked to take in a deep breath and, while holding the breath in, to bear down as though trying to move the bowels. This maneuver forces air against the closed glottis. A modified Valsalva maneuver is accomplished by having the patient pinch off the nose, close the mouth and try to blow his nose. The cheeks should expand outward as though the patient were blowing up a balloon.

A **Mueller maneuver** is performed by having the patient exhale and then try to inhale against a closed glottis.

(2) Water Test

The water test is done with the patient supine and turned up slightly on his left side. This slight LPO position will fill the fundus with barium. The patient is asked to swallow a mouthful of water through a straw. Under fluoroscopy, the radiologist closely observes the esophagogastric junction. A positive water test occurs when large amounts of barium regurgitate into the esophagus from the stomach.

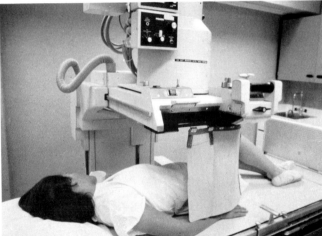

Water Test

Fig. 14-48

(3) Toe-touch Maneuver

The toe-touch maneuver is also performed to study possible regurgitation into the esophagus from the stomach. Under fluoroscopy, the cardiac orifice is observed as the patient bends over and touches his or her toes. Esophageal reflux and hiatal hernias are sometimes demonstrated using the toe-touch maneuver.

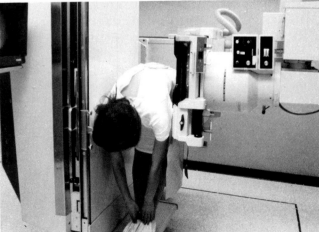

Toe-Touch Maneuver

Fig. 14-49

Post Fluoroscopy Imaging

Following the fluoroscopy portion of the esophagram, radiographs are obtained of the entire barium-filled esophagus. General positioning is similar to chest radiography but with higher centering. The area from the lower neck to the diaphragm must be visualized, requiring centering at the level of T5 or T6 (1 inch or 2.5 cm below sternal angle).

One to three spoonfuls of thick barium are fed to the patient before each exposure. The final spoonful is held in the patient's mouth until just before the exposure. The exposure is made after the bolus has been swallowed. It is usually unnecessary to have the patient stop breathing since respiration is suspended for approximately two seconds after deglutition.

The patient may be examined in either the recumbent or upright position. The thick barium will not descend as rapidly when the patient is lying down, and more complete filling of the esophagus will be accomplished.

Three positions or projections are considered routine for an esophagram or barium swallow. These include: (1) **RAO**, (2) **left lateral** and (3) **AP.**

Variations of the routine lateral are sometimes required. One variation is the soft tissue lateral position. When a foreign body is suspected high in the respiratory or digestive tracts, a soft tissue lateral is often the initial radiograph. Positioning is similar to an upright lateral of the cervical spine, although technical factors are adjusted so that approximately 10 kVp less is used. Radiopaque foreign bodies and some nonopaque foreign bodies can be demonstrated with this position. (A lower kVp is used to provide higher contrast and not overpenetrate small, less radiopaque foreign objects.)

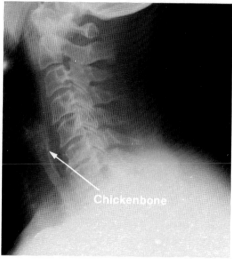

Fig. 14-50

Soft Tissue Lateral
(Demonstrates a chicken bone
lodged in esophagus)

Cardiac Series

The cardiac series is a radiographic examination very similar to the esophagram. The cardiac series consists of four views of the esophagus, well filled with a thick barium mixture. These are (1) a PA, (2) a left lateral, (3) a 45° RAO and (4) a 60° LAO. The filled esophagus indicates the size and configuration of the heart as seen on these four radiographs. The left lateral *(Fig. 14-51)* illustrates a massively enlarged heart. This patient suffered from rheumatic fever as a young person. Rheumatic fever attacks and damages the valves of the heart so that the myocardium or heart muscle has to work extra hard to pump adequate blood through the arteries. Whenever individual fibers of a muscle overwork, the result is an enlargement of the entire muscle, termed hypertrophy. This radiograph is an excellent demonstration of cardic hypertrophy.

The cardiac series, however, is rarely performed today because of the greater accuracy with other imaging modalities. One example is echocardiography, the use of ultrasound wave energy to study the heart. This is considered an ideal method to study the size of the heart and its components. It will measure accurately the ventricles, intraventricular septum, and demonstrate the heart valves.

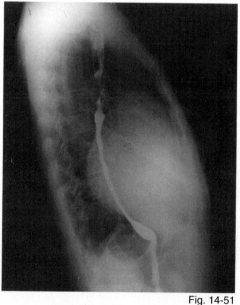

Fig. 14-51

Cardiac Series, Left Lateral

Upper GI Series

The second and very common radiographic procedure or examination of the upper gastrointestinal system involving contrast media is the **upper gastrointestinal series** (UGI).

Definition
Radiographic examination of the **distal esophagus**, **stomach**, and **duodenum** is termed an **upper GI series** (UGI).

Purpose
The purpose of the upper GI is to study radiographically the form and function of the distal esophagus, stomach, and duodenum, as well as to detect abnormal anatomical and functional conditions.

Clinical Indications
Some clinical indications for an upper GI series include:
- peptic ulcers
- hiatal hernia *(hi-a´tal her´ne-ah)*
- acute or chronic gastritis
- tumor, carcinoma and benign
- diverticula *(di´ver-tik´u-lah)*
- bezoars *(be´zor)*

Peptic ulcers which include gastric and duodenal ulcers are erosions of the stomach or duodenal mucosa due to various physiological or environmental conditions, such as excessive gastric secretions, stress, diet, and smoking. If untreated, the ulcer may lead to a perforation of the stomach or duodenum. The mucosal ulcer will usually fill with barium sulfate during the upper GI. A small peptic ulcer is demonstrated in *Fig. 14-52.*

A **hiatal hernia** is a condition where a portion of the stomach will herniate through the diaphragmatic opening. It may be a slight herniation or a severe form where a majority of the stomach is found within the thoracic cavity. A moderate size hiatal hernia is shown in *Fig. 14-53.*

Gastritis is inflamation of the lining or mucosa of the stomach. Gastritis may develop in response to various physiological and environmental conditions. **Acute gastritis** will present severe symptoms of pain and discomfort. **Chronic gastritis** is an intermittent condition that may be brought on by changes in diet, stress, or other factors.

Tumors in the stomach or duodenum may be either a carcinoma or benign. A **polyp** is a small mass growing from the mucosal wall. It could be either a cancerous or benign growth.

Diverticulae are a weakening and outpouching of a portion of the mucosal wall. Although benign they can lead to perforation if untreated. A double-contrast upper GI is best to diagnose any tumors or diverticulae. An air-filled, barium lined diverticulum of the duodenal bulb is shown in *Fig. 14-54.*

A **bezoar** is a mass of undigested material that gets trapped in the stomach. This mass is usually made up of hair, certain vegetable fibers, or wood products. The material builds up and may form an obstruction in time. Although a rare condition, it may be seen during an upper GI.

Contraindications
Contraindications for upper GI's apply primarily to the type of contrast media used. If the patient has a history of bowel perforation, laceration, or viscus rupture, the use of barium sulfate may be contraindicated. An oral water-soluble iodinated contrast media may be used in place of barium sulfate.

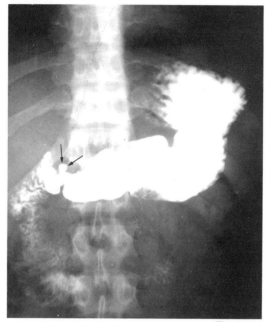

PA Projection – Peptic Ulcer   Fig. 14-52

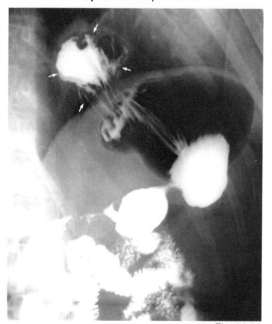

Obli. Projection – Hiatal Hernia   Fig. 14-53

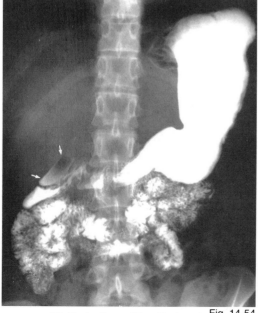

PA Projection – Diverticulum in Duodenum   Fig. 14-54

Upper GI Series continued

Patient Preparation

The goal of patient preparation for an upper GI series is for the patient to arrive in the radiology department with a completely empty stomach. For an examination scheduled in the morning hours, the patient should be NPO *(Non Per Os,* meaning nothing by mouth) from midnight until time for the examination. Food and fluids should be withheld for at least eight hours prior to the exam. The patient is also instructed not to smoke cigarettes or chew gum during the NPO period. These activities tend to increase gastric secretions and salivation.

The upper GI series is often a time-consuming procedure so the patient should be forewarned of the time the examination may take when the appointment is made. This is especially true if the UGI is to be followed by a small bowel series. The importance of an empty stomach should also be stressed when the appointment is made so that the patient will arrive properly prepared both physically and psychologically.

Pregnancy Precautions

If the patient is a female, then a menstrual history must be obtained. Irradiation of an early pregnancy is one of the most hazardous situations in diagnostic radiography.

X-ray examinations such as the upper GI series which include the pelvis and uterus in the primary beam and which include fluoroscopy should never be done on pregnant females unless absolutely necessary.

Any x-ray examination of the abdomen of a potentially pregnant female should be goverened by the "ten-day rule". Any female of child-bearing age should have such radiographic procedures **only** during the ten-day period after the start of menstruation. This is the only time when pregnancy can be ruled out with any certainty. Abdominal radiographs of a known pregnancy should be delayed at least until the third trimester, if done at all. This is especially important if fluoroscopy, which greatly increases patient exposure, is involved.

Room Preparation

Responsibilities of the radiographer prior to the patient's arrival include setting up the room for fluoroscopy. Room set-up for a UGI series is very similar to that for an esophagram. The thin barium sulfate mixture is the usual contrast medium necessary for an upper GI series. On occasion, thick barium may be used in addition to some type of gas-forming preparation. On rare occasions, water-soluble contrast media will be used in preference to the barium sulfate mixture.

The fluoroscopy table is raised to the vertical position, although with some very ill patients the exam must be started with the table horizontal. Therefore, the foot board should be placed at the end of the table. The room should be clean and tidy, and the control panel should be set for fluoroscopy. The spot film mechanism and the spot film camera should be properly loaded and in working condition. All cassettes for the entire exam should be provided. Lead aprons, lead gloves, and compression paddle should be provided for the radiologists, as well as lead aprons for all other personnel in the room. Any other equipment to be utilized during the examination should be readily accessible.

Prior to introduction of the patient and the radiologist, the examination procedure should be carefully explained to the patient and the patient's history should be obtained.

General Routine Procedure

General duties during fluoroscopy for an upper GI series are similar to those for an esophagram. The radiographer should follow the radiologist's instructions, assist the patient as needed and expedite the procedure in any manner possible. The fluoroscopic routine followed by radiologists varies greatly. The general routine of each physician may also vary since each patient and each examination is different. The fluoroscopy routine is usually begun with the patient in the upright position, as illustrated in *Fig. 14-57.* A wide variety of table moves, patient moves and special maneuvers follows until fluoroscopy is complete.

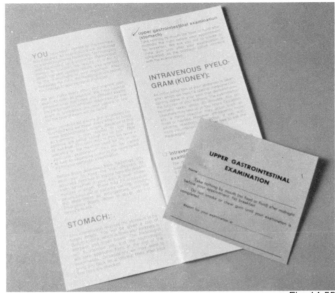

Fig. 14-55

Patient Preparation

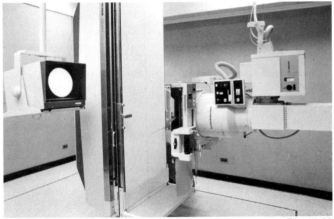

Fig. 14-56

Room Preparation

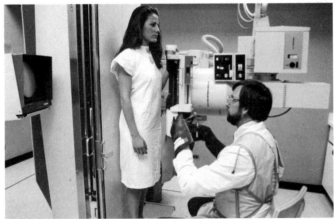

Fig. 14-57

Fluoroscopy

Upper GI Series continued

Table Moves

Since a large number of position changes are made during the fluoroscopic examination, the radiographer must help the patient with the barium cup, provide a pillow when the patient is lying down and keep the patient adequately covered at all times. The barium cup should be held by the patient in the left hand near the left shoulder whenever he (she) is upright. The cup must be taken from the patient when the table is tilted up or down.

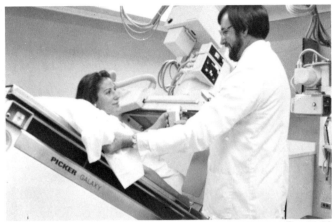

Fig. 14-58

Table Moves

Patient Moves

Various patient moves combined with table moves are made during the fluoroscopic procedure. The right anterior oblique position, illustrated in *Fig. 14-59,* allows barium to migrate toward the pyloric portion or distal stomach, while any air in the stomach will shift toward the fundus.

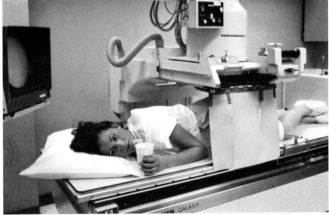

Fig. 14-59

Patient Moves

Post Fluoroscopy Routines

Following fluoroscopy, certain routine positions or projections are obtained to further document any tentative diagnosis concluded fluoroscopically. These overhead radiographs, such as the RAO shown being positioned in *Fig. 14-60,* must be obtained immediately following fluoroscopy, before too much of the barium meal has passed into the jejunum.

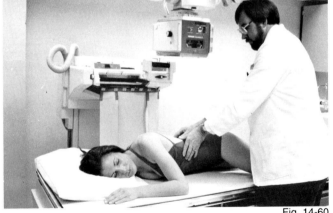

Fig. 14-60

RAO Positioning

Summary of Positioning Tips for Upper GI's

(1) **Clinical History**: Gain clinical history from the patient or his chart to determine clinical indications for the study and any past or recent abdominal surgery of the GI tract. Surgery or resection of the bowel or stomach will alter its normal position. Pay close attention to the flouro monitor to detect such differences which may affect positioning and centering on the post fluoroscopy filming.

(2) **Body Habitus**: Consider the body habitus of the patient. Remember the stomach will be high and transverse with the hypersthenic patient and low and vertical with the hyposthenic patient. The sthenic or average patient will have the duodenum bulb near the L2 region. Usually, L2 is located 1 - 2 in. (2.5-5 cm) above the lower lateral rib cage margin. Centering points in this text are designed for the average sthenic patient.

(3) **Fluoroscopy**: During fluoroscopy, identify the stomach on the fluoro monitor. Pinpoint surrounding structures to gain clues about location of the stomach and duodenum. For example, if the body of the stomach is adjacent to the iliac wing, then you need to center lower than the average or sthenic patient.

Part III Radiographic Positioning

National Survey

A survey of the operating procedures (department routines) was conducted throughout the United States. The following information was compiled from the survey indicating the national norm for basic and optional positions for esophagrams and upper GI's. The survey results were very consistent throughout all regions of the US. (The number in parenthesis in each box indicates the number of institutions responding to that part of the survey.)

Esophagram Routine

Esophagus	U.S. Average (522)	
	Basic	Optional
• RAO	88%	
• Left Lateral	55%	
• AP	48%	13%
• PA	30%	9%
• LAO		14%
• Soft Tissue Lateral		12%
• Fluoroscopy only		6%

Cardiac Series Routine

Cardiac Series	U.S. Average (334)	
	Basic	Optional
• RAO - 45°	91%	
• PA	87%	
• Left Lateral	84%	
• LAO - 60°	84%	

Upper GI Routine

Stomach and Duodenum	U.S. Average (529)	
	Basic	Optional
• RAO (Recumbent)	93%	
• PA (Recumbent)	85%	
• Right Lateral (Recumbent)	80%	
• LPO (Recumbent)	55%	14%
• AP (Recumbent)	50%	10%
• PA (Erect)	5%	12%
• Left Lateral (Erect)	4%	11%
• Double Contrast Techniques*	62%	13%

* Double Contrast techniques involve the use of both a positive (barium sulfate) and negative (usually carbon dioxide gas) contrast media.

Summary:

The **cardiac series** was included in the survey with routines as shown above. However it has been determined that this procedure is rarely performed anymore because of increased accuracy of other imaging modalities. Therefore this procedure is described on page 430 but not in the positioning pages which follow. However the procedure and positioning is very similar to that of the esophagram.

The **double contrast technique** for the upper GI is a common procedure as indicated on this survey. This procedure is described on page 425 under part II, radiographic procedure, but is not specifically described in the positioning pages which follow since generally the double contrast positioning routines are similar to the regular single contrast upper GI.

Basic and Optional Projections/Positions

Certain basic and optional positions or projections of the esophagus, stomach and duodenum are described and demonstrated on the following pages. The five positions or projections for the upper GI series are listed in order of suggested clinical usefulness.

While the routine of each radiologist or other clinical specialist may vary, the RAO and PA are considered a **minimum** series. The routine may also include other positions in addition to these five.

Esophagram
(Barium Swallow)
Basic
• RAO (35-40°)
• Left lateral
• AP (PA)
Optional
• LAO
• Soft tissue lateral

Upper GI Series
Basic
• RAO (Recumbent)
• PA (Recumbent)
• Right lateral (Recumbent)
• LPO (Recumbent)
• AP (Recumbent)

• RAO Position

Esophagram
Basic
• **RAO** (35-40°)
• Left Lateral
• AP (PA)

Structures Best Shown:
Esophagus between the vertebral column and heart.

Technical Factors:
• Film Size - 14 x 17 in. (35 x 43 cm), lengthwise.
• Moving or stationary grid.
• 100-125 kVp range.

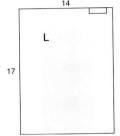

Patient Position:
• Recumbent or erect. Recumbent preferred because of more complete filling of esophagus (due to gravity factor with erect).

Shielding: Place lead shield over patient's pelvic region to protect gonads.

Part Position:
• Rotate **35-40°** from a PA with the right anterior body against film holder or table.
• Right arm down; left arm flexed at elbow and up by the patient's head.
• Flex left knee if recumbent.
• Align midline of thorax in the oblique position to midline of film holder and/or table.

Central Ray:
• CR **perpendicular** to film holder.
• Center to level **1 in.** (2.5 cm) **inferior** to **sternal angle** (T5 to T6 level).
• Minimum 40 in. (102 cm); or 72 in. (183 cm) SID if erect.

Collimation: Collimate the lateral borders to create two-sided collimation about 5 or 6 in. (12-15 cm) wide. Collimate end borders to film margins with L or R placed within collimation field.

Respiration: Suspend respiration and expose upon expiration. (See NOTE.)

NOTE: • Two or three spoonfuls of thick barium should be ingested and the exposure made immediately after last bolus is swallowed.
• For complete filling of the esophagus using thin barium, it may be necessary for the patient to drink through a straw with continuous swallowing and exposure made after 3 or 4 swallows without suspending respiration. (Patient will not be breathing immediately after a swallow.)

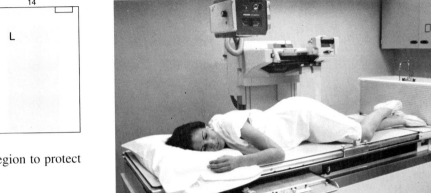

Fig. 14--61
RAO – Recumbent

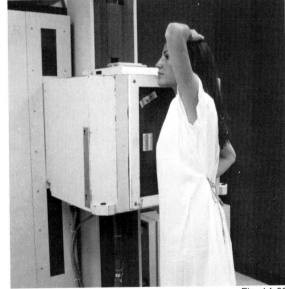

RAO – Erect
Fig. 14-62

Evaluation Criteria:
• Esophagus seen midway between heart and thoracic spine.
• The patient's upper limbs should not superimpose the esophagus.
• The entire esophagus is filled with contrast medium.
• Appropriate technique employed to clearly visualize borders of the contrast media filled esophagus.
• Patient ID information legible; R or L marker placed on lateral border visible without superimposing essential anatomy.

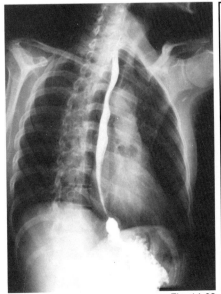

RAO
Fig. 14-63

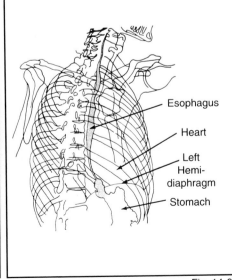

RAO
Fig. 14-64

Esophagus
Heart
Left Hemi-diaphragm
Stomach

• Left Lateral Position

Structures Best Shown:
Esophagus between the vertebral column and heart.

Technical Factors:
• Film Size - 14 x 17 in. (35 x 43 cm), lengthwise.
• Moving or stationary grid.
• 100-125 kVp range.

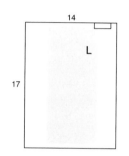

Patient Position:
• Recumbent or erect (recumbent preferred - see RAO) with left side against film holder.

Shielding: Place lead shield over gonadal area.

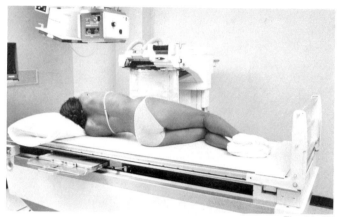

Left lateral – Recumbent   Fig. 14--65

Part Position:
• Arms placed over the head with the elbows flexed and superimposed; or arms crossed above head grasping opposite elbows.
• Align **mid-coronal plane to midline** of film holder and/or table.
• Insure shoulders and hips are in a **true lateral position**. (Midsagittal plane should be parallel to film.)

Central Ray:
• CR **perpendicular** to film holder.
• Center to mid-coronal plane **1 in.** (2.5 cm) **inferior** to **sternal angle** (T5-6 level).
• Minimum 40 in. (102 cm); or 72 in. (183 cm) SID if erect.

Collimation: Collimate along the lateral borders to create two-sided collimation about 5 or 6 in. (12-15 cm) wide.

Respiration: Suspend respiration and expose upon expiration.

NOTE: • Two or three spoonfuls of thick barium should be ingested and the exposure made immediately after last bolus is swallowed.
• For complete filling of the esophagus using thin barium, it may be necessary for the patient to drink through a straw with continuous swallowing and exposure made after 3 or 4 swallows without suspending respiration. (Patient will not be breathing immediately after a swallow.)

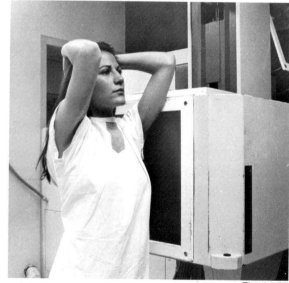

Left Lateral – Erect   Fig. 14-66

Evaluation Criteria:
• Esophagus seen between thoracic spine and heart.
• True lateral as indicated by direct superimposition of posterior ribs.
• The patient's arms should not superimpose the esophagus.
• The entire esophagus is filled with contrast media.
• Appropriate technique employed to clearly visualize borders of the contrast media filled esophagus.
• Patient ID information legible; R or L marker placed on lateral border visible without superimposing essential anatomy.

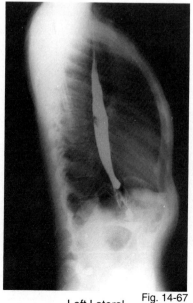

Left Lateral   Fig. 14-67

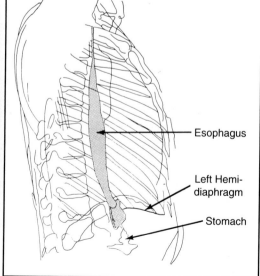

Esophagus

Left Hemi-diaphragm

Stomach

Left Lateral   Fig. 14-68

• AP (PA) Projection

Esophagram
Basic
• RAO (35-40°)
• Left Lateral
• **AP (PA)**

Structures Best Shown:
A frontal image of the esophagus.

Technical Factors:
• Film Size - 14 x 17 in. (35 x 43 cm), lengthwise.
• Moving or stationary grid.
• 100-125 kVp range.

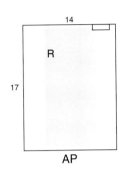

AP

Patient Position:
• Recumbent or erect (recumbent preferred), facing the x-ray tube with arms down at the patient's side.

Shielding:
Place lead shield over patient's pelvic region to shield gonads.

Part Position:
• Align **midsagittal plane to midline** of film holder and/or table.
• Insure shoulders and hips are **not rotated**.

Central Ray:
• CR **perpendicular** to film holder.
• Center to midsagittal plane, **1 in.** (2.5 cm) **inferior** to **sternal angle** (T5-6).
• Minimum 40 in. (102 cm); or 72 in. (183 cm) SID if erect.

Collimation:
Use tight side collimation to result in about 5 or 6 in. (12-15 cm) wide collimation field. Collimate end borders to film margins.

Respiration:
Suspend respiration and expose upon expiration.

Alternate PA:
This can also be taken as a PA projection with similar positioning, centering and CR locations.

NOTE: • Two or three spoonfuls of thick barium should be ingested and the exposure made immediately after last bolus is swallowed.
• For complete filling of the esophagus using thin barium, it may be necessary for the patient to drink through a straw with continuous swallowing and exposure made after 3 or 4 swallows without suspending respiration. (Patient will not be breathing immediately after a swallow.)

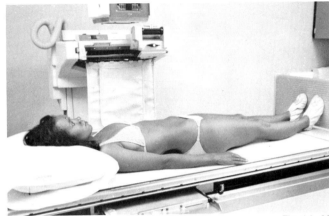

Recumbent AP

Fig. 14--69

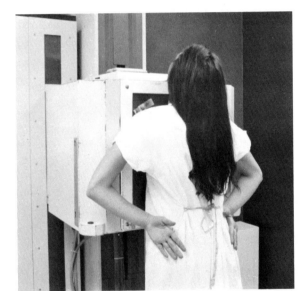

Erect (Alternate) PA

Fig. 14-70

Evaluation Criteria:
• The entire esophagus is filled with barium.
• No rotation of the patient's body evidenced by the symmetry of the sternoclavicular (SC) joints.
• Appropriate technique utilized to visualize the esophagus through the superimposed thoracic vertebrae.
• Patient ID information legible; R or L marker placed on lateral border should be visible without superimposing essential anatomy.

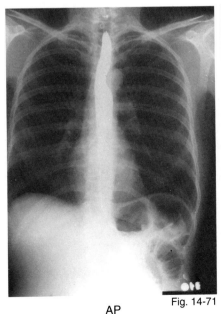

AP

Fig. 14-71

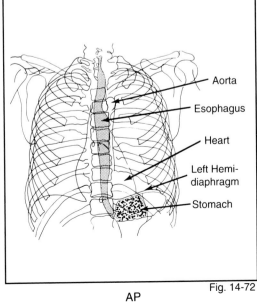

AP

Fig. 14-72

Aorta

Esophagus

Heart

Left Hemi-diaphragm

Stomach

Esophagram

• LAO Position

Esophagram
Optional
• **LAO**
• Soft Tissue
Lateral

Structures Best Shown:

Esophagus between the vertebral column and hilar region.

Technical Factors:

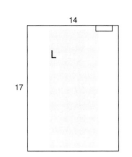

- Film Size - 14 x 17 in. (35 x 43 cm), lengthwise.
- Moving or stationary grid.
- 100-125 kVp range.

Patient Position:

- Recumbent or erect (recumbent preferred, see RAO), with body partially rotated into a LAO.

Shielding: Place lead shield over gonadal area.

Part Position:

- Rotate **35-40°** from a PA with the left anterior body against film holder or table.
- Left arm down by the patient's side, right arm flexed at elbow and up by the patient's head.
- Flex right knee if recumbent.

Central Ray:

- CR **perpendicular** to film holder.
- Center **1 in.** (2.5 cm) **inferior** to **level of sternal angle** (T 5-6 level).
- Minimum 40 in. (102 cm); or 72 in. (183 cm) SID.

Collimation: Collimate lateral borders to create two-sided collimation about 5 or 6 in. (12-15 cm) wide. Collimate end borders to film margins.

Respiration: Suspend respiration and expose upon expiration.

NOTE: • Two or three spoonfuls of thick barium should be ingested and the exposure made immediately after last bolus is swallowed.

- For complete filling of the esophagus using thin barium, it may be necessary for the patient to drink through a straw with continuous swallowing and exposure made after 3 or 4 swallows without suspending respiration. (Patient will not be breathing immediately after a swallow.)

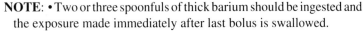

Evaluation Criteria:

- Esophagus seen between heart and thoracic spine.
- The patient's upper limbs should not superimpose the esophagus.
- The entire esophagus is filled with contrast medium.
- Appropriate technique employed to clearly visualize borders of the contrast media filled esophagus.
- Patient ID information legible; R or L marker placed on lateral border visible without superimposing essential anatomy.

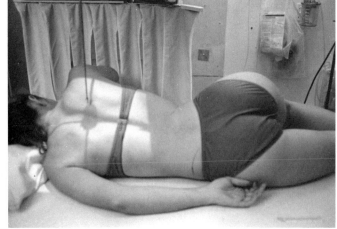

Recumbent LAO   Fig. 14-73

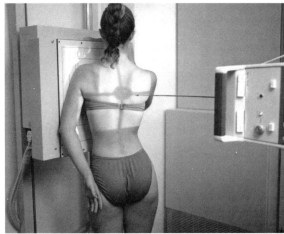

Erect LAO   Fig. 14-74

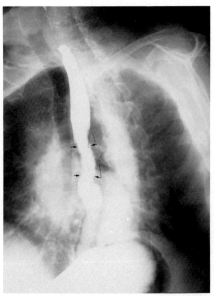

LAO   Fig. 14-75
(Demonstrates a constricted area of esophagus, probably carcinoma, see arrows)

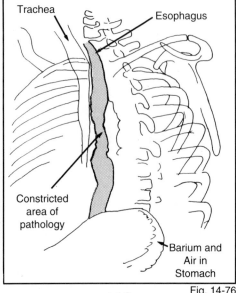

LAO   Fig. 14-76

(Labels in Fig. 14-76: Trachea, Esophagus, Constricted area of pathology, Barium and Air in Stomach)

• Soft Tissue Lateral

<table>
<tr><td>

Esophagram
Optional
• LAO
• **Soft Tissue Lateral**

</td></tr>
</table>

Structures Best Shown:

Laryngopharynx, larynx, upper esophagus and upper trachea.

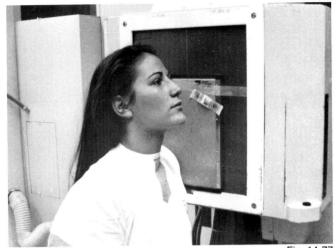

Fig. 14-77
Soft Tissue Lateral

Technical Factors:

• Film Size - 10 x 12 in. (24 x 30 cm), lengthwise.
• Moving or stationary grid.
• 60-70 kVp range.
• Short exposure time and small focal spot.

Patient Position:

• Erect if possible, seated or standing with arms down by side, in a left lateral position.

Shielding: Place lead shield over patient's pelvic region to protect gonads.

Part Position:

• Rotate entire body 90° from an AP/PA, with left shoulder against the film holder.
• Upper limbs down by patient's side with shoulders depressed.
• Extend or protract chin to remove ramus of mandible away from the laryngopharynx area.
• Adjust film height to place top of cassette at level of EAM (external auditory meatus).
• Position patient to center proximal airway and esophagus to center of film. (Proximal airway and esophagus lie anterior to cervical vertebrae.)

Central Ray:

• CR **perpendicular** to film holder.
• Center to **level of inferior margin of laryngeal prominence** (C6).
• Minimum 72 in. (183 cm) SID if possible to minimize magnification and increase definition.

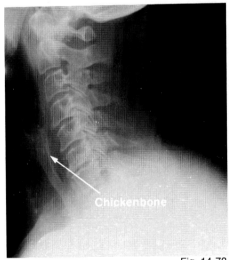

Fig. 14-78
Soft Tissue Lateral
(Positive - Chicken Bone)

Collimation: Closely collimate along the anteroposterior borders of the proximal airway and esophagus.

Respiration: See NOTE.

NOTE: • Exposure should be made during a slow deep inspiration to insure filling trachea and proximal airway with air. • In case of radiolucent foreign bodies, additional material such as shredded cotton soaked in barium is swallowed. • Expose after last bolus of contrast medium is swallowed.

Evaluation Criteria:

• The entire proximal airway and esophagus is filled with contrast media (with barium and/or air).
• No rotation of the cervical spine.
• Ramus of mandible not superimposed over proximal airway.
• Appropriate technique utilized to demonstrate the soft tissues of the pharynx and proximal esophagus. (Margins of the air-filled proximal airway should be visible.)
• Patient ID information legible; R or L marker placed on lateral border visible without superimposing essential anatomy.

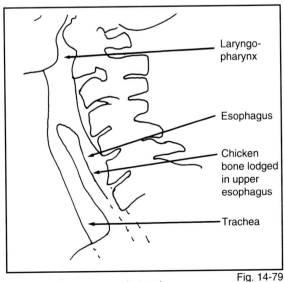

Laryngo-pharynx

Esophagus

Chicken bone lodged in upper esophagus

Trachea

Lateral

Fig. 14-79

• RAO Position

M97

Upper GI Series
Basic
• **RAO**
• PA
• R Lateral
• LPO
• AP

Structures Best Shown:
Stomach and C-loop of the duodenum. A profile image of the duodenum bulb.

Technical Factors:
• Film Size - 10 x 12 in. (24 x 30 cm), lengthwise.
      or   11 x 14 in. (30 x 35 cm).
• Moving or stationary grid.
• 100-125 kVp range.
   (80-100 kVp for double-contrast study)

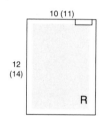

Patient Position:
• Recumbent with the body partially rotated into a RAO position, provide pillow for head.

Shielding: Place lead shield over patient's pelvic region to protect gonads without covering pertinent anatomy.

Part Position:
• From a prone position rotate **40-70°** with right anterior body against film holder or table. (Average body type - 45° oblique, heavy hypersthenic, - 70°, thin asthenic - 40°).
• Right arm down, left arm flexed at elbow and up by the patient's head.
• Flex left knee for support.

Central Ray:
• CR **perpendicular** to film holder.
• Average body type - center CR and film to duodenal bulb at **level of L 2** (1-2 in. or 2.5 to 5 cm above lower lateral rib margin), **midway between spine and lateral border of abdomen**. (See NOTE for body variations.)
• Minimum 40 in. (102 cm) SID.

Collimation: Collimate on four sides to outer margins of film, or to area of interest on larger film.

Respiration: Suspend respiration and expose upon expiration.

NOTE: • The stomach on a **hypersthenic** (heavy set) type is located high and transverse requiring 1 or 2 in. (2.5-5 cm) **higher centering** and **more rotation** on the oblique. The very slender **asthenic** has a low but vertical stomach near the midline, thus requiring about 2 in. (5 cm) **lower** centering **nearer the midline** with **less rotation** on the oblique.

Evaluation Criteria:
• Entire stomach and C-loop of duodenum is visualized.
• Body and pylorus of stomach is filled with contrast medium.
• Duodenal bulb is in profile.
• Appropriate technique employed to clearly visualize the gastric folds without overexposing other pertinent anatomy.
• Patient ID information legible; R or L marker placed on lateral border visible without superimposing essential anatomy.

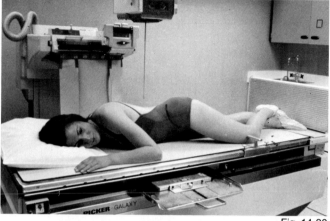

RAO   Fig. 14-80

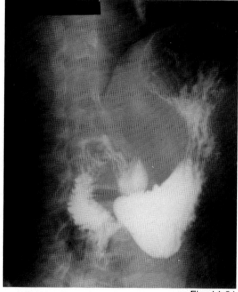

RAO   Fig. 14-81

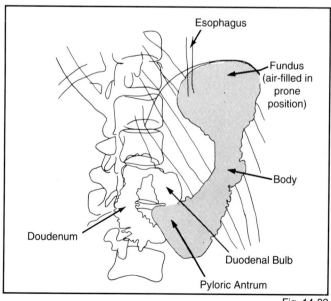

RAO   Fig. 14-82

•PA Projection

Structures Best Shown:
Stomach and duodenum with barium in the body and pylorus of the stomach.

Technical Factors:
- Film Size - 10 x 12 in. (24 x 30 cm), lengthwise.
  - or   11 x 14 in. (30 x 35 cm)
  - or   14 x 17 in. (35 x 43 cm) if small bowel is to be included.
- Moving or stationary grid.
- 100 to 125 kVp range.
  (80-100 kVp range for double-contrast study)

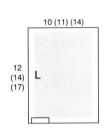

Patient Position:
- Patient prone with arms up beside head, provide pillow.

Shielding:
Place lead shield over patient's pelvic region to protect gonads without covering pertinent anatomy.

Part Position:
- Align midsagittal plane to midline of table.
- Insure there is **no body rotation.**

Central Ray:
- CR **perpendicular** to film holder.
- Average body type - center CR and film to duodenal bulb at level of **L 2** (1-2 in. or 2.5-5 cm above lower lateral rib margin), and **1 or 2 in. (2.5-5 cm) left of the vertebral column**.
  Hypersthenic - center about 2 in. or 5 cm higher;
  Asthenic - center about 2 in. or 5 cm lower and nearer midline.
- Minimum 40 in. (102 cm) SID.

Collimation:
Collimate on four sides to outer margins of film, or to area of interest on a larger film.

Respiration:
Suspend respiration and expose upon expiration.

Alternate PA Axial: The position of the high transverse stomach on a **hypersthenic** type patient causes almost an end on view with much overlapping of the pyloric region of the stomach and the duodenal bulb with a 90° PA projection. Therefore, a **35 to 45° cephalic angle** of the central ray separates these areas for better visualization. The greater and lesser curvatures of the stomach are also better visualized in profile.

Evaluation Criteria:
- Entire stomach and duodenum is visualized.
- Body and pylorus of the stomach is filled with barium.
- Appropriate technique employed to visualize the gastric folds without overexposing other pertinent anatomy.
- Patient ID information legible; R or L marker placed on lateral border visible without superimposing essential anatomy.

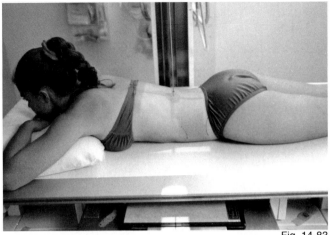

PA   Fig. 14-83

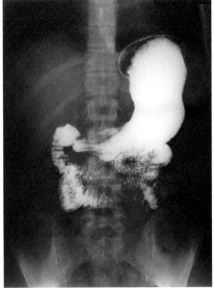

Fig. 14-84
PA

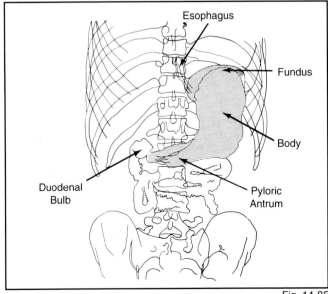

PA   Fig. 14-85

•Right Lateral Position

Upper GI Series
Basic
• RAO
• PA
• **R Lateral**
• LPO
• AP

Structures Best Shown:
Stomach and duodenum with a view of the retrogastric space with barium primarily in mid and distal stomach and duodenum.

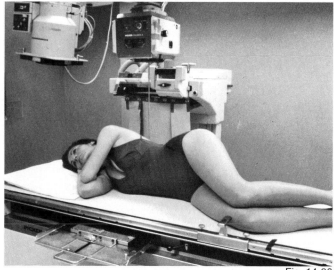

Right Lateral Position   Fig. 14-86

Technical Factors:
- Film Size - 10 x 12 in. (24 x 30 cm), lengthwise.
  - or   11 x 14 in. (30 x 35 cm)
- Moving or stationary grid.
- 100 to 125 kVp range.
  - (80-100 kVp range for double-contrast study)

10 (11)
12 (14) R

Patient Position:
- Recumbent in a right lateral position. Provide pillow for head. Arms up by the patient's head and knees flexed.

Shielding: Place lead shield over patient's pelvic region to protect gonads without covering pertinent anatomy.

Part Position:
- Insure shoulders and hips are in a true lateral position.
- Bottom of cassette should be about at level of iliac crest.

Central Ray:
- CR **perpendicular** to film holder.
- Average body type - center CR and film to duodenal bulb at level of **L 1** (midway between xiphoid tip and lower lateral margin of ribs) and **1 to 1.5 in. or 2.5-4 cm anterior to midcoronal plane** (midway between anterior border of vertebrae and the anterior abdomen).

- Hypersthenic - center about 2 in. or 5 cm higher; asthenic about 2 in. or 5 cm lower.)
- Minimum 40 in. (102 cm) SID.

Collimation: Collimate on four sides to outer margins of film, or to area of interest on larger film.

Respiration: Suspend respiration and expose upon expiration.

NOTE: Stomach is located about one vertebra higher in this position than in PA or oblique positions.

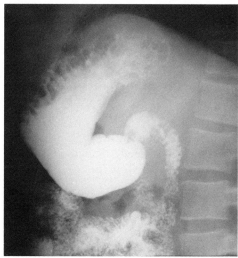

Right Lateral   Fig. 14-87

Evaluation Criteria:
- Entire stomach and duodenum is visualized.
- Demonstration of the retrogastric space.
- Pylorus of stomach and C-loop of duodenum should be visualized well on hypersthenic type patients.
- Vertebral bodies should be seen for reference purposes. The intervertebral foramen should be open indicating a true lateral position.
- Appropriate technique employed to visualize the gastric folds without overexposing other pertinent anatomy.
- Patient ID information legible; R or L marker placed on lateral border visible without superimposing essential anatomy.

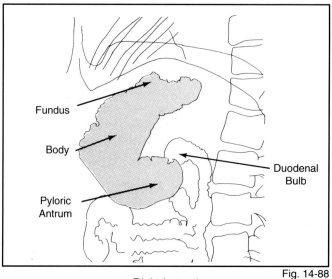

Fundus

Body

Duodenal Bulb

Pyloric Antrum

Right Lateral   Fig. 14-88

•LPO Position

<table>
<tr><td>Upper GI Series
Basic
• RAO
• PA
• R Lateral
• LPO
• AP</td></tr>
</table>

Structures Best Shown:
Stomach with barium filled fundus and duodenum with a profile image of the duodenal bulb.

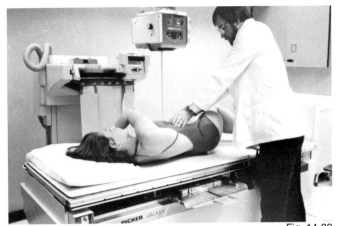

LPO   Fig. 14-89

Technical Factors:
• Film Size - 10 x 12 in. (24 x 30 cm), lengthwise.
    or   - 11 x 14 in. (30 x 35 cm)
• Moving or stationary grid.
• 100 to 125 kVp range.
  (80-100 kVp range for double-contrast study)

Patient Position:
• Recumbent with the body partially rotated into a LPO position. Provide pillow for head.

Shielding: Place lead shield over patient's pelvic region to protect gonads without covering pertinent anatomy.

Part Position:
• Rotate **30-60°** from supine position with left posterior against film holder or table. (Average body type - 45°, heavy hypersthenic - 60°, thin asthenic - 30°.)
• Flex right knee for support.
• Extend left arm away from body and raise right arm high across chest to grasp end of table for support (do not pinch fingers when moving Bucky).
• Bottom of cassette should be about at level of iliac crest.

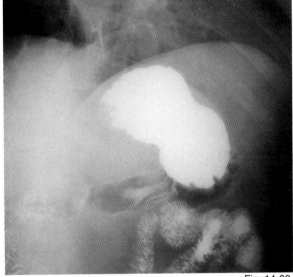

LPO   Fig. 14-90

Central Ray:
• CR **perpendicular** to film holder.
• Average body type - center CR and film to **level of L 1** (about midway between xiphoid tip and lower lateral margin of ribs), and **midway between vertebral spinous processes** and **left lateral margin** of abdomen.
• Hypersthenic - center about 2 in. or 5 cm higher; asthenic about 2 in. or 5 cm lower and nearer to midline.
• Minimum 40 in. (102 cm) SID.

Collimation: Collimate on four sides to outer margins of film, or to area of interest on larger film.

Respiration: Suspend respiration and expose upon expiration.

NOTE: Stomach is located higher in this position than in the lateral; therefore, center one vertebra higher than on PA or RAO positions.

Evaluation Criteria:
• Entire stomach and duodenum is visualized.
• An unobstructed view of the duodenal bulb without superimposition by the pylorus of the stomach.
• The fundus should be filled with barium.
• With a double contrast procedure the body and pylorus and occasionally the duodenal bulb are air filled.
• Appropriate technique employed to visualize the gastric folds without overexposing other pertinent anatomy.
• Patient ID information legible; R or L marker placed on lateral border visible without superimposing essential anatomy

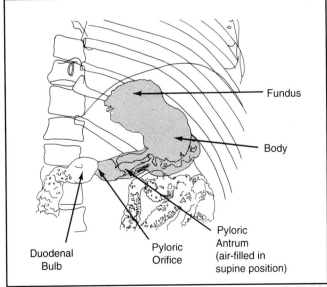

LPO   Fig. 14-91

Fundus
Body
Pyloric Antrum (air-filled in supine position)
Pyloric Orifice
Duodenal Bulb

•AP Projection

Upper GI Series
Basic
• RAO
• PA
• R Lateral
• LPO
• **AP**

Structures Best Shown:
Stomach and duodenum with barium concentrated in the fundus of the stomach. Hiatal hernia demonstrated in Trendelenburg position.

Technical Factors:
• Film Size - 11 x 14 in. (30 x 35 cm), lengthwise.
    or 14 x 17 in. (35 x 43 cm)
• Moving or stationary grid.
• 100 to 125 kVp range.
  (80-100 kVp range for double-contrast study.)

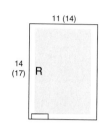

Patient Position:
• Patient supine, arms at sides; provide pillow for head.

Shielding: Place lead shield over patient's pelvic region to protect gonads without covering pertinent anatomy.

Part Position:
• Align **midsagittal plane to midline** of table.
• Insure there is **no body rotation**.
• Bottom of 11 x 14 in. (30 x 35 cm) cassette should be about at level of iliac crest.

Central Ray:
• CR **perpendicular** to film holder.
• Average body type - center CR and film to **level of L 1** (about midway between xiphoid tip and lower margin of ribs), **midway between midline and left lateral margin** of abdomen.
• Hypersthenic - center about 1 in. or 2.5 cm higher; asthenic about 2 in. or 5 cm lower and nearer to midline.
• Minimum 40 in. (102 cm) SID.

Collimation: Collimate on four sides to outer margins of film, or to area of interest on larger film.

Respiration: Suspend respiration and expose upon expiration.

Alternate AP Trendelenburg: A partial Trendelenburg (head down) position may be necessary to fill the fundus on a thin asthenic patient. A full Trendelenburg angulation facilitates the demonstration of hiatal hernia. (Install shoulder braces for patient safety.)

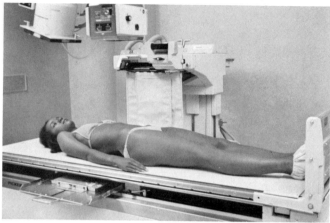

AP   Fig. 14-92

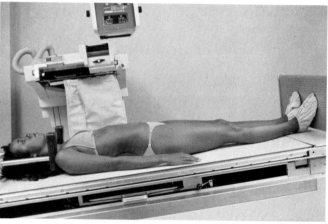

Alternate: AP Trendelenburg   Fig. 14-93

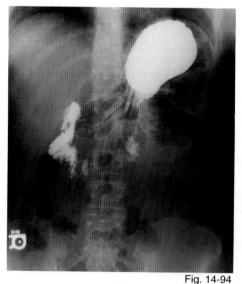

Fig. 14-94
AP

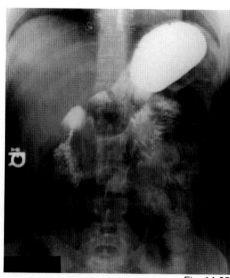

Fig. 14-95
AP Trendelenburg

Evaluation Criteria:
• Entire stomach and duodenum is visualized.
• Diaphragm and lower lung fields are included for demonstration of possible hiatal hernia.
• Fundus of the stomach is filled with barium.

• Appropriate technique employed to visualize the gastric folds without over-exposing other pertinent anatomy.
• Patient ID information legible; R or L marker placed on lateral border visible without superimposing essential anatomy.

Chapter 15
Radiographic Anatomy and Positioning
of the
Lower Gastrointestinal System

Contributions by: John Lampignano, M Ed, RT (R)
Barry T. Anthony RT (R)

Contents

Part I Radiographic Anatomy

Digestive System

The first five parts of the alimentary canal (through the stomach and first part of the small intestine, the duodenum) were described in the preceding chapter.

This chapter continues with the alimentary canal of the digestive system beyond the stomach beginning with the **small intestine** (small bowel). If the entire small bowel were removed from the body at autopsy, separated from its mesenteric attachment, uncoiled and stretched out, it would average 7 meters or 23 feet in length. During life, with good muscle tone, the actual length of the small intestine is shorter, measuring between 4.5 and 5.5 meters or 15 to 18 feet. Tremendous individual variation does exist, however. In one series of one hundred autopsies, the small bowel varied in length from 15 to 31 feet.

The **large intestine** (large bowel) begins in the lower right quadrant near its connection with the small intestine. The large intestine extends around the periphery of the abdominal cavity to end at the **anus.** The large intestine is about 1.5 meters or 5 feet long.

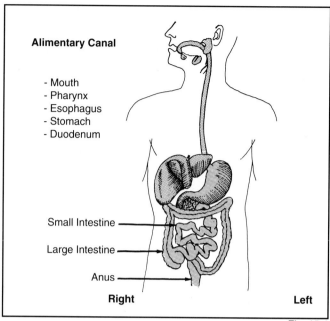

Alimentary Canal

- Mouth
- Pharynx
- Esophagus
- Stomach
- Duodenum

Small Intestine

Large Intestine

Anus

Right **Left**

Digestive System Fig. 15-1

Common Radiographic Procedures

Two common radiographic procedures involving the lower gastrointestinal system are presented in this chapter. Both of these procedures involve administration of a contrast medium.

1. **Small Bowel Series** (SBS)
- Study of small intestine

Radiographic examination specifically of the small intestine is termed a **small bowel series** or SBS. This examination is often combined with an upper GI series and, under these conditions, may be termed a small bowel follow-through. A radiograph of the barium-filled small bowel is shown in *Fig. 15-2.*

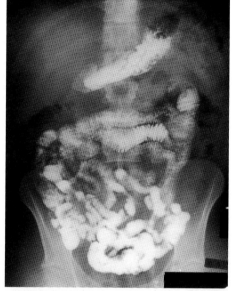

Small Bowel Series – PA Fig. 15-2

2. **Barium Enema** (BE, Lower GI Series, Colon)
- Study of large intestine

The radiographic procedure designed to study the large intestine is most commonly termed a **barium enema**. Alternate designations include BE, lower GI series or colon. *Fig. 15-3* demonstrates a large bowel or colon filled with a combination of air and barium, referred to as a double-contrast barium enema.

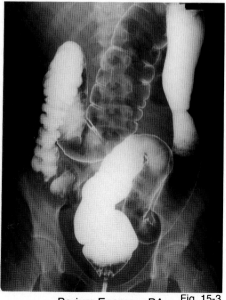

Barium Enema – PA Fig. 15-3

Small Intestine

The small intestine is located primarily in the central portion of the abdominal cavity. Beginning at the pyloric valve of the stomach, the three parts of the small intestine, in order, are **duodenum** *(du"o-de´num)*, **jejunum** *(je-joo´num)* **and ileum** *(il´e-um)*. The duodenum or first part of the small intestine is the shortest, widest and most fixed portion of the small bowel. Since the jejunum and ileum are much longer than the duodenum, and since the duodenum is posteriorly located, the many loops of small bowel shown in *Fig. 15-4* are jejunum and ileum. The location of the three parts of the small intestine in relationship to the abdominal regions is shown in *Fig. 15-5*.

Duodenum

The **duodenum** measures a fairly constant 10 inches (25 centimeters) in length and is much shorter than the other two sections of the small intestine. The usual position of the duodenum is outlined with small x's in *Fig. 15-5*.

The site of the **duodenojejunal flexure** is firmly held in position by a fibrous muscular band, the **ligament of Treitz** *(Fig. 15-6)*. This relatively fixed site of the small bowel becomes a radiographic reference point for certain small bowel studies.

Jejunum

The **jejunum** is located primarily to the left of midline in the upper and lower quadrants of the abdomen, making up about **two-fifths** of the small bowel remaining after the duodenum. The normal region of the jejunum is illustrated by the light gray portion in *Fig. 15-5*.

Ileum

The **ileum** is located primarily in the right and mid abdomen and pelvis. Approximately **three-fifths** of the small bowel remaining after the duodenum is ileum. The usual area of the ileum is illustrated by the dark gray area in *Fig. 15-5*. The terminal ileum ascends from the pelvis to join the large intestine at the ileocecal valve in the right lower quadrant.

Sectional Differences: The various sections of small intestine can be identified radiographically by their location and appearance. The C-shaped **duodenum** is fairly fixed in position. The proximal duodenum with its **bulb or cap** is unique and can be easily recognized on radiographs of the duodenum. The internal lining of the second portion (descending) of the duodenum is thrown into circular folds.

The circular folds continue throughout the remainder of the duodenum and are found in the jejunum as well. Radiographically, when the distal duodenum and the **jejunum** contain air, and especially when the bowel is distended, the internal lining of the duodenum and jejunum resemble a **coiled spring** or a stack of coins. When it contains barium, the appearance is described as **feathery**. While there is no abrupt end to the circular folds, the **ileum** tends not to have these indentations. Consequently, the internal lining of the ileum as it appears on a radiograph is **smoother** and does not have the feathery appearance.

A final observable difference in the three sections of small intestine is that the **internal diameter gets progressively smaller** from duodenum to ileum.

Radiographs demonstrating these sectional differences are shown in the anatomy review page which follows this section.

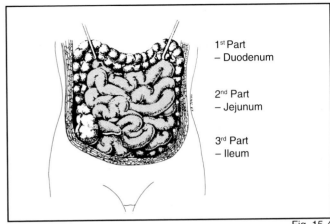

Fig. 15-4
Small Intestine (Cut Away Drawing)

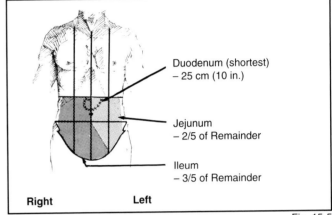

Fig. 15-5
Small Intestine

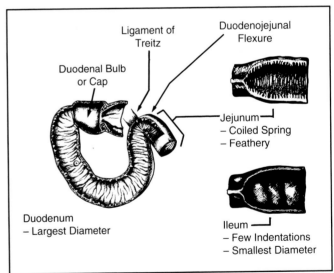

Fig. 15-6
Small Intestine (Cut Away Drawing)

Large Intestine

The large intestine begins in the lower right quadrant just distal to the **ileocecal valve.** That portion of the large intestine distal to the ileocecal valve is a saclike area termed the **cecum.** The **appendix** is a relatively long, narrow, blind tube at the distal end of the cecum.

The vertical portion of the large intestine superior to the cecum is the **ascending colon,** which continues as the **transverse colon** after the **right colic** *(kol'lik)* (hepatic) **flexure.** The **descending colon** continues from the transverse colon after another sharp bend termed the **left colic** (splenic) **flexure.** The descending colon continues as the S-shaped **sigmoid** *(sig'moid)* **colon** in the lower left quadrant.

The final segment of the large bowel is the **rectum.** The distal rectum contains the anal canal which ends at the **anus.**

Alternate names for certain parts of the large bowel are given in *Fig. 15-7.* **Colic valve** is an alternate name for the more common ileocecal valve. The more common appendix may be referred to as the **vermiform process.** The right colic flexure may be referred to as the **hepatic flexure,** while the left colic flexure may be called the **splenic flexure.** The distal portion of the descending colon is sometimes called the **iliac colon,** while the sigmoid colon may be termed the **pelvic colon.**

Large Intestine vs. Colon

Large intestine and colon are NOT synonyms, although many persons use these terms interchangeably. The **colon** consists of **four parts** and does not include the cecum and rectum. The four parts of the colon are (1) the **ascending colon,** (2) the **transverse colon,** (3) the **descending colon,** and (4) the **sigmoid colon.** The right and left colic flexures thus are also included as part of the colon. The cecum and rectum, however, (which are considered part of the large intestine), are not part of the colon.

The large intestine which includes the colon also consists of **four parts,** (1) **cecum,** (2) **colon,** (3) **rectum** and (4) **anal canal.** Each of these parts will be described beginning with the cecum.

1. Cecum

The **cecum** is a large, blind pouch located inferior to the level of the ileocecal valve. The cecum, with its attached **appendix,** is the most proximal portion of the large bowel. The internal appearance of the cecum and **terminal ileum** is shown in *Fig. 15-8.* The most distal part of the small intestine, the ileum, joins the cecum at the **ileocecal valve.** The ileocecal valve consists of two lips that extend into the large bowel.

The ileocecal valve acts as a sphincter to prevent the contents of the ileum from passing too quickly into the cecum. A second function of the ileocecal valve is to prevent reflux, or a backward flow of large intestine contents, into the ileum. The ileocecal valve does only a fair job of preventing reflux since some barium can almost always be refluxed into the terminal ileum when a barium enema is performed. The cecum is the widest portion of the large intestine and is fairly free to move about in the lower right quadrant.

Appendix: The **appendix** or **vermiform process** is a long (2-20 cm), narrow, wormshaped tube extending from the cecum. The term, vermiform, in fact, means wormlike. The appendix is usually attached to the posteromedial aspect of the cecum and commonly extends toward the pelvis. It may, however, pass posterior to the cecum.

Since the appendix has a blind ending, infectious agents may enter an appendix which cannot empty itself. The result is appendicitis. An inflamed appendix may require surgical removal, termed an appendectomy, before the diseased structure ruptures and causes peritonitis. Peritonitis is inflammation of the lining of the abdomen.

Occasionally, fecal matter or barium sulfate from a GI tract study may fill the appendix and remain there indefinitely.

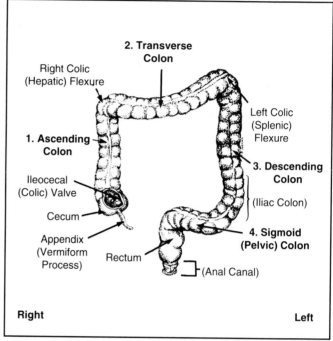

Large Intestine (Includes Colon)   Fig. 15-7

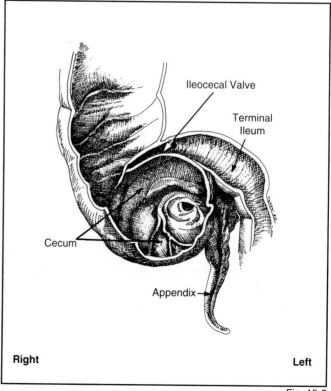

Terminal Ileum, Cecum and Appendix   Fig. 15-8

Large Intestine continued

2. Colon

The second part of the large intestine is the **colon.** The four parts of the colon are smaller in diameter than is the **cecum. The transverse colon** is the longest part of the colon and possesses considerable up and down movement. It normally loops downward beyond the right colic (hepatic) flexure as it passes to the left along the anterior surface of the abdominal cavity. Since the liver is such a large, solid organ, the **right colic (hepatic) flexure** usually lies lower in the abdomen than does the **left colic (splenic) flexure** which lies beneath the inferior pole of the spleen near the level of L1. The **ascending** and **descending colon** are within the retroperitoneum as will be described and illustrated later in this chapter.

The **sigmoid colon** normally lies in the pelvis, but does possess a wide freedom of motion. The sigmoid colon and the cecum are the two parts of the large intestine that possess the widest freedom of motion. The sigmoid colon finally passes posteriorly and inferiorly along the curve of the sacrum to continue as the **rectum.**

The location and position of these components of the colon will be important to remember during the barium enema procedure.

3. & 4. Rectum and Anal Canal

The third and fourth parts of the large intestine are the **rectum** and the **anal canal.** The **rectum** extends from the sigmoid colon to the **anus.** The rectum begins at the level of S3 and is about 4.5 inches (12 cm) long. The final 1-1.5 in. (2.5-4 cm) of large intestine is constricted to form the **anal canal.** The anal canal terminates as an opening to the exterior, the anus. The rectum closely follows the sacrococcygeal curve as demonstrated in *Fig. 15-10.*

The **rectal ampulla** is a dilated portion of the rectum located anterior to the coccyx. The initial direction of the rectum along the **sacrum** is down and back; however, in the region of the rectal ampulla, the direction changes to down and forward. A second abrupt change in direction occurs in the region of the anal canal, which is directed downward and backward. Therefore, the rectum presents **two anteroposterior curves.** This fact must be remembered when a rectal tube or enema tip is inserted into the lower GI tract.

Characteristics (Differences) of the Large Intestine

Three characteristics readily differentiate the large intestine from the small intestine. First, the **internal diameter** of the large intestine is usually greater than the diameter of the small bowel.

The longitudinal muscle fibers of the large bowel form three bands of muscle called **taeniae coli** which tend to pull the large intestine into pouches. Each of these pouches or sacculations is termed a **haustrum.** Therefore a second primary identifying characteristic of the large bowel is the presence of haustra.

The third differentiation is the **relative positions** of the two structures. The **large intestine** extends around the **periphery** of the abdominal cavity, while the **small intestine** is more **centrally** located.

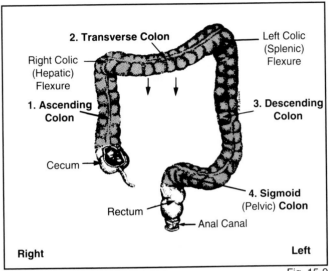

Colon – Four Parts

Fig. 15-9

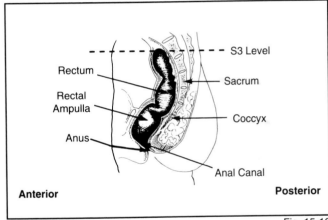

Rectum

Fig. 15-10

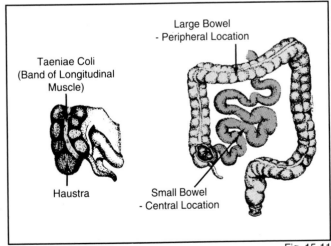

Intestine Differences
(Large vs. Small Intestine)

Fig. 15-11

Radiographs
(Anatomy Review)

Small Bowel

Three parts of the small bowel are demonstrated in *Figs. 15-12 and 13b*, a 30 min. and a 2 hour small bowel radiograph (taken 30 min. and 2 hours after ingestion of barium). Note the characteristic feathery-appearing section of jejunum (C), and the smoother appearance of the ileum region (D). The terminal ileum, the ileocecal valve (E) and the cecum of the large intestine are best shown on a spot film of this area *(Fig. 15-13a)*. A spot film using a compression cone is frequently taken of the ileocecal valve area at the end of a small bowel series to best visualize this region.

- A. Duodenum
- B. Area of ligament of Treitz (site of duodenojejunal flexure, superimposed by stomach on these radiographs)
- C. Jejunum
- D. Ileum
- E. Area of ileocecal valve

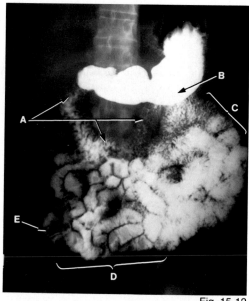

PA, 30 Min. Small Bowel   Fig. 15-12

Barium Enema

Anteroposterior (AP), lateral and right anterior oblique (RAO) rectum radiographs of a barium enema exam illustrate the key anatomy of the large intestine. Identify the structures labeled on the three radiographs below:

- a. Cecum
- b. Ascending colon
- c. Right colic (hepatic) flexure
- d. Transverse colon
- e. Left colic (splenic) flexure
- f. Descending colon
- g. Sigmoid colon
- h. Rectum

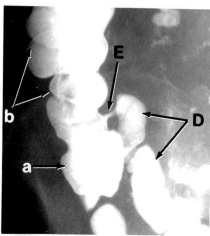

Fig. 15-13a
Spot Film of Ileocecal Valve
(courtesy of Jim Sanderson, RT)

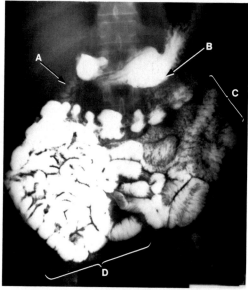

Fig. 15-13b
PA, 2 Hr Small Bowel

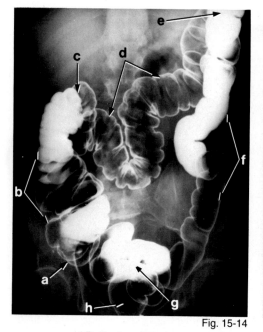

Fig. 15-14
AP, Barium Enema
(Double Contrast)

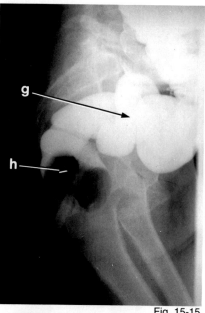

Fig. 15-15
Lateral Rectum, Barium Enema

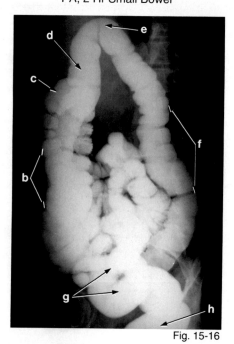

Fig. 15-16
RAO, Barium Enema
(Single Contrast)

Abdominal Cavity

Peritoneum

The abdominal cavity contains many organs. Not only does this largest of all cavities contain the major portion of the gastrointestinal system and its accessory organs, but it also contains certain organs of the endocrine, circulatory and urogenital systems. Most of these structures, as well as the wall of the abdominal cavity in which they are contained, are covered to varying degrees by an extensive serous membrane termed the **peritoneum** *(per"ĭ-to-ne'um)*. In fact, the total surface area of peritoneum is about equal to the total surface area of the skin covering the entire body.

A simplified transverse section of the abdominal cavity is shown in *Fig. 15-17.* There are two layers of the peritoneum; the parietal and the visceral. Peritoneum adhering to the cavity wall is termed **parietal peritoneum,** while that portion covering an organ is termed **visceral peritoneum.** The parietal and visceral layers form one continuous sheet.

Inside this peritoneal lining is a cavity, the **peritoneal cavity,** which is mainly filled with various organs. If all the loops of bowel and the other organs of the abdominal cavity were drawn in, there would be very little actual space left in the peritoneal cavity.

Mesentery

The simplified cross section of the abdominal cavity illustrated in *Fig. 15-18* demonstrates three important facts. **First,** there is a **double fold of peritoneum** extending anteriorly from the region in front of the vertebral body at this level. This double fold of peritoneum completely envelops a loop of small bowel. The specific term for a double fold of peritoneum connecting the posterior abdominal wall to an organ is **mesentery** *(mes'en-ter"e).*

Second, a layer of parietal peritoneum **partially covers** certain organs. At this level, both the ascending colon and the descending colon are partially covered.

Third, some structures, such as the aorta and inferior vena cava, are located **completely behind or posterior** to the parietal peritoneum. Organs or other structures located behind the peritoneum are termed **retroperitoneal structures.**

Greater Sac, Lesser Sac and Transverse Mesocolon

The midsagittal sectional drawing of an adult female, *Fig. 15-19,* shows peritoneum partially or completely covering various abdominal organs, as well as lining the abdominal cavity itself. The major portion of the peritoneal cavity, shown in dark gray, is termed the **greater sac.**

A smaller portion of the peritoneal cavity located posterior to the stomach is termed the **lesser sac.**

In this drawing, **mesentery** is seen connecting a loop of small bowel (ileum) to the posterior abdominal wall.

Mesentery also connects the transverse colon to the posterior abdominal wall. This specific double fold of peritoneum is termed the **transverse mesocolon.**

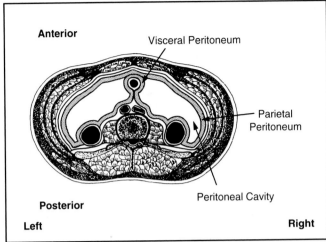

Fig. 15-17

Cross Section – Abdominal Cavity
(demonstrates peritoneum)

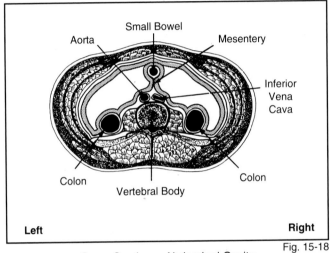

Fig. 15-18

Cross Section – Abdominal Cavity
(demonstrates mesentery)

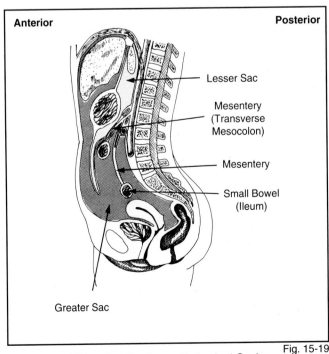

Fig. 15-19

Midsagittal Section – Abdominal Cavity
(demonstrates greater and lesser sacs
and transverse mesocolon)

Abdominal Cavity continued

Omentum

A different type of double fold of peritoneum, termed **omentum** *(o-men´tum)*, is shown in *Fig. 15-20*. Omentum is a term applied to a **double fold of peritoneum extending from the stomach to another organ**.

The **lesser omentum** extends superiorly from the stomach to portions of the liver. The **greater omentum** connects the transverse colon to the stomach inferiorly. The greater omentum drapes down from the sternum over the small bowel to form an apron along the anterior abdominal wall. It then folds back on itself and connects to the transverse colon.

Note that certain structures such as the rectum, bladder and uterus lie beneath the parietal peritoneum within the true pelvis.

Greater Omentum

The drawing on the left in *Fig. 15-21* demonstrates the abdominal cavity with the anterior abdominal wall, muscles and parietal peritoneum removed. The first structure encountered beneath the parietal peritoneum is the **greater omentum.** Varying amounts of fat are deposited in the greater omentum, which serves as a layer of insulation between the abdominal cavity and the exterior. A portion of the greater omentum has been omitted from this drawing to reveal the organs beneath.

This drawing also illustrates the apron-like construction of the greater omentum. The bottom edge of the greater omentum could be lifted, as shown, to expose the small bowel beneath and to show the connection between the greater omentum and the transverse colon.

The **transverse mesocolon,** is again seen connecting the transverse colon to the posterior abdominal wall.

Anatomical Relationships

This section describes the location and relationship of certain organs to others.

Retroperitoneal and Pelvic Organs

Figure 15-22 illustrates the abdominal cavity after removal of all structures either partially or completely covered by visceral peritoneum. Organs that have been removed are the liver, gallbladder, spleen, stomach, jejunum, ileum, cecum and the entire colon. The remaining organs are considered either **retroperitoneal** or **pelvic,** that is, those structures lying entirely behind the peritoneum are retroperitoneal, and those under the parietal peritoneum are pelvic organs.

Retroperitoneal Organs: Structures that are retroperitoneal are the **kidneys** and **ureters**, **adrenal glands**, **pancreas**, **duodenum**, **ascending** and **descending colon**, **rectum** and the **large blood vessels**. Two structures very often confused and erroneously thought to be located within the abdominal or peritoneal cavity are the **pancreas and duodenum.** These two structures are retroperitoneal.

Pelvic Organs: Located beneath the peritoneum in the **true pelvis** are the **rectum, urinary bladder** and **reproductive organs.**

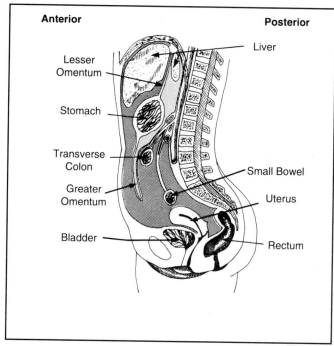

Cross section – Abdominal Cavity
(demonstrates omentum)

Fig. 15-20

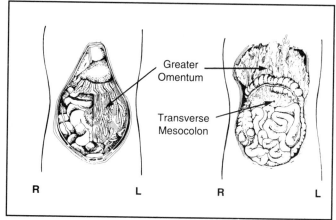

Greater Omentum

Fig. 15-21

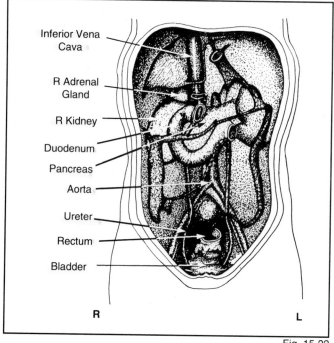

Retroperitoneal and Pelvic Organs

Fig. 15-22

Anatomical Relationships continued

Abdominopelvic Cavity (from left side)

The relative locations of various abdominal organs, as seen from the **left side,** are shown in *Fig.* 15-23. The **stomach** lies just inferior to the diaphragm, with its **fundus** much more posterior than the **body.**

The spleen of the circulatory system nestles between the stomach and the posterior abdominal wall. The spleen is ordinarily protected by the lower posterior rib cage.

The **transverse colon** lies underneath the greater omentum. The transverse colon is far anterior in the abdominal cavity, while its continuation, the **descending colon,** lies against the posterior abdominal wall. The S-shaped **sigmoid colon** first extends toward the anterior, then loops back posteriorly to continue as the rectum.

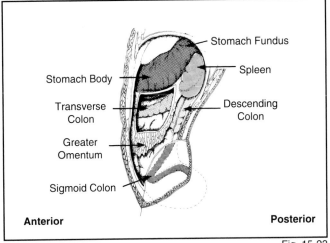

Fig. 15-23

Abdominopelvic Cavity
(Left Side)

Abdominopelvic Cavity (from right side)

The **abdominopelvic cavity** as seen from the **right side** is shown in *Fig. 15-24.* The large **liver** occupies most of the upper abdominal cavity on this side. Lying beneath the liver, but anterior to the midaxillary line, is the **gallbladder.** The right **kidney,** right **adrenal gland, duodenum and head of the pancreas** are retroperitoneal structures.

The **transverse colon** is far anterior compared to the **cecum** which lies against the posterior abdominal wall. The **appendix** extends inferiorly from the **cecum.** The cecum and appendix lie below the level of the **iliac crest.** The relative positions of various abdominal organs, both side to side and front to back, are important for the radiographer to know.

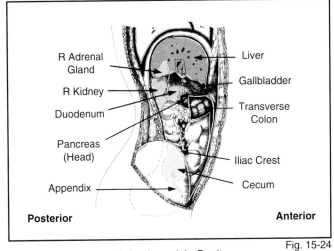

Fig. 15-24

Abdominopelvic Cavity
(Right Side)

Relative Locations of Air and Barium in Stomach and Intestine

The simplified drawings in *Fig. 15-25* represent the stomach and large bowel in both the **prone and supine positions.** If the stomach and large intestine were to contain both **air and barium sulfate,** the air would tend to rise and the barium would tend to sink due to gravity. The displacement and ultimate location of air is shown as dark gray.

When a person is supine, air rises to fill those structures that are most anterior, which are the transverse colon, sigmoid colon, and the body and distal end of the stomach. The barium sinks to fill primarily the fundus of the stomach, the duodenal portion of the small bowel, and both the ascending and descending portions of the colon and the rectum.

When a patient is prone, barium and air reverse positions. The drawing on the right illustrates the prone position, hence, air has risen to fill the rectum, ascending colon, descending colon, fundus and duodenal bulb. This spatial relationship is important both during fluoroscopy and during radiography when performing the barium enema or stomach examinations.

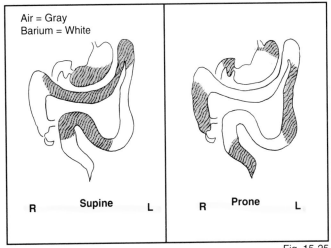

Fig. 15-25

Barium Vs. Air

Digestive Functions

Digestive Functions of the Intestines

Four primary digestive functions which are accomplished largely by the small and large intestines are:

1. **Digestion** (chemical and mechanical)
2. **Absorption**
3. **Reabsorption** of water, inorganic salts, vitamin K and amino acids
4. **Elimination** (defecation)

Most **digestion** and **absorption** take place within the small bowel. Also the majority of the salts and H_2O are **reabsorbed** in the small bowel. Approximately 95% of H_2O is reabsorbed in the small bowel. Some minimal reabsorption of H_2O and inorganic salts also occurs in the large bowel along with the elimination of unused or unnecessary materials.

The primary function of the large intestine, however, is the elimination of feces. Feces consist normally of 40 percent water and 60 percent solid matter, such as food residues, digestive secretions and bacteria. Other specific functions of the large bowel are some absorption of water, absorption of inorganic salt, and absorption of vitamin K in addition to certain amino acids. These vitamins and amino acids are produced by a large collection of naturally occurring microorganisms (bacteria) found in the large intestine.

Responsible Component	Function
Small Intestine - Duodenum - Jejunum (primarily)	1. **Digestion**, Chemical and mechanical 2. **Absorption**, nutrients, H_2O, salts and proteins 3. **Reabsorption** of H_2O and salts
Large intestine	(Some reabsorption) - Vitamins K Produced - Amino acids by bacteria 4. **Elimination** (defecation)

Summary: Lower Digestive System Functions

Movements of Digestive Tract

Of the various digestive functions of the intestine, digestive movements, sometimes referred to as mechanical digestion, is best demonstrated and evident on radiographic studies.

Small Intestine: Digestive movements throughout the length of the small bowel consist of (1) **peristalsis** *(per"i-stal'sis)* to propel intestinal contents along the digestive tract, and (2) **rhythmic segmentation** to thoroughly mix digested food and facilitate absorption.

Large Intestine: In the large intestine, digestive movements continue with (1) **peristalsis**, (2) **haustral** *(haws'tral)* **churning**, (3) **mass peristalsis** and (4) **defecation** *(def"e-ka'shun)*. Mass peristalsis tends to move the entire large bowel contents into the sigmoid colon and rectum, usually happening once every 24 hours. Defecation is a so called bowel movement or emptying of the rectum.

Small Intestine	1. Peristalsis 2. Rhythmic segmentation
Large Intestine	1. Peristalsis 2. Haustral churning 3. Mass peristalsis 4. Defecation

Summary: Digestive Movements and Elimination

Part II Radiographic Procedure

Lower Gastrointestinal System

The plain abdominal radiograph shown in *Fig. 15-26* is of a healthy, ambulatory adult. The many meters of small intestine are not visible in the central portion of the abdomen. In the average ambulatory adult, any collection of gas in the small intestine is considered abnormal. Without any gas present, the small bowel simply blends in with other soft tissue structures.

Due to variable amounts of gas and fecal matter normally present in the large intestine, this structure is grossly, but inadequately, visualized on the plain radiograph. Therefore, radiographic examination of the alimentary canal distal to the stomach and duodenum requires the introduction of contrast media for diagnostic visualization.

Small Bowel Series

Definition

A **radiographic study specifically of the small intestine** is termed a small bowel series or **SBS**. The upper GI and the small bowel series are often combined. Under these circumstances, the small bowel portion of the exam may be termed as a small bowel follow-through. A radiopaque contrast media is required for this study.

Purpose

The purpose of the small bowel series is **to study the form and function of the three components of the small bowel**, as well as **detect any abnormal conditions**.

Since this study also examines function of the small bowel, the procedure must be timed. The time should be noted when the patient finished drinking the last of the contrast media.

Clinical Indications

Some clinical indications for a small bowel series include:

- Enteritis or gastroenteritis
- Neoplasms
- Malabsorption syndromes
- Ileus

Enteritis *(en"ter-i'tis)* is a term describing the inflamation and/or infection of the small bowel. When the stomach is also involved, the condition is described as **gastroenteritis**.

Neoplasm *(ne'o-plazm)* is a term describing "new growth". This growth may be benign or malignant (cancerous). The small bowel series may demonstrate a stricture or blockage due to the neoplasm.

Malabsorption syndromes are conditions where the patient's GI tract is unable to process and absorb certain nutrients. During the small bowel series, the mucosa may appear to be swollen or thickened due to the constant irritation.

Ileus *(il'e-us)* is an obstruction of the small intestine as seen in *Fig. 15-27* wherein the proximal jejunum is markedly expanded with air. There are **two types** of ileus: (1) adynamic or paralytic, and (2) mechanical. Adynamic or paralytic ileus is due to the cessation of peristalsis. Without these involuntary, wave-like contractions, the bowel is flaccid and unable to propel its contents forward. Causes for adynamic or paralytic ileus include infection such as peritonitis or appendicitis, presence of certain drugs, or a post-surgical complication.

A mechanical obstruction is a physical blockage of the bowel. It may be due to tumor, adhesions, or hernias.

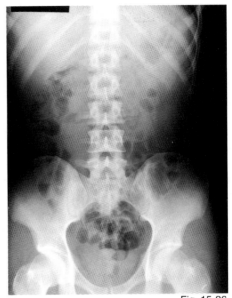

Fig. 15-26
Plain Abdominal Radiograph
(some gas seen in large intestine)

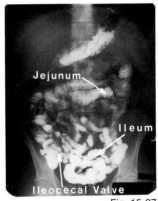

Fig. 15-27
Ileus (obstruction) of Small
Bowel

Contraindications

There are two strict contraindications to contrast media studies of the intestinal tract. **First,** presurgical patients and patients suspected of having a **perforated, hollow viscus** should **not** receive barium sulfate. The water-soluble, iodinated media should be used instead. With young or dehydrated patients, care must be given when using a water-soluble contrast media. Because of their hypertonic nature, they tend to draw water into the bowel leading to increased dehydration.

Second, barium sulfate by mouth is contraindicated in patients with a possible **large bowel obstruction**. An obstructed large bowel should first be ruled out with an acute abdominal series and a barium enema.

Small Bowel Procedures

Four methods are used to study the small intestine radiographically. Methods 1 and 2 are the more common methods. Methods 3 and 4 are special small bowel studies done if methods 1 and 2 are unsatisfactory, or if they are contraindicated.

1. UGI–small bowel combination
2. Small bowel only series
3. Enteroclysis
4. Intubation Method

1. Upper GI–Small Bowel Combination

For an upper GI–small bowel combination procedure, a routine upper GI series is done first. After the routine stomach study, progress of the barium is followed through the entire small bowel. During a routine upper GI series, the patient should have ingested one full cup or 8 ounces of barium sulfate mixture. For any small bowel examination, the exact time that the patient initially ingested barium should be noted because timing for sequential radiographs is based on the first ingestion of barium.

After completion of fluoroscopy and routine radiography of the stomach, the patient is given one additional cup of barium to ingest. The time that this is done should also be noted. The second cup of barium may be difficult for the patient to down since that amount of barium is a lot to swallow. Thirty minutes after the initial barium ingestion, a PA radiograph of the proximal small bowel is obtained. This first radiograph of the small bowel series (marked "30 minutes") is usually obtained about 15 minutes after completion of the UGI series.

Radiographs are obtained at specific intervals throughout the small bowel series until the barium sulfate column passes through the ileocecal valve and progresses into the ascending colon. For the first 2 hours in the small bowel series, radiographs are usually obtained at 15-30 minute intervals. If it becomes necessary to continue the examination beyond the 2-hour time frame, then radiographs are usually obtained every hour until barium passes through the ileocecal valve.

Inspection of Radiographs: As soon as each radiograph in the small bowel series is processed, it should be inspected by the radiologist. The physician may wish to examine any suspicious area under the fluoroscope or request additional radiographs.

Fluoroscopic Study: The region of the terminal ileum and ileocecal valve is generally studied fluoroscopically. Spot filming of the terminal ileum usually indicates completion of the examination.

The patient shown in Fig. 15-28 is in position under the compression cone, which may be utilized to spread out loops of ileum to better visualize the ileocecal valve.

Delayed Radiographs: The radiologist may request delayed radiographs in order to follow the barium through the entire large bowel. A barium meal given by mouth usually reaches the rectum in 24 hours.

2. Small Bowel Only Series

The second possibility for study of the small intestine is the small bowel only series as summarized on the right. For every contrast medium examination, including the small bowel series, a plain radiograph should be obtained before introduction of the contrast medium. If a routine abdomen was not obtained previously, it would be the first radiograph of any series depicting the small bowel.

For the small bowel only series, 2 cups of barium are ingested by the patient, and the time is noted. Depending on departmental protocol, the first radiograph is taken either 15 or 30 minutes after completion of barium ingestion. This first radiograph includes high centering to include the diaphragm. From this point on, the exam is exactly like the follow-up series of the UGI. Half-hour radiographs are taken for 2 hours, with one-hour radiographs thereafter, until barium is well into the

ascending colon. In the routine small bowel series, regular barium sulfate ordinarily reaches the large intestine within 2 or 3 hours.

Fluoroscopy with spot filming using a compression cone may again be an option to better visualize the ileocecal valve.

PROCEDURE

1. **Upper GI–Small Bowel Combination**
   Basic:
   - Routine UGI first.
   - Note time patient ingested first cup (8 oz) of barium.
   - Ingest second cup of barium.
   - 30-minute PA radiograph (center high for proximal SB).
   - Half-hour interval radiographs, centered to iliac crest, until barium reaches large bowel (usually 2 hrs).
   - One-hour interval radiographs, if more time is needed after two hours.

   Optional:
   - Fluoroscopy and spot filming of ileocecal valve and terminal ileum (compression cone may be used).

Summary

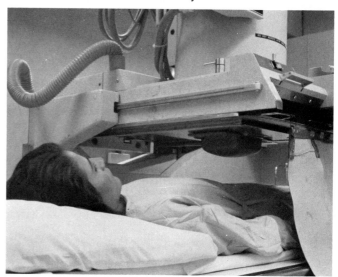

Fig. 15-28
Fluoroscopy of ileocecal region with compression cone

PROCEDURE

2. **Small Bowel Only Series**
   Basic:
   - Plain abdomen radiograph (scout).
   - 2 cups (16 oz) of barium ingested (note time).
   - 15-30 minute radiograph (centered high for proximal SB).
   - Half-hour interval radiographs until barium reaches large bowel (usually 2 hrs).
   - One-hour interval radiographs, if more time is needed.

   Optional:
   - Fluoroscopy with compression may be required.

Summary

Special Small Bowel Procedures

In certain situations, a more comprehensive evaluation of the small bowel is required. The **enteroclysis** procedure is a double contrast method of evaluating the small bowel. The **intubation method** provides for the direct introduction of contrast media into the small bowel.

3. Enteroclysis

Enteroclysis *(en″ter-ok′li-sis)* is a term describing the injection of a nutrient or medicinal liquid into the bowel. In the context of a radiographic small bowel procedure, it refers to a study wherein the patient is intubated under fluoroscopic control with a special enteroclysis catheter which passes into the region of the duodenojejunal junction (ligament of Treitz). A high density suspension of barium is injected through this catheter. Then either air or methylcellulose is injected into the bowel to distend it and provide a double contrast effect. Methylcellulose is preferred since it adheres to the bowel while distending it. This double contrast effect dilates the loops of small bowel while increasing visibility of the mucosa. This leads to increased accuracy of the study.

The disadvantages of enteroclysis are increased patient discomfort, longer examination time compared to a standard small bowel series, and the possibility of bowel perforation during catheter placement.

Enteroclysis is considered ideal for patients with a clinical history of small bowel obstruction, Crohn's disease, or malabsorption syndrome.

Upon proper filling of the small bowel with the contrast media, the radiologist will take the appropriate fluoro spot films. The radiographer may be asked to produce various projections of the small bowel to include AP, PA, obliques, and possibly erect projections.

After the procedure is completed, the catheter is removed and the patient is encouraged to increase water intake and possibly laxatives.

The radiograph seen on *Fig. 15-29* is an example of an enteroclysis. The end of the catheter is seen in the distal duodenum, not yet reaching the duodenojejunal junction (ligament of Trietz). The introduction of the methlycellulose dilates the lumen of the bowel, while the barium coats the mucosa.

4. Intubation Method

Gastrointestinal intubation *(in″tu-ba′shun)* is a technique whereby a nasogastric tube is passed through the patient's nose and through the esophagus, stomach, duodenum and into the jejunum *(Fig. 15-30).* This radiograph demonstrates the end of the tube still in the stomach, having not yet passed into the duodenum.

This procedure is performed for both diagnostic and therapeutic purposes. The **diagnostic intubation** procedure may be referred to as a small bowel enema. A single lumen tube is passed into the proximal jejunum. Placing the patient into a RAO position may aid in passing the tube from the stomach into the duodenum by gastric peristaltic action. Either a water-soluble iodinated agent or a thin barium sulfate suspension is then injected through the tube. Radiographs are taken at timed intervals similar to a standard small bowel series.

The **therapeutic intubation** procedure is often performed to relieve postoperative distention or decompress a small bowel obstruction. A double lumen cathether is advanced into the stomach. Mercury may be instilled on the outer lumen to aid in the advancement of the catheter. Through peristalsis, the catheter is advanced into the jejunum. The radiographer may be asked to take radiographs at timed intervals to determine if the catheter is advancing. Gas and excessive fluids can be withdrawn through the catheter.

An optional part of this study may include flouroscopy wherein the tube can be guided into the duodenum by the use of compression and manual manipulation.

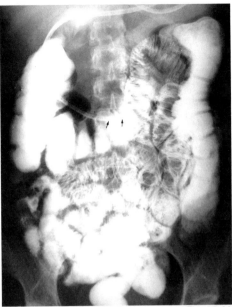

PA Radiograph – Enteroclysis Fig. 15-29

3. **Enteroclysis – Small Bowel Series**
   Basic:
   - Intubation into the duodenum.
   - Barium sulfate suspension is instilled.
   - Air or methylcellulose is instilled.
   - Fluoroscopic spot films and conventional radiographs are taken.
   - Upon successful completion of exam, intubation tube is removed.

Summary

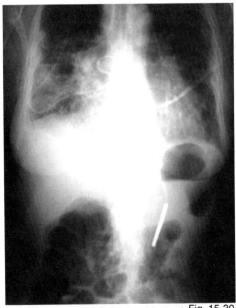

AP Abdomen – Intubation Method Fig. 15-30

4. **Intubation Method – Small Bowel Series**
   Basic:
   - Nasogastric tube inserted.
   - Contrast media instilled.
   - Note time that contrast media is instilled.
   - 15 to 30-minute radiographs.
   - Radiologist will specify filming sequence after two hours.
   Optional:
   - Fluoroscopy with compression may be required.

Summary

Small Bowel Series Procedure continued

Patient Preparation

Patient preparation for a small bowel series is identical to that for an upper GI series. In fact, the most common method of small bowel study is a combination of the two examinations into one long examination with the small bowel series following the UGI series.

The goal of patient preparation for either the upper GI series or the small bowel series is an **empty stomach**. Food and fluid must be withheld for at least **8 hours** prior to these exams. In addition, the patient should not smoke cigarettes or chew gum during the NPO period.

Pregnancy Precautions

If the patient is a female, then a menstrual history must be obtained. Irradiation of an early pregnancy is one of the most hazardous situations in diagnostic radiography.

X-ray examinations such as the small bowel series or the barium enema which include the pelvis and uterus in the primary beam and which include fluoroscopy, should **never** be done on pregnant females unless absolutely necessary.

Any x-ray examination of the abdomen of a potentially pregnant female should be governed by the "ten-day rule". This is the only time when pregnancy can be ruled out with any certainty. Abdominal radiographs and fluoroscopy of a known pregnancy should be delayed at least until the third trimester, if done at all.

Radiographic Room Preparation

Radiographic room preparation depends on the type of small bowel series to be performed. For the upper GI-small bowel combination, room preparation is exactly the same as for an upper GI series. One additional full cup (8 ounces) of barium sulfate mixture is needed. Initial radiographs for both the small bowel series can be made in any general radiographic room, unless the radiologist wishes to fluoroscope the patient's abdomen prior to ingestion of the barium sulfate mixture. Most of the sequentially timed radiographs in any small bowel series are performed in a general radiographic room.

For the enteroclysis and intubation methods, a general fluoroscopic room is necessary since a nasogastric tube must be advanced to the proximal small bowel.

Method of Imaging

Imaging for any overhead radiograph during a small bowel series is done on 14 x 17 in. (35 x 43 cm) film in order to visualize as much of the small intestine as possible. Spot filming of selected portions of the small bowel is done on smaller sized film.

The prone position is usually used during a small bowel series, unless the patient is unable to assume that position. The prone position allows abdominal compression to separate the various loops of bowel and create a higher degree of visibility.

For the 30-minute radiograph, the film is placed high enough to include the stomach on the finished radiograph. This requires longitudinal centering to the duodenal bulb and side-to-side centering to the midsagittal plane. Approximately three-fourths of the film should

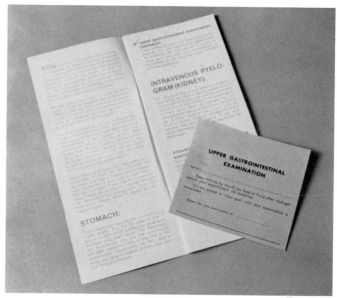

Patient Preparation   Fig. 15-31

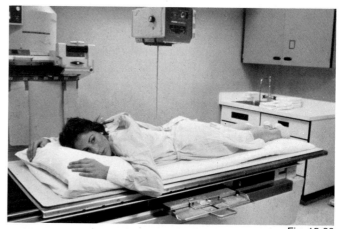

Fig. 15-32

Room Preparation

extend above the iliac crest. Since most of the barium will be in the stomach and proximal small bowel, a high kVp technique should be utilized on this initial radiograph.

All radiographs after the initial 30-minute exposure should be centered to the iliac crest. For the one-hour and later radiographs, medium kilovoltage techniques may be used since barium is spread through more of the alimentary canal and not concentrated in the stomach. Spot filming of the terminal ileum usually completes the examination.

Barium Enema (BE or Lower GI Series)

Definition
The **radiographic study of the large intestine** is commonly termed a barium enema. It requires the use of a contrast media to demonstrate the large intestine and its components. Alternate designations include BE and the lower GI series.

Types of Lower GI Examinations (Procedures)
There are three types of radiographic examinations of the large intestine which will be described and demonstrated in this chapter.
(1) Single contrast barium enema
(2) Double contrast barium enema
(3) Defecogram

Purpose
The purpose of the barium enema is to **study radiographically the form and function of the large intestine**, as well as to **detect any abnormal conditions**. Both the single contrast and the double contrast barium enema include a study of the entire large intestine, while the defecogram is a functional study of the distal portion, namely the anus and rectum.

Clinical indications for the barium enema include:
- Colitis   - Volvulus
- Diverticulosis/diverticulitis   - Intussusception
- Neoplasms   - Appendicitis

Colitis *(ko-li´is)*, is an inflammatory condition of the large intestine which may be caused by many factors including bacterial infection, diet, stress, and other environmental conditions. A severe form of colitis is **ulcerative colitis**. It is a chronic condition often leading to coin-like ulcers developing within the mucosal wall. These ulcers may be seen during the barium enema.

A **diverticulum** *(di″ver-tik´u-lum)* is an outpouching of the mucosal wall resulting from a herniation of the inner wall of the colon. Although a relatively benign condition, it may become wide-spread throughout the colon. The condition of having numerous diverticula is termed **diverticulosis**. If these diverticula become infected, the condition is now referred to as **diverticulitis**. A patient may develop peritonitis if a diverticulum perforates through the mucosal wall.

Diverticula will appear as small circular densities on the colon wall.

Neoplasms or tumors are common in the large intestine. While benign tumors do occur, carcinoma of the large intestine is a leading cause of death in both males and females. These cancerous tumors often encircle the lumen of the colon. The radiographic appearance leads to descriptive terms such as "apple core" or "napkin ring" lesions. Both benign and malignant tumors may begin as **polyps** *(pol´ips)*. A polyp is a small growth extending from the mucosal wall. (These are not the same as diverticulum described above.) The double contrast barium enema is valuable in detecting polyps.

Volvulus *(vol´vu-lus)* is a twisting of a portion of the intestine on its own mesentery. Blood supply to the twisted portion is compromised leading to obstruction and necrosis or localized death of tissue. While a volvulus may be found in portions of the jejunum or ileum, the most common sites are the cecum and sigmoid colon.

Intussusception *(in″tus-sus-sep´shun)* is the telescoping of one part of the bowel into another. It is often seen with infants. The barium enema may play a therapeutic role in re-expanding the involved bowel. Intussusception must be resolved quickly or it may lead to obstruction and necrosis of the bowel.

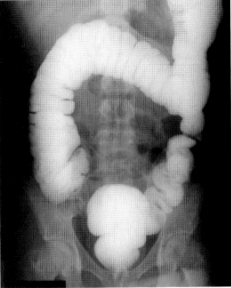

BE, Single Contrast   Fig. 15-33

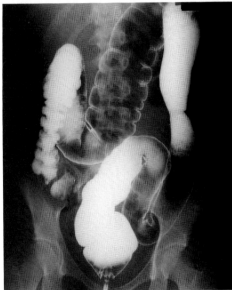

BE, Double Contrast   Fig. 15-34

Appendicitus: A barium enema may be performed to rule out appendicitis. Appendicitis may be caused by infection or a blockage of the blood vessels that feed the appendix. Sometimes a fecal mass may develop near the proximal aspect of the appendix cutting off the blood supply to it. This mass is termed an appendolith. The barium enema may be helpful in identifying a possible appendolith or an inflamed appendix.

Contraindication
The contraindications for the barium enema are similar to those described for the small bowel series. A careful review of the patient's chart and clinical history may help prevent problems during the procedure.

It is important to review the patient's chart to determine if the patient had a sigmoidoscopy or colonoscopy prior to the barium enema. If a biopsy of the colon was performed during these procedures, the involved section of the colon wall may be weakened, which may lead to perforation during the barium enema. The radiologist must be informed of this situation prior to beginning the procedure.

BE Procedure

Patient Preparation

Preparation of the patient for a barium enema is more involved than is preparation for the stomach and small bowel. The final objective, however, is the same. The **section of alimentary canal to be examined must be empty**. Thorough cleansing of the entire large bowel is of paramount importance to the satisfactory contrast medium study of the large intestine.

Contraindications to Cathartics   *(kah-thar'tiks)*

Certain conditions contraindicate the use of very effective cathartics or purgatives needed to thoroughly cleanse the large bowel. These exceptions are: (1) gross bleeding, (2) severe diarrhea, (3) obstruction and (4) inflammatory lesions such as appendicitis.

A cathartic or purgative is a substance that produces frequent, soft or liquid bowel movements. These substances increase peristalsis in the large bowel, and occasionally in the small bowel as well, by irritating the sensory nerve endings in the intestinal mucosa. This increased peristalsis dramatically accelerates intestinal contents through the digestive system.

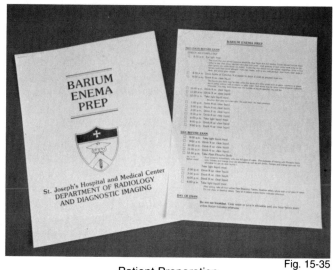

Patient Preparation   Fig. 15-35
(Courtesy of St. Joseph's Hospital and Medical Center)

Two Classes of Cathartics

Two different classes of cathartics may be prescribed. First are the irritant cathartics such as castor oil; and second are the saline cathartics such as magnesium citrate or magnesium sulfate. For best results, bowel cleansing procedures should be specified on patient instruction sheets for both inpatients and outpatients. A radiographer should be completely familiar with the type of preparation used in each radiology department. The importance of a clean bowel for a barium enema, and especially for a double-contrast barium enema, cannot be overstated because any retained fecal matter may obscure the normal anatomy or give false diagnostic information.

Radiographic Room Preparation

The radiographic room should be prepared in advance of the patient's arrival. The fluoroscopic room and examination table should be clean and tidy for each patient. The control panel should be set for fluoroscopy with the appropriate technical factors selected. The fluoroscopy timer should be set at its maximum, usually 5 minutes. The spot film mechanism should be in proper working order and a supply of spot film cassettes should be handy. The appropriate number and size of conventional cassettes should be provided. Protective lead aprons and lead gloves should be provided for the radiologist, as well as lead aprons for all other personnel to be in the room. The fluoroscopic table should be placed in the horizontal position, with waterproof backing or disposable pads placed on the table top. Waterproof protection is essential in case of premature evacuation of the enema.

The footboard is generally not necessary for the BE and may be removed. The Bucky tray must be positioned at the foot end of the table if the fluoroscopy tube is located beneath the table top. Place the radiation foot control switch appropriately for the radiologist or prepare the remote control area. Tissues, towels, replacement linen, bedpan, extra gowns, a room air freshener and a waste receptacle should be readily available. Prepare the appropriate contrast medium or media, container, tubing and enema tip. A proper lubricant should be provided for the enema tip. The type of barium sulfate used and the concentration of the mixture varies considerably depending on radiologist preferences and the type of examination to be performed.

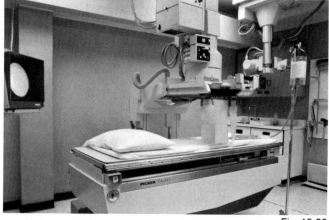

Room Preparation   Fig. 15-36

BE Procedure continued

Barium Enema Containers

A closed system type enema container is used to administer the barium sulfate or barium sulfate and air combination during the barium enema (*Fig. 15-37*). This closed type disposable barium enema bag system has replaced the older type open system for convenience and to reduce the risk of cross infection.

This system seen in the photograph demonstrates the disposable enema bag with a pre-measured amount of barium sulfate. Once mixed, the suspension travels down its own connective tubing and flow is controlled by a plastic stopcock. An enema tip is placed on the end of the tubing which is inserted in the patient's rectum.

After the examination, much of the barium can be drained back into the bag by lowering the system below table top level. The entire bag and tubing are disposed of after a single use.

Enema Tips

Various types and sizes of enema tips are available (*Fig. 15-38*). The three most common enema tips are (A) the plastic disposable, (B) the rectal retention, and (C) air contrast retention enema tips. All of these are considered single use, disposable enema tips.

Rectal disposable retention tips (B) and (C) (sometimes called retention catheters) are used on those patients who have a relaxed anal sphincter or who, for any reason, cannot retain the enema. These rectal retention catheters consist of a double lumen tube with a thin rubber balloon at the distal end (2). This balloon can be carefully inflated with air through a small tube (3) to assist the patient in retaining the barium enema. These retention catheters should be **fully inflated only with fluoroscopic guidance by the radiologist** because of the potential dangers of intestinal rupture. Due to the discomfort to the patient, the balloon should not be fully inflated until the fluoroscopy procedure begins.

A special type of rectal tip (C) is needed to inject air through a separate tube (5) which mixes with the barium tube (4) as it passes into the colon for a double contrast BE exam.

Contrast Media Preparation

The preparation of the contrast media for a closed system barium enema kit is specified by the manufacturer. The mixing instructions as supplied by the manufacturer should be followed precisely.

A debate has evolved over the temperature of the water that is used to prepare the barium sulfate suspension. Some experts recommend the use of cold water (40 to 45 degrees F) in the preparation of the contrast media. The cold water is reported to have an anesthetic effect on the colon and increase retention of the contrast media. Critics have stated that the cold water may lead to colonic spasm.

Room-temperature water is recommended by others to produce a more successful examination with maximum patient comfort. The radiographer should NEVER use hot water to prepare the contrast media. The hot water may scald the mucosal lining of the colon.

Since the barium sulfate produces a colloidal suspension, it is important to shake the enema bag prior to tip insertion to prevent separation of the barium sulfate and water.

Glucagon is a drug that is often given to control colonic spasm. It should be kept in the department for these situations.

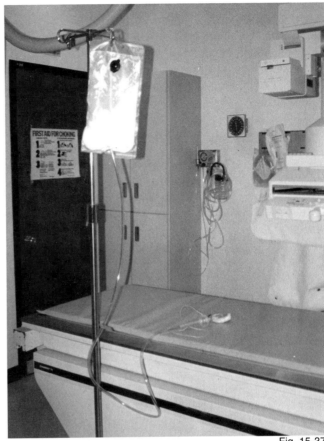

Closed System Enema Container   Fig. 15-37

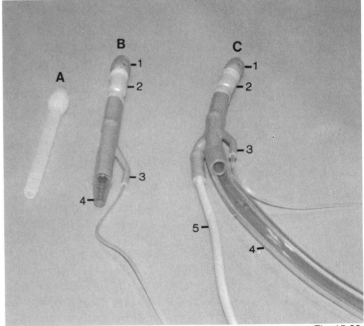

Enema Tips   Fig. 15-38

Description of Above:
A. Plastic enema tip
B. Rectal retention tip
   1. Enema tip with side and end holes
   2. Inflatable retention balloon
   3. Air tube for inflating balloon
   4. End attaching to enema bag tubing to introduce barium
C. Air contrast retention tip
   1 - 4. Same as above
   5. Tube to introduce air into colon

BE Procedure continued

Procedure Preparation

A barium enema patient is examined in an appropriate hospital gown. A cotton gown with the opening and ties in the back is preferable. Never use the type of gown that must be pulled over the patient's head to remove. Sometimes the gown will become soiled during the examination. The outpatient is instructed to remove all clothing, including shoes and socks or hose. Disposable slippers should be provided in case some barium is lost on the way to the restroom.

After the fluoroscopic room is completely prepared and the contrast medium is ready, the patient is escorted to the examination room. Prior to insertion of the enema tip, a pertinent history should be taken and the examination should be carefully explained. Since complete cooperation is essential, and since this examination can be somewhat embarrassing, every effort should be made to reassure the patient at every stage of the exam.

Any previous radiographs should be available for the radiologist. The patient is placed in the Sims position prior to insertion of the enema tip.

Sims Position

The Sims position is shown in *Fig. 15-40*. The patient is asked to roll onto the left side and to lean well forward. The right leg is flexed at the knee and hip, and is placed in front of the left leg. The left knee is comfortably flexed. The Sims position relaxes the abdominal muscles and decreases pressure within the abdomen.

During the procedure, each phase of the rectal tube insertion must be explained to the patient. Prior to rectal tube insertion, the barium sulfate solution should be well mixed. Before insertion, a little of the barium mixture should be run into a waste receptacle to insure that no air remains in the tubing or enema tip.

Rectal Tube

The radiographer wears a rectal glove and enfolds the enema tip in several sheets of paper toweling. The rectal tip is well lubricated with a water-soluble lubricant. Before the examination, the patient should be instructed to (1) keep the anal sphincter tightly contracted against the rectal tube to hold it in position and prevent leakage, (2) relax the abdominal muscles to prevent increased intra-abdominal pressure and (3) concentrate on breathing by mouth to reduce spasms and cramping. The patient must be assured that barium flow will be stopped during cramping.

Enema Tip Insertion

To insert the enema tip, adjust the opening in the back of the patient's gown to expose only the anal region. The rest of the patient should be well covered when inserting the rectal tube. Protect the patient's modesty in any way you can during the barium enema examination. The right buttock should be raised to open the gluteal fold and expose the anus. The patient should take in a few deep breaths prior to actual insertion of the enema tip. If the tip will not enter with gentle pressure, the patient should be asked to relax and assist if possible. The tip should **NEVER** be forced in such a manner which could cause injury to the patient. Since the abdominal muscles relax on expiration, the tip should be inserted during the exhalation phase of respiration.

The rectum and anal canal present a double curvature, therefore the tube is first inserted in a forward direction approximately 1-1.5 inches (2.5-4 cm). This initial insertion should be aimed toward the umbilicus. After the initial insertion, the rectal tube is directed superiorly and slightly anteriorly to follow the normal curvature of the rectum. The total insertion of the tip should not exceed 3 to 4 centimeters to avoid possible injury to the wall of the rectum. The rectal tube may be taped in place or held to prevent it from slipping out while the patient turns back into

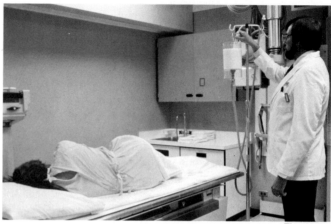

Procedure Preparation   Fig. 15-39

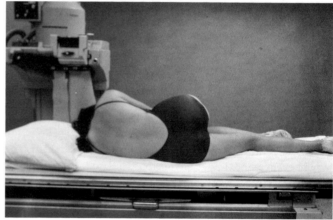

Sims Position   Fig. 15-40

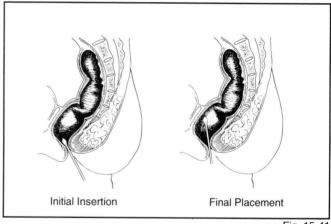

Initial Insertion   Final Placement

Enema Tip Insertion   Fig. 15-41

a supine position for fluoroscopy. This position is usually supine, but may be prone depending on the preference of the radiologist.

If the retention type tip is necessary, most departments allow the radiographer to instill one or two puffs of air into the balloon end to help hold it in place. The bulb should be filled to its maximum, however, only under fluoroscopic control as the fluoroscopy procedure begins.

BE Procedure continued

Fluoroscopy Routine

The radiologist is summoned to the radiographic room when all room and patient preparations are completed. Following introduction of the physician and patient, the patient's history and the reason for the examination are discussed.

During barium enema fluoroscopy, the general duties of the radiographer are to follow the radiologist's instructions, to assist the patient as needed and to expedite the procedure in any way possible. The radiographer must also control the flow of barium and/or air, and change fluoro spot cassettes. The flow of barium will be started and stopped several times during the BE. Each time the radiologist asks that the flow be started, the radiographer should say "barium on" after the clamp or hemostat is released. Each time the radiologist requests that the flow be stopped, the radiographer should say "barium off" after the tubing is clamped.

Many changes in patient position are made during fluoroscopy. These positional changes are made to better visualize superimposed sections of bowel, as well as to aid in advancement of the barium column. Areas of the large intestine best studied by positional changes include the rectosigmoid area, the two flexures and the cecal area. The radiographer may need to assist the patient with positional moves, and make sure that the tubing is not kinked or accidentally pulled out during the examination.

The fluoroscopic procedure begins with a general survey of the patient's abdomen and chest. If the retention type enema tip is required, the air balloon is inflated under fluoroscopic control at this point. Various spot radiographs are obtained of selected portions of the large intestine as the barium column proceeds in retrograde fashion from rectum to cecum. At the end of the fluoroscopic procedure, a little barium is refluxed through the ileocecal valve and fluoro spots are obtained of that area. Moderate discomfort is usually experienced when the large bowel is totally filled, so the examination must be concluded as rapidly as possible. Routine overhead radiographs are obtained with the bowel filled.

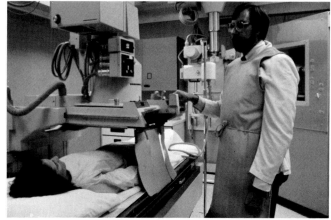

Fluoroscopy

Fig. 15-42

Types of Lower GI Examinations (Procedures)

Three specific types of radiographic examinations or procedures of the lower GI are as follows:
    (1) Single-contrast Barium Enema
    (2) Double-contrast Barium Enema
    (3) Defecogram

(1) Single-contrast Barium Enema Procedure

The single-contrast barium enema utilizes only a positive contrast medium. In most cases the contrast material is barium sulfate in a thin mixture. Occasionally, the contrast medium will have to be a water-soluble contrast material. If the patient is to be taken to surgery following the BE, then a water-soluble contrast medium must be used. An example of a single-contrast barium enema utilizing barium sulfate as the contrast medium is shown in *Fig. 15-43*.

(2) Double-contrast Barium Enema Procedure

Radiographic and fluoroscopic procedures for a double-contrast barium enema are somewhat different in that both air and barium must be introduced into the large bowel. Figure 15-44 is a double contrast BE radiograph taken in the right lateral decubitus position. An absolutely **clean large bowel is essential** to the double-contrast study, and a **much thicker barium mixture is required**. Although exact ratios depend on the commercial preparations utilized, the ratio approaches a one-to-one mix so that the final product is like heavy cream.

Two-Stage Procedure: One preferred method of coating the bowel is to utilize a two-stage, double-contrast procedure. Initially, the thick barium is allowed to fill the left side of the bowel. (The purpose of the thick barium mixture is to facilitate adherence to the mucosal lining.) Air is then instilled into the bowel, pushing the barium column through to the right side. The patient is then allowed to evacuate as much of the barium as possible.

The second stage consists of inflating the bowel with a large amount of air which moves the main column of barium forward leaving only the barium adhering to the mucosal wall. These steps are carried out under fluoroscopic control since the air column cannot be allowed to get in front of the barium column.

This procedure demonstrates neoplasms which may be forming on the inner wall of the bowel projecting into the lumen or opening of the bowel. These generallly would not be visible during a single-contrast, full column barium enema study.

Single-Stage Procedure: A single stage, double contrast procedure may also be used wherein the barium and air are instilled in a single procedure which reduces time and radiation exposure to the patient. With this method some high density barium is first instilled into the rectum with the patient in a slightly Trendelenberg position. The barium tube is then clamped, and with the table in a horizontal position the patient is placed into the various oblique and lateral positions following the addition of various amounts of air with the double-contrast procedure.

Spot Films (During Fluoroscopy): With both the single-contrast and the double-contrast studies, spot radiographs are obtained to document any suspicious area. The patient may be asked to rotate several times to distribute the barium and air better with the double-contrast procedure.

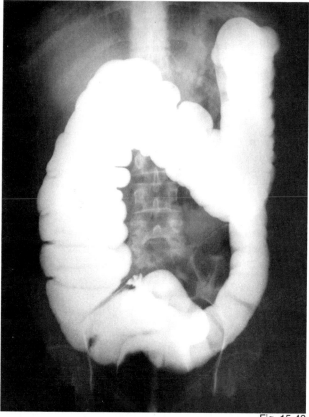

Fig. 15-43
Single-Contrast Barium Enema

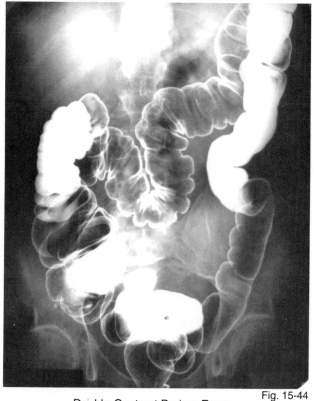

Double-Contrast Barium Enema   Fig. 15-44

Post Fluoroscopy Radiographs

After fluoroscopy and before the patient is allowed to empty the large bowel, one or more radiographs of the filled bowel should be obtained. The standard enema tip can be removed prior to these radiographs since this may make it easier to hold in the enema. However, some departmental routines keep the enema tip in during the overhead filming procedure. The retention type tip, however, is generally not removed until the large bowel is ready to be emptied when the patient is placed on a bed pan or on the commode.

Figure 15-45 demonstrates the most common position for a routine barium enema. This is the PA projection with a full-sized 14 x 17 in. cassette centered to the iliac crest. The PA projection with the patient in a prone position is preferred over an AP in a supine position because compression of the abdomen in the prone position results in a more uniform radiographic density of the entire abdomen.

The film and cassette should be centered to include the rectal ampulla on the bottom of the finished radiograph. This positioning will usually include the entire large intestine with the exception of the left colic flexure. It may be acceptable to cut off the left colic flexure on the radiographs if this area is well demonstrated on a previously obtained spot film. Some departmental routines however may include a second film centered higher to include this area on larger patients.

Other positions or projections are also obtained prior to evacuation of the barium. These radiographs must be obtained as rapidly as possible since the patient may have difficulty retaining the barium.

Once the routine pre-evacuation radiographs and any supplemental radiographs have been obtained, the patient is allowed to expel the barium. For the patient who has had the enema tip removed, a quick trip to a nearby restroom is necessary. For the patient who cannot make such a trip, a bedpan should be provided. For the patient who is still connected to a closed system, simply lowering the plastic bag to floor level and allowing most of the barium to drain back into the bag is helpful. Department protocol determines how a retention tip should be removed. One way is to first clamp off the retention tip, then disconnect it from the enema tubing and container. Once the patient is safely on a bedpan or commode, air is released from the bulb and the tip is removed.

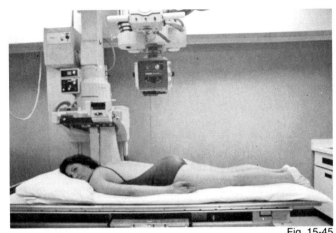

Fig. 15-45
Post Fluoroscopy Radiography – PA Projection

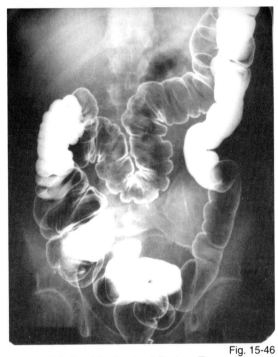

Fig. 15-46
PA, Double-Contrast Barium Enema

Post Evac Radiograph

After most of the barium has been expelled, a post evacuation radiograph is obtained. The post evac radiograph is usually taken prone, but maybe taken supine if needed. Most of the barium should have been evacuated. If too much barium is retained, the patient is given more time for evacuation and a second post evac film is taken.

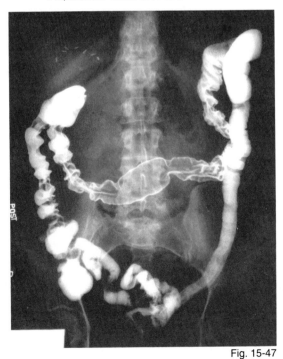

Fig. 15-47
PA, Post Evac

(3) Defecography

A third type of radiographic study involving the lower GI tract is defecography. This is a newer type of procedure being performed in many departments, especially on children or younger patients.

Definition and Purpose

The defecogram is **a functional study of the anus and rectum during the evacuation and rest phases of defecation** (bowel movement).

Clinical Indications

Clinical indications for defecography include **rectoceles**, **rectal intussusception**, and **prolapse of the rectum**. The rectocele, a common form of pathology, is a blind pouch of the rectum due to weakening of the anterior or posterior wall. These rectoceles may retain fecal material even after evacuation.

Special Equipment

A special commode is required for this study *(Fig. 15-48)*. It consists of a toilet seat built onto a frame which contains a waste receptacle, or a disposable plastic bag (A). The commode demonstrated has wheels or casters (B) so it can be rolled into position over the extended foot board and platform (C) attached to the table top (D). The entire commode with patient can then be raised or lowered by raising the table top with the attached footboard and commode during the procedure (see arrows). Clamps should be used (not shown in these visuals) to secure the commode to the foot board platform for stability during the procedure. The clamps allow the commode to be attached to the footboard to be raised as needed to utilize the table bucky and fluoroscopy unit. The seat is often cushioned (E) for patient comfort. The filters found beneath the seat (not shown) compensate for tissue differences and help maintain acceptable levels of density and contrast.

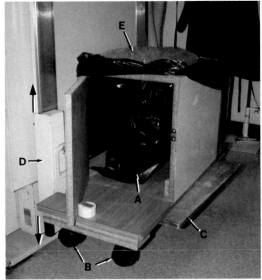

Commode for Defecogram   Fig. 15-48

Contrast Media

To study the process of evacuation, a very high density barium sulfate mixture is required. Some departments will produce their own contrast media by mixing barium sulfate with either potato starch or commercially produced additives. The potato starch thickens the barium sulfate to produce a mashed potato consistency. The normal barium sulfate suspension evacuates too quickly to detect any pathology.

A ready-to-use contrast media, **Anatrast®**, is available *(Fig. 15-50)*. This contrast media is premixed and packaged in a single use tube. Some departments will also introduce a thick liquid barium, such as **Polibar Plus®**, prior to the Anatrast to determine the appearance and alignment of the rectum.

Applicator

The mechanical applicator *(Fig. 15-50)* resembles a caulking gun similar to that used in the building industry. The premixed and prepackaged tube of Anatrast is inserted in the applicator and a flexible tube with an enema tip is attached to the opened tip of the tube (B-1).

The thick liquid Polibar is drawn into a syringe and inserted through a rectal tube and tip. In this example an inner plastic tube (C) is being used, inserted in an outer rectal tube (D) to which the enema tip is attached. The syringe is then used to instill the thick liquid Polibar Plus® contrast media. The inner plastic tube is attached to the syringe filled with the Polibar and inserted within the rectal tube to which is attached a standard enema tip for insertion into the rectum.

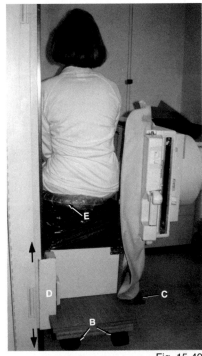

Patient in Position   Fig. 15-49

Labelled Parts:

A. Mechanical applicator
B. Tube of Anatrast (B-1 tip to be opened)
C. Inner plastic tube (for insertion of syringe or tube of Anatrast)
D. Rectal tube (to which enema tip is attached, D-1)
E. Syringe

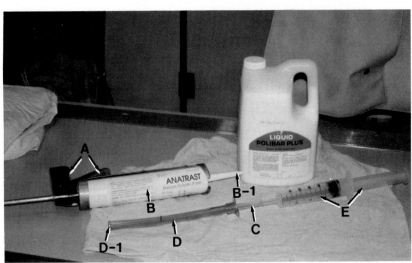

Applicator   Fig. 15-50

Defecography continued

Procedure

With the patient in a lateral recumbent position on a cart, the contrast media is instilled into the rectum with the applicator. The patient is quickly placed on the commode for filming during defecation. Fluoroscopy spot films and standard radiographic projections are taken during the study. The lateral rectum projection is usually preferred by most radiologists.

It is vital that the anorectal angle is demonstrated during the procedure. This angle is the alignment between the anus and rectum that shifts between the rest and evacuation phases. The radiologist will measure this angle during these phases to determine if any abnormalities exist. A lateral post evac radiograph is taken as the final part of this procedure.

Summary of Procedure

1. Place radiographic table vertical and attach commode with clamps.
2. Prepare contrast medium according to department specifications.
3. Set up imaging equipment (fluoroscopy, 105 mm spot film camera, spot cassette, or video recorder).
4. Have patient remove all clothing and change into a hospital gown.
5. Take a scout film using conventional x-ray tube (scout film must include the region of the anorectal angle).
6. Place patient in a lateral recumbent position on a cart and instill contrast medium.
7. Position patient on the commode and film patient in the rest and strain phases. Patient is in a lateral position and filmed using conventional x-ray tube.
8. Using fluoroscopy imaging devices or video recorder, patient is filmed while defecating.
9. Post evacuation film is taken.

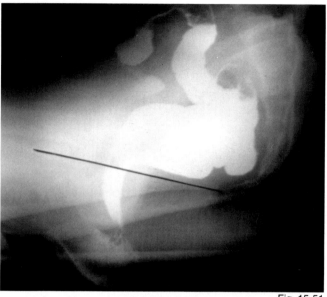

Lateral Defecogram
(during strain or evacuation)

Fig. 15-51

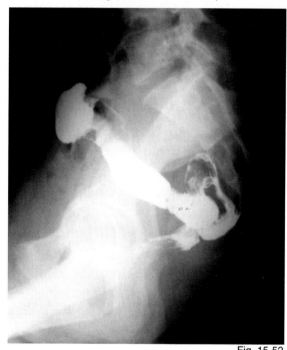

Lateral Defecogram
(same patient as above – post evac)

Fig. 15-52

Summary of Safety Concerns During the Barium Enema Procedure

Safety during the barium enema procedure is of utmost importance. A summary of these important safety concerns are as follows:

(1) **Review the patient's chart**. Note any pertinent clinical history on the exam requisition and inform the radiologist if the patient had a sigmoidoscopy or colonoscopy prior to the barium enema, especially if a biopsy was performed.

(2) **Never force an enema tip into the rectum**. This may lead to a perforated rectum. The radiologist will insert the enema tip under fluoroscopy guidance if needed.

(3) **The height of the enema bag should not exceed 24 inches above the table**. This distance should be maintained prior to

the beginning of the procedure. The radiologist may wish to raise bag height during the procedure based upon the rate of flow of the contrast media.

(4) **Verify the water temperature of the contrast media**. Too hot or cold water may injure your patient or compromise the procedure.

(5) **Escort the patient to the restroom**. A barium enema can be very stressful for certain patients. Patients have been known to faint during or after evacuation.

National Survey

A survey of the operating procedures (department routines) was conducted throughout the United States. The following information was compiled from the survey indicating the national norm for basic and optional positions for small bowel and barium enema series. The results were very consistent throughout all regions of the US. (Approximately 530 institutions responded to this part of the survey.)

Small Bowel Series Routine

Small Bowel Series	(533) U.S. Average	
	Basic	Optional
• PA (1/2 hr to 2 hrs, hourly after 2 hrs.)	85%	
• Ileocecal spots	79%	
• Enteroclysis procedure	12%	25%
• Intubation method	4%	17%

Summary

The survey indicated that **ileocecal spots** are routinely included as part of a small bowel series (79%). This however does not indicate whether this includes fluoroscopy along with spot films or just localized overhead radiographs of this area.

The survey indicated that **both** the **double-contrast** and the **single contrast** barium enema are considered basic or routine in most departments in the US, with the double contrast receiving a slightly higher indication.

The **Chassard-Lapine axial** is included in this chapter because of the percentage of survey respondents who indicated it as basic or optional. However because of the high gonadal dose, this is not a preferred projection for younger patients; and older patients have difficulty with sphincter control in this position.

Barium Enema Routine

Barium Enema	(533) U.S. Average	
	Basic	Optional
• Double-contrast	76%	14%
• Single-contrast	72%	16%
• PA	86%	
• L lateral rectum	77%	
• R lateral decub.	73%	
• L lateral decub.	73%	
• RAO	58%	
• LAO	56%	
• PA post-evac.	71%	
• AP	21%	
• LPO & RPO	18%	10%
• R lateral rectum	18%	7%
• AP axial (butterfly)	18%	7%
• LPO axial (butterfly)	15%	6%
• PA axial (butterfly)	15%	4%
• Chassard-Lapine axial	13%	11%

Basic and Optional Projections

Certain basic and optional projections or positions of the small and large intestine are demonstrated and described on the following pages. The radiologist and radiographer must closely coordinate their efforts during both the small bowel series and the barium enema. A great deal of individual variation exists among radiolo-gists. The routine or basic positions or projections listed may vary from hospital to hospital. The radiographic routine for the barium enema, in particular, must be thoroughly understood by the radiographer in advance of the examination since any radiographs needed must be obtained as rapidly as possible.

Small Bowel Series
Basic
• PA (every 15 to 30 min)
Optional
• Enteroclysis
• Intubation

Barium Enema
Basic
• PA and/or AP
• Lateral Rectum
• R and L Lat Decub
   (double-contrast)
• RAO and/or LAO
• PA Post Evac

Barium Enema
Optional
• AP and LPO Axial (Butterfly)
• PA and RAO Axial (Butterfly)
• Chassard-Lapine Axial
• LPO and RPO

• PA Projection

Small Bowel Series
Basic
• **PA** (every 15 to 30 min)
Optional
• Enteroclysis
• Intubation

Structures Best Shown:
Contrast-filled small intestine.

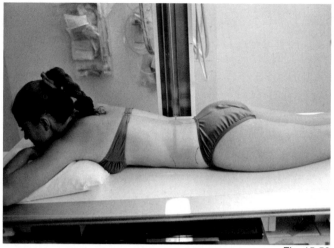
PA, 15 or 30 Min. – Centered Higher   Fig. 15-53

• **Upper GI-Small bowel combination:**
The small bowel series is commonly done in combination with the upper GI wherein additional barium is ingested following completion of the upper GI. (See page 456.)

• **Small bowel only series:**
Includes a scout abdomen radiograph followed by ingestion of barium and timed interval radiographs. (See page 456.)

• **Enteroclysis and intubation procedures:**
(See descriptions on page 457.)

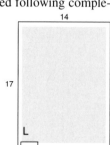

Technical Factors:
• Film Size - 14 x 17 in. (35 x 43 cm), lengthwise.
• Moving or stationary grid.
• 100 -125 kVp range.
• Time markers to be used.

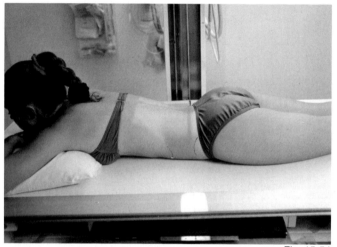
PA, Hourly – Centered to Iliac Crest   Fig. 15-54

Patient Position:
• Prone (or supine if necessary for AP projection), pillow for head.

Shielding: Place lead shield over pelvic region to protect gonads without covering pertinent anatomy.

Part Position:
• Align **midsagittal plane to midline of table** and/or film.
• Arms up beside head, legs extended with support under ankles.
• Assure there is **no rotation**.

Central Ray:
• CR **perpendicular** to film holder.
  (1) **15 or 30 min**: Center CR and mid point of film to about **2 in.** (5 cm) **above iliac crest.** (See NOTE.)
  (2) **Hourly:** Center CR and mid point of film to **iliac crest**.
• Minimum 40 in. (102 cm) SID.

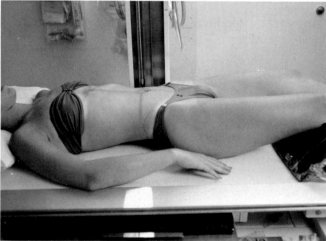
AP, Supine (if Necessary)   Fig. 15-55

Collimation: Collimate on four sides to outer margins of film.

Respiration: Suspend respiration and expose on expiration.

NOTE: • Timing begins with first ingestion of barium.
• Timed intervals of radiographs are dependent on transit time of specific barium preparation used and upon departmental protocol.
• First 30 minute radiograph: center high to include entire stomach. (Some departmental routines include the first radiograph at fifteen minutes, then each 30 minutes thereafter.)
• 30 minute interval radiographs taken until barium reaches large bowel (usually 2 hours).
• 1 hour intervals if more time is needed after 2 hours.
• Fluoroscopy and spot filming of ileocecal valve and terminal ileum after barium reaches this area is a common part of SBS routine. This however is determined by radiologist preference and departmental routines.

PA Projection continued

Evaluation Criteria:

- Entire small intestine is demonstrated on each radiograph with the stomach included on the first 15 and/or 30 minute radiograph.
- No rotation evident by symmetry of iliac wings and lumbar vertebra.
- Appropriate technique employed to visualize the contrast-filled small intestine without overexposing those parts that are only partially filled with barium.
- Patient ID info, time interval markers and R or L marker are visible without superimposing essential anatomy.

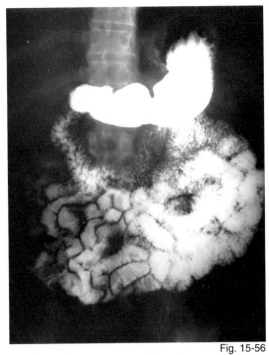

Fig. 15-56

PA SBS (30 min.)
(Most of barium in stomach, duodenum and jejunum)

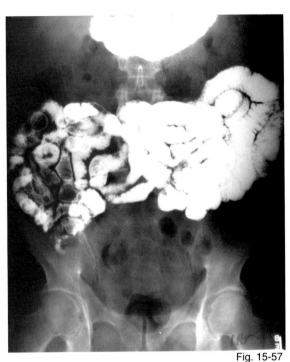

Fig. 15-57

PA SBS (1hr.)
(Most of barium in jejunum)

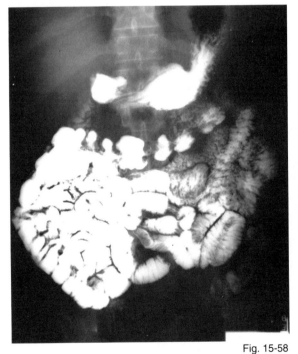

Fig. 15-58

PA 2 hr.
(Most of barium in ileum)

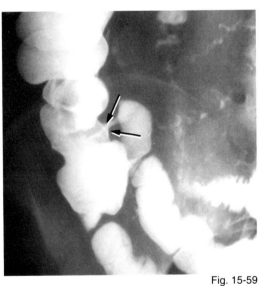

Fig. 15-59

PA (Ileocecal Spot)
(Barium in ileum and in cecum of large intestine and ascending colon. Ileocecal valve demonstrated by arrows.)

(Courtesy of Jim Sanderson, RT)

• PA and /or AP Projection

Barium Enema
Basic
• **PA and/or AP**
• L Lateral Rectum
• R and L Lat Decub
(double-contrast)
• RAO and/or LAO
• PA Post Evac

Structures Best Shown:
Entire contrast-filled large intestine. (Exception may be colic flexure, see NOTE below.)

Both PA and AP are generally taken with **double-contrast study.**

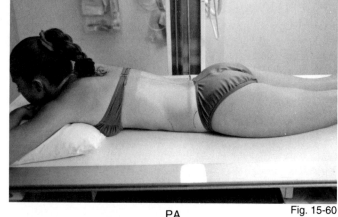

PA   Fig. 15-60

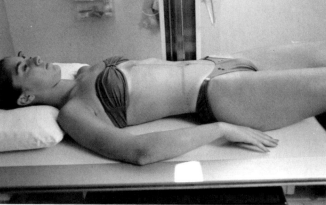

AP   Fig. 15-61

Technical Factors:
- Film Size - 14 x 17 in. (35 x 43 cm), lengthwise.
- Moving or stationary grid.
- 100-125 kVp range (single-contrast)
  80-90 kVp range (double-contrast)

Patient Position:
- Prone or supine, pillow for head.

Shielding:
Place lead shield over pelvic region to protect gonads without covering pertinent anatomy.

Part Position:
- **Midsagittal plane aligned to midline** of table.
- **No body rotation**.

Central Ray:
- CR **perpendicular** to film holder.
- CR and center of film to **iliac crest.**
- Minimum 40 in. (102 cm) SID.

Collimation:
Collimate on four sides to outer margins of film.

Respiration:
Suspend respiration and expose on expiration.

NOTE: • Proceed as rapidly as possible.
- For most patients the enema tip can be removed before overhead filming, unless a retention type tip is being used which should generally not be removed until the patient is ready to evacuate.
- Table may be tilted 10-15° Trendelenburg for double-contrast study.
- Include rectal ampula at lower margin of radiograph.
- Determine departmental policy regarding inclusion of the left colic flexure on all patients if this area is adequately included in spot films during fluoroscopy (most adult patients require 2 films if this area is to be included).
- For hypersthenic patient use 2 ea 14 x 17 films placed crosswise to include entire large intestine.

Evaluation Criteria:
- Entire large intestine should be demonstrated with the possible

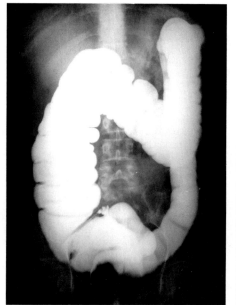

Fig. 15-62
PA

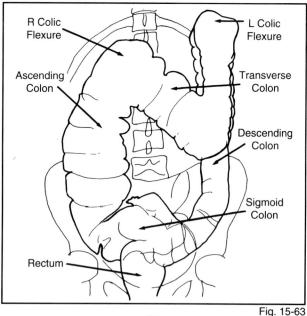

Fig. 15-63
PA

exception of the left colic flexure. (See NOTE above.)
- No rotation as evidenced by symmetry of hips and iliac wings.
- The transverse colon should be primarily barium filled on the PA, and air filled on the AP with a double-contrast study.
- Appropriate technique should visualize the entire air and barium filled large intestine without overexposing the mucosal outlines of those sections of primarily air-filled bowel on a double-contrast study.
- Patient ID info and R or L markers are visible without superimposing essential anatomy.

Barium Enema

• Left (Right) Lateral Rectum Position

Barium Enema
Basic
• PA and/or AP
• **L Lateral Rectum**
• R Lat Decub
• L Lat Decub
• RAO and/or LAO
• PA Post Evac

Structures Best Shown:
Lateral view of the rectosigmoid region.

Left and/or right lateral of rectum may be taken to demonstrate this area.

Technical Factors:
• Film Size - 10 x 12 in. (24 x 30 cm), lengthwise.
• Moving or stationary grid.
• 100-125 kVp range (for both single and double contrast studies).
• A compensating or wedge filter may be used for more uniform density.

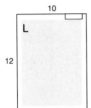

Patient Position:
• Lateral recumbent position, pillow for head.

Shielding:
Place lead shield over pelvic region to protect gonads without covering pertinent anatomy.

Part Position:
• **Align midaxillary plane to midline** of table and/or film.
• Flex and superimpose knees; arms up in front of head.
• Insure **no rotation**, superimpose shoulders and hips.

Central Ray:
• CR **perpendicular** to film holder.
• CR and center of film to level of **ASIS** and centered to **midaxillary plane.**
• Minimum 40 in. (102 cm) SID.

Collimation:
Collimate on four sides to outer margins of film.

Respiration:
Suspend respiration and expose on expiration.

Evaluation Criteria:
• Contrast-filled rectosigmoid region is demonstrated centered to film.
• No rotation as evidenced by superimposed hips.
• Appropriate technique employed to visualize both the contrast-filled rectum and sigmoid regions, with adequate penetration to demonstrate these areas through the superimposed pelvis and hips.
• Patient ID info and R or L markers are visible without superimposing essential anatomy.

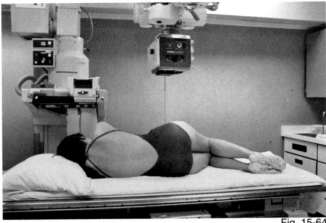

Fig. 15-64
Left Lateral Rectum

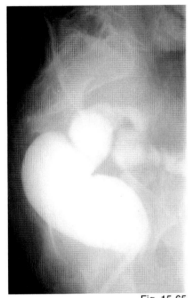

Fig. 15-65
Left Lateral Rectum

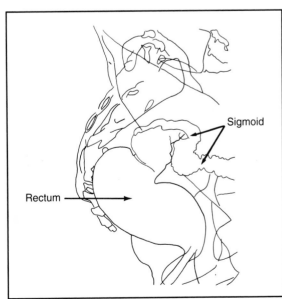

Fig. 15-66
Left Lateral Rectum

Barium Enema (Double Contrast)

• Right Lateral Decubitus Position

Barium Enema
Basic
• PA and/or AP
• L Lateral Rectum
• **R Lat Decub**
• L Lat Decub
• RAO and/or LAO
• PA Post Evac

Structures Best Shown:

Entire contrast-filled large intestine, especially helpful in demonstrating polyps. Best demonstrates the up side or air-filled portions of the large bowel.

Both right and left decubitus position are generally taken with double-contrast study (see following page).

Technical Factors:

• Film Size - 14 x 17 in. (35 x 43 cm), lengthwise with patient.
• Bucky or grid cassette.
• 89-90 kVp range (double-contrast study) (100-125 kVp range if single-contrast study).

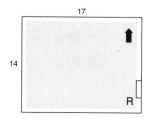

Patient Position:

• Lateral recumbent position, pillow for head, lying on **right** side on a radiolucent pad. (If on a cart, **lock wheels** or secure cart to prevent patient from falling.)
• Arms up, knees flexed.

Shielding:
Place lead shield over pelvic region to protect gonads without covering pertinent anatomy.

Part Position:

• **Align midsagittal plane to midline** of table or film holder.
• Position patient and/or film so that **iliac crest is to center of film.**
• Insure **no rotation,** superimpose shoulders and hips from above.

Central Ray:

• CR **horizontal,** perpendicular to film holder.
• CR centered to **level of iliac crest** and **midsagittal plane.**
• Minimum 40 in. (102 cm) SID.

Collimation:
Collimate on four sides to outer margins of film.

Respiration:
Suspend respiration and expose on expiration.

NOTE: • Proceed as rapidly as possible.
• For hypersthenic patient use 2 ea 14 x 17 in. (35 x 43 cm) films placed crosswise to include all of large intestine.

Evaluation Criteria:

• Entire large intestine is demonstrated with air-filled left colic flexure and descending colon.
• No rotation as evidenced by symmetrical appearance of pelvis and rib cage.
• Appropriate technique used to visualize borders of entire large intestine including barium-filled portions but to not over penetrate the air-filled portion of the large intestine. Mucosal patterns of air-filled colon should be clearly visible.
• Patient ID info , R or L marker and decub marker are visible without superimposing essential anatomy.

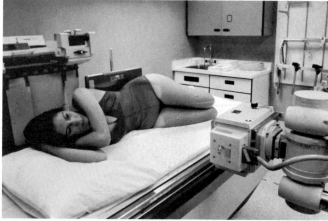

Right Lateral Decubitus (AP)　　　Fig. 15-67

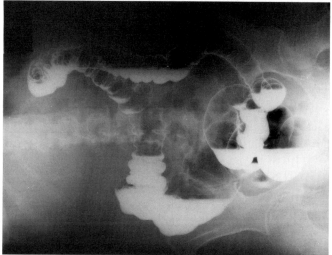

Right Lateral Decubitus　　　Fig. 15-68

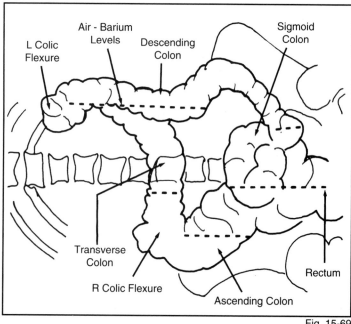

Right Lateral Decubitus　　　Fig. 15-69

• Left Lateral Decubitus Position

Structures Best Shown:
Entire contrast-filled large intestine, especially helpful in demonstrating polyps. Best demonstrates the up side or air-filled portions of the large bowel.

Both right and left decubitus position are generally taken with double-contrast study (see NOTE).

Technical Factors:
• Film Size - 14 x 17 in. (35 x 43 cm), lengthwise with patient.
• Bucky or grid cassette.
• 80-90 kVp range (double-contrast study). (100-125 kVp range if single-contrast).

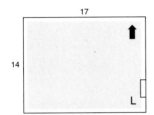

Patient Position:
• Lateral recumbent position, pillow for head, lying on **left** side on a radiolucent pad. (If on a cart, **lock wheels** or secure cart to prevent patient from falling.)
• Arms up, knees flexed.

Shielding:
Place lead shield over pelvic region to protect gonads without covering pertinent anatomy.

Part Position:
• Align **midsagittal plane to midline** of table or film holder.
• Position patient and/or film so that iliac crest is to center of film.
• Insure **no rotation**, superimpose shoulders and hips from above.

Central Ray:
• CR **horizontal,** perpendicular to film holder.
• CR centered to **level of iliac crest** and **midsagittal plane.**
• Minimum 40 in. (102 cm) SID.

Collimation:
Collimate on four sides to outer margins of film.

Respiration:
Suspend respiration and expose on expiration.

NOTE: • Since most double contrast BE studies include both R and L lateral decubitus positions, it is generally easier to take one as an AP projection with the back against the table or film holder, and the other as a PA with the abdomen against the table or film holder rather than sitting the patient up and turning them end to end on the cart or table.
• For hypersthenic patient use 2 ea 14 x 17 in. films placed crosswise to include all of large intestine.
• Proceed as rapidly as possible.

Evaluation Criteria:
• Entire large intestine is demonstrated with air-filled right colic flexure ascending colon and cecum.
• No rotation as evidenced by symmetrical appearance of pelvis and rib cage.
• Appropriate technique used to visualize borders of entire large intestine including barium-filled portions but to not over penetrate the air-filled portion of the large intestine. Mucosal patterns of air-filled colon should be clearly visible.
• Patient ID info, R or L marker and decub marker are visible without superimposing essential anatomy.

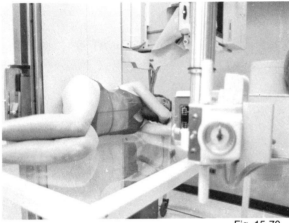
Left Lateral Decubitus (AP)　　Fig. 15-70

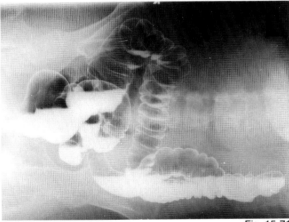
Left Lateral Decubitus　　Fig. 15-71

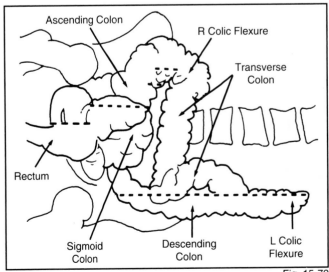
Left Lateral Decubitus　　Fig. 15-72

• RAO Position

Structures Best Shown:
Best demonstrates the **right colic** (hepatic) **flexure**, the cecum and the ascending and sigmoid colon.

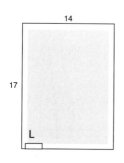

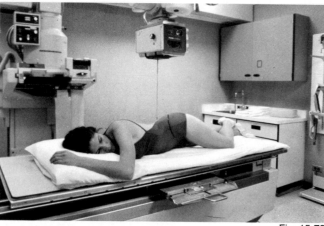

RAO   Fig. 15-73

Technical Factors:
• Film Size - 14 x 17 in. (35 x 43 cm), lengthwise.
• Moving or stationary grid.
• 80-90 kVp range (double-contrast study) (100-125 kVp range if single-contrast study).

Patient Position:
• Semiprone, rotated into a 35 to 45° right anterior oblique.
• Provide pillow for head.

Shielding: Place lead shield over pelvic region to protect gonads without covering pertinent anatomy.

Part Position:
• Align **midsagittal plane along long axis of table**, with right and left abdominal margins equal distance from center line of table.
• Left arm up on pillow, right arm down behind patient, left knee partially flexed.
• Check posterior pelvis and trunk for **35-45° rotation**.

Central Ray:
• CR **perpendicular** to film holder to a point about **1 in.** (2.5 cm) **to the left** of midsagittal plane.
• CR and center of film to **level of iliac crest.** (see NOTE).
• Minimum 40 in. (102 cm) SID.

Collimation: Collimate on four sides to outer margins of film.

Respiration: Suspend respiration and expose on expiration.

NOTE: • Proceed as rapidly as possible.
• Insure that rectal ampulla is included on lower margin of film. This may require centering 1 or 2 in. (5 - 10 cm) below the iliac crest on larger patients and taking a second film centered 1 to 2 in. (5 - 10 cm) above the crest to include the right colic flexure (Figs. 15-74a and 74b).
• A hypersthenic patient may require two films crosswise to include all the large intestine.

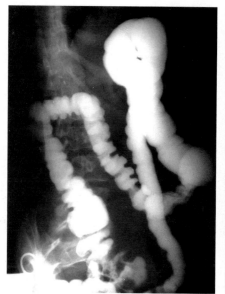

RAO   Fig. 15-74a
(Centered high to include R and L Colic Flexures)

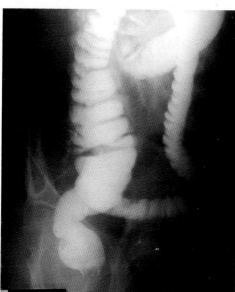

RAO   Fig. 15-74b
(Centered low to include rectal ampulla)

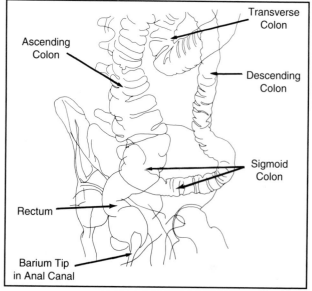

RAO – to include rectal ampulla   Fig. 15-75

Evaluation Criteria:
• Entire large intestine is included with the possible exception of the left colic flexure which is best demonstrated in LAO position.
• The right colic flexure and the ascending and sigmoid colon are seen "open" without significant superimposition.
• The rectal ampulla should be included on lower margin of radiograph.

• Appropriate technique should visualize the contrast-filled large intestine without significant overexposure of any portion.
• Patient ID info and R or L markers are visible without superimposing essential anatomy.

• LAO Position

Structures Best Shown:
Best demonstrates the **left colic** (splenic) **flexure** and the descending colon.

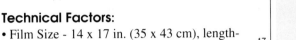

Technical Factors:
• Film Size - 14 x 17 in. (35 x 43 cm), length-wise.
• Moving or stationary grid.
• 100-125 kVp range (single-contrast).
  80-90 kVp range (double-contrast).

Patient Position:
• Semi prone, rotated into a 35-45° left anterior oblique.
• Provide pillow for head.

Shielding:
Place lead shield over pelvic region to protect gonads without covering pertinent anatomy.

Part Position:
• Align **midsagittal plane along long axis of table**, with right and left abdominal margins equal distance from center line of table.
• Right arm up on pillow, left arm down behind patient, left knee partially flexed.
• Check posterior pelvis and trunk for **35-45° rotation**.

Central Ray:
• CR **perpendicular** to film holder to a point about **1 in.** (2.5 cm) **to the right** of midsagittal plane.
• CR and film centered to **1 to 2 in.** (2.5-5 cm) **above iliac crest** (see NOTE).
• Minimum 40 in. (102 cm) SID.

Collimation:
Collimate on four sides to outer margins of film.

Respiration:
Suspend respiration and expose on expiration.

NOTE: • Proceed as rapidly as possible.
• Most adult patients require about 2 inches (5 cm) higher centering to include the **left colic flexure**, which will generally cut off lower large bowel; then a second film centered 2 or 3 inches (5-7.5 cm) lower is required to include the rectal area.

Evaluation Criteria:
• Entire large intestine should be included. (See NOTE.)
• The left colic flexure should be seen as open without significant superimposition.
• Descending colon should be well demonstrated.
• Appropriate technique should visualize the contrast-filled large intestine without significant overexposure of any portion.
• Patient ID info and R or L markers are visible without superimposing essential anatomy.

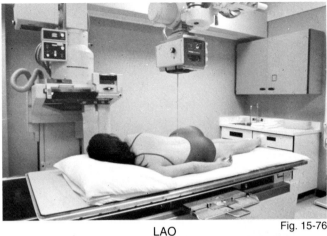

LAO   Fig. 15-76

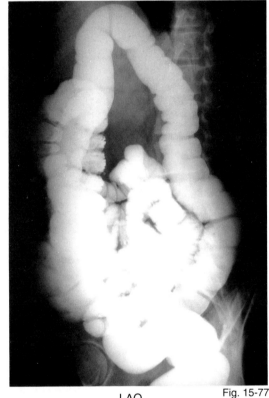

LAO   Fig. 15-77
(Centered high to include L colic flexure)

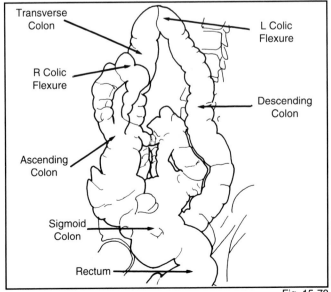

LAO   Fig. 15-78

Barium Enema

• PA (AP) Projection, Post Evac

Barium Enema
Basic
• PA and/or AP
• L Lateral Rectum
• R Lat Decub
• L Lat Decub
• RAO and/or LAO
• **PA Post Evac**

Structures Best Shown:
Mucosal pattern of large intestine with residual contrast media.

Most commonly taken prone as a PA, but may be taken with patient supine as an AP if necessary.

Technical Factors:
• Film Size - 14 x 17 in. (35 x 43 cm), lengthwise.
• Moving or stationary grid.
• 80-90 kVp range.
• Use post-evac marker.

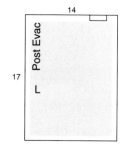

Patient Position:
• Prone or supine, pillow for head.

Shielding: Place lead shield over pelvic region to protect gonads without covering pertinent anatomy.

Part Position:
• **Midsagittal plane aligned to midline** of table.
• **No body rotation.**

Central Ray:
• CR **perpendicular** to film holder.
• CR and center of film to **iliac crest.**
• Minimum 40 in. (102 cm) SID.

Collimation: Collimate on four sides to outer margins of film.

Respiration: Suspend respiration and expose on expiration.

NOTE: • Taken after patient has had sufficient time for adequate evacuation.
• If radiograph shows insufficient evacuation to clearly visualize mucosal pattern, the patient can be given hot tea or coffee to stimulate further evacuation after which this radiograph should be repeated.
• Include rectal ampula on lower margin of radiograph.
• Lower kVp is used to prevent over-penetration with only the residual contrast media remaining in large bowel.

Evaluation Criteria:
• Entire large intestine should be visualized with only a residual amount of contrast media.
• No rotation as evidenced by symmetry of ilia wings and parts of the lumbar vertebrae.
• Appropriate technique employed to visualize outline of entire mucosal pattern of the large intestine without overexposure of any parts.
• Patient ID info, R or L marker and post evac markers are visible without superimposing essential anatomy.

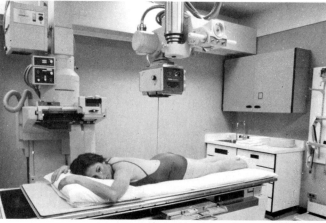

PA Post Evac   Fig. 15-79

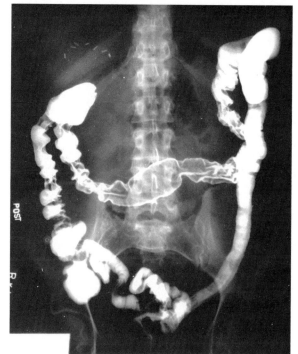

PA Post Evac   Fig. 15-80

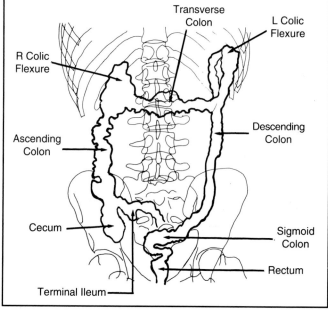

PA Post Evac   Fig. 15-81

- ## AP Axial Projection
- ## LPO Axial Position

("Butterfly" Positions)

Barium Enema
Optional
• **AP & LPO Axial**
• PA & RAO Axial
• Chassard-Lapine
• LPO and RPO

Structures Best Shown:
Elongated views of the rectosigmoid segments of large intestine.

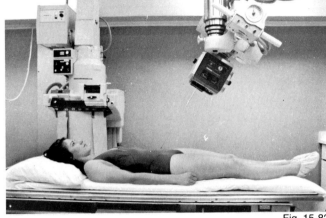

Fig. 15-82

AP Axial

Technical Factors:
- Film Size - 14 x 17 in. (35 x 43 cm), lengthwise.
    or   11 x 14 in. (28 x 35 cm), lengthwise.
- Moving or stationary grid.
- 100-125 kVp range for single-contrast,
    (or 90-100 kVp range, double-contrast).

14 (11)

17 (14) L

Patient Position:
- Supine or partially rotated into a LPO position.
- Provide pillow for head.

Shielding: Place lead shield over pelvic region to protect gonads without covering pertinent anatomy.

Part Position:
AP • Patient supine, **align midsagittal plane to midline** of table.
⁃ Extend legs, arms down by patient's side; insure **no rotation**.
LPO • Rotate patient **30 to 40°** into LPO (left posterior side down).
  • Raise right arm, left arm extended, right knee partially flexed.

Central Ray:
- CR angled **30-40° cephalad**.
AP • CR **2 in.** (5 cm) **inferior** to **level of ASIS**, and to **midsagittal plane**.
LPO • CR **2 in.** (5cm) **inferior** and **2 in.** (5 cm) **medial to right ASIS**.
  • Center film holder to CR.
  • Minimum 40 in. (102 cm) SID.

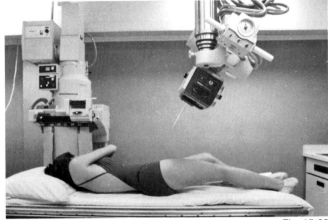

Fig. 15-83

LPO Axial

Collimation: Collimate on four sides to outer margins of film.

Respiration: Suspend respiration and expose on expiration.

NOTE: • Proceed as rapidly as possible.
- Similar views can also be obtained with a **PA axial** and **RAO** with **30-40° caudal** CR angle (see following page).

Evaluation Criteria:
AP • Adequate CR angulation evidenced by elongation of rectosigmoid segments of large intestine.
  • No rotation as evidenced by symmetrical appearance of pelvis.
LPO • Adequate CR angulation and patient obliquity evidenced by elongation and less superimposition of rectosigmoid segments of large intestine.
  • Appropriate technique used to visualize outlines of all rectosigmoid segments of large intestine. With air-contrast study, the kVp should be decreased so as not to over penetrate the air-filled outlines of these segments of large bowel.
  • Patient ID info and R or L markers are visible without superimposing essential anatomy.

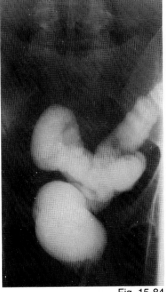
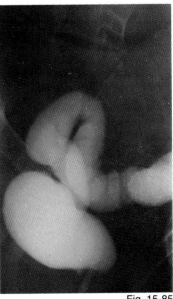

AP Axial   Fig. 15-84   LPO Axial   Fig. 15-85

Barium Enema

• PA Axial Projection
• RAO Axial Position

("Butterfly" Positions)

Barium Enema
Optional
• AP & LPO Axial
• **PA & RAO Axial**
• Chassard-Lapine
• LPO and RPO

Structures Best Shown:
• Elongated views of the rectosigmoid segments of large intestine.

Technical Factors:
• Film Size - 14 x 17 in. (35 x 43 cm), lengthwise.
    or   10 x 12 in. (24 x 30 cm), lengthwise.
• Moving or stationary grid.
• 100-125 kVp range for single-contrast,
  (or 90-100 kVp range, double-contrast).

14 (10)

17 (12)   L

Patient Position:
• Prone or partially rotated into a RAO position.
• Provide pillow for head.

Shielding: Place lead shield over pelvic region to protect gonads without covering pertinent anatomy.

Part Position:
PA • Patient prone, align midsagittal plane to midline of table.
    • Arms up beside head or down by sides away from body.
    • **No rotation** of pelvis or trunk.
RAO • Rotate patient **35 to 45°** into **RAO** (right anterior side down).
    • Left arm up, right arm down by side, left knee partially flexed.

Central Ray:
• CR angled **30-40° caudad**.
  PA • CR to exit at **level of ASIS** and to **midsagittal plane**.
  RAO • CR to exit at **level of ASIS** and **2 in.** (5 cm) to **left of lumbar spinous processes.**
• Center film holder to CR.
• Minimum 40 in. (102 cm) SID.

Collimation: Collimate on four sides to outer margins of film.

Respiration: Suspend respiration and expose on expiration.

NOTE: • Proceed as rapidly as possible.
• Similar views of rectosigmoid region as AP and LPO with 30-40° cephalad angle as described on preceding page.

Evaluation Criteria:
PA • Adequate CR angulation evidenced by elongation of rectosigmoid segments of large intestine.
• No rotation as evidenced by symmetrical appearance of pelvis.
RAO • Adequate CR angulation and patient obliquity evidenced by elongation and less superimposition of rectosigmoid segments of large intestine.
• Appropriate technique used to visualize outlines of all rectosigmoid segments of large intestine. With air-contrast study, the kVp should be decreased so as not to over penetrate the air-filled outlines of these

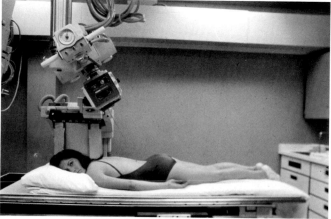

PA Axial   Fig. 15-86

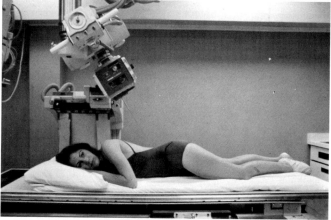

RAO Axial   Fig. 15-87

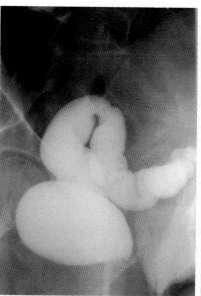
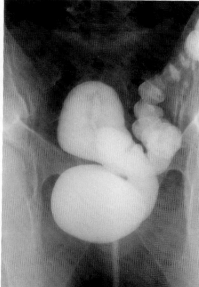

RAO Axial   Fig. 15-88   PA Axial   Fig. 15-89

segments of large bowel.
• Patient ID info and R or L markers are visible without superimposing essential anatomy.

• Chassard–Lapine Axial Position

Barium Enema
Optional
• AP & LPO Axial
• PA & RAO Axial
• **Chassard-Lapine**
• LPO and RPO

Structures Best Shown:
Rectosigmoid portion of large intestine.

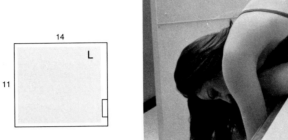
C – L Axial   Fig. 15-90

Technical Factors:
• Film Size - 11 x 14 in. (30 x 35 cm) crosswise to patient (lengthwise to table).
• Moving or stationary grid.
• 110-125 kVp range.

Patient Position:
• Patient seated on side of table, leaning forward.

Shielding: No gonadal shielding is possible.

Part Position:
• Have patient sit well back on table; then lean forward **as far as possible** grasping ankles.
• Abduct the thighs to help the patient lean forward further.

Central Ray:
• CR **perpendicular** to film holder, passing through a line midway between greater trochanters.
• Minimum 40 in. (102 cm) SID.

Collimation: Collimate on four sides to film borders.

Respiration: Suspend respiration and expose on expiration.

NOTE: • This projection is not commonly taken on younger patients because of high radiation dose to the gonads.
• Should only be attempted on patients with excellent sphincter control (or may be done after partial evacuation).

Evaluation Criteria:
• An axial view of the rectosigmoid region should be visible centered to the film.
• The sigmoid segments should appear in profile with minimal superimposition.
• Appropriate technique should visualize the rectosigmoid segments of the large intestine.
• Patient ID info and R or L markers are visible without superimposing essential anatomy.

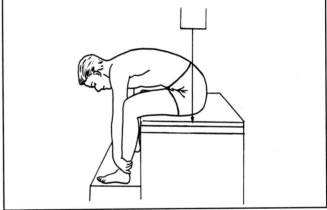
C – L Axial   Fig. 15-91

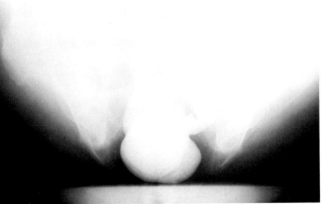
C – L Axial   Fig. 15-92

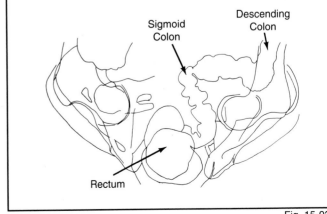
C – L Axial   Fig. 15-93

Descending Colon
Sigmoid Colon
Rectum

• LPO and RPO Positions

Structures Best Shown:
Contrast-filled large intestine.
LPO: Best demonstrates **right colic** (hepatic) **flexure**, ascending, cecum and sigmoid portions (similar to RAO position).
RPO: Best demonstrates **left colic** (splenic) **flexure** and descending portion (similar to LAO position).

Technical Factors:
• Film Size - 14 x 17 in. (35 x 43 cm), lengthwise.
• Moving or stationary grid.
• 100-125 kVp range (single-contrast)
 80-90 kVp range (double-contrast)

Patient Position:
• Semisupine, rotated 35-45° into right and left posterior obliques.
• Provide pillow for head.

Shielding: Place lead shield over pelvic region to protect gonads without covering pertinent anatomy.

Part Position:
• Flex elevated side elbow and place in front of head, place opposite arm down by patient's side.
• Partially flex elevated side knee for support to maintain this position.
• Align **midsagittal plane along long axis of table** with right and left abdominal margins equal distance from centerline of table.

Central Ray:
• CR **perpendicular** to film holder.
• CR and center of film to level of **iliac crests** and about **1 in.** (2.5 cm) **lateral to elevated side** of midsagittal plane. (see NOTE).
• Minimum 40 in. (102 cm) SID.

Collimation: Collimate on four sides to outer margins of film.

Respiration: Expose on expiration.

NOTE: • Proceed as rapidly as possible.
• Insure that rectal ampulla is included.
• Most adult patients require a second film centered 2 or 3 in. (5-7.5 cm) higher on the **RPO** if the left colic (splenic) flexure is to be included.
• A hypersthenic patient may require two films crosswise to include all of large intestine.

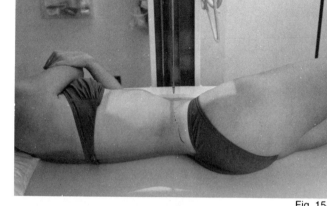

LPO — Fig. 15-94

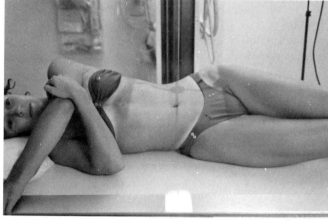

RPO — Fig. 15-95

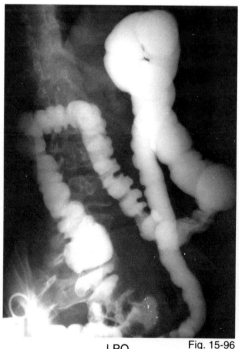

LPO — Fig. 15-96

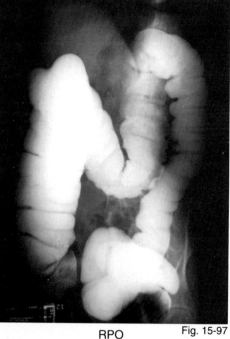

RPO — Fig. 15-97

(centered high to include both right and left colic flexures)

Evaluation Criteria:
• Entire contrast-filled large intestine including the rectal ampulla should be included (see NOTE).
• Appropriate technique should visualize the contrast-filled large intestine without significant overexposure of any portion.
 LPO: The **right colic** (hepatic) **flexure, ascending** and **rectosigmoid portions** should appear "open" without significant superimposition.

RPO: The **left colic** (splenic) **flexure** and the **descending portions** should appear "open" without significant superimposition. (A second film centered lower to include the rectal area is required on most adult patients if this area is to be included on these post-fluoroscopy overhead radiographs, see NOTE.)

Chapter 16
Radiographic Anatomy and Positioning of the Gallbladder and Biliary Ducts

Contributions by: John Lampignano, M Ed, RT (R)
Barry T. Anthony, RT (R)

Contents

Part I Radiographic Anatomy

Liver, Gallbladder and Biliary Ducts

Liver

Radiographic examination of the biliary system involves studying the manufacture, transport and storage of bile. Bile is manufactured by the liver, transported by the various ducts and stored in the gallbladder. In order to understand radiographic examination of the biliary system, one should understand the basic anatomy and physiology of the liver, gallbladder and connecting ducts.

The liver is the largest solid organ in the human body and weighs 3 or 4 pounds (1.5 kg), or one thirty-sixth of the total body weight in an average adult. It occupies most of the upper right quadrant. Of the nine abdominal regions, it occupies almost all of the right hypochondrium, a major part of the epigastrium and a significant part of the left hypochondrium.

As viewed from the front in *Fig. 16-1,* the liver is triangular in shape. The upper border is the widest part of the liver (approximately 8 to 9 inches or 20-23 cm) and is convex to conform to the inferior surface of the right diaphragm.

The right border of the liver is its greatest vertical dimension, approximately 6 to 7 inches or 15 to 17.5 cm. In the average person it extends to slightly below the lateral portion of the tenth rib just above the right kidney. The liver is fairly well protected by the lower right rib cage. Since the liver is highly vascular and easily lacerated, protection by the ribs is very necessary.

Gallbladder

The distal end of the gallbladder extends slightly below the anterior, inferior margin of the liver. The rest of the gallbladder lies along the inferior surface of the liver.

Lobes of the Liver

The liver is incompletely divided into two major lobes and two minor lobes. As viewed from the front in *Fig. 16-2,* only the two major lobes can be seen. A much larger **right lobe** is separated from the smaller **left lobe** by the **falciform** *(fal'si-form)* **ligament.** The two minor lobes can be seen only when viewing the visceral or inferior surface of the liver and are not shown on this drawing. The first of these is the **small quadrate lobe** located on the inferior surface of the right lobe between the gall-bladder and the falciform ligiment. Just posterior to the quadrate lobe is the second minor lobe, the **caudate lobe** which extends posteriorly to the diaphragmatic surface.

Function: The liver is an extremely complex organ and is absolutely essential to life. The liver performs over 100 different functions, but the one function most applicable to radiographic study is the production of large amounts of bile. It secretes from 800 to 1,000 ml, or about 1 quart of bile per day.

The major function of bile is to aid in the digestion of fats by emulsifying or breaking down of fat globules and absorption of fat following their digestion. Bile also contains cholesterol which is made soluble in the bile by the bile salts.

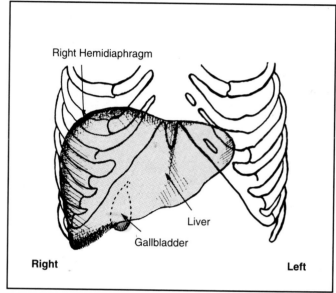

Liver and Gallbladder (Anterior View)   Fig. 16-1

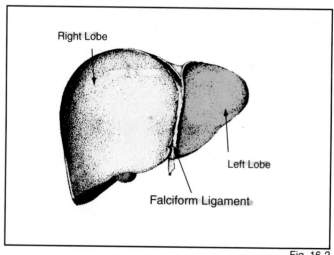

Liver (Anterior View)   Fig. 16-2

Gallbladder and Biliary Ducts

The gallbladder and the biliary ducts located outside of the gallbladder are shown in *Fig.* 16-3. Bile is formed in small lobules of the liver and travels by small ducts to either the **right or left hepatic duct.** The right and left hepatic ducts join to continue as the **common hepatic duct.** Bile is either carried to the **gallbladder** via the **cystic duct** for temporary storage or poured directly into the **duodenum** by way of the **common bile duct.**

Gallbladder and Cystic Duct

The gallbladder and cystic duct are shown in *Fig.* 16-4. The gallbladder (GB) is a pear-shaped sac composed of three parts— **fundus, body and neck.** The fundus is the distal end and the broadest part of the gallbladder. The main section of the gallbladder is termed the body. The narrow proximal end is termed the neck, which continues as the **cystic duct.** The cystic duct is 3 to 4 centimeters long, containing several membranous folds along its length. These folds are termed the **spiral valve**, which functions to prevent distension or collapse of the cystic duct.

The normal gallbladder is from 7 to 10 centimeters long, about 3 centimeters wide and normally holds 30 to 40 cc's of bile.

Functions of the Gallbladder

The **three** primary functions of the gallbladder are to **store** and **concentrate** bile, and to **contract when stimulated. First,** if bile is not needed for digestive purposes, it is stored for future use in the gallbladder.

Second, bile is concentrated within the gallbladder due to hydrolosis (removal of water). In the abnormal situation, if too much water is absorbed or if the cholesterol becomes too concentrated, gallstones (choleliths) may form in the gallbladder. (Cholesterol coming out of solution forms gallstones.)

As a **third** function, the gallbladder normally contracts when foods such as fats or fatty acids are in the duodenum. These foods stimulate the duodenal mucosa to secrete the hormone cholecystokinin (CCK). Increased levels of CCK in the blood cause the gallbladder to contract and the terminal opening of the common bile duct to relax. In addition, CCK causes increased exocrine activity by the pancreas.

Common Bile Duct

The common hepatic duct draining the liver joins with the cystic duct of the gallbladder to form the **common bile duct.** The common bile duct averages about 7.5 centimeters in length and has an internal diameter about the size of a drinking straw. The common bile duct descends behind the superior portion of the duodenum and the head of the pancreas to enter the second or **descending portion of the duodenum.**

The end of the common bile duct is closely associated with the end of the **main duct** of the **pancreas (duct of Wirsung)** as shown in *Fig. 16-5, (Ver'soongz).*[1]

In about 40% of individuals these two ducts remain separated by a thin membrane as they pass into the duodenum. In the remaining 60%, the common bile duct joins the pancreatic duct to form an enlarged chamber just proximal to the terminal opening termed the **hepatopancreatic ampulla (ampulla of Vater)** *(fah' terz).*[2] Near this terminal opening, the duct walls contain circular muscle fiber, termed the **hepatopancreatic sphincter (sphincter of Oddi)** *(Od'ez)*.[3] This spinchter relaxes when there are increased levels of CCK in the bloodstream. The presence of this ring of muscle causes a protrusion into the lumen of the duodenum. This protrusion is termed the **duodenal papilla,** which is the narrowest part of this passageway and therefore a common site for impaction of gallstones.

---

[1] Wirsung, German physician, 17th century.
[2] Abraham Vater, German anatomist, 1684-1751.
[3] Ruggero Oddi, 19th century Italian Physician.

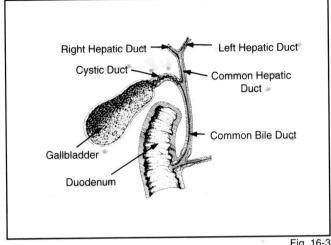

Fig. 16-3

Gallbladder and Extrahepatic Biliary Ducts

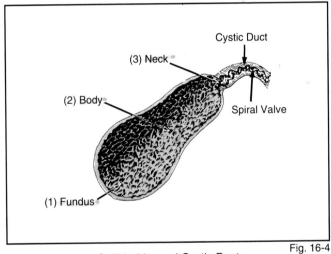

Fig. 16-4

Gallbladder and Cystic Duct

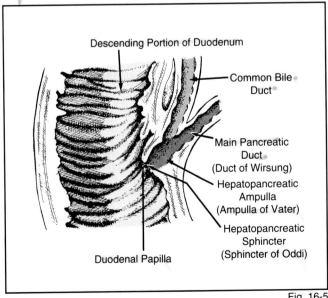

Fig. 16-5

Common Bile Duct

Gallbladder and Biliary Ducts.

The simplified lateral drawing in *Fig.* 16-6 illustrates the arrangement of the **liver, gallbladder and biliary ducts** as seen from the right side. The gallbladder is anterior to the midaxillary plane, while the duct system is about midway between the front and the back. This spatial relationship influences optimal positioning of either the gallbladder or the biliary ducts. If it were necessary to place the gallbladder as close to the film surface as possible, the prone position would be much better than the supine position. If the primary purpose is to drain the gallbladder into the duct system, the patient would be placed supine to assist this drainage.

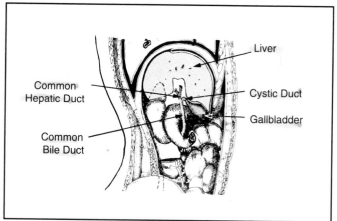

Gallbladder and Biliary Duct   Fig. 16-6

Gallbladder Location Variation

The usual position of the gallbladder varies according to the body build of the patient. In the **hypersthenic** body habitus, the gallbladder is usually located higher and more lateral than average.

In the average body build, which includes the **sthenic and hyposthenic** types, the gallbladder is usually located halfway between the xiphoid tip and the lower lateral rib margin.

In the **asthenic** body habitus, the gallbladder is much lower and more medial than average.

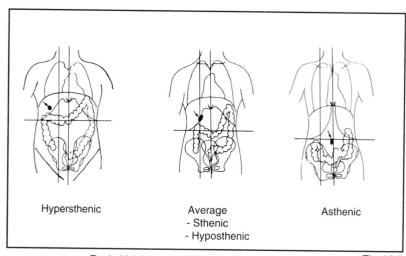

Body Habitus and Gallbladder Variation   Fig. 16-7

Radiographs (Anatomy Review)

Radiographs of the Gallbladder

(Cholecystogram)

This PA projection of the gallbladder demonstrates the cystic duct and the three major divisions of the gallbladder as labeled:

A. Cystic Duct
B. Neck
C. Body
D. Fundus

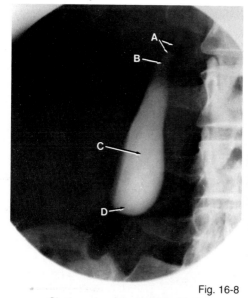

Fig. 16-8
Cholecystogram (Gallbladder)
(Courtesy of Bill Collins, RT)

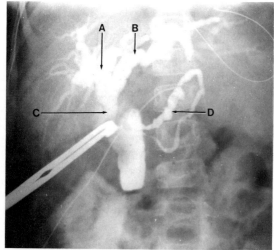

Fig. 16-9
Biliary Ducts

Radiographs of the Bilary Ducts:

Radiograph *16-9* demonstrates the various divisions and components of the biliary tract. This was taken during a surgical procedure wherein contrast media was injected via a catheter directly into the biliary ducts. This does not represent normal duct positions but visualizes certain identifiable duct components and demonstrates the complexity of the biliary system.

A. Right hepatic duct
B. Left hepatic duct
C. Common hepatic duct

D. Pancreatic duct (duct of Wirsung). This demonstrates an unusual and extra long loop of this duct.

The common bile duct and the hepatopancreatic ampula (ampulla of Vater) cannot be definitely determined from this radiograph alone.

Part II Radiographic Procedures

Gallbladder and Biliary Duct Radiography

Since the liver is such a large, solid organ, it can be easily located in the upper right quadrant on abdominal radiographs. The gallbladder and biliary ducts, however, blend in with other abdominal soft tissues and in most cases cannot be visualized without the addition of contrast media. Only about 15 percent of all gallstones contain enough calcium to be visualized on a plain abdominal radiograph.

Cholecystography

Terminology

Radiographic examination of the gallbladder and bilary ducts is referred to by different terms. It is important to identify a specific examination by the correct term.

Radiographic examination specifically of the gallbladder is termed **cholecystography** *(ko"le-sis-tog'rah-fe). Chole- (ko'le)* is a prefix denoting a relationship to bile. *Cysto-* means sac or bladder. Therefore, chole combined with cysto literally translates as bile sac or gallbladder.

Cholangiogram is a radiographic examination of the **biliary ducts**. There are a number of techniques to study the bile ducts and these techniques will be discussed in a later section.

A study of both the **gallbladder** and **biliary ducts** is termed a cholecystocholangiogram *(ko"le-sis"to-ko-lan'je-o-gram).* Through the use of contrast media, both components are demonstrated.

Oral Cholecystogram

Since the contrast media is ingested orally, for a **cholecystogram** *(ko'le-sis-to-gram),* this procedure is termed an oral cholecystogram, abbreviated, OCG *(Fig. 16-10).*

The most common way to get contrast media into the biliary system is orally (by mouth). Most cholecystography is accomplished following ingestion of four to six tablets or capsules during the evening preceding the examination. These oral contrast media for visualization of the gallbladder are termed **cholecystopaques**.

Purpose

The purpose of the oral cholecystogram is to study radiographically the anatomy and function of the biliary system. The oral cholecystogram measures: (1) the functional ability of the liver to remove the orally administered contrast medium from the bloodstream and to excrete it along with the bile, (2) the patency and condition of the biliary ducts and (3) the concentrating and contracting ability of the gallbladder.

Contraindications

Contraindications to cholecystography are few, but do include: (1) advanced hepatorenal disease, especially those with renal impairment; (2) active gastrointestinal disease such as vomiting or diarrhea, which would prevent absorption of the oral contrast medium and (3) hypersensitivity to iodine containing compounds.

Clinical Indications

A variety of abnormal conditions may be demonstrated during the oral cholecystogram. They include:
- Cholelithiasis *(ko"le-li-thi'ah-sis)* or biliary calculi (gallstones)
- Cholecystitis *(ko"le-sis-ti'tis)* acute or chronic
- Neoplasms *(ne'o-plazm)*
- Biliary stenosis *(ste-no'sis)*
- Congenital anomalies *(ah-nom'ah-les)*

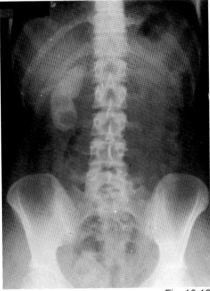

Fig. 16-10

Oral Cholecystogram (OCG)
(with gallstones – cholelithiasis)

Cholelithiasis is the condition of having gallstones. Cholelithiasis is the most common abnormality diagnosed during an OCG. Increased levels of bilirubin, calcium, or cholestrol may lead to the formation of gallstones. Female and obese patients are at a higher risk of developing gallstones. Ninety percent of all gallbladder and duct disorders are due to cholelithiasis. Symptoms of cholelithiasis include right upper quadrant pain usually after a meal, nausea, and possibly vomiting.

Although drugs have been developed that will dissolve these stones, most patients will have their gallbladder removed. A new laproscopic technique for removing the gallbladder (cholecystectomy) has greatly reduced the convalescence of the patient.

Cholecystitis is inflamation of the gallbladder. In acute cholecystitis, a blockage of the cystic duct restricts the flow of bile into the common bile duct. After a period of time, the bile begins to irritate the inner lining of the gallbladder and it becomes inflammed. Gas-producing bacteria may lead to a gangrenous gallbladder. The gallbladder with **acute cholecystitis** rarely becomes radiopaque during an OCG. Stenosis of the cystic duct prevents the contrast media from entering the gallbladder.

Chronic cholecystitis is almost always associated with gallstones, but may be an outcome of pancreatitis or carcinoma of the gallbladder. Symptoms of right upper quadrant pain, heartburn, and nausea may occur following a meal.

Neoplasms are new growths which may be benign or malignant. Malignant or cancerous tumors of the gallbladder can be aggressive and spread to the liver, pancreas, or GI tract.

Bilary stenosis is a narrowing of one of the biliary ducts. The flow of bile may be restricted by this condition. In the case of gallstones, the stenosis may prevent the passage of the small gallstones into the duodenum leading to obstruction of the ducts. Cholecystitis may result from biliary stenosis.

Congenital anomalies of the gallbladder are conditions that the patient possesses at birth. While most are benign, some may affect the production, storage, or release of bile.

NOTE: The number of oral cholecystograms being ordered has declined due to the increased use of ultrasound. Ultrasound of the gallbladder provides a noninvasive means to study the gallbladder and the bilary ducts. Small stones (choleliths) can be detected without the use of contrast media.

Oral Cholecystogram Procedure

Patient Preparation

Patient preparation for the oral cholecystogram blends nicely with preparations for an upper GI series, so these exams are usually scheduled on the same morning. If the patient has been on a fat-free diet, he should eat some fats for one or two days before the gallbladder examination. Ingestion of fats causes the gallbladder to contract. By making sure that the gallbladder has emptied prior to the administration of contrast medium, chances are increased that the newly formed bile, with contrast medium added, will be stored in the gallbladder.

Laxatives are to be avoided during the 24-hour period before the exam. The evening meal before the examination should be a light one and should not contain any fats or fried foods. When combined with an upper GI, the patient must be NPO (*Non Per Os*, meaning nothing by mouth) for at least eight hours, and must refrain from chewing gum or smoking until after the exams.

Depending on the contrast medium used, either four or six tablets or capsules are taken after the evening meal, but before 9 p.m. The usual cholecystopaques are most effective taken 10 to 12 hours before the exam. No breakfast is permitted and the patient reports to radiology in the early a.m. The exact patient prep and amount of contrast medium utilized will vary from hospital to hospital.

When the patient arrives in the radiology department for oral cholecystography, all clothing should be removed from the chest and abdomen, and the patient should put on a hospital gown.

Patient Preparation   Fig. 16-11

Patient Interview

Before the scout radiograph, the patient must be questioned about taking the contrast medium. The patient should **first** be asked how many pills were taken and at what time. It may be necessary to have the patient describe the capsules or tablets to confirm that they were the correct ones.

Second, the patient should be questioned regarding any reaction from the pills. Nausea followed by vomiting would prevent adequate absorption, as would active diarrhea. Any anaphylactoid or hypersensitivity reactions should be noted.

Third, it should be determined that the patient has not had breakfast.

Fourth, make sure that the patient still has a gallbladder. There is no need to do a cholecystogram on those rare occasions when the patient has already had the gallbladder surgically removed.

Cholecystogram Scout

After appropriate questioning, a scout radiograph is taken on a 10 x 12 or 14 x 17 inch film depending on departmental routines. The scout radiograph is made with the patient prone, as shown in *Fig. 16-13*. Since iodine is the major radiation-absorbing component of the contrast medium, a kilovoltage near 70 should be used. The scout radiograph must be checked to determine the presence or absence of an opacified gallbladder.

If the gallbladder shadow is present, the radiographer should determine (1) its exact location, (2) if there is overlap by intestine or bone, (3) if there is sufficient concentration for additional imaging and (4) if the exposure factors were optimal. If the gallbladder did not opacify adequately for imaging, the patient needs to be questioned again in detail about his preparation and, especially, about his diet for the past 24 hours.

Nonvisualization on the first day may result in a two-day study with a second dose of contrast medium or, perhaps, a trip to the ultrasound department for cholecystosonography.

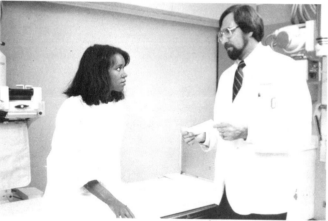

Patient Interview   Fig. 16-12

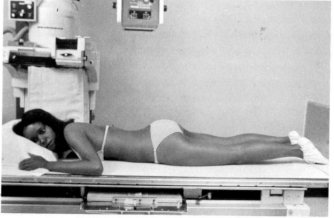

Cholecystogram Scout   Fig. 16-13

Oral Cholecystogram Procedure continued

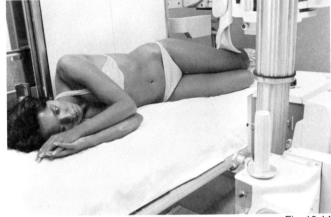

Fig. 16-14

Radiography – Right Lateral Decubitus

General Routine Procedures
One or more positions may be utilized if the gallbladder visualizes adequately on the scout radiograph. At least one erect position or a projection utilizing a horizontal beam is essential. A wide range in both the location and the pathology of the gallbladder make cholecystography an individual examination.

The right lateral decubitus position, as shown in *Fig. 16-14* or the upright position is utilized to stratify or layer out gallstones. This is the reason for at least one horizontal beam radiograph. Depending on the density of the stones in relation to the specific gravity of bile, stones may sink, rise or layer out in these two positions. Additionally, these positions allow the gallbladder to assume a different position in the abdomen and, perhaps, allow better visualization.

Method of Imaging
Many radiologists request fluoroscopy and spot films of the gallbladder in the upright position in addition to a variety of conventional radiographs. Spot filming allows use of compression and small positional changes to optimally visualize the gallbladder. A model is shown in position for upright fluoroscopy of the gallbladder in *Fig. 16-15.* If an upper GI series is scheduled in addition to the oral cholecystogram, the patient would then be in position for ingestion of barium.

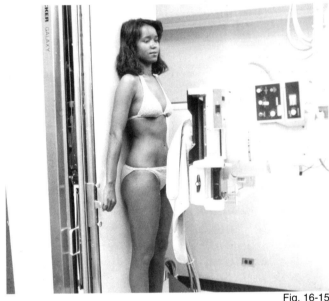

Fig. 16-15

Fluoroscopy

With Fatty Meal or CCK
Occasionally, after adequate imaging of the filled gallbladder, the radiologist may wish to test the ability of the gallbladder to contract and to study the extrahepatic biliary ducts. Gallbladder contraction may be accomplished in one of two ways.

First, administration of a "fatty meal" will stimulate the duodenal mucosa to produce CCK (cholecystokin) which, in turn, will cause the gallbladder to contract. Commercially available fatty meal substitutes are administered for this purpose. The patient is placed in an RPO position after the fatty meal (*Fig. 16-16*) so that the gallbladder can best drain. Radiographs are obtained in the same RPO position every 15 minutes until satisfactory visualization of the duct system is obtained.

The second method for gallbladder stimulation and contraction is much faster and more direct. Either cholecystokin (CCK) or a synthetic substitute is injected into the patient's venous system. This usually causes contraction of the gallbladder in five to ten minutes.

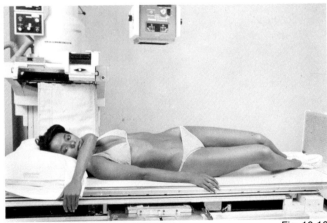

Fig. 16-16

Gallbladder Drainage Position – RPO

NOTE: This procedure is rarely done anymore as indicated in the survey results on page 496. It is more common today to utilize an ultrasound examination if a conventional oral cholecystogram does not result in sufficient diagnostic information.

This procedure should not be ordered or performed if stones are present.

Intravenous Cholangiogram

The intravenous cholangiography (IVC) is also rarely performed today due to the high incidence of contrast media reactions. With this added risk of possible reaction to contrast media, other diagnostic procedures are safer and more accurate. More common use of other procedures such as ultrasound, percutaneous transhepatic cholangiography, and endoscopic retrograde cholangiopancreatography (ERCP) have almost eliminated the need to perform IVC's.

The intravenous cholangiogram demonstrates the biliary ducts to determine if an obstruction exists due to calculi or other pathology.

The IVC is performed on patients with a history of (1) a nonvisualized gallbladder during an oral cholecytogram, (2) a cholecystectomized patient, (3) or severe vomiting or diarrhea which prevented the absorption of the contrast media prior to an OCG.

After the patient receives a bowel preparation, a drip infusion of contrast media is used. The usual adult dose is 100 milliliters slowly infused over a period of 30 to 40 minutes. Infusion must be slow to lessen the likelihood of nausea and subsequent vomiting.

Once infusion of the contrast media is begun, serial radiographs are obtained every 20 minutes until optimal visualization of the biliary ducts is achieved.

A 30 to 45 degree right posterior oblique (RPO) position is utilized to cast the biliary ducts away from the spine. Tomography may be helpful in demonstrating faint ductal shadows. (See *Figs. 16-17* and *16-18.*)

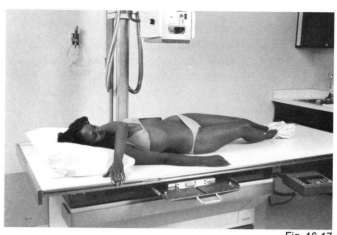

IV Cholangiogram – RPO Position   Fig. 16-17

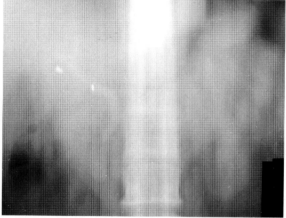

IVC – AP Tomogram   Fig. 16-18

Percutaneous Transhepatic Cholangiography

Percutaneous Transhepatic Cholangiography (PTC) is another type of cholangiography that demonstrates the biliary ducts. It is more invasive than other forms of cholangiography, but it gives the radiologist more options in the diagnosis and treatment of biliary conditions.

The PTC involves a direct puncture of biliary ducts with a needle. Once within a duct, iodinated contrast media is injected under fluoroscopic control. Fluoroscopic spot films and conventional radiographs are taken during the procedure.

Purpose
The PTC is performed for various clinical indications. The most common indications include:

(1) **Obstructive jaundice**: If the patient is jaundiced and the ducts are suspected to be dilated, an obstruction of the biliary ducts may be the cause. The obstruction may be due to calculi or biliary stenosis.

(2) **Stone extraction and biliary drainage**: PTC allows the radiologist to diagnose the condition and, using specialized equipment, remove the stone or dilate the restricted portion of the biliary tract. Excess bile may be drained during a PTC to decompress the biliary ducts.

Procedure
There is a certain amount of risk associated with the PTC due to the needle puncture into the liver tissue. The liver may hemorrhage internally or bile may escape into the periotoneal cavity.

While the percutaneous transhepatic puncture is performed by the radiologist, the radiographer has specific responsibilities. These responsibilities include:
(1) Prepare the fluoroscopic suite.
(2) Set up the sterile tray and include the long, thin-walled needle used for the puncture. (The needle is a Chiba or "Skinny" type. It has a flexible shaft that allows for easy manipulation of the needle during the puncture.)
(3) Select and prepare the contrast media. Determine if the patient is hypersensitive to iodinated contrast media.
(4) Take the appropriate scout films to verify position and technique.
(5) Monitor the patient during the procedure.
(6) Change fluoro spot films as needed.

The site of the puncture is surgically prepared. After the local anesthetic is given, the radiologist inserts the needle into the liver in the approximate location of the biliary ducts. More than one puncture may be necessary to locate the appropriate duct. Under fluoroscopic view, the radiologist adjusts the needle while slowly injecting the contrast media.

Once the ducts are filled, fluoroscopic spot films and conventional radiographs are taken.

Following the procedure, a chest radiograph may be ordered. Since the liver is near the right hemidiaphragm, the needle puncture may result in a pneumothorax. Both during and after the procedure, the patient's vital signs are closely monitored to detect deterioration.

In addition to studying the biliary ducts, the PTC may serve as a therapeutic procedure to extract stones or decompress dilated ducts.

A larger needle may be inserted into a duct containing a stone. A special basket catheter is passed over a guide wire and is positioned near the stone. Under fluoroscopic control, the stone can be extracted from the duct.

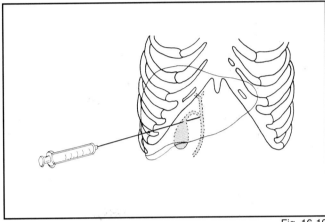

PTC Puncture   Fig. 16-19

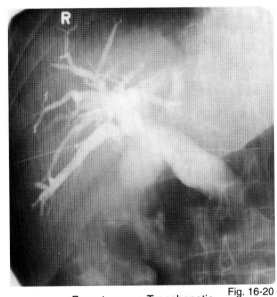

Fig. 16-20
Percutaneous Transhepatic
Cholangiogram (PTC)

Operative or Immediate Cholangiogram

The operative or immediate cholangiogram is performed during surgery, usually during a cholecystectomy. The surgeon may suspect that residual stones are located in one of the bilary ducts. After the gallbladder is removed, a small catheter is inserted into the remaining portion of the cystic duct. Iodinated contrast media is injected and conventional radiographs are taken. Most operative cholangiograms require the use of a high mA portable x-ray unit and grid cassettes.

Purpose
Operative cholangiograms are performed to:
(1) Investigate the patency of the biliary tract
(2) Determine the functional status of the hepatopancreatic ampulla
(3) Reveal any choleliths not previously detected
(4) Demonstrate small lesions, strictures or dilatations within the biliary ducts.

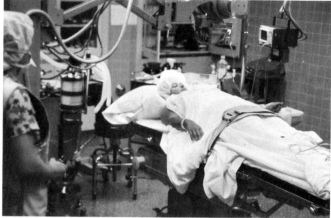
Scout Operative Cholangiogram   Fig. 16-21

Procedure
Proper planning and preparation is essential for a successful cholangiogram. But many operative cholangiograms may be scheduled at the last moment and the technologist doesn't have the opportunity to even take a scout film. In these situations, the technologist must be resourceful to produce quality radiographs.

In the ideal situation, the following steps should occur:
(1) The radiographer changes into surgical attire and insures that the portable unit is functional and clean.
(2) Before the patient is surgically prepared, take a scout film. Note the distance the film is advanced from the head of the table. A special ruler-and-tray set-up may be used in the positioning of the cassette.
(3) Process the scout film and adjust technique and film location accordingly.
(4) Once the catheter is in place, the surgeon will inject between 6 to 8 cc's of contrast media.
(5) Radiographs are obtained with the cooperation and synchronization of the surgeon, anesthesiologist, and radiographer. The anesthesiologist controls the breathing of the patient.
(6) Films are processed and may need to be reviewed by a radiologist. The radiographer may provide a written or oral report to the surgeon.

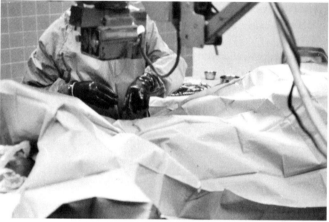
Proper CR Centering   Fig. 16-22

At least two, and preferably three radiographs are obtained in slightly different positions. Each exposure is preceded by a fractional injection of contrast medium. Positions may include an AP, a slight RPO, and a slight LPO. The RPO is helpful in projecting the biliary ducts away from the spine, especially with a hyposthenic patient.

Notes:
(a) Protective aprons must be provided to those persons remaining in the room.
(b) Some surgeons will dilute the contrast media with saline to reduce the risk of spasm of the biliary ducts. Biliary duct spasm may mimic biliary stenosis or obstruction. Also too dense of a contrast media may obscure small stones.
(c) If the OR table is tilted for the oblique positions, place the grid cassette **crosswise** to avoid objectionable grid cutoff.

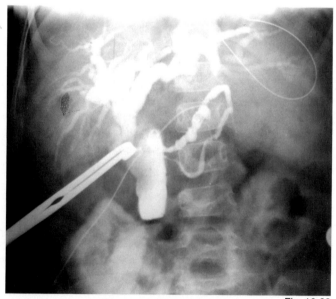
Operative Cholangiogram   Fig. 16-23

Centering Point
The surgeon should indicate the proper centering point on the sterile sheet covering the incision or, at least, indicate appropriate landmarks such as the xiphoid tip. In *Fig. 16-22*, the surgeon has twisted the sterile drape to identify the centering point.

Each fractional injection consists of 6 to 8 cc's of contrast medium. The exposure is made after the injection, after the surgeon steps back and after the anesthesiologist has stopped patient respiration.

T-tube, Postoperative, or Delayed Cholangiography

T-tube cholangiography, also termed postoperative or delayed cholangiography, is usually performed in the radiology department following a cholecystectomy. The surgeon may be concerned about residual stones in the biliary ducts that went undetected during the surgery. If these concerns exist, the surgeon will place a special T-tube cathether into the common bile duct. The catheter will extend to the outside of the body and is clamped off.

Purpose

T-tube cholangiograms are performed to:
(1) Visualize any residual or previously undetected choleliths.
(2) Evaluate the status of the biliary duct system.
(3) Demonstrate small lesions, strictures or dilatations within the biliary ducts.

Procedure

On the average, the T-tube cholangiogram is performed 1 to 3 days following surgery. In certain cases, the patient may be discharged from the hospital and brought back for the study as an outpatient. The procedure requires the use of fluoroscopy. Spot films are generally also taken. Conventional radiographs may be taken during the course of the study.

The following steps are taken in the performance of a T-tube cholangiogram:
(1) Prepare the fluoroscopic suite.
(2) Set up examination tray.
(3) Select and prepare the contrast media. Determine if the patient is hypersensitive to iodinated contrast media.
(4) Take the appropriate scout films to verify position and technique.
(5) Monitor the patient during the procedure.
(6) Change fluoro spot films as needed.
(7) Produce conventional radiographs as requested.

Since the T-tube catheter has been clamped off, drainage of excess bile is performed at the beginning of the procedure. An emesis basin should be provided for this task. Follow universal precautions when handling bile.

After duct drainage and under fluoroscopic control, the iodinated contrast media is injected fractionally and fluoro spot films are taken.

If residual stones are detected, the radiologist may elect to remove them. Similar to the PTC, a basket catheter may be passed over a guide wire and the stones are removed.

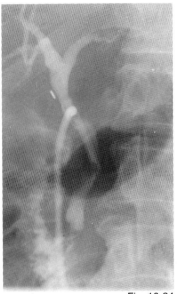

Fig. 16-24
T-tube Cholangiogram

Endoscopic Retrograde Cholangiopancreatography (ERCP)

A popular procedure of the biliary and main pancreatic ducts is Endoscopic Retrograde Cholangiopancreatography, or simply ERCP. The ERCP is an endoscopic procedure where a small catheter is passed through the hepatopancreatic ampulla and a contrast media is injected in a retrograde fashion into the biliary ducts. The procedure is usually performed by a gastroenterologist.

Purpose
The ERCP is performed to:
(1) Investigate the patency of the biliary/pancreatic ducts.
(2) Reveal any choleliths not previously detected.
(3) Demonstrate small lesions, strictures or dilatations within the biliary/pancreatic ducts.

Procedure
The ERCP is primarily a fluoroscopic procedure. Fluoroscopy is needed to aide with the cannulation of the hepatopancreatic ampulla and to provide spot films of the anatomy.

The ERCP may involve the following steps:
(1) Prepare the fluoroscopic suite.
(2) Set up the examination tray.
(3) Select and prepare the contrast media. Determine if the patient is hypersensitive to iodinated contrast media.
(4) Take the appropriate scout films to verify position and technique.
(5) Assist the gastroenterologist with fluoroscopy for the placement of the catheter.
(6) Monitor the patient during the procedure.
(7) Change fluoro spot films as needed.
(8) Produce conventional radiographs as requested.

The gastroenterologist will spray an oral anesthetic in the patient's throat to suppress the gag reflex while the fiberoptic endoscope is advanced into the duodenum (Fig. 16-25). Once the hepatopancreatic ampulla is isolated, a small catheter is passed through it and the contrast media is fractionally injected.

The radiographer may be asked to perform fluoroscopy during the procedure to identify the location of the tip of the endoscope in relationship to the ampulla. A radiologist may be present to take the spot films during the injection of contrast media.

Notes:
(a) Since the patient's throat is anesthetised during the procedure, they should remain NPO for at least one hour (or more) following the procedure. This will prevent aspiration of food or liquid into the lungs.
(b) Review the clinical history of the patient to determine if the patient has pancreatitis or, specifically, a pseudocyst of the pancreas. Injecting contrast media into a pseudocyst may lead to a rupture.
(c) Insure that all persons in the fluoroscopy room wear protective aprons.

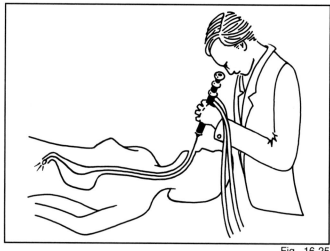

Endoscopy   Fig. 16-25

Endoscopy
Endoscopy (en-dos´ko-pe) is inspection of any cavity of the body by means of an endoscope, an instrument that allows illumination of the internal lining of an organ. Various fiberoptic endoscopes are available to examine the interior lining of the stomach, duodenum, and colon. Certain fiberoptic endoscopes allow cannulation and injection of contrast medium into small ducts such as the common bile duct or pancreatic duct as in an ERCP procedure.

Summary of Radiographic Procedures

Biliary System Radiography

In summary, **cholecystography and cholangiography** may be categorized by the method of contrast medium administration. Contrast medium is usually administered orally for cholecystography (gallbladder exam). For cholangiography, the biliary ducts are usually studied following intravenous infusion or direct injection of contrast medium.

Administration of Contrast Medium

(1) By mouth (oral) – **cholecystography** (Gallbladder).
(2) By intravenous infusion – **intravenous cholangiography** (IVC).
(3) By direct injection of ducts
    - During fluoroscopy – **percutaneous transhepatic cholangiography**
    - During surgery – **operative or immediate cholangiography**
    - Through indwelling drainage tube – **T-tube, post-op or delayed cholangiography**
    - Through catheter – **endoscopic retrograde cholangiopancreatography (ERCP)**

Part III Radiographic Positioning

National Survey:

A survey of the operating procedures (department routines) was conducted throughout the United States. The following information was compiled from the survey indicating the national norm for basic and special routines for oral cholecystography and operative cholangiography. (Numbers in parenthesis in each region represent the number of institutions responding to this part of the survey.)

Oral Cholecystogram (Gallbladder) Routine

Gallbladder	U.S. Average (528)	
	Basic	Optional
• PA Scout	78%	
• LAO	63%	
• Right Lateral Decubitus	31%	30%
• Fluoroscopy only	30%	12%
• PA Erect	19%	13%
• Fatty Meal or CCK-PZ injection	20%	24%

Operative Cholangiogram Routine

OR Cholangiogram	U.S. Average (499)	
	Basic	Optional
• AP	87%	
• RPO	28%	16%
• LPO	5%	7%

Survey Questions on Possible Discontinued Procedures:

The national survey included questions on (I) the **expected trend** in the next three or four years, (II) the **quantity** of specific exams done in their departments during the past year, and (III) whether or not **the procedure should still be taught and included** in a basic student textbook. The results were as follows:

Responses for Oral Cholecystograms (Gallbladder conventional overheads)

Gallbladder	U.S. Average (362)	East (136)	Midwest (171)	West (55)
I. Trend				
a. Increase	10%	12%	9%	2%
b. Decrease	55%	48%	59%	51%
c. No change	35%	40%	32%	47%
II. Annual Quantity				
a. 0-10	20%	15%	17%	27%
b. 11-89	43%	39%	41%	49%
c. 90-201	21%	24%	23%	16%
d. 202 +	17%	21%	19%	8%
III. Be Included				
a. Yes	89%	91%	86%	57%
b. No	11%	9%	14%	43%

Responses for Oral Cholecystograms (Gallbladder) (post fatty meal or CCK-PZ injection)

Gallbladder with fatty meal	U.S. Average (262)	East (97)	Midwest (117)	West (48)
I. Trend				
a. Increase	7%	12%	4%	2%
b. Decrease	43%	41%	40%	51%
c. No change	51%	47%	55%	47%
II. Annual Quantity				
a. 0-4	55%	38%	67%	60%
b. 5-24	26%	31%	23%	23%
c. 25-74	10%	17%	4%	12%
d. 75 +	8%	15%	5%	4%
III. Be Included				
a. Yes	53%	68%	40%	57%
b. No	47%	32%	60%	43%

Responses for T-Tube Cholangiograms

T-Tube Cholang.	U.S. Average (368)	East (135)	Midwest (167)	West (62)
I. Trend				
a. Increase	15%	22%	11%	15%
b. Decrease	17%	19%	17%	10%
c. No change	68%	59%	72%	76%
II. Annual Quantity				
a. 0-11	18%	16%	16%	27%
b. 12-36	41%	41%	41%	42%
c. 37-63	21%	22%	22%	16%
d. 64 +	20%	20%	21%	15%
III. Be Included				
a. Yes	97%	96%	97%	98%
b. No	3%	4%	3%	2%

Responses for Intravenous Cholangiograms

IVC	U.S. Average (251)	East (95)	Midwest (111)	West (45)
I. Trend				
a. Increase	2%	3%	3%	0%
b. Decrease	34%	29%	34%	42%
c. No change	64%	68%	64%	58%
II. Annual Quantity				
a. 0-3	81%	77%	85%	80%
b. 4-11	10%	13%	6%	14%
c. 12 +	9%	11%	9%	7%
III. Be Included				
a. Yes	31%	33%	26%	36%
b. No	69%	67%	74%	64%

Summary

The expected trends for all of these procedures are in general a **decrease** or **no change**, apparently due to the new imaging modalities which are largely replacing these procedures. This is more evident in the western states than in the east. However the survey results suggest that at least three of these procedures, **oral cholecystogram**, **operative cholangiogram**, and **T-tube cholangiogram** still are commonly done throughout the U.S. and need to be taught and included in this text.

Two of the procedures, **IVC** and **GB with fatty meal** are being done only occasionally and therefore are described in the procedure portion of this chapter but are no longer included in the positioning section.

Basic and Optional Projections/Positions

Certain basic and optional projections or positions of the gallbladder and biliary ducts are demonstrated and described on the following pages. The radiologist and radiographer must closely coordinate their efforts during examinations of this part of the body. Individual variations exist among radiologists, and the routine or basic positions or projections listed may vary from hospital to hospital.

Gallbladder
(Oral Cholecystogram)
Basic
• PA Scout
• LAO
Optional
• Right Lat. Decub.
• PA Erect

OR Cholangiogram
Basic
• AP
Optional
• RPO and/or LPO

Percutaneous transhepatic cholangiography, endoscopic retrograde cholangiopancreatogram and T-tube cholangiography are included as part of the basic positions/projections as listed below; however, these exams are performed by the radiologist, not the radiographer, so they are not described in the positioning pages of this chapter.

Percutaneous Transhepatic Cholangiogram
• Fluoro Spots
• Radiography optional

T-tube Cholangiogram
• Fluoro Spots
• Radiography optional

Endoscopic Retrograde Cholangiopancreatogram (ERCP)
• Fluoro Spots
• Radiography optional

• PA Projection – Scout

Gallbladder
(Oral Cholecystogram)
Basic
• PA Scout
• LAO
Optional
• Right Lat. Decub.
• PA Erect

Structures Best Shown:
General survey of opacified gallbladder.

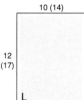

Technical Factors:
• Film Size - 10 x 12 in. (24 x 30 cm), lengthwise.
• Moving or stationary grid.
• 70-76 kVp range.
Exception: Some departmental routines include a
full abdomen scout on a 14 x 17 in. (35 x 43 cm),
with positioning as for a PA abdomen centered to level of
iliac crest or slightly above.

Patient Position:
• Patient prone, pillow for head, arms up beside head, legs
extended with support under ankles.

Shielding: Place lead shield over gonadal area, not ob-
scuring area of interest.

Part Position:
• Align midsagittal plane to long axis of table with right half
of abdomen centered to midline of table and/or film holder
for sthenic type patient (see NOTE).
• No rotation of pelvis or trunk.

Central Ray:
• CR **perpendicular** to film holder.
• For average sthenic patient, CR to **level of L 2** (which is
about .5 to 1 in. or 1.25 to 2.5 cm above lowest margin of rib cage)
about 2 in. or 5 cm **to right of midsagittal plane.** (See NOTE on
body habitus).
• Center film holder to CR.
• Minimum 40 in. (102 cm) SID.

Collimation: Collimate on four sides to film margins.

Respiration: Suspend respiration upon **expiration.**

NOTE: • The PA scout is taken to determine presence and location of
gallbladder, adequate concentration of contrast media and adequacy
of exposure factors.
• Body habitus variation: **Hypersthenic** (broad) - gallbladder more
horizontal, 2 inches (5 cm) higher and more lateral. **Asthenic** (thin)
- gallbladder vertical, 2 inches (5 cm) lower, near the midline.
• CR point should be marked on patient's skin for precise centering on
additional projections of gallbladder.

Evaluation Criteria:
• Entire opacified gallbladder and area of cystic duct is demonstrated.
• No motion of gallbladder or abdominal contents is evident.
• Appropriate technique used with short scale contrast to clearly visu-
alize gallbladder, even through overlying rib if present. Choleliths
(gallstones) may be visible as indicated by arrows in *Fig. 16-28*.
• Patient ID info and R or L marker should be visible without superim-
posing essential anatomy.

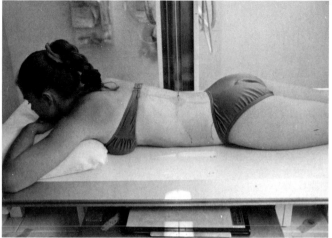

PA Scout (Sthenic Type)   Fig. 16-26

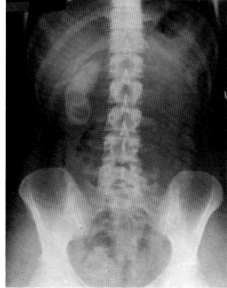

PA Scout (14 x 17)   Fig. 16-27

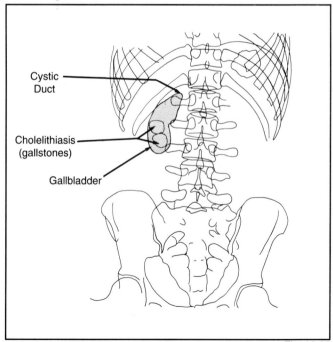

Cystic Duct

Cholelithiasis
(gallstones)

Gallbladder

PA Scout   Fig. 16-28

• LAO Position

Gallbladder
(Oral Cholecystogram)
Basic
• PA Scout
• **LAO**
Optional
• Right Lat. Decub.
• PA Erect

Structures Best Shown:
Opacified gallbladder projected away from vertebral column.

Technical Factors:
• Film Size - 10 x 12 in. (24 x 30 cm, lengthwise.
  or   8 x 10 in. (18 x 24 cm), lengthwise.
• Moving or stationary grid.
• 70-76 kVp range.

Patient Position:
• Patient semiprone, left anterior side down.
• Pillow for head, right arm up, left arm down, right knee partially flexed to maintain this position.

Shielding:
Place lead shield over gonadal area, not obscuring area of interest.

Part Position:
• Rotate patient **15 to 40°** (less rotation on broad hypersthenic, more rotation on thin asthenic type).
• Align midsagittal plane to long axis of table, approximate right half of abdomen to midline of table and/or film holder (determine from scout and resultant marking on skin).

Central Ray:
• CR **perpendicular** to film holder.
• CR to gallbladder as determined from scout.
• Center film holder to CR.
• Minimum 40 in. (102 cm) SID.

Collimation:
Four sided collimation to area of interest. (More collimation borders should be visible on larger film.)

Respiration:
Suspend respiration upon **expiration.**

NOTE: Accurate centering and collimation should be possible with skin marking from preceding scout film.

Evaluation Criteria:
• Entire opacified gallbladder and area of cystic duct is included centered to film.
• Gallbladder is seen in profile without self superimposition and is not superimposed upon vertebral column.
• No evidence of motion.
• Appropriate technique used with short scale contrast to clearly visualize gallbladder.
• Patient ID info and R or L marker should be visible without superimposing essential anatomy.

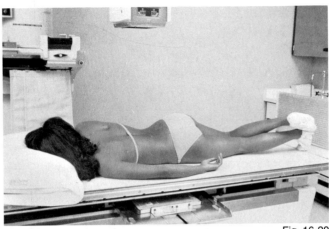

LAO
Fig. 16-29

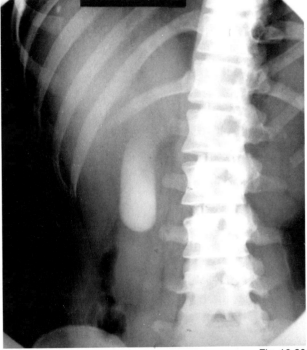

LAO
Fig. 16-30
(Courtesy of Bill Collins, RT)

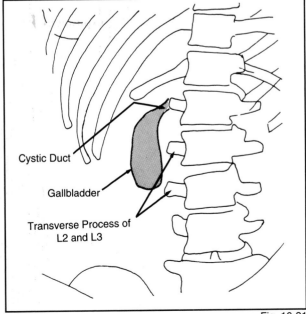

Cystic Duct
Gallbladder
Transverse Process of L2 and L3

LAO
Fig. 16-31

• Right Lateral Decubitus Position
PA (AP) Projection

<table>
<tr><td>

Gallbladder
(Oral Cholecystogram)
Basic
• PA Scout
• LAO
Optional
• **Right Lat. Decub.**
• PA Erect

</td></tr>
</table>

Structures Best Shown:
Opacified gallbladder projected away from the vertebral column with stratification of possible choleliths (gall stones).

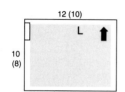

Technical Factors:
• Film Size - 10 x 12 in. (24 x 30 cm, lengthwise.
    or   8 x 10 in. (18 x 24 cm), lengthwise.
• Moving or stationary grid.
• 70-76 kVp range.
• Use decubitus marker.

Patient Position:
• Patient on radiolucent pads, lying on right side facing the table and/or film holder. (Separate pads for hips and shoulders allows gallbladder to move more freely.)
• Pillow for head, arms up above head, knees flexed one on the other.
• Secure cart wheels so patient will not fall.

Shielding: Place lead shield over gonadal area, not obscuring area of interest.

Part Position:
• Adjust cart and/or film holder to center gallbladder (GB) to film. (GB location determined from scout radiograph.)
• No rotation - insure that hips and shoulders are in a true lateral position.

Central Ray:
• CR **horizontal**, directed to GB, location determined from scout radiograph.
• Center film holder to CR.
• Minimum 40 in. (102 cm) SID.

Collimation: Four sided collimation to area of interest. (More collimation borders should be visible on larger film.)

Respiration: Suspend respiration upon **expiration**.

NOTE: • May be taken as an AP if necessary but a PA projection is preferred due to the more anterior location of GB.
• Decubitus position provides for "dropping" of GB away from spine, and for stratification of gall stones wherein the heavier than bile stones layer out or separate from those lighter than bile stones *(Fig. 16-33)*. Stones may not be visible on other projections.

Evaluation Criteria:
• Entire opacified gallbladder and area of cystic duct is included centered to film.
• Gallbladder is seen without motion, located below vertebral column.
• Stratification lines of choleliths should be visible if present.
• Appropriate technique used with short scale contrast to clearly visualize gallbladder without over penetrating and burning out possible choleliths.
• Patient ID info and a decubitus marker along with R or L marker should be visible without superimposing essential anatomy.

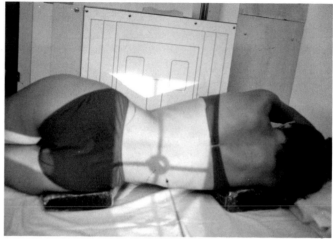

Right Lateral Decub. (PA)   Fig. 16-32

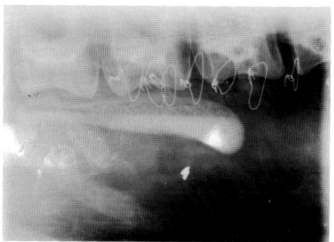

Right Lateral Decub.   Fig. 16-33

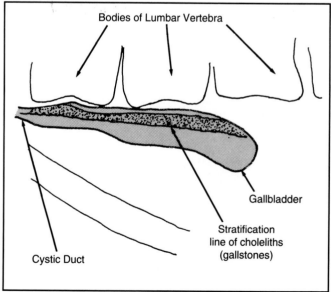

Right Lateral Decub.   Fig. 16-34

• PA Projection – Erect

Gallbladder
(Oral Cholecystogram)
Basic
• PA Scout
• LAO
Optional
• Right Lat. Decub.
• **PA Erect**

Structures Best Shown:
Opacified gallbladder with stratification of possible choleliths (gall stones).

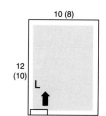

10 (8)

12 (10)

L

Technical Factors:
• Film Size - 10 x 12 in. (24 x 30 cm), lengthwise.
  or   8 x 10 in. (18 x 24 cm), lengthwise.
• Moving or stationary grid.
• 70-76 kVp range.
• Use erect marker.

Patient Position:
• Patient erect, facing the table and/or film holder.
• Arms at side.

Shielding: Place lead shield over gonadal area, not obscuring area of interest.

Part Position:
• Align a point on abdomen about **2 in.** (5 cm) **to right of midsagittal plane to midline of erect table** and/or film holder.
• Spread feet and distribute body weight evenly on both legs for stabilization.

Central Ray:
• CR **horizontal**, directed to GB, which will be 1 to 2 in. (2.5-5 cm) more inferior than on scout radiograph taken recumbent.
• Center film holder to CR.
• Minimum 40 in. (102 cm) SID.

Collimation: Four sided collimation to area of interest. (More collimation borders should be visible on larger film.)

Respiration: Suspend respiration upon **expiration.**

NOTE: • May be taken as an AP if necessary but the PA projection is preferred because of the more anterior location of GB.
• Change centering as needed for extremes of body habitus.
• Erect position with horizontal beam provides for stratification of possible gall stones similar to that of decubitus position. (Decubitus may be taken instead of erect if patient cannot stand.)
• May be taken as a spot film with fluoroscopy.

Evaluation Criteria:
• Entire opacified gallbladder and area of cystic duct is included centered to film.
• Gallbladder is seen without motion, located 1 to 2 in. (2.5-5 cm) more inferior than in recumbent position.
• Stratification lines of choleliths should be visible if present.
• Appropriate technique used with short scale contrast to clearly visualize gallbladder without over penetrating and burning out possible choleliths.
• Patient ID info, an erect marker along with R or L marker should be visible without superimposing essential anatomy.

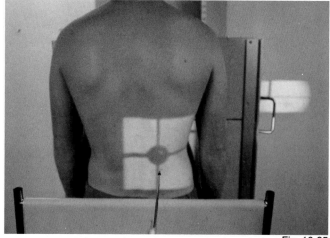

PA Erect   Fig. 16-35

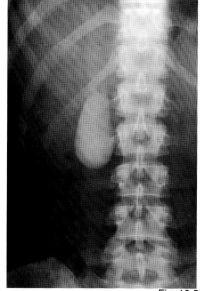

Fig. 16-36

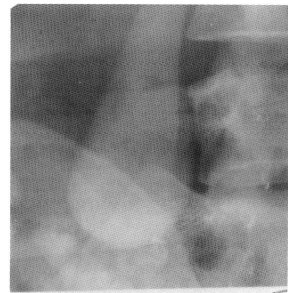

AP Erect Fluoro Spot   Fig. 16-37

• AP Projection
• LPO and/or RPO Positions

OR Cholangiogram
Basic
• **AP**
Optional
• **LPO or RPO**

Structures Best Shown:
Biliary duct system, drainage into duodenum and any retained gall stones.

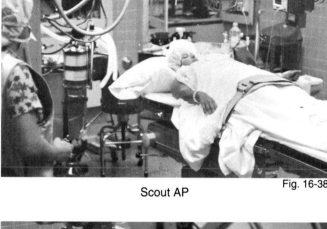

Scout AP   Fig. 16-38

Technical Factors:
• Film Size - 10 x 12 in. (24 x 30 cm), lengthwise (AP).
• Place grid **crosswise for oblique position** to prevent grid cutoff.
• Stationary grid.
• 70-80 kVp range.

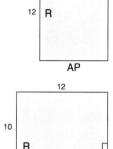

AP

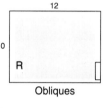

Obliques

Shielding: Due to sterile surgical field, gonadal shielding generally not used.

Patient and Part Position:
• Patient supine on surgery table.
• Table is tilted slightly for each oblique position.
• Communicate with surgical team regarding patient position, film placement and CR location.

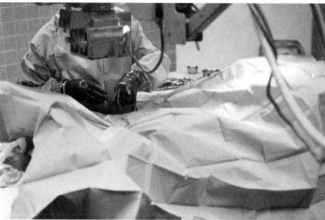

AP (centering point indicated by surgeon)   Fig. 16-39

Central Ray:
• Center midway between right lower rib cage margin and xiphoid tip, or **to where surgeon indicates**.
• Minimum 40 in. (102 cm) SID.

Collimation: Collimate to approximate film borders.

Respiration: Expose after surgeon injects contrast media and anesthesiologist stops patient motion.

Optional RPO and LPO:
• The RPO and LPO provide a different perspective of the biliary ducts. The RPO is the most helpful in projecting the ducts away from the spine. The surgeon will instruct whether or not these are to be taken.

NOTE: When possible, take a scout film prior to the beginning of surgery.

Evaluation Criteria:
• Entire biliary duct system filled with contrast media is demonstrated.
• No motion evident on radiograph.
• Appropriate technique employed to visualize the biliary duct system.
• Patient ID info and R or L marker should be visible without superimposing essential anatomy.

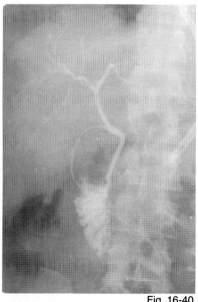

AP   Fig. 16-40

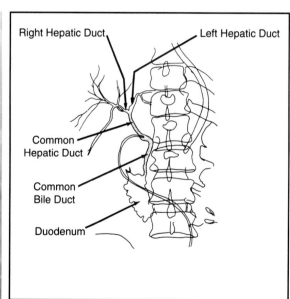

Right Hepatic Duct   Left Hepatic Duct

Common Hepatic Duct

Common Bile Duct

Duodenum

AP   Fig. 16-41

Chapter 17
Radiographic Anatomy and Positioning
of the
Urinary System

Contributions by: John Lampignano, M Ed, RT (R)
Barry T. Anthony, RT (R)

Contents

Part I Radiographic Anatomy

Part II Radiographic Procedures

Part III Radiographic Positioning

Part I   Radiographic Anatomy

Urinary System

Radiographic examinations of the urinary system are among the most common contrast medium procedures performed in radiology departments. The urinary system consists of two **kidneys, two ureters** (*u-rē'ter*), **one urinary bladder** and one **urethra** (*u-rē'thrah*).

The two kidneys are organs lying in the retroperitoneal space. These two bean-shaped organs lie on either side of the vertebral column in the most posterior part of the abdominal cavity. The right kidney is generally slightly lower or more inferior than the left due to the presence of the liver. Near the upper part of each kidney is an **adrenal gland**. These important glands of the endocrine system are located in the fatty capsule surrounding each kidney.

Each kidney connects to the single urinary bladder by its own ureter. Waste material, in the form of urine, travels from the kidneys to the bladder via these two narrow tubes, termed ureters. The saclike urinary bladder serves as a reservoir to store urine until it can be eliminated from the body via the urethra.

The Latin designation for kidney is *ren*, and *renal* is a common adjective referring to kidney.

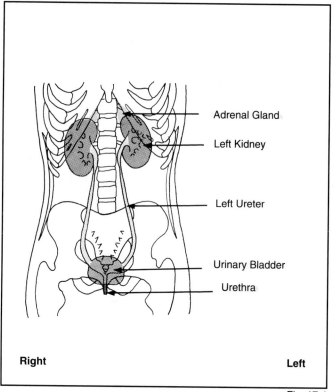

Urinary System   Fig. 17-1

Kidneys

The various organs of the urinary system and their relationship to the bony skeleton are shown from the left side in *Fig. 17-2*. The posteriorly placed **kidneys** lie on either side of the vertebral column in the upper abdomen. The lower rib cage forms a protective enclosure for the kidneys.

Ureters

Most of each **ureter** lies anterior to its respective kidney. The ureters follow the natural curve of the vertebral column. Each ureter initially curves forward following the lumbar lordotic curvature and then curves backward upon entering the pelvis. After passing into the pelvis, each ureter follows the sacrococcygeal curve before entering the posterolateral aspect of the bladder.

Urethra

The **urethra** connects the bladder to the exterior. The urethra exits from the body inferior to the symphysis pubis.

The entire urinary system is either posterior to or below the peritoneum. The **kidneys and ureters are retroperitoneal structures**, while the **bladder and urethra are infraperitoneal structures**.

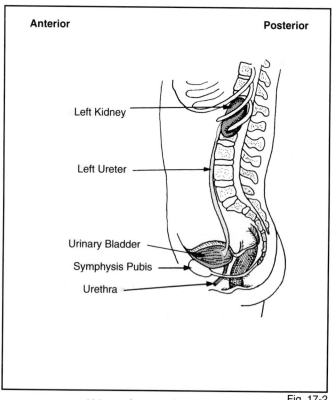

Urinary System (Lateral View)   Fig. 17-2

Kidneys

The average adult kidney is fairly small, weighing about 150 grams. The measurements are 4 to 5 inches (10-12 cm) long, 2 to 3 inches (5-7.5 cm) wide and 1 inch (2.5 cm) thick. The left kidney is a little longer but narrower than the right. Despite their small size, at least one functional kidney is absolutely essential for normal well-being. Failure of both kidneys, unless corrected, means inevitable death.

Kidney Orientation

The usual orientation of the kidneys in the supine individual is shown in *Fig. 17-3*. The large muscles on either side of the vertebral column cause the longitudinal plane of the kidneys to form a vertical angle of about 20 degrees with the midsagittal plane. These large muscles include the two **psoas** *(so'es)* **major muscles.** These muscle masses get larger as they progress inferiorly from the upper lumbar vertebrae. This gradual enlargement causes the 20° angle wherein the upper pole of each kidney is closer to the midline than its lower pole *(Fig. 17-3)*.

These large posterior abdominal muscles also cause the kidneys to rotate backward within the retroperitoneal space. As a result, the medial border of each kidney is more anterior than is the lateral border of each kidney *(Fig. 17-4)*.

The kidneys are located fairly close to the posterior aspect of the **diaphragm.** Since the kidneys are only loosely attached within the retroperitoneal space, they will move up and down with breathing movements of the diaphragm.

Cross Sectional View

A transverse section through the level of L2 is shown in *Fig. 17-4*. This visual illustrates the usual amount of backward rotation of the kidneys. The normal kidney rotation of about **30 degrees** is due to the midline location of the vertebral column and the large muscles on either side.

When posterior oblique positions are utilized during radiographic studies of the urinary system, each kidney, in turn, is placed parallel to the film plane. The body is rotated about 30 degrees in each direction to place one kidney, and then the other, parallel to the film plane. A 30° LPO will position the right kidney parallel to the film, and a 30° RPO will position the left kidney parallel.

Each kidney is surrounded by a mass of fatty tissue termed the **adipose capsule or perirenal fat.** It is the presence of these fatty capsules around the kidneys that permits radiographic visualization of the kidneys on plain abdominal radiographs. There is sufficient density difference between fat and muscle to visualize the outline of each kidney on a technically satisfactory, abdominal radiograph.

Normal Kidney Location

Most abdominal radiographs, including urograms, are performed on expiration with the patient supine. The combined effect of expiration and a supine position allow the kidneys to lie fairly high in the abdominal cavity. Under these conditions, the kidneys normally lie **halfway between the xiphoid tip and the iliac crest.** The left kidney normally lies about 1 centimeter more superior than does the right one. The top of the left kidney is usually at the level of the **T11 - T12 interspace.** The bottom of the right kidney is most often level with the upper part of **L3**. Each renal pelvis is usually near or slightly below the **transpyloric plane**, at the level of L1 - L2.

Kidney Movement: Since the kidneys are only loosely attached within their fatty capsule, they tend to move up and down with movements of the diaphragm and with position changes. When one inhales deeply or stands upright, the kidneys normally drop about one lumbar vertebra or 2 inches (5 cm). If the kidneys tend to drop more than one lumbar

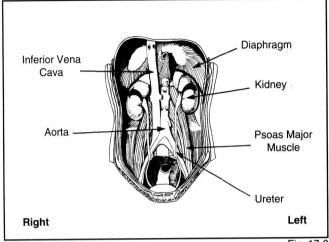

Kidney Orientation

Fig. 17-3

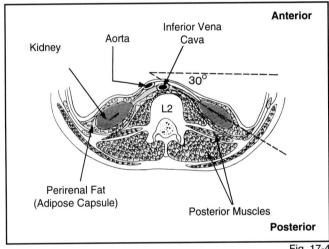

Kidney Orientation
(cross section, bottom view)

Fig. 17-4

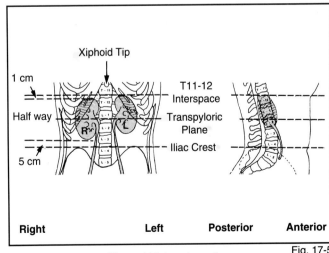

Normal Kidney Location

Fig. 17-5

vertebra, a condition termed **nephroptosis** *(nef"rop-to'sis)* is said to exist. Any excessive downward displacement of the kidneys is termed nephroptosis. With some very thin patients, in particular, the kidneys may drop dramatically and end up within the pelvis, which may create problems from a "kinking" or twisting of the ureters.

Large quantities of blood pass through the kidneys daily. Large **renal blood vessels** enter and leave the medial aspect of each kidney. One **ureter** also leaves each kidney medially near the location of the large renal blood vessels. Each kidney is arbitrarily divided into an upper part and a lower part, termed the **upper pole** and the **lower pole.**

Functions

The primary function of the urinary system is the production of urine and its elimination from the body. During production of urine, the kidneys:

   (1) remove nitrogenous wastes

   (2) regulate water levels in the body

   (3) regulate acid-base balance and electrolyte levels of the blood

Nitrogenous waste products such as urea and creatinine are formed during the normal metabolism of proteins. Buildup of these nitrogenous wastes in the blood results in the clinical condition termed uremia.

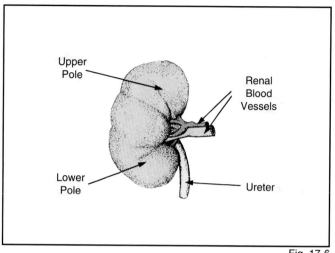

Kidney   Fig. 17-6

Urine Production

The average water intake for humans during each 24-hour period is about 2.5 liters. This water comes from ingested liquids and foods, and from the end products of metabolism. These 2.5 liters of water eventually end up in the bloodstream. Vast quantities of blood are filtered every 24 hours. At rest, more than one liter of blood flows through the kidneys every minute of the day, which results in about 180 liters of filtrate being removed from the blood every 24 hours. Over 99 percent of this filtrate volume is reabsorbed by the kidneys and returned to the bloodstream. During the reabsorption process, the blood pH and amounts of various electrolytes such as sodium, potassium and chloride are regulated.

From the large amount of blood flowing through the kidneys daily, about 1.5 liters or 1,500 cc's of urine are formed. This is an average amount that varies greatly depending on fluid intake, amount of perspiration and other factors.

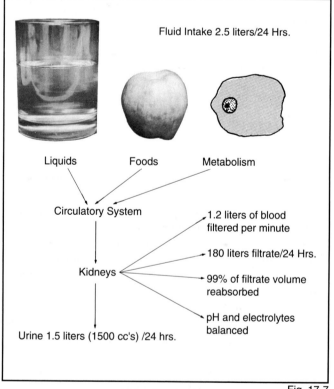

Urine Production   Fig. 17-7

Kidneys continued

Renal Blood Vessels

Large blood vessels are needed to handle the vast quantities of blood flowing through the kidneys daily. At rest about 25 percent of the blood pumped out of the heart with each beat passes through the kidneys. Arterial blood is received by the kidneys directly from the **abdominal aorta** via the left and right renal arteries. Each **renal artery** branches and rebranches until a vast capillary network is formed in each kidney.

Since most of the blood volume entering the kidneys is returned to the circulatory system, the **renal veins** must also be large vessels. The renal veins connect directly to the large **inferior vena cava** to return the blood to the right side of the heart.

Along the medial border of each kidney is a centrally located, **longitudinal fissure** termed the **hilum** *(hi'lum)*. The hilum serves to transmit the renal artery and renal vein, lymphatics, nerves and the ureter.

Macroscopic Structure

The macroscopic internal structure of the kidney is shown in *Fig. 17-9*. Directly under the **fibrous capsule** surrounding each kidney is the **cortex,** forming the peripheral or outer portion of the kidney substance. The internal structure termed the **medulla** is composed of from 8 to 18 conical masses termed **renal pyramids.** The cortex periodically dips between the pyramids to form the **renal columns**, which extend to the **renal sinus**. The renal pyramids are primarily a collection of tubules.

Each renal pyramid ends in a **minor calyx** *(ka'liks)*. Calyces appear as hollowed flattened tubes. There are from 4 to 13 minor calyces which unite to form 2 to 3 **major calyces.** The major calyces unite to form the **renal pelvis**, which appears in the shape of a flattened funnel. Each expanded renal pelvis continues as the **ureter.** Thus, urine formed in the microscopic or nephron portion of the kidney finally reaches the ureter by passing through the various collecting tubules, to a minor calyx, to a major calyx and then to the renal pelvis.

The term **renal parenchyma** *(par-eng'ki-mah)* is a general term used to describe the total functional portions of the kidneys such as those which are visualized during an early phase of an intravenous urogram procedure.

Microscopic Structure

The structural and functional unit of the kidney is the microscopic **nephron.** There are over one million nephrons in each kidney. One such nephron is shown in *Fig. 17-10*. Small arteries in the kidney cortex form tiny capillary tufts, termed **glomeruli** *(glo-mer'u-li)*. Blood is initially filtered through the many glomeruli.

Afferent arterioles supply blood **to** the glomeruli and **efferent** arterioles **away** to a secondary capillary network in close relationship to the straight and convoluted tubules. Each glomerulus is surrounded by a **Bowman's capsule**[1], which is the proximal portion of each nephron connecting filtrate. (The glomerulus is also part of the nephron which is made up of the glomerulus **and** the long tubules.) The glomerular filtrate travels from the Bowman's capsule to a **proximal convoluted tubule,** to the **descending** and **ascending limbs** of the **loop of Henle**[2] *(Hen'lez)*, to a **distal convoluted tubule,** to a **collecting tubule** and, finally, into a **minor calyx.** The filtrate is termed urine by the time it reaches the minor calyx. Between Bowman's capsule and minor calyces, over 99 percent of the filtrate is reabsorbed into the kidney's venous system.

Microscopically, the glomeruli, Bowman's capsules and the proximal and distal convoluted tubules of the many nephrons are located within the cortex of the kidney. The loop of Henle and the collecting tubules are

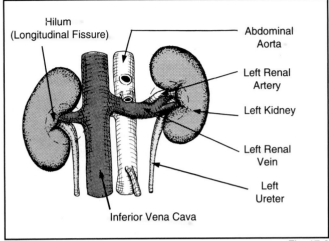
Renal Blood Vessels

Fig. 17-8

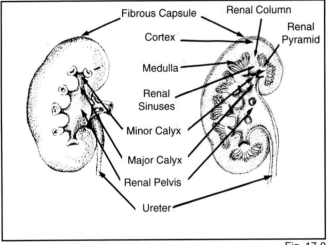
Renal Structure

Fig. 17-9

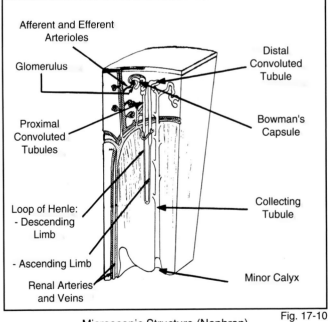
Microscopic Structure (Nephron)

Fig. 17-10

located primarily within the medulla. The renal pyramids within the medulla are primarily a collection of tubules.

---

[1] *Bowman*, Sir William, an English physician 1816-1892.

[2] *Henle*, Fredrich Gustav Jakob, a German anatomist 1809-1885.

Ureters

The ureters convey urine from the kidneys to the urinary bladder. Slow peristaltic waves along with gravity force urine down the ureters. The renal pelvis leaves each kidney at the hilum to become the **ureter.** The ureters vary in length from 28 to 34 centimeters, with the right one being slightly shorter than is the left. As the ureters pass inferiorly, they lie on the anterior surface of each psoas major muscle. Continuing to follow the curvature of the vertebral column, the ureters eventually enter the posterolateral portion of each side of the **urinary bladder.**

Prior to any pelvic surgery, the exact course of the ureters should be determined radiographically. The ureters are very narrow tubes and closely resemble surrounding tissue, therefore care must be exercised during surgery to leave the ureters intact. This is especially true during hysterectomies since the ureters are located close to the uterus.

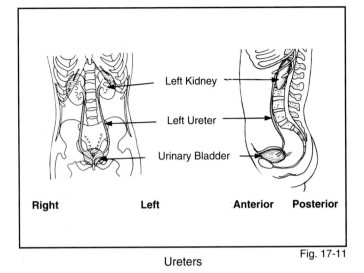

Right   Left   Anterior   Posterior

Ureters   Fig. 17-11

Ureter Size and Points of Constriction

The ureters vary in diameter from 1 millimeter to almost 1 centimeter. Normally, there are three constricted points along the course of each ureter. Should a kidney stone attempt to pass from kidney to bladder, it would have trouble passing these three spots.

The first point is the **ureteropelvic** *(u-re´ter-o-pel-vic)* **junction,** the second is near the **brim of the pelvis** where the iliac blood vessels cross, and the third is where the ureter joins the bladder termed the **ureterovesical** *(u-re˝ter-o-ves´i-kal)* **junction,** or UV junction. Most kidney stones passing down the ureter tend to hang up at the UV junction, but once the stone passes this point it will have little trouble passing through the bladder and urethra to the exterior.

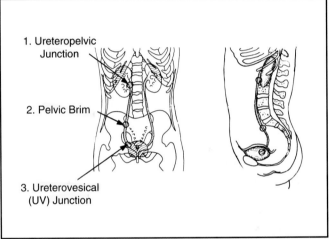

1. Ureteropelvic Junction

2. Pelvic Brim

3. Ureterovesical (UV) Junction

Fig. 17-12

Three Possible Points of Constriction
(possible sites for kidney stone lodging)

Urinary Bladder

The urinary bladder is a musculomembranous sac that serves as a reservoir for urine. The empty bladder is somewhat flattened and only assumes the more oval shape as in this drawing when partially or fully distended.

The triangular portion of the bladder along the inner, posterior surface is termed the **trigone** *(tri´gon)*. The trigone, shaded in *Fig. 17-13*, is the muscular area formed by the entrance of the two **ureters** from behind and the exit site of the **urethra.** The trigone is firmly attached to the floor of the pelvis. As the bladder fills, the top of the bladder expands upward and forward toward the abdominal cavity.

The gland surrounding the proximal urethra is the **prostate gland.** Only males possess a prostate gland so this drawing represents a male bladder, although the internal structure of the bladder in both sexes is similar.

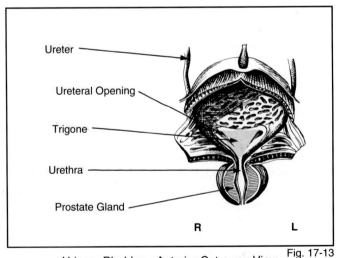

Ureter

Ureteral Opening

Trigone

Urethra

Prostate Gland

R   L

Urinary Bladder – Anterior Cut-away View   Fig. 17-13

Urinary Bladder continued

Bladder Functions

The **bladder** functions as a reservoir for urine and, aided by the urethra, it expels urine from the body. There is normally some urine in the bladder at all times, but as the amount reaches 250 milliliters there is a desire to void. The act of voiding is termed urination or micturition. Normally, urination is under voluntary control and the desire to void may pass if the bladder cannot be emptied right away. The total capacity of the bladder varies from **350 milliliters** to **500 milliliters**. As the bladder becomes fuller and fuller, the desire to void becomes more and more urgent. If the internal bladder pressure rises too high, involuntary urination will occur. Involuntary urination, whether due to excessive pressure or to organic problems, is termed **incontinence**.

Size and Position of the Bladder: The size, position and functional status of the bladder depends somewhat on surrounding organs and on how full the bladder is. When the rectum contains fecal matter, the bladder is pushed up and forward. A term pregnancy, as shown in *Fig. 17-14*, exerts tremendous pressure on the bladder.

Note: This drawing is only to show anatomy and the location of the urinary bladder in relationship to the fetus. Remember there are **no** radiographic urinary system exams or procedures done during pregnancy unless in special cases wherein the benefits outweigh the risks as determined by a physician.

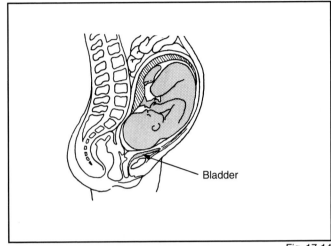

Term Pregnancy

Fig. 17-14

Male Pelvic Organs

The male pelvic organs are shown in midsagittal section in *Fig. 17-15*. When the **urinary bladder** is empty, most of the bladder lies directly posterior to the upper margin of the symphysis pubis. As the bladder distends, as it would during a cystogram or radiographic study of the bladder, more and more of the bladder will lie above the level of the symphysis pubis.

The male **urethra** extends from the internal urethral orifice to the external urethral orifice at the end of the penis. The urethra extends through the **prostate gland** and through the length of the penis. The male urethra averages 17.5 to 20 centimeters in length and serves two functions. Not only does the male urethra serve as the distal portion of the urinary tract, helping to eliminate urine stored in the bladder, but it also is the terminal portion of the reproductive system, serving as a passageway for semen.

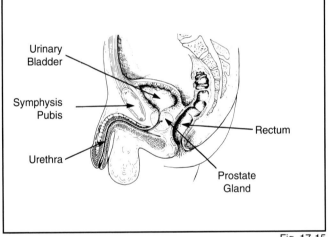

Male Pelvic Organs

Fig. 17-15

Female Pelvic Organs

The female pelvic organs are shown in midsagittal section in *Fig. 17-16*. The **urinary bladder** lies behind or above the upper margin of the symphysis pubis, depending on the amount of bladder distension. The female **urethra** is a narrow canal, about 4 centimeters long, extending from the internal urethral orifice to the external urethral orifice. The single function of the female urethra is the passage of urine to the exterior.

There is a close relationship between the urethra and bladder, and the **uterus and vagina.** The urethra is imbedded in the anterior wall of the vagina. The spatial relationship of the three external openings becomes important during certain radiographic procedures. The anal opening is most posterior, the urethral opening is most anterior, and the vaginal opening is in between.

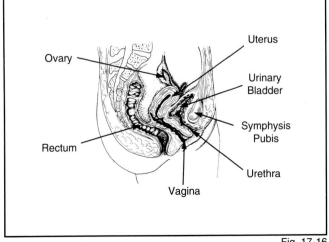

Female Pelvic Organs

Fig. 17-16

Anatomy Review (Radiographs)

Excretory Urogram

An AP radiograph of an excretory or intravenous urogram (IVU) is demonstrated below (*Fig. 17-17*) with certain anatomy of the urinary system labeled A-H. Contrast media injected intravenously allows these parts of the urinary system to be visualized on a radiograph.

A. Minor calyces
B. Major calyces
C. Renal pelvis
D. Ureteropelvic junction (UPJ)
E. Proximal ureter
F. Distal ureter
G. Ureterovesical junction (UVJ)
H. Urinary bladder

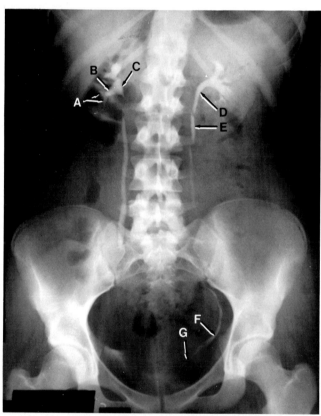

Excretory (Intravenous) Urogram   Fig. 17-17

Retrograde Pyelogram

The same anatomy is also labeled on this retrograde pyelogram (*Fig. 17-18*) wherein contrast media is being injected through a catheter inserted up (retrograde) through the urethra, bladder and the ureter to the level of the renal pelvis.

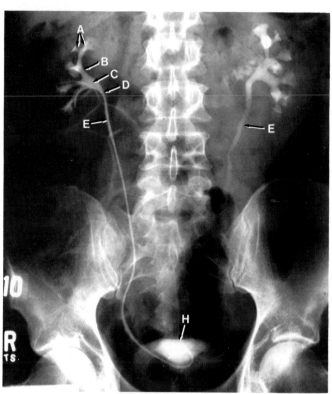

Retrograde Pyelogram   Fig. 17-18
(catheter in right ureter)

Voiding Cystourethrogram

Anatomy is labeled on this radiograph (*Fig. 17-19*) of the urinary bladder and urethra taken as the young male patient is voiding the contrast media.

A. Distal ureters
B. Urinary bladder
C. The trigone area of bladder
D. Area of prostate gland
E. Urethra

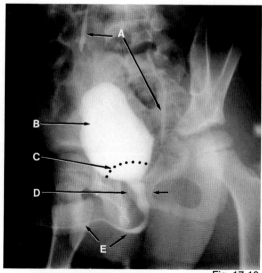

Voiding Cystourethrogram – RPO   Fig. 17-19
(Male)

Part II Radiographic Procedures

Kidney, Ureter and Bladder (KUB)

The plain abdominal radiograph or KUB shown in *Fig. 17-20* demonstrates very little of the urinary system. The gross outlines of the kidneys are generally demonstrated due to the fatty capsule surrounding the kidneys. In addition, the generalized gray area in the pelvis represents the urine-filled, urinary bladder. The rest of the urinary system blends in with the other soft tissue structures of the abdominal cavity. Therefore contrast media must be utilized to visualize the internal, fluid-filled portion of the urinary system radiographically.

Urography

Radiographic examination of the urinary system, in general, is termed urography *(u-rog′rah-fe)*. Uro is a prefix denoting a relationship to urine or to the urinary tract. The contrast media utilized to visualize the urinary tract are introduced into the human system in one of two ways. First, the contrast medium may be introduced into the bloodstream. This process is most often accomplished by intravenous injection.

The second requires some form of catheterization so that the contrast medium can be delivered directly into the structure to be studied radiographically (see *Fig. 17-18*). Radiographic examinations of the urinary system utilizing these two methods of contrast delivery are discussed in the remainder of this chapter.

Contrast Media

Various contrast media are used to visualize the different parts of the urinary system radiographically. Various brands of contrast media are available for use in urography.

The two major types of iodinated contrast media are ionic and nonionic. The chemical structure of the two types are somewhat different and behave differently in the body. It has been reported that patients experience less reactions with non-ionics. Both types contain organically bound iodine. The basic molecule for each of the different types of urographic contrast media is the tri-iodobenzoic acid molecule, which contains three organically bound iodine atoms per molecule. This basic iodine-containing molecule is found in those contrast media that are injected directly into the bloodstream, as well as in those media that are delivered directly into a hollow structure via catheterization.

Complications may follow administration of any contrast medium, but the majority of side effects and reactions occur following an intravascular injection. Since most studies of the kidneys require an intravenous injection, complications should be expected. Adverse reactions to contrast media cannot be predicted. Both the radiologist and the radiographer must be prepared for a reaction whenever contrast medium is injected.

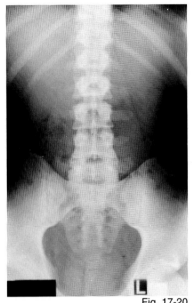

Fig. 17-20
Abdominal Radiograph
(KUB)

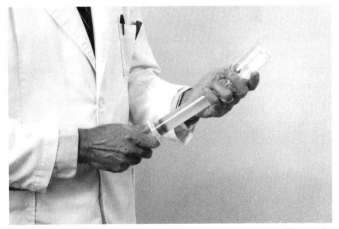

Contrast Media for Injection   Fig. 17-21

Contrast Media continued

Common Side Effects

Side effects occur in many patients as an expected outcome to the injected iodinated contrast media. They are brief and self-limiting.

Two common side effects following an intravenous injection of iodinated contrast media are a **temporary hot flash** and a **metallic taste in the mouth**. Both the hot flash, particularly in the face, and the metallic taste in the mouth usually pass quickly. Discussion of these possible effects and careful explanation of the examination will help to reduce patient anxiety and help to prepare the patient psychologically.

Patient History: A careful patient history may serve to alert the medical team to a possible reaction. Patients with a history of allergy are more likely to experience adverse reactions to contrast media than those who have no allergies. Questions to ask the patient should include:
1. Are you allergic to anything?
2. Have you ever had hay fever, asthma or hives?
3. Are you allergic to any drugs or medications?
4. Are you allergic to iodine?
5. Are you allergic to seafood or shellfish?
6. Are you allergic to other foods?
7. Have you ever had an x-ray examination that required an injection into an artery or vein?

A positive response to any of these questions will alert the injection team to an increased probability of reaction.

Selection and Preparation of Contrast Media

Selection and preparation of the correct contrast medium are important steps prior to injection. Since labels on various media containers are similar, one should always read the label three times. In addition, the empty container should be shown to the radiologist or other person making the actual injection. Whenever contrast medium is withdrawn into a syringe, be certain to maintain sterility of the medium, the syringe and the needle.

Preparation for Possible Reaction

Since contrast medium reaction is possible and unpredictable, a fully stocked emergency cart must be readily available whenever an intravenous injection is made. In addition to emergency drugs, the cart should contain cardiopulmonary resuscitation equipment, portable oxygen, suction and blood pressure apparatus, and possibly a defibrillator and monitor.

Reactions to Contrast Media

Most reactions to contrast media occur rapidly if they are going to happen, but, on occasion, a delayed reaction may occur. Reactions to contrast media can be classed as **mild, moderate or severe.** Mild reactions are usually self-limiting and require no medication for relief of symptoms. A moderate reaction is one that requires treatment for both the symptoms and the comfort of the patient. Any reaction that produces life-threatening symptoms requiring vigorous, active treatment is classed as a severe reaction. Any reaction, regardless of how minor it may seem, deserves careful observation. Mild reactions sometimes signal a more serious reaction to follow.

The patient should never be left alone following an intravenous injection. As the necessary radiographs are produced, observe the patient and question the patient regarding any changes. The radiologist or other responsible physician should remain within immediate reach for five minutes following an injection, and within easy reach for one hour thereafter. The physician must be summoned immediately for any moderate or severe reaction.

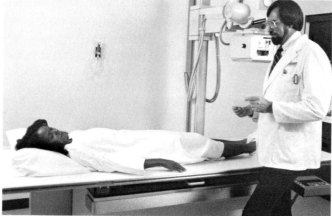

Discussion of History   Fig. 17-22

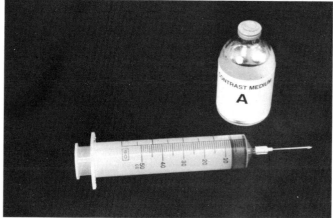

Possible Adverse Reactions   Fig. 17-23

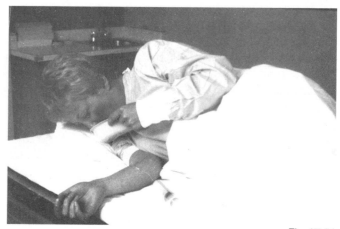

Mild Reaction   Fig. 17-24

Reactions to contrast media continued

Mild Reactions

The majority of reactions to contrast media are mild, usually requiring no treatment other than support and verbal reassurance. Mild reactions such as **nausea and vomiting** are fairly common. One should not forewarn the patient of their possible occurrence, however. Sometimes the power of suggestion is enough to bring on this type of reaction. Have an emesis basin handy in case of vomiting and a cold towel for the forehead in case of nausea. Take care that the patient does not vomit while supine. Either sit the patient up or turn the patient onto the left side, as shown in *Fig. 17-24* on preceding page.

Other mild reactions include **hives** or **urticaria** *(ur″ti-ka′re-ah),* **itching** and **sneezing**. These reactions cause some concern because they may signal a more severe response.

Mild reactions may also occur at the injection site, particularly if some of the contrast medium leaks out of the vein into the surrounding tissue. Such leakage is termed **extravasation** *(eks-trav″ah-sa′shun).* Pain, burning or numbness may result when extravasation occurs. A warm towel over the injection site may speed absorption of the contrast material.

Another mild reaction is a response to fear termed the **vasovagal** *(vas″o-va′gal)* **response**. Sometimes the sight of a needle or the sensation of a needle stick may trigger a vasovagal reaction. Symptoms include a sensation of weakness or dizziness, sweating and the feeling that precedes fainting. Explanation of the procedure and a confident injection team often deter this type of reaction. The patient's blood pressure should be taken during a vasovagal reaction since a marked drop in pressure indicates a more serious reaction.

Technologist Responsibilities:
(1) Monitor and comfort patient.
(2) Provide warm towel for extravasation.
(3) Document patient reaction.

Moderate Reactions

Moderate reactions require administration of some type of **medication** while the patient is still in radiology. Moderate reactions include **excessive urticaria** (hives), **tachycardia** *(tak″e-kar′de-ah)* or rapid heartbeat, **giant hives** and **excessive vomiting.** These symptoms usually respond rapidly and completely to the appropriate medication.

Technologist Responsibilities:
(1) Call for medical assistance (nurse, radiologist, etc.).
(2) Monitor and comfort patient.
(3) Document patient reaction.

Severe Reactions

Severe reactions are **life-threatening** and require **immediate, intensive treatment**. Very **low blood pressure, cardiac or respiratory arrest, loss of consciousness, convulsions, laryngeal edema, cyanosis, difficulty in breathing** and **profound shock** are examples of severe reactions. Delayed or inappropriate treatment for any of these symptoms or conditions could result in the patient's death. If a moderate or severe reaction is suspected, get help and summon the physician immediately.

Technologist Responsibilities:
(1) Call for immediate medical assistance.
(2) Remove any physical obstacles (tube, monitors, etc.) that may impede the medical staff.
(3) Assist medical staff in treating patient.

Mild Reactions

• Reaction examples
- Nausea and vomiting
- Hives (urticaria)
- Itching
- Sneezing
- Extravasation: burning or numbness at injection site
- Vasovagal response (fear): weakness, dizziness, sweating, feeling of passing out

Summary

Moderate Reactions

• Require medication
• Reaction examples
- Excessive urticaria (hives)
- Tachycardia (rapid heartbeat)
- Giant hives
- Excessive vomiting

Summary

Severe Reactions

• Life-threatening – require **immediate** treatment
• Reaction examples
- Very low blood pressure
- Cardiac or respiratory arrest
- Loss of consciousness
- Convulsions
- Laryngeal edema
- Cyanosis
- Difficulty in breathing
- Profound shock

Summary

Execretory Urography
(Intravenous Urogram – IVU)

The excretory or intravenous urogram (IVU) is the most common radiographic examination of the urinary system. This examination has often been referred to as an IVP or intravenous pyelogram. *Pyelo*, however, refers only to the renal pelves, since the execretory urogram normally visualizes more anatomy than just the renal pelvis, the term IVP should not be used. The excretory (intravenous) urogram or the IVU exam as it will be commonly referred to in this text, visualizes the **minor** and **major calyces**, **renal pelves**, **ureter**s and **urinary bladder** following an intravenous injection of contrast medium.

The IVU is a true functional test since the contrast medium molecules are rapidly removed from the bloodstream and are excreted completely by the normal kidney.

Purpose: The two-fold purpose of an excretory urogram (IVU) is to (1) **visualize the collecting portion of the urinary system** and (2) **assess the functional ability of the kidneys**.

Clinical Indications

The IVU is one of the most common contrast media examinations performed in the radiology department. The major clinical indications for the IVU include:
(1) Abdominal or pelvic mass
(2) Renal or ureteral calculi (kidney stones)
(3) Kidney trauma
(4) Flank pain
(5) Hematuria or blood in the urine
(6) Hypertension
(7) Renal failure
(8) Urinary tract infections (UTI)

The above includes certain conditions such as (2) **renal** or **ureteral calculi** which is a very common indication for the IVU. Renal calculi (kidney stones) are insoluble stones formed from crystals of salts found in the urine. These result from conditions such as an excessive intake of mineral salts combined with an insufficient intake of water, an abnormal alkaline or acid urine and overactivity of the parathyroid glands. They generally form in the pelvis of the kidney where they cause severe pain as they attempt to pass into or through the ureter where they may become lodged. This is a very painful condition that may require surgery or other invasive procedures to remove the obstruction.

(6) **Hypertension** or, more specifically, renal hypertension will often require an alteration of the normal IVU routine. The filming sequence for the study will allow for shorter spans of time between films. This procedure will be explained more completely in a later section.

(8) **Urinary tract infections** or **UTI** may be a chronic or acute condition. Bacteria entering the normally sterile urinary system may be difficult to control and eliminate. The most common bacteria is **Escherichia Coli** or **E. Coli**. The bacteria enters in a retrograde fashion through the bladder and may involve the ureters and kidney. **Pyelonephritis** is inflammation of the collecting system due to bacteria invasion. During the intravenous urogram, the calyces become enlarged and asymmetrical with chronic pyelonephritis.

An IVU prior to pelvic surgery will confirm the location of the urinary system structures and their function.

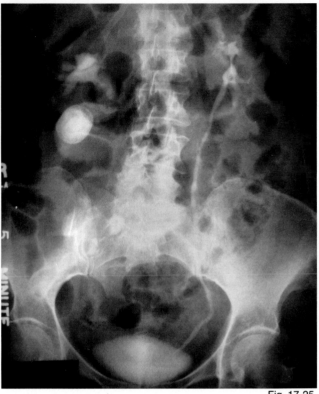

AP IVU   Fig. 17-25
Demonstrates unusually large calculus (stone) in right ureter
(Courtesy of Gateway Community College)

Contraindications

Even though present-day contrast media are considered to be relatively safe, the technologist must take extra care in obtaining patient history. Through the patient history, the technologist may become aware of certain conditions that will prevent the patient from having an IVU. The major contraindications include:
(1) Hypersensitivity to iodinated contrast media
(2) Anuria *(ah-nu' re-ah)* or absence of urine excretion
(3) Multiple myeloma
(4) Diabetes, especially mellitus
(5) Severe hepatic or renal disease
(6) Congestive heart failure
(7) Pheochromocytoma *(fe-o-kro" mo-si-to'mah)*
(8) Sickle cell anemia

This list includes certain conditions such as (3) **multiple myeloma** and (7) **pheochromocytoma**. Multiple myeloma is a malignant condition of the plasma cells of the bone marrow; and a pheochromocytoma is a rare tumor of the kidney. Research indicates that these patients are at greater risk during the IVU. Since (8) **sickle cell anemia** can compromise the function of the kidney, these patients are also at a higher risk.

It is important to interview the patient completely prior to the procedure. Some departments require the technologist to review the in-patient chart and note BUN and creatinine levels. Both are indications of renal function.

A patient with one of the above contraindications may need to be examined using some other imaging modality. Certain high-risk patients may still have the IVU after a series of premedication or therapy have been given.

Patients with a suspected sensitivity toward the contrast medium may receive steroids, benadryl, or diuretics prior to the procedure. While many departments stress dehydration prior to the procedure, it is reported that a hydration therapy of a saline IV drip and diuretic prior to the procedure, may reduce the risk for patients with multiple myeloma, diabetes mellitus, and other conditions.

Intravenous Urogram continued

Patient Preparation

Patient preparation for both the IVU and barium enema is similar. The intestinal tract should be free of gas and fecal material for both examinations. If both examinations are to be performed on the same patient, they can be done on the same day. The IVU is done first with the BE to follow.

The general patient preparation for the IVU includes:

(1) Light evening meal prior to the procedure
(2) Bowel-cleansing cathartic
(3) NPO after midnight
(4) Enema morning of the examination

Many patient preparation routines exist among departments. Certain pediatric and emergency-situation adult patients may receive no bowel preparation. Become familiar with your department's protocol.

Prior to the excretory urogram, all clothing except shoes and socks should be removed and replaced with a shortsleeved hospital gown. The opening and ties should be in the back. Always make certain that the patient scheduled for this examination or any other radiographic procedure is the correct patient. Double check the inpatient identification band and verify the outpatient with appropriate questions.

The patient should void just prior to the examination for two reasons: (1) a bladder that is too full could rupture, especially if compression is applied early in the exam, and (2) urine already present in the bladder dilutes the contrast medium accumulating there.

Pregnancy Precautions

If the patient is a female, then a menstrual history must be obtained. Irradiation of an early pregnancy is one of the most hazardous situations in diagnostic radiography.

X-ray examinations such as the IVU which include the pelvis and uterus in the primary beam, should **never** be done on pregnant females unless absolutely necessary and where the benefits exceed the risk.

Any x-ray examination of the abdomen of a potentially pregnant female should be governed by the "ten-day rule". Any female of child-bearing age should have such radiographic procedures **only** during the 10-day period after the start of menstruation. This is the only time when pregnancy can be ruled out with any certainty. Abdominal radiographs of a known pregnancy should be delayed at least until the third trimester, if done at all.

Radiographic Room Preparation

Equipment needed for urography, in addition to a suitable radiographic room, are: (1) correct type and amount of contrast medium drawn up in an appropriate syringe, (2) the empty container of contrast medium to show the physician or assistant doing the injection, (3) a selection of sterile needles to include a 19-gauge butterfly needle and tubing, (4) alcohol sponges or wipes, (5) tourniquet and (6) towel or sponge to support the elbow. Items also needed are (7) male gonadal shield, (8) emesis basin, (9) lead numbers, minute marker, and R and L markers, (10) emergency cart handy, (11) epinephrine or benadryl ready for emergency injection, (12) ureteric compression device (if used by department) and (13) a cold towel for the forehead or a warm towel for the injection site, if necessary.

These items should be assembled and ready before the patient is escorted to the radiographic room. Be certain that the room is clean and tidy for each patient, and make sure that the patient has voided prior to placing the patient on the radiographic table.

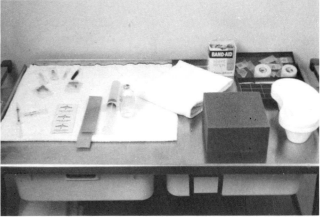

Excretory Urography Equipment   Fig. 17-26

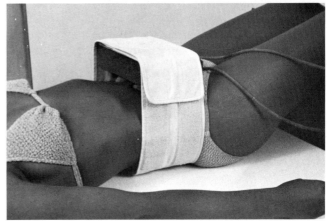

Ureteric Compression   Fig. 17-27

Ureteric Compression

A method utilized to enhance filling of the pelvicalyceal system and proximal ureters is ureteric compression. Furthermore, ureteric compression allows the renal collecting system to retain the contrast medium longer for a more complete study. One such compression device is shown on the model in *Fig. 17-27.* It is a velcro band that wraps around two inflatable pneumatic paddles. These paddles are held in place by a piece of plexiglass and sponge.

Prior to injection of the contrast medium, the device is placed on the patient with the paddles deflated. It is vital that the paddles are placed at the pelvic brim to allow for compression of the ureters. Without proper placement of the paddles, the contrast medium will be excreted at its normal rate.

Once the contrast media is introduced, the paddles are inflated and will remain in place until the radiologist orders the release of compression.

Contraindications to uteric compression: Certain conditions exist that will contraindicate the use of ureteric compression. These include:

(1) **Possible ureteric stones**. It may be difficult to distinguish between the effects of compression versus the appearance due to a stone.
(2) **Abdominal mass**. A mass may also present the same radiographic appearance as ureteric compression.
(3) **Aortic abdominal aneurysm**. The compression device may lead to leakage or rupture of the aneurysm.
(4) **Recent abdominal surgery**.
(5) **Severe abdominal pain**.
(6) **Acute abdominal trauma**.

Alternate Trendelenburg: The Trendelenburg position (wherein the head end of the table is lowered about 15°) will provide some of the same results as the compression procedure without as much risk to the patient with those symptoms that contraindicate ureteric compression.

General IVU Procedure

Department routine will vary for the intravenous urogram. This section will introduce a generic procedure for the IVU. The department supervisor should be consulted for specific differences from the following description.

Scout Film and Injection

The patient's clinical history and other pertinent information is discussed with the radiologist prior to injection. The radiographs should be checked for technique, location of the kidneys and signs of motion. These scout radiographs should be shown to the radiologist prior to injection. If the patient has a catheter in place, it should be clamped prior to injection.

When the injection is made, one should note the exact starting time and the length of injection. Timing for the entire series is based on the start of the injection, not on the end of it. The injection usually takes between 30 seconds to one minute to complete. As the examination proceeds, carefully observe the patient regarding any physical changes. Note in the chart the amount and type of contrast medium given to the patient.

After the full injection of contrast medium, radiographs are taken at specific time intervals. Each film must be marked with a lead number indicating the time interval when the radiograph was taken.

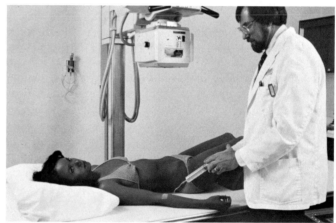

IVU Injection   Fig. 17-28

Basic Filming Routine

A basic routine for an IVU might include:

(1) **Nephrogram** or **Nephrotomogram**: Taken immediately after completion of injection (or one minute after start of injection) to capture the early stages of the contrast medium entering the collecting system. (Additional description on following page.)

(2) **Five Minute**: A full KUB to include the entire urinary system. The supine position (AP) is the preferred position.

(3) **Fifteen Minute:** A full KUB to include the entire urinary system. Once again, the supine position (AP) is most commonly requested.

(4) **Twenty Minute Obliques**: The LPO and RPO positioning will provide a different perspective of the kidneys and remove the ureters from the spine.

(5) **Post-void**: The post-void radiograph is taken after the patient has voided. The positions of choice may be a prone (PA), or an erect AP. Insure that the bladder is included on this final radiograph.

IVU Basic Routine

(1) Clinical history taken
(2) Scout radiograph taken
(3) Injection of contrast media
    (Note starting time of injection and type and amount of contrast media injected.)
(4) Basic filming routine
    - 1 minute Nephrogram or Nephrotomogram
    - 5 minute AP supine
    - 15 minute AP supine
    - 20 minute posterior obliques
    - Post-void (prone or erect)

Summary

IVU Procedure continued

Alternates to Routine

Many variations or alternates to the basic routine exist and the radiologist may order specific positions at any time during the study. Some common variations include:

(1) **Trendelenburg Position:** Some departmental routines include the Trendelenburg position for the early series radiographs to enhance the filling of the pelvic calyceal system. For this the head end of the table is tilted down about 15 degrees so that the contrast medium in the urine will tend to stay in the kidneys longer. Shoulder braces should be used to help the patient feel more secure.

(2) **Post-release or "Spill" Procedure with Ureteric Compression:** A full-size radiograph is taken after the release of compression. Explain to the patient what will be done, then release the air pressure as illustrated in *Fig. 17-30*. The spill radiograph or any other delayed imaging is usually done in the supine position.

 To assess for asymmetric renal function, compression should be applied immediately after the 5 minute film is exposed (unless contraindicated), then removed immediately prior to the 15 minute film.[1]

(3) **Erect Bladder Projection:** If the patient has history of prolapse of the bladder or enlarged prostate gland, the erect bladder position taken before voiding may confirm these conditions.

(4) **Delayed Radiographs:** Often with urinary calculi, the filling of the involved ureter is slow. The patient may be brought back to the department on a one or two hour basis. Insure that the radiology staff is aware of when the next radiograph is due before leaving the department for the day.

After the completion of the usual IVU series, a postvoid radiograph is often obtained in either the prone or upright position. By emptying the bladder, small abnormalities of the bladder may be detected. The upright position, will demonstrate any unusual movement of the kidneys.

 Present all radiographs to the radiologist before releasing the patient from the department.

Nephrogram or Nephrotomogram

Radiographs taken very early in the series are termed **nephrograms** *(nef'ro-grams)*. The renal parenchyma or functional portion of the kidney consists of many thousands of nephrons. Since individual nephrons are microscopic, the nephron phase is a blush of the entire kidney substance. This blush results from contrast medium throughout the many nephrons, but not into the collecting tubules as yet. The usual nephrogram is obtained with a radiograph at one minute after the start of injection. Ureteric compression, if used, tends to prolong the nephron phase to as long as five minutes in the normal kidney.

 With a nephrotomogram, *(Fig. 17-31)*, three separate focal levels are commonly taken during this phase of the study.

 Since the primary interest in nephrography is the two kidneys, centering and film size should be confined to the kidneys. Center halfway between the iliac crest and the xiphoid process unless a better centering point is determined after viewing the scout radiograph.

 Timing is critical on this radiograph so be certain that the exposure is made exactly 60 seconds after the start of the injection. The table, film and control panel must be in readiness even before the injection is begun since the injection will sometimes take nearly 60 seconds to complete.

Hypertensive IVU

Purpose

One special type of intravenous urogram is the **hypertensive urogram**. This examination is done on patients with high blood pressure (hypertension) to determine if the kidneys are the cause of the hypertension.

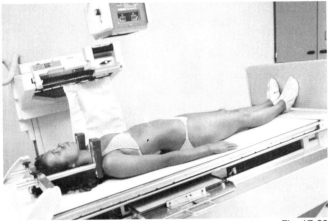

IVU – Trendelenburg Position   Fig. 17-29

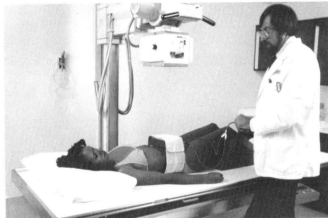

Post-release or "Spill" Procedure   Fig. 17-30

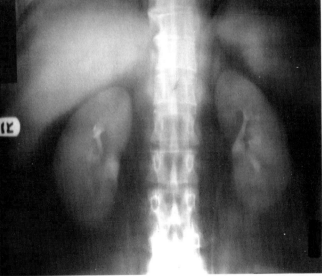

Nephrotomogram – 1 min.   Fig. 17-31

Procedure

During the hypertensive urogram, several early radiographs must be obtained. It is important that all cassettes are available and marked with lead numbers to reflect the time sequence of each film. Once the procedure begins, radiographs must be taken at a set interval.

 The hypertensive study will include, at least, one, two, and three-minute radiographs with the possibility of additional radiographs every 30 seconds. In most cases, timing begins at the start of injection.

 After the very early radiographs, the film sequence may be similar to a standard IVU with imaging of the ureters and bladder.

---

[1]Elkin, Milton, Radiology of the Urinary Tract, Vol. 1, P6, 1980

Retrograde Urography

Purpose

Retrograde urography is a **nonfunctional examination of the urinary system** during which contrast medium is introduced directly into the pelvicalyceal system **via catheterization** by a urologist during a minor surgical procedure. Retrograde urography is nonfunctional since the patient's normal physiologic processes are not involved in the procedure.

Procedure

Surgery personnel place the patient on the combination cystoscopic-radiographic table, usually located in the surgery department. The patient is placed in the modified lithotomy position, which requires that the legs be placed in stirrups as illustrated in *Fig. 17-32*. The patient is usually either sedated or anesthetized for this examination. The urologist inserts a cystoscope through the urethra into the bladder. After examining the inside of the bladder, the urologist inserts ureteral catheters into one or both ureters. Ideally, the tip of each ureteral catheter is placed at the level of the renal pelvis.

After catheterization, a **scout radiograph** is exposed. The scout radiograph allows the radiographer to check technique and positioning, and allows the urologist to check catheter placement. The **second radiograph** in the usual retrograde urographic series is a pyelogram. The urologist injects 3 to 5 cc's of any of the urographic contrast media directly into the renal pelvis of one or both kidneys. Respiration is suspended immediately after injection, and the exposure is made.

The **third and final** radiograph in the usual series is a ureterogram. The head end of the table may be elevated for this final radiograph. The urologist withdraws the catheters and simultaneously injects contrast material into one or both ureters. The urologist indicates when to make the exposure. This examination is used to directly visualize the internal structures of one or both kidneys and ureters.

The catheter is shown in place in *Fig. 17-33* with contrast media being injected into the right kidney. The left kidney and proximal ureter also show residual contrast media present.

Retrograde Cystography (Cystogram)

Purpose

Retrograde cystography is another **nonfunctional** urinary system examination. A cystogram *(sis'to-gram)* is a radiographic examination of the **urinary bladder** following instillation of an iodinated contrast medium via a urethral catheter.

Procedure

There is no patient preparation for this examination, although the patient should empty the bladder prior to catheterization. After routine bladder catheterization under aseptic conditions, the bladder is drained of any residual urine. The bladder is then filled with dilute contrast medium as illustrated in *Fig. 17-34*. The contrast material is allowed to flow in **by gravity only**, using an asepto syringe or drip infusion. One should never get in a hurry and attempt to introduce the contrast medium under pressure. Bladders have been ruptured through the use of unnecessary pressure.

After the bladder is filled, which may require 150 to 500 cc's, either fluorographic spot radiographs are taken by the radiologist or various overhead positions are exposed by the radiographer.

Routine positioning for a cystogram includes an **AP with a 15-degree caudal angle** and **both posterior obliques**.

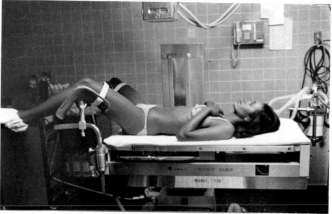

Retrograde Urogram
(Scout Position)

Fig. 17-32

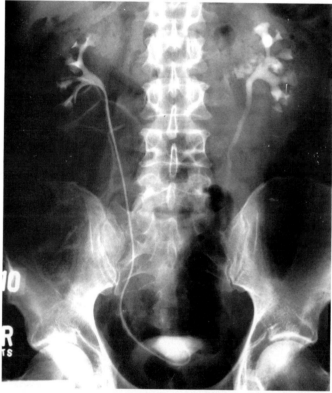

Retrograde Urogram

Fig. 17-33

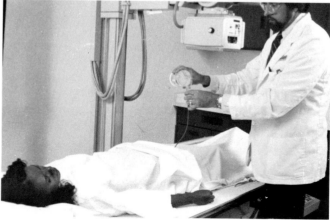

Cystogram – Instilling
Contrast Media

Fig. 17-34

Voiding Cystourethrography

Purpose

Voiding radiographs may be taken after the routine cystogram. When combined in this manner, the examination would be termed a cystourethrogram *(sist"o-u-re'thro-gram)* or voiding cystourethrogram (VCU). It will provide a study of the urethra and evaluate the patient's ability to urinate. Trauma or involuntary loss of urine are common clinical indications. The voiding phase of the examination is best done utilizing fluoroscopic control and a spot film camera.

Procedure

The procedure is sometimes done with the patient supine, although the upright position makes it easier to void. The key to a good voiding study is to gently remove the catheter from the bladder and urethra. First remove any liquid from the balloon portion of the catheter, if this type of catheter was used, and ever so gently remove the catheter. The urethra can be traumatized if care is not exercised.

The female is usually examined in the AP or slight oblique position, as shown on the radiograph in *Fig. 17-35*.

The male is best examined in a 30-degree right posterior oblique position. An adequate receptacle or absorbent padding must be provided for the patient.

After voiding is complete and adequate imaging is obtained, a post-voiding AP may be requested.

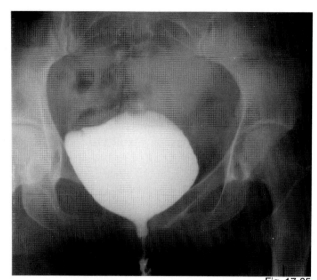

Fig. 17-35

Female Voiding Cystourethrogram

Retrograde Urethrography

Purpose

A retrograde urethrogram is sometimes performed on the male patient to demonstrate the full length of the urethra. Contrast medium is injected into the distal urethra until the entire urethra is filled in retrograde fashion.

Procedure

Injection of contrast material is sometimes facilitated by a special device termed a **Brodney clamp**, which is attached to the distal penis. A **30-degree right posterior oblique** is the position of choice; and centering is to the symphysis pubis. The tip of the syringe is inserted into the distal urethra and the injection is made. Ample contrast medium is used to fill the entire urethra and exposures are made. An RPO retrograde urethrogram on a male patient is shown in *Fig. 17-36*. Ideally, the urethra is superimposed over the soft tissues of the right thigh. This prevents superimposition of any bony structures except for the lower pelvis.

This procedure is rarely done today and therefore is also not included in the positioning section of this chapter. The voiding cystourethrogram, as described above, provides much of the same diagnostic information. This procedure is described and demonstrated in the positioning section which follows.

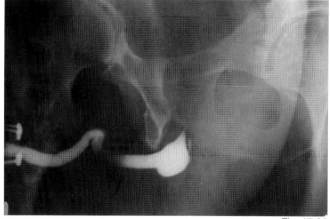

Fig. 17-36

Male Retrograde Urethrogram

Metallic Bead-chain Cystourethrography

Purpose

A special type of voiding cystourethrogram is performed on females with a diagnosis of stress incontinence or involuntary loss of urine. This examination is termed the metallic bead-chain cystourethrogram and is done to determine the anatomical relationship of the bladder and the urethra. This procedure was first described in 1937. It is rarely performed today.

Procedure

Four radiographs are taken with this metallic bead-chain procedure. **Two upright AP's** and **two upright laterals** are taken. First the physician inserts a flexible, metallic bead chain into the bladder. The distal end rests on the floor of the bladder, while the proximal end is taped to the patient's thigh. A catheter is then introduced and about 60 cc's of contrast medium are instilled in the bladder. After removing the catheter and standing the patient up, an AP and lateral are exposed while the patient is relaxed. A second set of radiographs is taken while the patient bears down or strains. A towel placed between the thighs will help the patient apply full pressure on straining. She may fear involuntary urination, otherwise.

Summary of
Urinary System Radiographic Procedures

Urographic procedures may be categorized by the method of contrast medium administration. Contrast medium is introduced either (1) into the circulatory system, or (2) directly into the structure to be studied.

(1) **Into the bloodstream**
   (usually intravenous injection)
   • Intravenous (Excretory) Urography (IVU)

(2) **Directly into the structure to be studied**
   (requires catheterization)
   • Retrograde Urography
   • Retrograde Cystography (Cystogram)
   • Voiding Cystourethrography
   • Retrograde Urethrography (rarely performed today)
   • Metallic bead-chain Cystourethrography (rarely performed today)

Part III Radiographic Positioning

National Survey:

A survey of the operating procedures (department routines) was conducted throughout the United States. The following information was compiled from the survey indicating the national norm for basic and special routines for intravenous urography and cystography. (The number by each region indicates the number of responding institutions)

Intravenous Urogram Routine

IVU	U.S. Average (509)		East (197)		Midwest (238)		West (74)	
	Basic	Optional	Basic	Optional	Basic	Optional	Basic	Optional
• AP (Scout & Series)	99%		99%		98%		100%	
• Nephrotomography	77%	13%	73%	13%	75%	13%	95%	2%
• LPO & RPO (30 degree)	70%		72%		64%		79%	
• AP Post-void (erect)	51%	21%	35%	12%	34%	12%	58%	18%
• PA Post-void (prone)	38%	15%	40%	14%	36%	16%	33%	24%
• AP Ureteric Compression	33%	19%	35%	12%	33%	15%	43%	13%
• AP Trendelenburg	3%	14%	3%	12%	2%	7%	7%	16%

Cystogram Routine

Cystogram	U.S. Average (499)	
	Basic	Optional
• AP (no angle)	85%	
• LPO and RPO (60 degrees)	70%	7%
• Lateral	51%	13%
• Fluoroscopy*		7%
• AP Post-void*		5%
• AP Voiding*		3%

* Write-ins by survey respondents

Summary

The survey responses for these two procedures were very consistent throughout the U.S. except for the IVU **nephrotomogram** and the **AP post-void erect.** A significantly higher number of respondents in the western states indicated these to be basic compared to the midwest and the east.

The **AP Trendelenburg** responses indicate this to be a relatively uncommon projection and it will no longer be described separately in the positioning section of this text.

Survey Questions on Possible Discontinued Procedures:

The national survey included questions on (I) the **expected trend** in the next three or four years, (II) the **quantity** of specific exams done in their departments during the past year, and (III) whether or not **the procedure should still be taught and included** in a basic student textbook. The results were as follows:

Responses for Retrograde Urograms

Retrograde Urograms	U.S. Average (354)	East (129)	Midwest (164)	West (55)
I. Trend				
a. Increase	24%	32%	20%	17%
b. Decrease	13%	16%	12%	13%
c. No change	63%	52%	68%	70%
II. Annual Quantity				
a. 0-19	18%	13%	14%	37%
b. 20-99	42%	43%	44%	45%
c. 100-200	21%	20%	24%	9%
d. 201 +	19%	24%	18%	9%
III. Be Included				
a. Yes	97%	98%	97%	95%
b. No	3%	2%	3%	5%

Responses for Voiding Cystourethrograms

Voiding Cystourethrograms	U.S. Average (353)	East (124)	Midwest (164)	West (65)
I. Trend				
a. Increase	17%	26%	13%	13%
b. Decrease	17%	19%	16%	19%
c. No change	66%	55%	71%	68%
II. Annual Quantity				
a. 0-9	18%	18%	16%	25%
b. 10-45	42%	42%	37%	57%
c. 46-102	19%	21%	22%	10%
d. 103 +	21%	19%	25%	8%
III. Be Included				
a. Yes	96%	95%	98%	97%
b. No	4%	5%	2%	3%

Responses for Cystograms

Cystograms	U.S. Average (362)	East (134)	Midwest (163)	West (62)
I. Trend				
a. Increase	16%	22%	12%	12%
b. Decrease	15%	18%	13%	13%
c. No change	69%	60%	75%	75%
II. Annual Quanity				
a. 0-9	16%	10%	17%	25%
b. 10-47	44%	47%	44%	44%
c. 48-99	20%	19%	18%	23%
d. 100 +	20%	24%	21%	8%
III. Be Included				
a. Yes	93%	96%	93%	92%
b. No		4%	7%	8%

Summary

These results indicate in general a trend of either an **increase** or **no change** for each of these three procedures. The increase in all cases was highest in the eastern states.

The difference in the increases between the various regions was significant. The percentage of increases in the east were about double of that in the west and midwest.

The overall quantity of these exams was relatively high throughout the U.S. indicating these are still common procedures and should be taught and included in the positioning section of this text.

The intravenous urogram (IVU) was not included in this part of the survey because it is known to be a very common procedure throughout all regions of the U.S.

Basic and Optional Projections/Positions

Certain basic or optional projections or positions of the urinary system are demonstrated and described on the following pages. The radiologist and radiographer must closely coordinate their efforts during examinations of this portion of the anatomy.

Intravenous (Excretory) Urography - IVU	**Retrograde Urography**	**Cystography**	**Voiding Cystourethrography**
Basic	Basic	Basic	Basic (Male)
• AP (Scout and Series)	• AP (Scout)	• AP (10-15° caudad)	• RPO (30°)
• Nephrotomogram	• AP (Pyelogram)	• Both Obliques (45-60°)	Basic (Female)
• LPO and RPO (30°)	• AP (Ureterogram)	Optional	• AP
• Erect AP - Post-void		• Lateral	
Optional:			
• AP Ureteric Compression			

• AP Projection (Scout and Series)

<table>
<tr><td>

Intravenous (Excretory) Urography - IVU
Basic
• **AP (Scout and Series)**
• Nephrotomogram
• LPO and RPO (30°)
• Erect AP - Post-void

</td></tr>
</table>

Structures Best Shown:
Collecting system of the kidneys, ureters, and urinary bladder filled with contrast medium.

See pages 516 and 517 for basic IVU procedure routines.

Tchnical Factors:
• Film Size - 14 x 17 in. (35 x 43 cm), lengthwise.
For nephrogram: 10 x 12 in. (24 x 30 cm), or
11 x 14 in (28 x 35 cm), crosswise.
• Moving or stationary grid.
• 70-75 kVp range.
• Include minute markers where applicable.

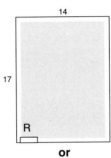

or

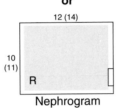

Nephrogram

Patient Position:
• Patient supine, pillow for head, arms at sides away from body.

Shielding: Shield gonads on males (females generally cannot be shielded without obscuring area of interest).

Part Position:
• Align midsagittal plane to center line of table and/or film holder.
• Flex and support knees to reduce lordotic curvature.
• Insure **no rotation** of trunk or pelvis.
• Include symphysis pubis on bottom of cassette. (A second smaller film of bladder area may be necessary on large patients.)

Central Ray:
• CR **perpendicular** to film holder.
• **For entire urinary system:** Center CR and film to **level of iliac crest**, and to midsagittal plane.
  For nephrogram: See following page.
• Minimum 40 in. (102 cm) SID.

Collimation: Collimate to film size or smaller if possible.

Respiration: Suspend respiration and expose upon expiration.

NOTE: • Have patient empty bladder immediately before beginning exam.
• Explain procedure and obtain clinical history prior to injection of contrast medium.
• Be prepared for possible reaction to contrast medium. (See page 513.)
• Check scout film for optimum technique and position of kidneys.

Evaluation Criteria:
• Entire urinary system is visualized from upper renal shadows to distal urinary bladder. The symphysis pubis should be included on lower margin of the film.
• Only a portion of the urinary system may be opacified on a specific radiograph in the series.
• No rotation evidenced by symmetry of iliac wings and rib cage.

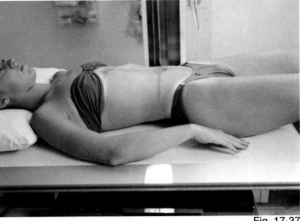

IVU Scout and Series   Fig. 17-37

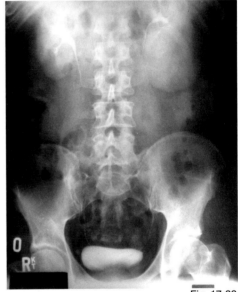

IVU (10 min.)   Fig. 17-38

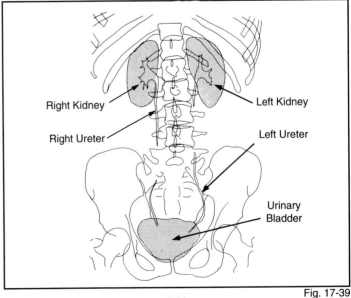

Right Kidney   Left Kidney

Right Ureter   Left Ureter

Urinary Bladder

IVU   Fig. 17-39

• No motion due to respiration or movement.
• Appropriate technique with short scale contrast should visualize the urinary system.
• Minute markers along with R or L markers should be visible on all series radiographs.

• Nephrotomography

Intravenous (Excretory)
Urography - IVU
Basic
• AP (Scout and Series)
• **Nephrotomogram**
• LPO and RPO (30°)
• Erect AP – Post-void)

Structures Best Shown:
Renal parenchyma during early stages of IVU.

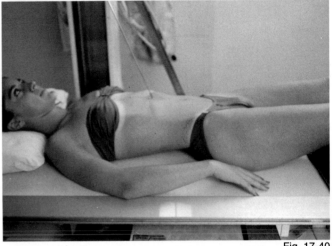
Nephrotomogram
Fig. 17-40

Technical Factors:
• Linear or multidirectional tomography
• Film Size - 10 x 12 in. (24 x 30 cm), crosswise.
  or 11 x 14 in. (28 x 35 cm) crosswise.
• Moving or stationary grid.
• 70-75 kVp range.
• Select the correct exposure angle:
  - 10 degrees or less angle produces larger section of tissue in relative focus.
  - 40 degree exposure angle produces thinner sections of tissue in relative focus.
  - If only three tomograms are to be taken, use a 10 degree or less angle (actually known as **zonography).**

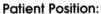

Patient Position:
• Patient supine, pillow for head, arms at side away from body.

Shielding: Place lead shield over gonadal area.

Part Position:
• Align midsagittal plane to center line of table.
• Flex and support knees to reduce lordotic curvature.
• Insure **no rotation** of trunk or pelvis.

Central Ray:
• Center **midway between xiphoid tip and iliac crest.**
• 40 in. (102 cm) SID (or distance as required by specific equipment).

Collimation: Collimate to film size or smaller if possible.

Respiration: Suspend respiration and expose upon expiration.

NOTE: • Explain tomographic procedure to reduce anxiety for patient. Obtain clinical history prior to injection of contrast medium.
• Remind patient to remain immobile between exposures.
• Check scout film to verify focus level, optimum technique and position of kidneys.
• Review tomography procedures in chapter 20 if unsure of the equipment setup and procedure.

Evaluation Criteria:
• Entire renal parenchyma is visualized with some filling of collecting system with contrast medium.
• No motion due to respiration or movement.
• Appropriate technique employed to visualize renal parenchyma.
• The specific focus level markers should be visible on each radiograph along with R or L markers.

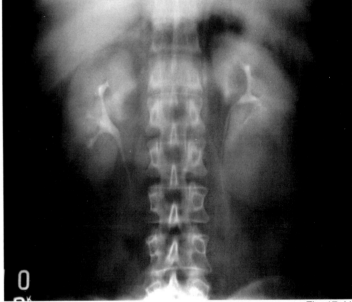
Nephrotomogram
Fig. 17-41

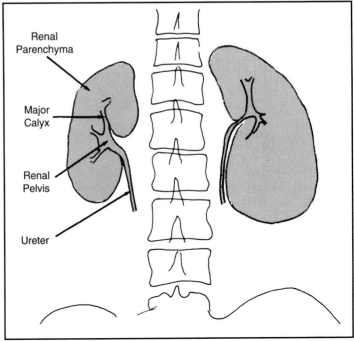
Nephrotomogram
Fig. 17-42

• LPO and RPO

Intravenous (Excretory) Urography - IVU
Basic
• AP (Scout and Series)
• Nephrotomogram
• **LPO and RPO (30°)**
• Erect AP – Post-void

Structures Best Shown:
The kidney on **elevated side** is placed in profile or parallel to the film and is best demonstrated with each oblique. (See anatomy *Fig. 17-9.*)

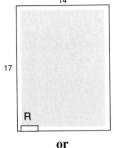

or

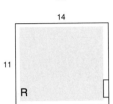

Technical Factors:
• Film Size - 14 x 17 in. (35 x 43 cm), lengthwise.
  or   11 x 14 in. (28 x 35 cm), crosswise. (See NOTE.)
• Moving or stationary grid.
• 70-75 kVp range.
• Include minute marker.

Patient Position:
• Patient supine and partially rotated toward the right or left posterior side.

Shielding:
Shield gonads on males. (Females generally cannot be shielded without obscuring area of interest.) (See NOTE.)

Part Position:
• Rotate body into a 30° posterior oblique for both R and L positions.
• Flex elevated side knee for support of lower body.
• Raise arm on elevated side and place across upper chest.
• Center vertebral column to midline of table and/or film.

Central Ray:
• CR **perpendicular** to film holder.
• Center CR and film holder to **level of iliac crest** and vertebral column.
• Minimum 40 in. (102 cm) SID.

Collimation:
Collimate to film size or smaller if possible.

Respiration:
Suspend respiration and expose upon expiration.

NOTE: Some departmental routines include a smaller film placed crosswise to include the kidneys and proximal ureters thus allowing gonadal shielding for both males and females. Centering would be midway between xiphoid and iliac crests.

Evaluation Criteria:
• The elevated side kidney is parallel to plane of film, not superimposed by vertebral column.

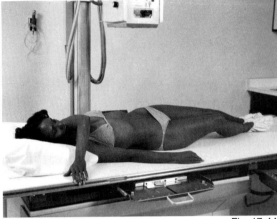

LPO – 30°   Fig. 17-43

RPO – 30°   Fig. 17-44

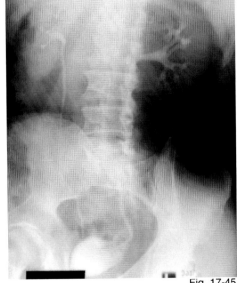

RPO   Fig. 17-45

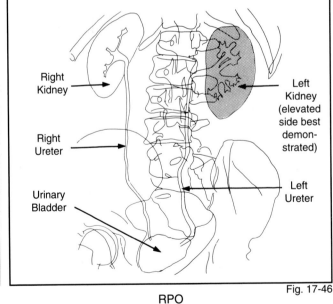

Right Kidney

Left Kidney (elevated side best demonstrated)

Right Ureter

Urinary Bladder

Left Ureter

RPO   Fig. 17-46

• The down side ureter is free of superimposition of the spine.
• Entire urinary system is visualized.
• Upper margin of kidneys should be included, as well as bladder and lower ureters if size permits. (See NOTE for exception.)
• No motion due to respiration or movement.
• Appropriate technique with short scale contrast employed to visualize the urinary system.
• Minute markers along with R or L markers should be visible.

• Erect AP – Post-void

<table>
<tr><td>
Intravenous (Excretory)
Urography - IVU
Basic
• AP (Scout and Series)
• Nephrotomogram
• LPO and RPO (30°)
• **Erect AP - Post-void**
</td></tr>
</table>

Structures Best Shown:
Kidneys (positional change) and nearly empty bladder.

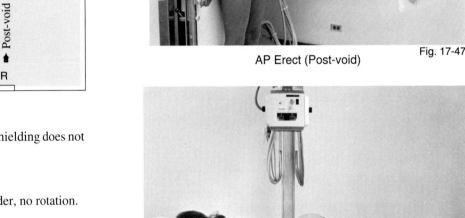
AP Erect (Post-void)   Fig. 17-47

Technical Factors:
• Film Size - 14 x 17 in. (35 x 43 cm), lengthwise.
• Moving or stationary grid.
• 70-75 kVp range.
• Use erect and/or post-void markers.

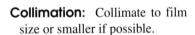

Patient Position:
• Patient in erect position, back against table or prone position.

Shielding: Use gonadal shielding only if such shielding does not obscure area of interest.

Part Position:
• Midsagittal plane to center of table or film holder, no rotation.
• Position arms away from body.
• Insure symphysis pubis is included on bottom of cassette.
• Center low enough to include prostate area, especially on older males.

Central Ray:
• CR **perpendicular** to film holder.
• Center to level of **iliac crest** and midsagittal plane.
• Minimum 40 in. (102 cm) SID.

Collimation: Collimate to film size or smaller if possible.

Respiration: Suspend respiration and expose upon expiration.

Alternate PA Prone: This may also be taken as a PA projection in the prone position with centering similar to that described above.

NOTE: • Erect position will demonstrate nephroptosis (positional change of kidneys).
• Erect post-void position may demonstrate an enlarged prostate gland pushing up on the floor of the bladder.

Alternate: PA (Post-void)   Fig. 17-48

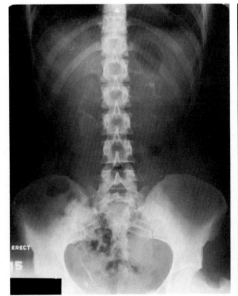
Fig. 17-49

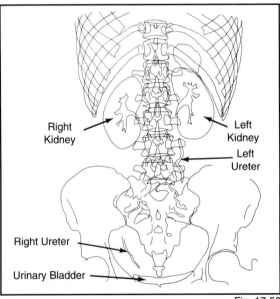
Right Kidney — Left Kidney — Left Ureter — Right Ureter — Urinary Bladder
AP Erect (post-void)   Fig. 17-50

Evaluation Criteria:
• Entire urinary system is included with only residual contrast media visible.
• All of symphysis pubis (to include prostate area on males) is included on radiograph.
• No rotation evident by symmetry of iliac wings.
• No motion due to respiration or motion.
• Appropriate technique employed to visualize residual contrast media in the urinary system.
• Erect and /or post-void markers along with R or L markers are visible.

• AP Projection – Ureteric Compression

Intravenous (Excretory)
Urography - IVU
Optional
• AP Ureteric Compression

Structures Best Shown:
Renal pelvis and calyces with enhanced pelvic calyceal and proximal ureter filling.

Warning: Compression should **NOT** be used with acute problems, abdominal masses or recent surgery. (A Trendelenberg position with 15° tilt which approximates the same effect can be used for such patients.)

Technical Factors:
• Film Size - 14 x 17 in. (35 x 43 cm),
         lengthwise
  or   11 x 14 in. (30 x 35 cm),
         crosswise. (See NOTE.)
• Moving or stationary grid.
• 70-75 kVp range.

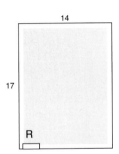

or

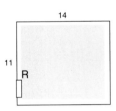

Patient Position:
• Patient supine with compression device over lower abdomen.

Shielding: Place lead shield over gonadal area unless it obscures area of interest.

Part Position:
• Align midsagittal plane to center line of table.
• Flex and support knees.
• Position arms away from body.
• Insure symphysis pubis is included on lower margin of film holder.

Central Ray:
• CR **perpendicular** to film holder.
• Center to **level of iliac crest** and midsagittal plane.
• Minimal 40 in. (102 cm) SID.

Collimation: Collimate to film size or smaller if possible.

Respiration: Suspend respiration and expose upon expiration.

NOTE: • Alternate centering with a smaller film placed crosswise is midway between xiphoid and iliac crests to center to kidneys and proximal ureters. (This allows gonadal shielding and tighter collimation for both males and females, which also results in better image quality.)
• Place compression paddles at level of ASIS.

Evaluation Criteria:
• Entire urinary system visualized with enhanced pelvic calyceal filling.
• No rotation evident by symmetry of iliac wings.
• No motion due to respiration or movement.
• Appropriate technique employed with short scale contrast to visualize the urinary system.
• Patient ID info and R or L marker should be visible.

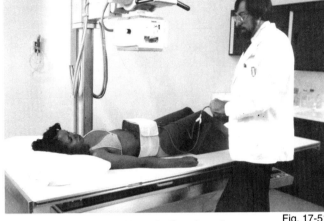

AP – Ureteric Compression   Fig. 17-51

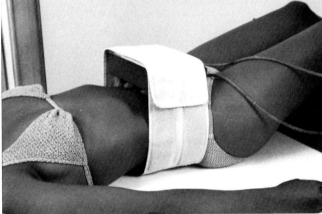

AP – Ureteric Compression   Fig. 17-52

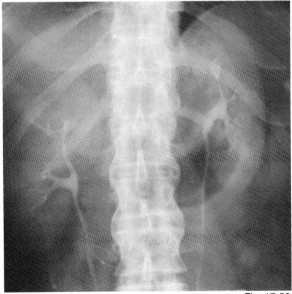

AP – Ureteric Compression   Fig. 17-53

• AP Projection – (Scout, Pyelogram, Ureterogram)

> **Retrograde Urography**
> Basic
> • AP (Scout)
> • AP (Pyelogram)
> • AP (Ureterogram)

Structures Best Shown:
Contrast-filled renal pelvis, major and minor calyces, and ureter(s).

This is considered an operative procedure carried out by a urologist under aseptic conditions. (See page 518 for procedure details.)

Technical Factors;
• Film Size - 14 x 17 in. (35 x 43 cm), lengthwise.
• Moving or stationary grid.
• 70-75 kVp range.
• Taken with special cystoscopic radiographic equipment.

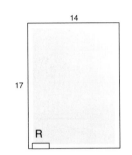

Patient Position:
• Modified lithotomy position with knees flexed over adjustable leg supports.

Shielding: Because of anatomy studied and sterile surgical field, gonadal shielding generally isn't practical.

Part Position:
• Insure symphysis pubis is included on bottom of cassette.
• **No rotation** of pelvis or trunk.

Central Ray:
• CR **perpendicular** to film holder.
• Center CR and film holder to **level of iliac crest** and midsagittal plane.
• Minimum 40 in. (102 cm) SID.

Collimation: Collimate to film size or smaller if possible.

Respiration: Expose after anesthetist suspends respiration if patient is under general anesthesia. The urologist generally indicates when to make exposure.

NOTE: • Take scout film after insertion of catheters but prior to injection of contrast media.
• Pyelogram demonstrates the renal pelvis, major and minor calyces.
• Ureterogram demonstrates the ureter.
• Ureterogram exposed as catheters are withdrawn.

Evaluation Criteria:
• Contrast-filled renal pelvis, major and minor calyces, and ureters visualized.
• No rotation evident by symmetry of iliac wings and rib cage.
• No motion due to respiration or movement.
• Appropriate technique with short scale contrast to visualize urinary system.
• Patient ID info and R or L marker should be visible.

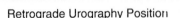

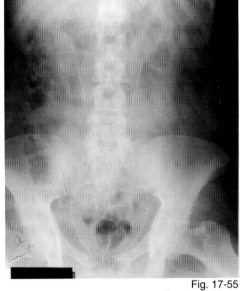

Fig. 17-54
Retrograde Urography Position

Fig. 17-55
Retrograde Urogram Scout
(catheters in place)

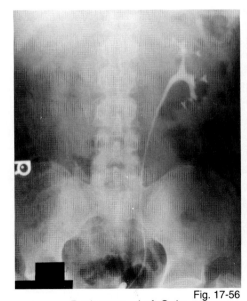
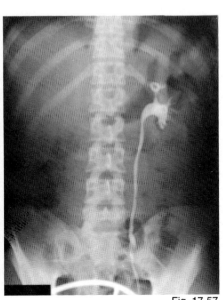

Fig. 17-56
Pyelogram – Left Only

Fig. 17-57
Ureterogram – Left Only
(catheter withdrawn)

Cystography

Cystography

- **AP Projection**
- **LPO and RPO Positions**
- **Lateral Position**

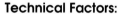

Cystography
Basic
• **AP**
• **Both Obliques (60°)**
Optional
• **Lateral**

Structures Best Shown:
Contrast-filled urinary bladder and distal ureters for possible reflux, prostate and proximal male urethra.

See page 518 for detailed procedure descriptions.

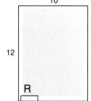

Technical Factors:
- Film Size - 10 x 12 in. (24 x 30 cm), lengthwise.
- Moving or stationary grid.
- 70-75 kVp range.
  (80-90 kVp for lateral)

Patient and Part Position:
AP
- Supine, with legs extended, midsagittal plane to center of table.

Posterior Obliques
- 45 to 60° body rotation. (Steep obliques are used to visualize posterolateral aspect of bladder, especially UV junction.)
- Partially flex downside leg for stabilization.
  Note: Do not flex elevated side leg to prevent superimposition of leg over bladder.

Lateral (Optional due to large gonadal radiation dose.)
- True lateral (no rotation).

Central Ray:
AP
- Center **2 in.** (5 cm) **superior to symphysis pubis** with **10-15° cauda**d tube angle (to project symphysis pubis inferior to bladder.)

Posterior Obliques
- Center **2 in.** (5 cm) **superior to symphysis pubis** and **2 in.** (5 cm) **medial to ASIS**.

Lateral
- Center **2 in.** (5 cm) **superior to and posterior to symphysis pubis**.

Collimation: Collimate to film size or smaller if possible.

Respiration: Suspend respiration and expose upon expiration.

NOTE: • Unclamp and drain bladder prior to filling with contrast medium.
- Contrast medium should **never** be injected under pressure but allowed to fill slowly by gravity in presence of an attendant.
- Include prostate area just distal to pubis on older males.

Evaluation Criteria:
- Distal ureters, urinary bladder and proximal urethra on males should be included.
- Appropriate technique employed to visualize the urinary bladder.
- **AP:** Urinary bladder is **not** superimposed by pubic bones.
- **Posterior Obliques**: Urinary bladder is **not** superimposed by partially flexed elevated side leg.
- **Lateral**: Hips and femurs are superimposed.
- Patient ID info and R or L marker should be visible.

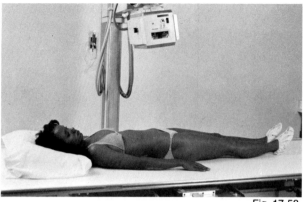

AP (10-15° Caudal)   Fig. 17-58

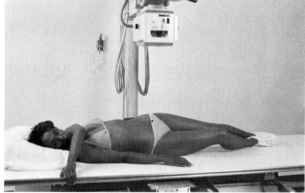

RPO (45-60°)   Fig. 17-59

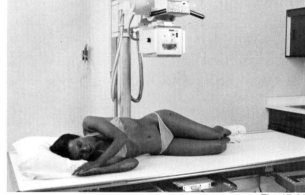

Right Lateral (Optional)   Fig. 17-60

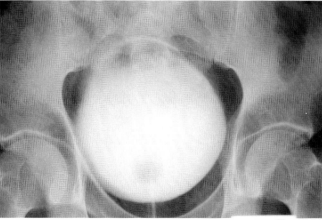

AP (10-15° Caudal)   Fig. 17-61

- **RPO (30°) – Male**
- **AP Projection – Female**

Voiding
Basic (Male)
• **RPO** (30°)
Basic (Female)
• **AP**

See page 519 for detailed procedure descriptions.

Structures Best Shown:
Functional study of the urinary bladder and urethra with possible ureteral reflux.

Technical Factors:
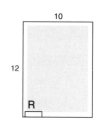

- Film Size - 10 x 12 in. (25 x 35 cm), lengthwise.
- Moving or stationary grid.
- 70-75 kVp range.

Patient Position:
- May be taken **recumbent or erect.**

Shielding:
Since bladder and urethra are primary area of interest, gonadal shielding isn't possible.

Part Position:
Male
- Oblique body **30° to the right** (RPO).
- Superimpose urethra over soft tissues of right thigh.

Female
- Supine or erect.
- Center midsagittal plane to table or film holder.
- Extend and slightly separate legs.

Central Ray:
- CR **perpendicular** to film holder.
- Center CR and film holder to **symphysis pubis.**
- Minimum 40 in. (102 cm) SID.

Collimation:
Collimate to film size or smaller if possible.

Respiration:
Suspend respiration and expose upon expiration.

NOTE: • Fluoroscopy and spot filming is best for this procedure.
- Catheter must be gently removed prior to voiding procedure.
- Provide radiolucent receptacle or absorbent padding for patient.

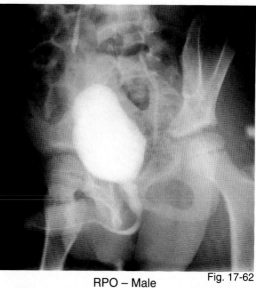

RPO – Male   Fig. 17-62

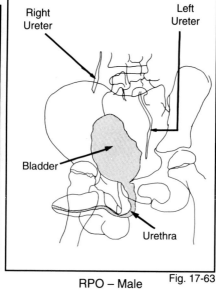

RPO – Male   Fig. 17-63

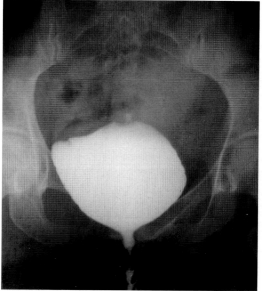

AP – Female   Fig. 17-64

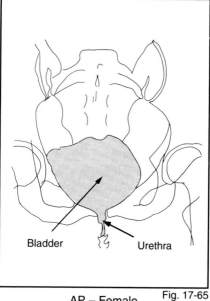

AP – Female   Fig. 17-65

Evaluation Criteria:
- Contrast-filled urinary bladder and urethra is visualized.
- Appropriate technique employed to visualize the urinary bladder without overexposing the male prostate area and the contrast-filled urethra of either male or female.
  - **RPO:** Male urethra containing contrast medium is superimposed over soft tissues of right thigh.
  - **AP:** Female urethra containing contrast medium is demonstrated inferior to the symphysis pubis.
- Patient ID info and R or L marker should be visible.

Chapter 18
Radiographic Anatomy and Positioning of the Mammary Gland

Contributions by: Nancy L. Dickerson, RT (R) (M)
Eugene D. Frank, MA, RT (R), FASRT

Contents

Mammography

Part 1 Radiographic Anatomy

Introduction

Breast cancer is the primary cause of death in women between the ages of 35 and 54. Currently 1 in 9 American women will develop breast cancer sometime in their life. The best defense against the disease is to have regular mammograms so that early detection is possible.

Accurate and careful positioning of the breast during mammography is imperative in diagnosing breast cancer. The **maximum** amount of breast tissue must be demonstrated on each view. Mammography images must contain maximum subject contrast, superb resolution, and have no artifacts. Mammographers should be certified through professional training, experience, and continuing education in mammography.

The technical aspects of mammography must be tightly controlled. Mammography should be performed on a dedicated mammography unit. The x-ray machine, processor, screens, and cassettes must be state-of-the-art and monitored regularly through an intensive quality control program. Every mammography unit should be accredited by the American College of Radiology.

Anatomy of the Breast

In the adult female, each of the mammary glands or breasts is a conical or hemispherical eminence located on the anterior and lateral chest wall. There is a great deal of variation in breast size from one individual to another and even in the same woman, depending on her age and the influence of various hormones. However, the usual breast extends from the anterior portion of the **second rib** down to the **sixth** or **seventh rib,** and from the lateral border of the sternum well into the axilla.

The surface anatomy includes the **nipple,** a small projection containing a collection of duct openings from the secretory glands within the breast tissue. The pigmented area surrounding the nipple is termed the **areola,** defined as a circular area of different color surrounding a central point. The junction of the inferior part of the breast with the anterior chest wall is called the **inframammary crease.** The **axillary tail** is a band of tissue that wraps around the pectoral muscle laterally, *(Figs. 18-1 and 18-2).*

The width of the breast on most patients is greater than the vertical measurement, from top to bottom. The vertical measurement, which may be described as the **craniocaudad diameter,** averages from 12 to 15 centimeters at the chest wall. The radiographer must realize that there is more breast tissue than the tissue that extends obviously from the chest. There is mammary tissue overlying the costocartilages near the sternum and breast tissue extending well up into the axilla. The breast tissue extending into the axilla is called the **tail of the breast** or the **axillary prolongation** of the breast.

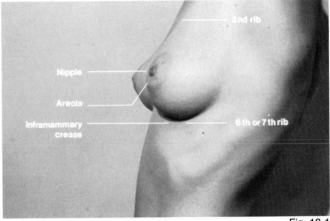

Surface Anatomy   Fig. 18-1

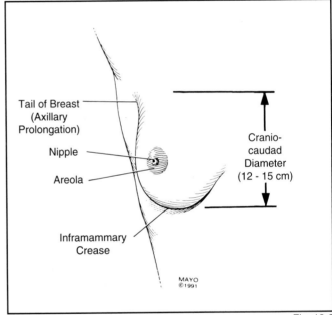

Surface Anatomy   Fig. 18-2
(Courtesy of Mayo Clinic)

Methods of Localization

Two methods are commonly used to subdivide the breast into smaller areas for localization purposes. The **quadrant system**, shown in *Fig. 18-3* is easiest to use. Four quadrants can be described by using the nipple as the center. These quadrants are the **UOQ** (upper outer quadrant), the **UIQ** (upper inner quadrant), the **LOQ** (lower outer quadrant), and the **LIQ** (lower inner quadrant).

A second method, shown on the right in *Fig. 18-3*, compares the surface of the breast to the face of a clock. A problem with the clock method arises when a medial or lateral portion of either breast is described. What is described at 3 o'clock in the right breast has to be described at 9 o'clock in the left breast.

If either the referring physician or the patient has felt a mass of any suspicious area in either breast, one of these methods is used to describe the area of special interest to radiology personnel.

Breast (Sagittal Section)

A sagittal section through a mature breast is illustrated in *Fig. 18-4*, showing the relationship of the mammary gland to the underlying structures of the chest wall. On this drawing the **inframammary crease** is at the level of the seventh rib, but a great deal of variation does exist among individuals.

The large **pectoralis major muscle** is seen overlying the bony thorax. A sheet of fibrous tissue surrounds the breast below the skin surface. A similar sheet of tissue covers the pectoralis major muscle. These two fibrous sheets connect in an area termed the **retromammary space.** This retromammary space must be demonstrated on at least one projection during the radiographic study of the mammary gland. Since the connections within the retromammary space are fairly loose, the normal breast exhibits considerable mobility on the chest wall.

The relative position of glandular tissue versus adipose tissue is illustrated in *Fig. 18-5*. The central portion of the breast is primarily **glandular tissue.** Varying amounts of **adipose** or **fatty tissue** surround the glandular tissue. Size variation from individual to individual is due primarily to the amount of adipose or fatty tissue in the breast. The amount of glandular tissue is fairly constant from one female to another.

Since the primary function of the mammary gland is lactation, or the secretion of milk, the amount of glandular and fatty tissue or the size of the female breast has no bearing on the functional ability of the gland.

The skin covering the breast is seen to be uniform in thickness, except in the area of the areola and nipple where the skin is somewhat thicker.

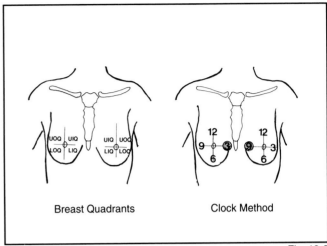

Breast Localization

Fig. 18-3

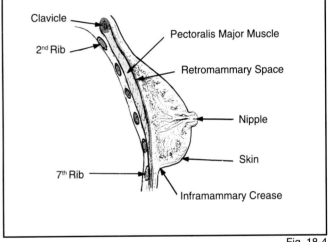

Breast Sagittal Section

Fig. 18-4

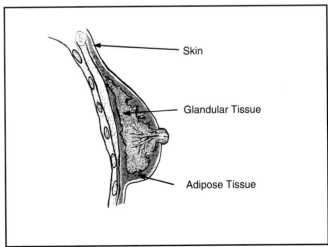

Breast Sagittal Section

Fig. 18-5

Radiographic Anatomy continued

Breast (Frontal)

The glandular tissue of the breast is divided in **15** or **20 lobes** arranged like the spokes of a wheel surrounding the nipple *(Fig. 18-6)*.

The glandular **lobes**, made up of a number of individual **lobules,** are not clearly separated, but are grouped in a radial arrangement as shown on this drawing. Distally the smallest lobules consist of clusters of rounded **alveoli.** Upon glandular stimulation, peripheral cells of the alveoli form oil globules in their interior, which when ejected into the lumen of the alveoli constitute milk globules. The clusters of alveoli which make up the lobules are interconnected and drain by individual **ducts.** Each duct enlarges into a small **ampulla** which serves as a reservoir for milk just prior to terminating in a tiny opening on the surface of the **nipple.**

The various subdivisions of these ducts and associated ampullae are activated during pregnancy to prepare for lactation and following birth, to produce milk for the newborn.

A layer of adipose tissue just under the skin surrounds and covers the glandular tissue. Lobular mammary fatty tissue, **subcutaneous fat,** is interspersed between the glandular elements. **Interlobular connective** or fibrous tissues surround and support the lobes and other glandular structures. Band-like extensions of this fibrous tissue are known as **Cooper's** (suspensory) **ligaments** of the breast, and function to provide support for the mammary glands.

Each breast is abundantly supplied by blood vessels, nerves, and lymphatic vessels. The veins of the mammary gland are usually larger than the arteries, and are located more peripherally. Some of the larger veins can usually be seen distinctly on a mammogram, a radiographic study of the breast. The term **trabeculae** is used by radiologists to describe various small structures seen on the finished radiograph such as small blood vessels, fibrous connective tissues, ducts, and other small structures that cannot be differentiated.

Breast Tissue Types

One of the major problems in radiography of the breast is that the various tissues are of general similar density. Breast tissue can be divided into three main types of tissues: (1) **glandular,** (2) **fibrous** or **connective,** and (3) **adipose** *(Fig. 18-7)*. Since these tissues are all "soft tissues," there is no bone or air-filled tissue to provide contrast. The fibrous and glandular tissues are of similar density—that is, radiation is absorbed by these two tissues in a similar fashion.

The major difference in the breast tissues is the fact that adipose or fatty tissue is less dense than either the fibrous or glandular tissue. This difference in density between the fatty tissue and the remaining tissues provides for the photographic density differences apparent on the finished radiograph.

Summary

Three types of breast tissue:
1. Glandular
2. Fibrous or connective } Similar density
3. Adipose ------------------ Less dense

The final mammogram radiograph *(Fig. 18-8)* demonstrates differences in tissue densities. These differences provide the basis for the radiographic image of the breast.

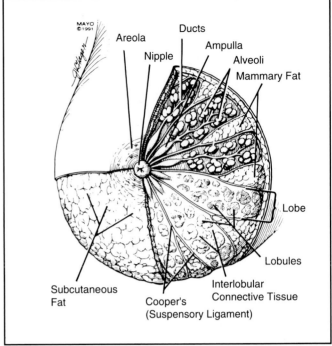

Breast, Anterior View (Glandular Tissue) Fig. 18-6
(Courtesy of Mayo Clinic)

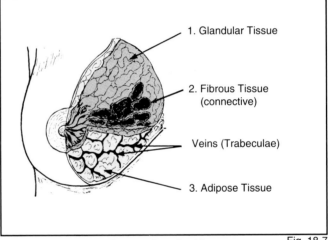

Breast, Anterior View Fig. 18-7
(Three Tissue Types)

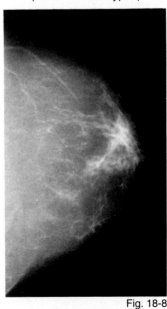

Fig. 18-8
Film-Screen
Mammogram

Breast Classifications

Technical radiographic factors for any one part of the body are determined mainly by the thickness of that particular part. A large elbow for example, will require greater exposure factors than a small elbow. In mammography however, **both** the **compressed breast thickness** and the **tissue density** contribute to technique selection. The breast size or thickness is easy to determine but breast density is less obvious and requires additional information.

The relative density of the breast is primarily affected by the patient's inherent breast characteristics, hormone status, age, and pregnancies. The mammary gland undergoes cyclic changes associated with the rise and fall of hormonal secretions during the menstrual cycle, changes during pregnancy and lactation, and gradual changes that occur throughout a woman's lifetime.

Generally speaking, however, breasts can be classified into **three broad categories**, depending on the relative amounts of fibro-glandular tissue versus fatty tissue.

(1) Fibro-Glandular Breast

The first category is the fibro-glandular breast. The younger breast is usually quite dense, since it contains relatively little fatty tissue. The common age grouping for the fibro-glandular category is postpuberty to about age thirty. However, those females over the age of 30 who have never given birth to a live infant will probably also be in this general grouping. Pregnant or lactating females of any age are also placed in this grouping because they possess a very dense type of breast.

(2) Fibro-Fatty Breast

A second general category is the fibro-fatty breast. As the female ages and more changes occur in the breast tissues, there is a gradual shift from low amount of fatty tissue to a more equal distribution of fat and fibro-glandular tissue. Therefore, in a 30- to 50-year-old group the breast is not quite as dense as in the younger group.

Radiographically, this breast is of average density and requires less exposure than the fibro-glandular type of breast.

Several pregnancies early in a woman's reproductive life will accelerate her breast development toward this fibro-fatty category.

(3) Fatty Breast

A third and final grouping is the fatty breast that occurs following menopause, commonly age 50 and above. Following a female's reproductive life, most of the glandular breast tissue atrophies and is converted to fatty tissue in a process called involution. Even less exposure is required on this type of breast than is required on the first two types of breasts.

The breasts of children and most males contain mostly fat in small proportions and, therefore, fall into this category also. While most mammograms are performed on the female patient, it is well to realize that between one and two percent of all breast cancer is found in the male; therefore, mammograms will occasionally be performed on a male.

(1.) Fibro-Glandular Breast

- Common age group - 15 to 30 years (and childless females over age 30)
- Pregnant or lactating females
- Radiographically dense
- Very little fat

(2.) Fibro-Fatty Breast

- Common age group - 30 to 50 years
- Young women with 3 or more pregnancies
- Average density, radiographically
- 50% fat - 50% fibro-glandular

(3.) Fatty Breast

- Common age group - 50 years and over
- Postmenopausal
- Minimal density, radiographically
- Atrophic
- Breast of children and males

Summary – Breast Classifications   Fig. 18-9

Summary:

In summary, in addition to breast size or thickness upon compression, the average density of the tissues of the breast will determine exposure factors. The most dense breast is the fibro-glandular type. The least dense is the fatty type, and the breast with equal amounts of fatty and fibro-glandular tissue is termed fibro-fatty.

Part II   Radiographic Procedure and Positioning

Breast Positioning and Compression

In mammography, the great variability of the breast, with respect to the proportion of fatty tissue to fibroglandular tissue, presents certain technical difficulties. In producing a superior quality mammogram, the shape and contour of the normal breast poses additional problems to the radiographer.

The **base** of the breast is that portion near the chest wall, while the area near the nipple is termed the **apex**. In either the cranio-caudad or the mediolateral projection, the base of the breast is much thicker and contains much denser tissues than the apex.

To overcome this anatomical difference, compression is used in combination with a specific shaped cone so that the more intense central portion of the x-ray beam (CR) penetrates the thicker base of the breast. The less intense filtered divergent beam passes through the outer periphery or apex to provide a more overall uniform density. (See long arrows in *Fig. 18-10*.)

Correct positioning using a dedicated mammography unit for the craniocaudad projection is illustrated in this visual.

Imaging Modalities

Various modalities for studying the tissues of the breast have been developed. **Film-screen mammography, xeromammography** and **sonography** or ultrasonography are currently the primary imaging modalities used. Film-screen mammography however remains the most important and widely used. Light scanning and thermography are generally no longer used in diagnosis. In a modern mammography department, film-screen mammography and sonography are used together to diagnose breast disease.

Today, the type of mammography a radiologist chooses is a matter of individual preference based on the evaluation of positive and negative features, but each type can provide diagnostic studies if done properly by qualified radiographers and diagnosed by board-certified radiologists.

Mammography

Mammography is the x-ray examination of the breast involving the first two imaging modalities, film-screen mammography and xeromammography. Many factors contribute to the overall quality of a mammogram. Some of these are the x-ray machine characteristics such as focal spot size, target material, beam filtration, kVp and mAs selection, film or other material selection, intensifying screens, breast position and compression, image processing, and the training and qualifications of the operator.

Film-screen Mammography

Film-screen mammography is the standard in current breast radiography. A dedicated free standing mammography unit with a small focal spot (0.3 mm or less), molybdenum target, suitable beam filtration, variable low kVp and mAs settings, use of automatic exposure control (AEC), a film/intensifying screen combination, grid, and firm breast compression provides the best breast image. Grids are commonly used for the majority of mammograms. Film image quality depends on these factors as well as careful film processing. A high quality image has exceptional contrast, superb resolution and detail.

The greatest benefit of the film-screen system is an **excellent image with a low radiation dose** to the breast allowing women to have this examination regularly. The ability to see **fine detail**, **edge sharpness**, and **soft densities** is a hallmark of a good film mammogram. An example of a good film mammogram is *Fig. 18-11*.

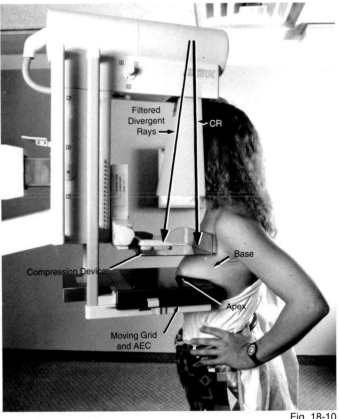

Fig. 18-10

Correct placement on a dedicated mammography unit
(Compression not firmly applied for this photo)

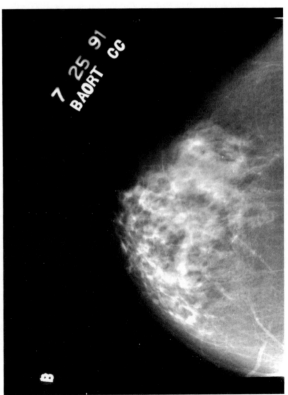

Film-Screen Mammogram   Fig. 18-11

Imaging Modalities continued

Xeromammography

Another mammographic procedure that has been widely accepted, but is used less than film-screen mammography, is xeroradiography. X-rays are used to produce the image, but a photoelectric recording method is used rather than silver halide film. A simplified explanation of this system appears in *Fig. 18-12*.

The xeroradiographic plate has an aluminum base with a thin layer of vitreous selenium, as shown in the upper drawing in *Fig 18-12*. The construction of the plate allows an electrical charge to be placed and held in the selenium layer.

Steps of Processing a Xeroradiograph: Step 1 of this process involves charging the plate in a special conditioning device. The selenium on the plate is termed a photoconductor. Electrical charges are neutralized by x-radiation passing through the breast, forming a latent image of the pattern of the breast tissues. This is demonstrated in step 2 on the center drawing, showing the x-ray exposure and the formation of the latent image.

Step 3 is carried out in a special processor. In the processor the latent image is first sprayed by a blue, finely divided, charged powder, producing a visible image on the surface of the plate. Using a heat transfer, the image on the plate is then transferred to a plastic coated paper.

Xeroradiograph: An example of a xeroradiograph is shown in *Fig 18-13*. In actual practice, xeroradiographs are various shades of blue rather than black, gray and white. However, since this example is printed in black and white, the blue color is not visualized. On the original xeroradiograph the dark gray areas were dark blue and the light gray areas were a lighter shade of blue.

Xeroradiographs are usually positives rather than negatives. The thick parts of the breast appear dark blue, while the thin parts appear as a lighter blue. The negative xeroradiograph is just the opposite. The negative would be similar to the film-screen mammogram and could be produced with less dose to the patient.

Comparison with Film-Screen Mammogram: Film-screen mammograms and xeromammograms have similar detail, edge sharpness and resolution characteristics. The border between any two density regions shows up better using xeroradiographic methods than do the same borders on a film-screen mammogram. This concept is known as **edge enhancement** and serves to accentuate the small differences in breast tissues.

Film-screen mammography, however, in general provides **better visualization of soft densities** (due to low kVp and film characteristics) that are lost on the xeromammogram.

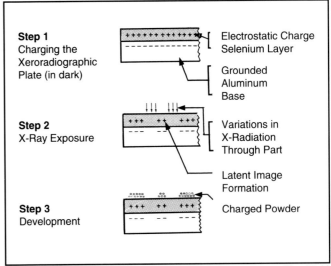

The Xeroradiographic Process   Fig. 18-12

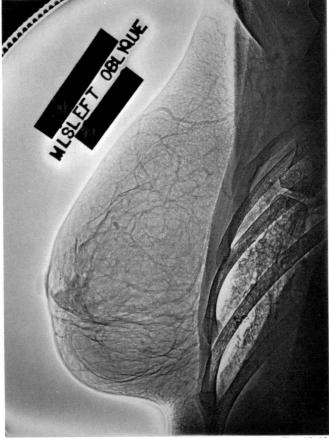

Xeroradiograph   Fig. 18-13

Sonography

Sonographic (ultrasound) imaging of the breast can be done two ways, with a dedicated breast sonographic scanner or with a conventional scanner and hand-held transducer.

Dedicated Sonographic Scanner: With the dedicated unit *(Fig. 18-14)*, the patient lies prone on a special couch and the whole breast is immersed in water and imaged in sections. A breast sonogram taken in this manner is shown in *Fig. 18-15*. Many dedicated sonographic units are currently being used, however, the manufacture of such units has ceased.

Conventional Scanner and Hand Held Transducer: With a conventional scanner *(Fig. 18-16)* the patient is supine or rolled-up slightly on a side. The hand held transducer is placed on a palpable mass or an area noted on a mammogram. *Fig. 18-17* shows an image on such a scanner. Sonographic imaging is not recommended for routine screening but is sometimes used as a follow-up procedure for additional information.

Additional New Breast Imaging Techniques

Magnetic Resonance Imaging and Digital Mammography

New techniques on the horizon are magnetic resonance imaging (MRI) of the breast and digital mammography (computerized image production). Many believe that one or both of these two newer modalities have much to offer in the future of clinical diagnosis of breast disease.

Summary

The various techniques of imaging the mammary glands can be used in conjunction with self-examination, and physician consultation and palpation. Breast cancer is the number one type of carcinoma found in the female. With the use of available high quality imaging methods and qualified operators and physicians, breast carcinoma can generally be detected and successfully treated.

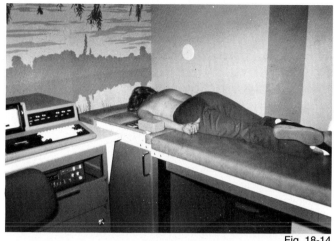

Fig. 18-14
Dedicated breast sonography scanner with water bath

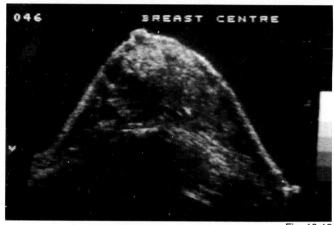

Fig. 18-15
Breast sonogram done on water bath unit

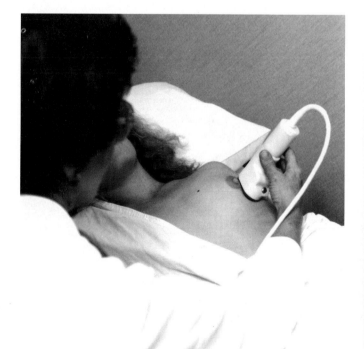

Fig. 18-16
Conventional scanner with hand-held transducer

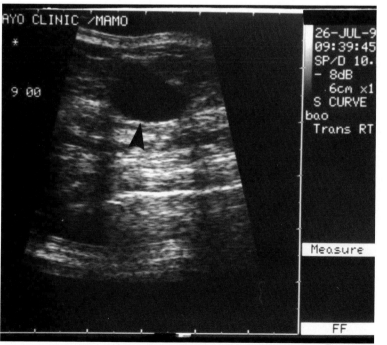

Fig. 18-17
Breast sonogram obtained with conventional scanner showing a cyst (arrow)

Basic and Optional Projections/Positions

Basic and Optional Projections

The most **basic or** primary screening views currently performed in mammography are the **craniocaudad** (CC) and **mediolateral oblique** (MLO). In addition, the **exaggerated-lateral craniocaudad** (XLCC) is described because of its frequent use. Also, because of the increasing number of patients who have breast implant procedures, the **Eklund technique** procedure is included.

Mammogram
Basic
• Craniocaudad (CC)
• Mediolateral Oblique (MLO)
Optional
• Exaggerated-Lateral Craniocaudad (XLCC)
• Implant procedure
  (Eklund Technique)

Additional Optional Projections

Additional projections which may be used to supplement the standard mammograms in order to better characterize or clarify findings include the following: (These will not be described in detail in this chapter.)

Axillary: For lymph nodes and other axillary content. Also done to obtain a view of a post-mastectomy surgical site. Compression is difficult to apply for this view.

Exaggerated- medial craniocaudad: Performed like the exaggerated lateral, with emphasis on the medial aspect of the breast. It is done when the exaggerated-lateral craniocaudad does not show that the lesion is in the lateral aspect of the breast. The patient is placed in the **CC** position and rotated so the **medial** part of the breast is on the film.

Magnification: 1.5 to 2 times enlargement of specific areas of interest such as nodules or microcalcifications. Performed with a microfocal spot (0.1 mm) and basic x-ray magnification principles. A magnification device attaches to the unit which raises the breast above the film, thereby magnifying the part. Most mammographic views can be performed with the magnification unit in place.

Mediolateral (true lateral): The x-ray tube is positioned horizontally 90° to obtain an exact location of a lesion for localization purposes or superimposition. The view also demonstrates fluid levels. The x-ray tube is at the **medial** aspect of the breast.

Lateromedial (reverse lateral): The x-ray tube is positioned horizontally 90° in the true lateral position. The tube is at the **lateral** side of the breast. This view shows fluid levels and lesions in medial part of the breast.

Lateromedial oblique (reverse oblique): Positioning for this view is the opposite of the mediolateral oblique described in this chapter. The x-ray tube is angled toward the **lateral** side at 40° to 60°. This view better visualizes lesions in the medial part of the breast. It also visualizes areas of concern in the IUQ and LOQ from a different projection.

Spot compression: Utilizes a small size compression device, which is placed over a specific area of the breast, to spread the breast tissue. The spot compression enables the borders of nodules to be defined better. The compression device can be used for most of the routine views.

Cleopatra: Performed to identify deep lesions in the axilla and tail of the upper outer quadrant. Positioning is similar to the exaggerated-lateral craniocaudad but emphasis is on the axillary tail. This view is moderately difficult to perform on dedicated mammography units. It is best done with the patient seated because the patient has to lean backwards and laterally.

• Craniocaudad Projection (CC)

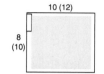

> **Mammogram**
> Basic
> • **Craniocaudad (CC)**
> • Mediolateral Oblique (MLO)

Structures Best Shown:
Entire breast tissue.

Both breasts are generally imaged on separate film for comparison.

Technical Factors:
- Film size - 8 x 10 in. (18 x 24 cm), crosswise or 10 x 12 in. (24 x 30 cm), crosswise.
- Moving or stationary grid (some breast types nongrid).
- 25 to 30 kVp (Xerox 55 kVp).

Patient Position:
- Standing; if not possible, seated.

Shielding: Waist apron.

Part Position:
- Film tray height is determined by **lifting the breast** to achieve a 90° angle to the chest wall. The tray will be at the level of the inframammary crease **at its upper limits**.
- The breast is pulled forward onto the film holder centrally with the nipple in profile.
- The arm on the side being imaged is relaxed and the shoulder is back out of the way.
- The head is turned away from the side being imaged.
- Wrinkles and folds on the breast should be smoothed out and compression applied until taut.
- The marker is always placed on the **axillary side**.

Central Ray:
- Perpendicular to the film and phototimer over the center of the breast at the chest wall.
- SID: Fixed, varies with manufacturer, about 60 cm (23.6 in).

Collimation: Collimate closely if dedicated unit allows, otherwise use appropriate cone.

Respiration: Suspend breathing.

Evaluation Criteria:
- The central, subareolar, and medial breast should be visualized (sometimes pectoral muscle is included).
- Tissue thickness is distributed evenly on the film.
- Optimum compression is noted.
- Dense areas are adequately penetrated.
- High tissue contrast and optimal resolution noted.
- Absence of artifacts.
- Marker is in proper position and patient identification is accurate with date included.

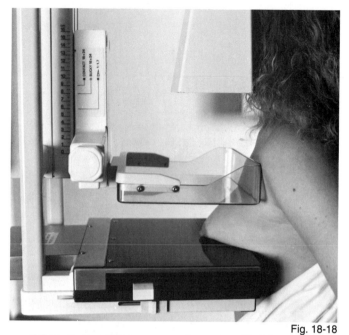

Fig. 18-18

CC Projection (Firm compression not applied for photo)

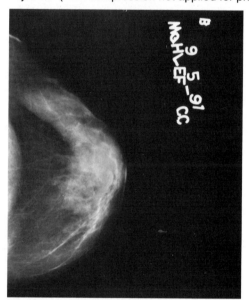

CC Projection   Fig. 18-19

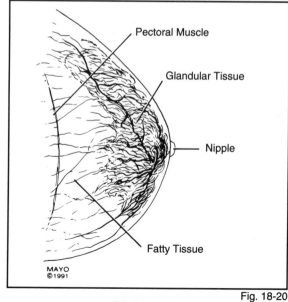

Pectoral Muscle

Glandular Tissue

Nipple

Fatty Tissue

MAYO ©1991

Fig. 18-20

CC Projection

•Mediolateral Oblique (MLO)

(Formerly referred to as lateral oblique, or just oblique)

> **Mammogram**
> Basic
> • Craniocaudad (CC)
> • **Mediolateral Oblique (MLO)**

Structures Best Shown:
Entire breast tissue.
Both breasts are generally imaged on separate films for comparison.

Technical Factors:
• Film size - 8 x 10 in. (18 x 24 cm), crosswise.
    or   10 x 12 in. (24 x 30 cm), crosswise.
• Moving or stationary grid (some breast types nongrid)
• 25 to 30 kVp (Xerox 55 kVp)

Patient Position:
• Standing; if not possible, seated.

Shielding: Waist apron.

Part Position:
• Tube and film holder remain at right angles to each other as CR is angled about 45°. CR enters the breast **mediolaterally, perpendicular** to the patient's pectoral muscle.
- Heavy and large-breasted women, angle 40-60° from vertical.
- Thin and small-breasted women, angle 60-70° from vertical.
• Adjust film height so top of film will be at the level of the axilla.
• With the patient facing the unit and feet forward exactly like CC view, place the arm of the side being imaged forward and the hand on the bar toward the front.
• Pull breast tissue and pectoral muscle **anteriorly** and **medially away from chest wall**. Push the patient slightly toward the angled film holder until the inferolateral aspect of the breast is touching the film holder. The nipple should be in profile.
• Apply compression slowly with the breast held **away from the chest wall and up**, to prevent sagging.
• The upper edge of the compression device will rest under the clavicle and the lower edge will include the inframammary fold.
• Wrinkles and folds on the breast should be smoothed out and compression applied until taut.
• If necessary, have patient gently retract opposite breast with other hand to prevent superimposition.
• The marker should be placed high and at the axilla.

Central Ray:
• Perpendicular to the film and phototimer over the center of the breast at the chest wall.
• SID: Fixed, varies with manufacturer, about 60 cm (23.6 in).

Collimation: Collimate closely if dedicated unit allows, otherwise use appropriate cone.

Respiration: Suspend breathing.

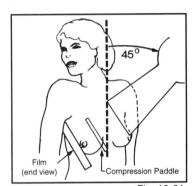

MLO Projection   Fig. 18-21

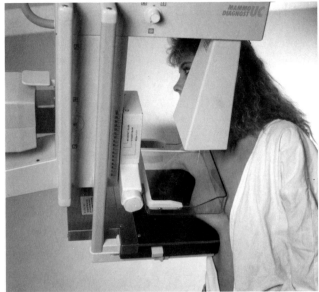

Fig. 18-22

MLO Projection (firm compression not applied for this photo)

(Note x-ray tube/ film unit angled about 45°, see *Fig. 18-21*.)

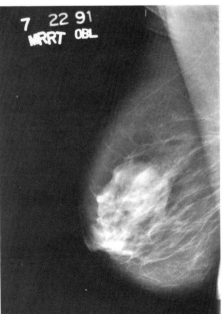

Fig. 18-23
MLO Projection

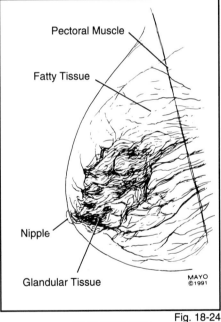

Fig. 18-24
MLO Projection

NOTE: To show **all** of the breast tissue on this view with a large breast, two films may be needed, one positioned higher to get all of the axillary region and a second film positioned lower to include the main part of the breast.

Evaluation Criteria:
• A good MLO will show pectoral muscle to the level of the nipple.
• Breast must be shown to be pulled out and away from the chest so as not to droop.
• Optimum compression is noted.
• Dense areas are adequately penetrated.
• High tissue contrast and optimal resolution noted.
• Absence of artifacts.
• Marker is in proper position and patient identification is accurate with date included.

• Exaggerated-Lateral Craniocaudad (XLCC)

Mammogram
Basic
• Craniocaudad (CC)
• Mediolateral Oblique (MLO)
Optional
• **Exaggerated-Lateral Craniocaudad (XLCC)**
• Implant procedure (Ekland Technique)

Structures Best Shown:
Breast tissue with emphasis on the **axillary tissue**.

This is the most frequently requested optional projection. It is done, if the CC projection does not show all the axillary tissue. In addition it is usually requested when a lesion is seen on the MLO but not on the CC.

Technical Factors:
• Film size - 8 x 10 in. (18 x 24 cm), crosswise,
  or   10 x 12 in. (24 x 30 cm), crosswise.

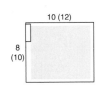

• Moving or stationary grid (some breast types nongrid).
• 25 to 30 kVp (Xerox 55 kVp).

Patient Position: Standing. If not possible, seated.

Shielding: Waist apron.

Part Position:
• Begin as if to do a CC projection but **rotate the body** slightly and position patient to include more of the **axillary** aspect of breast. *(Fig. 18-25.)*
• Put the patient's hand on the bar toward the front and relax the shoulder. (Some recommend angling the tube 5° mediolaterally.)
• The head is turned away from the side being imaged.
• The breast is pulled forward onto the film holder, wrinkles and folds should be smoothed out, and compression applied until taut.
• The marker is always placed on the axillary side.

Central Ray:
• Perpendicular to the film and phototimer over the center of the breast at the chest wall.
• SID: Fixed, varies with manufacturer, about 60 cm (23.6 in).

Collimation: Collimate closely if dedicated unit allows, otherwise use appropriate cone.

Respiration: Suspend breathing.

NOTE: • If a lesion is deeper, do a Cleopatra view.
• If a lesion is not found on lateral aspect of breast, do **exaggerated-medial** craniocaudad view.

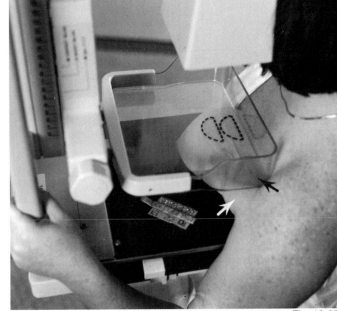

Fig. 18-25

XLCC Projection (firm compression is applied for photo)

Note: Patient is turned so axillary tissue (arrows) is included on the image. Note arm and hand is forward for ease in turning body.

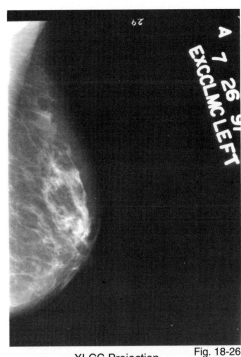

XLCC Projection   Fig. 18-26   XLCC Projection   Fig. 18-27

Evaluation Criteria:
• Evaluation criteria from CC projection also applies to this projection.
• The axillary aspect of the breast should be better visualized.
• May see pectoral muscle.
• Marker is in proper position and patient identification is accurate with date included.

• Implant Procedure with the Eklund Technique[1]

> **Mammogram**
> Basic
> • Craniocaudad (CC)
> • Mediolateral Oblique (MLO)
> Optional
> • Exaggerated-Lateral
>   Craniocaudad (XLCC)
> • **Implant procedure**
>   **(Eklund Technique)**

Patients who have breast implant procedures done for size and shape enhancement require routine mammography also because their breast tissue remains intact. However, a slightly different technique is used.

Standard CC and MLO Projections:
Standard CC and MLO projections, as previously described, are done first with the implant device in place *(Fig. 18-28).* Caution must be used with the compression device—firm compression cannot be accomplished.

Ecklund Technique:
The Eklund technique of "pinching" the breast *(Figs. 18-30 and 18-31)* is performed after the basic CC and MLO projections. During this procedure, the implant is pushed posteriorly to the chest wall so that the anterior breast tissue can be compressed and visualized in the usual manner *(Fig 18-29).*

Exception: The Eklund technique can be performed on most patients with implants, however, some implants become encapsulated and only the routine views with the implant in place can be done. An additional view such as the mediolateral or lateromedial may be helpful to demonstrate all the tissue.

Manual Exposure Techniques: For those views done with the implant in place, only **manual exposure techniques** can be set on the generator because the implant device will prevent the x-ray photons from reaching the phototimer sensor. This will cause **overexposure** of the breast and the phototiming system may possibly go to maximum backup time.

[1] Eklund, G.W., et. al. **Improved Imaging of the Augmented Breast.** AJR. 151:469-473, 1988.

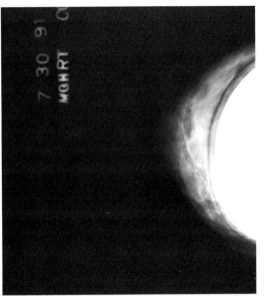

Fig. 18-28
Standard CC Projection with implant in place

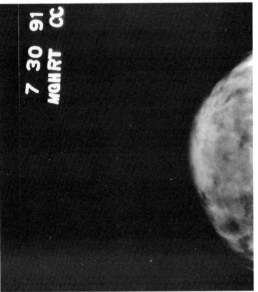

Fig. 18-29
Standard CC Projection with implant pushed back
(Same patient as in Fig. 18-28)

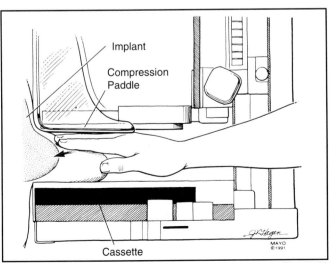

Fig. 18-30
Positioning with Eklund "pinch" technique
(Courtesy of Mayo Clinic)

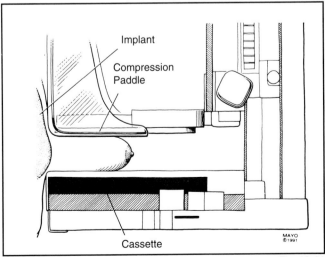

Fig. 18-31
Breast in place for CC Projection with implant pushed back
(Courtesy of Mayo Clinic)

Chapter 19

Pediatric Radiography

Contributions by: Claudia Calandrino, MPA, RT(R)
Jessie R. Harris, RT(R)

Contents

Part 1 Introduction and Principles

Introduction

The pediatric technologist sees children not just as adults in miniature but as very special human persons to be handled with care and special understanding. This requires patience and the necessary time to **talk to** and **make friends** with the child. Explaining instructions to the child in a way that they can understand is of great importance in developing trust and cooperation.

Age of Understanding and Cooperation

Children do not reach a sense of understanding at a specific predictable age. This varies greatly from child to child and the pediatric technologist must not assume that the small person lacks this capability. Generally however by the age of **two years**, most normal children can be talked through a diagnostic radiographic study without immobilization or parental aid. Most important is a sense of trust which begins at the first meeting between the patient and the technologist; the first impression the child has of this stranger is everlasting and forges the bond of a successful relationship.

Successful radiographic studies are dependent on two things. First and most important is the **technologist's attitude and approach to a child.** Second and also important is the **room's technical preparation**, which includes certain essential immobilization devices, as will be described and illustrated in this chapter.

Pre-exam Introduction and Child/Parent Evaluation

Self Introduction: At the first meeting, most patients are accompanied by at least one parent. It is important to:
• Introduce yourself as the technologist who will be working with this child.
• Find out what information the attending physician has given the parent and patient.
• Explain what you are going to do and what your needs will be.

Tears, fear and combative resistance are perfectly normal reactions for a young child. The technologist must take the time to communicate to the parent and child, in a language they can understand, exactly what they are going to do. They must try to build an atmosphere of trust in the waiting room before the patient is taken into the radiographic room. The technologist should discuss the necessity of immobilization as a last resort if the child's cooperation is unattainable.

Evaluate Parent's Role: This is also the time to evaluate the parent's role. There are three possibilities:
(1) Parent in room as an observer who lends support and comfort by their presence.
(2) Parent as a participator who assists with immobilization.
(3) Parent asked to remain in the waiting area and not accompany child into radiography room.

Many times children who act fearful and combative in the waiting room with the parent present will be much more cooperative without the parent. This is the time when the technologist's skills in communication are necessary. At this time the technologist should also try to convince the parent that he or she is capable of radiographing the patient **without** parental assistance.

This assessment of the parent's role is very important and requires an objective evaluation by the technologist. It may be determined that the parent's anxiety will interfere with the child's cooperation, then option (3) would be chosen. If option (2) is chosen, the parent must be instructed on the proper technique for holding the child immobile. Parents generally lack knowledge of how to position a patient properly and are often afraid of hurting their child. This can result in motion or rotation, thereby necessitating a repeat of the examination.

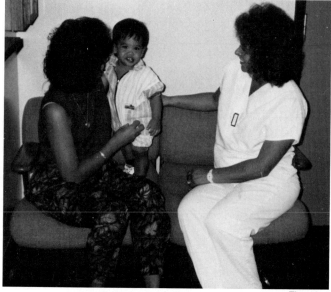

Technologist Introducing Herself   Fig. 19-1

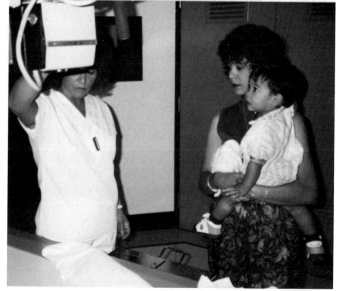

Talking to Patient and Developing Trust   Fig. 19-2

Reporting Child Abuse

Most medical facilities have a procedure in place to report suspected child abuse. In the past the term used for this was battered child syndrome (BCS). Today the acceptable term is **nonaccidental trauma (NAT).**

It is generally not the responsibility of the technologist to make a judgment as to whether or not child abuse has occurred, but rather to report the facts as they are seen or suspected. If NAT is suspected, the technologist should discuss this with the radiologist or such supervisor as determined by departmental protocol. State laws vary on technologists' responsibilities and it is most important that **every technologist know what their responsibilities are concerning this in the state in which they are working.**

Immobilization

There are immobilization devices on the market today which can be purchased. These can generally be found in a radiology supply catalog. Examples of these are the **Tam-em Board** and **Pigg-O-Stat** as demonstrated. The **Posi-Tot** is another type of immobilization device also available commercially. The cost effectiveness of these devices is dependent on how often the devices are utilized.

Tam-em Board

The **Tam-em Board** along with several short velcro straps for immobilizing the upper and lower limbs is shown in *Fig. 19-3*. This is a commercially available immobilization device that is easy to use and will be demonstrated in this chapter.

A **plexiglass hold-down paddle** is also shown in front of the Tam-em Board. This can be cut from a clear sheet of plexiglass of sufficient thickness for necessary rigidity. It can be used in various applications such as to hold down upper or lower limbs without obscuring essential anatomy. This can be an aid for parents to utilize in assisting with immobilization.

Pigg-O-Stat

The **Pigg-O-Stat** is a commonly used immobilization apparatus for erect chest and abdomen procedures on infants and small children up to the approximate age of two years. The infant or child is seated on the small bicycle type seat (A) with their legs placed down through the opening. This seat is adjustable in height. The arms are then raised above the head and the two clear plastic body clamps (B) are adjusted firmly against each side of the body to prevent movement. There are two sizes of these clamps which are easily interchangeable depending on the size of the child. The film holder is placed in the film mounting bracket (C).

The entire seat and body clamps are mounted on a swivel base (E) which can be rotated independent of the film holder. This places the patient into the desired position for erect AP, PA, lateral or oblique projections. The adjustable lead gonadal shield (D), is shown in position between the x-ray tube and patient. This shield also contains the necessary film markers. The entire Pigg-O-Stat device is mounted on a stand (F) with wheels and locks which allows it to be easily moved into position, and from room to room as needed.

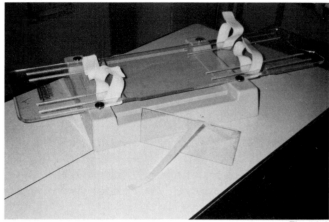

Tam-em Board
(Plexiglass hold-down paddle)
Fig. 19-3

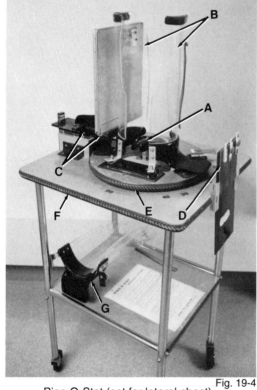

Fig. 19-4
Pigg-O-Stat (set for lateral chest)

A. Seat	E. Swivel base
B. Side body clamps	F. Mounting stand on wheels
C. Film holder mount	
D. Lead shield with markers	G. Extra set of smaller body clamps

Other Immobilization Forms

The simplest and least expensive form of immobilization is to utilize the paraphernalia that is commonly found in most departments. **Tape, sheets** or **towels, sandbags, covered radiolucent sponge blocks, compression bands, stockinette** and **ace bandages** if used correctly are very effective in immobilization.

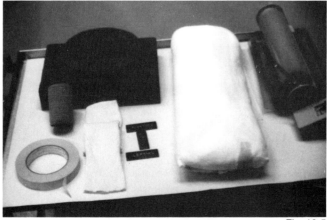

Immobilization Aids
Fig. 19-5

Immobilization continued

Sandbags

There are sandbags available for purchase. However most of these are used as weights for orthopedic patients. These bags are not as effective for immobilization of the pediatric patient as those bags that are made specifically for this purpose.

Strong canvas-type material and children's coarse sterilized playing sand should be utilized. Coarse sand is recommended because if the bag should break open the sand is easily cleaned up and the chance of causing artifacts on radiographs is minimized.

Two sandbag sizes are recommended, 8 x 18 in. (20 x 46 cm) and 13 x 20 in. (33 x 50 cm). The sandbags should not be overfilled with sand, so that the bag is stiff, rather the bag should be pliable so that when placed over a patient's limb it will mold to that part.

Tape

Masking or autoclave type tape is recommended. Adhesive tape will show on the radiograph and create an artifact that could obscure the anatomical part that the radiologist is evaluating. Also, there are numerous accounts of patients who have had an allergic reaction to adhesive tape. The fragile skin of infants can be injured by adhesive tape unless the tape is twisted so the adhesive surface is not against the skin. Gauze pads placed between skin and adhesive tape can also be used effectively.

Stockinette

If stockinettes are utilized, they should be tubular. They come in various sizes; 3 inch is recommended for small infants and 4 inch for larger children.

When using the stockinette, double the stockinette and place over the patient's arms covering the hands and arms to as close to the shoulder as possible. Not only does this serve to immobilize the arms, but it also serves as a pillow *(Fig. 19-7)*.

Ace Bandage

A four inch ace bandage is best for small infants and children while a 6 inch bandage works well for older children. These are best used for immobilizing the legs. When starting the wrapping process, begin at the patient's hips and wrap down to the patient's mid calf *(Fig. 19-8)*. Do not wrap so tightly that the circulation is cut off.

Compression Bands and Head clamps

Compression or **retention bands** are also valuable aids for immobilization. Compression bands, however, are more effective with pediatrics when used in combination with sandbags as will be demonstrated later in this chapter.

Various types of adjustable head clamps are also available which attach to the table top as shown in *Fig. 19-9*.

Weighted Angle Blocks as Head clamps

These are heavy steel angle blocks with thick radiolucent sponge pads attached *(Fig. 19-10)*. They are relatively inexpensive to have made compared to the cost of commercially available head clamps but are very effective and versatile in immobilization, especially when used in combination with sandbags and/or tape, or if the patient is mummified as shown in *Fig. 19-10*.

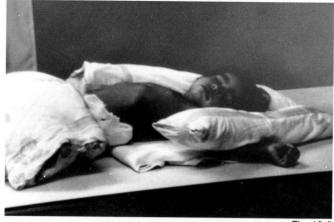

Effective Use of Sandbags   Fig. 19-6

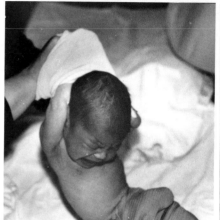 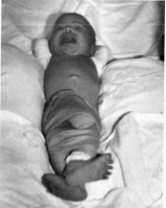

Fig. 19-7   Using Stockinette and Ace bandage   Fig. 19-8

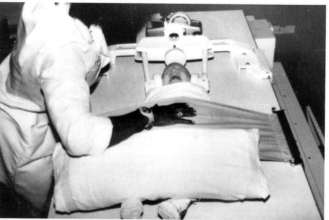

Compression Band and Head Clamps   Fig. 19-9

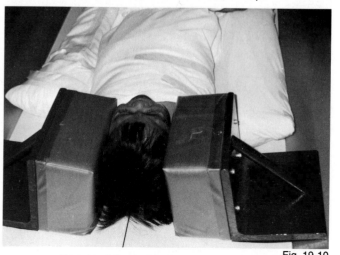

Weighted Angle Blocks as Head Clamps   Fig. 19-10
(Patient "mummified")

"Mummifying" or wrapping with Sheets or Towels

In addition to some type of head clamps, "mummifying" or wrapping is often necessary to immobilize the child for certain radiographic procedures such as head exams. This is very effective for immobilization if done correctly. Following is a five step method of how this is done:

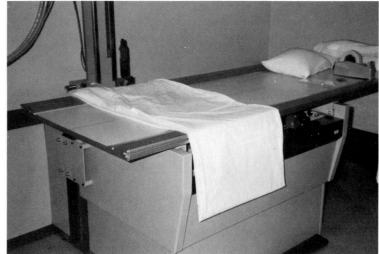

Step 1. Have the room set up and prepared before you bring in the patient. Place the sheet on the table folded in half or in thirds lengthwise, depending on the size of the patient.

Step 1   Fig. 19-11

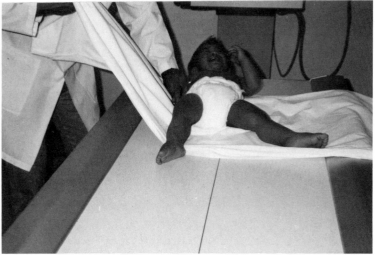

Step 2. Place the patient in the middle of the sheet, then place the patient's arm along side of his body. Take the end of the sheet closest to the technologist and pull the sheet across the patient's body tightly keeping the arm next to the patient's body.

Fig. 19-12

Step 2

Step 3. Place the patient's left arm along side of his body on top of the top sheet. Bring the free sheet over the left arm to the right side of the patient's body and around under the body as needed. Complete the wrapping process by pulling the sheet tightly enough so that the patient cannot free his arms.

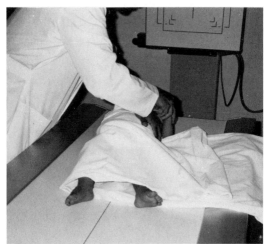

Fig. 19-13

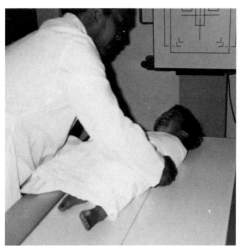

Fig. 19-14

Step 3

"Mummifying" or wrapping with sheets or towels continued

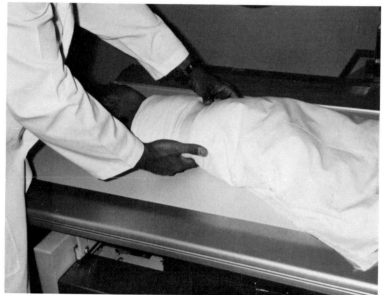

Step 4. Pull the sheet and tape the end of the sheet. Place a long piece of tape from the back of the right wrapped arm to the left wrapped arm over the sheet. This will prevent the patient from breaking out of the sheet.

Step 4   Fig. 19-15

Step 5. Place another piece of tape around the patient's knees. This will keep the patient's lower limbs from becoming free.

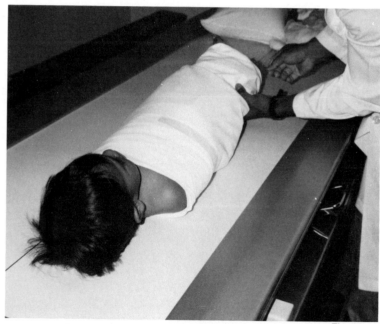

Step 5   Fig. 19-16

Bone Development (Ossification)

The bones of infants and small children go through various growth changes from birth through adolescence. The pelvis is an example where ossification changes are apparent in children. As shown in *Fig. 19-17*, the divisions of the hip bone between the ilium, ischium and pubis is evident. They appear as individual bones separated by a joint space, which is the cartilaginous growth region in the area of the acetabulum.

The heads of the femurs also appear to be separated by a joint space which should not be confused with fracture sites or other abnormalities. These are also normal cartilaginous growth regions.

Most primary centers of bone formation or ossification such as those involving the mid shaft area of long bones appear before birth. These primary centers become the **diaphysis** (D) of long bones (*Fig. 19-18* and *19*). Each secondary center of ossification involves the ends of long bones and is termed an **epiphysis** (E). This is demonstrated on the PA hand radiograph of a nine-year old in *Fig. 19-18*, and the lower limb of a 1 year old in *Fig. 19-19*. Note the epiphyses at the ends of the radius and ulna as well as the metacarpals and phalanges (see small arrows).

The epiphyses are the parts of bones which increase in size and appearance as a child grows, as shown on the growth comparison radiographs below. Note the change in size and shape of the epiphyses of the distal femur and proximal tibia and fibula from age 3 to age 12. Note also that the epiphysis at the proximal fibula is not apparent on the 3 year old (*Fig. 19-20*), but begins to appear slightly at age 4 (*Fig. 19-21*) and continues to increase in size and shape by ages 6 and 12 (*Figs. 19-22* and *23*).

The space between the diaphysis and epiphysis is made up of cartilage and is termed an **epiphyseal plate** (EP). These epiphyseal plates are found between each diaphysis and each epiphysis until skeleton growth is complete upon full maturity, which is normally at about twenty-five years. Growth charts are available which list and demonstrate normal growth patterns.

Radiographers need to be familiar with bone development in infants and children and recognize the appearance of these normal growth stages.

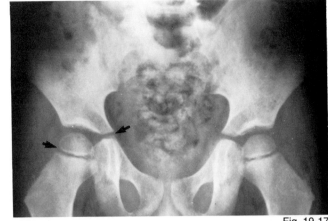

Fig. 19-17

Normal 3 Year-old Pelvis

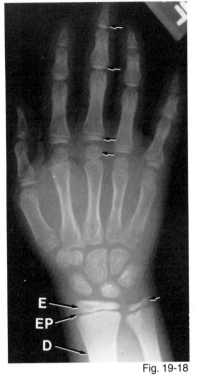

Fig. 19-18

Normal 9 Year-old Hand

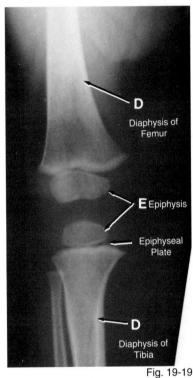

Fig. 19-19

Normal 1 Year-old Lower Limb

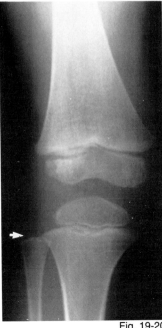

Fig. 19-20

3 Year-old

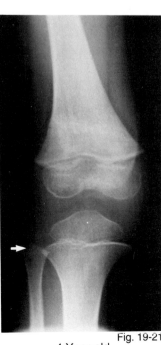

Fig. 19-21

4 Year-old

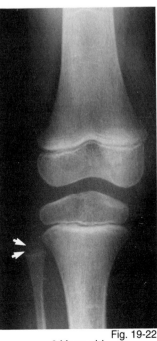

Fig. 19-22

6 Year-old

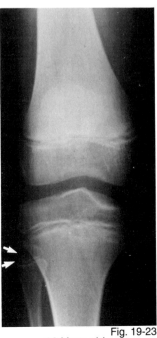

Fig. 19-23

12 Year-old

Radiation Protection

Gonadal Protection
Gonads of the child should **always** be shielded with contact type shields in addition to close collimation unless such shield obscures essential anatomy of the lower abdomen or pelvic area. Various shapes and sizes of contact shields are shown in *Fig. 19-24.*

Since parents will often request shielding for their child's gonads during the radiograph, they should also be aware of other safeguards used for radiation protection such as **close collimation**, **low dosage techniques**, and a **minimum number of films**. To relieve the parents' fears, the technologist should explain in as simple language as possible, the protection practices being used and why.

Parent Protection
If parents are to be in the room, they must be supplied with **lead aprons**. If they are immobilizing the child and their hands are near the primary beam, they should also be given **lead gloves.**

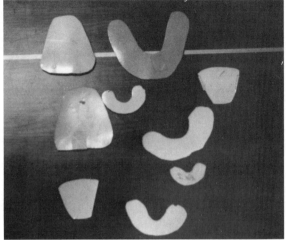
Contact Gonad Shields   Fig. 19-24

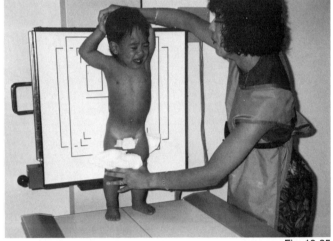
Fig. 19-25
Male Gonadal Shield in Place for Erect Abdomen

Pre-Exam Preparation

Before the patient is brought into the room the following should be completed:
- The necessary immobilization and shielding paraphernalia should be in place (sandbags, tape, Tam-em Board if used, sheets or towels, stockinette, ace bandages and shielding devices for patient and for parents if assisting).
- Cassettes and film markers should be in place and techniques set (if a solo technologist is performing the exam).
- The specific projections should be determined, which may require consultation with the radiologist.
- If two technologists are working together, they should discuss the role each will perform during the procedure. A suggested division of responsibilities is:
  - The assisting technologist sets techniques, makes exposures, changes the cassettes and processes the film.
  - The primary technologist positions the patient and instructs parents (if assisting), positions tube, collimation and required shielding.

Child Preparation: After the child is brought into room and the procedure explained to both child and parent's satisfaction, then due to the low dosage technique used, the parent or technologist must remove from the body parts to be radiographed any clothing, bandages and/or diapers. This is necessary to prevent such from casting shadows and creating artifacts on the radiograph.

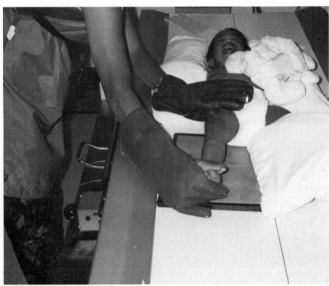
Fig. 19-26
Lead Aprons and Gloves for Parents

Patient Prep for Contrast Media Procedures

Patient history is very important for the pediatric patient. Many times the history will indicate what radiographic procedure is needed to help with the diagnosis and, most important, what prep is really necessary. The required prep may be very stressful on the parent as well as the patient. With infants and very young children who are on a regular feeding schedule, withholding a meal may prove to be very uncomfortable for the child. In these situations the child has a tendency to be very irritable and to start crying easily. The parent, unable to help the child, feels guilty.

Examinations that need the child to hold a feeding should be done early in the morning. For an upper GI the child who is truly hungry is more likely to cooperate and drink the contrast media that is needed to do the examination.

Commonly used patient prep for contrast media procedures are listed below. (These may vary in individual departments or when specifically altered by medical staff.)

Upper Gastrointestinal System

Infants and children to 2 years should be NPO (nothing by mouth) for two hours before any upper gastrointestinal examination. This includes water.

When explaining this to the parent, the simplest terms are best. "Absolutely nothing by mouth!"

For children 2 years and older, NPO or nothing to eat or drink from 12:00 midnight before the examination.

Lower Gastrointestinal System

For a lower gastrointestinal examination the patient history will determine what prep will be necessary.

Contraindications: Patients with the following history **do not** need a prep: **Hirschsprung's disease**, **constipation**, **extensive diarrhea**, possible **appendicitis**, **obstruction**, or those who **cannot withstand fluid loss**.

Instructions for all others who need to be prepared are as follows:

Infants and to age 2: NPO 4 hours prior to the examination.

Children 2 to 8 years: One ounce of an oral cleansing agent one day prior to the examination.

During the evening prior to the examination, the patient is to be given another ounce of an oral cleansing agent followed by 24 ounces of water. Dinner is to be clear liquid.

Adolescents (and Adults)**:** Two ounces of an oral cleansing agent one day prior to the examination. Clear liquid dinner and NPO after 12:00 midnight. At 2:00 a.m. another 2 ounces of the oral agent should be taken again followed by three 8 ounce glasses of water. Oral cleansing agents are more effective with the pediatric patient. Most parents are not proficient in administering cleansing enemas.

Finally, be prepared for a patient who might be both frightened and uncooperative and a parent who is very frustrated.

Intravenous Urogram (IVU)

No solid foods 4 hours prior to the study. May have clear liquids until 2 hours prior to the study.

Upper GI Prep

Infants - Age 2
- NPO 2 hrs before exam

2 yrs and older
- NPO after midnight

Summary

Lower GI Prep
(when not contraindicated)

Infants - Age 2
- NPO 4 hrs before exam

2 - 8 yrs
- 1 oz oral cleaning agent one day prior to exam
- Evening before, another oz of cleaning agent, 24 oz H_2O, clear liquid dinner

Adolescents (and Adults)
- 2 oz oral cleaning agent one day prior to exam
- clear liquid dinner
- NPO after midnight
- 2:00 a.m., 2 oz's oral cleaning agent followed by three 8 oz glasses of H_2O

Summary

IVU Prep

- No solid food 4 hrs before exam
- Clear liquids ok until 2 hrs before exam

Summary

• AP/PA Projection

Chest
Basic
• **AP**
• Lateral

Diagnostic Indications:

Asthma	Atelectasis
Adenopathy	Bronchitis
Cystic Fibrosis	Cough
CHF (Congestive Heart Failure)	Dyspena
Empyema	Embolus
Foreign Body	Heart Disease
Hemoptysis	Hyaline Membrane
Meconium Aspiration	Neoplasm
Metastases	Pleura Effusion
PFC (Persistent Fetal Circulation)	Pneumothorax

Technical Factors:
• Film Size - Determined by the size of patient.
• Film crosswise, if supine place cassette under patient.
• Grid not required.
• 65-70 kVp, shortest exposure time possible.

R

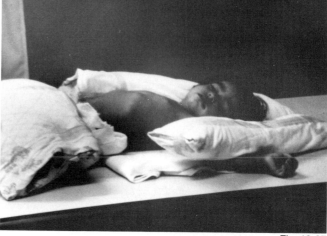

Supine, Immobilized with Sandbags   Fig. 19-27

Shielding: Contact lead shielding should be placed over the pelvic area with upper margin to level of iliac crests.

Patient Position:
• Generally taken supine unless a Pigg-O-Stat or similar erect immobilization device is available.
• Patient supine, arms extended to remove scapula from the lung fields.
• Arms are secured to the table with sandbags or velcro straps if using Tame-em Board.
• Legs extended to prevent rotation of pelvis. Hips and legs are secured by placing sandbags at the level of the hip to the top of the knee. If using Tame-em Board, hip and legs are velcro strapped to the board.
• If utilizing parental assistance:
  1. Have parent remove child's chest clothing.
  2. Provide parent with lead apron and gloves.
  3. Place child on cassette.
  4. Parent should extend child's arms over head with one hand while keeping head tilted back to prevent superimposing upper lungs. With other hand hold child's legs at level of the knees, applying pressure as necessary to prevent movement.
  5. Place parent in a position that will not obstruct technologist's view of patient while making exposure.
  6. Place lead gloves over the top of the parent's hands if parent is not wearing the gloves. (It may be easier to hold on to patient if not wearing the gloves.)

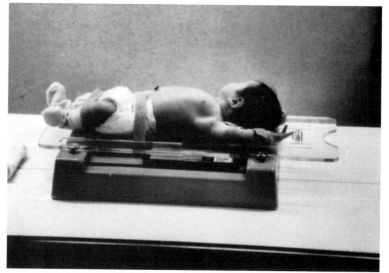

Immobilized with Tam-em Board   Fig. 19-28

Part Position:
• Place the patient in the middle of the cassette with the shoulders 2 in. (5 cm) below the top of the cassette.
• Insure that thorax is **not rotated**.

Central Ray:
• CR perpendicular to the film, centered to the midsagittal plane at the level of mid-thorax which is approximately at the mammillary (nipple) line.
• SID: 50-60 in. (127-212 cm). Tube raised as high as possible.

Collimation: Closely collimate on four sides to outer chest margins.

Respiration: Make exposure upon 2nd full inspiration. If child is crying, watch respiration and make exposure immediately after the child fully inhales.

AP/PA Projection continued

Erect PA Chest with Pigg-O-Stat

Patient Position:
- Patient placed on seat with legs down through center opening. Adjust seat to correct height so top of cassette is about 1 in. (2.5 cm) above shoulders.
- Arms are raised and side body clamps placed firmly against patient and secured by base adjustment and by adjustable strap.
- Lead shield raised to a level about an inch above iliac crest.
- Correct R and L markers and insp (inspiration) marker are set to be exposed on film.
- Insure no rotation.

Central Ray:
- CR **perpendicular** to film at **level of mid-thorax**.
- SID: 72 in. (180 cm).

Collimation: Collimate closely on four sides to outer chest margins.

Respiration: If child is crying, watch respiration and make exposure as child fully inhales and holds his breath. (Best inspiration occurs if patient is crying.)

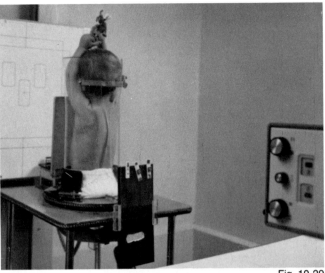

Immobilized by Pigg-O-Stat
Fig. 19-29

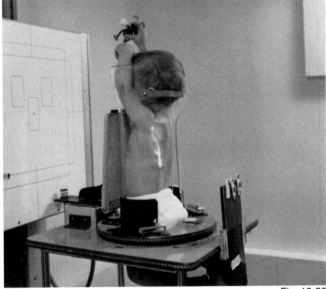

Immobilized by Pigg-O-Stat
Fig. 19-30

Evaluation Criteria:
- **No rotation**: Both sternoclavicular joints should be the same distance from the vertebral column. The distance from the lateral borders of the ribs to the spine should be the same on each side.
- The arms should be extended to remove the scapulae from the lung fields.
- Entire lungs which must be fully expanded.
- Collimation margins should be apparent on four sides.
- **No motion** should result in clear lung markings and sharp outlines of diaphragm and heart and rib borders.
- Correct penetration and exposure should faintly visualize outlines of vertebra and ribs through the heart shadow without over-exposing the fine vascular lung markings throughout lungs.
- Patient ID and right or left marker are placed correctly.

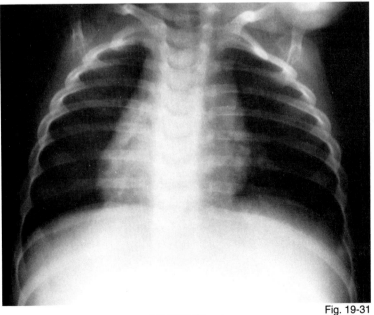

AP (PA) Chest
Fig. 19-31

• Lateral Position

Chest
Basic
• AP
• **Lateral**

Diagnostic Indications:
Same as for AP/PA chest.

Technical Factors:
• Film Size - determined by the size of patient.
• Film lengthwise under patient (unless crosstable is taken on Tame-em Board).
• Grid not required.
• 75-80 kVp, shortest exposure time possible.

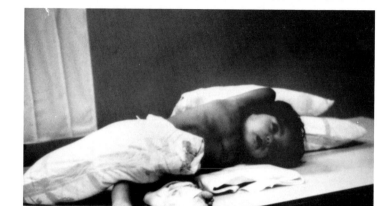

L

Shielding: Contact lead shielding should be placed directly over pelvic area with upper margin at the top of the iliac crest.

Patient Position:
• Patient lying on side in true lateral (generally left lateral) position with arms extended above head to remove arms from lung field. Bend arms at the elbows for patient comfort and stability with head placed between arms.
• Place one sandbag across arm that is closest to the film.
• Place a second sandbag over the top of the upside humerus .
• Place a third sandbag between the legs at the level of the knee while bending the legs forward.
• A fourth sandbag is placed across the top of the hips to further immobilize the patient.
• If using Tam-em Board, patient position does not change from the AP projection. Turn x-ray tube for crosstable projection and place vertical cassette against the lateral wall of the chest as shown *(Fig. 19-33)*.
• If utilizing parent assistance:
  1. Place patient on cassette in left lateral position (unless right lateral is indicated).
  2. Bring arms above the head and hold with one hand. Place the other hand across patient's lateral hips to prevent child from rotating or twisting.
  3. Place parent in a position that will not obstruct technologist's view of patient while making exposure.
  4. Place lead gloves over the top of parent's hand if parent is not wearing the gloves.

Part Position:
• Place the patient in the middle of the cassette with the shoulders about 2 in. (5 cm) below the top of cassette.
• No rotation, insure a true lateral position.

Central Ray:
• CR **perpendicular** to the film **centered to the midcoronal plane** at the level of the mammillary (nipple) line.
• When using Tam-em Board, center the x-ray tube in crosstable lateral position to mid-coronal plane of thorax at level of mammillary line.
• SID: 50-60 in. (127-212 cm).

Fig. 19-32

Recumbent Lateral Chest
(With immobilization aids)

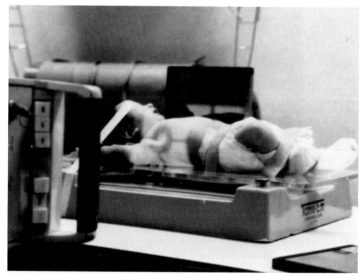

Fig. 19-33

Supine Crosstable Lateral Chest
(With Tam-em Board)

Collimation: Closely collimate on four sides to outer chest margins.

Respiration: Make exposure upon 2nd full inspiration. If child is crying, watch respiration and make exposure when the child fully inhales.

Lateral Chest continued

Erect Lateral Chest with Pigg-O-Stat

Can be used on infants and children up to approximately age 2 (age of this patient is 16 months). The larger size body clamps are being used on this patient and the seat is adjusted as low as it will go.

Patient Position:
• Patient placed on seat and adjusted to correct height so top of film holder is about 1 inch (2.5 cm) above shoulders.
• Arms are raised and side body clamps placed firmly against patient and secured by base adjustment and by adjustable strap.
• Lead shield raised to a level about an inch above iliac crest.
• Correct R and L markers and inspiration marker are set to be exposed on film.
• Insure no rotation.

Procedure if lateral follows PA Projection
If patient is already in position from the PA projecton, then patient and swivel base is turned 90 degrees to lateral position.

Lead shield remains in position and lead marker is changed to indicate correct lateral. Film cassette is placed in film holder mount.

Central Ray:
• CR **perpendicular** to film at **level of mid-thorax**.
• SID: 72 in. (180 cm).

Collimation: Collimate closely on four sides to outer chest margins.

Respiration: If child is crying, watch respiration and make exposure as child fully inhales and holds his breath.

Evaluation Criteria:
• **No rotation**: ribs posterior to the vertebral column should be superimposed.
• Lungs must be fully expanded.
• Arms should be elevated and not superimpose apices of lungs.
• All of lung fields should be included with collimation margins appearing on all four sides of the film. The center of the field should be at the level of the lower margin of the scapula.
• **No motion**: Lung markings and other structural outlines should appear sharp and not blurred.
• Correct exposure and penetration should visualize rib margins and lung markings through the heart shadow without overexposing other regions of the lungs.
• Patient ID and right or left marker are placed correctly.

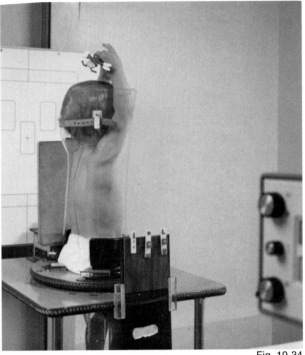

Pigg-O-Stat – Left Lateral

Fig. 19-34

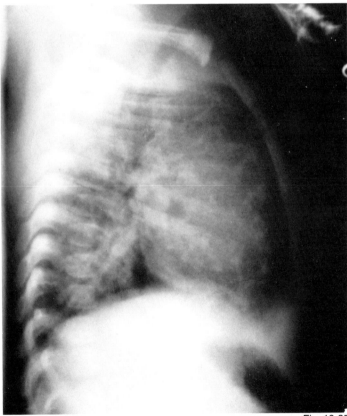

Lateral Chest

Fig. 19-35

• AP Projection (KUB)

Abdomen
Basic
• **AP** (KUB)
Optional
• AP erect

Diagnostic Indications:

Appendicitis	Foreign Body
Bleeding	Intussusception
Constipation	Hepatomegaly
Diarrhea	Mass
Distention	NEC (Necrotizing Enterocolitis)

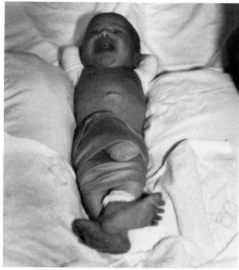

Fig. 19-36

Infant immobilized for AP Abdomen
(stockinette used for arms and ace
bandage for legs)

Technical Factors:
• Film Size - determined by the size of patient, film lengthwise.
• Moving or stationary grid, if more than 9 cm.
• 65-70 kVp, shortest exposure time possible.

Shielding:
• Use pediatric gonadal shield on all male patients. (Remember, for male patients gonads are just below the symphysis pubis.)
• Gonadal shielding may obstruct the necessary anatomy in the female patient. Consult with the radiologist before the film is taken.
• If gonadal shield is used for females, place shield below umbilicus.

Patient and Part Position:
• For an infant, immobilization can be achieved with stockinette for the arms above the head, and ace bandage for the lower limbs with sandbags on each side *(Fig. 19-36)*.
• Patient supine, aligned to midline of table and/or cassette.
• To prevent rotation with an uncooperative child, additional immobilization must also be utilized such as sandbags or a retention band *(Fig. 19-37)*.
• For the upper body, place sandbags over both arms at the level of the shoulder, and for the lower body place sandbags over mid-femurs.
• If utilizing parental assistance:
  1. Provide parent with lead apron and gloves.
  2. Position tube and film before placing child on table.
  3. Place parent in a position so as not to obstruct the vision of the technologist while radiographing the patient.
  4. Have parent hold both of the child's arms with one hand above the child's head and with the other hand apply pressure over child's knees.
  If parent is unable to completely immobilize the child, immobilization devices may also be used as described above.

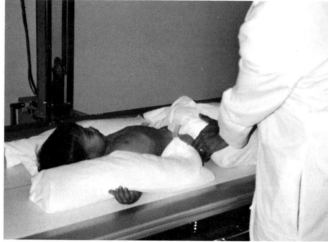

Child immobilized with sandbags for AP Abdomen   Fig. 19-37

Central Ray:
• Infants and small children: Center CR and film one inch (2.5 cm) above the umbilicus.
• Older children and adolescents: Center at the level of the umbilicus.
• Minimum 40 in. (102 cm) SID.

Collimation: Collimate closely on all four sides.

Respiration:
• For infants and small children who are not crying, watch the breathing pattern. When the abdomen is still, make the exposure.
• If the patient is crying, watch for the abdomen to be in full extension to make the exposure.

Evaluation Criteria:
• The vertebral column is lined to the center of the radiograph.
• The upper abdomen should include the diaphragm.
• The lower radiograph should include the symphysis pubis.
• **No rotation**: Pelvis and lumbar vertebrae should appear symmetrical.
• **No motion:** Diaphragm and outlines of gas patterns should appear sharp.

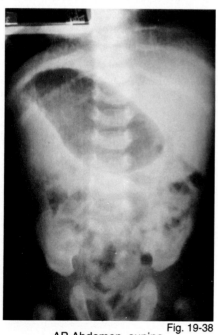

Fig. 19-38

AP Abdomen, supine

• Patient ID with date and Right or Left markers should be visible without superimposing abdominal structures.

• AP Erect

Abdomen
Basic
• AP (KUB)
Optional
• AP erect

Diagnostic Indications:
Same as AP Projection (KUB)

Technical Factors:
- Film Size - determined by the size of patient.
- Place cassette in film holder lengthwise.
- If child measures 9 cm or less, a grid is not required.
- 65-70 kVp, shortest exposure time possible.

Shielding:
- Use gonadal shielding on all patients, if such shielding does not obscure essential anatomy.

Patient Position:
- Patient in erect position, back against film holder.
- If utilizing parental assistance: (Infants and small children)
  1. Have parent put on lead apron and lead gloves.
  2. With infants and small children have parent bring both arms up above the patient's head, grasping patient's hands with one hand.
  3. Do not allow head to fall forward.
  4. Using the other hand grasp patient's knees to secure legs and prevent rotation.

Older Children:
- Seat child on stool with back against erect table or grid device.
- Have child reach up and back with arms and hold on to the top of the chest rack. If patient is unstable, have parent hold arms, or use retention band across upper body.
- Spread legs apart as far as the patient can to remove legs from the lower abdomen. (Demonstrated on radiograph, *Fig 19-41*.)

Tam-em Board:
- If utilizing Tam-em Board, secure patient to board with velcro straps.
- Secure patient and board firmly to table with compression band.
- Raise table to erect position.

Pigg-O-Stat: May be utilized for the projection as described earlier.

Central Ray:
- Infant and small children: CR centered 1 in. (2.5 cm) above the umbilicus.
- Older children and adolescents: CR at the level of the umbilicus.
- Minimum 40 in. (102 cm) SID.

Collimation: Collimate closely on four sides to area of interest.

Respiration:
- For infants and small children who are not crying, watch the breathing pattern. When the abdomen is still, make the exposure.
- If the patient is crying, watch for the abdomen to be in full extension to make the exposure.

Evaluation Criteria:
- The vertebral column is aligned to the center of the radiograph.
- **No rotation**: pelvis and lumbar vertebrae should appear symmetrical.
- **No motion**: Abdominal structures and gas pattern outlines appear clear and sharp.
- Patient ID including date, and Right or Left markers should be visible without superimposing abdominal structures.

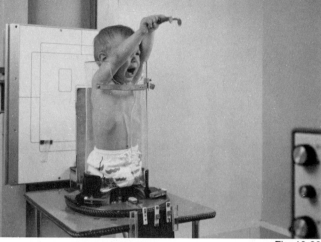

Ererct APAbdomen (with Pigg-O-Stat) Fig. 19-39
(Courtesy of Tyler D. Abraham)

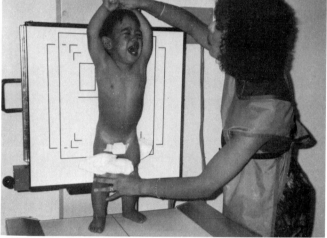

Fig. 19-40
Ererct APAbdomen (parent holding, with grid)

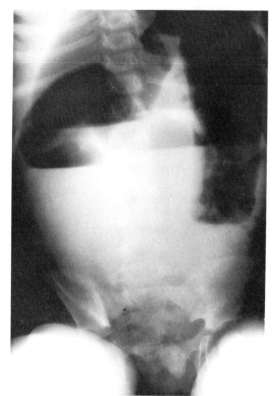

Fig. 19-41
Erect AP Abdomen
(demonstrates fluid levels and
distended air-filled large bowel)

• AP and Lateral

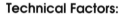

Upper Limbs
Basic
• AP
• Lateral

Diagnostic Indications:

Arthritis	JRA (Juvenile Rheumotoid Arthritis)
Avascular Necrosis	Neoplasm
Bone Dysplasis	Non Accidental Trauma
Bone Age	Osteodystrophy
Bowing	Osteoporosis
Congenital Anomaly	Rickets
Inflammation	Short Limbs
Infection	Trauma

Technical Factors:
• Film size is determined by the size of patient.
• Grid is not used for any body part under 9 cm.
• Use extremity/detail screen if available.
• 55-65 kVp, shortest exposure time possible.

Shielding:
• Secure or place lead shield over pelvic area.

Patient Position:
•Place patient in the supine position.
• Immobilize patient body part not to be radiographed either on the Tam-em Board or with sandbags before the part to be radiographed is positioned.
• When radiographing a long bone, place cassette under the limb to be radiographed including both proximal and distal joints.
• When radiographing a joint, place the cassette under the joint to be radiographed including a minimum of 1 to 2 in. (2.5-5 cm) of proximal and distal long bones.

Part To Be Positioned: AP/Lateral
• Align the part to be radiographed to the long axis of the film; or cross-cornered if necessary to include entire upper limb and both joints.
AP:
• Supinate the hand and forearm into the AP position.
Lateral:
• If patient is in the supine position, abduct the arm about 70° and turn the forearm and wrist into a lateral position.

Immobilization:
• Immobilize the hand, forearm, and humerus with either masking tape or compression band; or have parent immobilize wearing lead gloves.

Central Ray:
• CR perpendicular to the film directed to the mid point of the part to be radiographed.
• Minimum 40 in. (102 cm) SID.

Collimation: Collimate closely on four sides to area of interest.

NOTE: Older children may require an optional oblique on exams including joints such as the hand. If so, a **PA hand** (rather than an AP) should be taken along with the lateral and oblique.

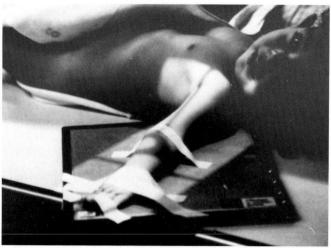

Fig. 19-42
AP Upper Limb (Secured with tape)

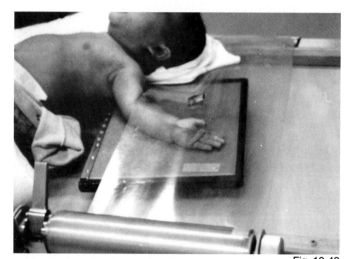

Fig. 19-43
AP Upper Limb (Secured with retention board)

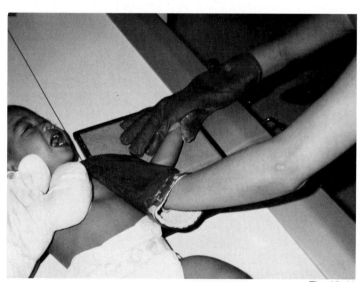

Fig. 19-44
Lateral Forearm and elbow
(Parent immobilizing)

Upper Limbs continued

Evaluation Criteria:

- **No motion**: Trabecular markings and bone margins should appear clear and sharp.
- Collimation borders should be evident on each side of upper limb without cutting off essential anatomy.
- Patient ID including date, should appear clear and legible, with correctly placed Right or Left markers without superimposing any body part pertinent to the diagnosis.

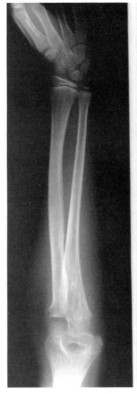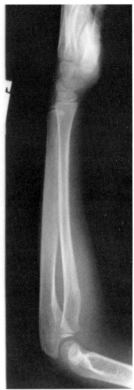

AP and Lateral Upper Limb

Fig. 19-45

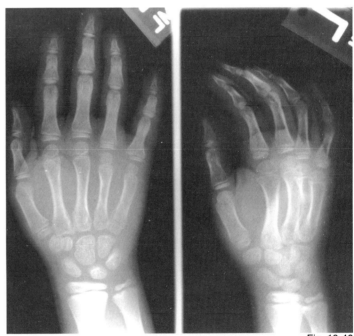

PA and Obli. Hand – 9 Year-old

Fig. 19-46

• AP and Lateral

For femur, knee, tibia-fibula and ankle.
(Foot may require separate projection of AP and lateral foot only)

Lower Limbs
Basic
• AP
• Lateral

Diagnostic Indications:

Arthritis
Avascular Necrosis
Blount Disease
CHD (Congenital Hip Dislocation)
Club Foot
Congenital Anomaly
Foreign Body
Fracture
Infection
Leg Perthes

Neoplasm
Osteomyelitis
Pes Cavas
Pes Planus
Post Reduction
Physiologic Bowing
Septic Arthritis
Slipped Epiphysis
Swelling
Trauma

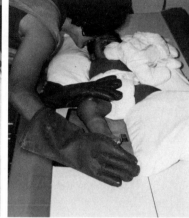

Fig. 19-47   AP   Lower Limb   Lateral   Fig. 19-48

Technical Factors:
• Film size is determined by the size of the body part to be radiographed.
• Grid not necessary for infants and small children.
• 55-65 kVp, shortest exposure time possible.

Shielding:
• Place lead gonad shield across pelvis, or over gonads, if proximal femurs are to be included.

Patient Position:
AP:
• With patient supine, immobilize arms and the leg not being radiographed.
• Place cassette under limb being radiographed, include entire limb from hips to feet. Align to cross-corners of cassette if needed to include all of limbs.
• Place femur as for a true AP projection rotating knee internally slightly until the interepicondylar line is parallel to plane of film. The feet and ankles should be in a true anatomical position.
• Immobilize the leg in this position with sandbag over the foot and compression band over the knee.
• If parent is being utilized for immobilization, have the parent hold the leg in this position with one hand firmly on the pelvis and the other holding the feet. A compression band may also be placed over the knees if necessary.

Lateral:
• Immobilize body parts not being radiographed.
• Place legs in a frog lateral position bending knees at an approximate 45 degree angle *(Fig. 19-50)*.
• If parent is being utilized for immobilization, have parent hold the feet and hips in position. The compression band may be placed over the knee area if needed.

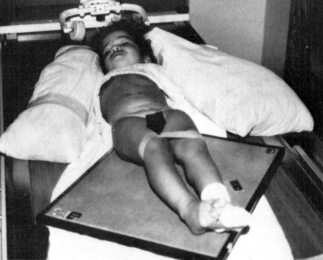

AP Lower Limbs   Fig. 19-49

Part To Be Positioned:
• Align patient body part to the center of the cassette.

Central Ray:
• Center the CR to middle of long axis of limb being radiographed.
• Minimum 40 in. (102 cm) SID.

Collimation: Collimate closely on four sides to area of interest.

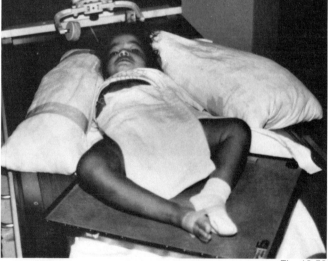

Lateral Lower Limbs   Fig. 19-50

Older Children:
• AP and lateral of femur and/or tibia/fibula may be taken separately as for adults with patient turned onto side for lateral position.

Lower Limbs continued

Evaluation Criteria:

- **No motion**: Trabecular markings and bone margins should appear clear and sharp.
- Patient ID information including date should be clear and legible with Right or Left markers not superimposing essential anatomy.

AP

- Lateral and medial epicondyles of distal femur should appear symmetrical and in profile.
- Tibia and fibula should appear alongside each other with minimal overlap.

Lateral.

- Medial and lateral condyles and epicondyles of distal femur should be superimposed.
- Tibia and fibula should appear mostly superimposed.

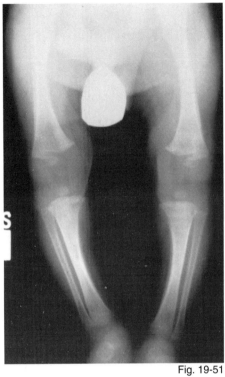

Fig. 19-51

AP Lower Limbs

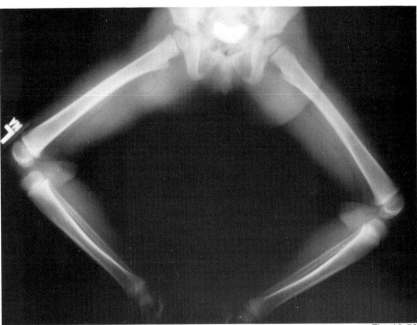

Fig. 19-52

Lateral Lower Limbs

• AP and Lateral

> **Pelvis & Hips**
> Basic
> • **AP**
> • **Lateral**

Diagnostic Indications:

Arthritis	Neoplasm
Avascular Necrosis	Osteomyelitis
Blount Disease	Pes Cavas
CHD (Congenital Hip Dislocation)	Pes Planus
Club Foot	Post Reduction
Congenital Anomaly	Physiologic Bowing
Foreign Body	Septic Arthritis
Fracture	Slipped Epiphysis
Infection	Swelling
Leg Perthes	Trauma

Technical Factors:
- Film size is determined by the size of body part to be radiographed, film crosswise.
- Use table Bucky or portable grid if more than 9 cm.
- 60-65 kVp, shortest exposure time possible.

Shielding:
- Before radiographing the patient discuss the examination with the radiologist. Patient's history may require that a gonad shield not be used.
- Female: Carefully shield the gonadal area. Place the female pediatric shield under the umbilicus and above the pubis. This will avoid covering the hip joints.
- Male: Carefully place the male pediatric shield at the level of the symphysis pubis.

Patient and Part Position:
- Align patient to center of table and/or film holder.
- Immobilize patient so that pelvis is not rotated.
- Immobilize arms with sand bags or Tam-em Board.

AP:
With patient in supine position, position hips for the AP projection by rotating knees and feet internally so that the anterior feet cross each other.
- Immobilize lower limbs in this position with tape and sandbags.

Lateral:
- "Frog" the legs by placing the soles of the feet together, knees bent and abducted. Bring patient heels as close to the distal pelvis as possible and tape soles of feet together.
- Keep the knees in the lateral position by securing tape to one side of the table crossing over both knees to the other side of the table. This can also be accomplished by using a compression band.

Central Ray:
- CR perpendicular to film, centered at the level of the hips.
- Minimum 40 in. (102 cm) SID.

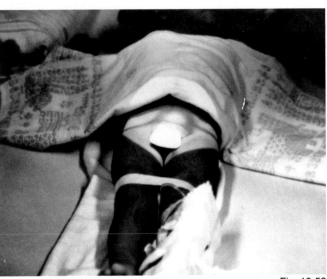

AP Pelvis

Fig. 19-53

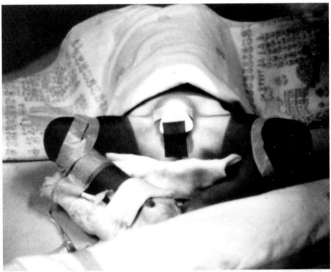

Lateral Hips and Proximal Femora

Fig. 19-54

Collimation: Collimate closely on four sides to area of interest.

Respiration:
- Infants and small children: Watch breathing pattern. When the abdomen is still make the exposure.
- If the patient is crying, watch for the abdomen to be in full extension.

Pelvis and Hips continued

Evaluation Criteria:

- **No rotation**: Both iliac crests should be equal in size and shape.
- Femoral heads should be perpendicular to the acetabula.
- **No motion**: Trabecular markings and margins of bones should appear clear and sharp.
- Correctly placed gonadal shielding should be evident on both male and female, without obscuring the hip joints (unless contraindicated by radiologist).
- Patient ID information including date should be clear and legible with correctly placed Right or Left markers not superimposing essential anatomy.

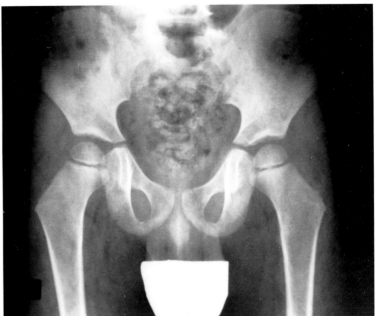

AP Hips and Proximal Femora (male) Fig. 19-55

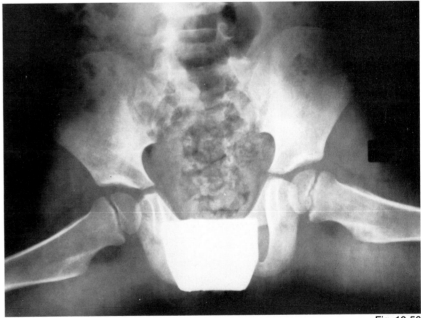

Lateral Hips and Proximal Femora (male) Fig. 19-56

• AP Projections

Skull (Head)
Basic
• **AP**
• Lateral

Diagnostic Indications:

Abnormal Sella
Congenital Anomalies
Croup
Epiglottitis
Headaches
Hearing Loss
Hydrocephalus
Mastoiditis
Post-Op

Shunt Check
Stridor
Sinugitis
Sidereal Synosto
Reconstruction
Retro Pharyngeal
Abscess
Trauma
Tumor

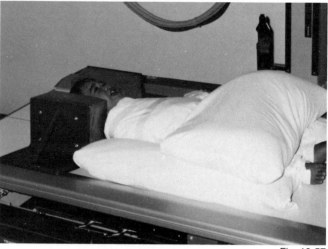

Patient mummified, sandbags and head supports in use
Fig. 19-57

Technical Factors:
• Film Size: Infants and small children
     - 8 x 10 in. (18 x 24 cm), crosswise.
   Children and young adolescents
     - 10 x 12 in (24 x 30 cm) crosswise.
• Use table Bucky, or portable grid.
• 65-70 kVp, shortest exposure time possible.

Shielding: Secure or place lead shield over pelvic area.

Patient Position:
• Mummify patient's body and limbs (necessary for most infants and small children).
• Patient supine, aligned to midline of table.
• If patient is combative, place sandbags over patient's legs and on each side of mummified body. Use compression band if needed.

Part Position:
• Position head with **no rotation.**
• Adjust chin so **orbitomeatal line is perpendicular to film.**
• Immobilize head with head clamps or head supports as demonstrated.
• Tape may also be used if necessary but turn adhesive side out over patient area so as not to adhere to skin.

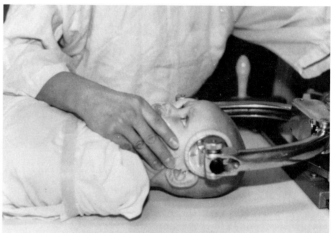

Patient mummified, head clamps in use
Fig. 19-58

Central Ray:
• CR **centered to glabella**, perpendicular to film for AP; a 15° cephalic for Caldwell; 30° caudal for axial (Towne).
• Center cassette to CR.
• Minimum 40 in. (102 cm) SID.

Collimation: Collimate closely on four sides to outer margins of skull.

NOTE: Generally holding by parent is **not** needed for exams of the head.

Evaluation Criteria:
• **No motion**, as evidenced by sharp margins of bony structures.
• **No rotation**, as evidenced by symmetrical orbits at equal distances from outer skull margins.
• Sufficient penetration and exposure should be evident to visualize the frontal bone and the petrous pyramids and dorsum sellae on the 30° axial.
• Patient ID information with Right or Left marker should be visible without superimposing essential anatomy.
AP with 15° cephalic angle:
• Petrous pyramids and internal auditory canals are projected into lower one-half to one-third of orbits.
AP with 30° cephalic angle:
• Petrous pyramids are projected below the inferior orbital rim, allowing vizualization of the entire orbital margin.
• Dorsum sella and posterior clinoids are projected into foramen magnum.

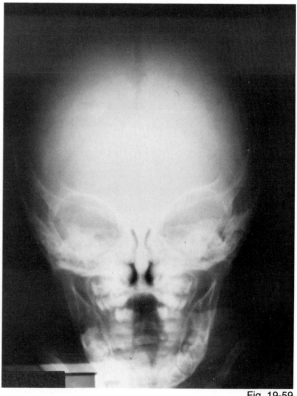

AP skull
Fig. 19-59

• Lateral Position

Skull (Head)
Basic
• AP
• **Lateral**

Diagnostic Indications
Same as AP projection on preceding page.

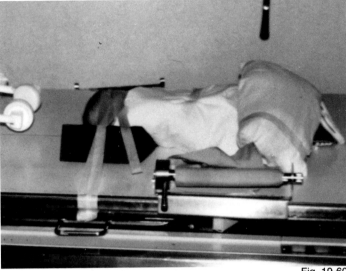

Lateral Skull – Infant　Fig. 19-60

Technical Factors:
• Film Size
  Infants and small children
  - 8 x 10 in. (18 x 24 cm) crosswise.
  Children and young adolescents
  - 10 x 12 in. (24 x 30 cm) crosswise.
• Use table Bucky or portable grid.
• 65-70 kVp, shortest exposure time possible.

10 (12)
8 (10) R

Shielding: Secure or place lead shield over pelvic area.

Patient Position:
• Mummify patient's body and limbs (necessary for most infants and small children).
• Patient in semiprone position, centered to midline of table. Place sandbags along patient's back and under elevated side of body.
• If patient is combative, place sandbag across buttocks with compression band across sandbags if needed.

Part Position:
• Rotate head into true lateral position and maintain by placing a sponge or folded towel under mandible.
• Place weighted support or sponge and sandbag behind head to prevent from pushing their head backward.
• Use compression band across head, or use tape by securing tape to each side of table and crossing patient's head with adhesive side up to prevent adhering to skin. Sandbags can also be placed over tape to prevent patient from lifting head from tabletop.

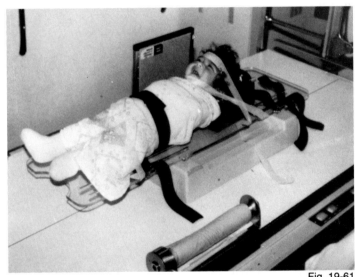

Crosstable Lateral with Tam-em Board – Infant　Fig. 19-61

Central Ray:
• CR perpendicular to film, centered midway between glabella and occipital protuberance.
• Center cassette to CR.
• Minimum 40 in. (102 cm) SID.

Collimation: Collimate closely on four sides to outer margins of skull.

NOTE: For infants the Tam-em Board can be used for skull exams with the lateral taken crosstable as shown in *Fig. 19-61* .

Evaluation Criteria:
• **No motion**, as evidenced by sharp margins of bony structures.
• **No rotation**, as evidenced by superimposed rami of mandible, orbital roofs and greater and lesser wings of sphenoid.
• Sella turcica and clivus are demonstrated in profile without rotation.
• Sufficient penetration and exposure should visualize parietal region and the lateral view outline of the sella turcica without overexposing perimeter margins of skull.
• Patient ID information with Right or Left marker should be visible without superimposing essential anatomy.

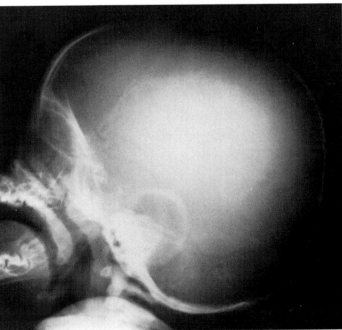

Lateral Skull　Fig. 19-62

Chapter 20

Conventional Tomography

Marianne Tortorici, RT(R), Ed.D.
Patrick Apfel, RT(R), M.Ed.

Contents

Drawings in Figs. 20-2, 20-6, 20-7, 20-8, 20-11, 20-12, 20-13, 20-14, 20-15 have been adapted with permission from: Tortorici, M,: Concepts in Medical Radiographic Imaging, Philadelphia: W. B. Saunders Co., 1992

National Survey Questions on Possible Discontinued Procedures:

A national survey included questions on the **quantity** of specific procedures such as conventional tomograms being done in their departments during the past year; the **expected trend** in the next three or four years; and whether or not the procedure **should still be taught and included** in a basic student textbook. The results were as follows: (The number of responding institutions is indicated in parentheses for each region.)

Conventional Tomograms	U.S. Average (349)	East (125)	Midwest (161)	West (58)
I. Trend				
a. Increase	16%	20%	12%	20%
b. Decrease	37%	41%	36%	28%
c. No change	47%	39%	52%	52%
II. Annual Quantity				
a. 0-24	18%	18%	17%	21%
b. 25-108	40%	40%	39%	53%
c. 109-249	20%	20%	22%	16%
d. 250 +	20%	22%	22%	10%
III. Be Included				
a. Yes	95%	97%	93%	93%
b. No	5%	3%	7%	7%

Summary:

These results clearly indicate that the newer imaging modalities such as CT and MRI have not replaced the basic conventional tomogram.

A good understanding of conventional tomography as presented in this chapter also helps in understanding principles and terminology of computerized tomography (CT) as described in later chapters.

Purpose

Tomography is a special type of imaging used to **obtain a diagnostic image of a specific layer of tissue or object, which is superimposed by other tissues or object(s)**. This is accomplished utilizing accessory equipment which allows the x-ray tube and film to move about a fulcrum point during film exposure. The resulting radiograph is called a **tomogram**, which demonstrates a clear image of an object lying in a specific plane while blurring the structures located above and below the specific plane. *Fig. 20-1* illustrates a patient in position on the x-ray table for a tomogram of the thoracic region. A basic linear tomographic equipment set-up is shown in position behind the patient connecting the x-ray tube to the Bucky tray. The basic principles of conventional tomography will be described beginning with terminology.

Terminology

Since the tomogram represents a section of the body, this type of filming is sometimes termed **body section radiography**. Other terms sometimes used to identify tomography are planigraphy, stratigraphy, and laminography. The International Commission on Radiological Units and Measures (ICRU) in 1962 established the term, **tomography**, to describe all forms of body section radiography.

Since terminology may differ, following is a list of terms and their definitions as used in this textbook:
- **Tomogram** - the radiograph produced by a tomographic unit.
- **Fulcrum** - the pivot point of the connecting rod between the x-ray tube and the film.
- **Fulcrum level** - distance, measured in centimeters or inches, from the table top to the fulcrum.
- **Objective plane** (focal plane) - the plane in which the object is clear and in focus.
- **Sectional thickness** - The thickness of the objective or focal plane. (This is variable, controlled by exposure angle and tube movement.)
- **Exposure angle** - the angle resulting from the x-ray beam movement *(Fig. 20-12 and 13)*.
- **Tube movement** (or shift) - the distance the tube travels.
- **Amplitude** - the amount of speed of tube movement measured in inches or centimeters per second.
- **Tube trajectory** - the geometric configuration or blurring pattern of tube movement *(Fig. 20-2)*.
- **Blur** - the area of distortion of objects outside the objective plane.
- **Blur margin** - the outer edge of the blurred object.

Each of these terms will be used and illustrated in this chapter beginning with tube trajectory.

Tube Trajectories

There are five basic types of trajectories for tube movement in tomography *(Fig. 20-2)*. These are listed from simplest to most complex:

(1) **Linear** --------- (unidirectional)
(2) **Elliptical**
(3) **Circular**　　　　 (multi-directional)
(4) **Spiral**
(5) **Hypocycloidal**

In linear trajectories (sometimes available as vertilinear and curvilinear) the tube moves in one direction. These trajectories are therefore identified as **"unidirectional"**.

The tube trajectories for elliptical, circular, spiral and hypocycloidal all move in several directions and are therefore identified as **multidirectional** (pluridirectional).

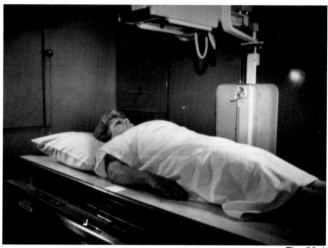

Linear Tomographic Unit　　　　Fig. 20-1

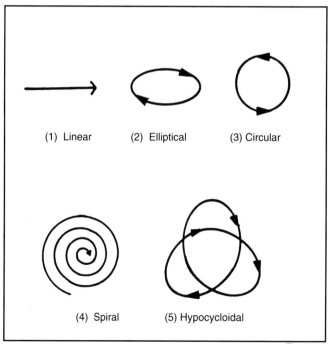

(1) Linear　　(2) Elliptical　　(3) Circular

(4) Spiral　　(5) Hypocycloidal

Five Basic Trajectories (Blurring Patterns)　Fig. 20-2

Unidirectional Tube Trajectories

Linear or unidirectional tomography involves the least complex type of equipment set-up *(Fig. 20-3)*. This utilizes a basic x-ray table with Bucky tray and overhead tube connected by a metal connecting arm or rod. This rod passes through an adjustable fulcrum level attachment (see *Fig. 20-4)*. This attachment is used to manually or electrically adjust the height of the fulcrum level.

Tube movement is achieved by a motor attached to the unit. Since the tube moves along the longitudinal axis of the table, the longitudinal tube lock must be opened (unlocked). The Bucky tray and tube angle locks must also be opened to permit these items to move freely.

Control Panel

The tomographic unit is operated by its own control panel. The options on the control panel vary from unit to unit. Common features of the control apparatus regulate the:
- tube travel speed (in inch or cm/sec) for those units with variable amplitude.
- objective plane (focal plane thickness, or sectional thickness).
- direction or type of tube trajectory or travel (on equipment with multidirectional capabilities).
- tube center.
- fulcrum level.

Some units are designed so that all features except the fulcrum level adjustment are on a control apparatus located in the x-ray room control area. In these units, it is common for the fulcrum level to be the adjustable type located directly on the fulcrum attachment connected to the x-ray table *(Fig. 20-4)*. Other units may also have the exposure angle selector located in x-ray table area rather than in the control booth area.

A large part of the object is parallel to the tube movement in unidirectional or linear tube trajectories. This limits the amount of blurring on the tomogram. It also creates an image having "streaks". The image clarity may be improved by maximizing the amount of perpendicular movement of the tube to the object. This is achieved by changing the type of tube trajectory to multidirectional. An example of multidirectional tomography is a specialized type of tomographic unit shown in *Fig. 20-5* used primarily for tomographic exams involving the skull.

Multidirectional Tube Trajectories

Of the four types of multidirectional movement, the least complex is the elliptical, which is a slight variation from the linear. The circular movement is "a step above" the elliptical pattern in complexity. The two most complex multidirectional movements are spiral and hypocycloidal. The more complex the multidirectional movement, the thinner the possible objective plane (see objective plane thickness section on a following page) and the clearer the image.

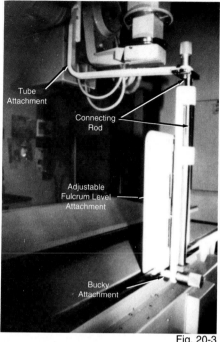

Fig. 20-3
Linear (unidirectional) Tomographic Equipment

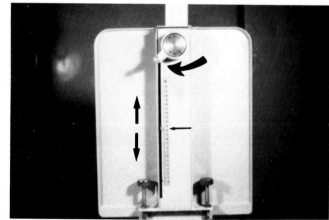

Adjustable Fulcrum Level Attachment   Fig. 20-4

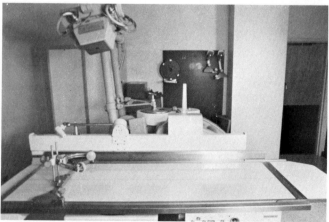

Multidirectional Tomographic Unit   Fig. 20-5

Fulcrum

The fulcrum is the pivot point through which the x-ray tube and film move. This pivot point is important because all structures located in its plane (objective plane) and parallel to the tube trajectory or travel remain sharp and in focus because they are in the same position (structures do not move) on the film during the exposure (see *B in Fig. 20-6*). Conversely, all objects located outside the objective plane, either above or below, are projected from one point on the film to another. For example see point A in *Fig. 20-6* as the tube and film move from position 1 to position 2. Point A starts out on the left edge of the film in position 1 but ends up on the right edge in position 2 resulting in movement or blurring of objects at point A.

Point C below the fulcrum level also in the same way is blurred as it is projected from one edge of the film to the other edge. (Point C is on the right edge of the film in position one, and finally ends up on the left edge of the film in position two.)

The amount of movement of these structures is determined by the distance the object is from the fulcrum. Consequently, the objects that remain stationary (do not move) appear well defined (sharp) on the tomogram while those objects above and below the fulcrum move and therefore are blurred. This is referred to as the **tomographic blurring principle**.

Variable Vs Fixed Fulcrum

The fulcrum level is used to determine the anatomical level of interest to be imaged. This may be achieved two ways. The most simple method utilizes a **variable fulcrum** (adjustable or movable). This is shown in *Fig. 20-7*.

A second method involves a **fixed fulcrum** and an adjusting height table *(Fig. 20-8)*. The fixed fulcrum adjusting height table is used most often with multidirectional or specialized tomographic units. In this system, the fulcrum level is changed by moving the patient and table up or down until the desired plane within the patient is at the level of the fixed fulcrum.

Determining Focal Level and Centering

To determine centering and where the fulcrum level should be, two 90° conventional radiographs are taken, such as a PA or AP and a lateral chest for a tomogram of a suspect area in the lungs. One radiograph, the PA, locates the object of interest relative to its lateral (right or left) position, e.g., 5 cm to the right of the spine. The lateral radiograph is used to determine the anterior/posterior location, e.g., 10 cm posterior to the sternum. Both radiographs are useful in determining the superior/inferior location of the object. By using the PA and lateral radiographs as well as knowledge of the basic location of organs, the technologist can approximate the site of the object or area of specific interest. The initial scout tomogram would be taken with the fulcrum set at the estimated level of the specific area of interest. Centering would be done by determining specific distances as measured on the PA and/ or lateral radiographs from known positioning landmarks.

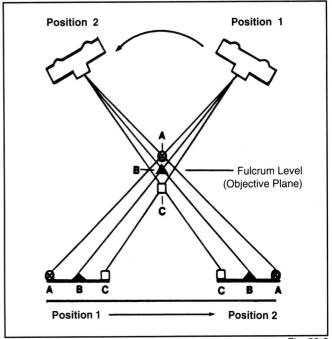

Tomographic "Blurring" Principle   Fig. 20-6

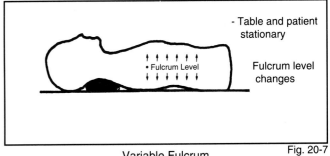

Variable Fulcrum   Fig. 20-7

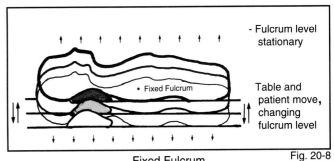

Fixed Fulcrum   Fig. 20-8

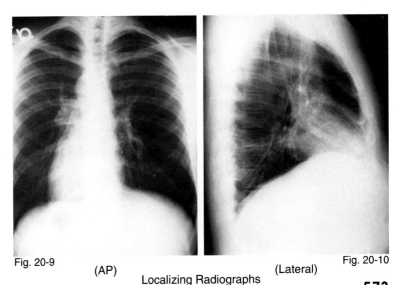

Fig. 20-9

(AP)   Localizing Radiographs   (Lateral)   Fig. 20-10

BLUR

Blur was defined as the **area of distortion of objects outside the objective plane**. In tomography the structures which superimpose the object of interest are blurred. These blurred objects or structures within the patient are either above or below the level of interest at the fulcrum level.

Influencing and Controlling Factors

There are four factors which determine the amount of blurring. They are:

(1) Distance the object is from the objective plane.
(2) Exposure angle (the degrees of angle of tube movement from position 1 to position 2).
(3) Distance the object is from the film.
(4) Tube trajectory (tube movement pattern).

The amount of blurring caused by the first two factors, (1) the distance the object is from the objective plane and (2) the exposure angle, is demonstrated in the following formula:

$$\text{Movement} = 2d \tan \Theta/2$$

Movement is a measurement of blurring wherein d is the distance of the object from the fulcrum, and Θ is the exposure angle. (Θ is the Greek symbol theta.)

(1) Distance of object from objective plane (d): The above formula reveals that if all factors except d remain constant, then as d increases, movement or blurring increases. This is demonstrated by comparing *Figs. 20-11* and *20-12* wherein the exposure angle remains constant at 30°, but "d" changes (distance from fulcrum plane to objects above and below). *Fig. 20-11*, with a greater "d" distance, has greater movement of objects A and C on the film from position 1 to position 2 therefore it has increased blurring.

This demonstrates that those objects within the body which are farther from the focal plane have greater movement and therefore increased blurring.

(2) Exposure angle (Θ): The formula also indicates that if only Θ (exposure angle) is increased and other factors remain constant, then the movement or blurring increases. This is demonstrated by comparing *Fig. 20-13* at a 60° exposure angle, with the 30° angle of *Fig. 20-12*. The 60° exposure angle increases the movement of objects A and C even if d remains fixed, thereby increasing the blurring.

Formula Summary: This formula demonstrates that as the **distance the object is from the objective plane increases** and/or as the **exposure angle is increased**, an increase in the amount of blurring occurs.

The net effect of this increased blurring is a **thinner focal plane** (objective plane) as described and demonstrated on the following page (*Fig. 20-15*).

(3) Object film distance: The third factor affecting blurring is the distance the object is from the film. **As the distance from the film increases, blurring increases**. This is not an adjustable or controlled variable but is determined by body part thickness, or by the general location or distance of the part being radiographed in relationship to the film.

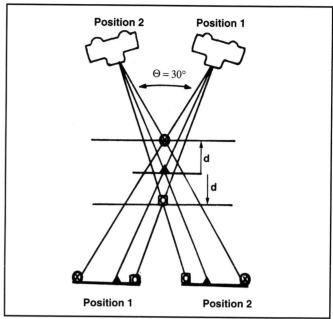

Fig. 20-11
Increase in "d" , Increase in Movement or Blurring

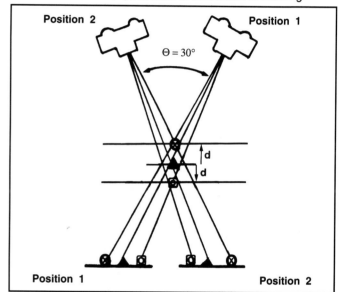

Fig. 20-12
Decrease in "d", Decrease in Movement or Blurring

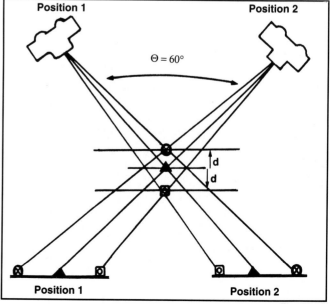

Fig. 20-13
Increase in Exposure Angle, Increase Movement and Increase in Blurring

Blur continued

(4) Tube trajectory or tube movement pattern: The fourth and last influencing or controlling factor determining the amount of blurring is tube trajectory or movement pattern. Maximum blurring of an object occurs **when the structure is perpendicular to the direction of tube movement.** In unidirectional or linear tube trajectories, the tube moves in only one direction. This results in a large portion of the object being parallel to the tube movement. Therefore **less overall blurring** occurs with unidirectional tube trajectory.

Conversely, multidirectional tube trajectories result in few parts of the object being parallel to the total tube movement. Therefore elliptical or circular tube movements result in a **greater amount of blurring.**

Maximum Blurring Patterns: The **spiral** and **hypocycloidal** movement patterns result in **maximum blurring** in that these include a vertical dimension as part of their multi-tiered movement resulting in maximum blurring of those structures that are both close and farther away from the focal plane. These movements are most useful in tomographic procedures involving the skull such as the small inner ear structures which require focal planes of 1 mm or less.

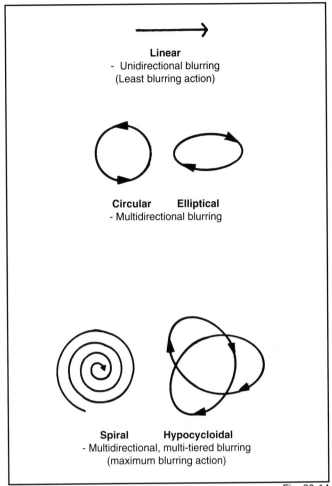

Linear
- Unidirectional blurring
(Least blurring action)

Circular   Elliptical
- Multidirectional blurring

Spiral   Hypocycloidal
- Multidirectional, multi-tiered blurring
(maximum blurring action)

Fig. 20-14
Summary of Tube Trajectories

Sectional Thickness (Objective Plane Thickness)

Blurring increases as the distance from the fulcrum level or objective plane increases as described above. This therefore results in a gradual process of blurring with those structures being the closest to the fulcrum level the least blurred, and those farthest away the most blurred. Also, the human eye is limited in its ability to distinguish blur from nonblur. Thus, the human eye accepts a certain amount of blur as being well defined. The amount of blur the eye accepts as well defined is subjective and varies from one individual to another. These combined factors result in what is defined as **sectional thickness**, or **objective plane "thickness".**

The **more blurring** that occurs, **the thinner the objective plane.** The primary factor affecting sectional thickness, and which is under the control of the operator, is the **exposure angle** *(Fig. 20-15).* It is advantageous to adjust the thickness of the objective plane to correspond to the object being imaged. Small objects are best imaged using a thin objective plane with greater exposure angle while large objects, such as the lung, should use a thick objective plane with less exposure angle.

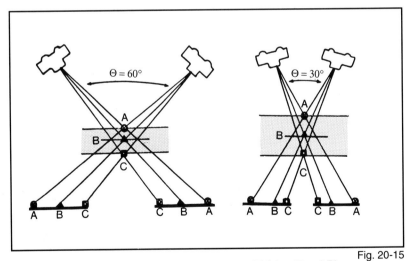

Fig. 20-15

Thinner Focal Plane   Thicker Focal Plane

Sectional Thickness
(Objective Plane Thickness)

Variations of Conventional Tomography

There are various techniques and imaging modalities which evolved from the fundamental principles of conventional tomography. The following is a brief discussion on several tomographic applications.

Autotomography (Breathing Technique)

In autotomography, the patient moves and the film and tube remain stationary. This is commonly termed a "breathing technique", which is easily performed on a regular conventional radiographic unit and requires no special equipment. The objective is to blur out structures (by having the patient move them) which superimpose the object of interest. Examples of autotomography are the sternal oblique *(Fig. 20-16)* and the transthoracic lateral of the proximal humerus. For these examinations, the patient breathes during the exposure which blurs the ribs and pulmonary markings.

Autotomography may also be a nonbreathing method such as a moving mandible to show the C spine as demonstrated in Chapter 9, *Fig. 9-71*, page 293.

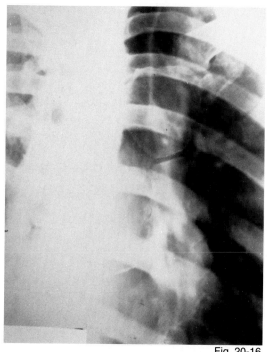

Fig. 20-16

Autotomogram - Sternum
(breathing technique)

Pantomography (Panorex)

Pantomography is used for curved body part, most commonly the mandible. An example of this is the panorex unit as illustrated in *Figs. 20-17 and 18*. In pantomography, the patient is stationary and the tube and film move. This is fully described and illustrated in chapter 12 on the mandible.

The beam restrictor of a pantomographic unit has a thin narrow slit (see arrows) which is essential for eliminating the diverging x-rays which normally produce penumbra blurring. This results in a pantomogram which has an image similar to a conventional radiograph *(Fig. 20-19)*.

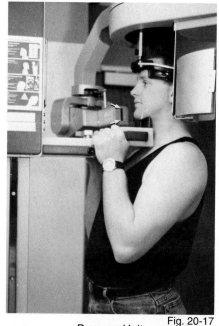

Fig. 20-17
Panorex Unit

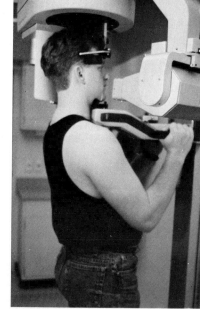

Fig. 20-18
Panorex Unit

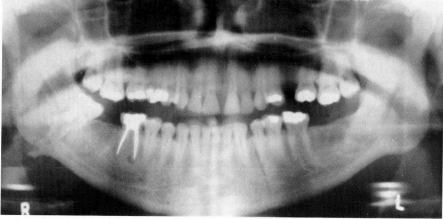

Pantomogram (panorex) of Mandible

Fig. 20-19

Variations of Conventional Tomography continued

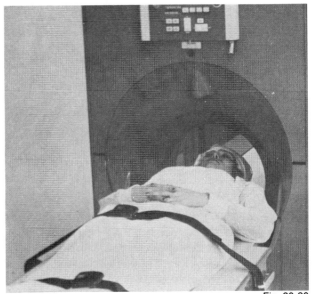

CT Unit   Fig. 20-20

Skip Tomography

Skip tomography is a tomographic technique in which the exposure stops during the center of the tube travel. This technique is most useful in body areas in which a dense object, e.g., bone, and object of interest are far apart, but overlay each other. Skip tomography is designed to "skip" or not expose, the dense object so it does not appear on the tomogram.

Computed Tomography (CT)

Computed tomography (CT) is similar to conventional tomography in that the tube and detectors (film in conventional tomography) move around a stationary patient. The primary difference is that CT does not use film to produce the image. Images are computer constructed via the detection of remnant radiation. The computer may be used to produce a "hard copy" of the image on film *(Fig. 20-21)*.

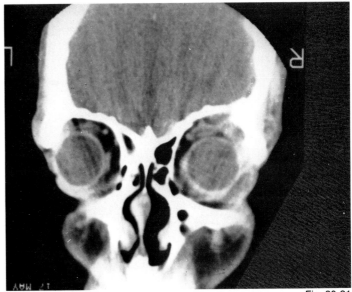

Computed Tomography of Orbits   Fig. 20-21

Chapter 21
Radiographic Anatomy and Positioning
of
Cranial Computed Tomography

Contributions by: Barry T. Anthony, RT (R)

Contents

21 Cranial Computed Tomography

Part I Radiographic Anatomy

Computed Tomography

The general principles of computed tomography (CT) are similar to conventional tomography as described in chapter 20 wherein the x-ray tube and the image receptors move about a focal point during the exposure. The primary difference, as described later in this chapter, relates to the use of computers to reconstruct the focused image or tomographic "slice" as received by the image receptors.

Prior to cranial computed tomography (CCT), direct imaging methods for the cranium could visualize very little except cranial bony anatomy. Occasionally a calcified structure, often the pineal gland, would visualize. Various brain tissues, cerebrospinal-fluid-filled spaces and blood vessels merged into a homogeneous gray shadow and could not be differentiated. Therefore, invasive special procedures utilizing some type of contrast medium were required to visualize the ventricles or blood vessels. A certain degree of risk was inherent in these special examinations.

The astounding success of CCT is based on the fact that direct information concerning the structure of normal and abnormal brain tissue can be obtained without subjecting the patient to painful and potentially fatal invasive procedures. Since individual anatomic structures can be visualized on computed tomograms, a good understanding of gross and radiographic anatomy is essential. Additionally, since CT's are viewed in sectional form, various coronal and axial sections are described in this chapter.

Anatomy of the Central Nervous System

The central nervous system can be divided into two main divisions: (l) the **brain or encephalon,** *(en-sef'ah-lon)* which occupies the cavity of the cranium, and (2) the **spinal cord or medulla spinalis,** *(me-dul'lah spi-na'lis)* which extends inferiorly from the brain and is protected by the bony vertebral column. The spinal cord terminates at the interspace of Ll and L2 with a tapered area called the **conus medullaris** *(ko'nus med'u-lar-is).*

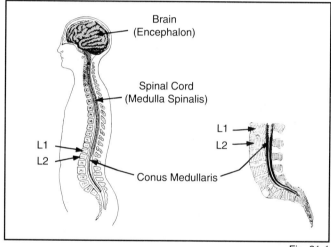

Central Nervous System

Fig. 21-1

Neurons

Neurons or nerve cells are the specialized cells of the nervous system that conduct electrical impulses. Each neuron is composed of an **axon, a cell body** and one or more **dendrites.** Dendrites are processes that conduct impulses toward the neuron cell body. The axon is a process leading away from the cell body.

A multipolar motoneuron is shown in *Fig. 21-2.* This type of neuron is typical of the neurons conducting impulses from the spinal cord to muscle tissue. A multipolar neuron is one with several dendrites and a single axon.

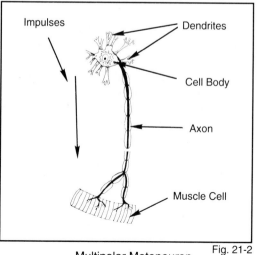

Multipolar Motoneuron

Fig. 21-2

Brain Coverings — Meninges

Both the brain and spinal cord are enclosed by three protective coverings or membranes termed meninges. The innermost of these membranes is the **pia mater,** *(pi'ah ma'ter)* literally meaning "tender mother". This membrane is very thin and highly vascular and lies next to the brain and spinal cord. It encloses the entire surface of the brain, dipping into each of the fissures and sulci.

The outermost membrane is the **dura mater** which means "hard" or "tough mother". This strong fibrous brain covering has an inner and an outer layer. The outer layer is tightly fused to the inner layer, except for spaces that are provided for large venous blood channels called **venous sinuses.** The outer layer closely adheres to the inner table of the **cranium** or skull.

Between the pia mater and dura mater is a delicate avascular membrane resembling a spider web and called the **arachnoid** *(ah-rak'noid).* Delicate threads attach the arachnoid to the pia mater.

Meningeal Spaces: Immediately exterior to each meningeal layer is a space or potential space. Exterior to the dura mater, between the dura and the inner table of the skull, is a potential space termed the **epidural** *(ep"i-du'ral)* **space.** Beneath the dura mater, between the dura and the arachnoid, is a narrow space called the **subdural** *(sub-du'ral)* **space** which contains a thin film of fluid. Both the epidural and the subdural space are potential sites for hemorrhage following trauma to the head.

Beneath the arachnoid, between the arachnoid and the pia mater, is a comparatively wide space termed the **subarachnoid** *(sub"ah-rak'noid)* **space.** The subarachnoid space is normally filled with cerebrospinal fluid (CSF).

Brain (Encephalon)

The brain can be divided into three general areas: (1) the **forebrain,** (2) the **midbrain,** and (3) the **hindbrain.** These three divisions of the brain are further divided into specific areas and structures. Understanding relationships between the structures in each of these three divisions helps in understanding the anatomy of the brain.

The forebrain consists primarily of the **cerebrum** *(ser'e-brum)* and involves two smaller portions called the **thalamus** *(thal'ah-mus)* and the **hypothalamus.** The hindbrain consists primarily of the **cerebellum** *(se"re-bel'um)* and includes the **pons** *(ponz)* **and medulla** *(me-dul'ah).* The midbrain connects the forebrain to the hindbrain. The combination of midbrain, pons and medulla is termed the **brain stem.**

Forebrain

The forebrain in humans is quite large and is located superiorly with the major portion being the cerebrum. The remainder of the forebrain is composed of structures located near the midline of the brain, including the thalamus and hypothalamus. Only the general areas of the thalamus and hypothalamus are demonstrated in *Fig. 21-4.* More detail on these portions of the brain is given later in this chapter.

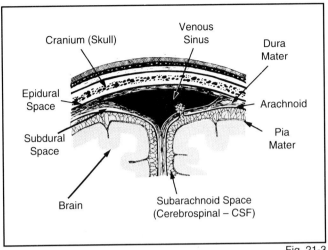

Meninges and Meningeal Spaces   Fig. 21-3

Brain Divisions

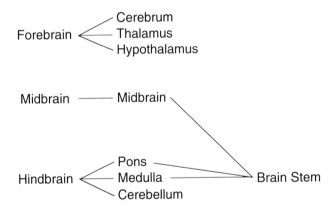

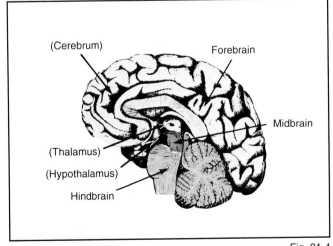

Brain (Midsagittal Section)   Fig. 21-4

Cerebrum

A sagittal section through the head and neck leaving the brain and upper spinal cord intact is demonstrated in *Fig. 21-5,* showing the relative size of the various structures. The cerebrum occupies the majority of the cranial cavity. The cerebellum lies inferior to the cerebrum and posterior to the brain stem. The spinal cord is continuous with the brain stem and is located inferior to the foramen magnum, the opening at the base of the skull.

Five Lobes of Each Cerebral Hemisphere: Each side of the cerebrum is termed a cerebral *(ser'e-bral)* hemisphere and is divided into five lobes. The four lobes seen in *Fig. 21-5* lie beneath the cranial bones of the same name. The frontal lobe lies under the frontal bone and the parietal lobe under the parietal bone. Similarly, the occipital lobe and the temporal lobe lie under their respective cranial bones. The fifth lobe is more centrally located and cannot be seen on a lateral view. The fifth lobe is termed the insula or central lobe.

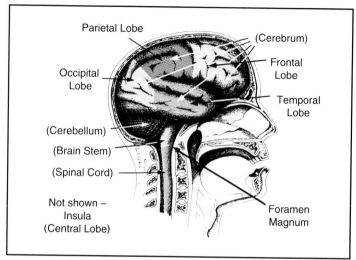

Brain and Upper Spinal Cord   Fig. 21-5

Cerebral Hemispheres

The top of the brain is shown in *Fig. 21-6.* The cerebrum is partially separated by a deep **longitudinal fissure** in the midsagittal plane. This fissure divides the cerebrum into a right and a left cerebral hemisphere. Parts of the **frontal, parietal and occipital lobes** are visualized.

The surface of each cerebral hemisphere is marked by numerous grooves and convolutions. Each convolution or raised area is termed a gyrus. Two such gyri, the **anterior central gyrus** and the **posterior central gyrus**, are shown in *Fig. 21-6.* Between any two gyri is either a shallow groove termed a sulcus or a deeper groove termed a fissure. An example of a sulcus is the shallow groove labeled **central sulcus.** The deeper separation between the two hemispheres, the longitudinal fissure, is an example of a fissure.

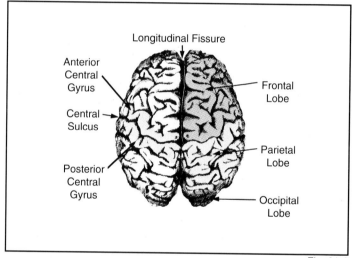

Brain (Top View)   Fig. 21-6

Cerebral Ventricles

Thorough understanding of the cerebral ventricles is important for cranial computed tomography. The ventricular system of the brain is connected to the subarachnoid space. There are four cavities in the ventricular system. These four cavities are filled with cerebrospinal fluid and interconnect through small tubes. The lateral drawing of the ventricular system in *Fig. 21-7* demonstrates the **right and left lateral ventricles, the third ventricle** and the fourth ventricle. The two lateral ventricles are located within the right and left cerebral hemispheres, while the third and fourth ventricles are midline structures.

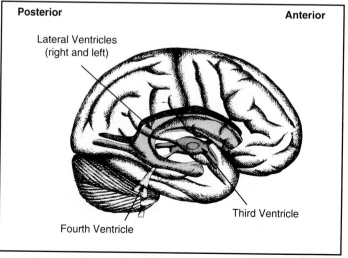

Cerebral Ventricles   Fig. 21-7

Lateral Ventricles

Each lateral ventricle is composed of four parts. The superior and lateral views in *Fig. 21-8* demonstrate that each of the lateral ventricles has a centrally located **body** and three projections or horns extending from the body. The **anterior or frontal horn** is toward the front. The **posterior or occipital horn** is toward the back, and the **inferior or temporal horn** extends inferiorly.

The two lateral ventricles are located on each side of the midsagittal plane within the cerebral hemispheres and are mirror images of each other. A space-occupying lesion or "mass lesion" would alter the symmetrical appearance of the ventricular system.

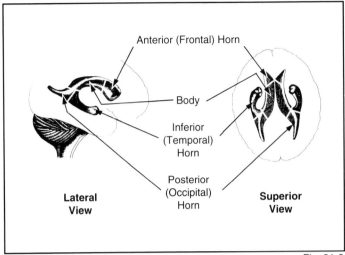

Lateral Ventricles   Fig. 21-8

Third Ventricle

Each of the lateral ventricles connects to the third ventricle through an **interventricular foramen or foramen of Monro.** The **third ventricle** is located in the midline and is roughly foursided in shape. It lies just below the level of the bodies of the two lateral ventricles. The **pineal gland** (pin′e-al) is located just posterior to the third ventricle and causes a recess in the posterior part of the ventricle.

Fourth Ventricle

The cavity of the third ventricle connects posteroinferiorly with the **fourth ventricle** through a passage known as the **cerebral aqueduct or aqueduct of Sylvius.** The diamond-shaped, fourth ventricle connects with a wide portion of the subarachnoid space called the **cisterna magna.** On each side of the fourth ventricle is a lateral extension termed the **lateral recess,** which also connects with the subarachnoid space through an opening or foramen.

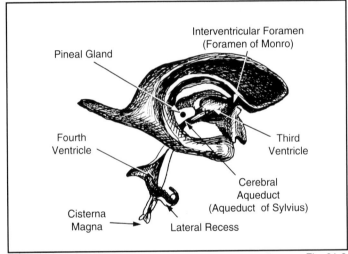

Ventricles (Lateral View)   Fig. 21-9

Superior View of Ventricles: A superior view of the ventricles is shown in *Fig. 21-10*. This view demonstrates the relationship of the **third and fourth ventricles** to the two **lateral ventricles.** The third ventricle is a narrow, slitlike structure lying in the midline between and below the bodies of the lateral ventricles. The **cerebral aqueduct** is clearly shown connecting the third ventricle to the fourth ventricle.

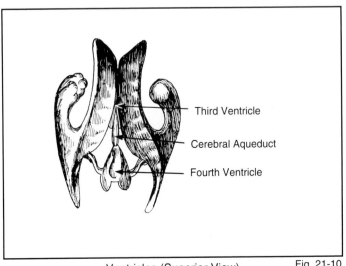

Ventricles (Superior View)   Fig. 21-10

Anterior View of Ventricles: An anterior view of the ventricles with the outline of the brain in place is shown in *Fig. 21-11*. The **interventricular foramina** connect the body of each lateral ventricle to the third ventricle. This view emphasizes the fact that the **third** and the **fourth ventricles** are midline structures. The **anterior horn, body and inferior horn** of each lateral ventricle are shown on this drawing as they would appear on a frontal projection of a cerebral pneumogram.

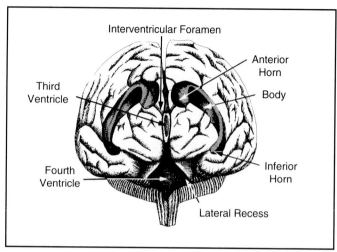

Ventricles (Anterior View) — Fig. 21-11

Subarachnoid Cisterns

Cerebrospinal fluid is normally manufactured within each ventricle. After cerebrospinal fluid leaves the **fourth ventricle,** it completely surrounds the brain and spinal cord by filling the subarachnoid space, as shown by the shaded area in *Fig. 21-12*. Any blockage along the pathway leading from the ventricles to the subarachnoid space may cause excessive accumulation of cerebrospinal fluid within the ventricles, a condition known as hydrocephalus.

There are several larger areas within the subarachnoid space or system called cisterns, the largest being the **cisterna magna.** These cisterns are usually named according to their locations. An example is the **cisterna pontis,** located just anterior to the **pons.**

The cerebrospinal-fluid-filled subarachnoid space and ventricular system are extremely important in computed tomography since these areas can be differentiated from tissue structures.

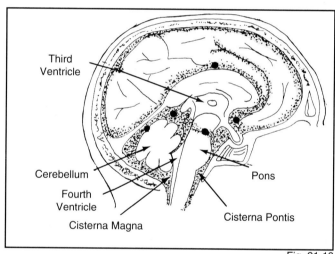

Subarachnoid Cisterns — Fig. 21-12

Other cisterns lie along the base of the brain and brain stem. The locations of these major cisterns around the base of the brain and the brain stem are shown in *Fig. 21-13*. Since the midbrain is totally surrounded by fluid-filled cisterns, this area can be well seen on a CT scan.

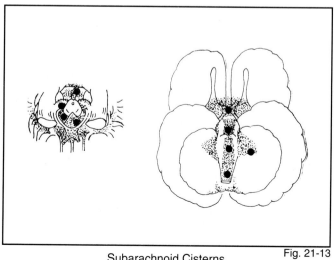

Subarachnoid Cisterns — Fig. 21-13

Hypothalamus

The third division of the **forebrain** is the hypothalamus. The lower border of the hypothalamus is shown in *Fig. 21-14.* Three parts of the hypothalamus labeled on this midsagittal section are the (1) **infundibulum** *(in″fun-dib′u-lum),* (2) **posterior pituitary gland** and (3) the **optic chiasma** *(ki-as′mah).*

The infundibulum is a conical process projecting downward and ending in the posterior lobe of the pituitary gland. The infundibulum plus the posterior pituitary are known as the **neurohypophysis** *(nu″ro-hi-pof′i-sis).*

The optic chiasma, so named because it resembles the Greek letter X (chi), is located superior to the pituitary gland and anterior to the third ventricle.

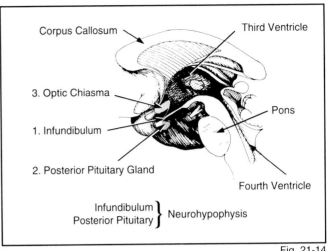

Fig. 21-14

Hypothalamus

Brain Divisions

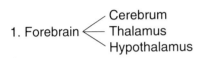

1. Forebrain — Cerebrum / Thalamus / Hypothalamus

2. Midbrain — Midbrain

3. Hindbrain — Pons / Medulla / Cerebellum → Brain Stem

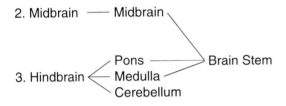

Midbrain

The midbrain is a short, constricted portion of the brain stem connecting the forebrain to the hindbrain.

Hindbrain

The hindbrain consists of the **cerebellum, pons and medulla.** As seen in the drawing in *Fig. 21-15,* the cerebellum is the largest portion of the hindbrain and the second largest portion of the entire brain.

Brain Stem: In addition to the pons and medulla, the brain stem includes the **midbrain.** The pons is a prominent swelling inferior to the midbrain. The medulla is the final portion of the brain stem, located at the level of the foramen magnum, the opening at the base of the skull. Thus, the **brain stem** is composed of **midbrain, pons and medulla,** and serves to connect the forebrain to the spinal cord.

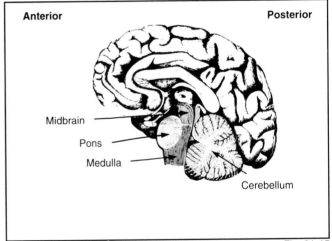

Fig. 21-15

Brain Stem and Hindbrain

Right Half of Brain

A midsagittal section of the brain shown in *Fig. 21-16* reveals the large **right cerebral hemisphere.** The **corpus callosum** is white brain tissue connecting the two cerebral hemispheres. The **thalamus and hypothalamus** are located centrally, beneath the cerebrum and corpus callosum.

Also shown on this midsagittal section of the brain are the three portions of the hindbrain, the **cerebellum, pons and medulla.**

Two important midline structures are demonstrated in *Fig. 21-16.* The **pituitary gland** is located just inferior to the hypothalamus, and the **pineal gland** is superior to the cerebellum.

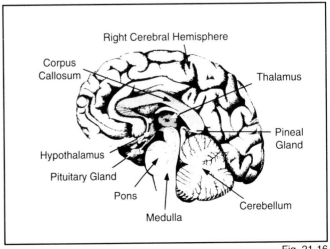

Fig. 21-16

Brain (Midsagittal Section)

Cerebellum

The second largest portion of the brain, the cerebellum, occupies the major portion of the posterior cranial fossa. In the adult, the size proportion between the cerebrum and cerebellum is about eight to one. The anterior and posterior surfaces of the cerebellum are shown in *Fig. 21-17.*

The cerebellum consists of two **hemispheres** united by a narrow median strip, the **vermis,** shown on the lower drawing of the anterior surface. Toward the superior end of the anterior surface is the wide, shallow **anterior cerebellar notch.** The fourth ventricle is located within the anterior cerebellar notch, separating the pons and medulla from the cerebellum.

Inferiorly, along the posterior surface, the cerebellar hemispheres are separated by the **posterior cerebellar notch.** An extension of the dura mater, termed the falx cerebelli, is located within the posterior cerebellar notch.

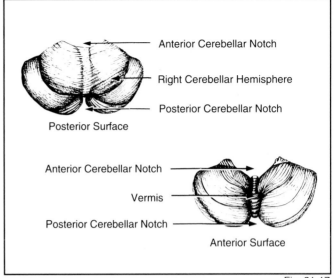

Cerebellum   Fig. 21-17

Gray Matter and White Matter

The central nervous system can be divided by appearance into white matter and gray matter. White matter in the brain and spinal cord is composed of tracts, which consist of bundles of myelinated axons. Myelinated axons are those wrapped in a myelin sheath, a fatty substance having a creamy-white color. Thus, axons comprise the majority of the white matter.

The gray matter is composed mainly of neuron dendrites and cell bodies. A section of brain tissue through the cerebral hemispheres is shown in *Fig. 21-18.* At this level of the brain, gray matter forms the outer **cerebral cortex,** while the more centrally located tissue is white matter. The underlying mass of white substance is termed the **centrum semiovale.** Deep within the cerebrum, inferior to this level, is more gray matter termed the **cerebral nuclei** or basal ganglia.

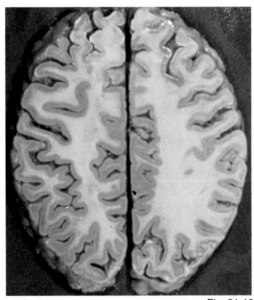

Brain Section   Fig. 21-18

Since a cranial computed tomographic scan can differentiate between white and gray matter, a section through the cerebral nuclei provides a wealth of diagnostic information. The horizontal or axial section of the right cerebral hemisphere shown in *Fig. 21-19* demonstrates those areas that can usually be visualized. Areas of white matter include the **corpus callosum** and the **centrum semiovale.** Gray matter areas include the **cerebral nuclei,** the **thalamus,** the **optic radiation** and the **cerebral cortex.** Any portion of the cerebrospinal-fluid-filled ventricular system provides an additional density and can be readily visualized.

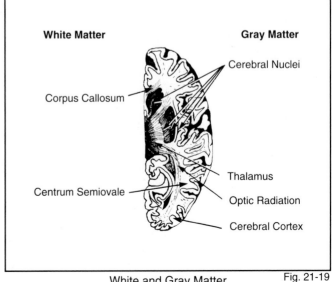

White and Gray Matter   Fig. 21-19

Cerebral Nuclei (Gray Matter)

The cerebral nuclei are collections of gray matter deep within the cerebrum, as demonstrated on the cutaway drawing *(Fig. 21-20)*. Four separate areas comprise the cerebral nuclei on each side. These are the (1) **caudate nucleus**, (2) the **lentiform nucleus**, composed of putamen and globus pallidus, (3) the **claustrum**, and (4) the **amygdaloid nucleus** or body.

The relationship of the **brain stem and cerebellum** to three of the cerebral nuclei and to the **thalamus** is shown in *Fig. 21-20*. The cerebral nuclei are bilaterally symmetrical collections of gray matter located on both sides of the third ventricle.

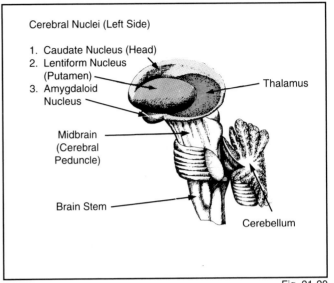

Cerebral Nuclei (Left Side)

1. Caudate Nucleus (Head)
2. Lentiform Nucleus (Putamen)
3. Amygdaloid Nucleus

Thalamus

Midbrain (Cerebral Peduncle)

Brain Stem

Cerebellum

Cerebral Nuclei

Fig. 21-20

Brain (Inferior Surface)

The inferior surface of the brain *(Fig. 21-21)* demonstrates the relationship of the hypothalamic structures to the other parts of the brain. The **infundibulum, pituitary gland and optic chiasma** are shown anterior to the pons and midbrain. Extending forward from the optic chiasma are the large **optic nerves,** and extending posterolaterally are the **optic tracts**. A portion of the corpus callosum is located deep within the longitudinal fissure.

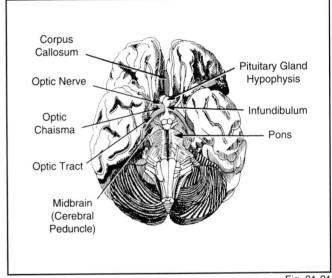

Corpus Callosum

Optic Nerve

Optic Chaisma

Optic Tract

Midbrain (Cerebral Peduncle)

Pituitary Gland Hypophysis

Infundibulum

Pons

Brain (Inferior Surface)

Fig. 21-21

Cranial Nerves

The twelve pairs of cranial nerves are shown on the drawing of the inferior surface of the brain in *Fig. 21-22*. The pairs shown are:

1. **Olfactory Nerve**
2. **Optic Nerve**
3. Oculomotor Nerve
4. Trochlear Nerve
5. **Trigeminal Nerve**
6. Abducens Nerve
7. Facial Nerve
8. Acoustic Nerve
9. Glossopharyngeal Nerve
10. **Vagus Nerve**
11. Spinal Accessory Nerve
12. Hypoglossal Nerve

The most important of the cranial nerves are numbers 1, 2, 5 and 10.

The familiar mnemonic, "On Old Olympus's Towering Tops, A Finn and German Viewed Some Hops," gives the first letter of each of the twelve pairs of cranial nerves and can be used to help remember these names.

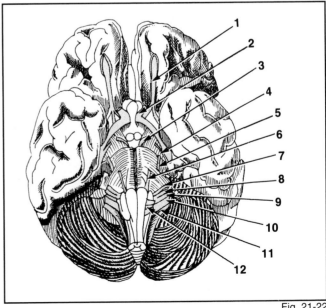

Cranial Nerves

Fig. 21-22

Orbital Cavity

The orbital cavities are often scanned as a routine part of cranial computed tomography. The orbital cavity as dissected from the front includes the **bulb** of the eye and numerous associated structures, as illustrated in *Fig. 21-23*. Orbital contents include the **ocular muscles**, **nerves** (including the large optic nerve), **blood vessels**, **orbital fat** and the **lacrimal gland**.

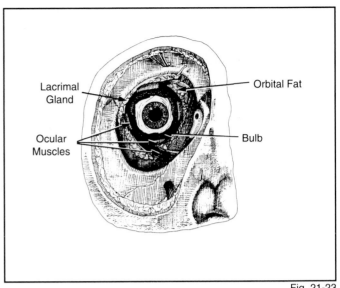

Orbital Cavity   Fig. 21-23

Orbital Cavities (superior view)

The orbital cavities are exposed from above in *Fig. 21-24* by removing the orbital plate of the frontal bone. The right orbit illustrates the normal fullness of the orbital cavity. The lacrimal gland in the upper outer quadrant, orbit fat, and ocular muscles help to fill the entire cavity. The internal carotid artery is seen entering the base of the skull. At this point, the internal carotid artery has already given off an artery that supplies the orbital contents.

The left orbital cavity, with fat and some muscles removed, illustrates the course of the **optic nerve** as it emerges from the bulb to course medially to the **optic chiasma.** Orbital tumors and foreign bodies can be readily detected through computed tomography of the orbits.

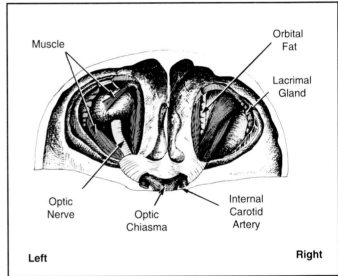

Orbital Cavities (Superior View)   Fig. 21-24

Visual Pathway

Axons leaving each eyeball travel via the **optic nerves** to the **optic chiasma.** Within the optic chiasma, some fibers cross to the opposite side and some remain on the same side, as shown in *Fig. 21-25*. After passing through the optic chiasma, the fibers form an **optic tract.** Each optic tract enters the brain and terminates in the thalamus.

In the thalamus, fibers synapse with other neurons, whose axons form the **optic radiations,** which then pass to the **visual centers** in the cortex of the occipital lobes of the cerebrum. Due to the partial crossing of fibers, sight can be affected in various ways depending on the location of a lesion in the visual pathway. An example is hemianopia, which causes blindness or defective vision in only half of the visual field of each eye.

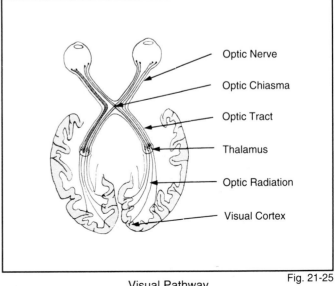

Visual Pathway   Fig. 21-25

Sectional Anatomy of the Brain

Familiarity with the gross structures of the central nervous system is important as well as the relative location of each because in CCT this anatomy is viewed primarily in cross-section. The rest of this part of the chapter on anatomy of the CNS now covers this anatomy viewed in various coronal and axial sections as seen on both drawings and CT scans.

Coronal Sections

Coronal Section 1

Cranial computed tomography displays thin, cross-sectional, gray-scale images of cranial structures. Understanding this type of radiographic information requires a good understanding of cranial anatomy displayed in sectional form.

Beginning with *Fig. 21-26,* seven coronal or frontal sections of the cranium are shown. The first coronal section presented is the most anterior, passing through the eyeballs and frontal lobes of the cerebrum. Those structures labeled in *Fig. 21-26* are:

A. Frontal bone
B. Falx cerebri
C. Cerebral cortex
D. Centrum semiovale of the frontal lobe
E. Crista galli of the ethmoid bone
F. Ocular muscle
G. Bulb or eyeball
H. Periorbital fat

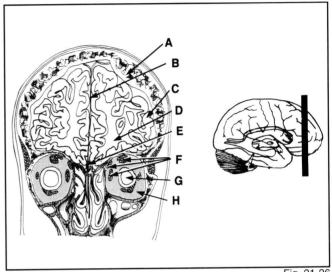

Coronal Section 1   Fig. 21-26

Coronal Section 2

Coronal section 2 is slightly posterior to the first coronal section. Those structures labeled are:

A. Superior sagittal sinus
B. Falx cerebri
C. Centrum semiovale of the frontal lobe
D. Corpus callosum
E. Anterior horn of the lateral ventricle
F. Temporal lobe
G. Optic nerve
H. Nasal septum
I. Maxillary sinus

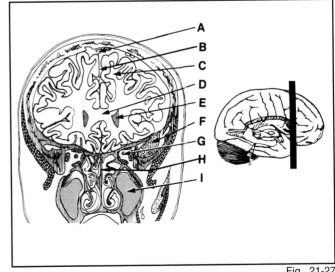

Coronal Section 2   Fig . 21-27

Coronal Section 3

Coronal section 3, represents a section through the pituitary gland. Those parts labeled are:
- A. Body of lateral ventricle
- B. Cerebral nuclei
- C. Pituitary gland
- D. Sphenoid sinus
- E. Greater wing of the sphenoid bone

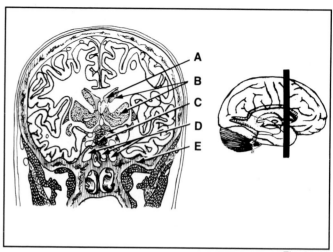

Coronal Section 3

Fig. 21-28

Coronal Section 4

The drawing in *Fig. 21-29* represents a coronal section through the main part of the thalamus. Those parts labeled are:
- A. Parietal lobe of the cerebrum
- B. Body of lateral ventricle
- C. Thalamus
- D. Inferior horn of lateral ventricle
- E. Pons
- F. Internal carotid artery
- G. Condyle of the mandible

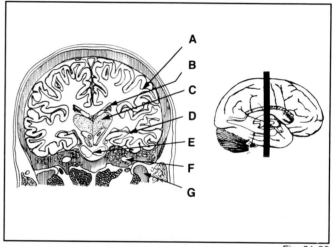

Fig. 21-29

Coronal Section 4

Coronal Section 5

The drawing in *Fig. 21-30* represents a coronal section through the posterior portion of the foramen magnum. Those labeled parts are:
- A. Superior sagittal sinus
- B. Inferior sagittal sinus
- C. Cerebellar hemisphere
- D. Midbrain
- E. Sigmoid sinus
- F. Mastoid process
- G. Medulla

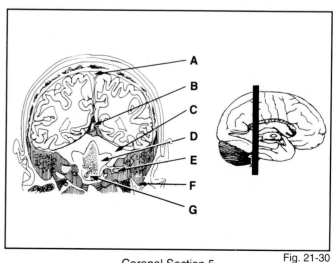

Coronal Section 5

Fig. 21-30

Coronal Section 6

The sectional drawing shown in *Fig. 21-31* depicts a section through the main substance of the cerebellum.
Labeled parts are:
- A. Superior sagittal sinus
- B. Parietal bone
- C. Falx cerebri
- D. Parietal lobe of cerebrum
- E. Inferior sagittal sinus
- F. Sigmoid sinus
- G. Cerebellar hemisphere
- H. Cerebellar tonsil

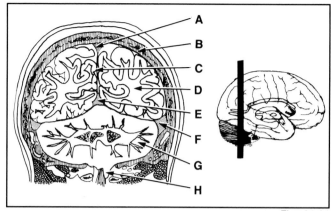

Coronal Section 6 Fig . 21-31

Coronal Section 7

The drawing in *Fig. 21-32* represents a coronal section through the confluence of the sinuses and is the most posterior of the sectional coronal slices. Labeled parts are:
- A. Occipital lobe of the cerebrum
- B. Occipital bone
- C. Confluence of sinuses
- D. Transverse sinus
- E. Cerebellar hemisphere

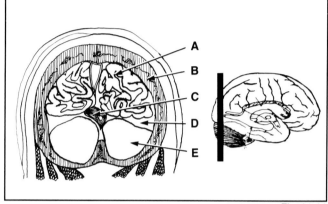

Coronal Section 7 Fig. 21-32

Axial Sections

Axial Section 1

Seven sectional drawings are now shown in axial orientation. Initial slices of the usual CCT scan are similar to the axial drawings. In computed tomography of the cranium, the patient's right is to the viewer's right. Axial section number 1, shown in *Fig. 21-33*, is the most superior of the axial sections and is termed the extreme hemispheric level. Parts labeled are:
- A. Anterior portion of the superior sagittal sinus
- B. Centrum semiovale (white matter of the cerebrum)
- C. Falx cerebri
- D. Central sulcus
- E. Cerebral cortex (gray matter of cerebrum)
- F. Posterior portion of superior sagittal sinus
- G. Cranium

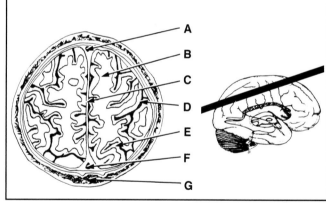

Axial Section 1 Fig. 21-33

Brain Tissue and CT – Extreme Hemispheric Level

An actual slice of brain tissue and a computed tomogram corresponding to the extreme hemispheric level are shown in *Fig. 21-34a and 34b*. Compare the brain tissue slice and the CT to the drawing in *Fig. 21-33*.

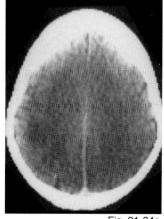
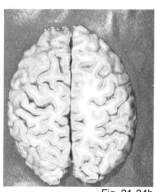

Fig. 21-34a
CT Section

Fig. 21-34b
Brain Tissue

Sectional Anatomy continued

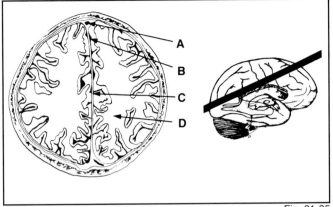

Axial Section 2   Fig. 21-35

Axial Section 2

Axial section number 2 *(Fig. 21-35) is* slightly caudad to axial section number 1. This level is superior to the ventricles and is termed the high hemispheric level. The anatomy shown in axial sections 1 and 2 is similar.

   A. Superior sagittal sinus
   B. and C. Longitudinal fissure with the Falx cerebri dipping
       down into the fissure.
   D.White matter of the cerebrum (centrum semiovale)

Brain Tissue and CT – High Hemispheric Level

A photograph of an actual slice of brain tissue and a computed tomogram corresponding to the high hemispheric level are shown in *Fig. 21-36a* and *36b*. This photograph and radiograph are at a similar level as the drawing in *Fig. 21-35.*

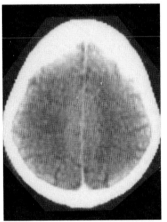
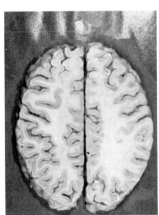

Fig. 21-36a   Fig. 21-36b
CT Section   Brain Tissue

Axial Section 3

Progressing farther toward the base of the brain, the sectional drawing in *Fig.* 21-37 progresses into the lateral ventricles. Those structures labeled are:

   A. Falx cerebri
   B. Anterior central gyrus
   C. Central sulcus
   D. Posterior central gyrus
   E. One lateral ventricle

The relationship of sulci and gyri are studied carefully by the neuroradiologist since the sulci are increased in size in cases of cerebral atrophy.

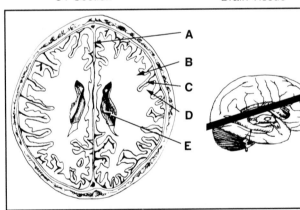

Axial Section 3   Fig. 21-37

CT – High Ventricular Level

A computed tomogram through the high ventricular level is shown in *Fig.* 21-38. Each lateral ventricle assumes a characteristic banana shape on the CCT scan at this level. The prominent cerebral sulci on this CCT scan indicate some atrophy of cerebral tissue.

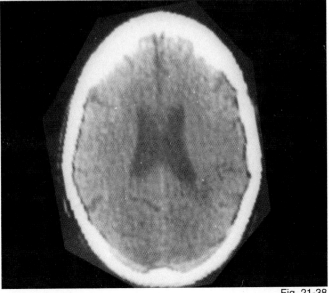

CT Section   Fig. 21-38

Axial Section 4

The drawing in *Fig.* 21-39 is of the mid-ventricular level. The deep-lying cerebral nuclei are visible at this level.

A. Corpus callosum
B. Anterior horn of the right lateral ventricle
C. Cerebral nuclei
D. Thalamus
E. Third ventricle
F. Pineal gland or body
G. Corpus callosum
H. Inferior horn of the right lateral ventricle
I. Straight sinus

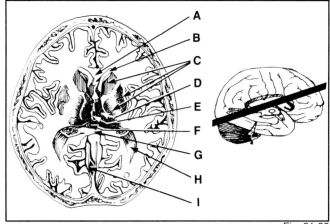

Axial Section 4   Fig. 21-39

Brain Tissue and CT – Mid-ventricular Level

The photograph of brain tissue and the computed tomogram in *Fig. 21-40a* and *40b* are at the level of the mid-ventricles. This brain tissue slice and radiograph compare to the drawing in *Fig. 21-39*.

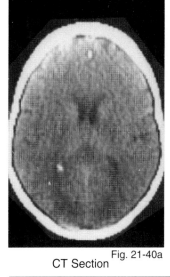
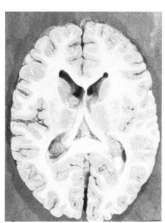

CT Section   Fig. 21-40a   Brain Tissue   Fig. 21-40b

Axial Section 5

The drawing in *Fig. 21-41*, titled Axial Section 5, represents a drawing of brain tissue through the mid-third ventricle. Cerebral nuclei are visible in addition to structures of the midbrain. Those parts labeled are:

A. Corpus callosum
B. Anterior horn and body of the right lateral ventricle
C. Cerebral nuclei
D. Third ventricle
E. Right sigmoid sinus
F. Cerebellar hemisphere
G. Internal occipital protuberance

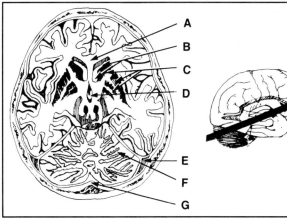

Axial Section 5   Fig. 21-41

Brain Tissue and CT – Mid-third Ventricle Level

A photograph of brain tissue and a computed tomogram through the mid-third ventricle level are shown in *Fig. 21-42a* and *42b*. This level corresponds to the drawing in *Fig. 21-41*.

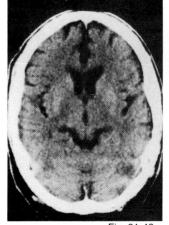
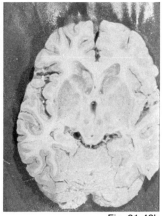

CT Section   Fig. 21-42a   Brain Tissue   Fig. 21-42b

Sectional Anatomy continued

Axial Section 6

The drawing in *Fig. 21-43* represents the tissue plane through the sella turcica. Parts labeled are:

A. Right frontal lobe of the cerebrum
B. Pituitary gland
C. Right temporal lobe
D. Petrous pyramid
E. Pons
F. Right sagittal sinus

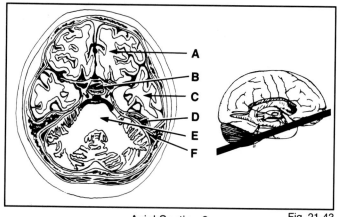

Axial Section 6   Fig. 21-43

Brain Tissue and CT – Sella Turcica Level

A photograph of actual brain tissue and a CCT scan through the level of the sella turcica are shown in *Fig. 21-44a* and *44b*.

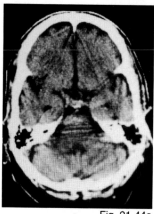
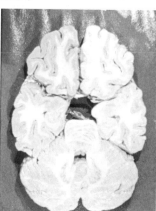

CT Section   Fig. 21-44a   Brain Tissue   Fig. 21-44b

Axial Section 7

Axial section number 7 represents a drawing of tissue in the orbital plane. Note in *Fig. 21-45* that a different angle is used to better visualize the orbital cavities. Those structures labeled are:

A. Ocular bulb or eyeball
B. Optic nerve
C. Optic chiasma
D. Temporal lobe
E. Midbrain
F. Cerebellum
G. Occipital lobe
H. Falx cerebri
I. Superior sagittal sinus

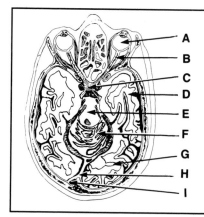

Axial Section 7   Fig. 21-45

CT – Orbital Level

A CCT scan through the orbital level is shown in *Fig. 21-46*. Compare the CT section through the orbital level with the drawing in *Fig. 21-45*. Note especially how clearly the ocular bulb and optic nerve are visualized.

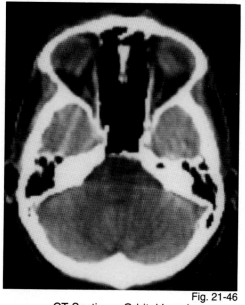

Fig. 21-46
CT Section – Orbital Level

Part II Basic Principles and Procedure

Definition

Cranial computed tomography (CCT) refers to radiographic examination of the cranium displayed as a thin, cross-sectional, grayscale, tomographic image representing a computer-assisted mathematical reconstruction of numerous x-ray absorption differences of the cranial contents.

Advantages over Conventional Radiography

Computed tomography has three distinct advantages over conventional radiography.

First, three-dimensional information is presented in the form of a series of thin slices of the internal structure of the part in question. Since the x-ray beam is closely collimated to that particular slice, the resultant information is not degraded by secondary and scatter radiation from tissue outside the slice being studied.

Second, the system is much more sensitive when compared to conventional radiography so that differences in soft tissue can be clearly delineated.

Third, CT measures x-ray absorption of individual tissues accurately, allowing the basic nature of tissue to be studied.

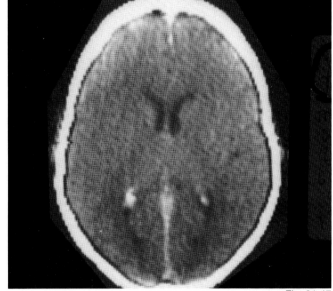

Cranial Computed Tomogram (Axial Section) Fig. 21-47

Computed Tomographic System

1. Scan Unit

All computed tomographic systems consist of four major elements. One major element is the **scan unit.** The scan unit provides large amounts of information to the computer. The scan unit is usually housed in a room by itself and is the part of the computed tomographic system seen by the patient. This room is often termed the treatment room or scanner room.

The scan unit consists of two parts: (1) the **patient table,** and (2) the **gantry.** The patient table or couch provides a fairly comfortable surface for the recumbent patient during the total scanning time. The gantry is a rigid support structure that encompasses the cranium within a central opening termed the **gantry aperture.** The depth to which the cranium is placed within the aperture determines the section to be studied. The gantry houses the x-ray tube or tubes and the radiation detector array.

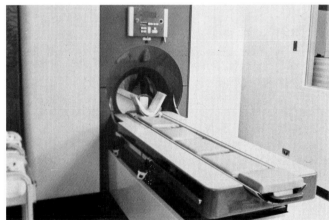

CCT Scan Unit Fig. 21-48

Scanning Position: The patient is shown in position in Fig. 21-49 for the first section or scan of a CCT. The tabletop is fitted with a cradle device to allow longitudinal movement of the patient. Once the patient is immobilized and positioned for the initial scan, the patient can be moved easily into and out of the gantry aperture using the cradle device. Once the patient is in correct position and the table height is set, the concentric point of the cranium coincides with the center of the x-ray beam geometry.

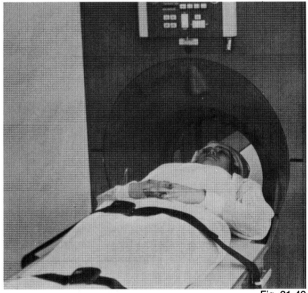

CCT Scanning Position Fig. 21-49

2. Processing Unit

A second element of any computed tomographic system is the **processing unit.** The processing unit or **computer** takes raw data and converts it into a meaningful picture form. It is the computer or processing unit that makes CT so different from conventional radiography and most other radiographic imaging modalities.

Huge amounts of raw data are received directly from the scan unit by the processor. This data consists of positional, reference and calibration information, in addition to all the individual absorption readings. The transmission readings alone can amount to more than 100 thousand bits of information. This mass of information is analyzed and converted to picture form for diagnosis. Modern ingenuity and computer technology allow the scanning and image reconstruction to be performed in a matter of seconds.

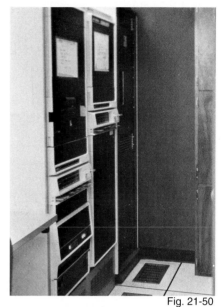

Fig. 21-50

Processing Unit or Computer

3. Display Unit

The third major element is the **display unit or direct-display console.** The reconstructed image produced by the computer is made visible by the display unit. Most systems project the picture on a gray-scale television screen. Various techniques are available to make the picture more easily interpreted. For example, portions of the picture can be enlarged, the contrast scale can be manipulated, and subtractions can be made to allow complete image analysis.

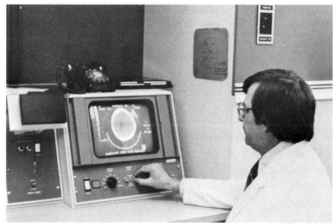

Display Unit   Fig. 21-51

Operator Console: The operator console is a part of the display unit and is located in the same room. Once the patient is properly positioned, all the necessary controls to proceed through each examination are located at the operator console. The radiographer communicates with the computer through a keyboard.

The operator console speeds the scanning procedure and minimizes errors by talking the operator through each step of the procedure. Several variables can be manipulated by the radiographer at the operator console under direction by the neuroradiologist.

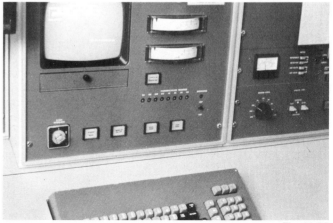

Operator Console   Fig. 21-52

4. Storage System

The fourth and final major element of all computed tomographic systems is a **storage system,** allowing individual computed tomograms to be viewed or reviewed at any time following the actual scan. Various types of storage are utilized, depending on the length of time the information must be held. Immediate storage is provided by the main memory of the computer system. Information is stored on a disc that holds a relatively small number of pictures. Immediate access is necessary to allow scans to be viewed while the patient is still on the table.

When full sets of scans are completed on several patients, the information is usually transferred to medium or long-term storage. The usual medium-term storage device is the floppy disc. For long-term storage, the information is placed on magnetic tape, as shown in *Fig. 21-53*.

Each of these storage devices—main memory, floppy disc and magnetic tape—store the complete picture information. When this information is retrieved, the image can be manipulated if necessary. Other forms of archival storage include radiographic or Polaroid film. These film methods only store what is seen on the display console.

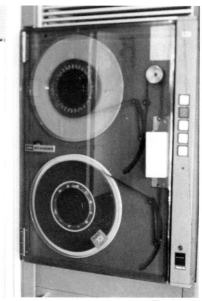

Fig. 21-53
Computer Main Memory

Basic Principle

The basic principle of computed tomography is that **the internal structure of any three-dimensional subject can be reconstructed from many different projections or views of that subject.** This necessitates the collection of large amounts of data in order to reconstruct an accurate picture of the original structure.

X-ray Transmission and Collection of Data

At least 180 different projections are required to obtain a diagnostically useful radiograph. This fact is demonstrated by assuming that the patient anatomy in question is a mass of homogeneous tissue with an air-filled cross in the center, as shown in *Fig. 21-54*. Several narrow beams of x-rays are directed through the section of tissue from right to left. All of the photons that pass through the tissue slice are collected on the left side of this "blockhead" illustration.

Due to the shape and configuration of the air-filled cross, more x-rays pass through the center of the slice than pass through either the top or the bottom. By plotting the intensity of radiation collected along the left side of the section, a profile of the emergent radiation is formed. If the x-ray beam were directed through the tissue at one-degree intervals until 180 readings were made, 180 different profiles would be formed. Collecting this large amount of transmission data for processing by the computer is the function of the scan unit.

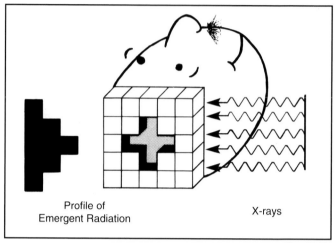

Profile of Emergent Radiation   X-rays

One Profile of Emergent Radiation   Fig. 21-54

Scanner Principles

Since the introduction of clinical CCT scanning in 1972, data gathering has progressed through four generations. The first generation scanners required about 4-1/2 minutes to gather enough information per slice of tissue. Each subsequent generation of scanner has decreased the amount of scan time necessary to gather the required volume of data. Fourth generation scanners require only 2 to 10 seconds per scan.

Fourth Generation Scanner

Fourth generation scanners possess a ring of 600 or more detectors, completely surrounding the patient in a full circle within the gantry. A single x-ray tube rotates through a 360-degree arc during data collection. Throughout the continuous rotary motion, short bursts of radiation are provided by a pulsed, rotating-anode x-ray tube.

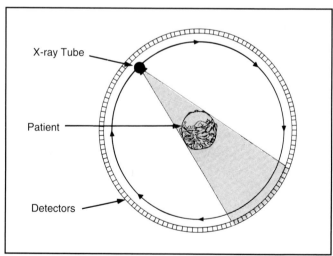

X-ray Tube

Patient

Detectors

Fourth Generation Scanner   Fig. 21-55

Source and Detector Collimation

In CCT, very close collimation is necessary to limit the radiation beam to the area of interest. The x-ray beam is actually collimated on both sides of the patient's head. The **source collimator** is located very close to the x-ray tube, and a **detector collimator** is located close to each detector in the detector array. The actual **thickness of the tomographic slice is controlled by the source collimator** and ranges from 1 to several millimeters. The detector collimators limit the amount of scatter radiation picked up by the detectors. Since each section is very thin, little secondary and scatter radiation escapes to neighboring tissue.

The location of the two collimators is shown diagrammatically in *Fig. 21-56*. The width and length of each individual transmission of radiation is limited by the collimators.

Volume Element (Voxel): After many transmissions of x-ray data, the reconstructed anatomy appears to be composed of a large number of tiny, elongated blocks. Each of the tiny blocks shown in the drawing of the "blockhead" represents a volume of tissue as defined by the opening in the source collimator. In CT language, each block is termed a **volume element,** which is shortened to **voxel.** Any CT slice is composed of a large number of voxels.

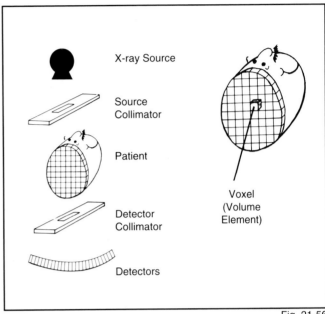

Fig. 21-56

Collimation and Volume Element (Voxel)

Principles of Image Reconstruction

The large amounts of data accumulated by the scan unit must be processed by the computer to provide a meaningful picture form. A simplified method of image reconstruction is shown in *Figs. 21-57* through *21-61* to demonstrate the principle utilized by computed tomography. The actual methods of reconstruction are much more complex and extensive than shown, but the basic principle is the same.

Exposure and Information Profile

Our subject is the "blockhead" with an air-filled cross located within a mass of homogeneous tissue. The total tissue volume of the slice in question is divided into a 5 x 5 system of **25 voxels,** as shown in Step A of *Fig. 21-57*. Step B of this illustration shows two beams of **x-radiation** directed through the slice of tissue in question. One beam is directed from right to left, while the second beam is directed from top to bottom. The collected data produces two **profiles** of information, as shown in Step C.

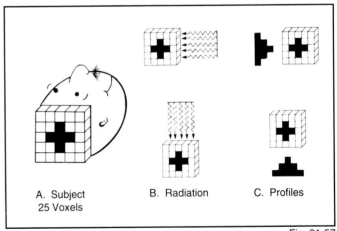

Fig. 21-57

Exposure and Information Profile

Principles of Image Reconstruction continued

Attenuation

Radiation is attenuated or absorbed more readily by the tissue surrounding the cross than by the air in the cross. Assume that each voxel of tissue absorbs one unit of radiation, and each airfilled voxel absorbs no radiation. This is represented in Step D of *Fig. 21-58* by assigning the **number 1 to each tissue voxel and O (zero) to each air-filled voxel.** Therefore, the two drawings in Step D represent relative attenuation values in very simplified form.

The next step, as shown by the two illustrations in Step E, is to **add the numbers in the direction of the two beams of radiation.** Each beam of radiation passes through a total of five voxels. The maximum number of 5 occurs along each border of the cross where the x-rays pass through five tissue voxels. Addition of numbers in the central portion of the cross results in the number 2 since only two voxels represent tissue in that direction. Addition of each row of numbers results in two profiles of radiation represented by the numbers, as shown in Step E of this illustration.

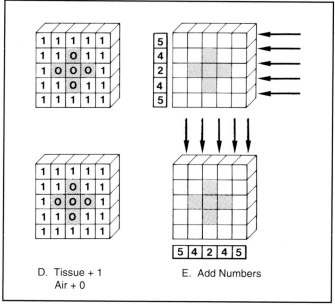

D. Tissue + 1
Air + 0

E. Add Numbers

Attenuation   Fig. 21-58

Summation

The next step involves **combining the two numerical profiles into one,** as shown in **Step F.** This is done by adding the numbers in each of the two directions. Therefore, the upper right voxel in Step F is represented by the number 10 since the transmission readings were 5 in each of the two directions. The sum for the lower voxel is 6, since 4 was obtained in one direction and 2 in the other direction.

The numerical composite, shown on the right in **Step G,** is the **sum of the numbers comprising each profile.** This addition process is essentially what the computer does with the large mass of transmission data accumulated by the scan unit.

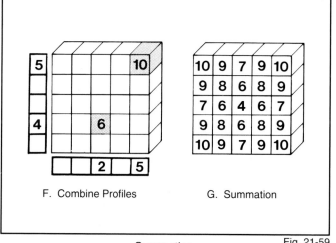

F. Combine Profiles   G. Summation

Summation   Fig. 21-59

Picture Reconstruction

The large amount of numerical data obtained by summation must now be transformed into a picture. This is done by **assigning various shades of gray, black or white to various numbers.** As shown in **Step H** of this illustration, the number 4 is assigned white and the number 10 is black. Any numbers between 4 and 10 are assigned darker and darker shades of gray, as shown in the table to the right in *Fig. 21-60.* A projection of this reconstruction as an image looks like the gray-scale drawing in **Step H.**

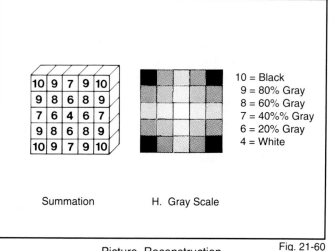

10 = Black
9 = 80% Gray
8 = 60% Gray
7 = 40%% Gray
6 = 20% Gray
4 = White

Summation   H. Gray Scale

Picture Reconstruction   Fig. 21-60

Principles of Image Reconstruction continued

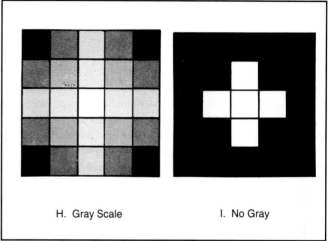

H. Gray Scale   I. No Gray

Image Manipulation   Fig. 21-61

Image Manipulation

Finally, the gray-scale image shown in Step H can be manipulated to give a more accurate reconstruction of the original image. Increasing the contrast or, in effect, removing the gray from the image results in a black and white image, shown in Step 1 of *Fig. 21-61*. This image results if any number equaling 6 or less is assigned white, and any number 7 or larger is assigned black. Basically, this describes cranial computed tomography. The internal structure of any three-dimensional structure can be reconstructed from many different projections of that subject.

Computed Tomographic Image

Degree of Attenuation of Each Voxel (Differential Absorption)

A computed tomographic image is shown in *Fig. 21-62*. Each voxel in the tissue slice is assigned a number proportional to the degree of x-ray attenuation of the entire chunk of tissue or voxel. Attenuation or differential absorption is defined as the reduction in the intensity of the x-ray beam as the beam passes through matter. X-ray photons are removed from the incident beam through absorption or scattering as a result of interaction with individual atoms or molecules comprising the matter. Many photons pass through the matter in question without any type of interaction.

Many variables affect the degree of attenuation. Variables include the energy of the x-ray beam, as well as the density, effective atomic number and number of electrons per gram of the subject matter. Generally, production of diagnostic images in radiology and in computed tomography depend entirely on the differential absorption or attenuation between adjacent tissues.

Converting Three-dimensional Voxels to Two-dimensional Pixels

Once the degree of attenuation of each voxel is determined, each three-dimensional tissue slice is projected on the television screen as a two-dimensional image. This **two-dimensional image** is termed the **display matrix** and is composed of tiny picture elements termed **pixels.** Each voxel is represented on the television screen as a pixel. The number of individual elements or pixels comprising the display matrix is determined by the manufacturer and may range from a fairly coarse matrix of 80 x 80 pixels to a very fine matrix of 512 x 512 pixels.

Computed Gray Scale

After the CT computer (through thousands of separate mathematical equations) determines a relative linear attenuation coefficient for each pixel in the display matrix, the values are then converted to another numerical scale involving CT numbers. Shades of gray are then assigned to the CT numbers. The end result is a gray-scale, computed tomographic image, as shown in *Fig. 21-62*.

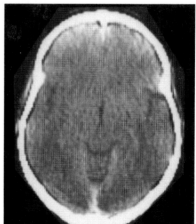

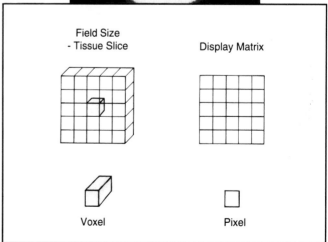

Field Size - Tissue Slice   Display Matrix

Voxel   Pixel

Computed Tomographic Image   Fig. 21-62

Cranial Computed Tomography Procedure

Purpose

The primary purpose of cranial computed tomography is to provide accurate diagnostic information, significantly improving the management of the patient. The ideal result is a definitive diagnosis that does not require collaborative tests for verification. CCT, in many instances, does provide this high degree of reliability. Acute trauma to the head, for example, may result in epidural or subdural hematoma formation. This type of lesion can be quickly, accurately and unequivocally diagnosed by CCT.

Indications

Virtually any suspected disease process involving the brain is an indication for cranial computed tomography. In the short time since the first patient was scanned on a prototype CCT unit in 1972, neuroradiologic emphasis has greatly changed. CCT has virtually eliminated the need for cerebral pneumography and echoencephalography. Furthermore, a substantial decrease in the number of cerebral angiograms and radionuclide brain scans has resulted.

Some of the more common indications for cranial computed tomography include **suspected brain neoplasms or masses, brain metastases, intracranial hemorrhage, aneurysm, abscess, brain atrophy, post-traumatic abnormalities** such as epidural and subdural hematomas, and **acquired or congenital abnormalities**.

Contraindications

Contraindications to cranial computed tomography are few. **About 50 percent of all CCT's do not require contrast enhancement**; consequently, these examinations are noninvasive. If the patient can be transported to the CT treatment room, the examination can be performed. With some very ill or massively injured patients, the transfer from patient room to treatment room and the transfer from patient bed to CT patient table may be the most hazardous part of the examination.

For the other 50 percent of all CCT's that require contrast enhancement, injection of an iodinated contrast medium is necessary. A very small percentage of persons may react adversely to an injection of iodinated contrast medium. A careful history must be taken prior to such an injection. Should the patient's history indicate a possible severe reaction, the patient's physician may choose to medicate prior to the examination or cancel the contrast-enhanced portion of the study.

Except for the patient with an actual history of severe reaction to iodinated contrast medium, and the nontransportable patient, there are no real contraindications to cranial computed tomography.

Patient Preparation

There is usually no patient preparation for a CCT. Unpleasant side effects such as nausea and/or vomiting may occur whenever iodinated contrast medium is introduced into the human circulatory system. For the contrast-enhanced examination, it is prudent to examine the patient with an empty stomach to prevent complications associated with premature gastric emptying.

Patient preparation may be necessary for the uncooperative type of individual. Patient motion during the scan is a serious impairment to the diagnostic CCT, so some cooperation is essential. Many circumstances may render the patient less cooperative than usual. Brain lesions may affect the patient in bizarre ways, depending on the location and amount of brain tissue involved.

Events prior to an acute head injury may include ingestion or inhalation of a variety of substances that may also alter normal behavior. Therefore, should sedation or anesthesia be necessary to allow scan completion without unwanted patient motion, appropriate medication must be administered by medical personnel. Preparation for resuscitative measures, including endotracheal tube placement capabilities, are mandatory for the sedated patient.

Contrast Media

The contrast media utilized for cranial computed tomography are identical to those used for excretory urography. These iodinated contrast media are usually administered as a bolus injection, but may be introduced via an intravenous infusion.

Complications

True anaphylactoid reaction to currently used iodinated contrast media is rare, but possible minor or major reactions must be foremost in the minds of radiology staff members whenever such injections are necessary. Complications arising from such injections are treated according to a well-established departmental protocol.

Postprocedure care includes careful observation since delayed reactions to contrast media are possible, although most reactions will occur within the first 5 minutes following injection if they are going to happen.

Scanner Room Preparation

Room preparation for a CCT is fairly simple. Basically, three steps need to be taken. First, the scanner or treatment room should be clean and tidy. All patients, as they are brought into the scanner room, should be made to feel that they are the first patient to utilize the equipment. Second, assemble any patient support items necessary. If oxygen, suction or IV pole are necessary, these should be provided. If the patient must be ventilated during examination or anesthetized prior to the procedure, the appropriate personnel must be assembled.

Finally, the operator console, direct display console and computer must be activated. The computer must be instructed via the typewriter to prepare for the appropriate procedure. If the examination is to be a contrast-enhanced procedure, then it is necessary to prepare for injection or infusion in the standard, sterile manner.

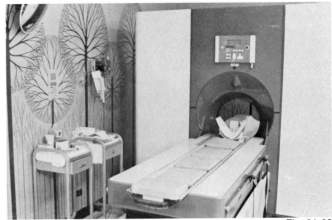

Room Preparation

Fig. 21-63

Cranial Computed Tomography Positioning

Basic Positioning

Routine positioning for cranial computed tomography is shown in *Fig. 21-64*. **The neck is flexed until a line 25 degrees to the IOML is parallel to the x-ray beam.** This positioning requires that the chin be depressed. An exact 25-degree angle is not absolutely necessary since both sides are seen on the finished reconstruction. More important is placement of the head so that no rotation and no tilt are detected on the scan.

The basic principles of skull positioning used in conventional radiography apply equally to computed tomography, with one major exception. In CCT, the **section of interest is placed parallel to the x-ray beam** rather than perpendicular to it. With accurate positioning, interested physicians can examine bilateral symmetry in the normal scan and asymmetry in the abnormal reconstruction.

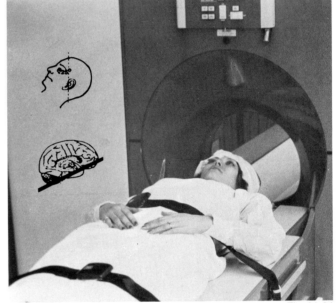

Routine CCT Positioning

Fig. 21-64

Alternate Positioning Method.

An alternate positioning method for routine cranial scanning is to use **a line connecting the** SOG (supraorbital groove) and the TEA (top of ear attachment). By placing this line parallel to the x-ray beam, similar results can be obtained when compared to the 25 degree to the IOML method. Positioning the head in this position allows most of the cerebellum to be visualized on the same slice as the area of the sella turcica.

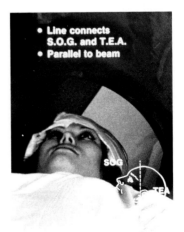

- Line connects S.O.G. and T.E.A.
- Parallel to beam

Fig. 21-65
Alternate Positioning

Procedure for Complete CCT

The procedure for a complete CCT scan may vary from facility to facility, but usually the initial sequence is six to ten scans. These **six to ten scans** cover the entire brain from base to vertex, in up to 13 millimeter sections. Depending on the scan unit in use, the sections may be thinner, such as 5, 8 or 10 millimeters.

The initial sequence is usually performed without contrast enhancement. Should enhancement be indicated, as determined by the provisional diagnosis and/or departmental routine, a second sequence is then performed. The same brain sections are again examined; but, for the second series, contrast medium is injected or infused.

CCT Scan

No Rotation: One of the axial sections in the cranial computed tomographic series is shown in *Fig. 21-66*. No rotation or tilt is detected on the section. The bilateral symmetry of the brain and cranial structures is demonstrated on this radiograph.

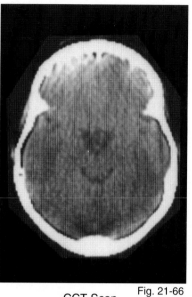

Fig. 21-66

CCT Scan
(Axial Section)

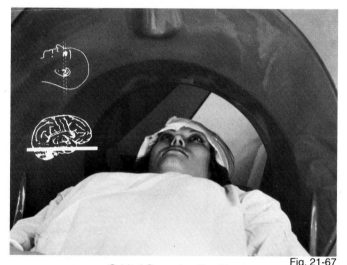

Orbital Scanning Position

Fig. 21-67

Orbital Scan Positioning

One variation to the basic CCT routine is **orbital scanning**. Some routines call for the automatic inclusion of approximately three sections through the orbits, utilizing a slightly different head position. The patient is shown in position for orbital scanning in *Fig. 21-67*. The head is in a neutral position so that the **radiation beam parallels the IOM line.** An alternative line used for the same result is one connecting the midlateral orbital margin and the TEA. This line is parallel to the IOML.

Orbital Scan

The radiograph in *Fig. 21-68* is an orbital scan utilizing the neutral head position. This radiograph clearly shows the orbital cavities, including the ocular bulbs and optic nerves.

Other positioning angles may be utilized to meet different needs. Certain scanners allow different positions to be assumed, including the basilar position for coronal sections. Certain units allow reconstruction of coronal sections based on axial section data stored in the computer.

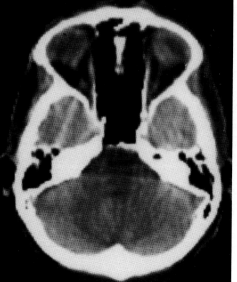

Fig. 21-68

Orbital Scan

Contrast Enhancement

The brain is well supplied with blood vessels that supply oxygen and nutrients. Oxygen must be in constant supply since total oxygen deprivation for the short time of 4 minutes can lead to permanent brain cell damage. Similarly, glucose must be continually available since carbohydrate storage in the brain is limited. Glucose, oxygen and certain ions pass readily from the circulatory blood into extracellular fluid, then into brain cells. Other substances found in the blood normally enter brain cells quite slowly. Still others, such as proteins, most antibiotics and contrast media, will not pass at all from the normal cranial capillary system into brain cells.

The brain is different from other tissues in that there is a natural barrier to the passage of certain substances. This natural phenomenon is termed the "blood-brain barrier." Contrast medium appearing outside the normal vascular system is an indication that something is wrong. A normal cranial computed tomograph is shown in *Fig. 21-69*, while the same level is shown in *Fig. 21-70* with contrast enhancement. Both are normal, without any disruption of the blood-brain barrier.

Examples of Positive CCT Images

Glioma

An example of a positive CCT is shown in *Fig. 21-71* and *72*. This particular lesion is a glioma *(gli-o´mah)*, a type of brain tumor. A noncontrast tomogram is shown in Fig. 21-71, and a contrast-enhanced version of the same slice in *Fig. 21-72*. Contrast enhancement is necessary for all suspected neoplasia due to possible breakdown of the normal blood-brain barrier.

Subdural Hematoma and Hydrocephaly

Two additional positive examples of cranial computed tomograms are illustrated in *Fig. 21-73* and *74*. A large bilateral, frontal, subdural hematoma of at least three weeks' duration is shown in *Fig. 21-73*. This type of lesion, whether acute or chronic, can be diagnosed without contrast enhancement.

Figure 21-74 demonstrates an example of hydrocephalus. Note the enlarged ventricles and how well they visualize on the CCT.

With well-maintained and properly functioning equipment, computed tomography of the head is not a difficult examination for the radiographer to perform, or for the neuroradiologist to interpret. CCT is an exciting, diagnostic, radiographic tool and is proving invaluable to the diagnosis of cranial disease.

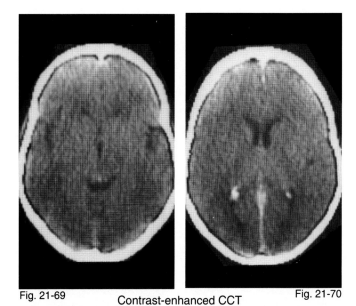

Fig. 21-69   Contrast-enhanced CCT   Fig. 21-70

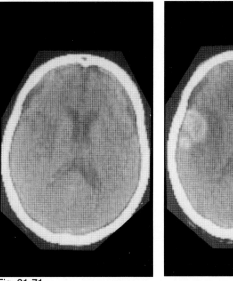

Fig. 21-71   Positive CCT (Gliomatous Tumor)   Fig. 21-72

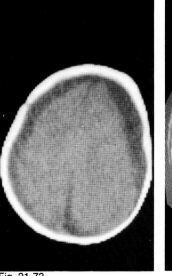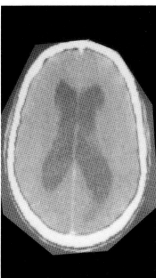

Fig. 21-73   Fig. 21-74
Subdural Hematoma   Hydrocephalus

Chapter 22
Radiographic Anatomy and Positioning
of
Thoracic, Abdominal and Pelvic
Computed Tomography

Contributions by: James D. Lipcamon, RT(R)

Contents

Introduction

Definition

Computed tomography refers to **a radiographic examination of a body cavity or body part in which x-rays and a computer are used to produce a cross-sectional slice of anatomy free of superimposed structures.** The images are representations of different shades of grays that correspond to the amount of x-ray which was absorbed as described in the preceding chapter on cranial computed tomography, (CCT). Axial or transverse sections of the thorax and abdomen are shown on the following pages.

Advantages Over Conventional Radiography

Computed tomography (CT) has become a well-accepted imaging device in diagnostic medicine. Excellent visualization of the site, free of superimposed structures, is the foremost advantage over conventional radiographic procedures. Its ability to discriminate differences in tissue densities (from .5 % to 1% in most scanners) make it a superior method. Because the x-ray beam is closely collimated and the scatter radiation reduced, excellent image quality is obtained.

Additionally, collected data can be manipulated and measured. By measuring the attenuation value, it is often possible to determine if a lesion is fat, fluid or calcium in nature. The extent and relationship of abnormal pathology to surrounding structures can be determined because the area can be visualized in two dimensions as shown in *Fig. 22-1*. Due to the utilization of the computer, software programs provide the capability of manipulating the acquired data into coronal and sagittal views.

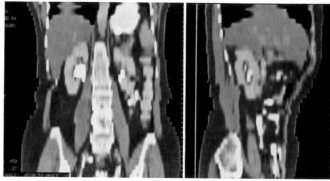

Coronal and Sagittal Reconstruction　　Fig. 22-1

Computed Tomographic System

Chapter 21 on cranial computed tomography explains not only the basic principles of computed tomography but also the various **components** of a computed tomographic system. These components include the **scan unit** (made up of the patient table or couch and the gantry), the **processing unit or computer, the display unit or console** and the **storage system.**

The earlier models of CT systems included a scanning unit with smaller apertures so that only smaller parts such as patients' heads could be scanned. Later model whole body scanners have larger apertures so entire bodies including chest, abdomen and pelvic area can be scanned, as described and illustrated in this chapter .

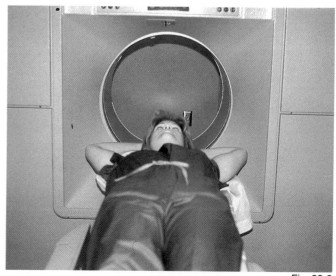

Whole Body Scanner　　Fig. 22-2
(Gantry and Table)

Part I Radiographic Anatomy

The anatomy of the thorax is covered thoroughly in **Chapter 2** on general chest anatomy, **Chapter 10** on the bony thorax and **Chapter 23** on the heart and circulatory system of the thorax. The anatomy from these chapters should be mastered before continuing with this study of sectional anatomy.

Thoracic computed tomography requires a thorough understanding of sectional anatomy of the thorax as viewed in **axial sections.**

Axial Sections of the Chest

Ten slices or sections of line drawings of the chest with corresponding CT scans of 10 mm thickness are shown in the axial orientation. The examination for these scans was obtained using bolus injections of intravenous contrast. The total volume used was 180 cc's. The patient's right is on the viewer's left as with conventional radiography.

Axial Section 1
Axial section number 1, shown in *Fig. 22-3*, represents a section at **the level of the sternal notch.** Parts labeled are:
  A. Right internal jugular vein
  B. Right carotid artery
  C. Left internal jugular vein
  D. Left subclavian artery
  E. Left carotid artery
  F. Right subclavian artery

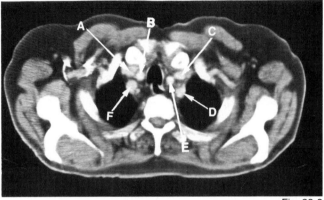

Axial Section 1   Fig. 22-3

Axial Section 2
Axial section 2 represents a section through the **superior portion of the manubrium.** Parts labeled are:
  A. Right brachiocephalic vein
  B. Right carotid artery
  C. Left carotid artery
  D. Left subclavian artery
  E. Esophagus
  F. Trachea
  G. Right subclavian artery

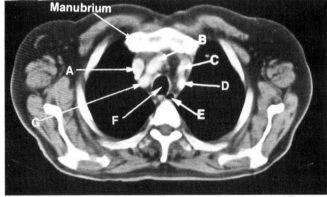

Axial Section 2   Fig. 22-4

Axial Section 3
Axial section 3 represents a section through the **inferior portion of the manubrium.** Parts labeled are:
  A. Right brachiocephalic vein
  B. Brachiocephalic artery (Innominate)
  C. Left brachiocephalic vein
  D. Left carotid artery
  E. Left subclavian artery
  F. Esophagus
  G. Trachea

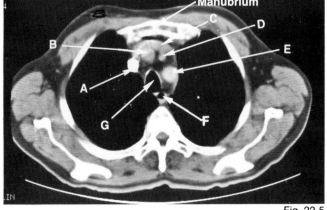

Axial Section 3   Fig. 22-5

Axial Sections of Chest continued

Axial Section 4

Axial section 4 represents a section at the level of the **aortic arch.**
The right and left brachiocephalic veins have united forming the
superior vena cava. Parts labeled are:
  A. Superior vena cava
  B. Aortic Arch
  C. Esophagus
  D. Trachea

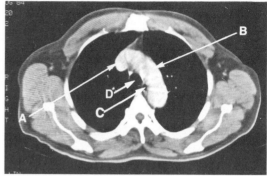

Axial Section 4   Fig. 22-6

Axial Section 5

Axial section 5 represents a section at the level of the
aortopulmonary window. The aortopulmonary window is a
space located between the ascending and descending aorta. Parts
labeled are:
  A. Superior vena cava
  B. Ascending aorta
  C. Aortopulmonary window
  D. Esophagus
  E. Descending aorta
  F. Trachea

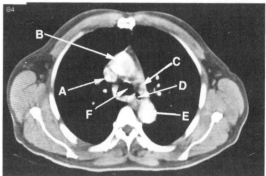

Axial Section 5   Fig. 22-7

Axial Section 6

Axial section 6 represents a section at the level of the **carina.** The
carina is the lower level of where the trachea divides into the
openings of the right and left bronchi (see Chapter 2, *Fig. 2-12*).
Parts labeled are:
  A. Superior vena cava
  B. Ascending aorta
  C. Mediastinal fat
  D. Main pulmonary artery
  E. Left pulmonary artery
  F. Left main stem bronchi
  G. Descending aorta
  H. Azygos vein
  I. Esophagus
  J. Right main stem bronchi
  K. Right pulmonary artery

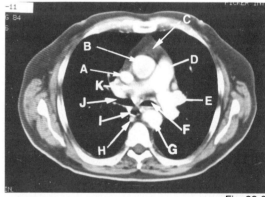

Axial Section 6   Fig. 22-8

Axial Section 7

Axial section 7 was taken at a level of 1 **cm below the carina.**
Parts labeled are:
  A. Superior vena cava
  B. Ascending aorta
  C. Main pulmonary artery
  D. Left pulmonary vein
  E. Left pulmonary artery
  F. Descending aorta
  G. Azygos vein
  H. Esophagus
  I. Right pulmonary artery

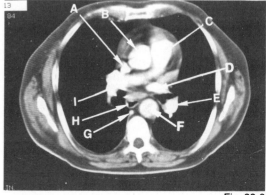

Axial Section 7   Fig. 22-9

Axial Sections of Chest continued

Axial Section 8

Axial section 8 is through the level of the **left atrium.**
Parts labeled are:
A. Right atrium
B. Aortic root
C. Pulmonary trunk
D. Left ventricle
E. Left pulmonary vein
F. Descending aorta
G. Azygos vein
H. Esophagus
I. Left atrium

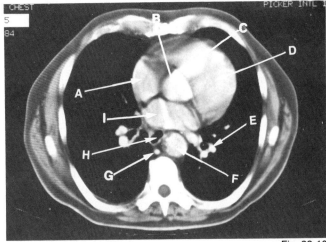

Axial Section 8

Fig. 22-10

Axial Section 9

In this section all **four cardiac chambers** are seen. The arrows pointing between the left atrium and left ventricle represent the approximate location of the mitral valve. Parts labeled are:
A. Inferior vena cava
B. Right atrium
C. Right ventricle
D. Interventricular septum
E. Left ventricle
F. Left atrium
G. Descending aorta
H. Azygos vein
I. Esophagus

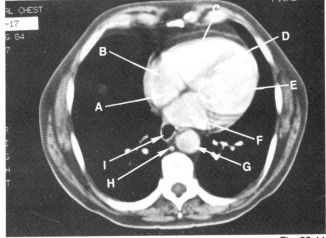

Axial Section 9

Fig. 22-11

Axial Section 10

At this level, **through the base of the heart,** the arrows between the right ventricle and right atrium are pointing to the area of the tricuspid valve. Parts labeled are:
A. Inferior vena cava
B. Right atrium
C. Pericardium
D. Right ventricle
E. Interventricular septum
F. Left ventricle
G. Left atrium
H. Descending aorta
I. Azygos vein
J. Esophagus
K. Right hemidiaphragm

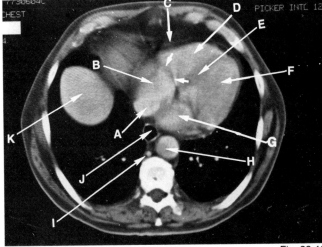

Axial Section 10

Fig. 22-12

Part II Radiographic Positioning and Procedure

Purpose

The primary purpose of thoracic computed tomography is to **serve as a diagnostic adjunct to conventional chest radiography.** However, because of its cost effectiveness, conventional chest radiography is still the primary screening tool in patients suspected of having chest disease. As a secondary purpose, CT serves as a valuable imaging modality in the staging and management of previously diagnosed conditions.

Indications

Most **mediastinal abnormalities** of the chest as documented on plain radiographs are an indication for computed tomography. This is demonstrated on the conventional chest radiograph in *Fig. 22-13* showing a **mediastinal mass**, as marked by the arrows. Compare this with the CT image in *Fig. 22-14* clearly defining the mediastinal mass; and the coronal and sagittal reconstruction in *Fig. 22-15* showing the true location and relative size of this mass.

Some of the more common indications for CT of the chest are **mediastinal and hilar lesions, aneurysms, abscess, cardiac and pericardial disease**.

The innovation of computed tomography has made conventional tomography of the thorax a procedure of the past in most departments.

Clinically suspected disease does not always appear on plain radiographs however. In fact, in many instances the radiograph will be negative. When the clinical history is suggestive of ongoing disease, CT can be a valuable diagnostic adjunct in such cases. Undetected or disguised abnormalities of mediastinal structures can be diagnosed before reaching advanced stages.

Another use of CT of the chest is in **the evaluation of pulmonary nodules where** CT can help to determine the benign or malignant nature of the node. Since benign nodes generally have evidence of calcium content, using thin collimation and measuring the attenuation value of the area can give an indication of the nature of the nodule.

Example of Thoracic Pathology

Figures 22-13 through *22-15* demonstrate how thoracic computed tomography can be used to provide diagnostic information on a mediastinal mass.

The AP radiograph *(Fig. 22-13)* of a 53-day-old male demonstrates mediastinal widening (arrows) of unknown cause. A CT axial scan *(Fig. 22-14)* shows a well circumscribed, homogeneous mass in the posterior mediastinum. Coronal and sagittal reconstructions *(Fig. 22-15)* give an additional 2 dimensions as to the mass's extent and relationship to adjacent structures. From the attenuation value of this mass, which is slightly above water, this mass was determined to be a bronchogenic cyst.

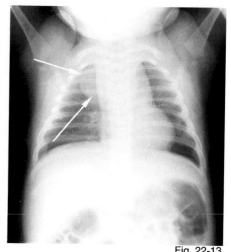

AP Radiograph   Fig. 22-13

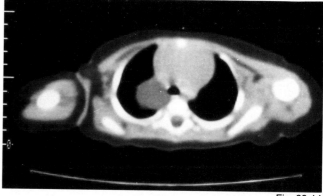

CT Image   Fig. 22-14

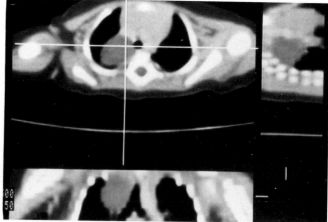

Coronal and Sagittal Reconstructions   Fig. 22-15

Contraindications

There are no major contraindications to computed tomography of the chest. One relative contraindication to CT however, as with any x-ray examination is **pregnancy**. In such cases, the benefits must be weighed against the risks.

With those patients who require a procedure with an injection of iodinated contrast media, a careful history must be taken in order to assess any possibility for **adverse reaction**.

Further, patients with a history of **renal failure**, **multiple myeloma**, **pheochromocytoma** or **diabetes** must be carefully evaluated. When the risk outweighs the benefit, the use of contrast media should be avoided.

Patient Preparation

There are no unusual patient preparation procedures to be followed for computed tomography examinations of the chest. To help reduce the incidence of nausea and/or vomiting following the introduction of intravenous contrast media, the patient should be examined with an empty stomach. To prevent the introduction of metal induced artifacts, patients are to change into clothing with cloth ties, and all opaque objects in the radiographic area of interest must be removed.

In order to obtain high quality examinations, patient cooperation is essential. Patient motion during the procedure seriously impairs the quality of the CT. Patients should be given brief instructions which are to the point and easy to understand. Factors such as breathing instructions and length of examination are important items to discuss.

Contrast Media

The identical contrast media used in excretory urography is utilized in computed tomography of the chest. Various methods are used for the administration of contrast media, including drip infusion, bolus injections, or combinations thereof. The method used is indicated by the clinical history or suspected site of the lesion.

Complications

The possibility of reaction to iodinated contrast material is ever present and although rare, has occurred after the administration of as little as 1 ml of contrast material.

Some common symptoms of minor anaphylactoid reaction are **urticaria** (hives), **nausea**, **vomiting**, and **flushing of the face**.

Moderate reactions include **urticaria**, **facial** and **laryngeal edema** and **hypotension**. Usually some treatment is required with moderate reactions.

Scanner Room Preparation

Proper preparation of the CT scanning room is essential. Particular emphasis should be placed on the readiness of equipment for emergency situations. Suction, blood pressure cuff, cardiac monitor, oxygen tanks and crash cart should be easily accessible. Emergency phone numbers should be placed near the phone and in easy to recognize colors.

The room should be clean. Contrast media, emesis, and blood should be cleaned immediately in order to reduce bacterial growth. All personnel working in the area should be trained in emergency procedures and be familiar with the workings of the unit.

Positioning for CT of the Chest

For routine examinations of the chest the patient is placed in a supine position with arms elevated above the head as shown in *Fig. 22-16*. Keeping the arms above the head will help reduce scan artifacts, particularly beam hardening artifacts from the humeral heads. Patients need to be instructed to keep their arms extended and close to the head so their elbows do not hit the sides of the gantry.

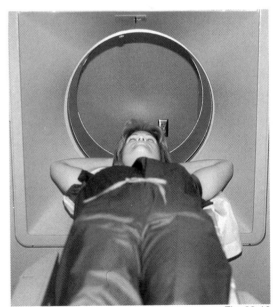

Fig. 22-16
Routine Patient Position for
Chest CT

Procedure for Complete CT of the Chest

For positioning of where slices are to occur for an examination, a pilot or localizing scan is used. A pilot or localizing scan is taken wherein the detectors and tube are stationary while the patient moves up through the gantry aperture on the patient couch *(Fig. 22-17). As* the patient moves through the gantry aperture, an exposure is made, the data is processed by the computer and an image is produced which looks similar to a conventional radiograph *(Fig. 22-18).*

Once this localizing radiograph *(Fig. 22-18)* is obtained, the location of the first slice is placed at the apices. Scanning continues to the level of the diaphragm in mediastinal pathology cases. If the primary concern is pulmonary malignancy, scanning continues to the level of the adrenal glands. This is done because a number of pulmonary malignancies will metastasize to the adrenal glands.

In routine CT examinations of the chest, a 10 mm slice thickness and couch incrementation is commonly used. Couch incrementation refers to how far the patient couch moves after each exposure is made. In instances of smaller lesions, smaller sections (3-5 mm) are used.

Soft tissue masses frequently constrict or compress the esophagus. To help distinguish the two, esophageal creams are used which help opacify the esophagus by coating the mucosa.

With the advent of third and fourth generation scanners with exposure times as fast as 1-2 seconds, motion artifact produced by respiratory and cardiac motion has virtually been eliminated. However, the patient should be instructed in suspended respiration at inspiration, expiration or at resting volume. It is critical that the same method be used throughout the examination so anatomical fluctuation is avoided.

Contrast Scales

When imaging and viewing chest scans from the display unit, two different contrast scales must be used. Mediastinal structures and lung parenchyma have differing attenuation values therefore necessitating two different mediastinal and lung contrast scales. **Mediastinal structures** are viewed and imaged using a **narrow contrast scale** as shown in *Fig. 22-19a.*

When viewing and imaging lung structures such as **pulmonary parenchyma**, a **wide contrast scale** is used as also demonstrated in *Fig. 22-19b.*

Contrast Enhancement

The use of intravenous contrast media can provide valuable information to chest examinations, particularly when the area of concern is the mediastinum. Contrast media has proven to be diagnostically useful in the separation of soft tissue lesions from vascular structures and in the distinction of a vascular from nonvascular lesion.

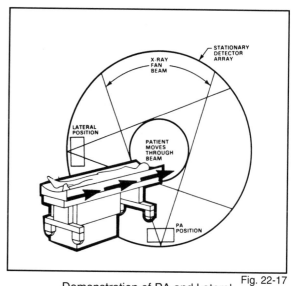

Fig. 22-17

Demonstration of PA and Lateral
Pilots or Localizing Scans for
Positioning of Slices
(Courtesy of Picker International)

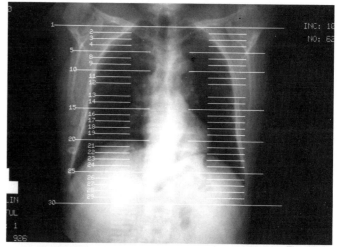

Fig. 22-18

Localizing Radiograph (Pilot Scan)

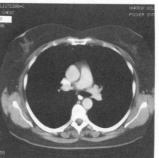 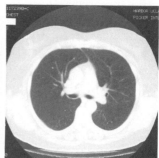

Fig. 22-19 a
Mediastinal (Narrow)
Contrast Scale

Fig. 22-19 b
Lung (Wide)
Contrast Scale

Part I Radiographic Anatomy

The anatomy of the abdomen and pelvis is covered in Chapters 3 and 7 respectively with additional anatomy of digestive, biliary and urinary systems in Chapters 14, 15 and 16. This anatomy from these chapters should be mastered before beginning this chapter on sectional anatomy of the abdomen and pelvis.

Axial Sections of the Abdomen

Nine sectional drawings of the abdomen are shown with corresponding CT in the axial orientation. A 10 mm slice thickness was used. The examination was obtained using a 50 cc bolus injection followed by a 100 cc drip infusion of intravenous contrast. An oral preparation of water-soluble contrast solution was used. Total volume was 900 ml. The patient's right is on the viewer's left. Axial section number 1 is shown in *Fig. 22-20*. The scan is through the **upper portion of the liver.** The liver is divided into 2 lobes, the right (A) and left (B) lobes. The labeled parts are:

    A. Right lobe of liver
    B. Left lobe of liver
    C. Stomach
    D. Spleen
    E. Aorta
    F. Inferior vena cava

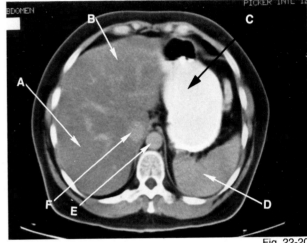

Axial Section 1

Fig. 22-20

Axial Section 2

This section represents the level of the **splenic hilus**. The splenic hilus is the area of the spleen where the splenic artery and vein enter and exit. Note that all four segments of the liver are easily seen. The right lobe is divided into anterior (B) and posterior (A) segments. The left lobe is divided into medial (C) and lateral (D) segments. Parts labeled are:

    A. Right lobe, posterior segment of liver
    B. Right lobe, anterior segment of liver
    C. Left lobe, medial segment of liver
    D. Left lobe, lateral segment of liver
    E. Stomach
    F. Splenic artery
    G. Spleen
    H. Aorta
    I. Inferior vena cava

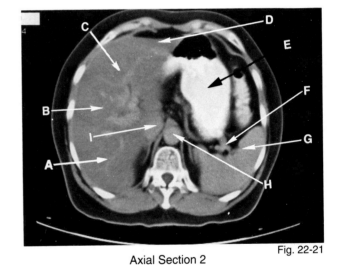

Axial Section 2

Fig. 22-21

Axial Sections of Abdomen continued

Axial Section 3

This scan is at the level of the **pancreatic tail** (G). The pancreatic tail is in its general position, anterior to the left kidney. Note the excellent visualization of the adrenal glands (I). The adrenal glands are most often seen as an inverted V shape. The parts as labeled are:

    A. Right lobe of liver (posterior segment)
    B. Gallbladder
    C. Right lobe of liver (anterior segment)
    D. Left lobe of liver (medial segment)
    E. Left lobe of liver (lateral segment)
    F. Stomach
    G. Pancreatic tail
    H. Spleen
    I. Adrenal glands

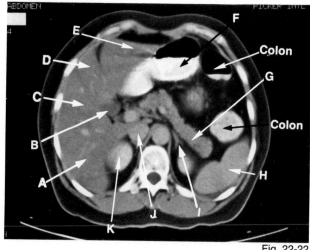

Axial Section 3   Fig. 22-22

Axial Section 4

This cross section is through **the body (F) and neck of the pancreas** (C). The splenic vein (G) runs posterior to the body and neck of the pancreas, joining the superior mesenteric vein (B) to form the portal vein. The parts as labeled are:

    A. Right lobe of liver (posterior segment)
    B. Superior mesenteric vein
    C. Neck of pancreas
    D. Left lobe of liver (lateral segment)
    E. Stomach
    F. Body of pancreas
    G. Splenic vein
    H. Spleen
    I. Aorta
    J. Inferior vena cava
    K. Right kidney

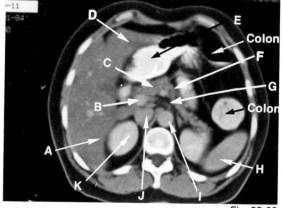

Axial Section 4   Fig. 22-23

Axial Section 5

This scan was taken at the level of the **second portion of the duodenum** (C). The head of the pancreas (I) is well outlined by the duodenum. If the second portion of the duodenum is inadequately opacified it can be confused for a pancreatic tumor. The parts as labeled are:

    A. Right lobe of liver (posterior segment)
    B. Gallbladder
    C. Second portion of duodenum
    D. Left lobe of liver (lateral segment)
    E. Stomach
    F. Left kidney
    G. Aorta
    H. Inferior vena cava
    I. Head of pancreas

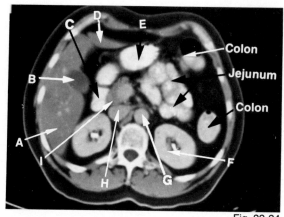

Axial Section 5   Fig. 22-24

Axial Sections of Abdomen continued

Axial Section 6
This cross-section is through the **uncinate process of the pancreas** (B). The uncinate process is a hooklike extension of the head of the pancreas. Note the left renal vein (E) which is coursing anterior to the aorta (G) and entering into the inferior vena cava (H). The left renal vein usually is longer than the right. The labeled parts are:
  A. Right lobe of liver
  B. Uncinate process of the pancreas
  C. Gallbladder
  D. Left lobe of liver
  E. Left renal vein
  F. Left kidney
  G. Aorta
  H. Inferior vena cava

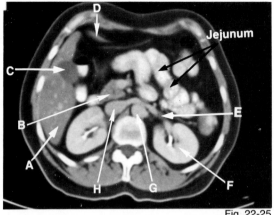

Axial Section 6

Fig. 22-25

Axial Section 7
This scan was taken through the **mid portion of the kidneys.** There is excellent visualization of the right and left renal pelvis (D). The parts as labeled are:
  A. Right lobe of the liver
  B. Uncinate process of the pancreas
  C. Gallbladder
  D. Left renal pelvis
  E. Aorta
  F. Inferior vena cava

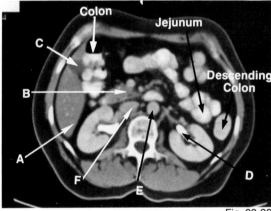

Axial Section 7

Fig. 22-26

Axial Section 8
This scan is 2 **cm caudal to the renal pelvis** and demonstrates the contrast filled ureters medial to the kidneys. The labeled parts are:
  A. Right lobe of the liver
  B. Left kidney
  C. Left ureter
  D. Aorta
  E. Inferior vena cava

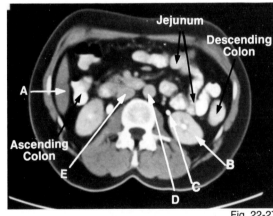

Axial Section 8

Fig. 22-27

Axial Section 9
This section is at the level of the **third portion of the duodenum** (B). The duodenum is seen crossing anteriorly to the inferior vena cava (G). The inferior poles of the kidneys are also seen. The labeled parts are:
  A. Right lobe of liver
  B. Third portion of the duodenum
  C. Left kidney
  D. Left ureter
  E. Aorta
  F. Right psoas muscle
  G. Inferior vena cava

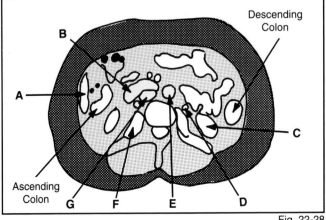

Drawing of Axial Section 9

Fig. 22-28

Axial Sections of the Pelvis

Male Pelvis

Ten sectional line drawings of the pelvis with corresponding CT scans of 10 mm slice thickness are shown in the axial orientation. The male pelvis was obtained using a 150 cc drip infusion of intravenous contrast. Intravenous contrast was not used for the female examination due to the patient being in renal failure. Gastrointestinal opacification was obtained by administering barium sulfate orally and by enema for both patients.

The patient's right is on the viewer's left. Axial section number 1 is shown in *Fig. 22-29*. This cross-section is 2 **cm caudal to the iliac crest.** This is a male pelvis. The labeled parts are:
- A. Gluteus medius muscle
- B. Right iliac wing
- C. Ascending colon
- D. Rectus muscle
- E. Psoas muscle
- F. Iliacus muscle

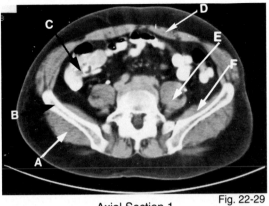

Axial Section 1   Fig. 22-29

Axial Section 2

This scan was taken at the level of the **sacroiliac joints** (H). This is a male pelvis. Parts labeled are:
- A. Gluteus maximus muscle
- B. Gluteus medius muscle
- C. Right iliac wing
- D. Cecum
- E. Rectus muscle
- F. Psoas muscle
- G. Iliacus muscle
- H. Sacroiliac joints
- I. Sacrum

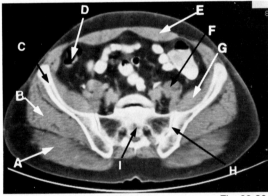

Axial Section 2   Fig. 22-30

Axial Section 3

At this level the **three gluteal muscles** are easily identified because of the excellent fat planes. The gluteal muscles assist in movement of the thigh. This is a male pelvis. Parts labeled are:
- A. Gluteus maximus muscle
- B. Gluteus medius muscle
- C. Gluteus minimus
- D. Rectus muscle
- E. Iliacus muscle
- F. Ilium
- G. Sigmoid colon

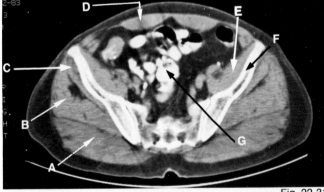

Axial Section 3   Fig. 22-31

Axial Section 4

This cross-section is at the level of the **ilium** (G). There is excellent visualization of the pyriformis muscles (I) which are located between the sacrum (J) and ilium (G). This is a male pelvis. The parts as labeled are:
- A. Gluteus maximus muscle
- B. Gluteus medius muscle
- C. Gluteus minimus muscle
- D. Iliopsoas muscle
- E. Rectus muscle
- F. Bladder
- G. Ilium
- H. Rectum
- I. Pyriformis muscles
- J. Sacrum

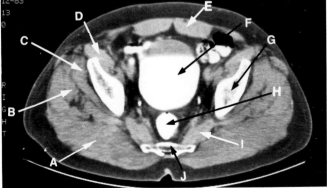

Axial Section 4   Fig. 22-32

Axial Sections of Pelvis continued

Axial Section 5

This section is at the level of the **acetabular roof** (B). The paired, oval shaped seminal vesicles (F) are seen posterior to the bladder (D). This obviously is a male pelvis. The labeled parts are:

A. Gluteus maximus
B. Acetabular roof
C. Rectus muscle
D. Bladder
E. Iliopsoas muscle
F. Seminal vesicles
G. Rectum

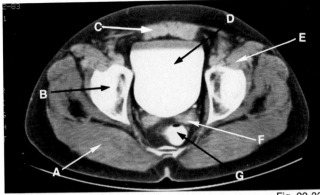

Axial Section 5   Fig. 22-33

Axial Section 6

At this level there is good demonstration of the **femoral heads** (C) **within the acetabulum** (D). Note also the greater trochanter (B). This is a male pelvis. The labeled parts are:

A. Gluteus maximus
B. Greater trochanter
C. Femoral head
D. Acetabulum
E. Bladder
F. Pubic bone
G. Rectum

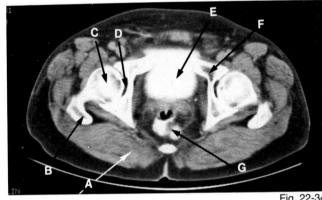

Axial Section 6   Fig. 22-34

Axial Section 7

This section, through the **symphysis pubis** (F) of this male pelvis, shows the prostate (L) between the symphysis (F) and the rectum (M). The size of the prostate varies with age. With progressive age the prostate increases in size. The labeled parts are:

A. Gluteus maximus
B. Femur
C. Femoral artery
D. Femoral vein
E. Pubic bone
F . Symphysis pubis
G. Pectineus muscle
H. External obturator muscle
I. Internal obturator muscle
J. Tensor fascia lata muscle
K. Ischial tuberosity
L. Prostate
M. Rectum
N. Ischiorectal fat

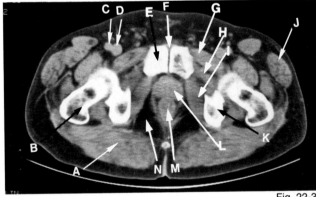

Axial Section 7   Fig. 22-35

Axial Section 8

This is a cross-section at the level of the **ischial ramus** (E). This is a male pelvis. The labeled parts are:

A. Gluteus maximus
B. Femur
C. Corpus cavernosum penis
D. Adductor muscles
E. Ischial ramus

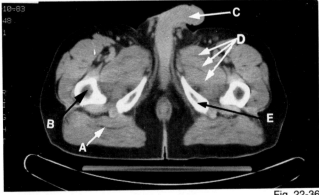

Axial Section 8   Fig. 22-36

Axial Sections of Pelvis continued

Female Pelvis

Axial Section 9

This scan is at the level of the **acetabulum** (C) of this female pelvis. There is good visualization of the uterus (H) which is bordered by the bladder (E) anteriorly and the rectum (I) posteriorly. The labeled parts are:

A. Gluteus maximus muscle
B. Femoral head
C. Acetabulum
D. Rectus muscle
E. Bladder
F. Iliopsoas muscle
G. Ischial spine
H. Uterus
I. Rectum

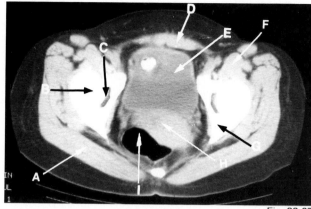

Axial Section 9

Fig. 22-37

Axial Section 10

This cross-section at the **symphysis pubis** (D) of this female pelvis gives excellent visualization of the vagina (I) due to insertion of a tampon. Other parts labeled are:

A. Gluteus maximus
B. Femoral neck
C. Pubic bone
D. Symphysis pubis
E. Pectineus muscle
F. External obturator muscle
G. Internal obturator muscle
H. Ischial tuberosity
I. Vagina
J. Rectum
K. Ischiorectal fat

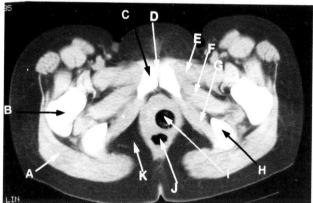

Axial Section 10

Fig. 22-38

Purpose

With the advent of computed tomography, the ability to diagnose abdominal and pelvic morphology has been significantly enhanced. Due to its speed and accuracy, CT has become an effective management and treatment tool for **abdominal and pelvic disease** and has been especially useful in the **cases of malignancies**. The use of standard diagnostic tests such as endoscopic retrograde cholangiopancreatography (ERCP) have been greatly reduced due to the completeness and cost effectiveness of CT examination.

Indications

Any abnormality of the abdomen and/or pelvis is an indication for computed tomography.

Abdomen: Some of the more common indications for computed tomography of the abdomen include suspected primary or **metastatic lesions of the liver, pancreas, kidney** or **spleen**. Computed tomography is a preferred choice for examination of suspected **adrenal gland pathology** and has replaced lymphangiography in detecting lymph-node malignancies. Other common indications are suspected **pancreatitis, abscesses** and **hepatic** or **splenic hematomas**.

Pelvis: In the region of the pelvis, computed tomography is primarily used to provide information on the **state of advancement of pelvic disease**. Computed tomography has proven valuable in the evaluation of **prostatic, cervix, urinary bladder,** and **ovarian carcinomas**. Other indications are evaluation of **soft-tissue masses** and diseases of the **pelvic muscles, suspected abscesses** and **evaluation of the hip joint**, especially in trauma patients as shown in *Fig. 22-40*.

Additionally, CT has been found particularly valuable in the exclusion or detection of occult disease (hidden or concealed).

Examples of Abdominal Pathology Visualized by CT

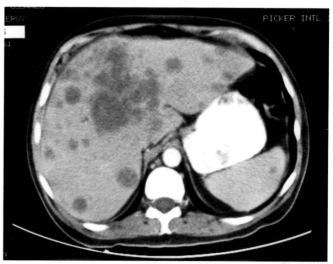

Fig. 22-39

Liver Metastasis

(There are multiple low density lesions of variable size within the liver tissue representing metastatic disease. Note the opacification of the aorta due to a bolus injection of contrast media.)

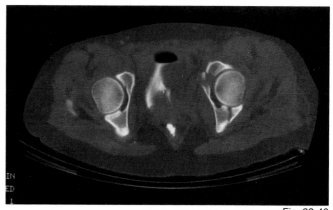

Fig. 22-40

Left Acetabular Fracture

(Scans of an 18-year-old female show fractures of the anterior and posterior segments of the acetabulum.)

Radiographic Positioning and Procedures continued

Contraindications

There are almost no contraindications to computed tomography of the abdomen and pelvis. Any patient who can be transported to the scanning unit can have the examination performed. However, as with any x-ray examination, **pregnancy** is a contraindication to CT. In each case, **the benefits must be weighed against the risks.**

For those patients who require a procedure with an injection of iodinated contrast media, a careful history must be taken in order to assess any **possibility for adverse reaction to the contrast media**. Furthermore, patients with a history of **renal failure**, **multiple myeloma**, **pheochromocytoma** or **diabetes must be carefully evaluated**. When the risk outweighs the benefit, the use of contrast media should be avoided.

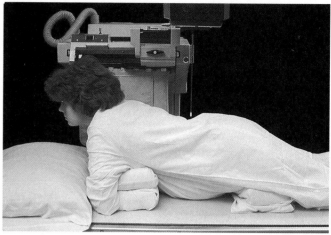

Warning: Benefits must outweigh the risks   Fig. 22-41

Patient Preparation

Proper patient preparation for computed tomography of the abdomen and pelvis is crucial. Inadequate or incorrect preparation may produce an inaccurate diagnosis.

The use of oral and rectal contrast media to opacify the gastro-intestinal tract is imperative for diagnostic examinations of the abdomen and pelvis. Unopacified portions of small and large bowel can be misdiagnosed as lymph nodes, abscesses or masses. This is demonstrated by comparing the scans in *Figs. 22-42* and *22-43* of the lower abdomen which show a questionable soft tissue mass on the left. After administering additional oral contrast media the mass is shown to be actually loops of small bowel. Questionable areas like this are seen frequently at the head or tail of the pancreas where unopacified loops of small bowel can be confused for pancreatic tumors.

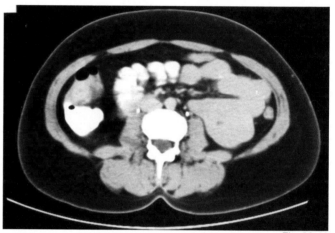

Pseudotumors of the Abdomen   Fig. 22-42

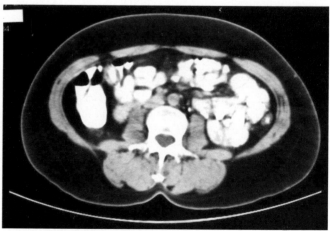

After administration of contrast media   Fig. 22-43

Types of Contrast Media

There are **two types** of positive contrast agents used to opacify the gastrointestinal tract. They are **barium sulfate suspensions** and **water-soluble solutions** (diatrizoate meglumine and diatrizoate sodium). Each has been proven effective, but in certain clinical situations only barium sulfate or water-soluble solutions can be used.

Barium Sulfate Suspensions

There are numerous flavored barium sulfate suspensions made especially for abdominal CT. In order to be useful in abdominal CT, barium sulfate suspensions must be of low concentrations to avoid streaking artifact due to beam hardening. Barium suspensions are effective, economical and, because they are premixed, are easy to administer.

The manufacturer's directions must be followed strictly when administering barium sulfate. Delays after ingestion allow water to be absorbed by the bowel which leaves residual barium and causes **beam hardening artifacts**, as shown by the scan in *Fig.* 22-44. Note the linear streaks arising from the stomach on this scan, which are examples of such beam hardening artifacts.

Water-Soluble Solutions

An alternative to barium sulfate suspensions for opacification of the GI tract is the use of water-soluble contrast agents. These agents are a valuable alternative when barium sulfate suspensions are not feasible. They provide good coating of the gastrointestinal tract and, because they increase peristaltic motion, they have a fast transit time. They can prove to be a disadvantage, however, in examinations requiring long exposure times (5 seconds or more) due to increased motion artifact.

Extreme care must be used in the preparation of water-soluble solutions.

Diatrizoate preparations containing 2-5% dilutions have been found to be generally safe and clinically useful. Preparations which contain 15-40% diatrizoate solution however are considered hypertonic. These may draw excessive amounts of fluid into the intestinal tract and may cause hypovolemia.

Other adverse reactions include diarrhea, nausea, and vomiting, occurring particularly when the solutions are used in large quantities and high concentrations. Urticaria (hives) may also occur.

Contraindications to Barium Sulfate

Barium sulfate is an insoluble material and therefore **should not be used in pre-operative patients** or patients suspected of having **gastrointestinal perforations.** Severe complications, such as barium peritonitis, can result from barium leakage into the abdominal and pelvic cavities.

Additional contraindications include patients with a **known hypersensitivity to barium sulfate** or patients with **diagnosed bowel obstruction.**

Contrast Media and Complications

The contrast media used and the possible complications due to reactions to iodinated contrast media is similar to that of intravenous urography as discussed in more detail in chapter 17.

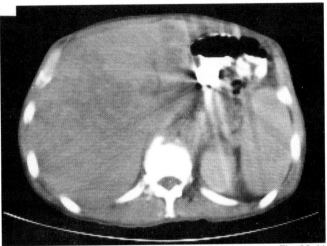

Beam Hardening Artifacts   Fig. 22-44

Recommended Oral and Rectal Contrast Media Volumes for Abdominal and Pelvic Scanning (Water-Soluble and Barium Sulfate Solutions)

The following **times** when the oral contrast is initiated, and the **volumes** given, are dependent on the parts of the gastrointestinal tract to be included in the scanning area.

Abdomen and pelvis (oral and by enema):
• 700-900 ml orally 30-45 minutes prior to scan
• 800-1000 ml enema immediately before scan
• 300 ml orally immediately before scan
• Patient in right decubitus position 3-5 minutes before scanning

Abdomen and pelvis (oral only):
• 1200-1500 ml 45-60 minutes prior to scan
• 300 ml immediately before scan
• Patient in right decubitus position 3-5 minutes before scanning

Upper abdomen only:
• 400-600 ml orally 15-30 minutes prior to scan
• 300 ml orally immediately before scan
• Patient in right decubitus position 3-5 minutes before scanning

Pelvis only:
• 700-900 ml orally 30-45 minutes prior to scan
• 800-1000 ml enema immediately before scan

Oral or Enema Method: The choice to use the oral and enema method, or the oral only method for preparation of the patient for abdominal and pelvic scans is strictly personal preference. However, in cases where the oral only method was used and the colon is not completely opacified an enema may be necessary.

Use of Tampon: To aid in easier anatomical localization of the vagina a tampon should routinely be used. Insertion of a tampon produces an entrapment of air. This is demonstrated in *Fig. 22-45.*

Patient Preparation
The abdominal tract should be as free from fecal matter as possible prior to examination. The patient should have taken a laxative and have had only clear liquids for supper the evening prior to exam. Fecal material restricts the flow of contrast and can also appear as a mass. Until the examination is performed the patient should continue to have clear liquids since solid food in the digestive tract can appear to be a gastric tumor.

Patients should change into clothing with cloth ties and all opaque objects in the radiographic area of interest must be removed.

In order to obtain high quality examinations, patient cooperation is essential. Patient motion during the procedure seriously impairs the quality of CT. Patients should be given brief instructions which are to the point and easy to understand. Items such as breathing instructions and length of examination are important to discuss.

Scanner Room Preparation
The room preparation, with equipment for possible emergency situations, room cleanliness, etc., is similar to that described earlier in this chapter on CT in the chest.

Positioning for CT of the Abdomen and Pelvis
Abdominal and pelvic examinations are routinely done in the supine position with arms elevated above the head. As with CT of the chest, keeping the arms elevated helps reduce the incidence of artifacts.

Sometimes a right decubitus position is used as explained on the following page.

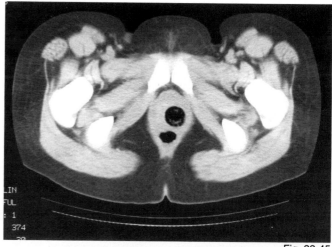

Fig. 22-45

Use of Tampon with Entrapment of Air
for Localization Purposes

Procedure for Complete CT of the Abdomen and Pelvis

Pilot or Localization

A localizing or pilot radiograph *(Fig. 22-46)* is obtained with the first slice starting at the xiphoid process. Scanning then continues to the symphysis pubis.

If only the upper abdomen is the area of interest, then scanning starts at the xiphoid process and continues to the iliac crest. If the pelvis is the only area of interest, then scanning starts at the iliac crest and continues to the symphysis pubis.

In certain examinations the decubitus position is valuable. This position frequently is used when the pancreas is the area of concern. Placing the patient in a right decubitus position immediately after drinking oral contrast causes the duodenum to fill because of gravitational flow. This technique helps eliminate false positives when pancreatic tumors are suspected.

Slice Thickness and Couch Incrementation

In routine examinations of the abdomen and pelvis a 10 mm thick slice is commonly used. The parameter used for couch incrementation will vary, depending on the clinical history. Couch incrementation refers to how far the couch or table moves after each slice. For most routine examinations a couch incrementation of 10 or 15 mm is used. A 20 mm incrementation occasionally will be used in detecting gross pathology and/or when a fast examination time is of importance. In certain instances small parameters (5-8 mm) may be used for detailed evaluation of organs such as the pancreas or kidney.

Exposure Times

Exposure times of **1-3 seconds** are needed for examination of the abdomen to reduce the effect of peristaltic and respiratory artifact on image quality.

Breathing Instructions

Suspended respiration is required in order to obtain high quality diagnostic images in abdominal examinations. It is essential that the same method of suspended respiration be used throughout the entire exam. Inconsistent suspended respirations can cause fluctuations in the exam by creating varying compressions of the diaphragm on abdominal organs.

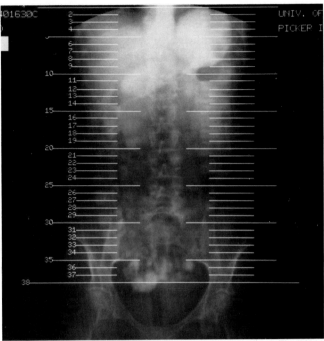

Fig. 22-46

Localizing (Pilot) Scan for
Abdomen and Pelvis
(solid white line represents the slice location)

Contrast Enhancement of Vascular Structures

Use of intravenous contrast is important in the evaluation of vascular structures of the abdomen and pelvis such as the abdominal aorta, inferior vena cava, portal vein and iliac arteries and veins.

Often lesions can be characterized and identified by their enhancement or by their attenuation when compared to normal enhanced adjacent tissue.

Occasionally, dual examinations will be performed with and without contrast. Some lesions may be isodense with normal tissue before or after contrast enhancement. This method is frequently used in evaluation of the liver and kidneys.

Intravenous contrast is also important for visualizing the ureters and bladder.

Chapter 23
Radiographic Anatomy and Positioning
of
Cerebral, Thoracic, Abdominal and Peripheral Angiography

Contributions by: Marianne Tortorici, RT(R), Ed.D.
Patrick Apfel, RT(R), M. Ed.
Barry T. Anthony, RT(R)

Contents

Survey Information

Survey Questions on Possible Discontinued Procedures

The national survey included questions on (I) the **expected trend** in the next three or four years, (II) the **quantity** of specific exams done in their departments during the past year, and (III) whether or not **the procedure should still be taught and included** in a basic student textbook. The results were as follows:

Peripheral Arteriograms	U.S. (314)	East (116)	Midwest (146)	West (52)
(upper and lower limbs)				
I. Trend				
a. Increase	33%	42%	28%	26%
b. Decrease	13%	16%	11%	13%
c. No change	54%	42%	61%	61%
II. Annual Quantity				
a. 0-9	20%	14%	21%	29%
b. 10-79	40%	37%	44%	33%
c. 80-163	23%	28%	17%	25%
d. 164+	17%	21%	18%	13%
III. Be Included				
a. Yes	91%	92%	90%	92%
b. No	9%	8%	10%	8%
Venograms	(357)	(132)	(165)	(60)
I. Trend				
a. Increase	28%	37%	23%	23%
b. Decrease	18%	17%	17%	25%
c. No change	54%	46%	60%	52%
II. Annual Quantity				
a. 0-29	17%	11%	15%	32%
b. 30-105	43%	41%	42%	48%
c. 106-177	20%	21%	22%	15%
d. 178+	20%	27%	21%	5%
III. Be Included				
a. Yes	98%	98%	98%	93%
b. No	2%	2%	2%	7%
Lymphangiograms	(277)	(98)	(127)	(52)
I. Trend				
a. Increase	4%	3%	5%	4%
b. Decrease	35%	36%	34%	35%
c. No change	61%	61%	61%	61%
II. Annual Quantity				
a. 0-4	65%	64%	68%	60%
b. 5-19	25%	27%	22%	28%
c. 20-54	6%	2%	7%	12%
d. 55+	4%	7%	3%	0%
III. Be Included				
a. Yes	58%	60%	56%	62%
b. No	42%	40%	44%	38%

Summary

The survey did not ask specific questions on **cerebral**, **thoracic** or **abdominal angiograms** because it is believed that these procedures will continue to be performed in sufficient numbers that they need to be taught and understood by student radiographers.

This is not as certain for peripheral angiography such as upper and lower limb arteriograms and/or venograms.

The survey however indicated that both **peripheral arteriograms and venograms** are being done in sufficient numbers to still be taught and included in a basic student textbook. The results in all regions of the U.S. do indicate that the majority of respondents expect **no change** in the number of these procedures over the next three or four years.

The quantity of **lymphangiograms** being done is very low in all regions with the majority of responding institutions doing less than four procedures per year. Therefore, this text does not include a specific section on this procedure, but it is briefly described in part I of the anatomy section.

Part I Radiographic Anatomy
(Cerebral, Thoracic, Abdominal and Peripheral)

Introduction

Definition

Angiography refers to the **radiographic examination of the blood vessels following injection of a positive contrast medium**. Since the various soft tissues of the body possess similar radiographic densities, a positive contrast medium must be added in order to study normal and abnormal distribution of the circulatory system. For example, the routine lateral skull radiograph in *Fig. 23-1* demonstrates none of the vessels of the cranial circulatory system, while the lateral carotid arteriogram in *Fig. 23-2* clearly differentiates between brain and blood vessels. This is also true for the circulatory system of other body regions such as the thorax, abdomen and the upper and lower limbs (peripheral). Angiography of these body parts will be studied in this chapter also wherein contrast media is injected into specific vessels of each of these regions.

A good understanding of the anatomy involved, as covered in part I of this chapter, is essential for performing angiography of any body region.

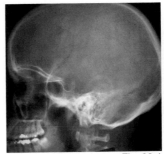

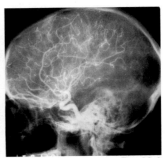

Fig. 23-1
Lateral Skull Radiograph

Fig. 23-2
Lateral Carotid Arteriogram

Circulatory System

Divisions or Components

The **circulatory system** consists of the **cardiovascular and lymphatic components.** The cardiovascular portion includes the heart, blood and vessels which transport the blood. The lymphatic element of the circulatory system is comprised of a clear watery fluid called lymph, lymphatic vessels, and lymphatic nodes. The cardiovascular and lymphatic components differ in the function and method of transporting the respective fluids within the vessels.

The **cardiovascular** or blood circulatory division may further be divided into the **cardio** (circulation within the heart) and **vascular** (blood vessel) components.

The vascular or vessel component is divided into the **pulmonary** (heart to lungs and back) and the general or **systemic** system (throughout the body).

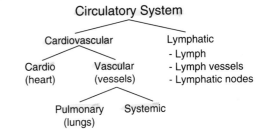

Circulatory System

Cardiovascular — Lymphatic
- Lymph
- Lymph vessels
- Lymphatic nodes

Cardio (heart) Vascular (vessels)

Pulmonary (lungs) Systemic

Cardiovascular System

The cardiovascular system (CVS) consists of the heart and vascular (blood and blood vessels) organs. The heart is the major organ of the cardiovascular system and functions as a pump to maintain circulation of blood throughout the body. The vascular component is a network of blood vessels which carry blood from the heart to body tissues and back to the heart again.

Functions: Functions of the cardiovascular system include:
1. Transportation of oxygen, nutrients, hormones and chemicals necessary for normal body activity.
2. Removal of waste products through the kidneys and lungs.
3. Maintenance of body temperature and water and electrolyte balance.
These functions are performed by the following blood components; red blood cells, white blood cells, and platelets suspended in plasma.

Blood Components: Red blood cells, or **erythrocytes**, are produced in the red marrow of certain bones and transport oxygen via the protein hemoglobin to body tissues.

White blood cells, or **leukocytes**, formed in both bone marrow and lymph tissue defend the body against infection and disease. **Platelets**, also originating from bone marrow, repair tears in blood vessel walls and promote blood clotting.

Plasma, the liquid portion of the blood, consists of 92% water and about 7% plasma protein and salts, nutrients, and oxygen.

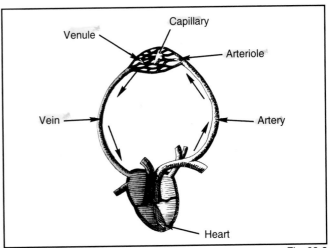

General Cardiovascular Circulation   Fig. 23-3

Venule Capillary Arteriole Artery Vein Heart

Systemic Circulation

Arteries: Vessels transporting oxygenated blood from the heart to tissues are called **arteries**. Arteries which originate directly from the heart measure approximately three centimeters in diameter. These arteries then subdivide and decrease in size as they extend from the heart to the various parts of the body. The smaller arteries are termed **arterioles.** As the blood travels through the arterioles, it enters the tissues via the smallest subdivision of these vessels, known as **capillaries** *(Fig. 23-3)*.

Veins: The deoxygenated blood returns to the heart through the venous system. The venous system extends from venous capillaries to venules to veins increasing in size as it nears the heart.
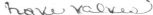 *(have valves)*

Pulmonary Circulation

The blood vessel circuit (veins, venules, capillaries, arterioles and arteries) which supplies blood to the lungs and back comprises the **pulmonary circulation** component of the cardiovascular system.

As previously noted, arteries generally carry oxygenated blood away from the heart to the capillaries. The exception to this are the **pulmonary arteries** which carry the **deoxygenated blood** to the lungs which has been returned to the heart through the venous system.

The superior and inferior vena cava empty the returning deoxygenated blood into the **right atrium** of the heart.

The heart pumps this deoxygenated blood from the **right ventricle** through the pulmonary arteries to the lungs where oxygen and carbon dioxide are exchanged through the small air sacs or alveoli of the lungs. The **oxygenated blood** then returns through the **pulmonary veins** to the **left atrium** of the heart (*Fig. 23-4*).

General Systemic Circulation

Heart

The heart is a muscular organ which pumps blood throughout the various parts of the body. Anatomically, the heart lies within the mediastinum, or middle area of the chest, and rests on the **diaphragm** (*Fig. 23-5*). Cardiac tissue differs from other muscle tissues of the body in its construction and is termed myocardium. The left side of the heart is responsible for the extensive systemic circulation, thus, the left muscle wall is about three times as thick as the right side.

The heart itself is divided into four chambers. These are the **right and left atria** and the **right and left ventricles.** Each chamber functions either to receive and/or pump blood. The blood circulation is a closed system by which unoxygenated blood enters the **right atrium** from all parts of the body, is reoxygenated in the lungs and returned to the body via the **left ventricle.**

Blood returning to the heart enters the right atrium through the **superior and inferior vena cava** (*Fig. 23-6*). Blood in the superior vena cava originates from the head, chest, and upper extremities. The inferior vena cava serves to deliver blood into the right atrium from the abdomen and lower extremities.

From the **right atrium,** blood is pumped to the **right ventricle** passing through the tricuspid valve. The right ventricle contracts moving the blood through the **pulmonary (pulmonary semilunar) valve** to the **pulmonary arteries** and on to the lungs. While in the lungs, the blood is oxygenated and then returned to the left atrium of the heart via the **pulmonary veins.** As the left atrium contracts, blood is transported through the **mitral (bicuspid) valve** to the left ventricle.

When the left ventricle contracts, the oxygenated blood exits the chamber via the **aortic (aortic semilunar) valve,** flows through the aorta and is delivered to the various body tissues by the remaining arterial vessels.

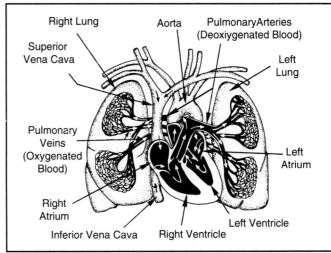

Pulmonary Circulation — Fig. 23-4

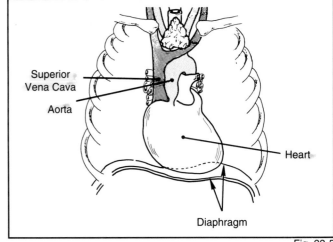

Heart and Mediastinal Structures — Fig. 23-5

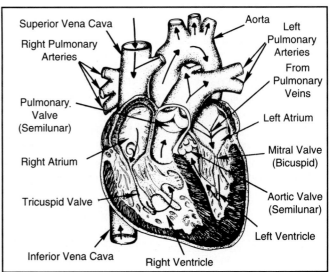

Cross-Section of Heart — Fig. 23-6

Cerebral Arteries

Blood Supply to the Brain

The brain is supplied with blood by major arteries of the systemic circulation. The four major arteries supplying the brain are: *(Fig. 23-7.)*

1. **Right common carotid artery**
2. **Left common carotid artery**
3. **Right vertebral artery**
4. **Left vertebral artery**

Major branches of the two common carotids supply the anterior circulation of the brain, while the two vertebrals supply the posterior circulation. Radiographic examination of the neck vessels and entire brain circulation is referred to as a "four-vessel angiogram" since these four vessels are collectively and selectively injected with contrast medium. Another common series is the "three-vessel angiogram" in which the two carotids and only one vertebral artery are studied.

Branches of the Aortic Arch

The aorta is the major artery leaving the left ventricle of the heart. There are three major branches arising from the **arch** of the **aorta**. These are *(Fig. 23-8)*:

1. **Brachiocephalic artery**
2. **Left common carotid artery**
3. **Left subclavian artery**

The brachiocephalic trunk is a short vessel which bifurcates into the right common carotid artery and the **right subclavian artery.** The right and left vertebral arteries are branches of the subclavian arteries on each side. Since the left common carotid artery rises directly from the arch of the aorta, it is slightly longer than the right common carotid artery.

In the cervical region, the two common carotids resemble one another. Each common carotid artery passes cephalad from its origin along either side of the trachea and larynx to the level of the upper border of the thyroid cartilage. Here, each common carotid artery divides into **external and internal carotid arteries.** The level of bifurcation of each common carotid is the level of the **fourth cervical vertebra.**

Neck and Head Arteries

The major arteries supplying the head, as seen from the right side of the neck, are shown in *Fig. 23-9*. The **brachiocephalic trunk artery** bifurcates into the **right common carotid artery** and the **right subclavian artery.**

The right common carotid artery ascends to the level of the fourth cervical vertebra to branch into the **external carotid artery** and the **internal carotid artery.** Each external carotid artery primarily supplies the anterior neck, the face and the greater part of the scalp and meninges (brain coverings). Each internal carotid artery supplies the anterior portion of the brain.

The **right vertebral artery** arises from the right subclavian artery to pass through the transverse foramina of C6 through C1. Each vertebral artery passes posteriorly along the superior border of C1 before angling upward through the foramen magnum to enter the cranium.

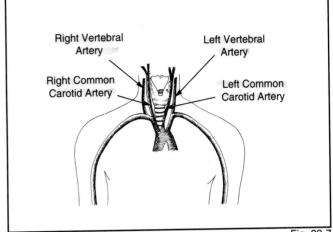

Blood Supply to Brain   Fig. 23-7

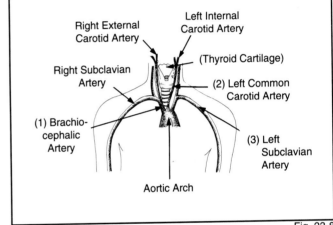

Branches of Aortic Arch   Fig. 23-8

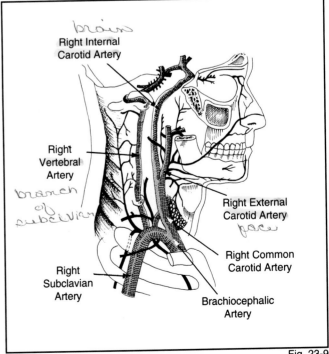

Neck and Head Arteries   Fig. 23-9

External Carotid Artery Branches

artograms not common

The four major branches of the external carotid artery are shown in *Fig. 23-10* These are:

1. **Facial artery**
2. **Maxillary artery** — *middle men.* < *ant. post.*
3. **Superficial temporal artery**
4. **Occipital artery**

The most important branch of the maxillary artery is **the middle meningeal artery, which** has an **anterior and a posterior branch.** This middle meningeal artery enters the cranial cavity and produces a groove along the inner table of the cranium. Trauma to the squamous portion of the temporal bone, sufficient to fracture the bone, may lead to a laceration of the middle meningeal artery and a subsequent epidural hemorrhage.

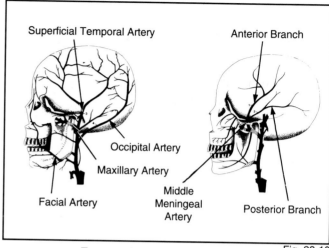

External Carotid Artery Branches   Fig. 23-10

Internal Carotid Artery

common (4 vessel) *foramen lacerum*

Each internal carotid artery ascends to enter the carotid canal in the petrous portion of the temporal bone. Within the petrous pyramid the artery curves forward and medially. Before supplying the cerebral hemispheres, each internal carotid artery passes through a collection of venous channels *sinuses* around the sella turcica. Each internal carotid artery passes through the dura mater, medial to each anterior clinoid process, to bifurcate into the cerebral branches.

The S-shaped portion of each internal carotid artery is termed the **carotid siphon** and is studied carefully by the neuroradiologist *(Fig. 23-11)*.

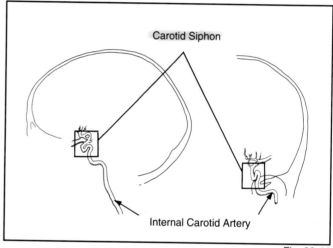

Internal Carotid Artery   Fig. 23-11

Anterior Cerebral Artery

w/in skull

The two end branches of each **internal carotid artery** are the **anterior cerebral** and the **middle cerebral arteries.** Each anterior cerebral artery and its branches supply much of the forebrain near the midline. The anterior cerebral arteries curve around the corpus callosum, giving off several branches to each cerebral hemisphere *(Fig. 23-12)*. Each anterior cerebral artery connects to the opposite one, as well as to the posterior brain circulation.

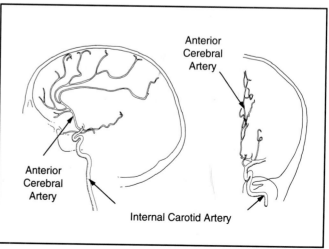

Anterior Cerebral Artery   Fig. 23-12

medial + anterior

Cerebral Arteries continued

Middle Cerebral Artery

The middle cerebral artery is the largest branch of each internal carotid artery. This artery supplies the lateral aspects of the anterior cerebral circulation. As the middle cerebral artery courses toward the periphery of the brain, branches extend upward along the lateral portion of the **insula or central lobe** of the brain. These small branches supply brain tissue deep within the brain *(Fig. 23-13).*

posterior +
lateral

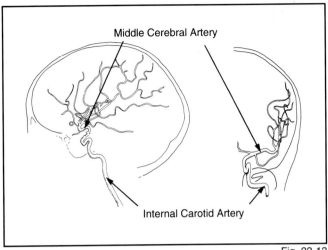

Fig. 23-13

Middle Cerebral Artery

Internal Carotid Arteriogram

When one internal carotid artery is injected with contrast medium, both the anterior cerebral artery and the middle cerebral artery fill. The arterial phase of a cerebral carotid angiogram is similar to the drawings in *Fig. 23-14.*

In the frontal view or anteroposterior projection, there is little superimposition of the two vessels since the anterior cerebral courses toward the midline and the middle cerebral extends laterally.

In the lateral position there obviously is some superimposition. Note that the internal carotid artery supplies primarily the anterior portion of the brain.

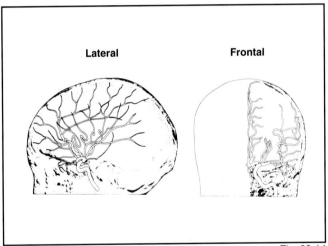

Fig. 23-14

Internal Carotid Arteriogram

Vertebrobasilar Arteries

The two **vertebral arteries** enter the cranium through the foramen magnum and unite to form the single **basilar artery.** The vertebral arteries and basilar artery and their branches form the vertebrobasilar system. By omitting much of the occipital bone in *Fig. 23-15,* these arteries are shown along the base of the skull. Several arteries arise from each vertebral artery prior to their point of convergence to form the basilar artery. These branches supply the spinal cord and the hindbrain. The basilar artery rests upon the **clivus,** the portion of the occipital bone anterior to the foramen magnum.

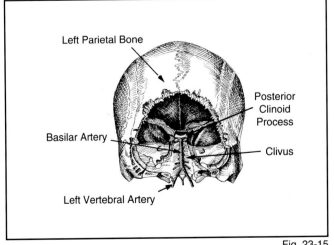

Fig. 23-15

Vertebrobasilar Arteries

Circle of Willis

The posterior brain circulation communicates with the anterior circulation along the base of the brain in the arterial circle, or circle of Willis (as shown in *Fig. 23-16*).

Not only are the anterior and posterior circulations connected, but also both sides connect across the midline. Therefore, an elaborate anastomosis interconnects the entire arterial supply to the brain. As the **basilar artery** courses forward toward the circle of Willis, it gives off several branches to the hindbrain and posterior cerebrum. The **posterior cerebral arteries** are two of the larger branches .

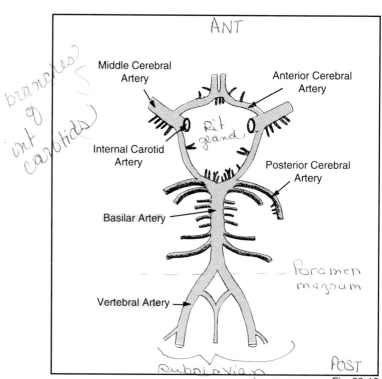

Circle of Willis   Fig. 23-16

Vertebrobasilar Arteriogram

A standard vertebrobasilar arteriogram appears similar to the simplified drawing in *Fig. 23-17*. The vertebral arteries, basilar artery and posterior cerebral arteries can be seen. The several branches to the cerebellum have not been labeled on this drawing.

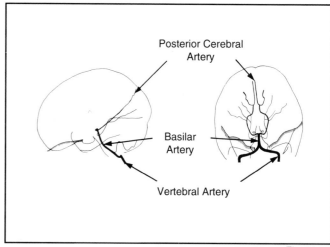

Vertebrobasilar Arteriogram   Fig. 23-17

Cerebral Veins

Great Veins of the Neck

The great veins of the neck drain blood from the head, face and cervical regions and are shown in *Fig. 23-18*. Each **internal jugular vein** drains the cranial and orbital cavities. In addition, many smaller veins join each internal jugular vein as it passes caudad to connect to the **brachiocephalic vein** on each side. The right and left brachiocephalic veins join to form the superior vena cava, which returns blood to the right heart.

The **external jugular veins** are more superficial trunks that drain the scalp and much of the face and neck. Each external jugular vein joins the respective **subclavian vein**. The **vertebral veins** form outside the cranium and drain the upper neck and occipital region. Each vertebral vein enters the transverse foramen of Cl, descends to C6 and then enters the subclavian vein.

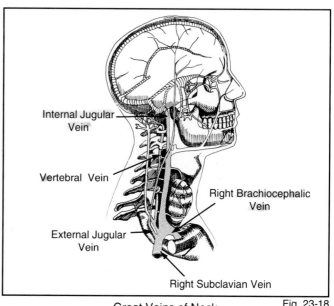

Great Veins of Neck   Fig. 23-18

Cerebral Veins continued

Dura Mater Sinuses

The sinuses of the dura mater are venous channels that drain blood from the brain *(Fig. 23-19)*. The sinuses are situated between the two layers of the dura mater.

The **falx cerebri** is a strong membranous portion of the dura mater extending down into the longitudinal fissure between the two cerebral hemispheres. A space between the two layers of the dura, along the superior portion of the longitudinal fissure, contains the **superior sagittal sinus.** The **inferior sagittal sinus** flows posteriorly to drain into the **straight sinus.** The straight sinus and the superior sagittal sinus empty into opposite transverse sinuses.

Each **transverse sinus** curves medially to occupy a groove along the mastoid portion of the temporal bone . The sinus in this region is termed the **sigmoid sinus.** Each sigmoid sinus then curves caudad to continue as the **internal jugular vein** at the jugular foramen.

The **occipital sinus** courses posteriorly from the foramen magnum to join the superior sagittal sinus, straight sinus and transverse sinuses at their confluence.

The **confluence of sinuses** is located near the internal occipital protuberance. Other major dura mater sinuses drain the area on either side of the sphenoid bone and sella turcica.

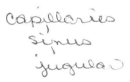

Cranial Venous System

The major veins of the entire cranial venous system are shown in *Fig. 23-20*. Only the most prominent veins are identified. One group not individually named is the external cerebral veins, which drain the outer surfaces of the cerebral hemispheres. Like all veins of the brain, the external cerebral veins possess no valves and are extremely thin since they have no muscle tissue.

Another important group is the deep cerebral veins that drain into the straight sinus along with the inferior sagittal sinus. These deep cerebral veins drain the area of the midbrain.

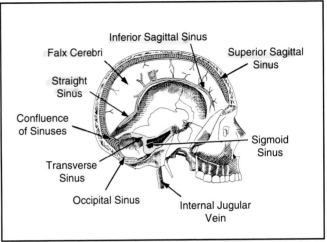

Dura Mater Sinuses   Fig. 23-19

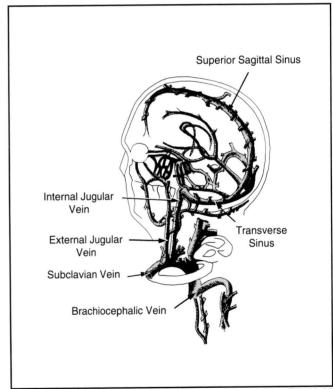

Fig. 23-20

Cranial Venous System

Thoracic Circulatory System

Thoracic Arteries

The **aorta and pulmonary arteries** are the major arteries located within the chest. The pulmonary arteries supply the lungs with blood (as shown earlier in *Fig. 23-4*).

The aorta extends from the heart to about the fourth lumbar vertebra and is divided into thoracic and abdominal sections. The **thoracic section** is subdivided into four segments (*Fig. 23-21*):
1. **Aortic bulb**
2. **Ascending aorta**
3. **Aortic arch**
4. **Descending aorta**

The bulb is at the proximal end of the aorta and is the area from which the coronary arteries originate. Extending from the bulb is the ascending portion of the aorta which terminates at approximately the second sternocostal joint and becomes the arch. The arch is unique from the other segments of the thoracic aorta because there are three arterial branches arising from it, the brachiocephalic artery, the left common carotid, and the left subclavian artery. (This is also shown on a previous page in *Fig. 23-8* under the cranial circulatory system.)

There are many variations of the aortic arch. Three more common variations sometimes seen in angiography, as shown in *Fig. 23-22,* are:
A. **Left circumflex aorta** (normal arch with the descending aorta downward and to the right)
B. **Inverse aorta** (arch is to the right)
C. **Pseudocoarctation** (arched descending aorta).

At its distal end, the arch becomes the descending aorta *(Fig. 23-21).* The descending aorta extends from the isthmus to the level of the twelfth dorsal vertebra. There are numerous intercostal, bronchial, esophageal, and superior phrenic arterial branches arising from the descending aorta, not shown in *Fig. 23-21.* These arteries transport blood to the organs for which they are named.

Thoracic Veins

The major veins within the chest are the **superior vena cava, azygos and pulmonary veins.** The superior vena cava returns the blood transported from the thorax to the right atrium. The azygos vein is the major tributary returning blood from the chest to the superior vena cava. *(Fig. 23-23).* The azygos vein enters the superior vena cava posteriorly. Blood from the chest enters the azygos vein from the intercostal, bronchial, esophageal, and phrenic veins.

The pulmonary veins return oxygenated blood from the lungs to the left atrium as previously shown in *Figs. 23-4* and *23-6.* The inferior vena cava returns blood from the abdomen and lower limbs to the right atrium as also shown in *Figs. 23-4* and *23-6.*

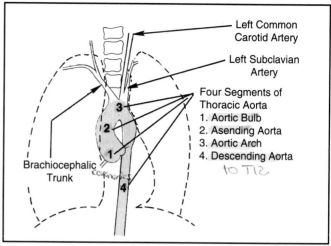

Left Common Carotid Artery
Left Subclavian Artery
Four Segments of Thoracic Aorta
1. Aortic Bulb
2. Asending Aorta
3. Aortic Arch
4. Descending Aorta
to T12
Brachiocephalic Trunk
coronaries

Thoracic Aorta   Fig. 23-21

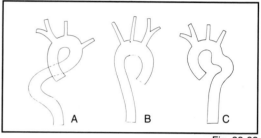

A   B   C

Variations of the Arch   Fig. 23-22

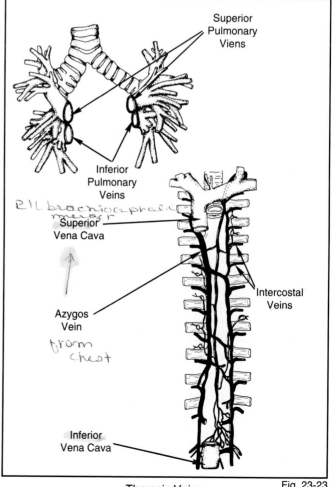

Superior Pulmonary Viens
Inferior Pulmonary Veins
R & L brachiocephalic major
Superior Vena Cava
Intercostal Veins
Azygos Vein
from chest
Inferior Vena Cava

Thoracic Veins   Fig. 23-23

Abdominal Circulatory System

Abdominal Arteries

The abdominal aorta is the continuation of the thoracic aorta. The abdominal aorta is anterior to the vertebrae and extends from the diaphragm to approximately L4 where it bifurcates into the right and left common iliac arteries. There are five major branches of the abdominal aorta that are of most interest in angiography. These are the **celiac axis, superior mesenteric artery, left renal artery, right renal artery and inferior mesenteric artery.** *(Fig. 23-24).* Any one of these branches may be selectively catheterized for study of a specific organ.

The **trunk** of the **celiac axis** arises from the aorta just below the diaphragm and about 1.5 cm above the origin of the superior mesenteric artery. Organs supplied with blood by the three large branches of the celiac trunk are the hepatic, splenic, and gastric.

The **superior mesenteric artery** supplies blood to the pancreas, most of the small intestine and portions of the large intestine, (cecum, ascending and about one-half of the transverse colon). It originates from the anterior surface of the aorta at the level of the first lumbar vertebra about 1.5 cm below the celiac artery.

The **inferior mesenteric artery** originates from the aorta at about the third lumbar vertebra (3 or 4 cm above the level of the bifurcation of the common iliac arteries). Blood is supplied to portions of the large intestine, (left half of transverse colon, descending colon, sigmoid colon and most of the rectum) by the inferior mesenteric artery.

The **right and left renal arteries** supplying blood to the kidneys originate on each side of the aorta just below the superior mesenteric artery at the level of the disc between the first and second lumbar vertebrae.

The distal portion of the abdominal aorta bifurcates at the level of the fourth lumbar vertebra into the **right and left common iliac arteries.** Each common iliac artery then divides into the **internal and external iliac arteries.** The internal iliac arteries supply the pelvic organs, (urinary bladder, rectum, reproductive organs, and pelvic muscles), with blood.

The lower extremities receive blood from the external iliac arteries. The external iliac artery is more significant in angiography than the internal iliac artery and is used to study each lower limb.

Abdominal Veins

Blood is returned from structures below the diaphragm (the trunk and lower limbs) to the right atrium of the heart via the **inferior vena cava.** There are several radiographically important tributaries to the inferior vena cava. These veins include the right and left **common iliacs, internal iliacs, external iliacs, renal veins,** *(Fig. 23-25)* and the **portal system** *(Fig. 23-26).* The iliacs drain the pelvic area and lower limbs, while the renal veins return blood from the kidneys.

The superior and inferior mesenteric veins return blood from the small and large intestine through the portal vein, hepatic vein and into the inferior vena cava. This is best shown in *Fig. 23-26.*

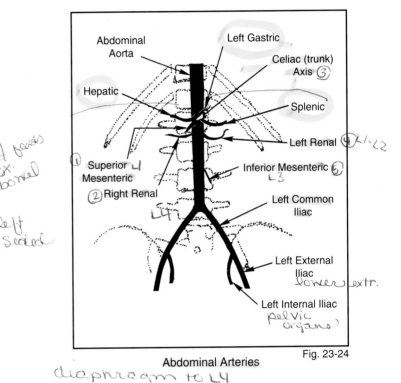

Abdominal Arteries

Fig. 23-24

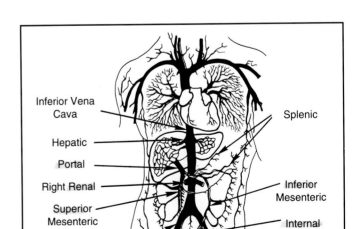

Abdominal Veins

Fig. 23-25

Portal System

The portal system includes all the veins which drain blood from the abdominal digestive track and from the spleen, pancreas and gallbladder. From these organs this blood is conveyed to the liver through the **portal vein.** While in the liver this blood is "filtered" and returned to the inferior vena cava by the hepatic veins. There are several major tributaries to the **hepatic vein** as shown in *Fig. 23-26.* The **splenic vein** is a large vein with its own tributaries which return blood from the spleen.

The **inferior mesenteric vein,** which returns blood from the rectum and from parts of the large intestine, usually opens into the splenic vein but in about 10% of cases it ends at the angle of union of the splenic and superior mesenteric veins. The **superior mesenteric vein** returns blood from the small intestine and parts of the large intestine. It unites with the splenic vein to form the portal vein.

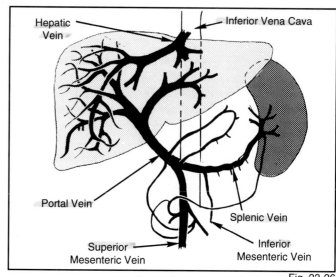

Portal System   Fig. 23-26

Peripheral Circulatory System

Upper Limb Arteries

The arterial circulation of the upper limb is generally considered to begin **at the subclavian** artery. The origin of the subclavian artery differs from the right to left side. On the right side the subclavian **arises from the brachiocephalic** artery, whereas the left subclavian originates directly from the aortic arch.

The subclavian continues to become the **axillary artery** which gives rise to the **brachial** artery. The brachial artery bifurcates into the **ulnar and radial** arteries at approximately the level of the neck of the radius. The radial and ulnar arteries continue to branch until they join together to form two palmar arches (deep and superficial). Branches of these arches supply the hand and fingers with blood *(Fig. 23-27).*

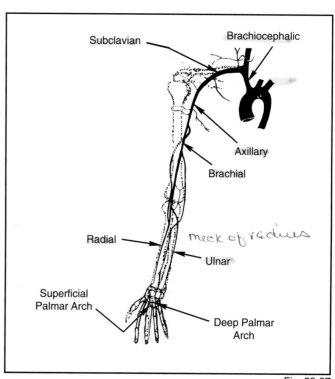

Upper Limb Arteries   Fig. 23-27

Upper Limb Veins

The venous system of the upper limb may be divided into two sets, the deep and the **superficial veins.** They communicate with each other at frequent sites and thus form two parallel drainage channels from any single region. The **cephalic and basilic veins** are the primary tributaries of the superficial venous system. Both veins originate in the arch of the hand. Anterior to the elbow joint is the **median cubital vein** (the vein most commonly used to draw blood) which connects the superficial drainage systems of the forearm. The upper basilic vein empties into the large **axillary vein** which then flows into the **subclavian** and eventually the **superior vena cava.** The lower basilic vein joins the median cubital vein continuing to the upper basilic vein *(Fig. 23-28).*

[handwritten: brachiocephalic forms svc]

The deep veins **include the two brachial veins which** drain the **radial vein, ulnar vein and the palmar arches.** The deep brachial veins join the superficial basilic to form the axillary vein, which empties into the subclavian and finally into the superior vena cava.

[handwritten: deep names go w/ art names]

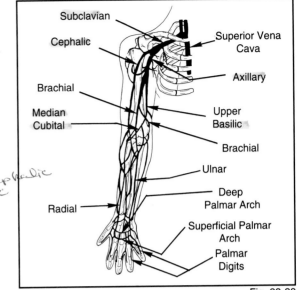

Upper Limb Veins   Fig. 23-28

Lower Limb Arteries

[handwritten: all fea beg femoral]

The arterial circulation of the lower limb begins at the **external iliac** artery and ends at the tarsal vessels *(Fig. 23-29).* The first artery to enter the lower limb is the **common femoral artery.** The common femoral artery divides into **the femoral and deep femoral** arteries. The femoral artery extends down the leg and becomes the **popliteal** artery at the level of the knee. Branches of the popliteal are the **anterior tibial, posterior tibial, and peroneal** arteries.

The **anterior tibial** artery continues as the **dorsalis pedis** artery with branches to the ankle and foot. The peroneal artery and the anterior tibial artery supply the calf and plantar surface of the foot.

[handwritten: trifurcation]

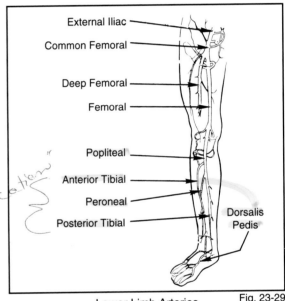

Lower Limb Arteries   Fig. 23-29

Lower Limb Veins

The veins of the lower limb are similar to the upper limb in that both have a **superficial and deep venous system.** The superficial venous system contains the **great and small saphenous** veins and their tributaries and the superficial **veins of the foot.**

The **great saphenous** vein is the longest vein in the body and extends from the foot, along the medial aspect of the leg to the thigh where it opens into the **femoral vein.** The **small saphenous** originates in the foot and extends posteriorly along the leg terminating at the knee where it empties into the **popliteal vein.**

The **major deep veins** are the **posterior tibial, peroneal, anterior tibial, popliteal and femoral.** The posterior tibial vein and the peroneal vein join after draining the posterior foot and leg. The posterior tibial extends upward and unites with the **anterior tibial** vein becoming the **popliteal** vein at the level of the knee. The popliteal continues upward to become the femoral vein before becoming the external iliac vein *(Fig. 23-30).*

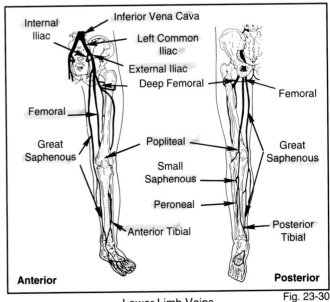

Lower Limb Veins   Fig. 23-30

Coronary Arteries

The coronary arteries are the vessels that deliver blood to the heart muscle. There are **two coronary arteries, the right and left.** Both coronary arteries originate from the **aortic bulb.** The right coronary artery arises from the right (anterior) sinuses of the aortic bulb, while the left coronary artery originates from the left (posterior) aortic bulb sinus. The right coronary artery supplies much of the **right atrium** and the **right ventricle** of the heart.

The left coronary artery supplies blood to both ventricles and the left atrium of the heart. There are many interconnections or anastomoses between the left and right coronary arteries. Blood returns to the right atrium of the heart via the coronary veins.

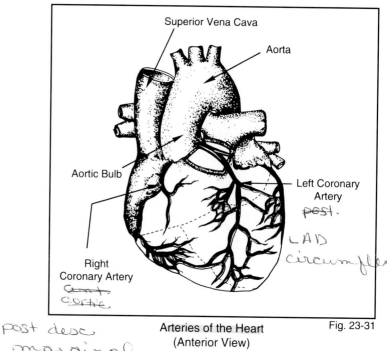

Arteries of the Heart
(Anterior View)

Fig. 23-31

Coronary Veins

The coronary sinus system returns blood to the right atrium for recirculation. The **coronary sinus** is a large vein on the posterior side of the heart between the atria and ventricles. The coronary sinus vein has three major branches: **the great, middle and small cardiac veins.** The great cardiac vein receives blood from both ventricles and the left atrium. The middle cardiac vein drains blood from the right ventricle, right atrium and part of the left ventricle. The small cardiac vein returns blood from the right ventricle. The coronary sinus drains most of the blood from the heart. Some small veins drain directly into both atria.

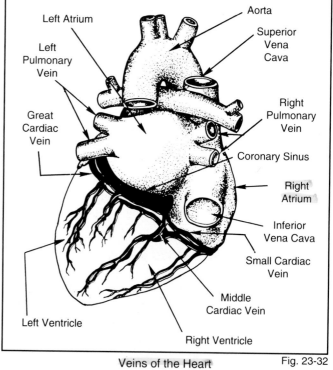

Veins of the Heart
(Posterior View)

Fig. 23-32

Summary of Major Arteries

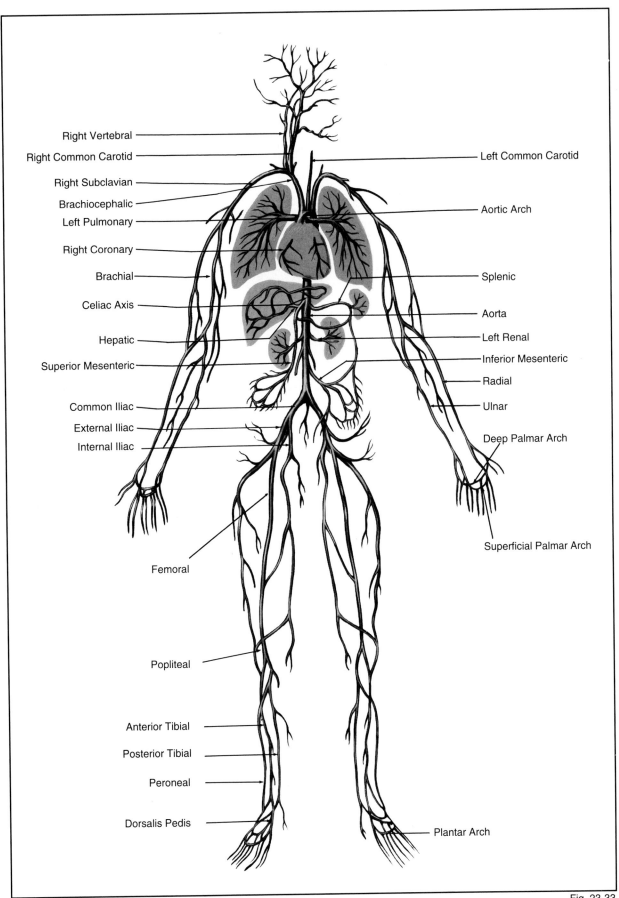

Right Vertebral

Right Common Carotid

Right Subclavian

Brachiocephalic

Left Pulmonary

Right Coronary

Brachial

Celiac Axis

Hepatic

Superior Mesenteric

Common Iliac

External Iliac

Internal Iliac

Femoral

Popliteal

Anterior Tibial

Posterior Tibial

Peroneal

Dorsalis Pedis

Left Common Carotid

Aortic Arch

Splenic

Aorta

Left Renal

Inferior Mesenteric

Radial

Ulnar

Deep Palmar Arch

Superficial Palmar Arch

Plantar Arch

Fig. 23-33

Angiography

Summary of Major Veins

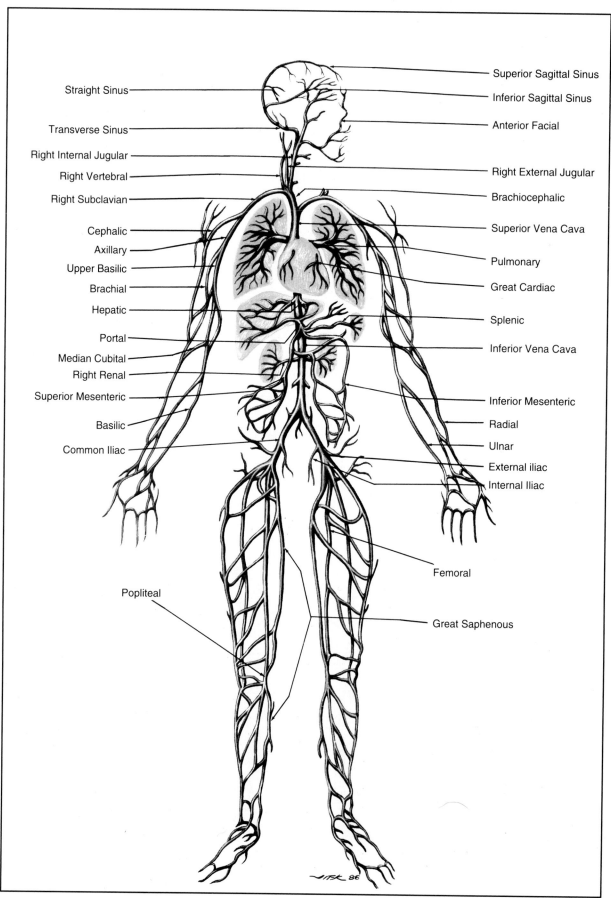

Straight Sinus

Transverse Sinus

Right Internal Jugular

Right Vertebral

Right Subclavian

Cephalic

Axillary

Upper Basilic

Brachial

Hepatic

Portal

Median Cubital

Right Renal

Superior Mesenteric

Basilic

Common Iliac

Popliteal

Superior Sagittal Sinus

Inferior Sagittal Sinus

Anterior Facial

Right External Jugular

Brachiocephalic

Superior Vena Cava

Pulmonary

Great Cardiac

Splenic

Inferior Vena Cava

Inferior Mesenteric

Radial

Ulnar

External iliac

Internal Iliac

Femoral

Great Saphenous

Fig. 23-34

Lymphatic System

Lymph Drainage

The lymphatic system serves to drain interstitial fluid (fluid in the spaces between the cells) and return it to the venous system. The fluid from the **left side of the body**, **the lower limbs**, **pelvis**, and **abdomen** enters the venous system via the **thoracic duct** (largest lymph vessel in body) which drains into the **left subclavian vein** near its junction with the left jugular vein.

The upper **right side of the body, upper limb**, **head** and **neck region** drain lymph fluid into the venous system at the junction of the **right jugular** and **right subclavian veins** via the **right lymph duct.** (See *Figs. 23-35* and *36.*)

Functions

Functions of the lymphatic portion of the circulatory system are:
1. Fight disease by producing lymphocytes and microphages
2. Return proteins and other substances to the blood
3. Filter the lymph in the lymph nodes
4. Transfer fats from the intestine to the thoracic duct and hence to the blood

The lymphatic system has no heart to pump lymph fluid to its destination. Fluid is transported by diffusion, peristalsis, respiratory movements, cardiac activities, massage and muscular activity. The transportation of lymphatic fluid is in one direction only; away from the tissues. The sequence of fluid movement is from lymphatic capillaries, to the different lymph vessels where the fluid enters the lymph nodes and is returned to the venous system by efferent lymphatic vessels.

Lymph nodes tend to form in clusters, although they may appear singularly. There are thousands of nodes throughout the body, some of which are identified in *Fig. 23-36.* The major collections of nodes which are seen radiographically are those in the thoracic, abdominal, pelvic and inguinal regions.

Lymphography

Lymphography *(lim-fog´rah-fe)* is the general term describing radiographic examination of the lymphatic vessels and nodes after injection of a contrast medium. The term **lymphangiography** is often used for a radiographic study of the **lymph vessels** following injection of contrast medium. This is done by injecting an oil-based contrast medium into a lymph vessel (usually in the feet or hands) then tracking its path by taking radiographs at timed intervals.

Since the rate of circulation of the lymphatic system is very slow, the required timed film sequences are also very slow. The lymph vessels are usually visualized within the first hour after injection and the lymph nodes 24 hours later.

With the advent of computed tomography and other newer imaging modalities which can readily visualize enlarged lymph nodes, fewer and fewer lymphography examinations utilizing contrast medium as described above are being performed.

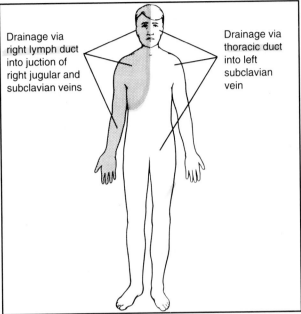

Drainage via right lymph duct into juction of right jugular and subclavian veins

Drainage via thoracic duct into left subclavian vein

Right and Left Lymph Drainage — Fig. 23-35

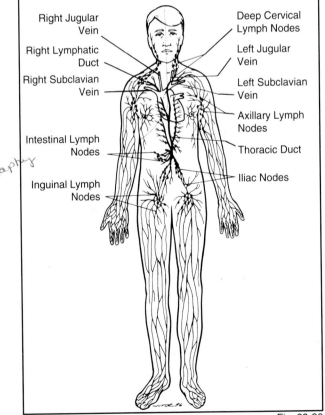

Right Jugular Vein

Right Lymphatic Duct

Right Subclavian Vein

Intestinal Lymph Nodes

Inguinal Lymph Nodes

Deep Cervical Lymph Nodes

Left Jugular Vein

Left Subclavian Vein

Axillary Lymph Nodes

Thoracic Duct

Iliac Nodes

Lymph Drainage — Fig. 23-36

Part II Radiographic Procedure and Positioning
(Cerebral, Thoracic, Abdominal and Peripheral)

The first part of this chapter covered the anatomy of the circulatory system which may be visualized radiographically with angiography following the injection of a positive contrast medium.

Part II of this chapter now covers the general procedure and the specific positioning required for angiography of the four anatomical regions, **cerebral**, **thoracic**, **abdominal** and **peripheral** (upper and /or lower limbs). Since angiographic procedures in each of these four body regions requires the injection of contrast medium, the introduction of a needle and/or catheter into the blood vessel is required. A common method for this is called the **Seldinger technique**.

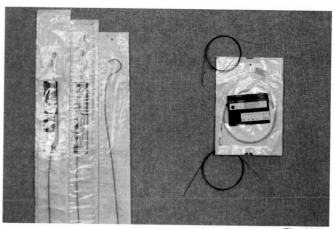

Seldinger Technique-
catheters and guide wires

Fig. 23-37

Seldinger Technique

The introduction of a catheter into a vessel requires puncturing through the skin, muscle, and tissue until the vessel of interest is reached. There are several methods that may be used to accomplish vessel puncture but the safest and most common method is the Seldinger technique. This technique was developed by Sven Seldinger in the 1950's and involves the use of specific catheters and guide wires. The catheters have different shapes at the distal end to permit easier access to the various vessels. The radiographer must be familiar with the various dimensions, types, construction, tip design and radiopacity of the catheters and guide wires in use in the radiology department.

Following is a step by step description of the Seldinger technique (as shown in *Fig. 23-38):*

Step 1, insertion of needle: The needle is placed in a small incision and advanced so that it punctures both walls of the vessel.

Step 2, placement of needle in lumen of vessel: Placement of the needle in the lumen of the vessel is achieved by slowly withdrawing the needle until a steady and vigorous blood flow returns through the needle.

Step 3, insertion of guide wire: When the desired blood flow is returned through the needle, the flexible end of a guide wire is inserted through the needle and advanced about 10 centimeters into the vessel.

Step 4, removal of needle: After the guide wire is in position, the needle is removed by withdrawing it over that portion of the guide wire remaining outside the patient.

Step 5, threading of catheter to area of interest: The catheter is then threaded over the guide wire and positioned to the area of interest under fluoroscopic control.

Step 6, removal of guide wire: When the catheter is located in the desired area, the guide wire is removed from inside the catheter. The catheter then remains as a connection between the exterior and the area of interest.

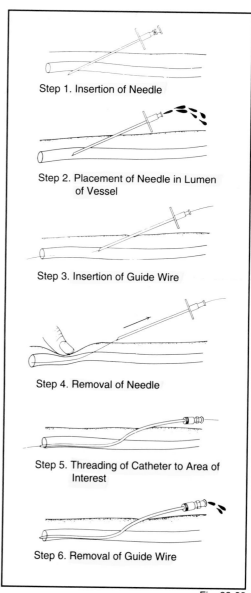

Step 1. Insertion of Needle

Step 2. Placement of Needle in Lumen of Vessel

Step 3. Insertion of Guide Wire

Step 4. Removal of Needle

Step 5. Threading of Catheter to Area of Interest

Step 6. Removal of Guide Wire

Seldinger Technique

Fig. 23-38

Angiography

Special Procedure Room

The special procedure room, shown in *Figs.* 23-39 and 23-40, is equipped for all types of angiographic procedures. The angiographic room is usually considerably larger than a conventional radiographic room. An adjoining room or adjacent alcove is often used to house control panels, generators and physiologic monitoring equipment. A scrub area, film processor, radiograph viewing area and adequate storage facilities should be readily accessible to the procedure room. The special procedure room should be close to, but somewhat isolated from, the general radiography department. The room location should be easily accessible to the emergency department, ambulance entrance, surgery and recovery rooms.

Equipment in Neuroangiographic Room

A modern neuroangiography suite generally includes the following:
1. Biplane film changers capable of rapid simultaneous or alternating exposures
2. Changers capable of serial uniplane filming and magnification techniques
3. Automatic, mechanical contrast media injectors
4. Image-amplified television fluoroscopy that can rotate to either frontal or lateral modes
5. Appropriate generators, controls and x-ray tubes
6. Island type table with floating top
7. Physiologic monitoring equipment

Additional equipment may include:
1. Stereo filming capabilities
2. Linear tomography
3. 70 or 90 mm. or larger cine
4. Video tape or disc recorder

The floor should be made free of any cables or wires by utilizing subfloor conduits for necessary circuitry. X-ray tubes, housings, collimators and certain other equipment can be placed on ceiling mounts and tracks to further clear the working area. Outlets for oxygen and suction should be located in the room walls.

Biplane Film Changers

The typical cerebral angiographic procedure utilizes biplane film changers in conjunction with two radiographic tubes. Each unit should be independent of the other, and the two should be easily placed at right angles to one another. This arrangement allows a series of radiographs in both the lateral position and the anteroposterior projection to be exposed with a single injection of contrast medium. Blood flow through the brain is rapid, usually passing from carotid artery to jugular vein in less than 8 seconds. Consequently, the biplane film changers must be capable of several radiographs per second, each with superb definition. There are three basic types of changers available. They include: (1) the roll film changer, (2) the cassette changer, and (3) the cut film changer. While each has advantages and disadvantages, the cut film changer, as illustrated in *Fig. 23-41*, is widely used for angiography.

The internal mechanism of the film changer moves film rapidly from the supply compartment to the exposure area intensifying screens, and finally to the receiving bin. A program selector operates the film changer during single or serial exposures, regulating film rate and the duration of each phase of the series. Therefore, the program selector controls the number of films per second as well as the total length of time that exposures are to be made. The program selector may be wired so that the contrast medium injector is synchronized with the imaging process.

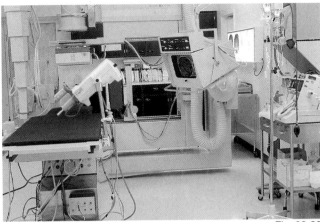

General Angiographic Room   Fig. 23-39

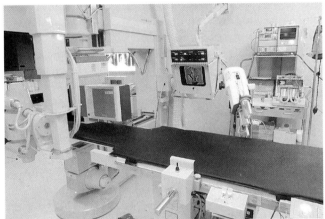

Neuroangiographic Room Equipment   Fig. 23-40

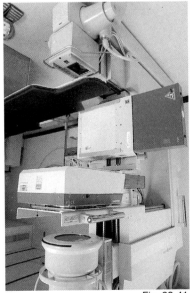

Biplane Film   Fig. 23-41
Changers

Equipment in Neuroangiographic Room continued

Automatic Contrast Medium Injector

As contrast medium is injected into the circulatory system, it is diluted by blood. The contrast material must be injected with sufficient pressure to overcome the patient's systemic arterial pressure and to maintain a bolus to minimize dilution with blood. In order to maintain the flow rates necessary for cerebral angiography, an automatic, mechanical injector must be used. The flow rate is affected by many variables, such as the viscosity of contrast medium, length and diameter of the catheter, and injection pressure. Depending on these variables and the vessel to be injected, the desired flow rate can be selected prior to injection.

A typical automatic contrast medium injector is shown in *Fig. 23-42*. Every injector has a syringe, a heating device, a high pressure mechanism and a control panel. The syringe may be reusable or disposable. Reusable syringes must be easily disassembled for sterilization. The heating device warms and maintains the contrast medium at body temperature, reducing the viscosity of the medium. The high-pressure mechanism is usually an electromechanical device consisting of a motor drive screw that drives a piston into or out of the syringe.

Some desirable features of an automatic mechanical injector other than safety, convenience and ease of use, and reliability of flow rate settings include: (1) an obvious ready light when armed and set for injection, (2) a squirt feature for test injections, and (3) controls to preclude inadvertent injection, or excessive pressure or volume injection.

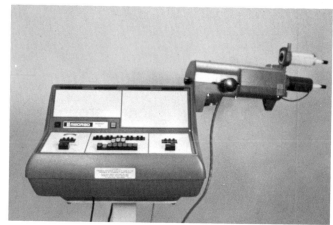

Automatic Contrast Media Injector   Fig. 23-42

Basic Radiographic Equipment

Island Table: A basic island radiographic table and two cut film changers are shown in *Fig. 23-43*. The island-type table is necessary for femoral catheterization techniques to allow the neuroradiologist to work from either side of the patient. A four-way floating top on a central pedestal permits the changers to be placed at either end of the table and still allow room for the image intensifier. The table height should be adjustable to permit magnification techniques.

X-ray Tubes: The need to visualize smaller and smaller blood vessels during angiography, and the use of magnification techniques, have resulted in specialized x-ray tubes. These x-ray tubes provide very small, effective focal spots that are the combined result of steep angle anodes and fractional focal spots.

Other modifications in the material composing the anode and focal track, as well as high-speed anode rotation, have increased the instantaneous loading capacity and the heat unit storage capabilities. The net result is an x-ray tube capable of (1) serial exposures with very high mA's and fast times and (2) superb definition production even during magnification techniques.

Collimators: Precise collimation is absolutely essential for neuroangiography. All shutters of the collimator must be in perfect alignment to prevent degradation of the image from off-focus radiation, or unwanted secondary and scatter radiation. Aperture diaphragms may also be used to further limit the field size.

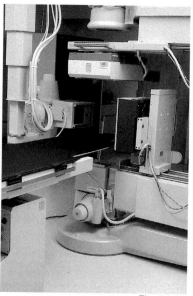

Fig. 23-43
Film Changers, Island Table
and X-ray Tubes

Sterile Supplies

Much of each angiographic procedure is carried out under aseptic conditions, and the entire exam must be carried out under clean conditions. The special procedures room and equipment must be scrupulously clean. The room should be fully stocked and prepared before the patient's arrival. All radiographic and electromechanical equipment must be checked and in working order. The appropriate sterile tray, catheters, guide wires and contrast medium must be assembled.

Basic Sterile Tray for Seldinger Catheterization

A sterile tray, such as the one shown in *Fig. 23-44*, contains the basic equipment necessary for Seldinger catheterization of a femoral artery. Basic sterile items include:
1. Hemostats
2. Control syringes with fingertip control for manual injection
3. Scalpel
4. Syringe and needle for local anesthetic
5. Medicine glasses and basins
6. Three-way stopcocks or a manifold mounting of multiple stopcocks
7. Gauze squares for skin preparation and cleansing
8. Sponge forceps
9. Draping material, towels and towel clips
10. Connecting tubing
11. Catheter to manifold adapter
12. Gowns, gloves and, on rare occasions, caps and masks

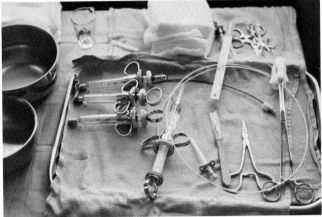

Basic Sterile Tray   Fig. 23-44

Items Added to Basic Sterile Tray

Sterile items that must be added to the basic tray are shown in *Fig. 23-45*. These include:
1. Appropriate catheter
2. Corresponding guide wire
3. Dilator
4. Arterial needle

The catheter shown in *Fig. 23-45* is a radiopaque, polyethylene tube that must be shaped at both ends by the neuroradiologist. These catheters may also be supplied pre-formed by various companies. The guide wire is a teflon-coated, safety wire with a J-shaped tip. The dilator shown is the same size as the catheter and is used whenever a non-teflon-coated catheter is used. The needle is a thin-walled needle of the Potts-Cournand design. These needles have a blunt tip with two different inserts, termed obturators. A sharp protruding obturator or a matching, blunt protruding obturator may be used when needed by the neuroradiologist.

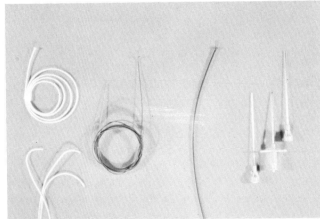

Additional Sterile Supplies   Fig. 23-45

Radiographic Procedure

Purpose

Cerebral angiography is the **radiographic examination of the blood vessels of the brain following injection of a positive contrast medium.** The primary purpose of cerebral angiography is to provide an exact vascular road map, enabling involved physicians to satisfactorily localize and diagnose certain abnormalities.

Indications

Cerebral angiography is indicated whenever surgical treatment is under strong consideration, and when other imaging modalities and nonradiographic studies have not provided a precise diagnosis. Cranial computed tomography is often performed prior to the angiographic study and, in many instances, provides sufficient information for diagnosis. **Vascular lesions, including arterial occlusions, aneurysms** and **arteriovenous malformations**, are best visualized by cerebral angiography.

Contraindications

There are few strict contraindications to cerebral angiography, although certain conditions make the examination more difficult for the neuroradiologist. These conditions include the young and the aged, advanced arteriosclerosis, and especially atherosclerosis, severe hypertension and severe cardiac decompensation. A history of anaphylactoid reaction to iodinated contrast media will cause some concern, as will a strong history of thromboembolism. One absolute contraindication to use of the femoral approach is **lack of pulsation of either femoral artery.** Serious illness exists in most cases requiring cerebral angiography; therefore, the procedure will be attempted in spite of most contraindications.

Contrast Media

Contrast media for cerebral angiography are various salts of organic iodide compounds. Cerebral angiography is usually performed using 100 percent meglumine salts at 60 percent weight-to-volume concentrations. Injectable meglumine salts tend to be less toxic than the sodium salts.

Reaction to the contrast medium or the premedication is a possibility and must be kept in mind. A vasovagal reaction initiated by fear may occur at any time. Genuine care and reassurance during the examination will be beneficial to all concerned.

Patient Placement

After transportation to the radiology department on a stretcher, the patient is placed in the supine position on a well-padded table. A pillow or sponge support placed under areas of strain, such as the small of the back and the knees, will add to patient comfort. Even though the patient is sedated, a burning sensation will be felt on injection. Restraints may be necessary to help prevent involuntary motion during this crucial phase of the examination. Wrist and knee restraints, and possibly a compression band across the pelvis, will be helpful. The skin surface of the femoral triangle on the side to be catheterized is shaved and prepared with a germicide. Appropriate sterile drapes are then placed over the prepared area, as shown in *Fig. 23-46.*

Patient Preparation

Patient preparation for cerebral angiography depends on patient condition, which dictates the amount of time available before the examination. The patient will be hospitalized and, ideally, should be NPO to prevent problems associated with premature evacuation of the stomach contents. Mild sedatives are generally prescribed so that the patient is relaxed, but able to fully cooperate. Adequate sedation lessens the intensity of burning pain felt along the pathway of the rapidly injected contrast medium. Certain patients may require general anesthesia or heavy sedation.

The patient must also be psychologically prepared to undergo the examination. Ideally, the neuroradiologist should visit the patient on the day prior to the examination to explain most of what will be done. This explanation must be done in language that the patient understands.

Prior to catheterization, both femoral artery pulses should be assessed and recorded. In addition, the dorsalis pedis and posterior tibial artery pulses are evaluated and recorded bilaterally before the procedure, just prior to catheter pullout and at the end of the procedure. Before, during and after the procedure, one member of the team should carefully note the patient's blood pressure, pulse and level of consciousness.

Consent Form: At the time of the neuroradiologist's visit, informed consent for the procedure is obtained from the patient or other legally authorized person. The examination is verbally described to the patient, and any complications that may occur are discussed. A printed sheet outlining relative risks and describing the procedure is presented to the patient for his signature. This informed consent sheet is then signed by the neuroradiologist, witnessed by an appropriate person and is placed in the patient's chart.

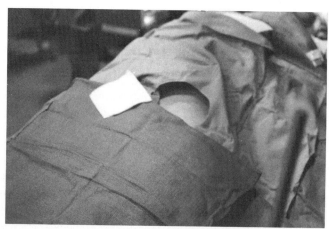

Patient Placement and Preparation   Fig. 23-46

Patient Ready for Neuroradiologist

Sterile items shown in *Fig. 23-47* are prepared for the arterial puncture by the neuroradiologist. The manifold shown on the lower part of the sterile sheet in this illustration is connected by lengths of tubing to (1) a transducer for vessel pressure readings, (2) a heparinized saline drip under pressure, and (3) an appropriate contrast medium. The syringe attached to the lower end of the manifold allows hand injection of contrast medium, while the upper end attaches to the positioned catheter.

Seldinger Catheterization Procedure

For cerebral angiography, the basic Seldinger technique is used to catheterize the femoral artery. The femoral approach is versatile in that any of the four vessels supplying the brain, as well as the arch of the aorta or the external carotids, can be injected directly.

Arterial Puncture and Insertion of the Catheter: After localization and assessment of the femoral artery, the neuroradiologist punctures the femoral artery with the special arterial needle. The arterial needle is placed in the femoral artery wherein blood will be ejected from the needle as shown in *Fig. 23-48*. The safety guide wire is immediately advanced through the needle cannula into the femoral artery, and up to the distal aorta, if possible. The cannula is removed and the vessel puncture site is dilated with the dilator. The dilator is removed and the catheter of choice is passed over the guide wire. Finally, the guide wire is removed and the catheter is flushed and attached to a saline drip.

The catheter is shown in place in *Fig. 23-49*. At this point the catheter is advanced to the ascending aortic arch and maneuvered into the vessel chosen for study. Proposed injection sites are always tested fluoroscopically following a hand injection of contrast medium. Once it is confirmed that the catheter is correctly placed, serial radiographic filming may proceed.

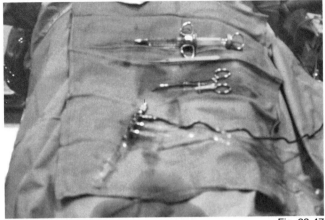

Ready for Neuroradiologist   Fig. 23-47

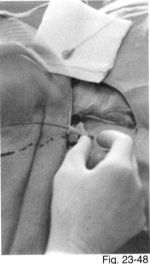
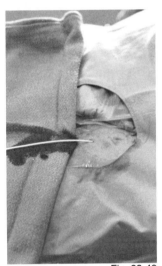

Fig. 23-48   Fig. 23-49
Arterial Puncture   Catheter in place

Positioning Routine and Examination Procedure

Scout Positioning for Internal Carotid (anterior circulation) Angiography

As soon as the patient is placed on the radiographic table, and prior to the catheterization process, scout radiographs are exposed. Scout radiographs are necessary whenever contrast medium is injected. If the primary interest is the internal carotid artery, or anterior brain circulation, an AP and a lateral scout are exposed.

Precise positioning is essential, so care must be taken to insure that the midsagittal plane is perpendicular to the frontal changer and parallel to the lateral changer. The infraorbitomeatal line (IOML) is placed perpendicular to the frontal changer, as shown in *Fig. 23-50*. The primary objective for the frontal projection is to superimpose the petrous ridge and the orbital plate on each side. This positioning projects the anterior and middle cerebral arteries above the floor of the anterior fossa. A line connecting the supraorbital groove (SOG) and the top of the ear attachment (TEA) should be parallel to the primary beam.

The central ray is directed 2 centimeters cranial (cephalad) to this line and passes through a line connecting the two concentric points. The lateral x-ray beam is centered to the concentric point. Both beams are tightly collimated.

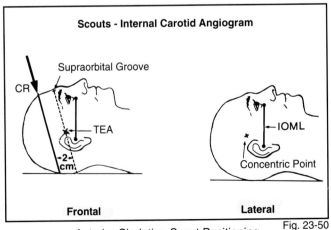

Anterior Cirulation Scout Positioning   Fig. 23-50

dim. to AP

Scout Positioning for Vertebrobasilar (posterior circulation) Angiography

If the primary interest is the posterior circulation or vertebrobasilar system, then slightly different positioning methods are utilized. The midbrain and hindbrain must be visualized when radiographically studying the vertebrobasilar system. The frontal position utilizes a caudal angulation of approximately 30 degrees to the IOML The central ray enters at about the hairline and exits at the level of the EAM. Parallax is a problem with extreme tube angles, and occasionally the neck must be hyperflexed (center illustration of *Fig. 23-51*) so that the central ray remains perpendicular to the frontal changer. This modification is especially necessary for magnification techniques. The 30-degree angle is maintained between the central ray and the IOML.

Laterally, the centering point is 2 centimeters posterior to and 1 centimeter superior to the EAM. Centering in this fashion corresponds to the area of the fourth ventricle.

Arch Aortography

In order to completely image the four major vessels leading to the brain, the neuroradiologist may elect to do an initial arch aortogram. Arch aortography allows the neuroradiologist to evaluate the major vessels for size, position, lumen status and anomalous origin. This position is rarely utilized during a three or four-vessel angiogram, but is included as one of several possibilities. The arch aortogram is described later in this chapter under thoracic angiography.

Position for Common Carotid Arteriography

A more likely beginning for a complete three- or four-vessel angiogram is two views of the neck to radiograph each common carotid artery. The position for a common carotid arteriogram is demonstrated in *Fig. 23-52*. Radiographs of the right common carotid artery in the AP and lateral positions are exposed to examine this artery and its bifurcation into internal and external carotid arteries. The area of bifurcation is studied carefully for occlusive disease. The left common carotid artery will be studied in a similar manner later in the examination.

Left Common Carotid Arteriograms

An AP and a lateral arteriogram of the left common carotid artery are shown in *Figs. 23-53* and *54*. The catheter has been placed in the most proximal portion of the common carotid artery. The area of bifurcation is of special interest to the neuroradiologist. On the AP projection, the internal carotid artery is located more laterally than the external carotid artery. On the lateral view to the right, the internal carotid artery courses anteriorly before ascending to the base of the brain.

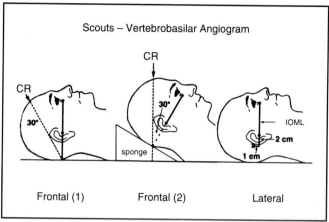

Scouts – Vertebrobasilar Angiogram

Frontal (1)   Frontal (2)   Lateral

Posterior Circulation Scout Positioning   Fig. 23-51

like Townes

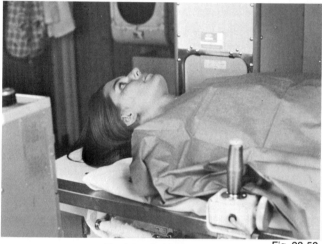

Position for Common Carotid Arteriography   Fig. 23-52

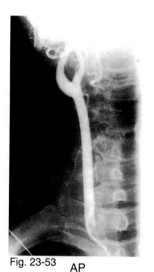
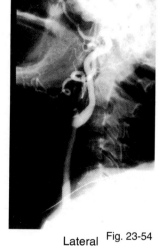

Fig. 23-53   AP   Lateral   Fig. 23-54

Left Common Carotid Arteriograms

Internal Carotid Angiography

Procedure and Position for Internal Carotid Angiography

Following injection of the right or left common carotid artery, the catheter is advanced into the respective internal carotid artery. Fluoroscopic control with hand injections of contrast medium assures the neuroradiologist of correct catheter placement. The anterior cerebral circulation is studied with a sufficiently long exposure run to visualize arteries, capillaries and veins. Assuming a normal circulation time, each plane is exposed at the rate of two exposures per second for 6 to 8 seconds.

Exposures usually alternate between frontal and lateral modes. Simultaneous firing of both x-ray tubes is usually not attempted due to the large amounts of cross-fogging and subsequent degradation of image quality.

Correct Positioning: Positioning for internal carotid angiography is demonstrated in *Figs. 23-55* and *56.* A cotton strap attached to a double-ratchet device is secured across the forehead for immobilization purposes.

For the AP projection, the frontal x-ray tube is angled caudad so that the central ray is parallel to the line connecting the SOG and TEA, and the central ray passes through a line connecting the two concentric points. Lateral centering is to the concentric point.

Explanation to Patient: After the patient is correctly positioned and the x-ray tubes and film changers are properly aligned, and immediately prior to injection, the neuroradiologist must explain to the patient the necessity of holding absolutely still even though a temporary burning sensation will be felt along the injection pathway. This warning cannot be minimized since, quite often, the burning sensation is intense.

Left Internal Carotid Arteriograms

Representative radiographs of the arterial phase of a left internal carotid angiogram are shown in these radiographs *(Figs. 23-57 and 58).* On the AP radiograph to the left, the floor of the anterior fossa and the petrous ridges superimpose. This allows visualization of the bifurcation of the internal carotid artery into the anterior and middle cerebral arteries.

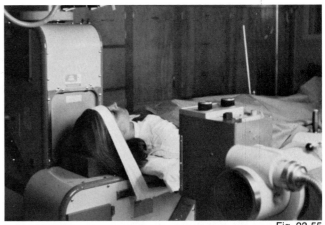

Position for Internal Carotid Angiography   Fig. 23-55

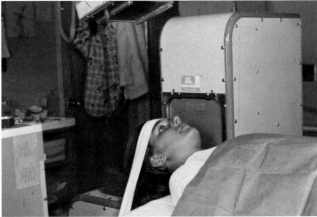

Position for Internal Carotid Angiography   Fig. 23-56

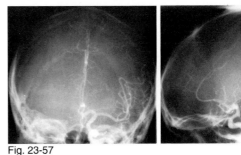

Fig. 23-57   Fig. 23-58

AP   Lateral

Left Internal Carotid Arteriograms

Magnification Radiography

Frontal Position (2X magnification)

The law of image magnification states that the width of the image is to the width of the object, as the distance of the image from the x-ray source is to the distance of the object from the x-ray source. In order to achieve 2X magnification in the frontal position, the patient's head needs to be positioned similar to the dry skull shown in *Fig. 23-59*. The center of the head is placed exactly halfway between the film and x-ray source. In 2X magnification, all anatomic structures equal to or larger than the effective focal spot size will be displayed twice their normal size on the finished radiograph.

Lateral Position (2X magnification)

Head placement to achieve 2X magnification in the lateral position is shown in *Fig. 23-60*. Again, the patient's head would be placed exactly halfway between the film and the x-ray source. If the object were placed even closer to the x-ray tube, there would be greater magnification of the image. Rarely will magnification factors greater than 2X be attempted using a focus-film distance of 100 cm. Due to the size of the collimator, the head must be placed very close to the exit port of the collimator in order to achieve magnification factors greater than 2X.

Another limiting factor is the size of the film used in the automatic changer. The maximum field size of the larger changers is 35 cm x 35 cm. Even at 2X magnification, the entire cranium barely fits on a 35 cm x 35 cm field.

Position for Magnification Angiography of Internal Carotid Artery

Figure 23-61 demonstrates patient positioning for a magnified, internal carotid angiogram. Due to the physical limitations of this particular x-ray table in relation to the frontal film changer, a focus-film distance of less than 100 cm is being utilized. Consequently, the frontal collimator is in close approximation with the forehead of the patient.

Air-gap Principle: A beneficial adjunct to magnification radiography is application of the air-gap principle. Whenever the image detection system is separated from the object by an appreciable distance, there is a remarkable decrease in the amount of secondary and scatter radiation that reaches the film surface. Much of the secondary and scatter radiation is directed away from the film. A large percentage of the weaker radiation emerging from the skull and directed toward the film is absorbed in the air and never reaches the film surface.

The advantage offered by utilization of the air-gap principle is that a stationary grid is no longer necessary for clean-up purposes. This reduces the amount of exposure necessary and decreases the radiation exposure to the patient. In addition, both x-ray beams should be closely collimated to further reduce radiation exposure to the patient. This close collimation is especially important because the short SID increases skin dosage to the radiation sensitive areas of the head and neck.

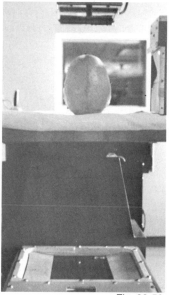

Fig. 23-59
Magnification Radiography
(Frontal)

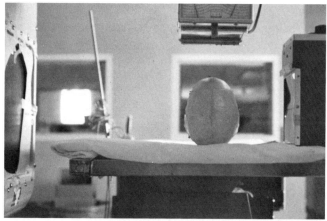

Magnification Radiography   Fig. 23-60
(Lateral)

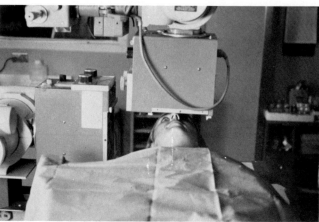

Internal Carotid Magnification   Fig. 23-61

Magnified Internal Carotid Arteriograms

Magnified radiographs of an internal carotid arteriogram are shown in *Figs. 23-62* and *63*. The AP radiograph to the left and the lateral radiograph to the right visualize arteries much smaller than those seen on a nonmagnified study. Patient motion must be minimized during magnification techniques since any unsharpness due to voluntary or involuntary movement will be accentuated. Any motion unsharpness will be proportionately enlarged, depending on the magnification factor.

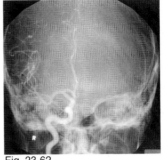 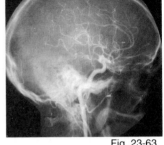

Fig. 23-62   Fig. 23-63

AP   Lateral

Magnified Internal
Carotid Arteriograms

Comparison of Conventional and Magnified Carotid Arteriograms. Two lateral internal carotid arteriograms are shown for comparative purposes in *Figs. 23-64* and *65*. The routine nonmagnified study is to the left, while the 2X magnified radiograph is to the right. The phase of circulation is similar for each of these radiographs. Small arteries that cannot be delineated on the routine study are readily apparent on the magnified view.

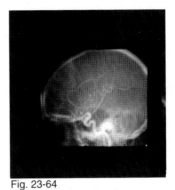 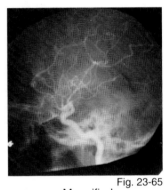

Fig. 23-64   Fig. 23-65

Conventional   Magnified

Conventional vs.Magnified
Carotid Arteriograms

Vertebrobasilar Angiography

Position for Vertebrobasilar Angiography

Following radiographic study of the neck and anterior circulation on both sides, the posterior circulation is studied, if necessary. Usually, the left vertebral artery is catheterized first. If injection volume and pressure are adequate to visualize certain branches of the opposite vertebral artery by reflux, then the right vertebral artery is usually not injected directly. Therefore, injection of both right and left internal carotid arteries and the left vertebral artery constitute the usual **three-vessel angiogram.** If both vertebral arteries are injected, the examination is termed a **four-vessel angiogram.**

Positioning for the vertebrobasilar angiogram is similar to positioning for the internal carotid angiogram. The patient's head is immobilized, and the IOML is adjusted perpendicular to the frontal changer. The more a patient can depress the chin, however, the better the results will be since less tube angulation is required. Frontal centering for the vertebrobasilar angiogram must include the area surrounding the fourth ventricle. Lateral centering is to the fourth ventricle, which is approximately 1 centimeter superior and 2 centimeters posterior to the EAM. Frontal positioning involves a modified semiaxial anteroposterior projection, maintaining a 30-degree angle between the central ray and the IOML. The central ray exits at the level of the EAM.

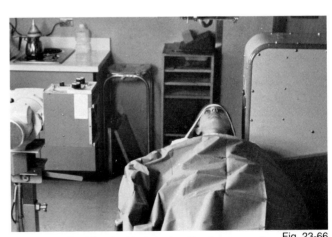

Position for Vertebrobasilar Angiography   Fig. 23-66

Left Vertebrobasilar Arteriogram

Representative vertebrobasilar arteriograms are shown in *Figs. 23-67* and *68.* The AP radiograph demonstrates a left-sided injection with adequate filling of the necessary branches of the right vertebral artery.

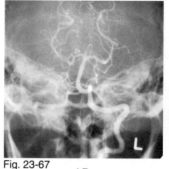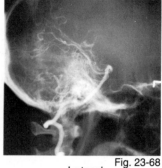

Fig. 23-67   AP   Lateral   Fig. 23-68

Left Vertebrobasilar Arteriorgrams

Position for Magnification Angiography of the Vertebrobasilar System

Patient position for magnification studies of the vertebrobasilar system is demonstrated in *Fig. 23-69.* The head is placed halfway between the focal spot and the film to achieve a 2X magnification. Rather than angle the x-ray tube and introduce an element of unsharpness due to parallax, the patient's head has been supported with polyurethane blocks to flex the neck so that no tube angulation is utilized. An angle of 30 degrees is maintained between the IOML and the central ray.

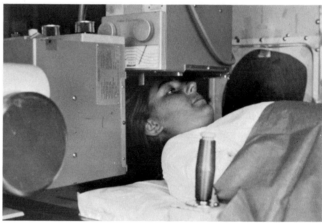

Vertebrobasilar Magnification   Fig. 23-69

Magnified Vertebrobasilar Arteriogram

Magnified vertebrobasilar arteriograms are shown in *Figs. 23-70* and *71.* The semiaxial anteroposterior projection to the left and the lateral radiograph to the right visualize a multitude of large and small arteries. Patient instructions, immobilization, close collimation and elimination of tube angulation all contribute to reduced unsharpness and, consequently, superior quality radiographs.

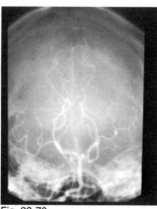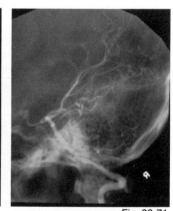

Fig. 23-70   AP   Lateral   Fig. 23-71

Magnified Vertebrobasilar Arteriogram

Aneurysm Arteriography

Special Oblique Positions

Occasionally, special oblique positions are necessary to fully evaluate aneurysms. A common site for aneurysm in the anterior circulation is near the bifurcation of the internal carotid artery into the anterior and middle cerebral arteries. The supraorbital oblique position, as shown to the upper left in *Fig. 23-72*, is identical to the frontal projection for the internal carotid artery, except that the head is rotated 30 degrees from the midsagittal plane.

The transorbital oblique position shown to the lower right in *Fig. 23-72* utilizes a 20-degree cephalic angulation in addition to the 30-degree rotation of the head. In most cases the head is rotated 30 degrees away from the side being injected.

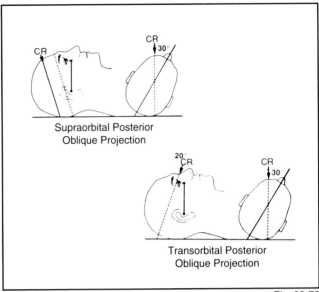

Supraorbital Posterior
Oblique Projection

Transorbital Posterior
Oblique Projection

Special Oblique Positions   Fig. 23-72

Oblique Position for Internal Carotid and Branches

The position for an oblique view of the left internal carotid artery and its branches is demonstrated in *Fig. 23-73*. This illustration could represent either oblique position, depending on tube angulation. An approximate 15-degree angulation to the feet would give the supraorbital oblique position, while a 20-degree cephalic angulation would produce the transorbital position. This oblique position is usually radiographed in both frontal and lateral planes. Since only the arterial phase needs to be visualized, a run of 3 to 4 seconds is usually adequate.

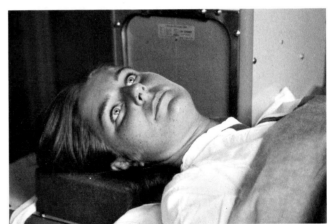

Oblique Position for Aneurysm   Fig. 23-73

Transorbital Oblique Radiography

An arteriogram utilizing the transorbital oblique position is shown in *Fig. 23-74*. A large aneurysm is evident at the bifurcation of the anterior and middle cerebral arteries.

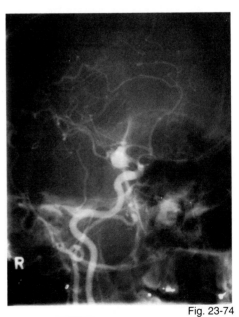

Fig. 23-74
Transorbital Oblique Position

Photographic Subtraction

Control and Injection Radiographs

Photographic subtraction is a technique that subtracts or cancels all structures common to both a scout radiograph and an injected radiograph. In theory, this technique will produce a radiograph that shows only the opacified vessels without interference from bony structures. Both the control radiograph and the injected radiograph, as shown in *Figs. 23-75* and *76,* are obtained during the exposure series. The control radiograph is exposed immediately prior to the injection and is the first radiograph of the series. There must be no motion and no contrast medium on the control radiograph .

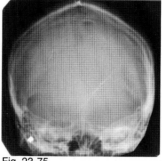 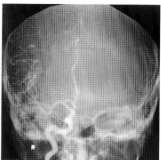

Fig. 23-75   Fig. 23-76

Control and Injection Radiographs

Positive Mask and Subtraction Radiographs

A standard radiograph, one in which bone and opacified vessels appear white, is a negative image. The simplest method of subtraction involves first producing an exact reversal of the control radiograph. This step is accomplished in the processing room by exposing a single-emulsion film through the control radiograph. The result is a positive image, termed a positive mask or diapositive.

A composite is then made by registration. A positive mask and any radiograph in the series containing contrast medium are precisely superimposed. All bony landmarks are placed in exact register and the two radiographs are taped together. A print is made of this composite. The positive and negative radiographs tend to cancel each other, leaving a radiograph showing only the opacified blood vessels.

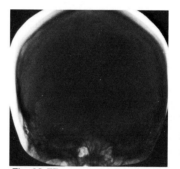 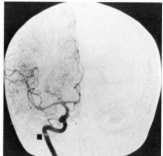

Fig. 23-77   Fig. 23-78

Positive Mask and Subtraction Radiographs

Subtraction Venogram

A magnified carotid venogram and a subtraction study of the same radiograph are shown in *Figs. 23-79* and *80.* It is apparent that more diagnostic information is made available to the neuroradiologist on the subtraction study. The two techniques of (1) direct roentgen enlargement or magnification and (2) composite mask subtraction greatly enhance the more routine methods of cerebral angiography. Techniques utilized in digital angiography allow electronic subtraction of the nonessential portion of the television image.

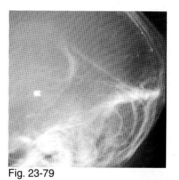 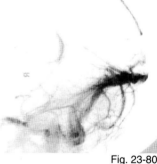

Fig. 23-79   Fig. 23-80

Regular Venogram Versus Subtraction

Radiographic Procedure

Purpose

Thoracic aortography *(a″or-tog′rah-fe)* is a **radiographic examination of the thoracic aorta following the injection of a radiopaque contrast medium**. The contrast medium outlines the contour of the aorta and its major branches. By observing the size, shape and possible displacement of the vessels, physicians are able to identify abnormalities. Abnormalities are frequently located in the aortic arch or its branches.

Indications

Thoracic aortography is indicated when patient symptoms suggest possible pathology of the aorta or its branches. This is especially true for patients with inconclusive preexaminations and persistent symptoms suggesting aortic pathology. Some specific pathologies which would indicate thoracic aortography are: **patent ductus arteriosus, aortic aneurysm, coarctation, aortic arch anomalies** or **aortic stenosis**.

Contraindications

The primary contraindication to thoracic aortography is **adverse reaction to the contrast medium**. Most patients having thoracic aortography are severely ill or have inconclusive previous test results. Thoracic aortography may be the only remaining test available to obtain conclusive evidence for proper diagnosis. This may necessitate thoracic aortography being performed under less than ideal situations, i.e. poor patient condition or possible reaction to contrast medium.

Patient Preparation

Patients having thoracic aortography are generally anxious and nervous about the procedure, thus, a mild sedative is recommended. The type and amount of medication given the patient is the decision of the attending physician. Atropine may be administered to lessen bradycardia.

Prior to the examination, a member of the angiography team should visit the patient to verbally explain the procedure and the risks involved. When the patient understands the procedure and potential complications, an informed consent is signed by the patient which outlines the risks of the procedure.

To assist in the diagnosis, preexamination tests should be performed. These would include an overpenetrated chest radiograph and the blood pressure differences between the right and left arms. The results of the tests are helpful in determining if there is any aortic pathology. If the patient has previous chest radiographs, the former radiographic diagnosis should be compared with the current diagnosis in order to determine possible changes.

Major Equipment

The major equipment ncedcd for thoracic aortography include:
1. Electromechanical injector
2. Single rapid serial film changer
3. Image intensifier with television monitor
4. Floating table top
5. Cineradiographic camera

The electromechanic injector is used to deliver the contrast medium to the area of interest. Placement of the catheter in the involved area is performed under fluoroscopy. The area of interest indicates the type of recording device to be used, i.e., a rapid serial film changer or cine camera. Cineradiography is utilized if the pathology is located in the aortic valve or left ventricle. To record the aortic arch and its branches, a rapid serial film changer is used. This type of filming is achieved by moving the floating table top over the serial film changer (see *Fig. 23-43*) in order to record the areas of interest.

Accessory and Optional Equipment

Additional equipment for thoracic aortography include:
1. Sterile angiographic tray
2. Vascular catheters
3. Electrocardiograph recorder
4. Emergency cardiopulmonary equipment (crash cart)

The sterile tray is used during insertion of the catheter in the vessel. The heart is monitored by attaching electrocardiographic leads to the patient's body. It is advisable to have an emergency cardiac cart either in the room or in the immediate vicinity should cardiopulmonary resuscitation become necessary.

Catheterization Method

The safest and most common method of catheterization of the aorta is through a puncture of the femoral artery using the Seldinger technique. After successful puncture of the femoral artery, a pigtail catheter or a closed-end catheter is inserted into the artery and positioned at the desired aortic location for contrast medium injection.

Contrast Medium

The amount of contrast medium used for thoracic aortography depends on the suggested pathology. Quantities ranging from 40 cc to 80 cc may be required. The larger dose would be injected when an aorta is dilated and when visibility of an entire arch is desirable. The smaller dose is advantageous in the case of a constricted aorta or when only a section of the aorta is to be visualized.

Reaction to the contrast medium or to the premedication is always a possibility as with any procedure using contrast medium and should be planned for in case it does occur.

Positioning Routine

The patient position for thoracic aortography depends on the pathology in question. Since the aorta courses posteriorly as well as to the left as it leaves the left ventricle of the heart, it is necessary to oblique the patient to open up the arch. Therefore, the positions most commonly used are a **right or left posterior oblique**. Regardless of the position, the radiograph should include the heart, arch and great vessels.

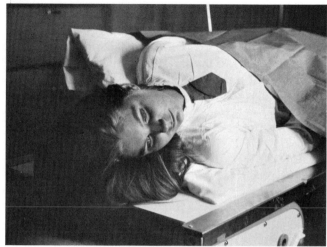

Fig. 23-81
Position (RPO) for Arch Aortography

Right Posterior Oblique

For a 30 to 45 degree right posterior oblique, the patient is positioned with the right side against the table, the left side angled upward 30 to 45 degrees while the head is in a lateral position *(Fig. 23-81)*. To stabilize the patient in this position, a radiolucent positioning block is placed between the patient's back and the table top while the head is similarly supported for comfort. This position is useful in visualizing arch or great vessel branch deformities *(Fig. 23-82)*.

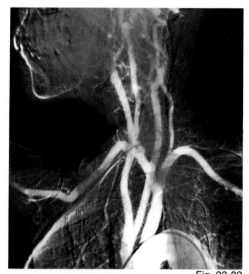

Fig. 23-82
Arch Aortogram (RPO)

Left Posterior Oblique

In a 30 to 45 degree left posterior oblique the patient is placed in a direction opposite to the right posterior oblique. The left side is down and the right side is facing upward at a 30 to 45 degree angle. This oblique is also used to demonstrate patent ductus arteriosus or coarctation.

Filming Rate: The filming rate for the rapid film changer should be 4 films/second for the first 2 seconds, followed by 2 films/second for 3 to 5 seconds. If cineradiography is employed, the rate of filming is 30 to 60 frames/second.

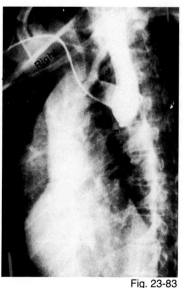

Fig. 23-83
Coarctation (RPO)

Radiographic Procedures

Purpose

Diagnostic abdominal angiography involves the **injection of contrast medium to demonstrate the contour, size and possible displacement of the abdominal aorta and its branches**. The shape, size and displacement of the vessels recorded on the radiographs are used by the physician to diagnose vascular disease.

Indications

Abdominal angiography is employed to detect **aneurysms**, **congenital anomalies**, **stenosis**, or **occlusions of the abdominal aorta**. Organs which receive blood directly from the abdominal aorta, i.e. kidneys, may be selectively catheterized to rule out any existing pathologies.

Contraindications

Abdominal angiography utilizing contrast medium should not be performed on patients having **known adverse reaction to contrast media** or allergic reactions to **iodine**. If there is an absence of a pulse in the vessel to be catheterized, a different vessel should be selected.

Patient Preparation

Patients should be premedicated prior to abdominal angiography. The type and amount of medication given the patient depends on the patient's condition. Most common prescriptions include drugs to protect against vasovagal reaction, and a mild sedative to relieve patient anxiety or stress. Anticoagulants should be withheld at least 4 hours before the procedure.

Prior to the examination, a member of the angiography team should visit the patient to verbally explain the procedure and risks involved. When the patient understands the procedure and potential complications, an informed consent is signed by the patient which outlines the risks of the procedure.

Major Equipment

The major equipment required for abdominal angiography includes:
1. Electromechanical injector
2. Single rapid serial film changer
3. Image intensifier with television monitor
4. Floating table top

The electromechanical injector is used to deliver the contrast medium to the area of interest. Image intensification is employed during catheter positioning. Images are recorded on the single plane rapid serial film changer. The floating table top serves to move the patient over the film changer for filming.

Accessory and Optional Equipment

The accessory equipment for abdominal angiography includes:
1. Sterile angiographic tray
2. Vascular catheters
3. Electrocardiograph recorder
4. Emergency cardiopulmonary equipment

Catheterization of the vessel is performed using the sterile tray. The type of catheter employed for abdominal angiography de-

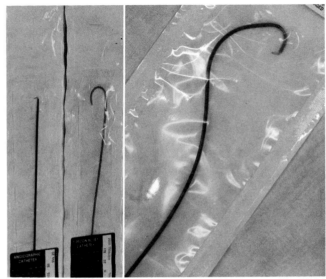

Abdominal Angiography Catheters   Fig. 23-84

pends on the area of interest. Figure 23-84 represents a variety of catheters that may be used for abdominal angiography .

The electrocardiograph recorder is used to monitor the patient's heart. Cardiopulmonary equipment should be in the room or immediately available if needed.

Catheterization Method

The most common approach to abdominal angiography is via puncture of the femoral artery using the Seldinger technique. The type and position of the catheter within the vessel depends on the area of interest.

For nonselective abdominal angiography, radiographs are taken of the abdomen. This requires the injection of a large bolus of contrast medium in a short period of time. A **straight end catheter** with side holes or a pig-tail is most advantageous for delivering large quantities of contrast medium and should be used for demonstration of the abdominal aorta and its branches.

Selective abdominal angiography pertains to the catheterization of one of the abdominal aortic branches. The most common branches catheterized are the renals and celiac axis. Since these vessels are small, as compared to the abdominal aorta, an end hole only catheter is used for injection of contrast medium.

Contrast Medium

The amount of contrast medium injected is relative to the size of the organ to be examined. For demonstration of the entire abdomen, 40 to 50 cc of a high concentration contrast medium is delivered at a rate of 25 cc/second. Selective abdominal angiography of the celiac axis requires 35 to 45 cc of a high concentration contrast medium injected at 8 to 12 cc/second, while selective renal angiography contrast volume range is 6 to 10 cc at a rate of 5 to 6 cc/second.

abd aorta / renals

translumbar puncture

Positioning Routine and Filming Procedure

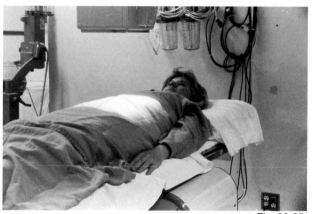

Position for Abdominal Angiogram   Fig. 23-85

Abdominal Angiography

Filming for abdominal angiography is performed with the patient supine utilizing an anterior-posterior projection. The area of interest governs the size of the field to be irradiated.

To demonstrate the abdominal aorta, the patient is positioned for an anterior-posterior projection as shown in *Fig. 23-85*. The midsagittal plane is perpendicular to the film. Care should be taken to insure that both the proximal and distal ends of the pathology are recorded on the radiographs *(Fig. 23-86)*.

Film Rate and Sequence: A common filming sequence involves fourteen radiographs. The rate used is 2 films/second for 4 seconds, followed by 1 film/second for 2 seconds and finally 1 film every other second for 8 seconds.

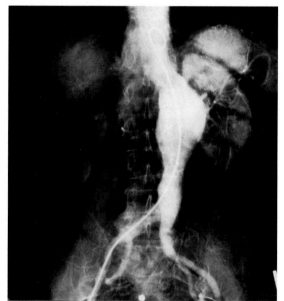

Abdominal Angiogram   Fig. 23-86

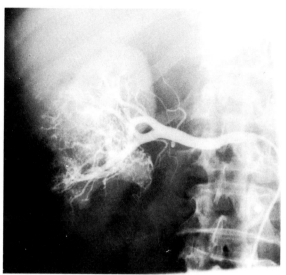

Renal Arteriogram Fig. 23-87

Renal Angiography

Renal angiography uses the supine position which demonstrates the kidney in an oblique position *(Fig. 23-87)*. The irradiated field in renal angiography differs from abdominal angiography in that the field is limited to the upper quadrant of the abdomen containing the kidney of interest *(Fig. 23-88)*.

Filming Rate: The filming rate is 2 to 3 films/second during injection, followed by 1 film/second for 2 seconds and 1 film every other second for 6 seconds.

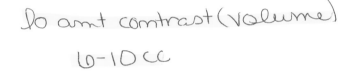

No amt contrast (volume)

6-10 cc

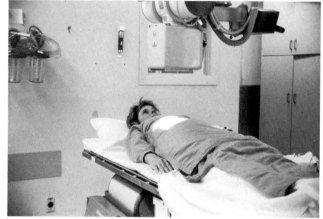

AP Projection for Renal Angiogram Fig. 23-88

Splenaportography

The anterior-posterior projection best demonstrates the liver and spleen. This projection should include the lower thoracic and upper abdominal regions during mid-inspiration. *(Fig. 23-89)*.

Filming Rate: The filming rate is 2 films/second for 4 seconds and 1 film/second for 16 to 20 seconds.

A post injection radiograph is taken to determine if there are any extrasplenic contrast medium deposits.

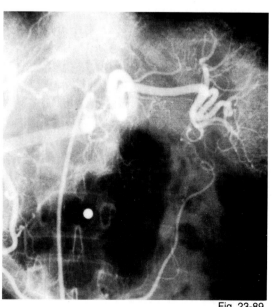

Splenaportogram Fig. 23-89

Radiographic Procedure

Purpose

Peripheral **angiography** is a radiographic examination of the vessels of the **upper or lower limbs following the injection of contrast medium**. Upper limb angiography includes arterial examination of the shoulder, upper arm, elbow, forearm, wrist, and hand areas. Lower limb angiography includes procedures to examine the arteries called arteriography. *(ar"te-re-og'rah-fe)* ; or procedures for the **veins** of the lower limb, called **venography** *(ve-nog'rah-fe)*. Lower limb procedures involve x-rays of the abdomen, thigh, knee and leg areas.

During peripheral angiography, contrast medium flows through the vessels of interest outlining their shape and location. By observing the degree of vessel opacity and flow of the contrast medium within the system, physicians are able to identify abnormalities.

Indications

Peripheral angiography is indicated in cases of **tumors**, **emboli**, **thrombus**, **arteriovenous malformations** and **occlusions**. The majority of peripheral angiograms are performed to investigate diseases having pathological origin. However, a large percent of arteriovenous malformations result from trauma.

Contraindications

The most common contraindication to peripheral angiography is **adverse reaction to contrast medium**. For lower limb arteriography, an examination should be done to assess the presence of bruits, scar tissue, or the absence of a femoral or iliac pulse at the puncture site. If any of these symptoms are present, then a puncture in that area should be avoided.

Caution is advised when performing lower limb venography on patients suspected of thrombosis, phlebitis, severe ischemic disease, local infection or a totally obstructed venous system as contrast medium extravasation can create complications.

Patient Preparation

Patients having peripheral angiography should be premedicated to reduce anxiety and stress. Anxiety can be alleviated by having a member of the angiographic team explain the procedure and risks involved to the patient. When the patient understands the procedure and potential risks, an informed consent is signed by the patient.

Prior to the examination, the pulses should be assessed to determine their strength and if bruits are present. Weak pulses or the presence of bruits require that an alternate vessel be catheterized. A mixture of 2% lidocaine with the contrast medium may be given to alleviate pain during the injection.

Major Equipment

The major equipment used for arteriography includes:
1. Rapid serial film changer
2. Image intensifier with television monitor device
3. Electromechanic injector

Placement of the catheter is accomplished by viewing the catheter with the image intensifier. The rapid film changer is used to record the image. Injection of the contrast medium is the function of the electromechanic injector.

Lower extremity arteriography also requires a stepping table. This table automatically moves a predetermined distance at varying intervals so that a different part of the patient is over the film changer for each table movement *(Fig. 23-90)*.

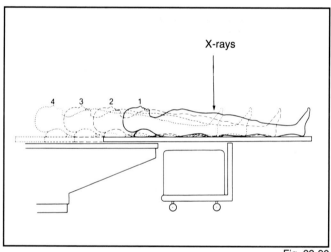

X-rays

Stepping Table   Fig. 23-90

Accessory and Optional Equipment

Additional equipment needed for peripheral (upper and lower limb) angiography includes:

1. Sterile angiographic tray
2. Vascular catheters
3. Emergency cardiopulmonary equipment

The sterile tray is used during insertion of the catheter. It is recommended that an emergency cardiac cart be immediately available should cardiopulmonary resuscitation be required.

When performing lower limb arteriography both lower extremities may be examined simultaneously. Concurrent injection of the iliacs requires the use of a Y luer lock.

Venography of the lower limb employs different accessory equipment than arteriography. The accessory equipment for venography includes a 50 cc syringe, small butterfly needle, extension tubing and a tourniquet. These items are used for a hand injection of the contrast medium.

Catheterization Method

Lower limb arteriography may include the abdomen and lower limbs or involve selective catheterization of the lower limbs. If abdominal angiography is to be performed, the catheter is placed at the level of the twelfth thoracic vertebra via a femoral artery. The type of catheter employed is a pigtail, ring or straight tip catheter having multiple side holes with the end hole occluded. These catheters allow for the delivery of a large bolus of contrast medium over a short period of time.

When visualization of the iliac and lower limbs arteries is performed, an end-hold, multiple side-hole catheter is placed at the level of the fourth lumbar vertebra following femoral artery puncture. Sometimes pathology is such that the contralateral side is catheterized in place of the involved side. In these cases a selective sharp, curved catheter is used to catheterize the vessel of interest *(Fig. 23-91)*.

Catheterization of the upper limb may be performed via the axillary, brachial or femoral arteries. The femoral approach is the safest and most common. The most common catheter used for upper limb angiography is a brachiocephalic end hole.

Contrast Medium

The amount of contrast medium for lower limb arteriography varies with the type of filming required. When abdominal radiographs are required, 40 to 60 cc of high concentration contrast medium is used at a rate of 10 to 15 cc/second. Selective lower limb arteriography employs a dose of 20 to 30 cc injected at a rate of 8 to 10 cc/second.

Often, patients having lower limb arteriography have poor circulation. To increase the rate of blood flow, certain drugs, i.e. tolazoline, may be administered prior to the injection of the contrast medium to dilate the vessels thereby increasing the blood flow rate. Other methods used to increase blood flow are blood pressure cuffs and exercise. Exercise decreases aortic pressure and facilitates the flow of blood to the distal parts of the body. A blood pressure cuff is used to increase blood flow by inflating it at a level above the knee for 3 minutes then deflating it which creates a rapid flow of blood toward the feet.

Upper limb arteriography requires 15 cc of a 45% to 60% concentration of contrast medium. The contrast medium is injected at a rate of 7 to 8 cc/second.

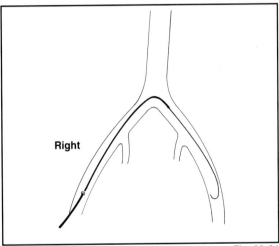

Fig. 23-91

Selective Contralateral Catheterization
of Common Iliac Artery

Lower Limb Arteriography

After catheterization and placement of the catheter in the appropriate vessel for arteriography, anterior-posterior projection radiographs are taken. The filming rate and centering for lower limb arteriography involving the abdominal aorta are the same as abdominal angiography. When radiographing the lower limbs, to insure a true anterior-posterior projection, the patient's feet are internally rotated 30 degrees. The feet may be taped together or otherwise supported to prevent movement during filming.

Filming Sequence

The actual filming of arteries of the lower limbs involves the sequencing of table top movement, radiographic technique changes, and proper exposure synchronization. The great variance in the thickness of the leg requires the correct use of the anode heel effect. Thus, the cathode end of the x-ray tube should be placed toward the thickest part, the thigh.

Stepping Table

Exposures are made of the thighs, knees and lower legs *(Fig. 23-92)*. This is achieved by activation of the stepping table top which moves the individual parts of the patient over the rapid serial film changer automatically.

Other methods that may be used to maintain the same density through the lower limb are wedge filters, special cones, or special cassettes with varying speed intensifying screens.

Upper Limb Arteriography

Upper limb arteriography is also performed with anteriorposterior projections. The patient's arm is placed diagonally on the rapid serial film changer *(Fig. 23-93)*.

Filming Rate: Filming Rate depends upon the area of interest. The rate for the proximal portion is 1 film/second for 20 seconds.

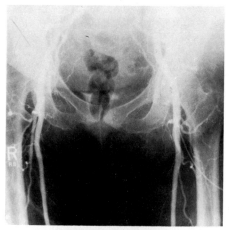
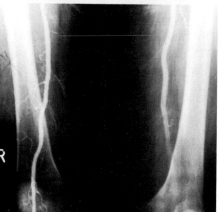
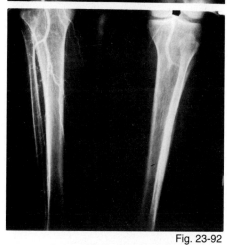

Fig. 23-92
Lower Limb Arteriogram

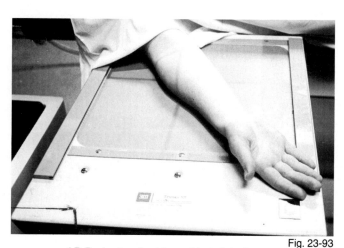

Fig. 23-93
AP Projection for Upper Limb Arteriogram

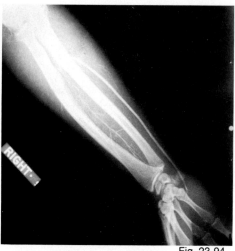

Fig. 23-94
Upper Limb Arteriogram

Lower Limb Venography

Lower limb venography is a contrast medium study of the deep veins from the ankle to pelvic area. As contrast media is injected, AP and lateral radiographs of the limb are taken. Filming is accomplished by utilizing fluoroscopic spot filming on 14 in. x 14 in. (35 x 35 cm) cassette or by high speed cameras employing a 105 mm roll or 100 mm precut film.

Filming Sequence: A typical filming procedure would include:
-AP and lateral of calf to include knee
-AP and lateral centered at knee
-AP and lateral of thigh
-AP of hip to include iliac crest
Fluoroscopic control insures that all levels of the venous circulation are visualized with contrast present.

Equipment and Procedure
In addition to a fluoroscopic unit with filming capabilities, a 90 degree tilting table with a foot board, and a small block is needed. The contrast medium is introduced through a superficial vein on the dorsum or anterior surface of the foot. The injection begins with the table and patient semi-erect (approximately 60 degrees). The patient stands on the block (resting on the footboard) with the unaffected leg. (See arrows, *Fig. 23-95*.) The affected leg is allowed to dangle (away from the block) so that it bears no weight.

As the contrast is injected, the distal aspect of the extremity is filmed. The table is slowly lowered in stages (to decrease the affect of gravity and allow flow of the contrast upward) and the mid and proximal portions of the extremity are filmed.

Filming of the hip area is performed with the table horizontal *(Fig. 23-96)*. When the exam is completed, a flushing solution (e.g. saline or 5% Dextrose in water) is used to force contrast from the lower extremity. This aids in preventing a possible phlebitis which may be caused by the irritating effect of the contrast on the lining of the veins.

Contrast Medium
Approximately 50 to 100 cc of a water soluble, iodine based contrast medium of relatively low density is used for venography. Since injection is into a distal superficial vein, 1 or 2 tourniquets are applied just above the ankle to compress the superficial system and direct the contrast medium into the deep system through interconnecting veins *(Fig. 23-99)*.

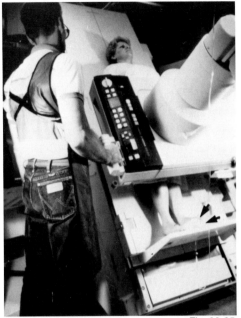

Fig. 23-95
AP Knee and Thigh Area Filming

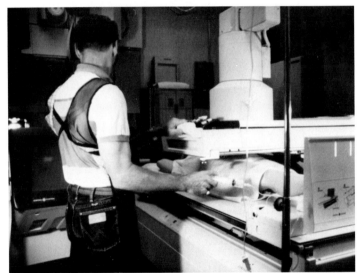

AP Hip Area Filming   Fig. 23-96

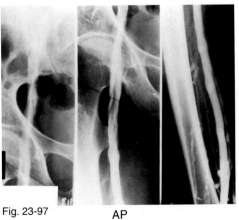

Fig. 23-97   AP
Lower Limb Venograms

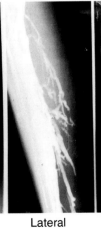
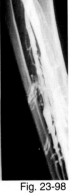

Lateral   Fig. 23-98

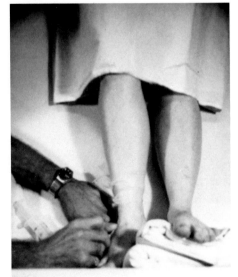

Fig. 23-99
Injection of Contrast Medium
(2 tourniquets applied)

Chapter 24
Arthrography and Myelography

Marianne Tortorici, RT(R) Ed. D.
Patrick Apfel, RT(R), M. Ed

Contents

Survey Information

Survey Questions on Possible Discontinued Procedures:

A national survey included questions on (I) the **quantity** of specific procedures being done in their departments during the past year; (II) the **expected trend** in the next three or four years; and (III)whether or not the procedure **should still be taught and included** in a basic student textbook. The results for arthrograms and myelograms were as follows: (The number of responding institutions is indicated in parentheses for each region.)

Arthrograms	U.S. Average (364)	East (134)	Midwest (171)	West (59)
I. Trend				
a. Increase	20%	23%	21%	15%
b. Decrease	36%	34%	37%	36%
c. No change	44%	43%	42%	49%
II. Annual Quantity				
a. 0-16	20%	21%	16%	24%
b. 17-50	22%	23%	19%	28%
c. 51-96	21%	23%	22%	10%
d. 96-199	20%	18%	22%	18%
e. 200 +	17%	13%	21%	18%
III. Be Included				
a. Yes	97%	96%	98%	98%
b. No	3%	4%	2%	2%
Myelograms	(360)	(132)	(169)	(59)
I. Trend				
a. Increase	17%	31%	15%	7%
b. Decrease	35%	27%	36%	47%
c. No change	46%	42%	49%	46%
II. Annual Quantity				
a. 0-21	17%	11%	19%	27%
b. 22-92	23%	23%	20%	32%
c. 93-174	19%	17%	21%	18%
d. 175-382	23%	27%	24%	8%
e. 383 +	18%	22%	16%	15%
III. Be Included				
a. Yes	99%	99%	99%	100%
b. No	1%	1%	1%	0%

Summary:

The survey clearly indicates that both **arthrograms** and **myelograms** are being done in sufficient numbers that they need to be included in the curriculum of educational programs. The survey suggests that myelograms are still commonplace in most radiology departments even though MRI procedures of the spinal cord are being done more and more frequently where such equipment is available.

A lower percent in the west indicated an increase in both of these procedures. Generally however the highest percent in all regions indicated **no change**, suggesting that at the time of this survey, MRI in general has not replaced either one of these diagnostic procedures (at least in those radiology departments affiliated with radiologic technology educational programs responding to this survey).

Part I Arthrography

Introduction

Arthrography *(ar- throg'rah-fe)* is a **contrast media study of synovial joints and related soft tissue structures.** The joints examined by this procedure include the hip, knee, ankle, shoulder, elbow, wrist and temporomandibular joints. This section is devoted to arthrography of the knee and shoulder.

It should be noted that although some physicians recommend arthrography as the method of choice for examination of the knee or shoulder joint, others prefer Magnetic Resonance Imaging (MRI) to evaluate these joints.

In considering arthrography as a whole, the technique of examination is similar for all the joints with variations occurring primarily due to anatomical differences. An example of arthrogram radiographs of a temporomandibular joint (TMJ) is seen in *Figs. 24-1* and *24-2* wherein contrast media is seen in the temporomandibular joint space in lateral open and closed mouth positions.

Arthrograms of the shoulder and knee are the most common of arthogram procedures being done today and will be described and illustrated in this chapter.

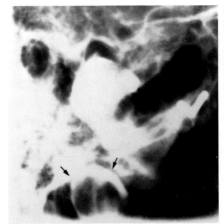
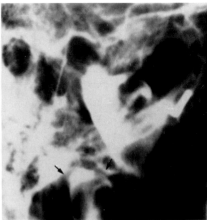

Fig. 24-1   Closed Mouth   Open Mouth   Fig. 24-2

TMJ Arthrograms

Knee Arthrography

Anatomy

The anatomical structures demonstrated during arthrography of the knee are presented in Chapter 6.

Purpose

Knee arthrography is performed to **demonstrate and assess the knee joint and associated soft tissue structures for pathology.** The structures of major interest include the **joint capsule**, **menisci** and the **collateral**, **cruciate** and other **minor ligaments**. These structures are visualized through the introduction of a contrast medium into the joint capsule with fluoroscopic spot filming and/or routine radiographic filming utilized to record a permanent image.

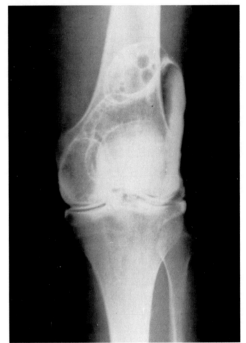

AP Knee Arthrogram   Fig. 24-3

Indications

Knee arthrography is indicated when **tears of the joint capsule, menisci or ligaments are suspected.** The knee is a joint which is subject to considerable stress especially during sports activities. Therefore, much of the pathology seen in the knee is due to trauma. An example of non traumatic pathology indicating arthrography is a Baker's Cyst which communicates with the joint capsule in the popliteal area.

Contraindications

In general, arthrography of any joint is contraindicated when the patient is known to be allergic to an iodine based contrast medium or to local anesthetics.

Patient Preparation

Any arthrographic procedure should be thoroughly explained before the examination proceeds to preclude unnecessary anxiety on the part of the patient. The patient should be advised of any complications, and must sign an informed consent form.

Major Equipment

The major equipment for knee arthrography varies with the method of filming. Filming may be accomplished by **fluoroscopic spot filming**, **conventional radiographic** (vertical or horizontal beam) **filming** or by a **combination of both**. If a conventional radiographic room is used, it must be equipped such that horizontal beam radiography can be accomplished.

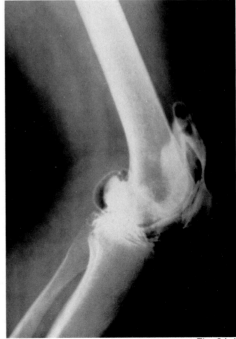

Fig. 24-4

Lateral Knee Arthrogram

Accessory and Optional Equipment

Accessory and optional equipment for examination of the knee will vary according to the method of filming, except for those items needed for the contrast injection and preparation of the injection site. These are basically the same for any arthrogram tray.

Arthrogram Tray: Generally, a **disposable tray** is used to prepare the site for injection which is an aseptic procedure. Such a tray should contain **prep sponges**, **gauze sponges**, a **fenestrated drape**, **one 50 cc** and **two 10 cc syringes**, a **flexible connector**, **several hypodermic needles** (usually **18, 20, 21 and 25 gauge**) and a **5 ml ampule of local anesthetic** such as xylocaine. Additionally, **sterile gloves**, and **antiseptic solution** (such as betadine), a **razor** and the **contrast media** are needed. For knee arthrography, a **2" to 3" wide ace bandage** is also required.

The injection site is prepared by shaving the area with a razor, and cleansing the site by using the prep sponges and basin containing the antiseptic solution. The area is dried with the gauze sponges and draped with the fenestrated drape. The positive contrast medium is drawn up for injection later (approximately 5 cc) with a 10 cc syringe and 18 gauge needle. The physician injects the skin, underlying tissues and the joint capsule with the local anesthetic using a 10 cc syringe with a 21 or 25 gauge needle.

Needle Placement and Injection Process

A retropatellar, lateral or medial approach may be used during needle placement. The actual site of injection is the preference of the physician.

With the site prepared, draped and anesthetized the physician introduces the 20 gauge needle, mounted on a 10 cc syringe, through the skin and underlying tissues into the joint space. All joint fluid is aspirated. If it is normal in appearance (i.e., clear and tinged yellow), it may be discarded. If it appears abnormal (cloudy) it should be sent to the laboratory for assessment.

With all of the fluid aspirated, the positive contrast medium (drawn up earlier) is injected into the joint through the 20 gauge needle, which has been left in place for the injection. If the study is a dual contrast exam, the 50 cc syringe is used to inject the negative contrast medium.

Once the contrast medium is injected, the needle is removed and the ace bandage is wrapped around the distal femur to obliterate the area of the suprapatellar bursae.

Contrast Media

Knee arthrography can be accomplished by utilizing a radiolucent (negative) medium, a radiopaque (positive) medium or a combination of both media (dual contrast). The dual contrast study seems to be the method of choice. For this study, a very small amount (approximately 5 cc) of a relatively low density positive medium (ex. trade name: Renografin M 60®) is used along with 80 - 100 cc of a negative medium such as carbon dioxide, oxygen or room air.

With the media injected, the knee is gently flexed which produces a thin, even coating of the soft tissue structures with the positive medium.

Fluoroscopic or Overhead Filming: Either fluoroscopic or overhead radiography is used for filming. The accessory filming equipment is minimal and basically the same. Film holders include 8" x 10" cassettes or, for fluoroscopy, 9" x 9" cassettes. A table mounted patient restraining device arranged as a sling around the knee area should be available. The sling is used to provide lateral or medial stress to "open up" the appropriate area of the joint to better visualize the meniscus during fluoroscopy. Overhead (vertical beam) radiography is the least used

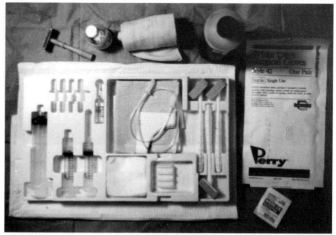

Arthrogram Tray   Fig. 24-5

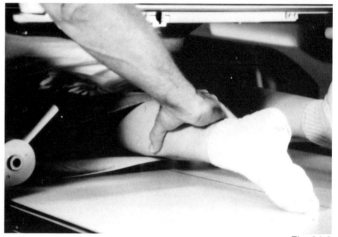

Knee Arthrogram   Fig. 24-6
(sling around knee in place)

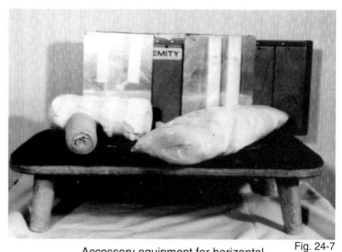

Fig. 24-7
Accessory equipment for horizontal
beam radiograph of knee

method for filming. Fluoroscopy is a more common method employed for filming and requires that the fluoroscopic tube have a small (fractional) focal spot to provide the detail necessary to adequately visualize the menisci.

Horizontal Beam Radiography: Horizontal beam radiography is another common form of filming as described and illustrated on a following page. This requires a 7 x 17 cassette, a lead diaphragm, a low small table or stand to support the knee, a firm pillow and a 5 lb. sandbag *(Figs. 24-7 and 24-12)*.

Knee Arthrography continued

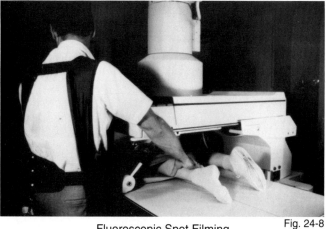

Fluoroscopic Spot Filming   Fig. 24-8
(left knee)

Positioning Routines

Radiographic Routines
The routine positioning and procedure for knee arthrography varies with the method of examination, i.e., fluoroscopy, conventional radiography or combination of both.

Fluoroscopy and Spot Filming
During fluoroscopy the radiologist usually takes a series of closely collimated views of **each meniscus**, rotating the leg approximately **20 degrees between each exposure**. The result is a spot film with nine exposures of each menisci which demonstrates the meniscus in profile throughout its diameter *(Fig. 24-9)*.

Evaluation Criteria:
- Each meniscus should be clearly visualized in profile on each of the nine collimated areas. Additional exposures may be necessary to demonstrate pathology.
- The meniscus being visualized should be in center of collimated field
- Correct exposure and adequate penetration should be evident to visualize the meniscus and contrast media.
- The meniscus under examination should be appropriately marked as M (medial) or L (lateral).
- Patient ID marker should be clear, and R or L marker should be visualized without superimposing anatomy.

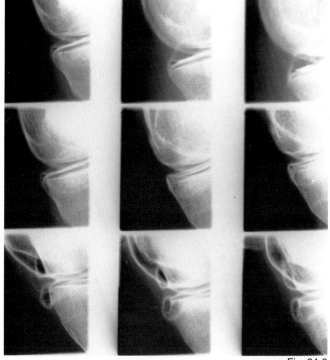

Fluoroscopic Spot Film   Fig. 24-9
(approx. 20° rotation between exposures)

Conventional "Overhead" Projections
In addition to the spot films, routine AP and lateral films of the entire knee, utilizing the radiographic tube, are usually included. These radiographs are taken after removing the ace bandage from the distal femur.

Evaluation Criteria
- The AP and lateral radiographs should demonstrate the entire articular capsule as outlined by the combination negative and positive contrast media.
- Positioning criteria should be similar to the conventional AP and lateral knee as described in chapter 6.
- Patient ID marker should be clear, and R or L marker should be visualized without superimposing anatomy.

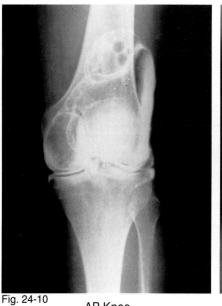

Fig. 24-10   AP Knee

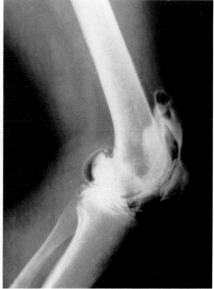

Lateral Knee   Fig. 24-11

Knee Arthrography continued

Horizontal Beam Projections

Horizontal beam radiography is another common method of filming for knee arthrography and requires some special equipment. This includes:

- A 7" x 17" cassette divided to accommodate six exposures.
- Lead diaphragm providing an opening limited to the size of the marked exposure sites on the cassette.
- Low, small table or stand used when radiographing the lateral meniscus; a firm pillow.
- 5 lb sandbag.

These last two items are used to open up the appropriate area of the joint space to visualize the lateral and medial menisci.

Each meniscus is radiographed on one film with the patient's leg **rotated 30 degrees between each exposure.** The resulting radiograph demonstrates **six views of each meniscus**, in profile, throughout its diameter.

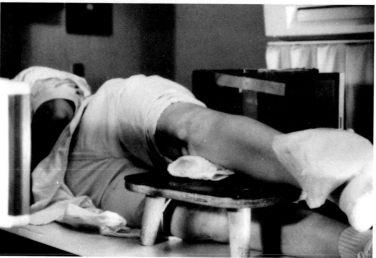

Horizontal Beam Projection

Fig. 24-12

Evaluation Criteria

- Each meniscus should be demonstrated in six exposures on the 7" x 17" film.
- Collimated fields should not overlap.
- The joint/meniscus should be centered to the collimated field.
- Correct exposure and adequate penetration to visualize the meniscus and contrast media.
- The meniscus under examination should be appropriately marked as M (medial) or L (lateral).
- Patient ID marker should be clear, and R or L marker should be visualised without superimposing anatomy.

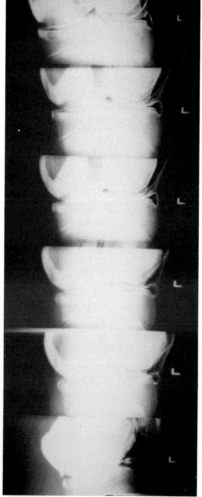

Fig. 24-13

Six views of lateral meniscus.
(AP on top to lateral on bottom)

Shoulder Arthrography

Purpose

Arthrography of the shoulder utilizes either a single or double contrast injection to **demonstrate the joint capsule, rotator cuff** (formed by conjoined tendons of four major shoulder muscles), **the long tendon of the biceps muscle** and **the articular cartilages.**

Equipment and Procedure

A radiographic/fluoroscopic room is needed for the procedure, similar to that of a knee arthrogram. Contrast injection is monitored under fluoroscopic control and conventional filming is done utilizing the overhead x-ray tube. Equipment and supplies needed includes a standard, disposable arthrogram tray and a 2.5 in. to 3.5 in. spinal needle.

Need Placement and Injection Process

The injection site, directly over the joint, is prepared as in any arthrographic procedure. Once the area is anesthetized, the physician uses fluoroscopy to guide the needle into the joint space. Since the joint is quite deep, a spinal needle must be used. A small amount of contrast medium is injected to determine if the bursa has been penetrated. Once the contrast medium has been fully instilled, filming begins.

Contrast Media

Arthrography of the shoulder can be accomplished utilizing either a single, positive contrast medium or a combination of positive and negative (dual) contrast media. For a single contrast study, 10 to 12 cc of a positive medium such as Renographin M-60® is used. For a dual contrast study, 3 to 4 cc of the positive medium and 10 to 12 cc of a negative medium (e.g. room air) are used.

A dual contrast study is believed by some to better demonstrate specific areas, such as the inferior portion of the rotator cuff, when the views are done with the patient upright.

Routine Positioning and Filming Sequence

Routine radiography varies and filming can be done with the patient upright or supine. A suggested filming sequence can include **scout AP projections,** with **internal and external rotation** as standard, and a **glenoid fossa, transaxillary** or **bicipital groove view** (per departmental routine or as indicated).

Once the contrast medium has been injected, the views are repeated. If the radiographs appear normal, the patient is directed to exercise the shoulder and the radiographs are repeated a second time. Caudal angulations of 15 to 23 degrees may be used on the AP projections per specific department routines.

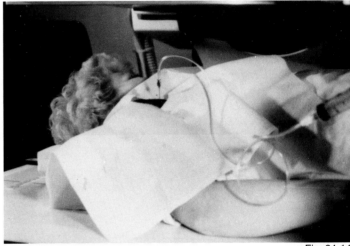

Fig. 24-14

Needle Placement

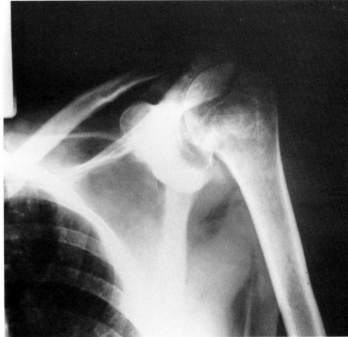

Fig. 24-15

AP Shoulder with Contrast Media

Part II Myelography - Radiographic Procedure

Anatomy

The anatomy related to myelography (mi"e-log'rah-fe) is covered in chapters 8 and 9 of the cervical, thoracic and lumbosacral spine, and the central nervous system in Chapter 21 on cranial computed tomography.

Purpose

A myelogram (mi'e-lo-gram) is a **radiographic study of the spinal cord and its nerve root branches**. In the past myelography was often considered a special procedure and filming was largely performed by special procedure technologists. However, with the advancement of technology and improvement of contrast media, myelography is considered more of a routine contrast media examination rather than a true special procedure.

The spinal cord and nerve roots are outlined by injecting a contrast medium into the subarachnoid space of the vertebral canal. The shape and contour of the contrast medium is assessed to detect possible pathology. Most pathology occurs in the lumbar or cervical spine regions, thus, myelography is most often performed in these areas.

Indications

Myelography is performed to **detect various lesions which may be present within the spinal canal or which may be protruding into the canal**. These lesions most commonly include **cancerous** or **benign tumors, cysts** and **herniated nucleus pulposus** (herniation of the inner portion of a spinal disc). If pathologies are present, myelography serves to discern the extent, size and level of the lesion. Another important feature of myelography is the ability to determine if multiple lesions exist. The most common pathological finding of myelography is a herniated nucleus pulposus (HNP).

Contraindications

Contraindications for myelography include **blood in the cerebrospinal fluid** (CSF), **arachnoiditis** (inflammation of the arachnoid membrane), **increased intracranial pressure** and **previous lumbar puncture performed within two weeks of the current exam**.

The presence of blood in the CSF indicates probable irritation in the vertebral canal which can be aggravated by contrast medium. Myelography is contraindicated in the case of arachnoiditis because performance of the examination may increase the severity of the arachnoiditis. Tapping the subarachnoid space when increased intracranial pressure exists may cause severe complications to the patient. Performing myelography on a patient who had a lumbar puncture two weeks prior to the myelography may result in contrast medium extravasating outside the subarachnoid space through the previous needle hole.

Patient Preparation

Patients having myelography tend to be apprehensive about the examination. To reduce anxiety and relax the patient, an injectable sedative/muscle relaxant is usually administered one hour prior to the examination. The type of medication used is determined by the physician.

As in the case of other examinations involving the injection of contrast medium, prior to the procedure the process should be explained to the patient. The patient should also be advised as to the possible complications of the procedure and an informed consent should be signed by the patient.

Major Equipment

The major equipment for myelography includes a radiographic/fluoroscopic room with a 90 degree tilting table, shoulder braces, and a footrest with myelography "boots." Shoulder braces are used to secure the patient when performing the study which requires that the patient be tilted Trendelenburg (head is lower than feet). Boots, attached to the footrest, may also be used to help maintain the patient in the Trendelenburg position. It is advisable to use both the boots (if available) and shoulder rests together rather than one or the other separately. The footrest is utilized when placing the patient in the upright position.

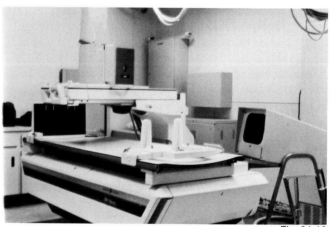

Fig. 24-16

Myelography Room

Accessory and Optional Equipment

The accessory equipment for myelography includes a grid cassette and a myelography tray. The number and sizes of grid cassettes used will depend on the area of the spinal canal being examined. Grid cassette holders are utilized for crosstable exposures made during the filming procedure.

The myelography tray is generally a prepackaged, sterilized unit prepared by a commercial company (*Fig. 24-17*). A typical myelography tray should contain the following: **disposable razor, basin** and **sponge; sterile drapes; sterile gauze; 2 cc syringe; 25 g and 22 g needles; 18 g spinal needle; local anesthetic; 2 to 3 test tubes** and **10 cc syringe.**

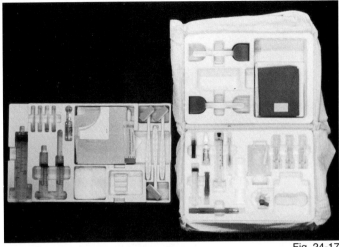

Myelogram Tray   Fig. 24-17

Needle Placement and Injection Process

Introduction of contrast medium for myelography is accomplished through a puncture of the subarachnoid space. There are generally two locations for the puncture site: the **lumbar** and **cervical** (C 1-2) areas. Of the two locations, the lumbar area is safer, easier on the patient, and more conducive to patient positioning and filming than the cervical region. A cervical puncture is indicated if the lumbar area is contraindicated or if pathology indicates a complete block of the vertebral canal obstructing the flow of contrast medium to the upper spinal region.

After the puncture site is selected, the physician should fluoroscope the patient to mark the center of the location on the back of the patient. This facilitates placement of the needle in the subarachnoid space. When the location is marked, the patient is placed in the proper position for the puncture. The position of the patient during a lumbar puncture is prone with a pillow or large positioning block placed under the abdomen to help straighten the normal lordotic curve in this area *(Fig. 24-18)*.

During a cervical puncture, the patient may be seated *(Fig. 24-19)*, or prone with the head flexed. In both types of punctures the injection site is prepared by shaving any hair present with the disposable razor and cleaning the skin using the basin, sponge and an antiseptic solution. The area is then dried with the gauze pad and draped with the sterile drapes. A local anesthetic is administered using the 2 cc syringe with either the 22 g or 25 g needle. The spinal needle is inserted through the skin and underlying tissues into the subarachnoid space.

The location of the needle in that space is verified by an unobstructed flow of cerebral spinal fluid (CSF) which generally is allowed to flow or drop out through the needle. (Allowing free flow of the CSF rather than drawing it out reduces the risk of trauma at the distal end of the needle within the canal.) A sample of CSF may be taken at this time and sent to the laboratory for analysis.

Once the needle is in the appropriate position, the contrast medium is drawn up in the 10 cc syringe to be injected into the subarachnoid space and filming begins as described on the following page. Sterile technique is maintained throughout the filming sequence.

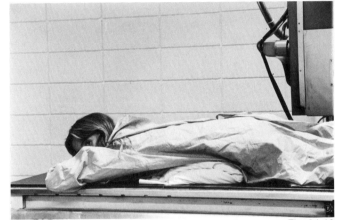

Position for Lumbar Puncture   Fig. 24-18

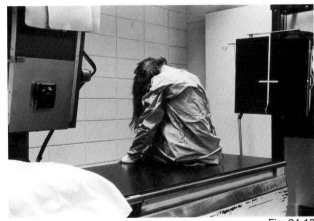

Position for Cervical (C1-2) Puncture   Fig. 24-19

Contrast Media

The best type of contrast medium for myelography is one that is miscible (mixes well) with the cerebrospinal fluid, is easily absorbed, non-toxic, inert (non-reactive) and has good radiopacity. No one type of contrast medium meets all the above criteria. The type of medium used is determined by the radiographic information needed and the health of the patient. The two main types of contrast media used for myelography are **oil-based** and **water soluble** media.

Oil Based: Oil contrast medium provides good radiopacity and has a history of few complications. Although the radiopacity is good, it does not demonstrate the root branches adequately. This type of medium is not readily absorbed by the body and should be removed from the subarachnoid space after the examination is completed. Consequently, the spinal needle is left in place during the procedure when using an oil medium which makes patient positioning difficult. Residual oil-based medium is absorbed by the body at a rate of 1 cc per year. Although few complications occur, residual oil-based medium has been known to cause arachnoiditis, meningitis, and osteomyelitis. An example of an oil-based cervical myelogram is shown in *Fig. 24-20*.

Water Soluble: Water soluble contrast medium is rapidly replacing the oil based type for myelography. Water soluble contrast media provide excellent radiographic visualization of the nerve roots and are absorbed quickly by the body. This is beneficial, since the spinal needle can be removed after injection of the contrast to facilitate patient positioning. Absorption begins within 30 minutes post injection and provides good visualization for about one hour post injection. After 4-5 hours, the contrast medium will have a hazy radiographic effect and is radiographically undetectable after 24 hours.

Dosage: Dosage for myelography contrast media will vary according to the area under examination. In general, the **cervical and lumbar areas require 12-15 cc of an oil-based medium** or **10 cc of a water soluble medium.** The **thoracic area** employs **25-30 cc of oil-based medium** or **12 cc of water soluble medium.**

Positioning Routines

Fluoroscopy and Spot Filming

Oil-based Contrast Medium: Spot filming routines during fluoroscopy may vary among institutions depending on physician preferences but usually when using an oil-based contrast medium, spot films are taken in the **prone position** and the **anterior oblique position.**

Water Soluble Contrast Medium: Water soluble contrast medium studies permit **either prone or supine** and **anterior or posterior oblique** positioning *(Figs. 24-21* and *24-22).*

During fluoroscopy the patient is moved from Trendelenburg to the erect position to facilitate the flow of contrast medium to all areas under examination. Spot films are taken of the areas under study. After fluoroscopy, the radiographer takes conventional overhead radiographs as described on the following page.

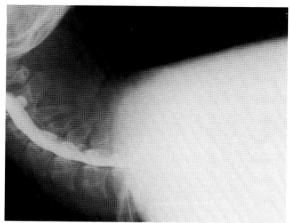
Fig. 24-20
Oil-based Cervical Myelogram

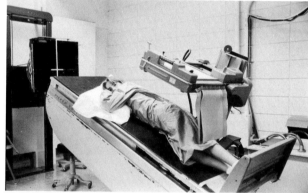
Fig. 24-21
Right Anterior Oblique for
Spot Filming of Lumbar Myelogram

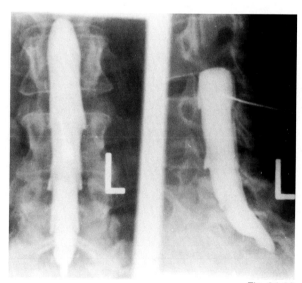
Fig. 24-22
Spot Films of Lumbar Myelogram
(PA and Oblique)

Conventional "Over head" Routines
(Following Flouroscopy)

Cervical Region

Transcervical lateral (crosstable): The patient is prone with the arms extended along the sides of the body and the shoulders depressed. The chin is extended and resting on a small positioning sponge or folded linen for comfort and to maintain extension. The central ray is directed to the level of C5. The field should be collimated to reduce scatter radiation. Respiration is suspended during the exposure.

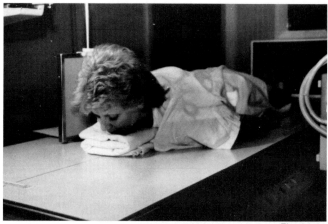

Transcervical (Crosstable) Lateral

Fig. 24-23

Swimmers (crosstable) lateral: The patient is prone with the chin extended. For a right lateral, the right arm is extended along the right side of the body with that shoulder depressed. The left arm is flexed (i.e., stretched superior to the head). The central ray is directed to the level of C-7. The field should be collimated to reduce scatter radiation. Respiration is suspended during the exposure.

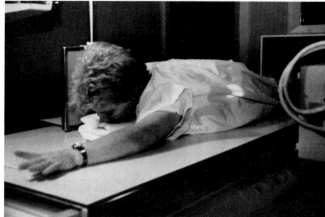

Swimmers (Crosstable) Lateral

Fig. 24-24

Thoracic Region

Right Lateral Decubitus: (AP or PA projection with a horizontal x-ray beam). The patient is positioned in a true right lateral with the right arm flexed, superior to the head. The left arm is extended and resting along the left side of the body. To maintain the alignment of the spine parallel to the table top, the patient may rest the head on the arm. If needed, a small positioning sponge or folded linen may be placed between the head and the arm to maintain alignment.

The central ray is directed to the level of T7. Collimate field to reduce scatter radiation. Respiration is suspended during the exposure.

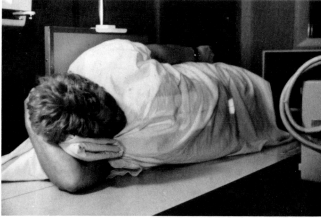

Right Lateral Decubitus
(AP Projection)

Fig. 24-25

Left Lateral Decubitus: (AP or PA projection with a horizontal x-ray beam). The patient is positioned in a true left lateral with the left arm flexed, superior to the head. The right arm is extended and resting along the right side of the body. Maintain alignment of the spine parallel to the table top as in Right Lateral Decubitus position.

The central ray is directed to the level of T7. Collimate closely to reduce scatter radiation. Respiration is suspended during the exposure.

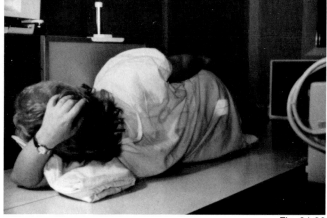

Left Lateral Decubitus
(PA Projection)

Fig. 24-26

Right or Left Lateral (vertical beam)

The patient is positioned in a **true lateral** with the knees flexed. Both arms are semi-flexed. The alignment of the spine should be maintained parallel to the table top. The patient may rest the head on the hands, or a small positioning sponge or folded linen may be placed between the hands and the head to maintain alignment of the spine. The central ray is directed to the level of T7. The field should be collimated to reduce scatter radiation. Respiration is suspended during the exposure.

NOTE: The reason a supine AP projection and a transthoracic lateral is not preferred for the thoracic region is that pooling of the contrast medium occurs in the mid thoracic region in the supine position due to the usual thoracic curvature. (This of course is more prominent in some patients.) This is especially true when using some water soluble contrast medium where only 7 to 15 cc of contrast medium is used rather than the 30 cc of oil-based medium. Therefore to demonstrate the entire spinal canal of the thoracic region, AP or PA projections are usually taken in both the right and left lateral decubitus positions, in addition to the vertical beam lateral projection.

Lumbar Region

Semi-erect transabdominal (crosstable) Lateral

The patient is positioned prone with the arms flexed, superior to the head. The table and patient are semi-erect. The radiologist, under fluoroscopic control, will adjust the angulation of the table to concentrate the contrast medium in the lumbar area.

The central ray is directed to L3. Collimate field to reduce scatter radiation. Respiration is suspended during the exposure.

Radiographs

Evaluation Criteria (for all levels of the spinal column)

• The appropriate level of the spinal column, with contrast present, should be demonstrated.
• Correct exposure and adequate penetration to demonstrate anatomy and contrast medium.
• Patient ID markers and anatomical markers (right or left) should be clearly visualized without superimposing anatomy.
• Collimation should be evident.

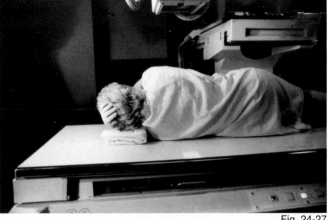

Left Lateral   Fig. 24-27

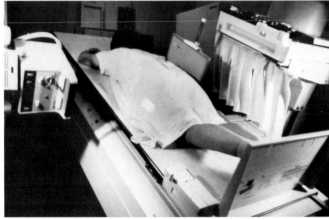

Semi-erect Transabdominal   Fig. 24-28

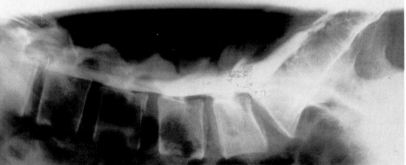

Lumbar – Transabdominal   Fig. 24-29

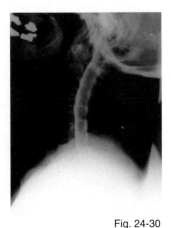

Fig. 24-30
Transcervical
(Crosstable Lateral)

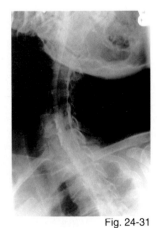

Fig. 24-31
Swimmers Lateral
(Crosstable Lateral)

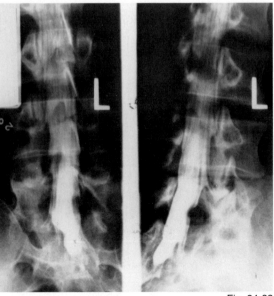

AP and Oblique, Lower Lumbar   Fig. 24-32

Additional Myelographic Special Procedures

Computed Myelography

Computed myelography is computer-enhanced radiographic examination of the vertebral column, spinal cord and spinal nerves following injection of a water-soluble contrast medium.

In addition, nonenhanced computed tomography of the vertebral column and its contents is often performed. An example of a computed myelogram is shown in *Fig. 24-33*.

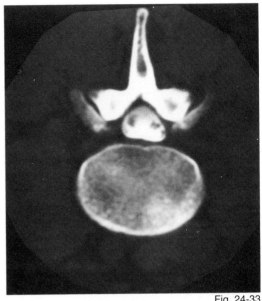

Fig. 24-33
Computed Myelogram
(Axial Section)

Discography

Discography *(dis-kog'rah-fe)* or nucleography is radiographic examination of individual intervertebral discs following injection of water-soluble, iodinated contrast medium into the center of the disc (nucleus pulposus). An example of a cervical discogram is shown in *Fig. 24-34*.

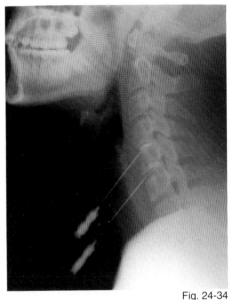

Fig. 24-34
Cervical Discogram

Epidural Venography

Epidural venography *(ve-nog'rah-fe)* is a radiographic examination of the collection of veins lining the spinal canal. This intricate plexus of veins is closely related to the intervertebral discs. This examination complements myelography in the diagnosis of intervertebral disc herniations. An example of an epidural venogram *(ve'no-gram)* is shown in *Fig. 24-35*.

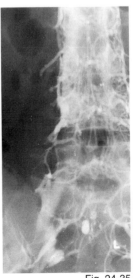

Fig. 24-35
Epidural Venogram

Chapter 25
Magnetic Resonance Imaging

Joan Radke, BS , RT(R)
E. Russell Ritenour, Ph.D.

Contents

Part I Physical Principles of Magnetic Resonance Imaging

Definition

Magnetic Resonance Imaging (MRI) refers to **the use of magnetic fields and radio waves to obtain a mathematically reconstructed image.** This image represents differences among various tissues of the patient in the **number of nuclei,** and in the **rate at which these nuclei recover** from stimulation by radio waves in the presence of a magnetic field.

Comparison with Radiography

X-rays are electromagnetic waves and as such can be described in terms of their wavelength, frequency, and the amount of energy that each "wave packet" or photon carries. A typical x-ray photon used in medical imaging may have a wavelength of 10^{-9} centimeters, a frequency of 10^{19} hertz (cycles/sec) and an energy of 60,000 electron volts *(Fig. 25-1).*

Imaging with x-rays is possible because the photon has enough energy to ionize atoms. Thus, some photons are removed from the total number sent into the patient. The pattern of photons transmitted through the patient constitutes a radiographic image which may then be captured by an image receptor such as film. The fact that x-ray photons have enough energy to ionize atoms implies that some small biological hazard is associated with a radiographic examination.

It is possible to obtain an image of the body through the use of electromagnetic waves having energies far below that required to ionize atoms thereby reducing if not eliminating the threat of biological harm to the patient. The technique of Magnetic Resonance Imaging (MRI) makes use of the **radio** portion of the electromagnetic spectrum wherein photons have relatively long wavelengths of 10^3 to 10^{-2} meters with frequencies of only 10^5 to 10^{10} hertz. A typical photon used in MRI has an energy of only 10^{-7} electron volts (a tenth of a millionth of an electron volt). See *Fig. 25-2.*

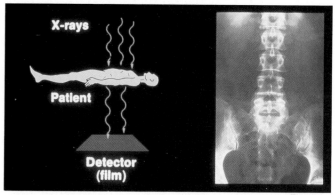

Typical X-ray – 60,000 eV Energy
(Implies some biological hazard)

Fig. 25-1

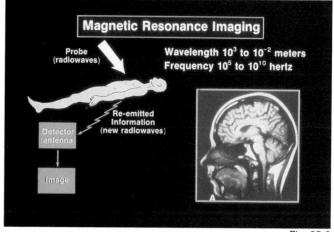

MRI – 0.0000001 eV Energy

Fig. 25-2

General Principles of MRI

Certain **nuclei** in the body will receive and re-emit radio waves of specific frequencies when those nuclei are under the influence of a magnetic field. These re-emitted radio signals contain information about the patient which is captured by a **receiver** or **antenna.** The electrical signal from the antenna is transmitted through an "analog-to-digital" (A to D) converter and then to a computer where an image of the patient is reconstructed mathematically.

The main components of the MRI system are shown in *Fig. 25-3* and are discussed in more detail later in this chapter. However, before beginning a study of the components or the equipment of an MRI system, the physical principles of MR imaging will be discussed.

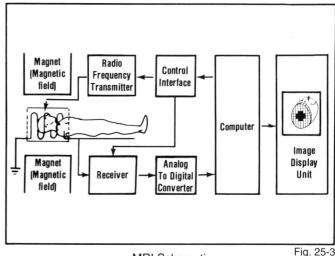

MRI Schematic

Fig. 25-3

The Interaction of Nuclei With Magnetic Fields

(The Basis of MR Imaging)

Radiographic imaging involves the interaction of x-rays with the electrons surrounding the nuclei of atoms whereas, magnetic resonance imaging involves the interaction of radio waves (and static magnetic fields) with the nuclei alone. Not all nuclei respond to magnetic fields. A list of the nuclei found in the body that are magnetic themselves (those having odd numbers of protons or neutrons) and thus suitable for magnetic resonance studies is shown in *Fig. 25-4*. Although there are in theory a number of such suitable nuclei, at present most imaging is performed with **hydrogen nuclei (single protons).**

One reason for this preference is that there is a great deal of hydrogen present in any organism. To convince ourselves of this fact we need only recall that there are two hydrogen atoms in each water molecule and that the body is roughly 85% water. Hydrogen is also contained within many other molecules. Thus, a typical cubic centimeter of the body may contain approximately 1,022 hydrogen atoms, each of which is capable of sending and receiving radio signals. Other nuclei do not exist in such abundance and therefore will not provide such a strong signal.

Precession

Magnetic Resonance Imaging is possible because a magnetic nucleus will **precess** about a strong **static (unchanging) magnetic field.** The phenomenon of precession **occurs whenever a spinning object is acted upon by an outside force.** Three examples of precession are shown in *Fig. 25-5*. A spinning top, when acted upon by the force of gravity, precesses or wobbles about the line defined by the direction of gravitational force. In MRI application, a spinning proton (hydrogen nucleus) precesses when placed in a strong magnetic field. A third example is the earth itself which precesses because of the interplay between the forces of the sun and the planets.

The **rate of precession** of a proton in a magnetic field **increases as the strength of magnetic field increases.** The rate of precession of protons in an MRI system is difficult to imagine. Protons in a low field system may precess at 5,000,000 cycles per second. (See *Fig. 25-5.*)

Sending a Radio Signal to Precessing Nuclei

After the static magnetic field has been applied, the precession of nuclei in the patient can be further influenced by radio waves since a radio wave contains a time varying magnetic field. One effect of the radio wave is to cause the nucleus to precess at a greater angle. **The longer the radio wave is applied to the patient the greater the angle of precession.** In the example shown in *Fig. 25-6*, the radio wave has been applied long enough to cause the nucleus to change from near vertical (parallel to the static magnetic field) to horizontal (at right angles to the static magnetic field). However, even this duration of the radio waves sufficient to change the precession of the nuclei to a near horizontal position seems short in relation to events in everyday life. We say that the radio wave is applied to the patient in a "pulse" that may last for a fraction of a second during the "send" phase of the MRI process. Pulse sequences are described in more detail later in this chapter.

Nuclei Suitable for MR	
$^{1}_{1}$H	- Hydrogen
$^{13}_{6}$C	- Carbon
$^{14}_{7}$N	- Nitrogen
$^{17}_{8}$O	- Oxygen
$^{39}_{19}$K	- Potassium
$^{19}_{9}$F	- Fluorine
$^{23}_{11}$Na	- Sodium
$^{31}_{15}$P	- Phosphorus

Fig. 25-4
Nuclei Potentially Suitable for MRI

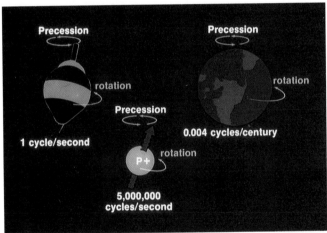

Examples of Precession   Fig. 25-5

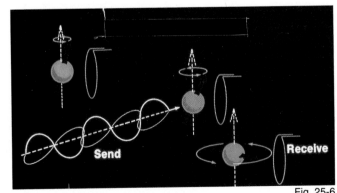

Radio Waves Increase Angle of Precession   Fig. 25-6

Resonance

Radio waves affect the precessing nuclei because the **time varying magnetic field** of the radio wave (i.e., the radio frequency part of the electromagnetic spectrum) changes at the same rate as the nuclei precess. This means that as the nucleus rotates, the magnetic field appears at just the proper time to have maximum effect in "pushing" the nucleus away from the static magnetic field. This timing of a force and a periodically changing system is an example of the concept of **"resonance."**

Another common example of resonance is the pushing of a child on a swing. When we push a child on a swing, we naturally push the child in "resonance." That is, we apply force to the swing at a frequency that matches the frequency with which the swing returns to us. We know that if we apply our energy at any other frequency there will be no useful effect. Thus, the principle of resonance explains why we use radio frequency waves applied in pulses for MR imaging. **Radio waves** (because of their specific wavelength) **are in resonance with the precessing nuclei.** (This explains the use of radio waves in MRI rather than other electromagnetic waves such as microwaves or visible light which, because of their wavelength, would not be in resonance with the precessing nuclei.)

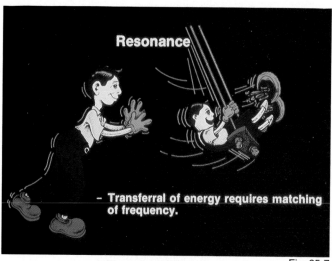

Example of Resonance   Fig. 25-7

Receiving the MRI Signal From Body Tissues

Because the nucleus is itself a tiny magnet, as it rotates it emits electromagnetic waves. These emitted waves from nuclei within body tissue are picked up by an antenna or **receiver coil during** the "receive" phase of the MRI process *(Fig. 25-8)*. This electrical signal obtained from the receiver coil is sent to a computer. The image of the patient is then reconstructed by the computer. Various mathematical techniques may be used to build up an image from the received radio waves. Some techniques are similar to those used in computed tomography.

The received signal is described relative to random superimposed signals or noise that is also picked up by the antenna. The signal to noise ratio (SNR or S/N) is used to describe the relative contribution of the true signal from the tissue and random noise.

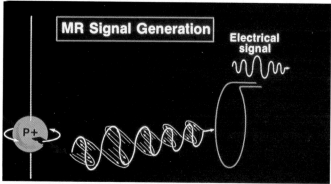

MRI Signal Generation   Fig. 25-8

Relaxation

When the radio frequency pulse that was sent to the nuclei is over, the nuclei are precessing together in phase. As soon as the radio frequency pulse is turned off, the nuclei begin to return to a more random configuration in a process called **relaxation**. As the nuclei relax, the MRI signal received **from** the precessing nuclei diminishes. The rate of relaxation gives us information about normal tissue and pathologic process in the tissues. Thus, relaxation influences the appearance of the MR image. Relaxation may be divided into two categories as shown in *Fig. 25-9*. These are commonly refered to as **T1** and **T2** relaxation.

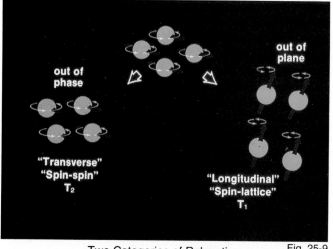

Two Categories of Relaxation   Fig. 25-9

Relaxation continued

T1 Relaxation: This relaxation category occurs when the spins begin to precess at **smaller and smaller angles,** that is from a near horizontal or transverse precession to a more vertical (see *Fig. 25-10).* This process, referred to as **longitudinal or spin lattice** type relaxation (T1) causes the MRI signal to **decrease in strength.** We define the time required for this signal to decrease to 37% of its maximum value as T1 (See *Fig. 25-10.)*

T2 Relaxation: When spins begin to precess **out of phase** with each other, the result is referred to as **transverse or spin-spin type** relaxation. This is called T2 relaxation. Note in *Fig. 25-11* that the nuclei along the top of the graph are shown to be "in phase" at the beginning but that they go out of phase as indicated by the direction of the arrows. As this T2 relaxation occurs, the MRI signal will **decrease in strength.** The time required for the MRI signal to decrease to 37% of its maximum value is defined as T2 (See *Fig. 25-11.)*

The rate of these two types of relaxation changes, T1 and T2 following exposure to the radio frequency (applied in resonance) constitutes the primary basis from which the MR image is reconstructed. However, a third factor, spin density, also plays a minor role in determining the appearance of the MR image.

Spin Density: A stronger signal will be received if the **quantity** of hydrogen nuclei that are present in a given volume of tissue **is increased.** However, this quantity, called the "proton density" or **"spin density"** is a minor contributor to the appearance of an MR image because the tissues imaged by proton (hydrogen nucleus) do not differ markedly in spin density. A more important consideration as discussed above, is that the nuclei that compose **different tissues** within the body, **respond at different relaxation rates,** T1 and T2.

Summary: The **MRI signal strength,** as received by an antenna or receiver coil, is used to define the **brightness of each point of the image of the patient.** Thus, the differences among T1, T2 and spin density of tissues produce differences in relative brightness of points in the image. The **three primary factors** which determine the signal strength and therefore the brightness of each part of the image or the image contrast are **spin density** and **T1 and T2** relaxation rates. Other factors such as flowing blood or the presence of contrast material also play a role, but are beyond the scope of this introductory discussion.

Magnetic Resonance Imaging is a fundamentally different way of looking at the body compared to other imaging modalities. For example, in radiography, the physical density (grams per cc) and atomic number of tissues determine the appearance of the image. The rate of recovery of atoms from their interactions with x-rays is not important in radiography. In MRI however, the rate of recovery of nuclei following the application of radio waves (relaxation rate) is the most important factor in determining the MR image. This provides the basis for the MR image as seen in *Fig. 25-12.* High tissue density such as in dense bone structure does **not** result in image contrast in **MR** imaging. Soft tissues such as grey and white matter of the brain, the brain stem and the corpus callosum however, are clearly visualized because of the response of nuclei in these tissues as described above.

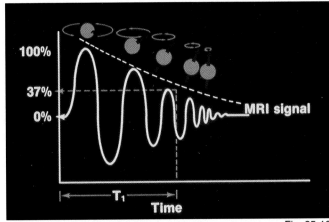

T1 Relaxation
(Longitudinal, spin - lattice)

Fig. 25-10

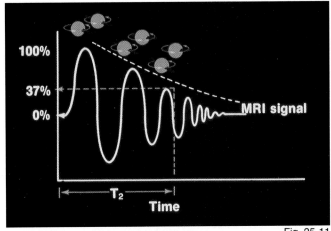

T2 Relaxation
(Transverse, spin - spin)

Fig. 25-11

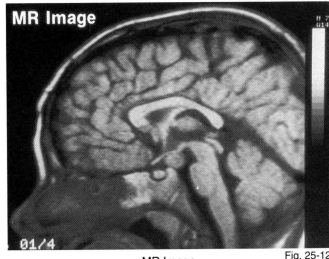

MR Image

Fig. 25-12

Gradient Magnetic Fields

To further understand the method of image reconstruction used in MRI, it is necessary to understand the concept of a **gradient, or a change of magnetic field strength through a certain region or "slice" of body tissue.** The gradient magnetic field is used to obtain information from specific regions or slices of body tissue. Knowledge of the exact location of origin of received MRI signals from within the patient allows the computer to reconstruct the MR image.

Earlier in this chapter it was shown that the strength of the magnetic field determines the **precession rate** of the nuclei. The precession rate determines the exact value of radio wave frequency that will be in resonance with the nuclei. The MRI system sends and receives radio waves from nuclei only when those nuclei are precessing at the same frequency as the frequency of the radio wave, i.e. at resonance frequency. Thus, an MRI system **changes the gradient** or **magnetic field strength through a certain region or slice of body tissue so that the system will only receive the MR signal from nuclei that precess within that region or slice.** The computer can decode this as well as other information such as spin density and T1 and T2 relaxation and can thereby, reconstruct the MRI image.

The use of gradient magnetic fields in MRI is similar in many ways to the use of x-ray collimators in CT (Computed Tomography) where information from specific slices of irradiated tissue is used to reconstruct the CT image. Gradient magnetic fields are produced by "gradient coils" located within the bore of the main system magnet.

The gradient magnetic fields are much weaker than the static magnetic field produced by the main MRI system magnet. The gradient field adds to or increases the strength of the static magnetic field over some regions of the patient and decreases the strength of the static field over other regions of the patient. Since the strength of the magnetic field determines the frequency of precession of nuclei, this in turn determines the frequency of the MRI signal produced from that region. Thus, gradient fields cause different regions of the patient to produce MRI signals at slightly different frequencies. (See *Fig. 25-13*.)

Summary: The strength of the MRI signal is determined by the number of nuclei per unit volume (spin density) and the orientation of the nuclei with respect to the static magnetic field (T1 relaxation) and with respect to each other (T2 relaxation). The **location of origin** within the patient of the MRI signal may be determined by the **frequency** of the MRI signal. The application of gradient magnetic fields assures us that the frequency of the MRI signal will vary from one location to another within the patient and that the computer may therefore, produce a unique image of the patient.

The frequency of the signal is a measure of how often it varies in strength. Other techniques are used to alter the "phase" of the MR signal, whether it is large or small at a specific time. By varying the frequency in one direction, and the phase in another direction, the location of origin of MR signal may be found for each point within a slice.

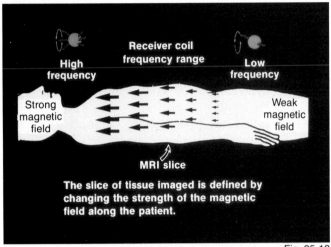

Gradient Magnetic Fields
(Basis of MRI "slice")   Fig. 25-13

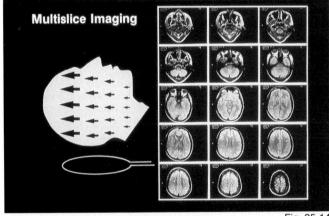

Multislice Images   Fig. 25-14

Multislice Imaging

Figure 25-14 demonstrates multislice MR imaging of the cranium. Note by the anatomical structures visualized on these various images that each image represents a reconstruction of data received by the computer through the receiving coils as the magnetic field strength was varied or changed through specific regions or slices of the body tissues.

Pulse Sequences

The image produced by an MRI system is critically influenced by the exact sequence of radio wave pulses used as well as the moment at which the signal emitted by the nuclei is sampled or received. Since the duration of the radio wave pulse that is sent into the patient determines the angle at which the nucleus precesses, **the length of the pulse is often specified in terms of the angle it will produce.** Figure 25-15 illustrates 90, 45, and 180 degree pulses.

Spin - Echo Pulse Sequence: A typical pulse sequence is diagrammed in *Fig. 25-16.* The sequence contains two pulses, a 90 degree pulse and a 180 degree pulse. Radiofrequency waves are sent into the patient during each pulse. The sequence is repeated again after a time TR, (repetition time) has elapsed. Typical TR values used in imaging may vary from 200 - 2000 millisec (0.2 - 2 sec). The pulse sequence changes the angle of precession of the nuclei and causes a radiofrequency wave called an "echo" to be emitted from the patient.

In MRI techniques, the receiver coil listens to an echo of the signal, rather than the initial signal, which is called the FID or free induction decay. The echo is intercepted by the receiver coils of the MR system and is used to construct an image of the patient. The echo occurs at a time TE (time-to-echo) after the initial pulse of the sequence. Typical TE values used in imaging vary from 10 - 100 milliseconds. Both TR and TE are technique variables that are selected by the operator of the MR system to optimize the appearance of an image and to allow acquisition of information weighted toward T1 or T2 relaxation rates.

Acquisition of an image requres that gradient magnetic fields be turned on and off at appropriate times during a pulse sequence. Gradients are used to vary the phase and frequency of precession of protons throughout the patient so that the origin of the MR signal (echo) may be assigned to the appropriate locations within the image. The complete pulse sequence timing diagram for a spin-echo pulse sequence is shown in *Fig. 25-17.* A spin-echo pulse sequence is a commonly used pulse sequence in clinical situations and is just one of the techniques available for imaging. Gradient-echo and inversion recovery are two other types of pulse sequences. (See definitions at end of chapter.) The slice select gradient, G slice, is turned on while pulses are sent into the patient. The frequency encoding gradient, G frequency, is turned on only while the echo signal is received. The phase encoding gradient, G phase, is turned on between pulses. The entire process is repeated with different values of the phase encoding gradient (indicated by the dotted lines for G phase in *Fig. 25-17*).

The three gradient directions (slice, phase and frequency) correspond to the three axes of the patient, x, y , z which may be identified with slice (plane) selection. The x, y and z gradients are explained in more detail later in this chapter.

[1,2]Hendee WR; Ritenour , ER; **Medical Imaging Physics**, 3rd ed. Mosby-Year Book, Chicago, 1992.

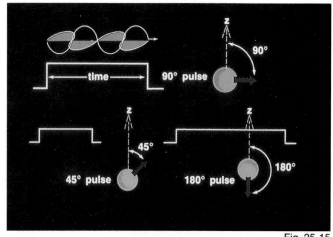

Pulse Sequences

Fig. 25-15

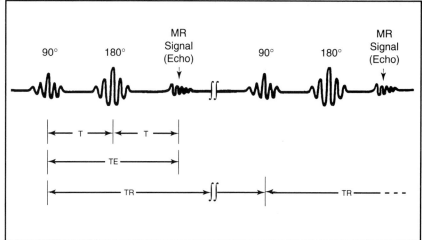

Spin-echo Pulse Sequence[1]

Fig. 25-16

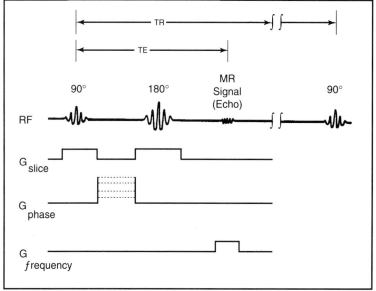

Fig. 25-17

A magnetic resonance image acquisition diagram showing a spin - echo pulse sequence along with gradient magnetic fields.[2]

Pulse Sequence continued

Pulse Sequence Timing Factors: At the present, several types of pulse sequences are used to accentuate one or more of the parameters that influence MR images. Figure 25-18 demonstrates the differences in the appearance of the image created by changing certain pulse sequence timing factors. Notice that some areas of the image change almost completely from white to black because of the change in pulse repetition time (TR), or the time between pulse sequences. The time between the initial pulse that is sent into the patient and the time that the MR signal is sampled from the patient, the time-to-echo (TE), also influence the image. Both the TR and TE are selected by the operator and have a profound influence upon contrast in the image.

Number of Signal Averages: Another variable that is set by the operator and that influences the appearance of the image is the number of signal averages. The entire pulse sequence is repeated several times and the MR signal value is then averaged. Signal averaging reduces the effects of spurious noise but increases the time required to complete a scan.

Summary: A good understanding of the physical principles of MR imaging involving the interaction of nuclei with magnetic fields as described in this chapter, provides a foundation for further study and understanding of all parameters of MRI.

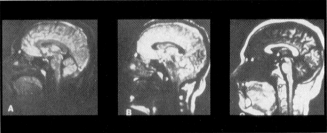

TR (pulse sequence) Variables   Fig. 25-18

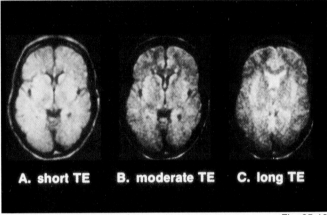

A. short TE   B. moderate TE   C. long TE

TE (time-to-echo) Variables   Fig. 25-19

Part II Equipment Components

MRI System Components

The application of the principle of magnetic resonance in the modern hospital requires an impressive collection of "state of the art" equipment. The six main components of the MRI system are shown in *Fig. 25-20* and are discussed in the following section. They are as follows:

- **Magnet**
- **Gradient coils**
- **Radiofrequency coils**
- **Electronic support systems**
- **Computer**
- **Display**

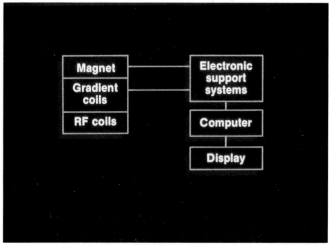

MRI Main Components   Fig. 25-20

Magnets

The most visible and probably the most often discussed component of the MRI system is the magnet. The **magnet provides the powerful static** (constant strength) **magnetic field** about which the nuclei precess. At the present time there are **three** types of MRI system magnets. Not one of the three is inherently superior to the others. Each have their own unique characteristics. They share a common purpose however, in creating a magnetic field that is measured in units of **Tesla** *(Tes´la)*[1]. Field strengths used clinically vary from .1 to 2.0 Tesla. In comparison, the earth's magnetic field is approximately 0.00005 Tesla *(Fig. 25-21)*.

Static field strengths surrounding the magnet, called fringe magnetic fields, are sometimes measured in **Gauss** *(Gous)*[2]. One Tesla equals 10,000 Gauss.

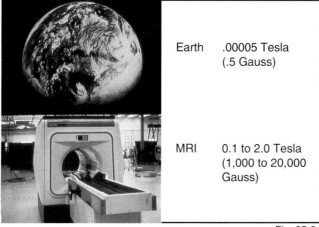

| Earth | .00005 Tesla (.5 Gauss) |
| MRI | 0.1 to 2.0 Tesla (1,000 to 20,000 Gauss) |

Magnetic Field Strength   Fig. 25-21

Resistive Magnets: The resistive magnet *(Fig. 25-22)* works on the principle of the **electromagnet,** wherein a magnetic field may be created by passing an electrical current through a coil of wire. Resistive magnets require large amounts of electrical power many times greater than that required for typical radiographic equipment, to provide the high currents necessary for the production of high strength magnetic fields. The cost of this electrical power must be considered as part of the cost of operation of the unit.

In addition, the high electrical currents produce heat which must be dissipated with a cooling system. The heat is produced by the resistance of the wire to the flow of electricity. This resistance acts as a type of "friction" which produces heat and ultimately limits the amount of current which can be produced. Typical resistive systems produce magnetic field strengths of up to **0.3 Tesla.**

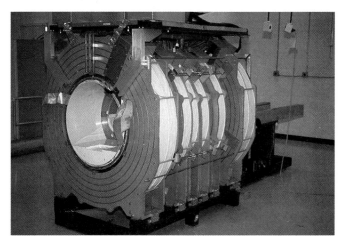

Resistive Magnet   Fig. 25-22
(Field strength to 0.3 Tesla)

---

[1] Nikola *Tesla*, 1856-1943, U.S. (born in Croata) researcher in electromagnetic phenomena . *Tesla* is a unit of magnetic flux density equal to one weber per square meter (SI unit of measurement).

[2] Karl F. *Gauss*, German physicist, 1777-1855, a measurement of magnetic flux density in lines of flux per square centimeter (GCS unit of measurement).

Permanent Magnets: The high operating costs associated with the other two types of magnets, namely the electrical power and cryogens, are avoided in the permanent magnet system *(Fig. 25-23)*. Certain materials can be given permanent magnetic properties. An example of a very small permanent magnet of this type is the magnet used to attach notes to refrigerator doors. For MRI use, certain very large permanent magnets may be made with field strengths up to **0.3 Tesla.**

The initial cost of the permanent magnet is somewhere between the above two types. Since no electrical power is needed for this magnet, the operating cost is nearly negligible. A disadvantage however, may be the inability to turn off the power of the magnetic field. If metal objects accidentally become lodged in the bore of the magnet, they must be removed against the full power of the magnetic field.

Superconducting Magnets: The superconducting magnet *(Fig. 25-24)* also uses the principle of the **electromagnet.** In addition, it uses a property that is demonstrated by some materials at **extremely low temperatures,** the property of **superconductivity.** A superconductive material is a material that has lost all resistance to electrical current. When this occurs, very large electrical currents may be maintained with essentially no use of electrical power. Thus, the electrical costs of running a superconducting magnet are negligible.

A significant factor however, is the cost of providing these very low temperature cooling materials, called "cryogens" *(kri'o-jen)*. The two cryogens currently employed are liquid nitrogen (-195.8° C), and liquid helium (-268.9° C). The cost of maintaining this intensive cooling system is of the same order of magnitude or even higher than the electrical costs of a resistive system. The initial cost is also the highest of the three types of magnets. Higher magnetic field strengths are possible with the superconducting magnet with values as high as **2 Tesla** for clinical use. These are currently a common type of magnet in clinical use because of their greater magnetic field strength.

Gradient Coils

In addition to the powerful magnets, a second major component of the MRI system is the gradient coil. The gradient magnetic fields **cause nuclei in different locations within the patient to precess at slightly different rates,** allowing the computer to determine the location within the patient from which the received MRI signal originated. This information is, of course, crucial to the reconstruction of an image of the patient. The **gradient fields are much weaker** than the static magnetic fields and can be produced by relatively simple coils of wire.

One typical configuration of the gradient coils is shown in *Fig. 25-25*. An MRI system may contain three sets of gradient coils, allowing a gradient to be applied in the three directions - x, y, and z. These coils, referred to as the x, y, and z gradient coils, are located within the bore of the main system magnet. By electronically adjusting the amount of current in these three sets of coils, it is possible to obtain a gradient in any direction. This flexibility allows a magnetic resonance imaging system to obtain images at any orientation within the patient.

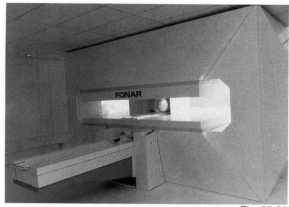

Fig. 25-23

Permanent Magnet
(Field strength to 0.3 Tesla)

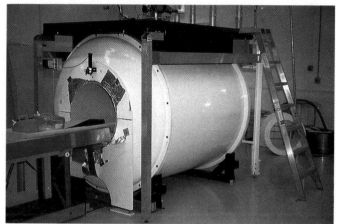

Fig. 25-24

Superconducting Magnet
(Field strength to 2 Tesla)

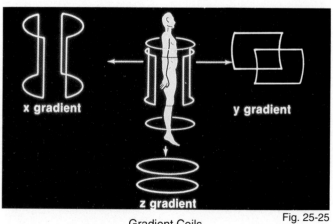

Fig. 25-25

Gradient Coils

MRI System Components continued

Radio Frequency RF Coils

A third key component of the MRI system is the radio frequency (RF) or "send and receive" coils. These RF coils act **as antennas to produce and detect the radio waves** that are referred to as **the MRI "signal."**

A typical RF coil is encased or enclosed in the gantry of the magnet and thus is not specifically visible. These encased RF coils, sometimes referred to as body coils, **completely surround the patient** including the table on which the patient lies as indicated by the arrows in *Fig. 25-26*.

Designs of RF coils vary from this large, enclosed **body coil** to separate smaller **circumferential whole-volume coils**, which also encircle the part being imaged. Examples of these are the head coil and the limb (extremity) coil *(Fig. 25-27)*.

Some **surface coils**, such as the shoulder coil, are placed on the area to be imaged. Generally, this type of surface coil is used to image more superficial structures.

These various coils will be described and demonstrated in use with specific MRI procedures later in this chapter. A display of an assortment of circumferential whole-volume and surface coils are shown in *Fig. 25-27*.

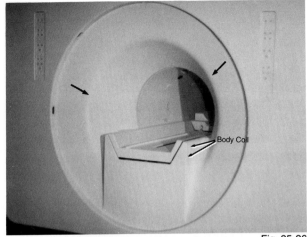
RF (Body) Coil in Gantry of Magnet   Fig. 25-26

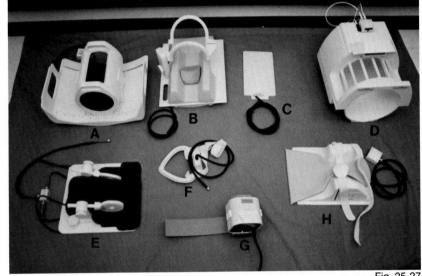
Display of Circumferential Whole-volume and Surface Coils   Fig. 25-27

A. Limb (extremity) coil   D. Head Coil
B. Volume neck coil   E. TMJ coil (bilateral)
C. Planar surface coil   F. Shoulder coil
   (License plate coil)   G. Wrist coil
                                H. Posterior C spine coil

Electronic Support System

The electronic support systems, making up the fourth component of the MRI system, can be divided into two parts. The first part, the **power supply**, provides voltage and current for all parts of the MRI system that require it, such as the gradient coils, the cooling system, the magnet, and the computer. The power usage varies in different MRI systems. For example, the cooling system and magnet requirements are negligible in permanent magnet systems, but they provide the heaviest load in resistive systems. Thus, the power consumption varies from about 25 kilowatts in permanent magnet systems to over 150 kilowatts in resistive systems.

The second major part of the electronic support system is the **RF transmitter and receiver.** This part of the system performs the same functions as broadcast radio communication transmitters and receivers. It sends the radio wave pulses into the patient and receives the MRI signals from the patient. (The RF send and receive coils, as described above, are part of this system.) The RF transmitter also contains amplifiers that boost the strength of relatively weak radio signals received from deep within a patient in the bore of the magnet.

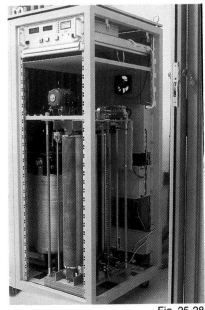
Fig. 25-28
Example of Power Supply
(25-150+ Kilowatts)

Computer

The fifth component of the MRI system is the computer, a key component of an MRI unit. It processes information from all parts of the MRI system. During a scan it controls the timing of pulses to coincide with changes in gradient field strengths. After a scan it reconstructs the image of the patient using techniques such as Fourier transforms that are similar to those used in computed tomography.

The computer contains both internal and external memory devices. Internal memory allows the computer to manipulate the millions of bits of information required to define an image of the patient. External memory includes the various types of magnetic storage media such as hard disks, optical disks, and tape cartridges which are used to store information for future use.

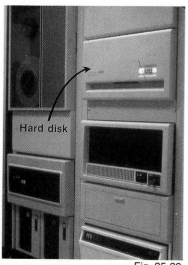

Fig. 25-29
MRI Computer

Display

The sixth and last component of the MRI system to be discussed is the display or workstation which allows the technologist to control the operation of the system and view images as they are reconstructed. A central or system workstation, as shown in *Fig. 25-30,* may contain the **controls** used by the technologist to **select pulse sequences, set the various operator adjustable parameters,** such as number of signal averages and pulse repetition time (TR), and to **initiate the scan.** Controls on the display allow **brightness and contrast to be altered** to bring out significant features in the image.

Independent display stations located away from the central display station (in a separate room) are often included to allow images to be viewed while other patients are being scanned. Image processing capability is sometimes available to allow enhancement operations such as digital filtering.

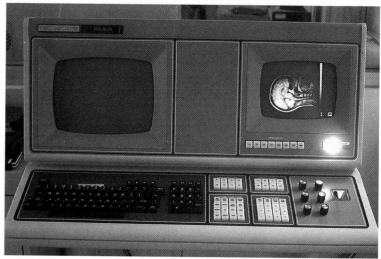

MRI Display Station   Fig. 25-30

Summary of MRI Imaging Process and System Components Used

Following is a five step summary of the entire MR imaging process identifying the component of equipment used and the results of each step:

Step	Component	Result
1. Apply static magnetic field	magnet	Nuclei align and precess
2. Select slice by applying gradient magnetic field (variation of magnetic field strength over patient)	gradient coils	Nuclei precess at a particular frequency
3. Apply RF pulses	RF sending coil or antenna	Nuclei in the slice area precess in phase at a greater angle
4. Receive RF signal	RF receiving coil or antenna	Electrical signal is received from nuclei and sent to computer
5. Convert signal to image	computer	Reconstructed image is displayed

Summary   Fig. 25-31

Part III Clinical Applications

It has become increasingly popular to refer to radiology departments as diagnostic imaging centers. This new terminology is due in part to the increased use of magnetic resonance imaging. The need for radiographers to have a basic knowledge of MRI continues to grow as MRI continues to improve in its ability to show disease processes.

With increases in the number of MR scanners available, radiographers will continue to be called upon to assume staff positions in the MRI section of radiology. Many students of radiologic technology will have the opportunity to observe and participate in patient examinations utilizing MRI.

Comparison with Computed Tomography

In clinical applications MRI is often compared to computed tomography (CT) because MRI, like CT, displays images in sections. CT scanners acquire data that is manipulated by the computer to form axial or transverse sections *(Fig. 25-32)*. Coronal, sagittal and 3D views can also be reconstructed from the data as described in chapter 22 *(Fig. 22-1)*.

MRI also has the diversity to image anatomy in axial or transverse, sagittal or coronal sections or planes *(Figs. 25-33,34,and 35)*. Oblique views of anatomical structures can also be obtained by using a combination of gradient coils.

MRI and CT technologists require an in-depth knowledge of anatomy (including sectional anatomy) for accurate viewing of images obtained from various planes or sections. A thorough knowledge of bony landmarks, organs and vessel placement will enable technologists to appropriately interpret images to determine if the scans have adequately covered the region of interest.

CT shows an improvement in soft tissue contrast over conventional screen-film imaging. This ability to show soft tissue contrast is referred to as **contrast resolution**. The MR imaging system is more sensitive to the molecular nature of tissue and thus allows excellent contrast resolution as shown on these MRI sections. For example, MRI is sensitive to the slight difference in tissue composition of normal gray and white matter of the brain. Therefore, MRI is replacing CT as the study of choice for diseases involving the CNS, especially for examination of white matter pathology.

While CT and conventional radiography measure the attenuation of the x-ray beam, MRI uses a technique that stimulates the body to produce a radio frequency signal and uses an antenna or receiver coil to measure this signal as already discussed in part 1 of this chapter. Technologists of MRI are required to have an understanding of how technical factors affect signal production. These technical factors impact the contrast and spatial resolution. Therefore, the technologist is required to utilize these technical factors for optimum image quality.

Diagnosis of diseases such as those involving the CNS can be made with MRI by making comparisons between the signal produced in normal tissue and the signal produced in abnormal tissue.

Unlike CT, nuclear medicine and radiography, no ionizing radiation is used in MRI. Therefore, MRI is deemed safer in terms of biological tissue damage. Even though the MRI scanner does not use ionizing radiation, there are safety considerations that must be identified and understood as demonstrated on the following pages.

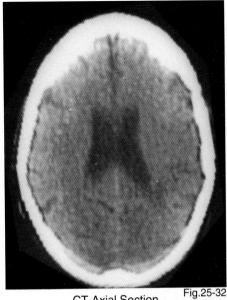

CT Axial Section   Fig.25-32

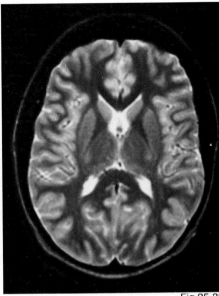

MRI Axial Section   Fig.25-33

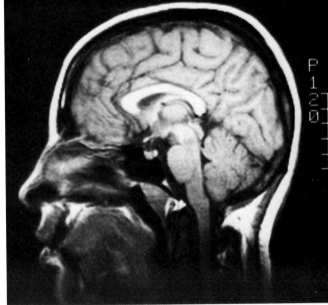

MRI Sagittal Section   Fig.25-34

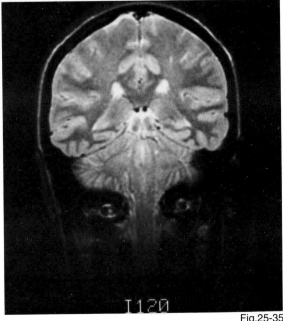

MRI Coronal Section   Fig.25-35

Basic Safety Considerations

Safety concerns for the technologist, patient and medical personnel must be recognized and are due to **the interaction of the magnetic fields with metallic objects and tissues.** During a MR scan, patients as well as other personnel in the immediate area are exposed to **static, gradient-induced** (time-varying) and **radio-frequency (RF) magnetic fields.**

Suggested maximum permissible field strengths for these fields are illustrated in *Fig. 25-36.* These values are to assist a hospital and review boards in assessing health consequences of operating an MR unit. It may be acceptable to operate an MR unit which exceeds these guidelines provided that the vendors of the MR equipment have shown to the satisfaction of the hospital or review board that the actual static, time varying and RF fields do not create a significant health risk.[1]

Safety concerns of MRI resulting from the interaction of these magnetic fields with tissues and metallic objects are as follows:

(1) Potential hazard of projectiles.
(2) Electrical interference with implants.
(3) Torquing of metallic objects.
(4) Local heating of tissues and metallic objects.
(5) Electrical interference with the normal function of nerve cells and muscle fibers.

Each of these five safety concerns will be discussed beginning with the potential hazards of projectiles.

(1) Potential Hazard of Projectiles

A static magnetic field surrounds the magnet and is referred to as the **fringe magnetic field.** Certain items are not allowed inside these fringe fields and monitoring is essential before allowing anyone to enter the magnet room. Warning posters and door security systems need to be in use to prevent unauthorized personnel from entering restricted areas within the fringe magnetic field.

The fringe magnetic fields are generally measured in Gauss (G). The fringe field strength is inversely proportional to the cube of the the distance from the bore of the magnet, therefore the danger of projectiles becomes greater as one moves closer to the magnet. For example on a 1.5 Tesla imaging system, a ferromagnetic object 3 feet away will have a force 10 times that of gravity; and at 7 feet it would equal that of gravity *(Fig. 25-38).* If a small ferromagnetic object were released close to the magnet, it could become lethal as it attains a terminal velocity of 40 miles per hour by the time it reaches the center of the magnet.[2]

In the event of a code (respiratory or cardiac arrest), the patient must first be removed from the scan room and all personnel advised of the routine procedure of response to eliminate the possibility of metallic objects becoming dangerous projectiles.

[1]Stark DD, Bradley, WG; **Magnetic Resonance Imaging**; CV Mosby; St Louis, MO: 1987

[2] Williams, K.D.; Drayer, B.P.; BNI Quarterly, Barrow Neurological Institute of St. Joseph's Hospital and Medical Center; Phoenix, AZ; 5:1 1989

Static Field:	2.0 Tesla
Time-varying Field:	3T/S
Radio-frequency Fields:	SAR of 0.4 W/kg (whole body)
	or
	2.0 w/kg (in any gram)

Fig. 25-36

Maximum permissable field strength guidelines
(Guidelines by Food and Drug Administration through the publication of National Center for Devices and Radiological Health (DHHS:1982)

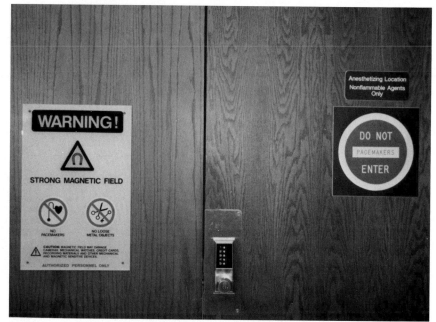

Fig. 25-37

Warning Posters and Door Security
(Courtesy of University of Iowa Hospitals and Clinics)

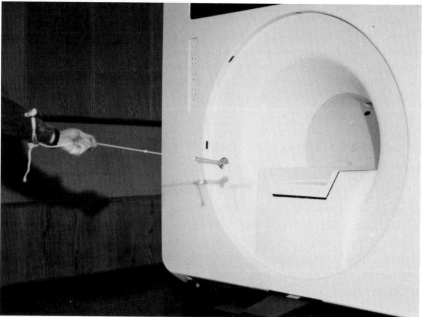

Demonstration of Potential Hazard of Projectiles Fig. 25-38
(Courtesy of University of Iowa Hospitals and Clinics)

(A metallic object is shown in midair suspension as it is strongly attracted towards the magnet. If not securely held back by the rope, it would become a dangerous projectile. This demonstration is not recommended without adequate precautions and safety measures)

Potential Hazard of Projectiles continued

As a rule, patient equipment such as O_2 tanks, IV pumps, patient monitoring equipment, wheelchairs, and carts are **not** allowed inside the **50 Gauss line,** although some special equipment has been designed to be used specifically in MRI.

Figure 25-39 below represents recommended minimum distances for various types of devices and/or personnel in relationship to the various Gauss line perimeters around the MRI system.

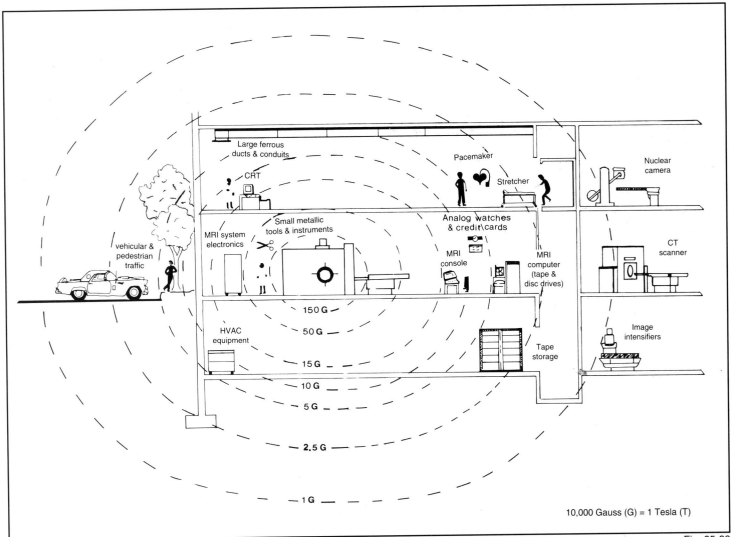

Recommended Minimum Distances – Based on a Non-magnetically Shielded System

(Courtesy of Picker International)

Fig. 25-39

(2) Electrical Interference with Electromechanical Implants

A second major concern is possible damage to electronic components and function of cardiac pacemakers therefore, these are not allowed within the **5 Gauss line**. Besides the static magnetic field causing possible damage to cardiac pacemakers, the RF pulses may induce voltage in the pacemaker leads.

Other devices that may be adversely affected by MRI are cochlear implants, neurostimulators, implanted drug infusion pumps and bone growth stimulators. Objects such as magnetic tapes, credit cards, and analog watches may also be affected and should therefore be kept outside the **10 Gauss line** as shown above.

Basic Safety Considerations continued

(3) Torquing of Metallic Objects

The third safety concern involves metallic objects such as surgical clips located inside or on the patient's body and their interaction with the static field. The magnetic field may cause torquing or a twisting movement of the object and damage to the tissue surrounding the surgical site.

The most important contraindication in this category is for patients with intracranial aneurysm clips. Various aneurysm clips have been shown to exhibit torquing when exposed to the static magnetic field used in MRI. Aneurysm clips would be considered a contraindication unless the exact type is known and has been proven to be nonferro-magnetic.[1]

Caution is recommended for all patients with recent placement of surgical clips . Stapedial replacement prostheses may be considered a contraindication. Patients with metallic foreign objects such as bullets, shrapnel and especially intraocular metallic objects must be carefully screened. Conventional screening radiographs may be indicated.

(4) Local Heating of Tissues and Metallic Objects

A fourth area of concern is with local heating of tissues and large metallic objects inside the patient's body. The RF pulses which pass through the patient's body cause tissue heating. This heating is measured in W/kg (watts per kilogram) and is referred to as the **SAR** or specific absorption ratio. Technologists must be concerned with SAR limits although MR scanners may be equipped to regulate the parameters so that SAR limits are not exceeded. (See *Fig. 25-36* on a preceding page.) Often the technologist must enter the patient's weight for this calculation to be made.

The amount of heat produced is dependent on the number of slices, the flip angle, the number of signal averages, the TR and the tissue type. The body is able to dispel the heat through the normal circulatory and evaporative processes. At the RF levels used in MR, no biologically detrimental tissue heating has been shown to occur.

This however, is one reason pregnant women are not routinely scanned. The increase in fetal temperature may be harmful. The effects of this for MRI have not been fully documented.

(5) Electrical Interference with Normal Functions of Nerve Cells and Muscle Fibers

Rapidly changing gradient-induced magnetic fields may cause electrical current in tissues. These may be great enough to interfere with the normal function of nerve cells and muscle fibers. Examples of this include sensations of flashes of light and ventricular fibrillation. The maximum gradient magnetic field change allowed in MR is at least ten times lower than the threshold value for fibrillation and has therefore, not been considered a serious problem .

Occupational Hazards

To date there have been no documented long term biological adverse effects for technologists working in the MRI department. As a precaution, some MRI centers have recommended that technologists who are pregnant remain outside the scan room when the gradients are pulsing. Radiobiologists continue to investigate the possibility and occurrence of adverse effects due to electromagnetic fields.

Summary: The primary concern is safety of the patient and medical personnel from dangers involving MRI due to interaction of the magnetic fields with tissues and metallic objects as described above. The absolute contraindications for patient scanning will be addressed in the following section.

Patient History

A thorough patient history must be obtained before scanning. When contrast is indicated, an allergy history must be obtained. A patient information form *(Fig. 25-40)* is given to the patient before the exam in preparation for the upcoming questions. The patient is questioned regarding surgical, accidental and occupational histories. If an implant is unknown, the exam may have to be delayed until an exact description can be obtained. Conventional radiographs may also need to be obtained first. Many limb prostheses are magnetic and must be removed before entering the scanning room. They may turn into projectiles. Permanent eyeliner and other types of eye makeup may contain metallic fragments and can cause discomfort.

MR Information Form

You have been referred to the Magnetic Resonance Imaging Center for an examination which your physician feels may provide useful diagnostic information about your physical condition. Magnetic resonance (MR) imaging is a technique which will provide pictures of the interior of your body. This examination consists of placing you inside a large magnet. Radio signals will be transmitted into your body. This will cause your body to emit weak radio signals which are picked up by an antenna and formed into a picture or image by a computer. The examination will take about an hour. The only discomfort will be from lying still in the confined center of the magnet for a length of time, and the examination is rather noisy.

Examining you could be hazardous if you have certain metal in your body from either surgery or an accident.

Please inform us if you have any of the following:
- *Cardiac pacemaker*
- *Electronic implant*
- *Aneurysm clip in the brain*
- *Inner ear surgery*
- *Metallic fragments*
- *Metal in and/or removed from your eye(s)*
- *Eye prostheses*
- *Pregnancy*

Nothing should enter the examination room that can be attracted to a magnet. You may or may not receive an injection of a contrast agent to improve the diagnostic capability of the examination. This agent is injected into one of your veins. Most patients experience no unusual effects from this injection.

Your radiologist will be happy to answer any specific questions you may have about the procedure, either before or at the time of the study.

At this time, please empty all of your pockets and remove your watch, earrings, necklaces, chains, and anything in your hair which contains metal. You may be asked to change into a hospital gown.

Your name:_____   Your weight:_____

Fig. 25-40

Sample Patient Information Form
(Courtesy of University of Iowa Hospitals and Clinics)

---

[1] Heiken, Jay P.; Brown, Jeffery J.; **Manual of Clinical Magnetic Resonance Imaging**, 2nd Ed.; Raven Press; 1991.

Patient History continued

Contraindications

There are certain absolute contraindications to patient MR scanning as shown in *Fig. 25-41*. Although not an absolute contraindication, pregnancy is also often considered a contraindication. When an MRI examination is indicated with pregnancy, an informed consent should be obtained and clinically documented.

Patient Preparation

Each person involved in patient scheduling and preparation plays a key role in a successful MR exam. A brief form or brochure explaining the exam may be given when the appointment is scheduled *(Fig. 25-42)*. Gaining the patient's confidence is a major concern because the more relaxed and comfortable the patient is, the more likely a successful exam. Sufficient time must be allowed to inquire about the patient's history, explain the exam in detail, removing all metal and assuring that the patient is comfortable. Information to be included when preparing a patient for an MR scan may include explanations of the following:

1. A description about the MR scanner.
2. The importance of lying still.
3. The knocking sound they will hear.
4. The length of time a sequence will last.
5. The two-way communication system and the monitoring that will take place.
6. The lack of ionizing radiation.
7. The importance of removing all metal.

Certain pulse sequences generate a high volume knocking noise that is associated with the gradient usage. The patient must be informed of this and ear protection may be required during these sequences.

Relieving Patient Anxiety

The aperture or bore of the magnet (gantry) into which the patient is positioned on the scanning couch or table for MR imaging is shown in *Fig. 25-43*. This may be a rather narrow and confining space and some patients with claustrophobic tendencies may become anxious or even alarmed by this. There is some controversy over whether to tell the patient they may experience claustrophobia but in general it is considered better to not mention the potential for claustrophobia. The MR technologist however, must be prepared if the patient mentions claustrophobia, in which case, steps can be taken to ensure the patient has as little anxiety as possible. Claustrophobia may occur quite spontaneously once the patient is in the magnet. The following options may be used to reduce anxiety and gain a successful examination:

(1) Music and relaxation techniques. Have the patient close his/her eyes and think of something pleasant.
(2) Move the patient slowly into the magnet.
(3) Allow a family member in the room during the exam. The family member can hold the patient's foot or hand reminding the patient that the scanner is open on both ends.

In some situations sedation may be required. The type of sedation and contraindications vary depending on department routines. The patient must be closely monitored if sedated and must not be allowed to travel home alone following sedation.

Summary

The major concerns in preparing a patient for an MRI examination are:

(1) Screening for contraindications
(2) Explaining the exam, (reducing patient anxiety and fear)
(3) Removing all metal
(4) Assuring patient comfort

[1]Shellock, F.G.; Crues JV; Safety Consideration in Magnetic Resonance Imaging; MRI Decisions; 2:25;1988.

Absolute Contraindications to MRI [1]
- Pacemakers
- Ferromagnetic aneurysm clips
- Metallic fragments in the eye
- Cochlear implants
- Starr-Edwards pre-6000 model prosthetic heart valve
- Internal drug infusion pumps
- Neurostimulators
- Bone-growth stimulators

Absolute Contraindications   Fig. 25-41

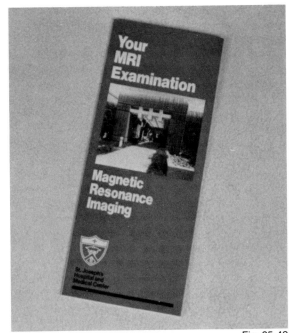

Patient Information Brochure   Fig. 25-42
(Courtesy of St. Joseph's Hospital and Medical Center)

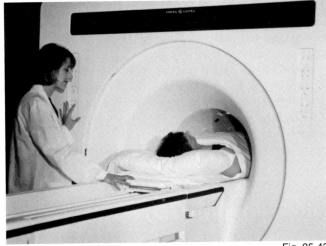

Relieving Patient Anxiety   Fig. 25-43
(Claustrophobia may occur)
(Courtesy of University of Iowa Hospitals and Clinics)

Patient Monitoring

Monitoring of the patient may require frequent reassurance during the scan or during the breaks between pulse sequences. If reassurance is given during the examination the patient must be reminded to not move or talk during data acquisition.

Monitoring of the sedated patient is difficult due to the length of the bore of the magnet. The key concerns are whether the patient is breathing and whether they have enough oxygen. Observing respirations is generally sufficient to ensure breathing but a pulse oximeter may be used to ascertain whether there is adequate exchange of 0_2 and $C0_2$. Magnetic field and RF interference can cause problems in the operation of such monitoring equipment and therefore, present some limitations.[1]

Contrast Agents

Contrast agents have become increasingly popular for MR examinations. The contrast agent that is most popular is **Gadolinium-DTPA (Gd-DTPA).**[2] It is currently given in a dose of .2 ml/kg with the injection rate not to exceed 10 ml/min. The injection may be followed by a saline flush. The patient may experience a sensation at the injection site and should be observed during and after the injection for possible reaction. Gd-DTPA has lower toxicity and has fewer side effects than iodinated contrast.

After injection , a sufficient level of contrast remains in the system for approximately 60 minutes which allows a great deal of latitude in scan time. The major route of excretion is through the kidneys, therefore renal failure would be a contraindication for its use. Pregnancy may also be a contraindication for the use of Gd-DTPA.

Gd-DTPA is considered a **paramagnetic agent** and **shortens the Tl and T2 relaxation time of water protons.** Overall Gd-DTPA quickens the rate at which water protons align with the main magnetic field. This results in greater MR signal and higher contrast, especially in areas where gadolinium crosses the blood brain barrier (BBB). (The blood brain barrier is the selective barrier separating the blood from the parenchyma of the central nervous system.) The contrast agent remains confined intravascularly for a period of time unless the BBB has been damaged by pathologic processes. Gd-DTPA is generally used with Tl-weighted pulse sequences.

Gd-DTPA improves visualization of small tumors and tumors of isointensity with normal brain. The most frequent use of Gd-DTPA is in evaluation of the central nervous system. Gd-DTPA is useful for evaluation of **meningionas**, **acoustic neuroma**, **Schwannomas**, **chordomas** and **pituitary tumors.** (See end of chapter for definitions.).

This contrast media often helps identify primary disease (tumor) from secondary effects (edema). Further, it helps in the evaluation of metastasis, infection, inflammatory processes and subacute cerebral infarcts. In the spine, Gd-DTPA increases sensitivity in detecting primary and secondary tumors and can help differentiate scarring from recurrent disc disease in the postoperative spine.

Contrast use may become increasingly important in abdominal, thoracic and limb (extremity) imaging. At the present time, Gd-DTPA has been FDA approved for evaluation of the brain and CNS. It is likely that approval will also be granted for evaluation of other areas of the body besides the CNS in the future. Oral contrast agents are still under investigation but have been used with limited success in research trials.

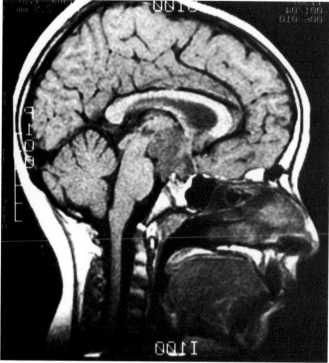

Fig. 25-44

Without Contrast Agent (T1-Weighted Image)
(Pathology appears gray)

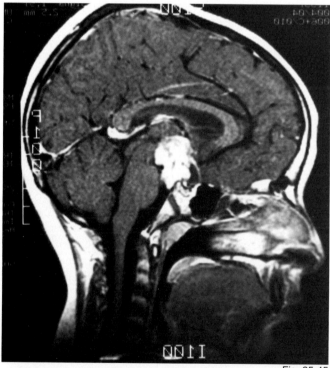

Fig. 25-45

With Contrast Agent, Gd-DTPA (T1-Weighted Image)
(Pathology appears as "bright" areas in central brain)

---

[1] Runge, Val, **Clinical Magnetic Resonance Imaging**; JB Lippincott Co. 1990; pp 506-507.

[2] **Gadolinium** (gad"o-lin'e-um) - a rare element which is metallic and very magnetic; symbol, Gd- DTPA (Diethylene-Triaminepentaacetic Acid).

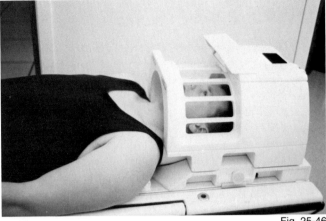

Head Coil in Place   Fig. 25-46

Positioning Considerations and Coil Selection

The patient lies in the bore of the magnet in the supine, prone, oblique or decubitus position. In most situations, the patient is supine with the anatomy of interest centered to the RF coil. The distinction between types of RF coils varies between manufacturers, but one way of classifying these coils is to divide them into two categories: (1) **circumferential whole-volume coils**, and (2) **surface coils**.[1]

Care must be taken when placing the coils. For safety reasons, the coil must be connected properly and the lines not looped as they extend from the magnet. This reduces the chance of electric "arcing" of sparks that may burn the patient.

Attention must be given to the orientation of the surface coil relative to the transmit coil. No signal will be detected unless the receiving coil **is perpendicular to the magnetic field established by the transmitter coil**. A slight tilt can result in significant loss of signal. For a superconductive system, the coil can be placed coronal or sagittal to the main magnetic field.

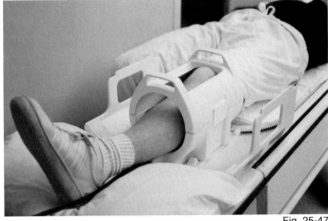

Knee Coil in Place   Fig. 25-47

(1) Circumferential Whole-volume

Three of the more common circumferential whole-volume coils which surround the part being imaged are the **body coil**, the **head coil**, the **limb** (extremity or knee) **coil** and the **volume neck coil**.

The performance of an RF coil is largely determined by its filling factor, which reflects the ratio of the total coil volume to the volume of the anatomic region within the coil.

S/N ratio is enhanced by selecting a coil that most closely approximates the size of the anatomic region being studied. Therefore, smaller surface coils are sometimes chosen over the whole-volume coils for small volume imaging.[2]

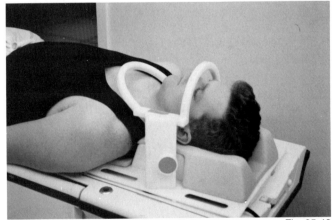

Volume Neck Coil in Place   Fig. 25-48

(2) Surface Coils

Surface coils are placed directly on the body part being imaged. The greatest SNR (signal-noise-ratio) is obtained near the surface of the structure to which the coil is applied, with a fall-off in signal occurring with increasing distance from the coil.[3] The anatomy of interest should be centered to the middle of the coil and the coil must be kept still during data acquisition. The main advantage of surface coils is the increase in SNR. The main disadvantage is the limited field of view.

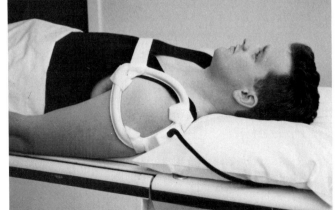

Shoulder Coil in Place (Surface Coil)   Fig. 25-49

[1,2,3] Heiken, Jay P.; Brown, Jeffery J.; **Manual of Clinical Magnetic Resonance Imaging**, 2nd Ed.; Raven Press; 1991.

Imaging Parameters

The MR imaging system employs many technical factors which must be considered, understood and sometimes modified at the control panel during the course of the examination. Many scanners allow these factors to be programmed into a protocol similar to CT protocol's programming. Pulse sequence parameters are designed to suppress artifacts and optimize the diagnostic quality of the specific anatomy and pathology.

The process of choosing parameters involves considerably more than selection of TR and TE. The initial decision also involves the **type of pulse sequence** to be used such as spin-echo, gradient echo or inversion recovery. Besides the type of pulse sequence, the other operator dependent choices include **matrix size, slice thickness, interslice gap, field of view, number of data acquisitions, RF flip angle, coil selection, single or multiple slice acquisition, multislice position** and **multislice excitation order**. These factors allow the examination to be tailored for a particular area of interest and abnormality. Many of these factors are interrelated individually as well as collectively. These relationships have an impact on the S/N ratio, contrast, spatial resolution and artifact production. These factors affect imaging time which in turn affects patient cooperation and management of scheduling.[1]

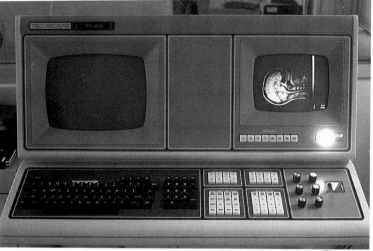

Control Panel and Display Station   Fig. 25-50

Subject Contrast

The contrast in MR arises from the relationship of operator-dependent options previously discussed and tissue factors including proton density, Tl and T2 relaxation times and tissue motion such as flow of CSF and blood. These tissue factors depend on the biochemistry of the tissue. By choosing certain pulse sequences, images can be produced that emphasize these tissue factors and allow visualization of the contrast seen in MR images.

Proton Density (Spin -Density) Images

A pulse sequence using a combination of long TR and short TE (TR 2000 ms and TE 20-30 ms) produces images with contrast resulting from the **proton density**, (sometimes referred to as spin density) with the contrast effects due to Tl and T2 relaxation having been decreased. Since Tl and T2 have been suppressed, pathology which can be demonstrated by the change in Tl and T2 relaxation times may be invisible on an image produced in this manner. The use of pulse sequences with varying amounts of Tl and T2 weighting help to identify anatomy and pathology.

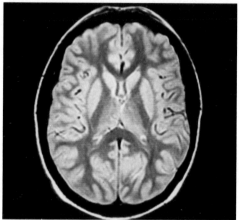

Proton Density Image   Fig.25-51

T1-Weighted Images

In order to maximize the difference in signal intensity based on Tl relaxation times, the TR in the pulse sequence is shortened. **A short TR, short TE sequence produces a Tl-weighted image** (TR 350-800 ms and TE of 30 ms or less). This allows structures with short T1 relaxation times to be bright (fat, proteinogenous fluids, subacute blood) and structures with long Tl to be dark (neoplasm, edema, inflammation, pure fluid, CSF). One aspect to remember with Tl-weighted imaging is that as the TR is shortened, the overall signal to noise decreases.

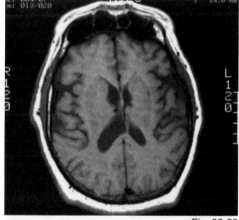

T1-Weighted Image   Fig. 25-52

T2-Weighted Images

T2-weighted imaging employs a long TR and long TE pulse sequence (TR 2000 ms and TE 60-80 ms). As the TE is lengthened the T2 contrast increases however, the overall signal to noise decreases. The structures on a T2-weighted image will show contrast reversal from the structures on the Tl-weighted image.

Structures with long T2 appear bright (neoplasm, edema, inflammation, pure fluid, CSF). Structures with short T2 appear dark (structures with iron such as blood breakdown products).

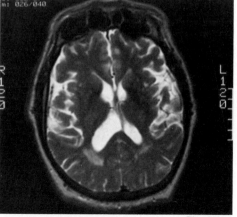

T2-Weighted Image   Fig. 25-53

[1] Brant-Zawadeki, Michael; Norman, David; **Magnetic Resonance Imaging of the Central Nervous System**; Raven Press; 1987; p43.

Imaging Parameters continued

Tissue	Proton Density	T1 (msec)	T2 (msec)
CSF	10.8	2000	250
Gray matter	10.5	475	118
White matter	11.0	300	133
Fat	10.9	150	150
Muscle	11.0	450	64
Liver	10.0	250	44

Fig. 25-54

Comparison of Representative Proton Density, T1 and T2 Values for Various Tissue Types at Midfield Strength [1]

Summary of T1 and T 2-Weighted Images

Although T1 and T2 relaxation occur simultaneously, they are independent of each other. The T1 of most biological tissue is in the range of 200 to 2000 msec. The T2 relaxation in most tissues fall in the 20 to 300 msec range, although water has a T2 in the range of 2000 msec. (See *Fig. 25-54*.)

Notice that the T1 is greater than or equal to the T2 relaxation times for any given tissue. The pulse sequences are generally chosen to accentuate the difference between the relaxation times of different tissues. Contrast between tissues is achieved in the final MR image by accentuating these differences. However, regardless of how the pulse sequence is changed, if there are few mobile hydrogen protons (as is the case for cortical bone and air), the image will be black.

Motion Reduction Techniques

MRI software techniques can reduce or eliminate problems related to involuntary motion and flow, or in some cases like MR angiography, enhance anatomy where flow is present. When motion causes problems that result in signal alterations, these signal alterations are referred to as **motion artifacts**.

Software methods which compensate for artifacts related to motion and flow are available, however, they usually require a tradeoff of longer imaging times. These techniques include **signal averaging**, **reordered phase encoding**, **gradient movement nulling** and **presaturation**. (See definition of terms at end of chapter.) These techniques may be used individually or in combination.

The other technique used to reduce problems related to motion is **physiologic gating.** One type, **respiratory gating,** employs bellows placed around the patient's chest. These are used either to trigger data acquisition by the patient's respirations, or only to accept data acquired during a certain phase of the respiratory cycle. Pulsatile arterial flow (motion related to cardiac movement) and CSF pulsations can be reduced by synchronizing the MR sequence with the cardiac cycle. This is called **cardiac gating**.

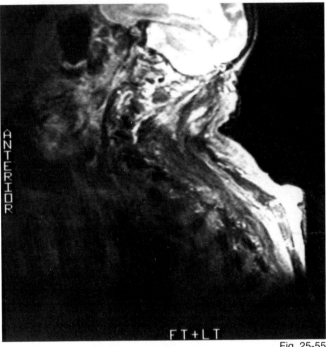

Fig. 25-55

MRI Image with Motion Artifacts
(Sagittal C spine, image quality severely degraded due to patient movement during data acquisition)

Rapid Imaging Techniques

Most MR imaging utilizes a multiacquisition spin echo technique, but rapid imaging techniques are continuing to develop. Currently the most widely used rapid imaging technique is gradient echo imaging (GE), also referred to as gradient recalled echo (GRE) imaging. This technique uses a single RF excitation pulse (10°-90°) and the echo is produced by reversal of the magnetic field gradient rather than a 180° RF pulse used in conventional spin echo imaging. This technique allows variations in the pulse sequence and can be manipulated to achieve T1, T2, and proton density weighting. Other methods for rapid image acquisition such as rapid spin echo technique, are currently being researched.

The major advantages of rapid imaging techniques are rapid acquisition time, reduced SAR, and motion artifact. These sequences allow acquisition of data during breathholding. The use of rapid imaging techniques is likely to continue to increase as techniques are further developed. The main disadvantages are low S/N ratio and an increase in other types of artifacts (besides motion artifact).

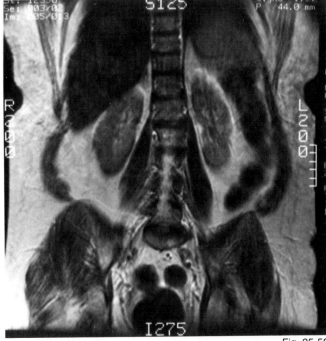

Fig. 25-56

Rapid Imaging Techniques
(Coronal section of abdomen using rapid data acquisition technique)

[1] Lufkin, Robert B.; **The MRI Manual**; Year Book Medical Publishers, Inc.; 1990; p 24.

Part IV MRI Examinations

The more common MRI examinations and guidelines for imaging will be described and discussed. There is an increasing number of software choices which are selected depending upon the patient and pathologic considerations. Both T1 and T2-weighted images are acquired, allowing for a complete examination and diagnosis. The main goal is **good quality images in an acceptable time limit**. When choosing software options, attention is given so that the scan time, resolution, S/N, and number of slices are within acceptable limits.

In all examinations, careful attention to patient comfort and to the positioning of the part with the magnet is of utmost importance.

The high cost of MR equipment requires that constant attention is given to efficient scheduling of patient exams. By choosing parameters carefully, positioning the patient accurately and maintaining patient comfort, the goal of good quality images within the scheduled time limit, usually one hour or less, can be achieved.

Brain Imaging
Routine Sections
• Sagittal
• Coronal
• Axial

Spine Imaging
Routine Sections
• Sagittal
• Axial

Limb & Joint Imaging
Routine Sections
• Sagittal
• Coronal
• Axial

Cardiovascular System Imaging
Routine Sections
• Sagittal
• Coronal
• Axial
• Obliques

Abdomen and Pelvis Imaging
Routine Sections
• Sagittal
• Coronal
• Axial

Angiography
• Time of Flight Method
• Phase Contrast Method
  - 2 D Images
  - 3 D Images

• Brain Imaging

Brain Imaging
Routine Sections
• Sagittal
• Coronal
• Axial

Structures Best Shown:
Gray matter, white matter, nerve tissue, basal ganglia, ventricles, brain stem.

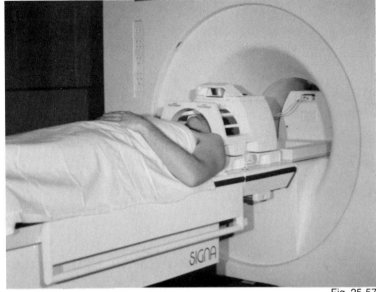

Fig. 25-57
Patient Positioned in Head Coil
(Patient and coil will be moved into magnet center.)

Pathology Demonstrated:
White matter disease, especially multiple sclerosis and other demyelinating disorders, neoplasm, infectious diseases including those associated with AIDS and herpes, hemorrhagic disorders, CVA and ischemic disorders

Contrast Agent:
• Gd-DTPA with T1-weighted images. Gd-DTPA has been proven to aid in the diagnosis for a large number of different brain abnormalities.

Technical Factors:
• Standard head coil
• Surface coils are used for smaller anatomical regions such as for an orbit or TMJ study.
• T 1-weighted sequence
• T 2-weighted sequence

Part Position:
• Patient supine, head first.
• Head rests comfortably in head coil.
• Head and coil centered to the main magnet.

T1-Weighted Images:
T1-weighted images are used to demonstrate anatomic structure. Gd-DTPA T1-weighted studies are best utilized to improve detection, and to characterize lesions identified on T1 and T2-weighted images.

T2-Weighted Images:
T2-weighted images are effective in demonstrating pathology and the edema which is associated with the abnormality. Conditions demonstrated on T2-weighted image include infarction, trauma, inflammation, degeneration, neoplasm and bleeding.

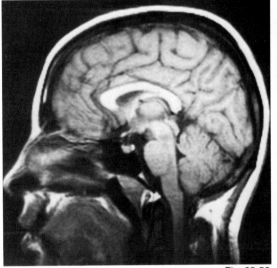

Fig. 25-58
Sagittal Section (T1)

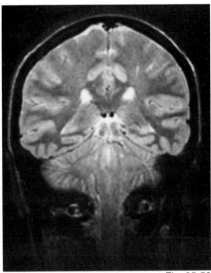

Fig. 25-59
Coronal Section (T2)

Comparisons with CT:
MRI has proven to have superior soft tissue contrast resolution, multi-planar imaging capabilities and no ionizing radiation as compared to CT. MRI is superior to CT in imaging of the posterior fossa and brainstem due to the lack of bone artifact, and in detecting small changes in tissue water content.

In cases where small calcifications are important to identify, CT is chosen over MRI because MRI is generally insensitive to small calcification. CT and conventional radiographs have remained the study of choice for brain imaging to diagnose fractures of the calvarium. The very ill patient with monitoring and life support equipment is often imaged in CT as is the trauma patient. This is due to the faster exam time, tolerance to patient motion, ability to monitor the patient adequately, the ability to show acute blood and fractures and the physical components of life support equipment.

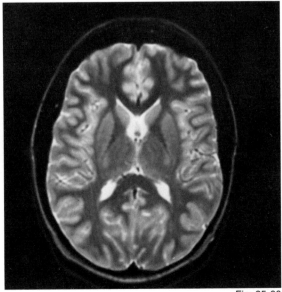

Fig. 25-60
Axial Section (T2)

• Spine Imaging

Spine Imaging
Routine Sections
• Sagittal
• Axial

Structures Best Shown:
Spinal cord, nerve tissue, intervertebral disks, marrow, facet joint spaces, basivertebral vein, ligamentus flavum.

Pathology Demonstrated:
Disc herniation and degeneration, bone and bone marrow changes, neoplasm, inflammatory and demyelinating disease, and congenital and developmental abnormalities.

Contrast Agent:
• Gd-DTPA with T1-weighted.
• These images are acquired through the abnormal area. Gd-DTPA enhances tumors and is useful postoperatively to help differentiate scarring from recurrent disc disease.

Technical Factors:
• C Spine: Planar, contour or quadrature surface coil
• T/L spine: Planar surface coil (see arrows).
• T1-weighted sequence
• T2-weighted sequence
• Cardiac gating (when myelopathy is suspected)

Part Position:
• Patient supine, head first for C spine, head or feet first for T spine and feet first for L spine.
• Anatomy of interest centered to the surface coil.
• Surface coil and patient centered to the main magnet.

T1-Weighted Images:
T1-weighted images are useful to show anatomic details such as nerve roots outlined by fat, information requiring discs, vertebra, facet joints and adaquacy of intervertebral foramina. Also useful in evaluation of cysts, syrinx, and lipomas.

T2-Weighted Images:
T2-weighted images are required in the evaluation of disc disease, cord abnormalities, tumor, and inflammatory changes. Gradient Echo (GE) or spin-echo images utilizing T2-weighting produce a myelographic effect showing sharp contrast between cord and CSF.

Comparison with CT: The major advantage of MR over CT includes the facts that it does not require the use of intrathecal (within a sheath) contrast material to evaluate the spinal cord and subarachnoid space, and it covers large areas of the spine in a single sagittal view. CT remains essential for evaluation of significant spinal trauma.

Even though the need for myelography has decreased, it is still useful in selected cases. Myelography combined with CT is useful when patient motion or severe scoliosis renders MR suboptimal.

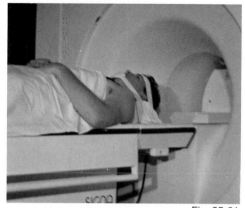

Fig. 25-61

Cervical Spine
(Posterior C spine coil in place, will be moved to magnet center)

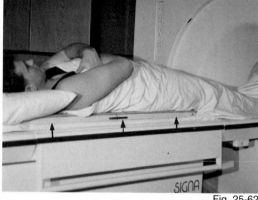

Fig. 25-62

Lumbar Spine
(Planar surface coil under patient, will be moved to magnet center)

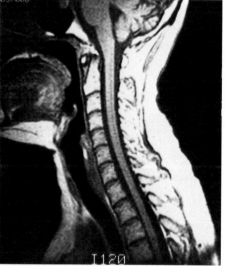

Fig. 25-63

C Spine, Sagittal Section (T1)

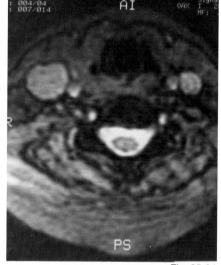

Fig. 25-64

C Spine, Axial Section (T1)

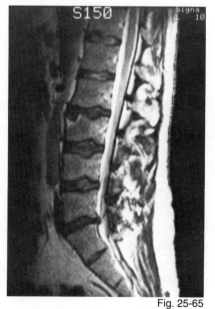

Fig. 25-65

L Spine, Sagittal Section (T2)

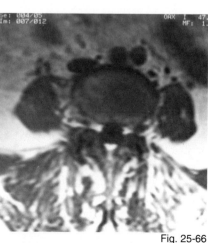

Fig. 25-66

L Spine, Axial Section (T1)

• Limb or Joint Imaging

<table>
<tr><td>

Limb or Joint Imaging
Routine Sections
• Sagittal
• Coronal
• Axial

</td></tr>
</table>

Structures Best Shown:

Fat, muscles, ligaments, tendons, nerves, blood vessels, marrow.

Pathology Demonstrated:

Bone marrow disorders, soft tissue tumors, osteonecrosis, ligament and tendon tears.

Technical Factors:

• Limb (extremity) coils
• T1-weighted sequence
• T2-weighted sequence
• If the region of interest is fairly deep, then a coil that surrounds the object is chosen. If the structure is superficial, then a coil that lies on top of the anatomy is chosen.

Part Position:

• Head or feet first. *(Fig. 25-67 and 68).*
• Supine or prone as most comfortable.
• Anatomy of interest centered to the coil.
• Coil centered to main magnet.

T1-Weighted Images:

T1-weighted images are useful for showing anatomic detail and for evaluating articular cartilage, ligaments and tendons. T1-weighted images are also useful in depicting osteonecrosis.

T2-Weighted Images:

T2-weighted images are useful to show tumors, inflammatory changes and the edema surrounding ligament and tendon tears. T2-weighted images are also useful for bone marrow disorders, bony tumors and to show the extent of lesions in muscles.

NOTE: MR is an increasingly effective imaging method for the musculoskeletal system. MRI is a primary method of evaluating internal derangements of the knee, meniscal abnormalities in the TMJ, avascular necrosis, soft tissue masses and bone marrow abnormalities.[1] Evaluation of shoulder disorders with MRI has proved useful.

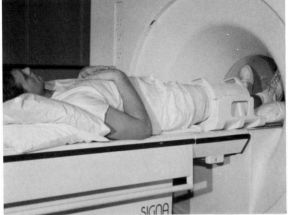

Fig. 25-67
Knee Coil Placement

Fig. 25-68
Shoulder Coil Placement
(Patient with coil in place will be moved to magnet center)

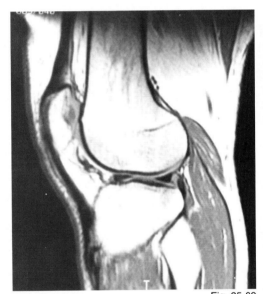

Fig. 25-69
Knee, Sagittal Section (Proton Density)

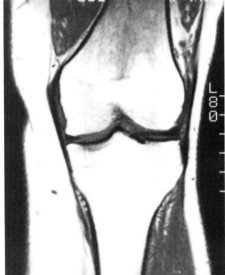

Fig. 25-70
Knee, Coronal Section (T1)

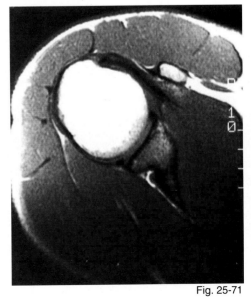

Fig. 25-71
Transaxial Shoulder (T1)

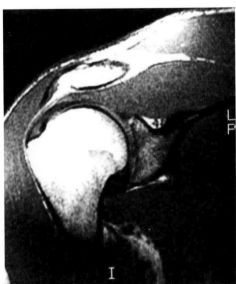

Fig. 25-72
Coronal Shoulder (T1)

[1] Runge, Val M.; **Clinical Magnetic Resonance Imaging**; J.B.Lippincott Co.; 1990; p 403.

• Cardiovascular System Imaging

> **Cardiovascular system Imaging**
> Routine Sections
> • Sagittal
> • Coronal
> • Axial
> • Oblique

Structures Best Shown:
Great vessels, fat, myocardium, skeletal muscles, static and moving blood, valves, pericardium, coronary arteries.

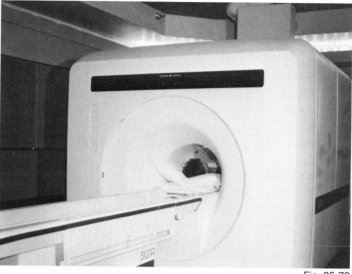

Fig. 25-73
Patient Positioned for Cardiovascular MRI

Pathology Demonstrated:
Congenital heart disorders, graft patency, cardiac tumors, thrombi, pericardial masses, evaluation of aortic dissection and aneurysm.

Technical Factors:
• Body coil
• T1-weighted sequence
• T2-weighted sequence (as needed)
• Cine (as needed)
• Gating (respiratory and cardiac)

Part Position:
• Supine (or prone) feet first.
• Nipple level at magnet center.

T1-Weighted Images:
T1-weighted images are useful for showing anatomic detail of the heart, great vessels and pericardium. Patent coronary artery bypass grafts, and thrombus are demonstrated with T1-weighted images.

T2-Weighted Images:
T2-weighted images are useful for detection of infarction, thrombus and pericardial effusions.

Cine:
Cine images allow evaluation of muscle thinning, previous infarction, wall motion and valve abnormalities. Volume measurements can be taken.

Gating:
The most widely used gating mechanism is the electrocardiogram. The heart's electrical activity bears a constant relationship to its mechanical activity. The R wave is often used to synchronize the MR sequence with the cardiac cycle. The recording of EKG is difficult due to the static and changing magnetic fields. The electrodes are placed to maximize the amplitude of the R wave. Special electrodes containing non-ferrous metals are used.

NOTE: MRI is unlikely to replace echo cardiography but can provide a 3D view of tumors and masses, especially as to the extent of growth. MRI used as an adjunct to CT, has proven helpful in assessing mediastinal pathology and in the evaluation of aortic dissection and aneurysm. Radiographs of the thorax will continue to be used as a first tool of assessment.

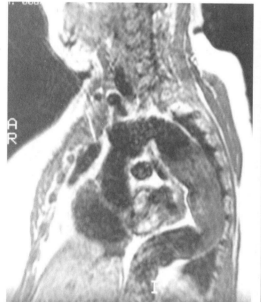

Fig. 25-74
Sagittal Section (T1)
(Demonstrates an aortic aneurysm)

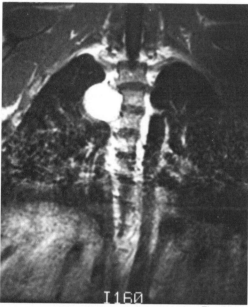

Fig. 25-75
Coronal Section (T1 with GD)
(Aorta shown posterior to heart, paraspinal mass demonstrated)

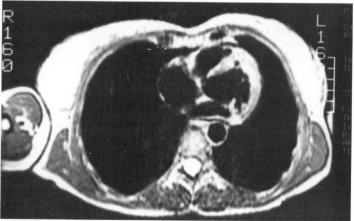

Fig. 25-76
Axial Section (T2)

Note: The above sections are not on the same patient.

• Abdomen and Pelvis Imaging

Abdomen & Pelvis Imaging
Routine Sections
• Sagittal
• Coronal
• Axial

Structures Best Shown:
Liver, pancreas, spleen, adrenals, gallbladder, kidney, vessels, reproduction organs.

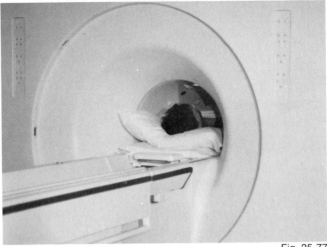

Patient positioned for abdominal MRI
Fig. 25-77

Pathology Demonstrated:
Tumor size and staging of tumors especially pediatric tumors such as neuroblastoma, and Wilm's tumor. Retroperitoneal structures and hemangioma of the liver are well demonstrated by MRI.

Pre-Exam Prep:
Patients may be asked to fast or only consume clear liquids 4 hours prior to scanning. Glucagon is often administered to reduce peristalsis of the bowel.

Technical Factors:
• Body Coil
• T1-weighted sequence
• T2-weighted sequence
• Respiratory gating
• Breathholding in upper abdomen
• Generally a standard body coil is utilized however, surface coils may be used for superficial structures. A transrectal coil may be used to image the prostate and reproductive organs.

Part Position:
• Supine, feet first for abdomen and pelvis.
• Area of interest centered to main magnet.

T1-Weighted Images:
T1-weighted images are useful for demonstrating anatomic detail. T1-weighted images also help identify tumors containing fat and hemorrhage.

T2-Weighted Images:
T2-weighted images are useful to demonstrate changes in water content in the tissue associated with tumors and other abnormalities.

Note: MRI evaluation of the abdomen has been limited due to artifacts caused by respiratory, cardiac and peristaltic motion. An acceptable oral contrast material remains a limitation in abdominal MRI. CT is still the primary method for evaluation of the liver due to motion artifacts. Ultrasound and CT will likely remain the imaging modality for renal cysts. MRI has proved useful in the evaluation of renal transplants.

Pelvic anatomy is well demonstrated by MRI. Ultrasound remains the screening tool for uterine, ovarian and scrotal abnormalities.

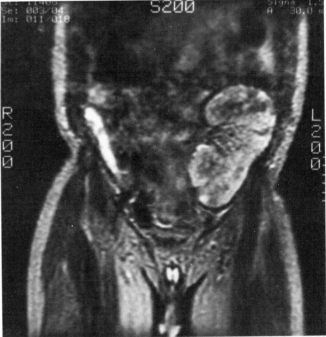

Coronal Section (T2)
(Post kidney transplant on left)
Fig. 25-78

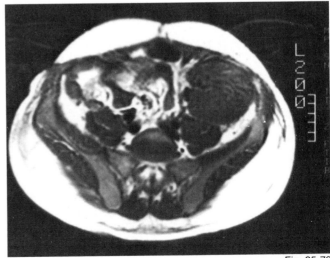

Axial Section (T1)
(Transplanted kidney on left)
Fig. 25-79

• Angiography

Pathology Demonstrated:

Aneurysm, AVM, stenotic disease, and graft patency detection.

Angiography

MR angiography is an imaging method that exploits the physical properties of blood to generate contrast and thus allows visualization of blood vessels. These physical properties include **blood velocity, pulsation of blood, turbulent flow** or **lack of turbulent flow** and **relaxation times**. The operator-dependent choices are complex and require an understanding of hemodynamics and software options which are supplied by the manufacturer.

In general, the imaging strategies can be broken down into two fundamental approaches. They are **Time-of-Flight** (TOF) and **Phase Contrast** angiography. Further, the information can be obtained as a series of 2D images or as a 3D data set.

Time-of-Flight (TOF)

TOF angiography generally relies on the inflow of fully magnetized blood into the imaging plane. This process is described as **flow-related enhancement**. Blood that flows into the slice will not have experienced RF pulses and will therefore, appear brighter than stationary tissue. This allows the moving and stationary spins to be distinguished and thus create MR angiograms.[1]

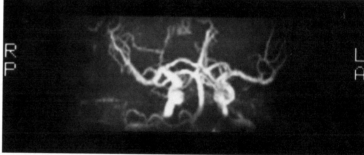

3D Time of Flight   Fig. 25-80

Phase Contrast

The phase contrast technique utilizes alterations in spin phase for image contrast. This imaging technique relies on velocity-induced phase shifts to distinguish flowing blood from stationary tissues. Two or more acquisitions with opposite polarity of the bipolar flow-encoding gradients are subtracted to produce an image of the vessels.[2]

2D Images

In general the 2D acquisition method will be used to image medium to slow flow areas and straight vessels. Specific applications include carotid arteries, basilar and vertebral arteries, and limbs.

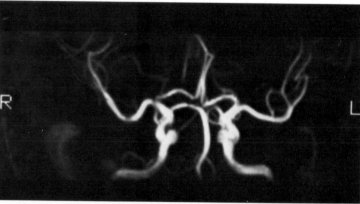

3D Phase Contrast   Fig. 25-81

3D Images

3D acquisition methods may best be used where flow is faster, especially through tortuous vessels. Both methods allow the images to be obtained in a sequential fashion, and post processing allows the images to be viewed from a variety of angles. This allows vessels to rotate around an axis and can then be viewed with reduced overlap.

NOTE: MR angiography is likely to become a common procedure in the screening and imaging of a known lesion. The biggest drawbacks include motion artifact and the turbulent flow which may give a false impression of a defect. Improvements in imaging techniques however, will continue to reduce these drawbacks.

[1,2.] GE Medical Systems, **Signal Applications Guide: Vascular Magnetic Resonance Imaging,** Vol.3, pp 46,48, Aug.1990

Definition of Terms

Pathological Terms

(Dorland's Illustrated Medical Dictionary, 27th ed)

Acoustic Neuroma *(nu-ro´mah)*: A tumor growing from nerve cells and nerve fibers involving the sense of hearing.

Chordoma *(kor-do´mah)*: A malignant tumor arising from the embryonic remains of the notochord (the rod-shaped body defining the primary axis of the embryonic body).

Meningioma *(me-nin-je-o´mah)*: A hard, slow growing vascular tumor occuring primarily along the meningeal vessels and superior longitudinal sinus invading the dura and skull causing erosion and thinning of the skull.

Osteonecrosis *(os˝te-o-ne-kro´sis)*: A death or necrosis of bone.

Pituitary Tumors: Tumors involving the pituitary gland.

Schwannoma *(shwon-no´mah)*: A new growth of the white substance of Schwann (nerve sheath).

Terms Related to MRI

Artifacts: False features of an image caused by patient instability or equipment deficiencies.[1]

Averaging (signal averaging): A SNR-enhancing technique in which the same MR signal is repeatedly acquired two or more times and then combined and averaged.[2]

Bipolar flow-encoding gradients: Gradients whose polarity is inverted in order to encode velocities as changes of phase–a technique used in phase contrast angiography.[2]

Cine: In magnetic resonance imaging, acquisition of multiple images at different times in a cycle, e.g. the cardiac cycle and subsequent sequential display of the images in a manner that simulates motion.[2]

Coil: Single or multiple loops of wire designed either to produce a magnetic field from current flowing through the wire or to detect a changing magnetic field by voltage induced in the wire.[1]

Contrast resolution: Ability of an imaging process to distinguish adjacent soft tissues from one another. This is the principal advantage of MRI.[1]

Cryogen: Atmospheric gases such as nitrogen and helium that have been cooled sufficiently to condense into a liquid.[1]

Field of view (FOV): The area (usually expressed in cm) of the anatomy being imaged; a function of acquisition matrix times pixel size.[2]

Filling factor: Measure of the geometric relationship of the RF coil and the body. It affects the efficiency of irradiating the body and detecting MRI signals, thereby affecting the signal-to-noise ratio. Achieving a high filling factor requires fitting the coil closely to the body.[1]

Flip angle: Amount of rotation of the net magnetization vector produced by an RF pulse, with respect to the direction of the static magnetic field B_o.[1]

Flow-related enhancement: A process by which the signal intensity of moving tissues, like blood, can be increased compared with the signal of stationary tissue. Occurs when unsaturated, fully magnetized spins replace saturated spins between RF pulses.[2]

Fourier transform (FT): Mathematical procedure to separate the frequency components of a signal from its amplitudes as a function of time. The Fourier transform is used to generate the spectrum from the FID and is essential to most imaging techniques.[1]

FOV: See field of view.

Free induction decay (FID): If transverse magnetization (Mxy) of the spins is produced, a transient NMR signal will result that will decay with a characteristic time constant T2. This decaying signal is the FID.[1]

Fringe field: Stray magnetic field that exists outside the imager.[1]

Gating: An MR technique, used to minimize motion artifacts, in which conventional electrocardiography or photopulse sensing is used to trigger the acquisition of image data. It times data acquisition to physiological motion.[2]

Gauss (G): Unit of magnetic flux density in the older CGS system. The currently preferred (SI) unit is the Tesla (T) (IT = 10,000 G).[1]

Gradient coils: Current-carrying coils designed to produce a desired gradient magnetic field. Proper design of the size and configuration of the coils is necessary to produce a controlled and uniform gradient.[1]

Gradient-induced magnetic field: A magnetic field that changes in strength in a given direction. These fields are necessary to select a region for imaging (slice selection) and for encoding the location of the MR signal.

Gradient moment nulling: Application of gradients to correct phase errors caused by velocity, acceleration or other motion. First-order gradient nulling is the same as flow compensation.[2]

Gradient pulse: Briefly applied gradient magnetic field.[1]

Inversion recovery (IR): RF pulse sequence for MRI wherein the net magnetization is inverted and returns to equilibrium with the emission of an NMR signal.[1]

Terms Related to MRI continued

Magnetic field gradient: Device for varying the strength of the static magnetic field at different spatial locations. This is used for slice selection and determining the spatial locations of the protons being imaged. Also used for velocity encoding, flow comp, and in place of RF pulses during gradient echo acquisitions to rephase spins. Commonly measured in Gauss per centimeter.[2]

Partial saturation (PS): Excitation technique applying repeated 90° RF pulses at times on the order of or shorter than Tl. Although partial saturation is also commonly referred to as saturation recovery, the latter term should properly be reserved for the particular case of partial saturation when the 90° RF pulses are far enough apart in time that the return of nuclear spins to equilibrium is complete.[1]

Phase contrast (PC) angiography: A 2D or 3D imaging technique that relies on velocity-induced phase shifts to distinguish flowing blood from stationary tissues. Two or more acquisitions with opposite polarity of the bipolar flow-encoding gradients are subtracted to produce an image of the vasculature.[2]

Phase encoding: The act of localizing an MR signal by applying a gradient to alter the phase of spins before signal readout. In reordered PE, the sequence if localizing the signal is altered.[2]

Pixel: Acronym for a picture element; the smallest discrete part of a digital image display.[1]

Precession: Comparatively slow gyration of the axis of a spinning body so as to trace out a cone, caused by the application of a torque tending to change the direction of the rotation axis.[1]

Presaturation: See saturation.[2]

Proton density: See spin density.[1]

Pulse sequences: Set of RF or gradient magnetic field pulses and time spacings between these pulses.[1]

Radio frequency (RF): Electromagnetic radiation just lower in energy than infrared. The RF used in MRI is commonly in the 10- to 100-MHz range.[1]

Radiofrequency (RF) pulse: A burst of RF energy which, if it is at the correct Larmor frequency, will rotate the macroscopic magnetization vector by a specific angle, dependent on the pulse's amplitude and duration.[2]

Receiver coil: Coil of the RF receiver; detects the NMR signal.[1]

Relaxation time: After excitation, the nuclear spins will tend to return to their equilibrium position, in accordance with these time constants.[1]

Rephasing gradient: Gradient magnetic field applied briefly after a selective excitation pulse, in the opposite direction to the gradient used for the selective excitation. The result of the gradient reversal is a rephasing of the spins, forming a spin echo.[1]

RF coil: Used for transmitting RF pulses and or receiving NMR signals.[1]

RF magnetic fields: Electromagnetic radiation just lower in energy than infrared. RF magnetic fields are applied during pulse sequences.

Saturation: Repeated application of radiofrequency pulses in a time that is short compared to the T1 of the tissue, producing incomplete realignment of the net magnetization with the static magnetic field.[2]

Saturation recovery (SR): Particular type of partial saturation pulse sequence in which the preceding pulses leave the spins in a state of saturation so that recovery to equilibrium is complete by the time of the next pulse.[1]

Signal averaging: Method of improving SNR by averaging several FIDs or spin echoes.[1]

Signal-to-noise ratio (SNR or S/N): Used to describe the relative contributions to a detected signal of the true signal and random superimposed signals or noise. The SNR can be improved by averaging several NMR signals, by sampling larger volumes, or by increasing the strength of the B_o magnetic field.[1]

Spin density (SD): Density of resonating nuclear spins in a given region; one of the principal determinants of the strength of the NMR signal from that region.[1]

Spin echo: Reappearance of an NMR signal after the FID has disappeared. The result of the effective reversal of the dephasing of the nuclear spins.[1]

Spin echo imaging: Any one of many MRI techniques in which the spin echo NMR signal rather than the FID is used.[1]

Static magnetic fields: The regions urrounding a magnet. A magnetic field produces a magnetizing force on a body within it.

Tl: Spin lattice or longitudinal relaxation time; the characteristic time constant for spins to tend to align themselves with the external magnetic field.[1]

T2: Spin-spin or transverse relaxation time; the characteristic time constant for loss of phase coherence among spins oriented at an angle to the main magnetic field owing to interactions between the spins. T2 never exceeds T1.[1]

TE echo time: Time between middle of 90° RF pulse and middle of spin echo.

Tesla (T): Preferred (SI) unit of magnetic flux density or magnetic field intensity. One Tesla is equal to 10,000 Gauss, the older (CSG) unit. One Tesla also equals one Newton/amp-m.[1]

Time-of-Flight (TOF) angiography: 2D or 3D imaging technique that relies primarily on flow-related enhancement to distinguish moving from stationary spins in creating MR angiograms. Blood that has flowed into the slice will not have experienced RF pulses and will therefore appear brighter than stationary tissue.[2]

Time-varying magnetic field: (See gradient-induced magnetic field.)

Terms Related to MRI continued

Torque: Force that causes or tends to cause a body to rotate. It is a vector quantity given by the product of the force and the position vector where the force is applied.[1]

TR: Repetition time. The time between successive excitations of a slice—i.e., the time from the beginning of one pulse sequence to the beginning of the next. In conventional imaging, it is a fixed value equal to a user selected value. In cardiac-gated studies, however, it can vary from beat to beat depending on the patient's heart rate.[2]

Turbulence: In a flowing fluid, velocity components that fluctuate randomly, causing spin dephasing and signal loss.[2]

Two-dimensional Fourier transform imaging (2DFT): Form of sequential plane imaging using Fourier transform imaging.[1]

Voxel: Volume element; the element of three-dimensional space corresponding to a pixel for a given slice thickness.[1]

---

[1] Bushong, Stewart C.; **Magnetic Resonance Imaging Physical and Biological Principles**; The C.V. Mosby Company; 1988.
[2] Signa Applications Guide; **Vascular Magnetic Resonance Imaging**; Vol 3; GE Medical Systems; Cat. # E8804DB; 1990.

References

Books:

Berquist, Ehman, Richardson; **Magnetic Resonance of the Musculoskeletal System**; Raven Press; 1987.

Brant-Zawadski, Michael; Norman, David; **Magnetic Resonance Imaging of the CNS**; Raven Press; 1987.

Bushong, Stewart C.; **Magnetic Resonance Imaging Physical and Biological Principles**; C.V. Mosby Co.; 1988.

Heiken, Jay P.; Brown, Jeffrey J.; **Manual of Clinical Magnetic Resonance Imaging**, 2nd Ed.; Raven Press; 1991.

Kaiser, Ramos; **MRI of the Spine: A Guide to Clinical Applications**; Theime Medical Publishers, Inc.; 1990.

Lufkin, Robert B.; **The MRI Manual;** Year Book Medical Publishers, Inc.; 1990.

Maravilla, Cohen; **MRI, Atlas of the Spine**; Raven Press; 1991.

Partain, et al; **Magnetic Resonance Imaging Volume 1 Clinical Principles**, 2nd ed.; W.B. Saunders; 1988.

Runge, Val M.; **Clinical Magnetic Resonance Imaging**; J.B. Lippincott Company;1990.

Stark DD, Bradley WG (Eds); **Magnetic Resonance Imaging**; C.V. Mosby; St. Louis, MO; 1987.

Periodicals:

BNI Quarterly; Barrow Neurological Institute of St. Joseph's Hospital and Medical Center; Phoenix, AZ; Vol. 5:1; Winter; 1989

Brant-Zawadski, M.D., Michael; **MR Imaging of the Brain**; Radiology; Jan 1988; Vol 166; Number 1.

G.E. Medical Systems; **Signa Applications Guide, Vascular Magnetic Resonance Imaging**; Vol. 3 ; Cat. # E8804DB; 1990.

Marqulis, Higgins, Kaufman, Crooks; **Clinical Magnetic Resonance Imaging**; Radiology Research and Education Foundation; San Francisco; 1983.

Shellock, F.G.; Crues, J.V.; **Safety Considerations in Magnetic Resonance Imaging**; MRI Decisions,2:25, 1988.

Shellock, Frank; Emanual, M.D.; **Policies, Guidelines, and Recommendations for MR Imaging Safety and Patient Management**; SMRI Report Journal of Magnetic Resonance Imaging; Vol 1; Number 1; Jan/Feb 1991.

Shellock, Frank; **MR Imaging of Metallic Implants and Materials: A Compilation of the Literature**; AJR; Oct. 1985.

Underwood, Richard,; Firmin, David; **Magnetic Resonance of the Cardiovascular System**; Blackwell Scientific Publications; London; 1991.

Bibliography

Abrams, H., editor. *Angiography*, ed. 2, vol. 1. Boston: Little, Brown and Co., 1971.

Ballinger, Phillip W. *Merrill's Atlas of Radiographic Positions and Radiologic Procedures*, ed. 7, vol. 1, 2, & 3. St. Louis: C. V. Mosby Co., 1991.

Becker, R.; Wilson, J.; Gehweiler, J. *The Anatomical Basis of Medical Practice*, ed. 1, Baltimore: The Williams & Wilkins Co., 1971.

Bushong, Stewart C. *Radiologic Science for Technologists*, ed. 4. St. Louis: C. V. Mosby Co., 1988.

Cahill, D.R; Orland, M.J. *Atlas of Human Cross-Sectional Anatomy*, Philadelphia: Lea & Febiger, 1984.

Christensen, E.; Curry, T.; Dowdey, J. *An Introduction to the Physics of Diagnostic Radiology*, ed. 2. Philadelphia: Lea & Febiger, 1978.

Clark, K. C. *Positioning in Radiography*, ed. 11. London: Ilford Ltd., William Heinemann Medical Books, Ltd., 1986.

Compere, W. *Radiographic Atlas of the Temporal Bone*, Book 1, ed. 1. St. Paul, Minnesota: H.M. Smyth Co., Inc., 1964.

Cullinan, Angeline M. *Optimizing Radiographic Positioning*, Philadelphia: J. B. Lippincott Co., 1992.

Egan, R. *Technologist Guide to Mammography*, ed. 1, Baltimore: The Williams & Wilkins Co., 1968.

Eisenberg, R.L.; Dennis, C.A.; May, C.R. *Radiographic Positioning*, Boston: Little, Brown and Co., 1989.

Etter, L. *Roentgenography and Roentgenology of the Middle Ear and Mastoid Process*, ed. 1. Springfield, Illinois: Charles C. Thomas, Publisher, 1965.

Gerhart, P.; Van Kaich, G. *Total Body Computed Tomography*, ed. 2. Stuttgart: Georg Thieme Publishers, 1979.

Gray, H. *Anatomy of the Human Body*, ed. 30. Philadelphia: Lea & Febiger, 1985.

Hendee, W.R.; Ritenour, E.R. *Medical Imaging Physics*, ed. 3; Chicago: Mosby - Year Book Inc., 1992.

Jacobi, C.; Paris, D. *Textbook of Radiologic Technology*, ed. 5. St. Louis: C. V. Mosby Co., 1972.

Kreel, L.; Steiner, R. *Medical Imaging*, ed. 1. Exeter, Great Britain: A. Wheaton & Co. Ltd., 1979.

Meschan, I. *An Atlas of Anatomy Basic to Radiology*, ed. 1. Philadelphia: Lea & Febiger, 1975.

Meschan, I. *Radiographic Positioning and Related Anatomy*, ed. 2 Philadelphia: W. B. Saunders Co., 1978.

New, P.; Scott, W. *Computed Tomography of the Brain and Orbit*, ed. 1. Baltimore: The Williams & Wilkins Co., 1975.

Norman, D.; Korobkin, M.; Newton, T., eds. *Computed Tomography*, ed. 1. St. Louis: C. V. Mosby Co., 1977.

Quinn, C.B. *Fuchs's Principles of Radiographic Exposure, Processing and Quality Control*; ed. 4. Springfield, Illinois: Charles C. Thomas; 1990.

Ramsey, R. *Advanced Exercises in Diagnostic Radiology, Computed Tomography of the Brain*, ed. 1. Philadelphia: W. B. Saunders Co., 1977.

Statkiewicz, M.A.; Ritenour, E.R. *Radiation Protection for Student Radiographers;* Denver: Multi-Media Publishing; 1983.

Taveras, J.; Wood, E. *Diagnostic Neuroradiology*, ed. 2, vol. 1, Baltimore: The Williams & Wilkins Co., 1976.

Tortora, G. R., Anagnostakos, N.P. *Principles of Anatomy and Physiology*. ed 4. New York: Harper & Row Publishers, 1984.

Valvassori, G. *Radiographic Atlas of the Temporal Bone*, Book 2, ed. 1. St. Paul, Minnesota: H.M. Smyth Co., Inc., 1964.

Woodburne, R.T., Burkel, W.E. *Essentials of Human Anatomy*, ed. 8 New York: Oxford University Press, 1988.

Index

Index

Index

Index

Index

Index

Index

Index

Index

Index

Index

Index

Index

Index

Urethra, 87
  female, 509
  male, 509
  radiographic anatomy of, 504, 508
Urethrography, retrograde, 519
Urinary system, 87, 503-530
  composition and functions of, 4
  contrast media and, 512-513
  cystography for, 529
  cystourethrography for, 529
  excretory urography and, 514-517
  hypertensive intravenous urography and, 517
  intravenous urography for, 523-527
  kidney, ureter, and bladder radiographs for, 511
  metallic bead-chain cystourethrography and, 519
  positioning for, 521-522
  radiographic anatomy of, 504-510
  retrograde cystography and, 518
  retrograde urethrography and, 519
  retrograde urography and, 518, 528
  urography and, 511-512
Urinary tract infection, 514
Urine, production of, 506
Urography
  excretory
    post-void anteroposterior projection for, 526
    procedures for, 514-517
    radiographic anatomy of, 87
  hypertensive intravenous, 517
  intravenous
    anteroposterior projection for, 523
    in child, 553
    hypertensive, 517
    indications and contraindications of, 514-515
    LPO and RPO positions for, 525
    preparation for, 515
    ureteric compression and, 527
    positioning for, 521
    procedures for, 516-517
    retrograde, 518
Urticaria, as reaction to contrast medium, 513
Uvula, 50

V

Valsalva maneuver, 429
Valve
  cardiac, 630
  ileocecal, 84
  pyloric, 417
Variable fulcrum, 573
Varices, esophageal, 427
Vasovagal response, as reaction to contrast medium, 513
Vater's ampulla, 485
Vein
  of breast, 534
  cerebral, 634-635
  coronary, 640
  definition of, 629
  of lower limb, 639
  portal, 638

Vein—cont'd
  pulmonary, 57, 630
  rib and, 299
  of upper limb, 639
Vena cava, 630
  in abdominal cross section, 86
Venogram, subtraction, 656
Venography
  epidural, 679
  of lower limb, 665
Venous sinus, 581
Ventral decubitus position, definition of, 20
Ventral surface, definition of, 15
Ventricle
  cardiac, 630, 640
  cerebral, 582-584
Vermiform process, 448
Vermis, 586
Vertebra; *see also* Spine
  cervicothoracic, 291
  as example of irregular bone, 8
  lumbar, 246-247, 250
  thoracic, 272-273
Vertebra prominens, 50, 274
  chest radiographs and, 63
  as landmark, 281
Vertebral arteries, 631
Vertebral column
  abdominal radiographs and, 81
  curvatures of, 245
  radiographic anatomy of, 244
Vertebral end of rib, 299
Vertebral notch, 246
Vertebrobasilar artery, 633
  angiography of
    positioning for, 653
    scout positioning for, 650
  arteriography of, 634
Vertex of skull, 315
Vertical portion of frontal bone, 318
Vertical section, definition of, 23
Vessel; *see also* Angiography; Artery; Vein
  abdominal and pelvic computed tomography and, 625
  of breast, 534
  great, 57
  lymphatic, 643
  renal, 507
Vestibular window, 396
Vestibule, 396
View, incorrect use of term, 29
Viewing of radiograph, 14
Visceral peritoneum, 451
Visceral pleura, 54
Visual pathway, 588
Voice box, 52
Voiding cystourethrography
  anatomy and, 510
  male and female, 530
  positioning for, 522
Volar surface, 15, 24
Voluntary motion, 34
Volvulus, 459
Vomer bone, 345
Vomiting, as reaction to contrast medium, 513
Voxel, 601

W

Water test, 429
Waters method
  modified, for orbit, 375
  for nasal bones, 366
  for paranasal sinus, 402, 404
  for zygomatic arch, 370
Waters projection, 354, 359, 360
Water-soluble contrast medium, 425
  abdominal computed tomography and, 623, 624
  for myelography, 676
Weighted angle block, 548
White blood cell, 629
White matter, 586
Whole body scanner, 608
Window
  aortopulmonary, 610
  oval, 396
Windpipe, 53
Wing, sphenoid, 320
Wirsung's duct, 485
Wrist, 100-103
  carpal bridge of, 129
  carpal canal of, 127-128
  joint classification of, 107
  lateral position for, 124
  movements of, 25
  oblique position for, 123
  posteroanterior projection for, 122, 132
  projections for, 48
  radial flexion, posteroanterior projection for, 125
  routine for, 110

X

Xeromammography, 537
Xeroradiography of breast, 537
Xiphoid, 298
Xiphoid process, 280
Xiphoid tip, 280, 281, 505
X-ray beam divergence, 35
X-ray tube, angiography and, 646

Z

Zygapophyseal joint
  cervical, 274, 275, 279
  sacral, 249
  thoracic, 273, 278
Zygapophyseal joint, lumbar, 247, 250, 252
Zygomatic arch
  anteroposterior axial projection for, 371
  lateral position for, 373
  oblique axial projection for, 372
  parietoacanthial projection for, 370
  parieto-orbital projection for, 374
  radiographic anatomy of, 344
  routines for, 355
  submentovertex projection for, 369
Zygomatic bone, 344
  orbit and, 349
Zygomatic process, 319, 343